DEVELOPMENTAL NEUROBIOLOGY

Third Edition

DEVELOPMENTAL NEUROBIOLOGY

Third Edition

MARCUS JACOBSON

The University of Utah School of Medicine
Salt Lake City, Utah

PLENUM PRESS • NEW YORK AND LONDON

Library of Congress Cataloging-in-Publication Data

Jacobson, Marcus, 1930-
    Developmental neurobiology / Marcus Jacobson. -- 3rd ed.
      p.   cm.
    Includes bibliographical references and index.
    ISBN 0-306-43797-X
    1. Developmental neurology.   I. Title.
    [DNLM: 1. Nervous System--embryology. 2. Nervous System--growth &
  development.   WL 101 J17d]
    QP363.5.J3 1991
    599'.0188--dc20
  DNLM/DLC
  for Library of Congress   91-3946
                                                             CIP

ISBN 0-306-43797-X

© 1991, 1978, 1969 Plenum Press, New York
A Division of Plenum Publishing Corporation
233 Spring Street, New York, N.Y. 10013

Printed in the United States of America

Contents

DEVELOPMENTAL NEUROBIOLOGY

Third Edition

1   Beginnings of the Nervous System

There is, it would seem, in the dimensional scale of the world a kind of delicate meeting place between imagination and knowledge, a point, arrived at by diminishing large things and enlarging small ones, that is intrinsically artistic.

Vladimir Nabokov (1899–1977), in
Speak Memory (1966,
revised edition)

1.1. Historical Orientation

*This was a theory of trial and error—of **conjectures and refutations**. It made it possible to understand why our attempts to force interpretations upon the world were logically prior to the observation of similarities. Since there were logical reasons behind this procedure, I thought that it would apply in the field of science also; that scientific theories were not the digest of observations, but that they were inventions—conjectures boldly put forward for trial, to be eliminated if they clashed with observations; with observations which were rarely accidental but as a rule undertaken with the efinite intention of testing a theory by obtaining, if possible, a decisive refutation.*

Karl R. Popper (1902–),
*Conjectures and Refutations:
The Growth of Scientific
Knowledge*, 1962

The history of neuroscience can be viewed as a gradual improvement of techniques with which complex organisms could be analyzed and reduced

Note to the reader: sections in bolder type throughout the book summarize the main concepts and observations to better enable rapid skimming of the large work.

to their constituent cells and molecules. This can be called the reductionist neuroscience research program.

The reductionist program was founded upon two main assumptions: Firstly, development is the assembly of elementary units in various combinations and configurations, advancing from simple to complex, each stage caused by the conditions of the immediately preceding stage. The second assumption underlying the reductionist program is that one of the main aims of embryology is to deduce the events of development and morphogenesis from the activities of elementary units.

The idea that living organisms are reducible to elementary components, invisible corpuscles and fibers, which were already in the 17th century sometimes termed molecules, was held by Pierre Gassendi (1592–1655) and Robert Boyle (1627–1691) among others (reviewed by Hall, 1979). This idea was one of the essential parts of a research program which culminated in what I have called the mechanization of the brain picture (see Section 11.1). As Popper states in the epigraph to this section, the idea leads, and the techniques and results follow, during construction of a scientific research program. Atomistic and molecular theories of living organisms were proposed in the 17th and 18th centuries, long before the cell theory was advanced in the 19th—reduction of organ-

1

isms to their constituent parts did not only occur in the logical order from larger to smaller components, from the top down, but also from the atoms and molecules to the macroscopic structures, from the bottom up. Modern theories of cellular structure echo the micromechanical models of the 17th and 18th century theorists. One of the consequences was that conjectures about molecular mechanisms were made that could not be tested experimentally until centuries later. Many examples can be given of such premature conjectures which were systematized and generalized to form premature theories.[1]

Methods to implement the reductionist program would remain unavailable for almost a century, though it was clearly perceived as the desired goal. Koelliker[2] prophetically states in the first English edition of his *Manual of Human Histology* (1853): *"If it be possible that the molecules which constitute cell membranes, muscular fibrils, axile fibres of nerves should be discovered, and the laws... of the origin, growth, and activity of the present so-called elementary parts, should be made out, then a new era will commence for histology, and the discoverer of the law of cell genesis, or, of a molecular theory, will be as much or more celebrated than the originator of the doctrine of all animal tissues out of cells."*

The cell theory, introduced by Schwann in 1839, defined cells as elementary units whose division, transformation, combination, and permutation to form complex organisms could be observed with the lately improved microscopes and histological methods. Because of its inclusivity, the cell theory permitted generalization from one form to all others, so that development of the nervous system was no longer considered to be governed by its own exclusive laws. The cell theory is a paradigm; the neuron theory emerged from it as an important special case. Sherrington says this in the opening sentence of *The Integrative Action of the Nervous System* (1906): *"Nowhere in physiology does the cell theory reveal its presence more frequently in the very framework of the argument than at the present time in the study of nervous reactions."*

From 1828 to 1839, the concept of epigenesis was established by Von Baer as a central theory of embryology: *"The general before the specific, and so on down to the smallest parts."* This theory opened the way for a causal analysis of development of organs and relatively gross structures. Epigenesis was interpreted by von Baer and most of his contemporaries in terms of homology and the unity of body plan of all animals. The theory of germ layers and the theory of segmentation were results of this interpretation of development.

Embryology was still practiced as a branch of morphology not requiring reference to histological structure. That changed after 1830, when the achromatic compound microscope made it possible to see fibers and globular bodies in the central nervous system. In 1837 Purkinje discovered the flask-shaped cells in the cerebellar cortex which now bear his name. He concluded that in all animals the nervous system is formed of three components, fluid, fibers, and globules. Such globules were at first thought to develop by precipitation out of a homogeneous fluid substance. This notion was consistent with the theory of epigenesis and it persisted for at least a decade after the introduction of the cell theory (see Sections 5.1 and 6.1).

Beginning in 1839 with the publication of Schwann's book on the cell theory, cells were shown to be the basic units of all multicellular organisms, and the primary roles of cells in heredity and development were very slowly revealed. There was an initial period of confusion, during which cells were still believed to originate by precipitation from a homogeneous "cytoblasteme" (Schwann's term, 1839) in addition to their production by mitosis (Flemming's term, 1860). However, by 1850–1855 Remak could give an account of vertebrate development in terms of cells originating

---

[1]The maturity of a theory relates the functions of the theory to the stage of construction of a scientific research program (M. Jacobson, *Conceptual Foundations of Neuroscience*, in preparation). A theory is mature when it fits into a progressing research program and operates effectively in guiding techniques to obtain new facts. A premature discovery, hypothesis, or theory may be true but cannot be accepted into a research program because it is too far in advance of the stage of construction of that program. Mendel's theory of inheritance is the best known example of a premature theory.

[2]Correctly spelled either Koelliker or Kölliker: he used both forms. In his *Entwicklungsgeschichte* (1879, second edition) the title page has Kölliker, the preface is signed Koelliker, and his signature is invariably in the latter form, which I have used in this book. For additional consideration of Koelliker, see Sections 5.1, 6.1, 10.1, and Figs. 6.2 and 10.3.

only from other cells, a concept that was finally generalized in the dictum *omnis cellula e cellula* (Virchow, 1858). Nevertheless, Darwin was able to write the *Origin of Species* over a period of about 20 years until its publication in 1859 without any reference to cellular structure. This I find one of the most remarkable facts of the history of science. It shows that scientists do not necessarily work under the influence of the spirit of the times (zeitgeist) or within a "paradigm," as defined by Thomas Kuhn (1962, 1970, 1974).

During the second epoch, particularly as the result of the work of Remak (1850–1855), Koelliker (1852), and Virchow (1858), nerve cells and neuroglial cells were shown to be the basic units of organization of the nervous system, and nerve fibers were recognized as parts of nerve cells (see Sections 5.1 and 6.1). By 1874 Wilhelm His could formulate a purely mechanistic theory of development of the nervous system in terms of cell division, migration, aggregation, differentiation, and changes in cell form and function. This is an indication of the rate of progress that occurred in understanding the behavior of cells following the first glimmerings of the cell theory in the minds of Schleiden (1838) and Schwann (1839). Apart from formulating a general cell theory, these two got almost everything else wrong, so that their original ideas about cells were almost totally overturned before 1870.[3]

The history of ideas about morphogenesis has an extensive literature (Russell, 1930; Radl, 1930; Needham, 1931, 1934; Meyer, 1939; Hughes, 1959; Adelmann, 1966; Hall, 1969, to cite only well-known

secondary sources). A sketch using broad strokes should be sufficient for the purposes of this historical orientation. Goethe, to whom we owe the term morphology, and his contemporaries and immediate successors, conceived of morphogenesis in terms of plastic transformations of tissues and organs driven by innate formative stimuli and molded by environmental forces. This concept was greatly advanced by Schwann and his successors, who could begin to understand morphology and morphogenesis in terms of cells. Morphogenesis of the nervous system was analyzed in terms of histogenesis, changes of cell shape, cell movements, and migrations (Remak, 1850–1855; Koelliker, 1852; His, 1868, 1887, see Section 2.1). Wilhelm His (1874, 1894) showed how changes in cell shape are involved in folding of tissues such as the neural plate (see Section 1.8). The concept of cell migration in the developing nervous system was also worked out by His, first from his observations on the origins of the peripheral nervous system from the neural crest (His, 1868), the migration of cells from the olfactory placode (His, 1889; Koelliker, 1890), and later from the discovery that the neuroblasts migrate individually from the ventricular germinal zone to the overlying mantle layer of the neural tube (His, 1889).

The revolutionary discovery of cell migration in the vertebrate central nervous system by His was at first greeted with skepticism, but the universality of this form of cellular behavior soon became apparent. In 1893 Loeb showed migration of pigment cells in *Fundulus,* a teleost, and migration of presumptive skeleton cells and mesenchyme cells in sea urchin embryos was discovered by Herbst (1894) and Driesch (1896). Mechanisms of cell migration were proposed by analogy with the locomotory movements of protozoa (Korschelt and Heider, 1903–1909), but there were no means for making progress along those lines at that time. Other cases of cell migration in the vertebrate central nervous system were also baffling. After discovery of the cerebellar external granular layer (Obersteiner, 1883; Herrick, 1891), several attempts were made to follow the migration of granule cells until the problem yielded to Cajal's definitive analysis in the 1890s, as discussed at length in Section 10.11 (Ramón y Cajal, 1911, pp. 80–87).

In this chapter we refer frequently to the germ layers—ectoderm, mesoderm, and endoderm.

---

[3] I agree with Schopenhauer that the will to criticize is stronger than the will to praise—malice is inherent, but one must be taught to be just, to praise, and to find satisfaction in the achievements of others. *"Not to prayse or disprayse: all did well"* (William Harvey) would be more polite but would not be a just estimate of the achievements of Schleiden and Schwann, as the reader may verify from their original works or from reliable secondary sources (Baker, 1955; Hughes, 1959; Hall, 1969). Yet they deserve as much credit for planting the original idea as the others who tended and pruned the tree of knowledge and profited from the fruits. It is noteworthy that so many of those who overturned the original misconceptions and who established the cell theory on secure grounds (Helmholtz, Henle, Koelliker, Reichert, Remak, M. Schultze, Virchow) were students of Johannes Müller, and it was through him that they were also among the first to apply the cell theory to neural development.

These terms are loaded with various shades of meaning acquired during almost two centuries of usage. Heinrich Christian Pander (1794–1865), the discoverer of the germ layers, recognized their interrelationships but also conjectured that each layer has a different developmental fate, as his description of the situation in the chick embryo shows: *"In reality there begins in each of these three layers a specific metamorphosis, and each strives to achieve its objective; only each is not yet sufficiently independent to produce by itself that for which it is destined; each one still needs the help of its companions, and thus all three, although destined for different purposes, work mutually together until each has attained its determined level"* (Pander, 1817). From the very beginning it was implied that there are distinct and recognizable embryonic tissues called the germ layers, namely, "the mesoderm", "the ectoderm," and "the endoderm." The defects of this notion were pointed out long ago (His 1874; Koelliker 1884; De Beer, 1947; Oppenheimer, 1967), but the terms were not abandoned.

The first challenge to the germ layer theory by His (1874) was indirect—he pointed out weaknesses in the gastrea theory of Haeckel (1866), according to which the three germ cell layers originate during phylogeny from an ancestral form, the gastrea, which is recapitulated during ontogeny in the form of a three-layered gastrula in all vertebrates. His showed that this theory does not apply to avian and mammalian embryos in which the layers develop by delamination. The epiblast contains cells that give rise to progeny in all three germ layers; therefore, His maintained, the physiological functions of the layers matter more than their embryonic origins. The first studies of cell lineages of the leech, *Clepsine*, by C. O. Whitman (1878, 1888) showed that the early cleavage cells are qualitatively different from one another and not only a means of producing enough cells to populate the germ layers, which Haeckel thought were the first to develop qualitative differences. Whitman (1878) provided the first evidence and other evidence was quick to follow (reviewed in E. B. Wilson, 1896, pp. 297–302) to support the theory of His (1874) that the egg cytoplasm contains predetermined substances that are destined to contribute to the formation of specific parts of the body.

The germ layer theory of vertebrate embryonic development received its first experimental refutation from the finding by Platt (1893) that visceral cartilage (a mesodermal tissue) originates from cranial neural crest (an ectodermal tissue) in the urodele, *Necturus*. This aroused a storm of protests from the dogmatists, but they were soon silenced by the corroboration of Platt's findings (von Kupffer, 1895; Dohrn, 1902; Brauer, 1904). Since that time the evidence has clearly shown that the neural crest, a so-called ectodermal tissue, contains pluripotential cells which give rise to progeny that populate all the classical germ layers (Table 4.1). When the terms ectoderm, mesoderm, and endoderm are used, we would be aware that: *"There is no invariable correlation between the germ layers and either the presumptive organ-forming regions or the formed structures. It follows that the germ layers are not determinants of differentiation in development, but embryonic structures which resemble one another closely in different forms although they may contain materials differing in origin and in fate. The germ-layer theory in its classical form must therefore be abandoned"* (De Beer, 1947).

Experimental analysis of the embryonic origins of the nervous system may conveniently be dated from 1918, with the first of a series of crucial experiments by Hans Spemann (1869–1941) in which he identified a region in the dorsal lip of the blastopore as the source of the stimulus for neural induction in amphibian embryos (Hamburger, 1988, review).

In 1918 Spemann reported that a piece excised from the region above the dorsal lip of the blastopore of an early gastrula of the newt *Triturus*, transplanted into the ventral side of another early gastrula of the same species, resulted in development of a second embryonic axis, joined to the belly of the host. To show the contribution of host and graft cells to the tissues of the second embryonic axis, Spemann and Mangold (1924) used two species of newts with different pigmentation and found that the second embryo was a mosaic derived from host and donor cells integrated in well-organized tissues and organs, including the central and peripheral nervous systems (Fig. 1.1). From this they deduced that the graft had "organized" a new body plan in the host tissue which was completely reprogrammed from ventral mesoderm and ectoderm.[4]

---

[4]Spemann's first result showing the action of the implanted dorsal blastoporal lip was reported in 1921 in a footnote to a paper already in press, and the term "organizer" was defined there. In the 1924 paper by Spemann and Mangold only five cases showing organiza-

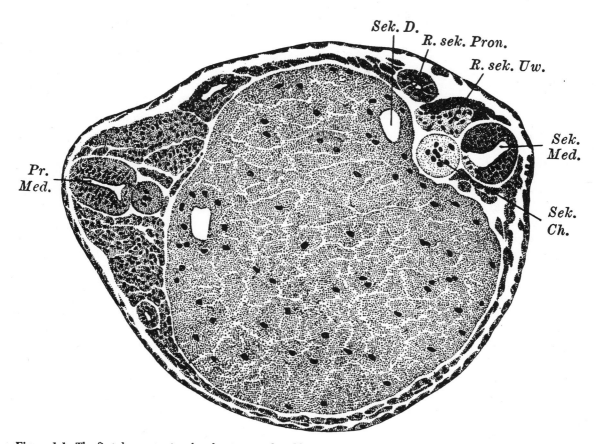

Figure 1.1. The first demonstration that the tissues induced by a grafted "organizer" are derived from both the host and the graft. Cross-section through a chimeric newt embryo which developed from a lightly pigmented host gastrula into which was grafted the dorsal blastoporal lip from a darkly pigmented species of newt. The secondary (induced) neural tube (Sek. Med.) and somite (R. sek. Uw.) are formed partly from the host and partly from the graft. Pr. Med. = primary neural tube; R. sek. Pron = secondary pronephric duct; Sek. Ch. = notochord; Sek. D. = endoderm. From H. Spemann and H. Mangold, *Arch. mikr. Anat. Entw. Mech.* **100**:599-638 (1924).

tion of a second neural tube were reported of the hundreds of grafts that were made, most of which died and were excluded from the final analysis. Hamburger (1988) gives a superb account, based on his personal recollections, of the events leading up to the celebrated Spemann–Mangold experiment. Hamburger (1988, p. 65) states that Spemann had little interest in theory and discounts the evidence that Spemann conceived of embryonic development in terms of a general vitalistic theory. Some evidence for Spemann's theoretical proclivity is provided in Section 11.1. For example, his intentions are revealed in the title of the German edition of his Silliman Lectures given at Yale University in 1933: *Experimentelle Beiträge zu Einer Theorie der Entwicklung* (1936). When that was translated into English, the title was changed to *Embryonic Development and Induction* (1938), but the vitalistic theory was retained.

The observation that host and graft cells fit together harmoniously in all parts of the new pattern assumed great significance when fate maps showed that the ventral region of the host is destined to form ventral mesoderm and epidermis, and the grafted tissue is fated to become chorda-mesoderm and not nervous system (Vogt, 1925, 1929; see Vogt's obituary notice by Spemann, 1941). Therefore, the cells of both graft and host change their fates when integrated into the secondary central nervous system. The region dorsal to the blastopore lip, which uniquely possesses the power to reorganize the developmental fates in ventral cells, is called the *organizer*.

The Spemann–Mangold experiment is one of

the most celebrated and provocative, not so much for what it succeeded in explaining but for what it left unexplained, namely, the mechanisms by which ventral cells are induced to adopt dorsal fates, in particular the mechanisms of induction of the second central nervous system (Nakamura and Toivonen, 1978, review). The results of that experiment have been repeatedly confirmed, most recently by using intracellular cell lineage tracers to show that the induced second nervous system originates mainly from ventral cells of the host embryo (Gimlich and Cooke, 1983; J. C. Smith and Slack, 1983; M. Jacobson, 1984). But the mechanisms by which the ventral cells, originally fated to form belly skin, vascular mesoderm, and endoderm, become reprogrammed to form central nervous system and somitic mesoderm remain enigmatic. This is discussed further in Section 1.4. The Spemann–Mangold experiment proves that the positions of the cells, and not their lineages, must be the overriding factors in determining their fates in amphibian embryos, and other evidence shows that this conclusion applies also to avian and mammalian embryos (see Section 1.3). Spemann expresses this idea picturesquely in his autobiography: *"We are standing and walking on parts of our body which we could have used for thinking if they had been developed in another position in the embryo"* (Spemann, 1924, p. 167).

1.2. Development of the Basic Plan of the Body

If we knew the complete genome sequence of an organism, we could not, from that evidence alone, be able to deduce its program of morphogenesis, or its final form and size; we could not answer the ontogenetic question of how gene expression results in the three-dimensional organism or the phylogenetic question of how genetic mutations result in evolution of phenotypes. How essentially the same gene products form a brain at one position and a spinal cord at another place is not given directly by the genome, but eventuates from a network of regulatory epigenetic processes that control the spatial pattern of gene expression that underlie cell differentiation and assembly into tissues: cell interactions, cell proliferation, cell movements and changes in shape, and cell death.

We may conceive of development in terms of hierarchies at many levels from multigene families to the phenotype, with groups of components interacting within and between levels (Whyte *et al.*, 1969; Pattee, 1973; Dressler and Gruss, 1988). It is not yet clear whether it will be possible to lump together all process of pattern formation and morphogenesis under one set of laws, as optimists have always hoped, e.g., the mechanical models of His (1874); entelechy of Driesch (1908); metabolic gradients of Child (1941); positional information of Wolpert (1969); catastrophe theory of Thom (1975); topobiology of Edelman (1988). Nor is it clear whether morphogenesis will be split into an increasing number of epigenetic systems governed by many different rules, as pessimists fear (c.f. Waddington, 1970, *"There cannot be any one general theory of morphogenesis, at a level more particular than the very abstract ideas. . . ."*). I do not agree with such a pessimistic prognosis because we already know that there are mechanisms of spatial patterning of gene expression, resulting in morphological and tissue patterns, which have been conserved in many animals of different phylogenetic status. On the other hand, certain regulatory mechanisms have evolved as adaptations of early development. We shall have to understand the mechanisms that have been conserved during evolution as well as those that have evolved separately during phylogeny, especially as expressed in early mammalian embryogenesis.

Pattern formation in embryos of multicellular animals requires development of polarity, bilateral symmetry, and segmentation. Many components of these processes have been identified by molecular genetic techniques, most successfully in the fly, *Drosophila* (Akam, 1987; Rubin, 1988; Ingham, 1988; Goto *et al.*, 1989; Struhl *et al.*, 1989; French, 1990), and increasingly in the frog, *Xenopus* (Dawid and Sargent, 1988) and the mouse (Dressler and Gruss, 1988; Wilkinson *et al.*, 1989b; Wilkinson, 1990). Our principal concerns are with understanding how the basic plan of the nervous system originates in the embryo. In order to do so, it is necessary to consider the antecedent processes in development of a fundamental body plan.[5]

[5]One is continually struck by the boldness with which nineteenth century biologists claimed to see affinities between body plans of quite disparate organisms. For exam-

Formation of a body plan in the vertebrates starts in the oocyte, continues immediately after fertilization and cleavage of the egg, and is essentially completed in the gastrula. There are at least three stages. First, establishment of polarity, i.e., the asymmetric distribution of one or more cytoplasmic properties, in the egg and early blastula (e.g. Davidson, 1986, Chapter 6, review). These regional differences in the egg and newly fertilized embryo are used to establish different cell lineages in blastomeres which inherit different cytoplasmic determinants during early cleavages and also to establish cellular differences which are initially required for cells to interact with one another. There is no reason for localization of determinants of terminally differentiated cell types, but determinants may be used by cells for setting up the body plan prior to commitment to cellular histotypes (M. Jacobson, 1985, review). Second, expression of regional inequalities as different cellular functions. Third, cell interactions (inhibitory as well as facilitatory, long range as well as short range) resulting in further regional differences. These processes form a hierarchical cascade at the end of which different programs of development are expressed in small groups of cells

---

ple, near the end of his 1849 paper *"On the Anatomy and the Affinities of the Family of the Medusae,"* T. H. Huxley casually remarks that the archetypal medusa is constructed on the same plan as the chick embryo! The history of the long quest for the basic plan of the nervous system can be found in von Kupffer (1906) and Kuhlenbeck (1973). Authorities agree that a primary morphological pattern of the vertebrate CNS develops before closure of the neural tube and that the pattern consists of the ventral median floor plate with bilaterally symmetrical longitudinal subdivisions extending to the rostral end of the floor plate. At that level a primary transverse boundary develops marking a division between mesencephalon and rhombencephalon (His, 1892; J. B. Johnston, 1902, 1905, 1906, 1909; Herrick, 1908; Kingsbury, 1920, 1922, 1930; M. Jacobson, 1978, 1980, 1985a,b). At later stages of development of the neural tube additional transverse boundaries form a neuromeric pattern which may well be secondary, resulting from inductive interactions with mesodermal segments. The place of comparative morphology, at the heart of biology, has lately been usurped by molecular genetics, but both are required for deciphering the laws of development, for not only does evolution determine morphology, but the reverse also holds, that morphology determines the possibilities for evolution.

arranged in a pattern. Functional differences between cells at different positions in the body plan are the preconditions for cell behaviors that result in morphogenetic movements such as gastrulation and neurulation.

Phylogenetic differences in the mechanisms by which the body plan is established in early embryos result from differences in the times at which components of the pattern-generating system are expressed; either during oogenesis, or at the time of fertilization, or during cleavage or later. In the tunicates, invertebrates which occupy an evolutionary position close to the origin of the vertebrates, molecular determinants in the oocyte, and thus under direct control of the maternal genome, are segregated into different parts of the fertilized egg and are distributed into different cell lineages of the embryo, where they determine development of specific anatomical structures (Whittaker, 1973, 1979; Jeffery, 1985). Although regular patterns of cleavage normally occur in embryos of this type, experiments have shown that cell determination is not a function of any fixed pattern of divisions of the cell nucleus, but only of partitioning of cytoplasmic components (Whittaker, 1980, 1982, 1983).

The mechanisms of formation of the body plan in the amphibia appear to be intermediate between tunicates and amniotes (reviewed by Gerhart, 1980). Maternal cytoplasmic determinants have been found to be localized in the frog oocyte. These are factors that may affect expression of the embryo's genome or they may produce regional differences in function by affecting ion fluxes or metabolism (Melton, 1987; Weeks and Melton, 1987). During the first cell cycle after fertilization, materials of maternal origin are relocated in relationship to the point of sperm entry which determines the anterior-posterior axis in *Xenopus* (Black and Gerhart, 1985; Vincent *et al.*, 1986; Rebagliati *et al.*, 1985; Melton, 1987; Mercola *et al.*, 1988; Yisraeli *et al.*, 1990). The dorsal–ventral axis develops in *Xenopus* as a result of inductive interactions which are considered later (J. C. Smith and Slack, 1983; J. C. Smith, 1989, reviews).

During the first few cleavage cycles in amphibian embryos, cytoplasmic materials are unequally distributed in separate lineages. This cytoplasm contains regulatory proteins (or their mRNAs) that initiate specific gene activity which results in functional differences between blastomeres (Wakahara, 1989, review). One of the differences between blastomeres is their ability to synthesize inductive molecules and receptors for them. This enables inductive interactions to commence during cleavage stages. Signaling between cells, certainly mediated by growth factors, although probably not limited to them, starts during early cleavage stages and continues through blastula and gastrula stages in *Xenopus* (reviewed by Dawid *et al.*, 1989; J. C. Smith, 1989). In the Amphibia, the cytoplasmic factors exert determinative activities very early to establish a spatial pattern of differential gene expression resulting in an early spatial pattern of cell differentiation which is necessary to accomplish gastrulation and to effect cell-to-cell interactions. The early spatial specification can be termed morphological specification, in contradistinction to histological specification, which occurs as a result of cell-to-cell signaling later in development (see Section 2.11). We can thus make a distinction between *morphoregulatory factors*, which must be expressed early in order to establish the embryonic axes, and *historegulatory factors*, which are expressed relatively late in order to establish patterns of histological differentiation (see Section 1.3). Therefore, removal of blastomeres at the 4- or 8-cell stage, or removal at a later stage of a number of cells equivalent to the progeny of one or more blastomeres of the 4-cell stage, results in reduction of a size of embryo, but not in ablation of any specific cell type. For example, Rohon–Beard neurons are not reduced in number after removal of the blastomere at the 16-cell stage that normally gives rise to most of the Rohon–Beard neurons (Fig. 1.2). Compensatory production of those neurons occurs from neighboring blastomeres from which Rohon–Beard neurons do not normally originate (M. Jacobson, 1981a,b). This also shows that Rohon–Beard neurons are not determined by a cell lineage mechanism, even though their very early origin, and precise regulation of their small population size, might suggest that they are so determined.

In amniotes, the meager evidence available shows that the body plan is determined by cell position and cell interactions and not by inheritance of cytoplasmic determinants or by cell lineage. In birds, the blastodisc is initially radially equipotential. The anterior–posterior axis of the blastoderm is oriented with respect to gravity late during cleavage as cells accumulate at the lowest end of the blastocoele, which becomes the head. This occurs during passage of the egg down the oviduct so that experimental rotation of the egg in the oviduct results in duplication of the embryonic axis and the production of twins (Clavert, 1960a,b; Eyal-Giladi, 1969, 1984). In mammals, embryonic polarity is established as a result of asymmetry produced by implantation of the embryo in the uterine endometrium (L. J. Smith, 1985). The subsequent mechanisms of development of the body plan in amniotes are not known. A good overview of theoretical models of biological pattern formation is provided by Meinhardt (1982).

In the fruit fly, *Drosophila*, analysis of many mutations that alter the body plan has revealed several classes of genes whose action specifies the metameric pattern of the embryo (reviewed by Scott and O'Farrell, 1986; Nusslein-Volhard *et al.*, 1987; Doe and Scott, 1988; Ingham, 1988; Rubin, 1988; French, 1990). These are maternal effect genes (the terminal, anterior, and posterior classes of genes) which are expressed very early and determine the separate domains of head, trunk, and tail; the segmentation genes, which act later, and control subdivision into separate segments (the gap, pair-rule, and segment polarity genes), and finally, the homeotic genes, which specify identity of individual segments. Some of these pattern formation genes have been cloned and the spatial domains of their expression have been demonstrated by *in situ* hybridization. Some of their gene products have been shown to bind to DNA, indicating that they may act as regulators of transcription.

Mutations in segmentation genes result in development of abnormalities of the number and axial polarity of segments (Hiromi *et al.*, 1985; Ingham *et al.*, 1986). Mutations in homeotic genes result in development of structures in a segment that properly belong to a different segment. The domains of expression of homeotic genes, which define developmental compartments, do not correspond exactly with histological patterns or with morphological segments (Morata and Lawrence, 1977). In the *Drosophila* embryo, each morphological segment is composed of two compartments, anterior and posterior, which are called parasegments (Martinez-Arias and Lawrence, 1985). The fact that the boundaries of domains of gene expression may not always correspond with morphological boundaries should be

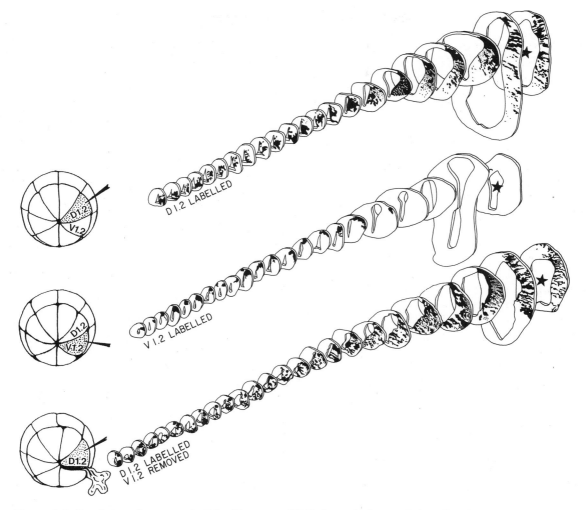

Figure 1.2. Regulation after removal of the blastomere (V1.2) from which most Rohon–Beard neurons originate in *Xenopus* embryos. Horseradish peroxidase was injected by means of a micropipette into a single identified blastomere of the 16-cell *Xenopus* embryo and the embryos were allowed to develop for 40–45 hours and were processed to show the labeled clones. Blastomere D1.2 gave rise to a clone in the dorsolateral parts of the brain and lateral parts of the spinal cord as shown in serial section reconstruction (A). Blastomere V1.2 gave rise to a clone restricted to dorsal rhombencephalon and spinal cord, including the majority of Rohon–Beard neurons (serial section reconstruction B). After removal of V1.2, blastomere D1.2 gave rise to a clone which was far more extensive than normal and included a normal number of Rohon–Beard neurons (serial section reconstruction C). From M. Jacobson, *J. Neurosci.* 1:923–927 (1981), copyright Society for Neuroscience.

kept in mind when assessing the significance of segmental patterns in the central nervous system.

Genes which specify segment identity in Drosophila (e.g., *Antennapedia*) have been found to contain a common element of 180 base pairs, called the homeobox (Gehring, 1987, review). The homeobox has been highly conserved in segmented animals, including insects and vertebrates (McGinnis, 1985;

Akam, 1989), and also in some nonsegmented invertebrates (Holland and Hogan, 1986). The homeobox is found in homeotic genes which are believed to specify positional values in the anteroposterior or rostrocaudal axis of the animals. In *Drosophila*, homeobox genes are clustered in two complexes termed *Antennapedia-C* and *Bithorax-C* which are adjacent on the right arm of chromosome 3 (Lewis,

1978; Kaufman et al., 1985). Clustering of homeobox genes is also found in the human (Boncinelli et al., 1988), mouse (Graham et al., 1988, 1989; Sharpe et al., 1988), the frog, Xenopus (Harvey et al., 1986), and zebra fish (Njolstad et al., 1988). In the mouse the homeobox genes are organized in four clusters named Hox-1, Hox-2, Hox-3, and Hox-5 located on chromosomes 6, 11, 15, and 2, respectively (Graham et al., 1988, 1989).

The spatial order of the homeobox genes in the clusters is the same as the order in which the genes are expressed in the anteroposterior axis in Drosophila (Harding et al., 1985; Akam, 1987) and in the rostrocaudal axis in the mouse (Graham et al., 1988, 1989). In the nervous system of Drosophila the anterior boundary of expression of Abdominal-B is at the sixth abdominal ganglion; Abdominal-A is expressed in the first abdominal ganglion; Ultrabithorax expression extends to the metathoracic ganglion; Antennapedia is expressed as far anterior as the prothoracic ganglion; expression of sex combs reduced reaches the second subesophageal ganglion; Deformed is expressed in the first subesophageal ganglion; and Labial expression extends more anteriorly.

In the frog and mouse, homeobox genes are expressed in the central and peripheral nervous system and in mesodermal tissues (somites, kidneys, lungs), but not in endodermal tissues (Feinberg et al., 1987; Krumlauf et al., 1987; Dressler and Gruss, 1988; Graham et al., 1988). The anterior boundary of homeobox gene expression is always more rostral in the CNS than in the mesodermal tissues (Dony and Gruss, 1987; Graham et al., 1988, 1989; Quant, 1988). This probably reflects the rostral displacement of the spinal cord in relation to the vertebrae that occurs during mammalian development.

A number of mouse homeobox genes that are expressed in the CNS have been characterized in some detail. Several mouse homeobox genes have been reported to be transcribed in the CNS: Hox 1.2 (Toth et al., 1987), Hox 1.3 (Odenwald et al., 1987), Hox 1.5 and Hox 2.1 (Ruddle et al., 1985), Hox 2.2 (Schughart et al., 1988), Hox 2.5 (Graham et al., 1988, 1989; Bogarad et al., 1989), and En-2 (Davis et al., 1988). Some of these continue to be expressed in the adult nervous system: Hox 1.3 protein is found in cerebellar Purkinje cells and pyramidal cells of the hippocampal dentate gyrus (Odenwald et al., 1987); Hox 3.1 protein is present in a variety of types of neurons in the spinal cord, and in dorsal root and sympathetic ganglia of adult mice (Awgulewitsch and Jacobs, 1990).

The Hox 3.1 locus maps to chromosome 15 and it is specifically expressed in the CNS at later stages of development and in the adult. Its expression in the CNS starts at E10.5 and persists in the adult in neurons of the cervical and rostral thoracic spinal cord, with the highest level of expression in the ventral half of the spinal cord (Awgulewitsch et al., 1986; Utset et al., 1987; Le Moullic et al., 1988). Hox 3.1 protein accumulates in the nuclei of neurons starting at E10.5 and persists in fully differentiated neurons in the adult mouse (Awgulewitsch and Jacobs, 1990). Its functions are at present unknown.

In the mouse, the Hox-2 complex on chromosome 7 consists of seven homeobox genes which are expressed in the central nervous system (Graham et al., 1988; Wilkinson et al., 1989). All these genes have the same 5'-to-3' orientation and are arranged in the same order on the chromosome as they are expressed in the rhombencephalon, and spinal cord. The rostral boundary of expression of the Hox-2.5 gene is in the spinal cord at the level of the third cervical vertebra, and the genes of the Hox-2 complex located 3' of Hox-2.5 have correspondingly more rostral boundaries of expression in the rhombencephalon as shown in Fig. 1.3 in the 12-day mouse embryo (Graham et al., 1989). The rostral boundaries of homeobox gene expression correspond with rhombomere anatomical boundaries (Wilkinson and Krumlauf, 1990, review). Anatomical boundaries may develop as a result of interactions in the regions of overlap of their domains of gene expression. Although they have different rostral levels of expression, all the genes of the Hox-2 complex are expressed to the caudal end of the spinal cord.

The function of the homeobox genes may be to specify positional values in the anteroposterior axis, independent of the development of segmentation (Hoey et al., 1986). Graham et al. (1989) suggest that the clustering of homeobox genes is related to regulation of the cluster by cis-acting regulatory elements in such a manner that each gene is controlled by several regulatory elements acting combinatorially.

Drosophila and mouse homeobox genes have been isolated and sequenced. Comparison between the sequences of mouse Hox-2 homeodomains and

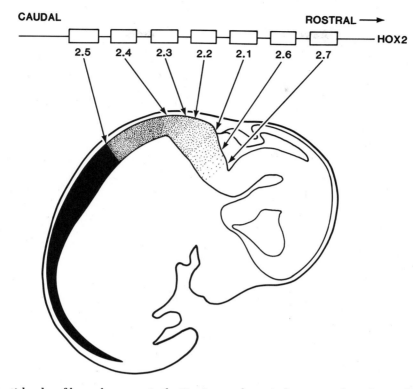

Figure 1.3. Spatial order of homeobox genes in the *Hox-2* gene cluster is the same as the order in which the genes are expressed in the rostrocaudal axis of the central nervous system of the mouse embryo. A parasagittal section of a 12.5 day mouse embryo showing the CNS (stippled) and the rostral boundaries of expression (arrows) of different genes of the Hox-2 complex as shown by *in situ* hybridization. From A. Graham, N. Papalopulu, and R. Krumlauf, *Cell* 57:367–378 (1989), copyright Cell Press.

those of the *Antennapedia-C* and *Bithorax-C* gene complexes (Fig. 1.4) shows considerable similarities. On the basis of this comparison *Hox-2* genes can be subdivided into eight subfamilies each of which is related to a different *Drosophila* homeotic gene. This comparison suggests that mouse homeobox genes and *Drosophila* homeotic genes originated from a common ancestor before separation of the arthropod and vertebrate phylogenies (Akam *et al.,* 1988; Graham *et al.,* 1989; P. W. H. Holland, 1990).

The most obvious feature of the body plan of the vertebrates is segmentation or metamerism, that is, serial repetition of homologous structures along the craniocaudal axis. Metamerism is an example of the efficient operation of the principles of modular construction and developmental parsimony. The same developmental program is used, repeated serially. Complexity is achieved by variations in expression of the program in each meta-

mer. Metamers are composed of parts called *meromes* (Lankester, 1911); e.g., the metamer may have nervous, skeletal, muscular, vascular, renal, integumentary, and alimentary meromes. A *meristic series* consists of a series of homologous meromes arranged in a linear pattern, such as myotomes, pronephric funnels, vertebrae, ribs, digits, teats. In the nervous system, neuromeres, cranial and spinal nerves, and their locally aggregated nerve cells are meromes that form distinct meristic series.

During vertebrate evolution the meromes within the same segment have varied independently of one another, showing that they are determined by different genes. Lewis (1965, 1978) proposes that homeotic genes of the bithorax complex in *Drosophila,* which specify the morphological identity of different body segments, have evolved by iteration of an ancestral gene. This would result in

```
                RKRGRQTYTRYQTLELEKEFHFNRYLTRRRRIEIAHALCLTERQIKIWFQNRRMKWKKENK

Hox2.5     SRKK-CP--K----------L--M----D--H-V-RL-N-S---V---------M--M--
Hox1.7     TRKK-CP--KH---------L--M----D--Y-V-RL-N-----V---------M--I--
Hox3.2     TRKK-CP--K----------L--M----D--Y-V-RV-N-----V---------M--M--
Hox5.2     TRKK-CP--K----------L--M----D--Y-V-RI-N-----V---------M--MS-
Abd-B      VRKK-KP-SKF---------L--A-VSKQK-W-L-RN-Q-----V---------N--NSQ

Hox2.4     -R------S-----------L--P---K----VS---G-----V--------------N
Hox3.1     -RS-----S-----------L--P---K----VS---G-----V--------------N

Hox2.3     --------------------Y-------------T----------------------
Hox1.1     ------------------------------------------------------H-

Hox2.2     GR------------------Y-----------------------------------S-
Hox1.2     GR------------------------------N-----------------------
Hox6.1     -R----I-S-----------------------N---------------------SN

Abd-A      -R--------F-----------H-----------------------L---LR
Ubx        -R-----------------T-H---------M---------------L---IQ
Antp       ------------------------------------------------------

Hox2.1     G--A-TA---------------------------------S---------------D--
Hox1.3     G--A-TA---------------------------------S---------------D--
Scr        T--Q-TS---------------------------------------------L---H-

Hox2.6     P--S-TA---Q-V--------Y---------V---------S-----------DH-
Hox1.4     P--S-TA---Q-V-------------------T---S---V------------DH-
Hox5.1     P--S-TA---Q-V-------------------T---P----------------DH-
Dfd        P--Q-TA---H-I--------Y----------T-V-S----------------D--

Hox2.7     S--A-TA--SA-LV-----------C-P--V-M-NL-N-S-------------Y--DQ-
Hox1.5     S----TA---P-LV----------M-P--V-M-NL-N---------------Y--DQ-
Hox4.1     S--A-TA--SA-LV----------FV-P--VQM-NL-N-S------------Y--DQ-
ZenZ1      L--S-TAF-SV-LV---N--KS-M--Y-T------QR-S-C---V--------F--DIQ
ZenZ2      S--S-TAFSSL-LI---R---L-K--A-T-----SQR-A-----V--------L--STN
Pb ?

Hox1.6     PNAV-TNS-TK-LT---------K----AA-V---AS-Q-N-T-V---------Q--RE-
Labial     NNS--TNF-NK-LT--------------A------NT-Q-N-T-V---------Q--RV-
```

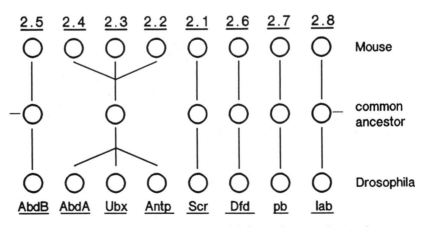

Figure 1.4. Amino acid sequence comparisons of mouse and *Drosophila* homeodomains, showing the existence of related subgroups. The *Antp* sequence at the top was used as the basis for all comparisons. Dashes represent identical amino acids. Separation into subgroups is based on sequence changes shared by the various members. The relative order of the *Drosophila* genes is shown on the left. At the bottom of the diagram is a possible scheme for evolution of mouse and *Drosophila* clusters from a common ancestral cluster. From A. Graham, N. Papalopulu, and R. Krumlauf, *Cell* 57:367–378 (1989), copyright Cell Press.

repetition of the same body segment unless gene expression is altered locally, for example, by interaction of genes with regionally localized, maternally derived cytoplasmic determinants (Nüsslein-Volhard and Wieschaus, 1980; Hiromi *et al.*, 1985). Another way in which variation of segmental pattern can occur is by duplication or transposition of a particular structure up or down the metameric series. Transpositions must be distinguished from homeosis, in which a merome is made in the likeness of a different one belonging to another metamer. In addition to local variation of meromes, there has been a phylogenetic tendency for serially arranged structures to be reduced in number by loss and by coalescence or fusion (tagmosis). Such changes have been rampant during evolution of the vertebrate nervous system. It is important to distinguish between changes that are primarily in the nervous system and those that are secondary, resulting from changes in peripheral structures, such as limbs.

It is also necessary to distinguish between two types of regional variations in segmentation: *heterosis* and *homeosis*. Heterosis includes increase or decrease in the number of segmentally arranged structures as a result of duplication or coalescence, displacement or ectopia. Homeosis (or homoeosis) was originally defined by Bateson (1894) as *"the assumption by one member of a meristic series of the form or characters proper to other members of the series."* True homeotic variations involve serially homologous structures either by development of a body part belonging to one member of the series in place of another or by development of such a part in a position in which it does not normally appear.

There are at least three diagnostic criteria by which heterosis can be distinguished from homeosis. The first distinguishing feature of homeosis is discontinuity in the morphological pattern. There are abrupt qualitative morphological changes without small intermediate variations. There are two different states which are stable, without a series of small intermediate variations. By contrast, heterosis is continuously variable and shows intermediate states in quality, quantity, and position. All cases of ectopic and misaligned neurons are examples of heterosis, for example, neurons that fail to complete their migration, because of mechanical obstacles or because of mutations which produce abnormalities in the cellular mechanisms of neuronal migration

(see Section 10.15). Secondly, homeosis is almost always expressed fully from an early stage of development, whereas heterosis may develop gradually. Thirdly, homeotically transformed tissues are innervated from the nearest available central nervous system, whereas heterotic tissue derives at least part of its innervation from the appropriate (original) level of the central nervous system. The lateral line organs provide a good example of lack of correspondence between segmental values of nerve and peripheral organs. Although the lateral line organs are finally positioned segmentally, they are not innervated by sensory nerves of their own segments but by branches of the vagus nerve, which is the segmental nerve associated with their original position.

In all cases of heterosis involving changes in relative positions of central nervous system and peripheral tissues, it is always the origins of the nerve supply which indicate the segmental value of the tissue or organ. For example, the diaphragm and the tongue retain their original innervation during and after displacement far from their original sites of development. The diaphragm changes its sites of bony attachment from upper cervical segments to finally become attached to thoracic ribs. Therefore, the nerve supply of muscles is generally a more reliable indication of homology than the sites of attachments of muscles to bones (homology means inferred common ancestry and not merely parallel evolution or functional similarity; C. Patterson, 1988). For example, in the teleost *Gadus*, the pelvic fins are innervated by spinal nerves 5–7 although positioned in front of the pectoral fins, which are innervated by spinal nerves 1–4 (Goodrich, 1913). This shows either that the nerves grow to their appropriate fins, or more likely, that the fins migrate after they have been contacted by the nerves, towing the nerves with them. Such towing of nerves by organs is well established by the cases of the tongue and the diaphragm. **The place of origin of the limbs, and their homologies, are shown by the segmental origins of their nerve supply: in heterosis the segmental origins of the limb and nerve supply are different, in homeosis they are the same.** This matter is taken up again in Section 9.4 in discussing innervation patterns of limbs.

There are different categories of segmentation. *Primary segments* are serially repeated parts of the body, that are serially homologous, and develop autonomously. Mesodermal somites in the vertebrates are primary segments. Serially homologous structures are not necessarily segments: they may secondarily take up segmental positions, as in the case of lateral line organs in fish and amphibians; they may arise by fusion of parts of two neighboring segments and are then termed *parasegments,* e.g., vertebrae; or they can arise in the intersegmental tissue, e.g., ribs. Cranial and spinal ganglia and nerves are not primarily segmental but they may be intersegmental or parasegmental, as discussed later in this section. *Secondary segmentation* develops under the influence of the primary mesodermal segmentation. The surface ectoderm and gut are primarily unsegmented, but they develop local specializations that may be serially repeated as in the skin appendages, under the influence of adjacent mesoderm. Neuromeres (Fig. 1.5) are serially repeated enlargements of the neural tube. They are transient and disappear at later stages. Whether they represent primary or secondary segments will be discussed below.

The evidence showing that mesoderm is segmented up to the front of the head and that serially repeated pattern of enlargements, called neuromeres, develops in the neural tube of vertebrates may be found in the standard texts (Gegenbauer, 1898; Johnston, 1905; von Kupffer, 1906; Neal, 1918; Delsman, 1922; Goodrich, 1930; De Beer, 1937; Vaage, 1969; Bergquist, 1952; Kuhlenbeck, 1973; Jarvik, 1980).

Nineteenth century neuromorphologists identified 11 neuromeres in all vertebrates arranged as a bilaterally symmetrical meristic series consisting of one prosencephalic, two diencephalic, two mesencephalic, and six preotic rhombencephalic neuromeres (Fig. 1.5). Additional rhombomeres may appear in some species depending on the number of spinal segments that become incorporated into the hindbrain. Other features that were recognized by the earlier workers are the low numerical density of cells in the boundary regions between neuromeres and the regular association of cranial nerve nuclei with certain neuromeres. Thus, the motoneurons supplying the first three branchial arches (V, VII, and IX) develop in rhombomeres 2, 4, and 6, respectively. These observations have been essentially confirmed and amplified by later investigators.

Recent evidence indicates that boundaries between rhombomeres in the chick embryo coincide with lines of clonal restriction of cell mingling during development (Fraser *et al.,* 1990; A. Lumsden, 1990, review). Those findings afford a subtle satisfaction to the originators of the idea and the discoverers of the significance of clonal restriction of cell mingling resulting in formation of clonal domains or morphological compartments in the vertebrate CNS (M. Jacobson, 1980, 1983, 1985a,b; Sheard and Jacobson, 1987, 1990; see Section 2.11). The strongest proof of the value of your ideas occurs when others sincerely believe that they have just invented them.

Correspondence between cranial neuromeres (encephalomeres, rhombomeres) and cranial mesodermal segmentation is not apparent in light microscopic histological preparations. Several authors have proposed that such a correspondence once existed in an ancestral form (Ziegler, 1908; Goodrich, 1918; Delsman, 1922). Recent evidence shows that there is such a correspondence during early stages of development in vertebrate embryos. In the mouse embryo the neuromeres develop exactly in correspondence with the underlying segmented mesenchyme, viewed by scanning electron microscopy (A. G. Jacobson and Tam, 1982). Viewed by means of stereo scanning electron microscopy, the cranial mesoderm of chick and mouse embryos develops bilateral compactions of mesoderm to form somitomeres (Fig. 1.6). The first pair of somitomeres appears to be related to the prosencephalon, another six appear to correspond with the rhombomeres (Meier, 1979, 1981, 1984; Meir and Tam, 1982; A. G. Jacobson, 1988, review). Somitomeres are formed in the paraxial mesoderm along the length of the embryo in cranial-to-caudal order during gastrulation, before development of the central nervous system. This, of course, makes it difficult to perform operations to alter the relationship between cranial mesoderm and the brain.

The question of whether the neuromeres are primary segments or secondary to mesodermal segmentation has been debated inconclusively for the past century (reviewed by von Kupffer, 1906; Vaage, 1969; Kuhlenbeck, 1973). Recent descriptive studies using immunocytochemistry and new techniques for labeling neurons show that there are groupings of neurons in the rhombomeres that relate to mesodermal segments of the branchial arch mesoderm, for example (Lumsden and Keynes, 1989). The somitomeres start forming at Stage 3 in the chick embryo, and all the cranial somitomeres have been formed by Stage 9, whereas the neuromeres only

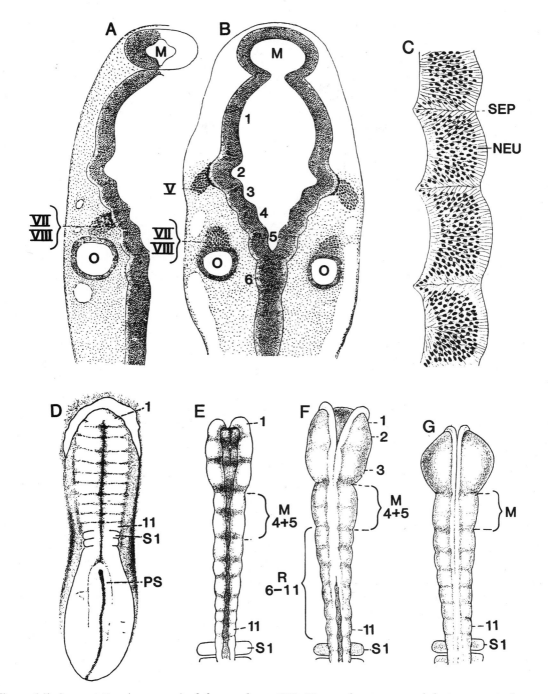

Figure 1.5. Segmentation (neuromery) of the vertebrate CNS. Nineteenth century morphologists recognized primary neuromeres in the open neural plate which give rise to 11 secondary neuromeres, consisting of cell clusters separated by transverse boundaries of low cell density in the neural tube: three in the prosencephalon, two in the mesencephalon and six in the rhombencephalon. (A) Duck embryo, beginning of 4th day, horizontal section through the hindbrain. (B) Same embryo as A, but 3 sections more ventral. M = mesencephalon; 1–6 = neuromeres of the rhombencephalon; O = otocyst; cranial ganglia V and VII/VIII are labeled. (C) Histological structure of hindbrain neuromeres of a human embryo showing the cell-poor boundaries (septa) between cell-rich neuromeres. (D–G) Chick embryos of 22, 24, 25.5, and 26 hours (two, five, six, and seven somites) showing development of 11 secondary neuromeres and their disappearance in rostrocaudal sequence: prosencephalic (1–3), mesencephalic (4 and 5), rhombencephalic (6–11). From K. von Kupffer, in *Handbuch der vergleichende und experimentelle Entwicklungslehre der Wirbeltiere*, R. Hertwig (ed.), Fischer Verlag, Jena, 1906.

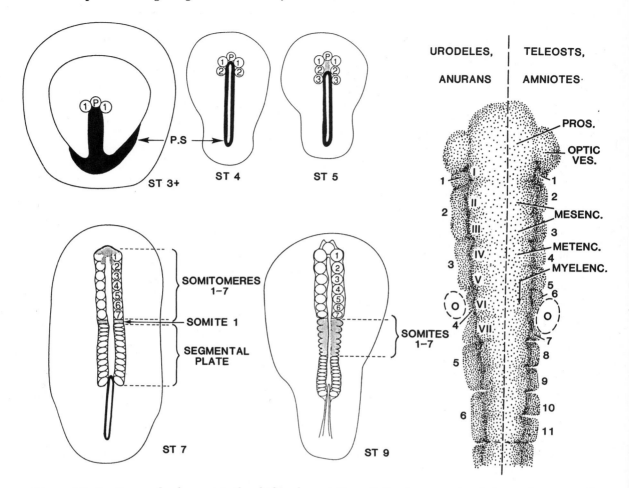

Figure 1.6. Somitomere development in the chick embryo at Stages 3–9 and a comparison between the pattern of somitomeres and neuromeres in amphibians, fish, and amniotes. In the chick embryo the first pair of somitomeres appears at Stage 3 (± 15 hours) on each side of the prechordal plate (P) at the anterior end of the primitive streak (P.S). Additional pairs of somitomeres form in the paraxial mesoderm on each side of Hensen's node at the anterior end of the primitive streak, until about 18 somitomeres have developed. The eighth somitomere condenses to form the first somite at St 7. Additional somites condense at the anterior end of the segmental plate. Neuromeres (Roman numerals) appear to correspond with the caudal somitomeres in teleosts and amniotes but not in amphibia. The arrangement in sharks is similar to that in the amphibia. The rostral neuromeres have disappeared by Stage 9 so that neuromere I in this figure probably corresponds with neuromere 3 in Fig. 1.5. Modified from A. G. Jacobson, *Development* **104** (Suppl.):209–220 (1988), copyright The Company of Biologists.

start developing at Stage 9. This sequence also indicates that the neuromeres are secondary to mesodermal segmentation, but the alternative opinion has been put forward, namely, that in the hindbrain the ectoderm is primarily segmented (C. D. Stern, 1990). However, to answer the question of whether the CNS segments are primary or only secondary to mesodermal segments will require an experimental analysis of the effects of altering the relations be-

tween mesoderm and CNS at different stages of development before and after development of the head mesoderm. Such an experimental analysis is difficult because head segmentation involves interactions between cells of cranial neural origin and craniofacial mesenchyme (Noden, 1983, 1988). Where such transplantations have been performed at trunk levels, the results show that segmentation in the spinal cord and peripheral ganglia is secondary to mesodermal segmentation and not an intrinsic property of the spinal cord (Detwiler, 1936, review; Keynes and Stern, 1988).

Detwiler's experiments done more than 50 years ago on *Amblystoma* embryos are still the most extensive analysis of the problem of the relationship between mesodermal and neural segmentation. They provide the best evidence that the segmentation of the spinal cord and peripheral nerves is secondary to mesodermal segmentation and that neither the neural tube nor the neural crest is intrinsically segmented (summarized in Detwiler, 1936, pp. 145–166). These conclusions were reached as a result of experimental grafting of parts of the spinal cord, grafting extra somites, and removal of somites. In all cases the spatial pattern of spinal nerves and ganglia corresponded with the segmentation of adjacent mesoderm.

Development of somite identity and autonomy occurs very early during embryonic development. In the chick embryo, ectopic grafts of pieces of somitic mesoderm develop into segments with the values that each would have expressed in the original position in the axial series (Pinot, 1969; Kieny *et al.*, 1972). In amphibians, from the time at which somites first become visible, they show regional differences in size and cell number. In the mouse, the initial number of cells in the most rostral trunk somite is 150–200, increasing progressively to 1000–1500 in the lumbosacral region and then decreasing rapidly in the caudal region (Tam, 1981). During vertebrate somitogenesis, new somites are added to the trunk by separation of mesoderm from the anterior border of the hindmost mesodermal segment (Bellairs, 1979). This occurs at the rate of one new somite every 60–75 minutes in *Xenopus* and every 100 minutes in the chick. Thus, there is a rostral-to-caudal gradient of formation and maturation of somites upon which further specializations are superimposed at later stages, for example, during development of somites that contribute to limbs. The cells of a single somite remain together, mingling very little with cells of neighboring somites, during migration of the somitic cells in the chick (Bagnall *et al.*, 1989). Segmental boundaries are thus maintained throughout development.

Although the problems of segmental patterning in the central and peripheral nervous systems and their relationship to mesodermal segmentation remain unresolved and controversial, it is not impossi-

ble to summarize the present state of understanding and the outstanding questions as follows.

The anatomical relationships between a particular segmental level of the central nervous system and related mesodermal segmental structures, somites, skull, vertebrae, and limbs are very variable. This is most marked in the head, so that some authors have denied that any correspondence exists between neuromeres in the head (encephalomeres) and head mesodermal segments (reviewed by Vaage, 1969). Any correspondence that might have originally existed in ontogeny and phylogeny has been distorted as a result of variations of the sense organs, mouth and branchial arches, and variable numbers of trunk segments that have been incorporated in the cranium in different vertebrates. Nevertheless, the variability of patterns of relationships between the CNS and head structures in different vertebrates does not completely obscure the homologies indicating a common ancestral pattern (van Wijhe, 1886; Gegenbauer, 1898; Ziegler, 1908; Goodrich, 1918; Delsman, 1922; Jarvik, 1980).

One of the main problems is to show conclusively whether correspondence between neural and mesodermal segments originates independently in the neurectoderm and mesoderm, or whether only the mesoderm is intrinsically and primarily segmented and it imposes a secondary segmental pattern on the adjacent neural tube and neural crest. If the latter occurs, are the serially repeated components of central and peripheral nervous system true segments, intersegments, or parasegments? In other words, how are serially repeated neural structures such as spinal nerve roots and spinal ganglia related to segmentation in the mesoderm?

There are no known cases of homeotic mutations in the vertebrate nervous system. One of the reasons for this may be that the nervous system is primarily unsegmented and only becomes segmented secondarily under influence of mesodermal segmentation.

1.3. Specification of Cell Fates

The term cell specification (synonymous with determination) denotes the processes by which the fates of the progeny of cleavage stage blastomeres are established in the normal embryo. Cells of different types normally develop in the embryo in a species specific spatial pattern. Therefore, specification is also associated with pattern formation, and underlying them both are regionally specific patterns of gene expression (Davidson, 1986, 1990, reviews).

There are two modes of establishing spatial patterns of differential gene activity: inheritance by blastomeres of cytoplasmic determinants that are regionally prelocalized in the egg; and positional specification by cell interactions mediated by morphogens, inductors, or growth factors. The first mode leads to determinative lineages in which cell fates are specified by the region of cytoplasm containing specific determinants inherited from the egg. The second mode leads to indeterminate probabilistic lineages in which specification of cell fate is contingent on cell position.

Indeterminate lineages enable cell specification to occur differently in different individuals of the same species. While both determinate and indeterminate cell lineages occur in embryos of all animals, only indeterminate lineages have been found in the vertebrate central nervous system (M. Jacobson, 1983, 1985, review; M. Jacobson and Moody, 1984; Kimmel and Warga, 1987; M. Jacobson and Xu, 1989), as we shall see in Section 2.11, which should be read in conjunction with this section. Much has been written about the relationship between variability of cleavage patterns and the type of cell fate specification (Davidson, 1986, 1989, 1990). In general, an invariant cleavage pattern is associated with determinate lineages, whereas variable cleavage patterns are always found in the vertebrates and are associated with indeterminate lineages. However, regardless of variability of cleavage, a group of blastomeres may inherit specific cytoplasmic determinants from a certain region of the egg cytoplasm. If these determinants start acting only after many cleavages, when the blastomeres are small, the prior pattern of cleavage will be irrelevant provided that the cells remain coherent before the specification of cell fates. The time of cell migration and cell mingling in relation to the time of specification of cell fates is critical (M. Jacobson, 1985, review). Lineage restrictions or commitments to parts of the body plan (requiring morphospecific gene activity) occur before cell migration in all vertebrates. By contrast, lineage

specification to individual cellular histotypes (involving histospecific gene activation) can occur either before or after cell migration—it occurs before cell migration in the determinate lineages, but after migration in the indeterminate lineages. Development of the central and peripheral nervous systems involve large scale cell migrations during which inductive cell-to-cell interactions occur which are necessary for specification of cell fates. The inductive interactions require prior specification of cells that produce inductive signals and those that are competent to receive them. The inductive interactions that determine whether competent ectodermal cells enter a neural differentiation pathway are considered in the following section.

1.4. Neural Induction and Determination

Close proximity between the archenteron roof (which later forms the notochord, somites, and prechordal plate) and the overlying ectoderm is the essential normal condition for development of the nervous system from that ectoderm. This effect is known as *neural induction*. The ectoderm is called the *induced tissue*, while the prospective chordamesoderm (tissue arising from the dorsal lip of the blastopore in amphibians and from the primitive streak in birds and mammals) is the *inducer* or *inductor* from which the inducing stimulus arises. After its induction, the neural plate is able to act as a neural inducer on competent ectoderm. This is called *homeogenetic induction* (Mangold and Spemann, 1927).

The capacity of a tissue to react to the influence of an inducer is known as its *competence*. Competence for neural induction is uniquely limited to the ectoderm of the gastrula—ectoderm from the blastula or from the neurula cannot respond to the primary inductive stimulus. Competence of the ectoderm could be a factor determining the size of the neural plate (Albers, 1987), or the main factor could be the area of contact between ectoderm and chordamesoderm (Nieuwkoop *et al.*, 1985). The ectoderm of the early gastrula has the ability, under the appropriate conditions, to differentiate along many different lines. The *prospective potency* of any embryonic tissue is its ability, under various conditions, to differentiate into a variety of tissues. The *prospec-*

tive significance or *prospective fate* of a tissue is its fate if left undisturbed during normal development. Prospective neurectoderm is that part of the ectoderm that will differentiate as neural tissue during normal development. The prospective neurectoderm gradually undergoes a progressive restriction of prospective potency. Pieces of prospective neurectoderm from the early gastrula, if grafted elsewhere in the embryo, can become epidermis, endoderm, or mesoderm, but toward the end of the period of gastrulation the prospective neurectoderm will differentiate only as neural tissue when translocated or when isolated *in vitro*. This restriction of prospective potency is known as *determination*. By the end of gastrulation the nervous system as a whole and the major parts of the nervous system—forebrain, midbrain, hindbrain, and spinal cord—have been determined. Some specific neuronal types, for example, the Rohon–Beard cells of the spinal cord and Mauthner's neurons of the medulla in frog embryos, are already determined by the end of gastrulation, and the progressive restriction of the prospective potency of parts of the neural plate continues throughout neurulation.

Determination of cell fates may occur in two ways: by a cell lineage mechanism or by inductive cell interaction, or by both. There is good evidence that both mechanisms operate during development of mesoderm in frog embryos. After fertilization, factors in the egg are displaced by cytoplasmic movements into the vegetal pole and become localized in vegetal blastomeres (Rebagliati *et al.*, 1985; Melton, 1987; Weeks and Melton, 1987). As a result of the activities of such factors, the vegetal cells induce mesodermal fates in the blastomeres of the marginal zone (Sudarwati and Nieuwkoop, 1975). Dorsal vegetal blastomeres induce dorsal mesoderm, which becomes the Spemann–Mangold organizer, located in the dorsal lip of the blastopore of amphibian embryos (Nieuwkoop, 1973). Mesoderm induction has to precede neural induction, so it is preferable to use the term "neural induction" rather than "primary neural induction" to denote the neural inductive action of chorda-mesoderm on the overlying ectoderm.

There is good evidence that cellular growth factors are directly involved in mesoderm induction (Smith, 1989, review): basic fibroblast growth factor (bFGF, Slack *et al.*, 1987; Slack and Isaacs, 1989;

Kimelman and Kirschner, 1987; Burgess and Maciag, 1989, review; Rifkin and Moscatelli, 1989, review), transforming growth factor-β:type 2 (TGF-β2, Kimelman and Kirschner, 1987; Rosa *et al.*, 1988), and XTC mesoderm-inducing factor obtained from a *Xenopus* cell line (J. C. Smith, 1987; Cooke *et al.*, 1987; J. C. Smith *et al.*, 1988; J. B. A. Green *et al.*, 1990). None of those factors have neural inductive activity. However, screening of a large number of cell lines for their neural inductive abilities has led to the discovery of a mouse macrophage cell line which secretes a factor that induces head structures, including brain and eyes (Sokol *et al.*, 1990; see Section 1.5).

The active component of XTC mesoderm-inducing factor is the *Xenopus* homologue of mammalian activin A (J. C. Smith *et al.*, 1990; van den Eijnden-Van Raaij *et al.*, 1990). Activins modulate the release of follicle-stimulating hormone from cultured anterior pituitary cells. This example illustrates the principle that the same factors can serve functions in the embryo which are entirely different from their roles in adults. There are qualitative differences in the types of mesoderm induced by these factors. TGF-β2 enhances synthesis of extracellular matrix molecules, especially during morphogenesis of tissues derived from embryonic mesoderm (reviewed by Roberts and Sporn, 1987; Heine *et al.*, 1988; Rizzino, 1988). XTC-MIF and activin-like proteins induce dorsoanterior mesoderm whereas bFGF induces ventroposterior mesoderm in competent animal pole cells (J. B. A. Green *et al.*, 1990; J. C. Smith *et al.*, 1990). Acting together these factors appear to be responsible for regionalization of the mesoderm including regionalization of the dorsal mesoderm required for neural induction (J. Cooke, 1989).

Experimental evidence shows that at early blastula stages the *Xenopus* embryo consists of presumptive ectoderm in the animal hemisphere and presumptive endoderm in the vegetal half (Jones and Woodland, 1986). During mesoderm induction a signal from the vegetal hemisphere induces cells to form mesoderm in the equatorial zone (J. C. Smith, 1989, review). According to the model of Slack and his collaborators, shown in Fig. 1.7 (J. C. Smith and Slack, 1983; J. C. Smith, 1989, review), two different signals pass from the vegetal to animal cells: on the dorsal side one signal induces notochord and some somitic muscle, on the ventral side another signal

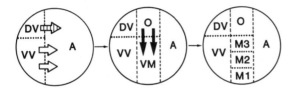

Figure 1.7. The three-signal theory to explain development of antero–posterior (animal–vegetal) and dorso–ventral polarity in the *Xenopus* embryo (Smith and Slack, 1983; Slack *et al.*, 1984; Smith *et al.*, 1985; Dale and Slack, 1987). Two mesoderm induction signals are assumed to originate from the vegetal hemisphere of the early blastula. The dorsal–vegetal (DV) signal induces dorsal mesoderm which becomes the "organizer" (O). The ventral vegetal signal (VV) induces ventral mesoderm (VM). The ventral mesoderm then receives a signal from the organizer which results in formation of somitic muscle (M3), and pronephros (M2), and the most distant mesoderm forms blood (M1).

induces blood and mesenchyme. A third signal originates from the newly induced dorsal mesoderm to dorsalize adjacent mesodermal cells to form muscle rather than blood. According to this concept, the Spemann organizer graft is the source of the third signal, inducing muscles in the ventral mesoderm which otherwise would have formed blood (J. C. Smith and Slack, 1983). The "third signal" is also presumed to act during normal gastrulation.

During gastrulation, as the archenteron roof moves forward from the dorsal lip of the blastopore, it exerts its inductive effect on progressively more anterior regions of the overlying ectoderm. This temporospatial progression of neural induction is thought to be one of the causes of the regional diversification of the neurectoderm. The more posterior regions of the neurectoderm are subject to the inductive stimulus for the longest time and, moreover, have a greater contact with the somitic mesoderm than the anterior part of the neurectoderm, which comes into contact with the prechordal plate mesoderm only for a relatively short time. For example, the entire prospective neurectodermal area is determined in less than 14 hours after first contact with the archenteron roof, in the newt *Triturus*, but while the posterior part is in contact with the inducer for that entire period, the anterior part is subject to induction only for 3 or 4 hours before it loses its competence to respond (Suzuki and Kuwabara, 1974).

The time of contact with the inducer tissue that is required to produce neural determination in com-

petent ectoderm has been studied by sandwiching inducing tissue between pieces of competent ectoderm and then separating the tissues after varying periods of contact. Using ectoderm of *Triturus*, weak induction is found after 1 hour of contact, whereas strong induction requires 3-4 hours (Johnen, 1964, Suzuki *et al.*, 1975). This technique is limited by the difficulty of completely separating the inducing tissue from the ectoderm, unless one of the interacting tissues is clearly marked with a fluorescent label, for example, and that was not possible until recently. Another limitation of such experiments is that early signs of neural differentiation in the ectoderm were very difficult to detect until the introduction of nerve cell specific markers, such as antibodies that recognize molecules appearing only in differentiating neural cells (Jones and Woodland, 1989), for example, the 180 kDa form of the neural cell adhesion molecule (N-CAM) as shown in Fig. 1.8 (Jacobson and Rutishauser, 1986; Levi *et al.*, 1987; Saint-Jeannet *et al.*, 1989), and N-CAM mRNA (Kintner and Melton, 1987). Antibodies that recognize molecules that disappear from the ectoderm after neural induction have also been useful for defining temporal and spatial parameters of neural induction (Akers *et al.*, 1986; Jones and Woodland, 1987).

The time at which neural determination occurs can now be assayed by the capacities of presumptive neural ectoderm to express nerve cell specific markers autonomously *in vitro*, after isolation of the ectoderm at different stages of development. Using antibodies to N-CAM as reagents for detecting neuralization of competent ectoderm, we showed that neural induction occurs in the ectoderm near the animal pole by 2.5-3 hours after the beginning of gastrulation in *Xenopus* embryos (Jacobson and Rutishauser, 1986). This is preceded by a rapid increase in N-CAM messenger RNA, starting at the beginning of gastrulation (Kintner and Melton, 1987; see Section 1.7). In *Xenopus*, development of the induction mechanism and of competence to respond does not require cell division or cell interactions before gastrulation: expression of a neural specific antigen occurs in *Xenopus* embryos with cell division blocked from the 128-cell stage (Jones and Woodland, 1989), and blastomeres dispersed from the 128-cell stage express N-CAM following reaggregation at Stage 9.5 (Sato and Sargent, 1989).

To find out how long the organizer maintains

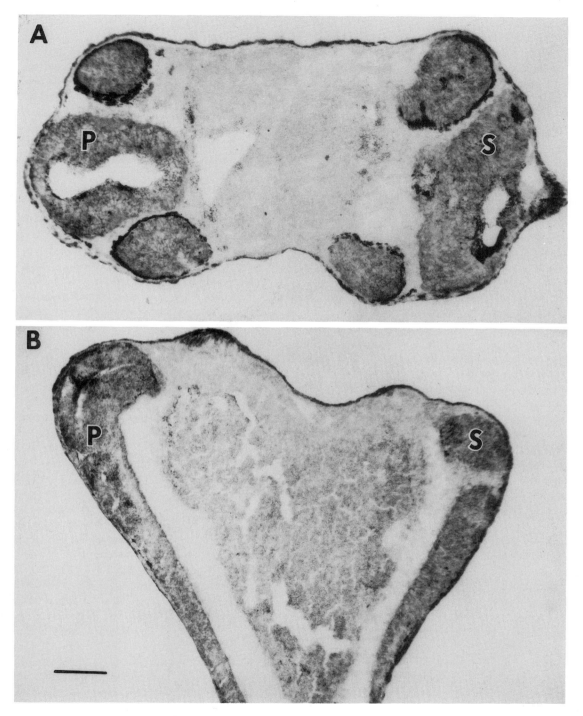

Figure 1.8. Neural cell adhesion molecule (N-CAM) is expressed strongly in an induced, secondary nervous system as well as in the primary central nervous system (see Figure 1.1). Tissue sections stained immunohistochemically for N-CAM. Wild-type *Xenopus* embryos at Stage 30 that had received a graft of dorsal blastopore lip in the ventral marginal zone at Stage 10. (A) Section cut coronally at the level of the eyes. (B) Section cut in the parasagittal plane. Greatly enhanced N-CAM reactivity is seen in the primary (P) or host nervous system, and secondary (S) or experimentally induced central nervous system. The dark pigment in the epidermis is melanin. Magnification bar = 100 μm. From M. Jacobson and U. Rutishauser, *Dev. Biol.* **116**:524–531 (1986), copyright Academic Press, Inc.

its neural inductive power and how long the ectoderm remains competent, experiments have been done in which the chordamesoderm and ectoderm, derived from embryos at different stages of development, are allowed to interact under controlled conditions. The results of such experiments show that the ectoderm loses competence relatively rapidly, before the end of gastrulation, whereas the inductive power of the chordamesoderm starts earlier and persists longer than the competence of the ectoderm (Gebhardt and Nieuwkoop, 1963).

How do regional differences in the nervous system develop? The evidence shows that the primary differences are in the mesoderm, not the ectoderm, at least with respect to specification of large-scale regional patterning of the nervous system. The mesoderm is regionally specified, as we have seen earlier in this chapter, and that may be a prior condition for regional specification of the nervous system. Classical experiments show that the chordamesoderm at the beginning of gastrulation induces brain and sense organs, and at later stages induces progressively more caudal structures. That this is not necessarily the result of differences in time of contact of the ectoderm with the inducer is shown by an elegant experiment of Holtfreter (1933, cited in Spemann, 1938, p. 293). Holtfreter showed that embryos cultured in high salt solution, without a vitelline membrane, gastrulate not inward, but outward to produce an inside-out embryo termed an exogastrula. When small pieces of competent ectoderm are placed on the endomesodermal part of a complete exogastrula, they undergo neural induction in accordance with the position of the chordamesoderm: ectoderm placed on the front end is induced to form brain, eyes, otic vesicles, and olfactory organs; on the middle the ectoderm is induced to form spinal cord; and posteriorly tail structures are formed.

How the regional determination of the neurectoderm occurs seems to have been resolved into two phases that overlap but are spatially and temporally almost separate at their extreme limits. One of the definitions of these two phases has been given by Nieuwkoop (1962, 1967a,b): first, *activation* of the ectoderm by the underlying chordamesoderm determines the size and form of the neural plate and results in the development of forebrain structures only; second, *transformation* of the already activated neurectoderm is brought about by interaction with

mesoderm and results in development of more caudal structures of the nervous system. Both activation and transformation are distributed as morphogenetic fields; that is, they have continuous, quantitative variation in space and time which, because the thickness of the neurectoderm is negligible compared with its length and width, results in mediolateral and anteroposterior (craniocaudal) differences in morphological development. From the point of view of the substances involved in these gradients, regional determination is seen as the result of at least two different agents acting on the neurectoderm: the neuralizing agent emanating from the anterior part of the archenteron roof and prechordal plate induces cranial structures in the nervous system such as forebrain and eyes, whereas mesodermalizing agent arising from the notochord and somites induces more caudal neural structures. These agents or other similar substances with the same effects, which have been identified as protein, have been isolated from various sources: the neuralizing agent from alcohol-treated liver and the mesodermalizing agent from alcohol-treated guinea pig bone marrow (Toivonen and Saxén, 1955a,b; T. Yamada, 1958; H. Tiedemann, 1968). The chick mesodermalizing agent is related to *Xenopus* XTC factor and to TGF-β2 (Grunz *et al.*, 1989). These factors are proteins and bind to plasma membrane receptors. Their roles in neural induction are indirect, via mesoderm which is the source of the neural induction stimulus. In addition to the induction stimulus, the mesoderm has a regionalizing action. Evidence that retinoic acid is a regionalizing factor, working in the anteroposterior axis of the *Xenopus* embryo, is discussed in Section 1.5.

The quantitative regionalizing effect of mesoderm on competent neurectoderm has been assayed by Saxén and Toivonen (1961) and Toivonen and Saxén (1968). They disaggregated neurectodermal cells of the forebrain region, mixed them in different ratios with trunk mesoderm cells, and reaggregated the mixtures. The aggregates were cultured for 14 days and then examined histologically. Only forebrain structures with nasal and optic rudiments developed in aggregates composed mostly of neurectodermal cells (ratio of ectodermal to mesodermal cells 10:1 or 5:1). It appeared as if the intrinsic tendency of the tissue was to develop as forebrain. Increasing the ratio of mesodermal cells to neurectodermal cells in the aggregates resulted in corresponding increases in caudal structures of the nervous system. Hindbrain and ear rudiments developed when the ratio of ectodermal to mesodermal cells was 5:2, and spinal cord developed when the ratio was 5:5 or less. Toivonen and Saxen (1968) concluded: *"During the initial stage of induction the cells are determined to become neural, but they acquire no stable regional character. This is subsequently controlled by the mesodermal cells and apparently in a quantitative way, since an increasing amount of mesoderm surrounding the neural cells shifts segregation in the caudal direction."* This effect may also be seen by grafting a fold of competent ectoderm onto the presumptive neural ectoderm of the preneurula (Nieuwkoop, 1952). The basal portion of such grafts differentiates into nervous structures like those in the host brain at the point of attachment of the graft, whereas the apical region of the graft always develops into forebrain structures.

1.5. Cellular Mechanisms of Neural Induction

From the time of discovery of the induction phenomenon, it has been tacitly implied that liberation of an inducer substance or substances occurs and that the site of origin, rate of diffusion, and stability will determine the "field" of action of the inducer. However, until very recently, no specific agent has been shown to be an authentic neural inducer whereas a variety of nonspecific physical and chemical agents may induce neural differentiation in competent ectoderm.

Isolated pieces of early gastrula ectoderm from *Ambystoma* and *Triturus* differentiate into neural structures when treated with a variety of chemicals (Holtfreter, 1944, 1945; T. Yamada, 1950) or even when subjected to changes in pH or to transient exposure to high concentrations of cations (Barth and Barth, 1969). It is generally believed that these multifarious inductive agents produce their effects indirectly either by release of the normal inducers by sublethal cytolysis or else by means of the second messengers cyclic AMP or inositol triphosphate. However, the possibility that specific neural inducers were present in the various heterologous inducers could not be ruled out.

Whether embryonic morphogenetic tissue interactions in general and neural inductions in particular are mediated by direct contact between the interacting cells or by diffusion of materials from one to the other has been a controversial topic for many years but is now being resolved with better techniques. The earlier studies of kidney tubule induction across a millipore filter led to the conclusion that a diffusible substance was involved (C. Grobstein, 1959; Koch and Grobstein, 1963). The first evidence to throw strong doubt on this was provided by Nordling *et al.* (1971), who found that a second millipore filter interposed between the spinal cord and metanephric mesenchyme increases the time for kidney tubule induction by about 12 hours. This is far too long for the increased diffusion time across the additional filter but is consistent with the increased time required for growth of fine cytoplasmic processes across the additional filter. The technique of interposing a filter between the interacting tissues had been used since 1961 to study neural induction, but there are limitations in the use of millipore filters for such studies: the millipore filter is an irregular mesh, and the possibility cannot be excluded that very fine cytoplasmic processes penetrate the filter by a tortuous path that cannot be seen with the electron microscope. The use of nuclepore filters which have pores of uniform dimensions has given different results, depending on the tissues that were used. Thus it now seems certain that induction of metanephric kidney tubules through a nuclepore filter requires direct cell contact (Wartiovaara *et al.*, 1974; Saxén *et al.*, 1976). It is known that metanephric tubules can be induced by direct contact with a number of embryonic tissues, including spinal cord and salivary mesenchyme. However, when a nuclepore filter with pore diameter 0.1 μm is interposed, only the spinal cord is effective, whereas either tissue is effective through a filter of 0.6 μm pore diameter. This correlates with the fact that spinal cord is able to send processes through 0.1 μm pores, whereas salivary mesenchyme requires a minimum pore diameter of 0.6 μm. Induction of kidney tubules is never seen when the interposed filter does not permit penetration of cytoplasmic processes between inductor cells and the responding mesenchyme. By contrast, evidence that the signal in neural induction is carried by diffusible substances was obtained by Toivonen *et al.* (1975). They separated newt gastrula dorsal lip mesoderm from competent surface ectoderm by means of nuclepore filters with pore diameters from 0.1 to 1.8 μm. Neural induction occurred in all cases, although electron microscopic examination did not reveal any cytoplasmic processes in the pores.

The evidence now shows that whereas intercellular contact is required for induction of kidney tubules in mouse metanephrogenic mesenchyme, the neural inductive signal can be transmitted by diffusion in amphibians. This is probably the case in the chick embryo also: at the time when neural induction is presumed to occur in the chick embryo before Stage 3 of the Hamburger and Hamilton (1951) series (Waddington, 1952; Abercrombie and Bellairs, 1954; Gallera et al., 1968), the presumptive neural ectoderm and chordamesoderm are not in direct contact but are separated by a basement membrane and extracellular matrix about 200–500 Å wide (Bellairs, 1959). Extracellular materials on the cell surfaces between the interacting tissues are most likely to play an important role during induction requiring direct contact, and this has been observed in mouse salivary gland (C. Grobstein, 1967; Bernfield and Wessells, 1970). Similarly, antibodies to cell surface glycoproteins have been shown to perturb epithelia-mesenchymal interactions (Sarida et al., 1988) in which direct contact between the interacting cells is required.

Embryonic inductions are now being viewed as special cases of cell-to-cell signaling which also include the better understood cases of action of hormones, neurotransmitters, and growth factors. Agonists such as steroid hormones, thyroid hormone, and retinoic acid diffuse into the cell and bind to intracellular receptors. Other agonists, including neurotransmitters and protein hormones, bind to specific receptors on the cell surface which are either directly coupled to other components of the plasma membrane or may be mediated by diffusible second messengers released from the plasma membrane into the cytoplasm. One class of agonists, including the well-understood case of norepinephrine, which binds to the β-adrenergic receptor, activates adenylate cyclase, which results in release of the second-messenger cyclic adenosine monophosphate (cAMP), which in turn activates protein kinase A. Another class of agonists includes the well-known cases of acetylcholine and transforming growth factor beta (TGF-β). These bind to specific receptors and activate phos-

pholipase C, which breaks down phosphatidyl inositol (4,5)-diphosphate to form diacyl glycerol and the second-messenger inositol 1,4,5-trisphosphate ($InsP_3$). The former activates protein kinase, the latter releases calcium from intracellular stores. The protein kinases (Nishizuka, 1988) phosphorylate many cellular proteins, and intracellular calcium also has a wide range of cellular actions, including modulation of ion conductance through plasma membrane ion channels, modulation of intercellular communication through gap junctions, control of phosphorylation of proteins via calmodulin, and control of mitosis.

The biochemical mechanisms of neural induction are not known at present, but are likely to be elucidated in the near future. There is growing evidence implicating growth factors in mesoderm induction, especially members of the TGF-β superfamily (Rosa et al., 1988) and bFGF (Kimelman and Kirschner, 1987; Slack and Isaacs, 1989), and activin-like proteins in determination of dorsal structures (J. C. Smith et al., 1990). However, none of those peptide growth factors so far tested induce neurectodermal derivatives in competent ectoderm. Recently a single protein factor named PIF (apparent molecular weight 28 kDa) secreted by a mouse macrophage cell line, has been shown to result in formation of an anterior–posterior axis and to induce anterior neural structures such as brain and eye in cultured presumptive ectoderm excised from Xenopus blastula (Sokol et al., 1990). Incubation of a small piece of presumptive ectoderm results in elongation of the tissue within about 6 hours, and in differentiation of anterior neural structures in about 1 day.

Evidence implicating protein kinase C in neural induction in Xenopus (Otte et al., 1988) may be a clue to the possible involvement of the second messenger Ins P_3 in neural induction, but the specific agonist(s) and receptor(s) remain to be demonstrated. It is not surprising, therefore, that many experimental conditions that may result in either mobilization of intracellular calcium or in activation of protein kinase C, or in both, may result in neural induction. By contrast with growth factors, which bind to plasma membrane receptors and work through second messangers, steroid hormones, thyroid hormone, and retinoic acid bind directly to intracellular receptors and work directly on the DNA.

They could, therefore, work during neural induction and regionalization of the neurectoderm in a manner analogous to their action on other organs.

All-*trans*-retinoic acid is a morphogen responsible for establishing the anterior–posterior axis of the limb in the chick embryo (Tickle *et al.,* 1982; Eichele and Thaller, 1987; Thaller and Eichele, 1987; Eichele, 1989, review). When an ion-exchange bead impregnated with retinoic acid is implanted at the anterior margin of the chick wing bud, opposite the zone of polarizing activity, it causes duplication of the limb pattern in low doses and truncation of the pattern in high doses. Retinoic acid binds to cellular retinoic acid-binding protein (Chytil and Ong, 1984; Giguere *et al.,* 1987; Petkovich *et al.,* 1987; M. Robertson, 1987) which belongs to a receptor superfamily including thyroid hormone and steroid hormone receptors (Evans, 1988, review). The retinoic acid–receptor complex binds to nuclear receptors for retinoic acid, which results in activation or repression of specific sets of genes (Mangelsdorf *et al.,* 1990). The retinoic acid-receptor complex may function to determine commitment of cells to specific lineages and to control differentiation of committed cells. High levels of cellular retinoic acid-binding protein are present in the chick neural tube, dorsal root ganglia, sympathetic ganglia, and enteric ganglia (Maden *et al.,* 1989). This indicates that these neurons require retinoic acid during development. Treatment of *Xenopus* embryos with low doses of retinoic acid (10^{-7} to 10^{-5} M) for 30 minutes at any stage from early cleavage until shortly after gastrulation results in suppression of anterior or transformation of anterior to posterior patterns of CNS development (Durston *et al.,* 1989). Retinoic acid does not prevent neural induction in recombinations of ectoderm and mesoderm *in vitro*. Its effects are on regional determination in the neurectoderm, resulting in suppression of differentiation of telencephalon, mesencephalon, olfactory organs, and eyes, but rhombencephalon, otic vesicles, and spinal cord are increased in size (Durston *et al.,* 1989). This may be compared with the action of retinoic acid on the chick wing bud. In the wing bud, retinoic acid acts on the mesenchyme in a dose-dependent manner: low doses give duplicated digit patterns, high doses truncations (Tickle *et al.,* 1989). In *Xenopus*, low doses of retinoic acid give truncations, namely, suppression of development of anterior regions of the nervous system, and this action is on the neurectoderm rather than the mesoderm (Durston *et al.,* 1989). At high doses retinoic acid and other retinoids are potent teratogens, producing developmental anomalies in various organs, including the nervous system (Wolf, 1984, review).

During normal development the conditions must be highly constrained by the specificity of binding of the putative inductor(s) and membrane and intracellular receptors, and by restricting the time of action of the components of the system. These restrictions may be affected by rapid breakdown of rate-limiting intermediates and by action of inhibitory components. No doubt the molecular machinery of neural induction will begin to be revealed within a few years. However, if we may generalize from the history of progressive elucidation of the mechanism of neural transmission at chemical synapses (Nicoll, 1988), after the basic mechanisms are first revealed, the picture will become increasingly complicated as the details are disclosed and as species- and tissue-specific variants are discovered.

From this mass of observations it now becomes clearer that **inductive tissue interactions have evolved in several ways in different tissues and in different species. Specificity of induction is a property of the mesoderm, but the time and spatial extent of induction are limited by the competence of the ectoderm. The tissues may interact by direct contact, or the interaction may be mediated by a diffusible agent or even by an agent packaged in vesicles. In all cases, the essence of the interaction is the transmission of a signal or signals from one tissue and the reception of the signal and its transduction as a change in the other tissue. Neural induction is probably mediated by a diffusible agent that binds to specific receptors on competent cells. Neural induction appears to be a multistep process in which the first step starts before the beginning of gastrulation (Jacobson and Rutishauser, 1986; Sharpe *et al.,* 1987; Savage and Phillips, 1989). Transduction events are likely to include breakdown of inositol phospholipid resulting in activation of protein kinase C and in release of the second-messenger inositol triphosphate which modulates intracellular calcium activity. Such events are likely to be triggered by a variety of agents resulting in nonspecific induction. Re-**

gionalization of neural differentiation requires additional diffusible morphogens, including retinoic acid, which can specify neural differentiation in a position-dependent manner.

1.6. Development of Polarity and Pattern in the Neural Plate[6]

One may think of the neural plate as a morphogenetic field of the central nervous system in the sense that it is the smallest unit of tissue that alone can form the entire central nervous system *in situ* or in isolation (Weiss, 1939). This definition can be extended to include the fact that the pattern cannot be completely restored after removal of an entire morphogenetic field, but after removal of parts of the field a whole pattern may reform within the residual cell population. This capacity for pattern regulation becomes progressively restricted topographically within the neural plate so that, as neurulation advances, separate fields emerge for the eyes, and probably for other regional subdivisions of forebrain, midbrain, and hindbrain. These regional or secondary fields contain elements that are uniquely determined as regards prospective cellular phenotypes. The first such phenotype determination occurs for Mauthner's neurons in the hindbrain and for Rohon–Beard cells in the neural folds, as dis-

cussed later in this section. As each region of the neural plate has a different prospective significance, that is, will give rise to different regions of central nervous system if left undisturbed, regional specificity of gene activation would seem to be essential, but it is not known how that might be controlled.

Detailed maps of the prospective brain regions in the neural plate have been made by the vital staining method invented by Goodale (1911) and applied to amphibians by Vogt (1925). In this method, small regions of the embryo have been stained with Nile blue sulfate or neutral red, and the stained parts have been identified at later stages of development. Maps have been made in this way of the presumptive eye region (Petersen, 1923; Woerdeman, 1929; Manchot, 1929), of the neural crest (R. C. Baker and Graves, 1939; Fautrez, 1942; Hörstadius, 1950), and of the entire neural plate of amphibian embryos (Nieuwkoop, 1955; C. O. Jacobson, 1959; von Woellwarth, 1960; Keller, 1976; Keller *et al.*, 1985). Prospective brain and spinal cord regions in the neural plate of the chick embryo have been mapped by marking cells with carbon particles (Spratt, 1959), and by grafting small pieces of quail embryo neural tube to the corresponding position in the chick embryo (Couly and Le Douarin, 1985, 1987; Schoenwolf *et al.*, 1989), as shown in Fig. 1.9.

Other methods of tracing cells during development include grafting polyploid cells in diploid embryos—the polyploid cells and the progeny can be recognized by their larger nuclei (M. Jacobson and Hirose, 1978; Turpen and Knudsen, 1982)—or grafting cells labeled with a heritable intracellular cell lineage tracer (reviewed by M. Jacobson, 1987, 1989) or with a lectin such as wheat germ agglutinin–colloidal gold conjugate (Smits-Van Prooije *et al.*, 1986; Tam and Beddington, 1987). These and other methods of tracing cell lineages are considered in more detail in Section 2.11.

Vital staining methods of fate mapping have serious limitations: the stains are applied to relatively large regions likely to contain cells with several different fates; the dyes fade, so that many progeny are likely to escape detection, especially single stained cells that have mingled with unstained cells. Embryonic surgical excision and transplantation experiments are notoriously liable to be misinterpreted in the light of insufficient knowledge of the normal developmental program of the excised

---

[6]A physical basis for tissue and organ polarity was first defined by Herbert Spencer in his *Principles of Biology* (1863). He there states that *"organic polarity can be possessed neither by the chemical units nor the morphological units, we may conceive it as possessed by certain intermediate units which we may term physiological."* This concept was elaborated by Ernst Haeckel in his concept of *"Promorphologie"* dealing with the level of organization between the cellular and the molecular. Haeckel thought of such subcellular organization as a basis for different kinds of symmetry in living organisms. The seductiveness of this concept of the paracrystalline organization of living matter is shown by the number of its adherents, notably Carl Nägeli and Ross Harrison, who expressed that concept in his final statement of the nature of symmetry in the embryo (Harrison, 1945). The notion that left–right symmetry is determined in the embryo *"by means of a mechanism in which a molecule, which itself has handedness, is aligned with respect to the anteroposterior and dorsoventral axes"* (N. A. Brown and Wolpert, 1990) is the most recent effort along those traditional lines.

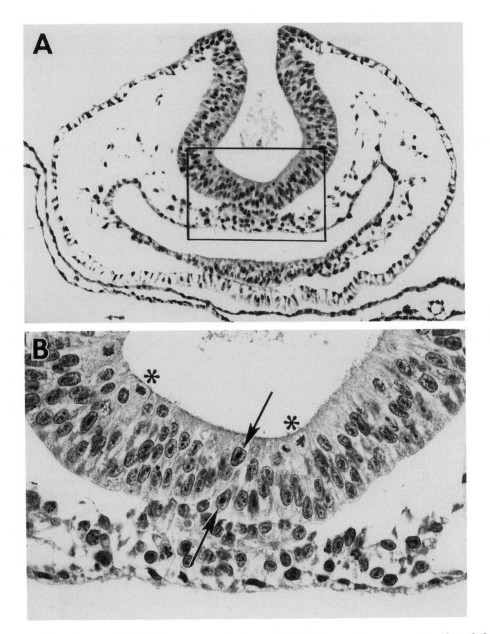

Figure 1.9. Analysis of neurepithelial cell rearrangement using quail-chick chimeras. Transverse section through the neural tube of a quail-chick chimera at the midbrain level (A). The area in the box is enlarged in B. Arrows point to quail cells. Asterisks indicate mitotic figures. Compare this with Figures 2.1 and 2.2. Quail cells were grafted just rostral to Hensen's node, and during transformation of the neural plate to the neural tube (a period of 24 hours) the cells divided a maximum of three times and extended caudally in the midline. The results show that shaping of the avian neural plate involves cell division and cell rearragements. From G. C. Schoenwolf and I. S. Alvarez, *Development* **106**:427–439 (1989).

tissue (e.g., M. Jacobson, 1968a, corrected by Holt *et al.*, 1986; Cooke, 1981, corrected by Cooke, 1985). Many other cases may be cited in which misattribution of the fates of regions of the embryo that were excised, transplanted, or cultured *in vitro* resulted in errors of interpretation of the results. Vital stains have now been superseded wherever possible by heritable cell lineage tracers injected directly into identified single embryonic cells (reviewed by M. Jacobson, 1987, 1990a).

Horseradish peroxidase or fluorescent labeled dextran, injected into individual blastomeres, has been used for fate mapping in the leech (Weisblat *et al.*, 1978; Weisblat and Shankland, 1985), ascidian (Nishida and Satoh, 1983), fish (Kimmel and Warga, 1986), frog (M. Jacobson and Hirose, 1978 , 1981; Hirose and Jacobson, 1979; M. Jacobson, 1980, 1981a,b, 1983, 1985a,b; Moody, 1987a,b; Sheard and Jacobson, 1987), and mouse (Balakier and Pedersen, 1982; Cruz and Pedersen, 1985; Winkel and Pedersen, 1988). These tracers, injected intracellularly, do not alter normal development, do not diffuse to neighboring cells, are transmitted to all the descendants of the initially injected cell, and can be detected in those progeny at much later stages of development. This method has the advantages of leaving the embryo intact and of not interfering seriously with normal development, and it provides fate maps at the level of resolution of single cells (Fig. 1.10). This is discussed at greater length in Section 2.11.

The main disadvantage of all methods of fate mapping is that they do not give any information about the degree of determination at the time of staining but show only the potential fate (i.e., the prospective significance) of different regions of the neural plate. However, fate maps are indispensable for showing changes of fates that may occur after surgical grafting or explantation of pieces of the embryo. The surgical methods of excision and transplantation interfere more or less with normal development but give information about the regulative capacity and the extent to which each region of the embryo is committed to the formation of specific parts of the final structure.

Several experimental methods—excision, transplantation, and explantation—have been used to map the prospective significance of different parts of the neurepithelium and to discover the time at which its axes of symmetry are fixed. Accurate fate

maps are needed with which to interpret such results. The degree of restitution that is possible after surgical excision of various parts of the neurepithelium at different stages of development provides clues to the time of determination of the parts that are not reconstituted and to the regulative capacity of the remaining parts (Du Shane, 1938; Aufsess, 1941: Detwiler, 1947; Pratt, 1949; Holtzer, 1951; Stefanelli, 1951; Watterson and Fowler, 1953; Corner, 1963, 1964). Excised pieces of neural plate or neural tube are replaced by regeneration from the sides or, in the case of unilateral excision, from the intact half and never from the cranial or caudal margin of the wound. Regeneration from the contralateral tissue occurs after unilateral excision of the neural plate (W. H. Lewis, 1910; Harrison, 1947; Corner, 1963), of the forebrain (Burr, 1916), of the midbrain (Detwiler, 1944; Harrison, 1947), and of the spinal cord (Detwiler, 1947; Holtzer, 1951).

Other investigators have studied the capacity of isolated pieces of neural epithelium to differentiate into parts of the central nervous system when transplanted to other parts of the embryo or when explanted *in vitro* (W. H. Lewis, 1910; Mangold, 1931, 1933; Aufsess, 1941; TerHorst, 1947; von Woellwarth, 1952; Waechter, 1953; Kälén, 1958; Corner, 1964). These studies show the remarkable self-differentiation capacity of small pieces of neural plate transplanted to other regions and of isolated pieces of the neural plate and neural tube to develop *in vitro* as if they had been left in the embryo.

Another strategy has been to make grafts to different positions in the neural plate or neural tube with or without reversal of the axis of the graft, at different stages of development. Reversal of the axes of the graft gives information about the time of axial polarization of the neurepithelium (Spemann, 1906, 1912; Detwiler, 1940, 1943, 1949, 1951; Roach, 1945; Sládecek, 1952, 1955; C. O. Jacobson, 1964).

The effects of reversing the axes of the neural plate were first tested in amphibians by Spemann (1906, 1912). He excised a large piece of the anterior part of the neural plate with the underlying mesoderm and reimplanted it with its anteroposterior axis reversed. The rotated piece of neurepithelium develops according to its original position; that is, it is inverted in the rostrocaudal axis. This was confirmed by Roach (1945), who showed that bilateral or unilateral anteroposterior inversion

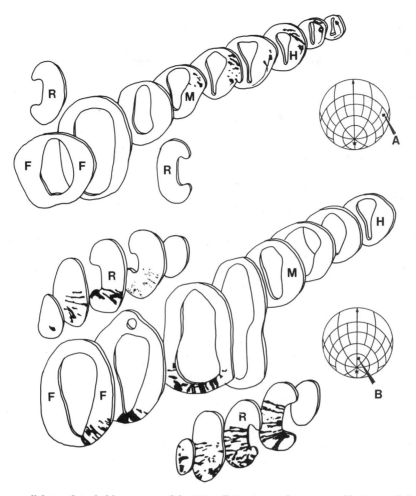

Figure 1.10. Nerve cell fates of single blastomeres of the 512-cell *Xenopus* embryo mapped by intracellular injection of a cell lineage tracer (horseradish peroxidase). The positions of the injected progenitor cells (A) and (B) are shown on a grid used to locate the blastomeres in relation to the animal pole (star) and dorsal midline (arrow) of the 512-cell embryo. The diameter of the embryo is about 1.2 mm. The positions of the labeled progeny in the nervous system are shown in reconstructions of every tenth serial section through the forebrain (F), midbrain (M), hindbrain (H), and retina (R). Other labeled progeny, not shown, were located outside the central nervous system. The progeny are located in a region of the embryo called a clonal domain. The invariant relationships between positions of progenitor cells and the locations of their clonal domains provide the data for construction of a fate map. Adapted from M. Jacobson, *J. Neurosci.* 3:1019–1038 (1983).

of the neurepithelium, with or without underlying mesoderm in the preneurula (Stages 13 and 14) of the salamander, results in anteroposterior inversion of the parts of the nervous system formed from the graft (Fig. 1.11). This shows that the anteroposterior polarity of the neurepithelium is already determined in the preneurula. However, different results were obtained by Sládecek (1955). He excised the anterior part of one side of the neural plate in sala-

mander neurula (Stages 14–16), rotated the piece 180 degrees, and reimplanted it with antero-posterior and mediolateral axes inverted. Complete regulation occurs in grafts made at Stage 14 and almost complete regulation in grafts made at Stages 15 and 16, resulting in development of a normal brain. Sládecek suggested that this occurs because his grafts are entirely within the neural folds, whereas grafts such as those made by Roach (1945)

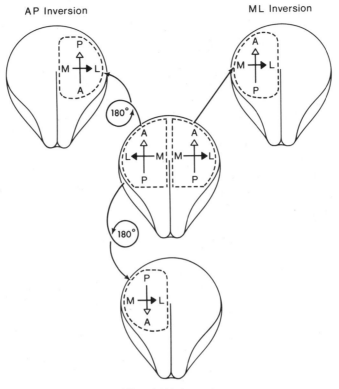

Figure 1.11. Method of producing axial inversion of the neural plate by unilateral grafts of neural ectoderm, either with or without underlying mesoderm, in the early neurula of the salamander. By this method, Roach (1945) and Sládecek (1952, 1955) showed that the anteroposterior axis of the neural plate is determined before the mediolateral axis.

do not regulate because part of the neural fold is included in the graft. Most likely, the differences are related to the size of the grafts. The tendency of small grafts of rotated neurepithelium to regulate and larger grafts not to regulate was observed by Alderman (1935), Nicholas (1957), and C. O. Jacobson (1964).

Inversion of the mediolateral axis only of the anterior part of the neural plate can be achieved by interchanging the left half of the neural plate of one salamander embryo with the right half of another (Roach, 1945; Sládecek, 1952), as is shown in Fig. 1.11. In Roach's experiments the grafts were made at Stage 14, and they subsequently developed according to their inverted position; that is, almost complete regulation occurred, resulting in a normal brain. This shows that the mediolateral polarity is not fixed in the neurepithelium at Stage 14. Sládecek (1952) found that the mediolateral axis is already fixed at Stages 15 and 16. That there may be regional differences in the time of polarization of the neurepithelium is shown by the results of inverting pieces of the presumptive hindbrain. Detwiler (1940, 1943, 1949, 1951) found that almost complete regulation occurred after anteroposterior inversion of the presumptive hindbrain of the salamander at Stages 19–26, and evidence of failure of regulation was seen only after inversion at Stage 27.

In the experiments described so far, attention is given only to the external morphology of the brain or to the large internal structures of the parts of the brain that develop from the grafts. When the gross morphology of the brain is normal, the graft is considered to have regulated; abnormalities of gross morphology were taken as evidence of determination of various brain structures. More convincing evidence of determination of neural connectivity may be obtained from detailed anatomical studies (Holtzer, 1951; C. O. Jacobson, 1964), studies of motor function (Székely, 1963; Straznicky, 1963; Straznicky and Székely, 1967), and electrophysiological mapping of neuronal projections (M. Jacobson, 1967, 1968a; R. Levine and M. Jacobson, 1974).

Holtzer (1951) found that after unilateral excision of the spinal cord of the salamander at Stages 18–24 the regeneration that occurs from the intact side is less complete when the excision is made at later rather than earlier stages. The cells that are not reconstituted at later stages are assumed to have been determined at earlier stages. Similar conclusions about the early determination of specific neurons were reached by Stefanelli (1951). He showed that Mauthner neurons, which differentiate in the medulla, are already determined in the neural plate at Stages 15–16 in the salamander. If the region of neural plate containing the prospective Mauthner cells is excised after Stage 16, Mauthner neurons fail to develop at later stages. In fact, Mauthner neurons originate as postmitotic cells in the gastrula, Stage 12 in the frog *Xenopus* (Vargas Lizardi and Lyser, 1974). Extirpation of parts of the neural fold has shown that the Rohon–Beard cells, which are the primary sensory neurons of the spinal cord of early larval amphibians, are already determined in the early neurula. Bilateral removal of the neural fold of the prospective trunk region of Stage 13 salamander embryos results in absence of Rohon–Beard cells from spinal segments 3–19, whereas from 10 to 20 Rohon–Beard cells normally develop in each spinal segment (Du Shane, 1938). Rohon–Beard cells originate as postmitotic neurons in the frog, *Xenopus*, over a period of about 6 hours, starting at late gastrula stages (Lamborghini, 1980). This indicates that commitment to differentiation of Mauthner and Rohon–Beard neurons is completed at or before these cells originate as postmitotic neurons and that this occurs during gastrulation.

C. O. Jacobson (1964) made a detailed histological study of the brain that develops after craniocaudal inversion of the prospective hindbrain region of the neural plate without underlying mesoderm, in the salamander neurula. Although the external morphology of the brain at later stages appears normal, there are significant deviations from normal histology which indicate that the structures in the graft develop in accordance with their origin. The most obvious abnormality is the development of primary motor nuclei in ectopic positions in reversed order in the cranio-caudal axis of the hindbrain. The motor roots emerge at the level of their nuclei and innervate adjacent muscles nonselectively. For example, eye muscles are innervated by cranial nerve VII, and hyoid muscles by cranial nerve V. This is in agreement with other evidence of nonselective innervation of muscles such as limb muscles innervated by cranial nerves (Braus, 1905; Detwiler, 1930a,b; Nicholas, 1933; Hibbard, 1965b), the nonselective reinnervation of skeletal muscles after cross union of motor nerves (review, Sperry, 1948), and the innervation of skeletal muscle by implanted foreign motor nerves (Aitken, 1950; H. Hoffman, 1951b). The selectivity of formation of neuromuscular connections is discussed in Section 9.3.

Sensory roots enter the rotated hindbrain nonselectively at the points of emergence of the motor roots (C. O. Jacobson, 1964). However, their central fibers form apparently normal longitudinal fiber tracts in the medulla regardless of the abnormal positions of entry of sensory roots. This is assumed to be the result of selective affinity between the sensory nerve fibers. The central connections of sensory nerves in the rotated hindbrain were not studied. It would be of great value to determine whether sensory nerves grow into inverted hindbrain to form connections congruent with their peripheral sense organs, as they appear to do after inversion of their peripheral sensory fields (Weiss, 1942; Kollros, 1943b; Sperry and Miner, 1949; Miner, 1956; Eccles *et al.*, 1962b; M. Jacobson and Baker, 1968, 1969; R. E. Baker and Jacobson, 1970; see Section 11.5). Evidence of the polarizing influences of the graft on the course of cranial nerve VIII was obtained by C. O. Jacobson (1964). In five of eight cases in which nerve VIII entered the inverted medulla, the course of the ascending and descending branches of nerve VIII was appropriate to the polarity of the graft; in one case both normal and repolarized branching occurred, and in two cases the branches grew according to their original polarity and contrary to that of the graft.

In summary, it appears that the motor neurons must already have developed stable position dependent properties (i.e., irreversibly specified) before the surgical inversion of the hindbrain anlage, and that those specificities are later expressed in accordance with the original position of the cells. Such precocious determination is apparently characteristic of large neurons with long axons, that is, principal neurons or Type I neurons (M. Jacobson, 1970a, 1975a; see Sections 2.12 and 10.2).

The rule that Type I neurons are programmed at a very early stage is illustrated by the Mauthner neuron, which comes into existence as a postmitotic cell in the late gastrula stage in amphibians (Stefanelli, 1951). The stem cell that gives rise to the Mauthner neuron in *Xenopus* undergoes its final DNA synthesis in the late gastrula (Stage 12) 3–4 hours after the beginning of neural induction (Vargas Lizardi and Lyser, 1974). The mitosis that gives rise to the Mauthner neuron occurs 1–2 hours later, at Stage 13. Stefanelli (1951) showed that extirpation of the medulla before Stage 13 can result in restoration of the missing part, including Mauthner neuron, whereas after Stage 13 the Mauthner neuron is missing, although the medulla may be largely or completely restored. Although the program for differentiation of Mauthner neuron is initiated at Stage 13, the Mauthner cell cannot be recognized histologically until Stages 29–30, about 20 hours later.

The polarity of the Mauthner neuron and the course of its axon were studied in inverted hindbrain grafts by C. O. Jacobson (1964). The polarity of Mauthner neuron conforms with that of the rostrocaudally inverted medulla if the graft includes the presumptive Mauthner neuron, which lies at the lateral margin of the neural plate. In 25 animals in which Mauthner axons initially grew toward the head instead of toward the tail, 16 ultimately reached the spinal cord, either by making a hairpin bend within the graft or by following a tortuous course through graft and normal brain. In cases where the Mauthner cell body is not included in the graft and is normally polarized, the majority of cases in which the Mauthner axon runs through the graft follow a course that conforms with the inverted polarity of the graft. Although C. O. Jacobson (1964) reached somewhat different conclusions, a plausible interpretation is that his results show that the initial direction of outgrowth of the Mauthner axon is de-

termined by the polarity of the cell body, but that the subsequent direction of axonal growth is highly influenced by the polarity of the central nervous system through which the axon grows. This interpretation is in agreement with conclusions reached by Stefanelli (1951) and Hibbard (1965a) from their observations of the growth adjustments of Mauthner nerve fibers, and by M. Jacobson and Huang (1985) and Huang and Jacobson (1986) from their observations of outgrowth of nerve fibers in *Xenopus* embryos, which are discussed more fully in Section 5.12. A discussion of whether the controlling factors are mechanical, chemical, or electrical or a combination of several factors appears in Chapter 5.

To summarize, there are at least three different causes of axial polarization of the central nervous system: the distribution of cell types varies over the tissue; groups of cells with different structures form in ordered sequence; individual cells have polarity and are aligned in one or more axes. All three causes operate in axial polarization of the neural plate and tube. Firstly, there is a nonuniform distribution of cell types in the neural plate. Commitment to different nerve cell types starts during gastrulation. In amphibians, several types of large neurons originate as postmitotic cells before the end of gastrulation, although they are not identifiable histologically until after formation of the neural tube. Secondly, it appears that founder cell populations are established in a specific pattern in the neural plate. The descendants of each founder cell group form morphological components of the central nervous system, such as retina, forebrain and midbrain, hindbrain, and spinal cord. Thirdly, metameric organization of the mesoderm imposes a segmental organization on the central nervous system, most easily seen in the correspondence between nerve roots and somites, but also evident in a segmental arrangement of the neuronal organization of the hindbrain and spinal cord. Because these three main causes of axial polarization of the neural plate and tube occur at different times and rates, the effects of surgical removal or transplantation of pieces of the neural plate or neural tube will depend on the time of the operation and on whether mesoderm is also included. In summary, such experiments seem to show that axial polarization of the neurepithelium of the neural plate occurs in the anteroposterior and mediolateral (dorsoventral) axes, sequentially and independently in the two axes, within a relatively short period of several hours in amphibian embryos.

1.7. Roles of Neural Cell Adhesion Molecules in Neural Morphogenesis

Cell adhesion is a well-recognized mechanism of morphogenesis (Holtfreter, 1939; Townes and Holtfreter, 1955; Moscona, 1956, 1957; P. Weiss and Taylor, 1960; Steinberg, 1970, 1974). From the early studies it was evident that different cell surface adhesion molecules can selectively mediate cell interactions, associations, and assembly into tissues. However, it was not until Gerisch (1977) first used adhesion-inhibiting antibodies that it became possible to characterize cell adhesion molecules by immunological and biochemical techniques and to show that cell adhesion can be inhibited with specific antibodies (Rutishauser et al., 1976; Thiery et al., 1977; Hyafil et al., 1980; Hoffman et al., 1982; Damsky et al., 1983; Rathjen and Schachner, 1984). Those investigations indicated that cell adhesion molecules are integral membrane glycoproteins with adhesive sites on the cell surface. Adhesion between different cells involves either binding between molecules of the same type (homophilic binding) or between different molecules (heterophilic binding).

Cell adhesion molecules can express a very wide range of functional specificities as a result of differences of their biochemical characteristics, quantity, spatial distribution, and time and duration of expression. These parameters may be independently regulated during development. Many cells express several different cell adhesion molecules simultaneously in different combinations. Cell adhesion molecules are not cell-type-specific. A few different cell adhesion molecules may be involved in a large variety of different morphogenetic processes (reviewed by Edelman, 1983, 1984a,b, 1985, 1989b; Takeichi, 1988; Rutishauser and Jessell, 1988; Linnemann and Bock, 1989). However, the possible repertoire of actions of cell adhesion molecules is limited to short-range interactions involving direct contact between cells forming coherent assemblies. Long-range signaling between cells is mediated by diffusible molecules, and usually involves cells that are separated by basement membranes or are in contact with substantial quantities of extracellular matrix, and also often involves migrating cells or motile parts of cells, like growth cones. Thus, side-to-side adhesion of axons to form bundles is mediated by cell adhesion molecules whereas adhesion of the growth cone to the substratum is mediated by substratum adhesion molecules and integrins. However, N-CAM may also function as a substratum adhesion molecule as it has heparin and fibronectin binding sites. **Cell adhesion molecules hold cells together for mechanical stability and to allow them to interact by means of other molecules. The neural cell adhesion molecules may also have more dynamic actions, for example, by altering cell shape and motility via the linkage between actin microfilaments and the cytoplasmic domain of the adhesion molecule.**

There are two large classes of cell adhesion molecules: those whose adhesivity is dependent on Ca^{2+} belong to the cadherin family (Takeichi, 1988, review); those whose adhesivity is independent of Ca^{2+} include several belonging to the immunoglobulin superfamily. The latter include various forms of the neural cell adhesion molecule (N-CAM), the L1 neural cell adhesion molecule, myelin-associated glycoprotein (MAG, see Section 3.15), and fasciclins (Table 1.1). Even a selective review of the immense literature on cell adhesion molecules is beyond our scope and their roles are considered where necessary at many places in this book.

Calcium-dependent cell adhesion molecules are a family of glycoproteins called cadherins (Shirayoshi et al., 1986). They have a molecular weight of 124–127 kDa, are composed of 723–748 amino acids, and have a sequence similarity of 50–65 percent. Cadherins have a transmembrane carboxyl terminus and an amino terminus carrying the extracellular adhesion site and calcium binding site. Cloning of cDNAs coding for cadherins (Gallin et al., 1987; Nagafuchi et al., 1987; Hatta et al., 1988) has made it possible to transfect cells with expression vectors carrying the full-length cDNA coding region of the cadherin molecule, under control of a suitable promoter. Such transfected cells express calcium-dependent adhesion that is blocked by specific monoclonal antibodies (Nagafuchi et al., 1987; Hatta et al., 1988). Transfected cells expressing E-cadherin do not adhere to those expressing

Table 1.1. Neural Cell Adhesion Molecules

Molecule	Species	M_r ($\times 10^3$)	Ligands	Tissue distribution	References
N-cadherin (similar or identical molecules: A-CAM; N-cal-CAM)	Chick, mouse	124	Homophilic	Embryonic mesoderm, neurectoderm, nerve cells, cardiac and skeletal muscle, primordial germ cells, adherens junctions	Hatta and Takeichi, 1986; Takeichi, 1988
N-CAM	Vertebrates, some invertebrates	180 140 120	Homophilic, heparin, fibronectin	Neurectoderm, neurons, glial cell, embryonic muscle, Schwann cells	Cunningham et al., 1987; Edelman, 1984; Rutishauser and Jessell, 1988
L1 (similar or identical molecules: Ng-CAM; NILE; 69A1)	Mouse, chick	200	Homophilic, heterophilic	Neurons, glial cells	Faissner et al., 1985; Moose et al., 1988; Grumet et al., 1988
MAG	Mouse, chick	100 (?)	Heterophilic	Oligodendrocytes	Poltorak et al., 1987
P_O	Mammals	29	Homophilic	Myelinating Schwann cells, axons, neurepithelium, body epidermis	Wood and Dawson, 1973; Martini et al., 1988
Fasciclins	Insects Fasciclin I Fasciclin II Fasciclin III	70 95 46,59,66,80			Patel et al., 1987

N-cadherin, whereas those expressing the same cadherin adhere to one another. Those findings show that cadherin molecules adhere to one another by a homophilic binding mechanism and that different cadherins, although structurally similar, have different specificities. E-cadherin has been shown to be involved in a variety of early morphogenetic events, including compaction of the 8- to 16-cell embryo (Hyafil et al., 1980, 1981; Shirayoshi et al., 1983; Damsky et al., 1983; M. H. Johnson et al., 1986), histogenesis of embryonic endoderm (Richa et al., 1985), and in cell movements during early morphogenesis (Thiery et al., 1984; Damjanov et al., 1986). Early in development all cells express E-cadherin but mesodermal and neural cells lose it and gain N-cadherin.

N-cadherin has been shown to play a role in side-to-side adhesion of mesodermal cells during formation of somites, and in morphogenesis of the mesonephros (Hatta and Takeichi, 1986; Hatta et al., 1987). N-cadherin appears in the neural plate neurepithelial cells at the same time as E-cadherin

disappears from them. N-cadherin is expressed on neurepithelial cells of the neural tube but is lost from differentiated neurons. Neural crest cells lose N-cadherin before they start migrating but start expressing N-cadherin after they reach their destinations. Outgrowing neurites possess N-cadherin, which enables axons to adhere homophilically to one another as well as to astrocytes (Tomaselli et al., 1988). Antibodies to N-cadherin perturb histogenesis of the chick embryo retina in vitro (Matsunaga et al., 1988).

N-CAM in the adult mammalian brain consists of three glycoproteins of 120, 140, and 180 kDa. It is encoded by a single gene and mRNAs for the three forms of N-CAM are produced by differential splicing. Evidence for the homophilic adhesive mechanism of N-CAM has been obtained by incorporating the molecule into liposomes and showing that they adhere to one another and to cell surfaces, and that the adhesion can be inhibited by specific antibodies (S. Hoffman and Edelman, 1983; Sadoul et al., 1983; Edelman, 1988, review). N-CAM polypeptide has three domains: the extracellular amino terminus, which contains the specific homophilic binding site; the carboxyl terminus, which is associated with the plasma membrane and cytoplasm; and an intermediate extracellular domain, to which are attached long, unbranched chains of polysialic acid. The quantity of polysialic acid is inversely related to the binding strength, and developmental regulation of the quantity of polysialic acid can result in significant functional changes. Lightly sialylated N-CAM is expressed in neurepithelial germinal cells and in terminally differentiated neurons where it results in strong side-to-side adhesion between cells. By contrast, migrating neurons and outgrowing dendrites and axons possess heavily sialylated N-CAM, whose adhesivity is low enough to permit cells to form temporary contacts with one another (Sunshine *et al.,* 1987; Rutishauser *et al.,* 1988).

N-CAM and N-cadherin are generally expressed simultaneously on the same neural cells, and their different mechanisms of adhesion allow a greater range of functional effects than would be possible with only one kind of neural cell adhesion molecule. N-CAM has been implicated in primary neural induction (Edelman, 1983, 1984a,b; but see M. Jacobson and Rutishauser, 1986), induction of feather rudiments (Chuong and Edelman, 1985a, 1985b), formation of axon bundles and tracts (Rutishauser *et al.,* 1978; Balak *et al.,* 1987), axonal guidance (Silver and Rutishauser, 1984), histogenesis of the CNS (Rutishauser *et al.,* 1978b; Buskirk *et al.,* 1980), histogenesis of the retina (Balak *et al.,* 1987; M. Jacobson, 1988), formation of neuromuscular connections (Grumet *et al.,* 1982; Rutishauser *et al.,* 1983; Balak *et al.,* 1987; M. Jacobson, 1988), and formation of the retinotectal map (Fraser *et al.,* 1984; M. Jacobson, 1988).

L1 is a calcium-independent neural cell adhesion molecule found in postmitotic neurons but not glial cells in mouse nervous system (Rathjen and Schachner, 1984; Faissner *et al.,* 1984 a,b, 1985; Moose *et al.,* 1988). L1 is a 200 kDa integral membrane glycoprotein. The same molecule in the chicken is called Ng-CAM (Grumet and Edelman, 1988). When incorporated into liposomes or covaspheres, Ng-CAM shows homophilic binding. Liposomes containing Ng-CAM also bind specifically to glial cells. Since the latter do not possess Ng-CAM, the binding to glial cells is heterophilic, involving another receptor (Grumet *et al.,* 1988). L1

has been implicated in migration of cerebellar granule cells (Lindner *et al.,* 1983, 1986) and in fasciculation of axons (Fischer *et al.,* 1986).

1.8. Morphogenesis of the Neural Tube

Folding of epithelial sheets as a basic feature of morphogenesis was first recognized by Wilhelm His (1894). Several intrinsic mechanisms have been shown to be involved, including localized or oriented cell division, oriented cell movements, differential cell adhesion, and changes in cell shape, especially apical constriction and basal expansion, converting cuboidal to wedge shaped cells (reviewed by Ettensohn, 1985). The ability of the isolated neural plate to fold over to form a tube was demonstrated by Roux (1895) in the chick embryo and Glaser (1914) in the amphibian. Elevation of the neural folds continues following excision of the neural plate (Hörstadius and Sellman, 1946; C. O. Jacobson, 1962; C. O. Jacobson and Jacobson, 1973). Extrinsic forces help to shape the neural tube and are involved in neurulation: attachment of the midline of the neural plate to the prechordal plate mesoderm and notochord, forming hinge point changes in the extracellular matrix surrounding the neural plate, and elevation of the somites (Brun and Garson, 1983; Smedley and Stanisstreet, 1985; Schoenwolf, 1988; Schoenwolf *et al.,* 1988).

Flexure of the neural plate occurs at the level of the rostral end of the notochord, starting before neural tube closure begins (A. G. Jacobson, 1981; A. G. Jacobson and Tam, 1982). The process of folding of the neural plate to form the neural tube is called *neurulation.* It may be subdivided in four main phases: formation, shaping, bending, and fusion (Schoenwolf and Smith, 1990, review). The first stage is formation of a thickened neurepithelium forming the neural plate consisting of elongated cells, at different phases of the mitotic cycle. This becomes shaped like a spoon, broad in front and narrow behind. Shaping is accomplished by forces intrinsic to the neurectoderm. The margins of the neural plate become raised to form the neural folds, and the midline region of the neural plate is depressed to form the neural groove. The neural folds are elevated, with the midline notochordal attachment forming a hinge as a result of wedging of the cells of the floor plate. A second hinge region develops on each side (Schoenwolf, 1982, 1985). As the dorsal part of the neurepithelium bends inward, the neural folds meet dorsally and fuse in the dorsal midline to form a tube. Fusion of the neural folds starts at one point in the region of the future hindbrain, followed by fusion at the rostral and caudal ends and progression rostrally and caudally from those points (Sakai, 1989, review). The neurepithelium detaches or delaminates from the lateral ectoderm, which moves toward the dorsal midline during the process of neurulation and fuses dorsally over the neural tube (Martins-Green, 1988). The cells at the margin of the neural folds and the lateral ectoderm move into the space between the dorsal part of the neural tube and the overlying ectoderm, where they form the neural crest, which is considered in Chapter 4.

Formation of a tube by elevation and folding of the margins of the neural plate is called *primary neurulation* to distinguish it from the process of *secondary neurulation* by which the lumbosacral region of the spinal cord is formed in the tail bud of birds and mammals (Criley, 1969; Schoenwolf and De-Longo, 1980; Costanzo *et al.*, 1982) and the entire neural tube is formed in teleost fish embryos (Ishii, 1967; Miyayama and Fujimoto, 1977; Nakao and Ishizura, 1984). Secondary neurulation occurs by cavitation of an initially compact mass of cells called the medullary cord. Whether the cavitation occurs as a result of cell death or secretion of extracellular materials, or by both processes, is not known.

It is not known whether primary or secondary neurulation is the phylogenetically more ancient mode. At the end of his 1876 paper *"On the Development of the Spinal Nerves in Elasmobranch Fishes,"* F. M. Balfour slips in the remark *"that the embryonic mode of formation of the spinal canal, by folding of the external epiblast, is the very method by which I have supposed the spinal canal to have been formed in the ancestors of the vertebrates."* In those days the biologist could hardly make a discovery without staring evolution in the face. After a long period of neglect, the problem of the evolution of neurulation now seems ready for reinvestigation.

The cells of the neurepithelium undergo characteristic movements toward the midline of the embryo during formation of the neural plate. This displacement was originally shown by observing the

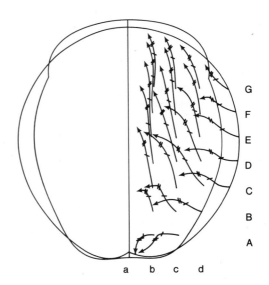

Figure 1.12. Trajectories of cells displaced in the neural plate of the newt followed with time-lapse cinematography. The cells were at the origin of the arrows at embryonic Stage 13; had reached the position of the single transverse bar at Stage 14; were at the position of the double transverse bar at Stage 14.5; and had arrived at the points of the arrows at Stage 15. Meanwhile, the embryo had changed its shape from the wider outline at Stage 13 to the narrower outline at Stage 15. From B. Burnside and A. G. Jacobson, *Dev. Biol.* 18:537–552 (1968), copyright Academic Press, Inc.

movement of groups of cells that had been marked by a vital stain (Goerttler, 1925; Vogt, 1929; Manchot, 1929; C. O. Jacobson, 1962) or by following movements of pigmented cells (Burnside and Jacobson, 1968), as shown in Fig. 1.12 in the newt neural epithelium. Cell displacement in the chick embryo neurepithelium during neurulation has been traced by microinjection of a fluorescent tracer into the neurepithelium (Schoenwolf and Sheard, 1989). Displacement of cells in the neural plate of the rat may be due to differential cell proliferation; for example, lengthening of the neural plate and tube may be caused by oriented mitoses producing new cells in the rostrocaudal axis (Tuckett and Morriss-Kay, 1985). In the chick, shaping of the neural plate involves rapid cell rearrangement and cell division, with the latter occuring in both mediolateral and rostrocaudal axes (Schoenwolf and Alvarez, 1989).

During shaping of the neural plate the cells do not more independently of each other: time lapse cinematography of amphibian embryos shows that the neural epithelium moves as a whole, with different parts moving at different speeds (C. O. Jacobson, 1962; Burnside and Jacobson, 1968). Cells retain their contacts with their neighbors while they are migrating at speeds ranging from 4 to 95 μm per hour for distances up to 896 μm in the neural plate of a 2.5 mm newt embryo (Burnside and Jacobson, 1968), as shown in Fig. 1.12. Independent movement of cells is limited because the cells of the neural plate (P. C. Baker and Schroeder, 1967) and neural tube (Duncan, 1957; Bellairs, 1959) are bound together at their apices by intercellular junctions. Some rearrangement may occur as a result of mitosis: cells lose their basal contacts and round up near the apex during metaphase, and the plane of the mitotic spindle may be specifically oriented so as to position the daughter cell preferentially with respect to the longitudinal or transverse axes of the neurectoderm (Tuckett and Morriss-Kay, 1985). A model of cell movements in epithelial sheets has been proposed by A. G. Jacobson *et al.* (1986). Called the "cortical tractor model," it proposes that basal-to-apical flow of the cortical cytoplasm, carrying membrane components from the base to the apex of the cell, can result in changes of cell shape and cell motility without breaking the apical intercellular junctions.

More than a century ago Wilhelm His noticed numerous mitotic figures in the neurepithelium of the chick embryo and he suggested that rapid cell proliferation plays a role in shaping and bending of the neural plate and neural tube (His, 1868, 1874). Rapid cell proliferation has been observed in the neurepithelium of the chick, mouse, and rat (Jelineck and Friebova, 1966; S. L. Kauffman, 1968; D. B. Wilson, 1982; Schoenwolf, 1985; Tuckett and Morriss-Kay, 1985; J. L. Smith and Schoenwolf, 1988; Schoenwolf and Alvarez, 1989), whereas few mitotic figures are seen in the neural plate of the amphibia. Gillette (1944) has shown that there is a relatively small increase in the number of cells in the neural plate of the salamander, from 113,000 at Stage 13, just before formation of the neural plate, to 139,000 at Stage 19, after closure of the neural tube. By contrast, in the chick embryo, there is a high mitotic rate in the neural plate and neural tube (cell cycle length 6–12 hours; Table 2.1) and as the duration of neurulation is about 24 hours, the number of neurepithelial cells could triple during neurulation (Schoenwolf, 1985).

Another important problem is the formation

and maintenance of the lumen in the neural tube, the neurocele, which ultimately forms the ventricular system (Jelínek and Pexeider, 1970). The composition of the fluid in the neurocele, and its functions, also require further investigation. Transient complete occlusion of an extensive segment of the neural tube is a normal occurrence in chick (Desmond and Jacobson, 1977; Desmond and Schoenwolf, 1985, 1986), mouse (Kaufman, 1983), rat (Freeman, 1972), and human (Desmond, 1982), and it has been suggested that occlusion may play a role in enlargement of the brain as a result of increased hydrostatic pressure in the lumen.

Wilhelm His anticipated modern conceptions of neural plate folding when he wrote in 1894: "*Suppose we have a sheet of cells, the elements of which are as wide at their bases as they are at the free surface. If now, as a result of internal forces, the cells are all induced to become thicker at their bases and thinner at their free ends, the result will be that the sheet bends and folds together to form a hollow structure.*" Much progress has been made in understanding how the neurectodermal cells constrict at the apex but less is known about how they may expand at the base (J. L. Smith and Schoenwolf, 1988). And the way in which changes in cell shape are regionally or locally regulated remains in the realm of hypothesis.

The neural plate of urodeles and the chick embryo is a single layer of columnar cells forming a pseudostratified epithelium, whereas that of anurans is already two cells thick before neurulation starts (Schroeder, 1970). Cell elongation results in a reduction in the area and an increase in the thickness of the neural plate. Characteristic changes in the shape of neurepithelial cells occur during neurulation. The cells of the early neural plate are cuboidal, and they become progressively more elongated and narrower at the apex and ultimately become wedge shaped in the newt (Burnside, 1971, 1973, 1975), axolotl (Brun and Garson, 1983), *Xenopus* (Schroeder, 1970), and the chick (Karfunkel, 1971, 1972, 1974; Schoenwolf and Franks, 1984).

Wedging of cells is mainly restricted to the dorsolateral and ventral median hinge points in the chick embryo (Schoenwolf and Franks, 1984), as shown in Fig. 1.13. Schoenwolf (1988) calculates that only about 10 percent of cells in the chick neural plate become wedge shaped during neurulation.

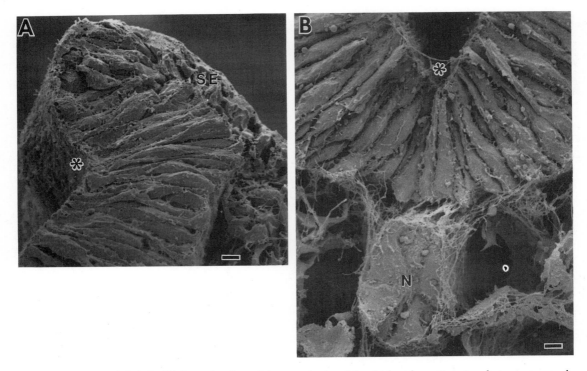

Figure 1.13. Neurepithelial cells during bending of the neural tube of the chick embryo. Scanning electron micrographs showing the changes in shapes of neurepithelial cells at the dorsolateral (A) and median (B) hinge points in the future hindbrain of a Stage 8 (26–29 hour) chick embryo. Asterisks = hinge points; N = notochord; SE = surface ectoderm; magnification bar = 5 μm. Figures provided by G. C. Schoenwolf and J. L. Smith.

Evidence that microfilaments are not necessarily involved is that treatment of neurulating chick embryos with cytochalasin D does not prevent shaping of the neural plate and elevation of the neural folds, and wedging of cells in the floor plate forming the median hinge occurs despite the absence of apical microfilament bands in those cells (Schoenwolf *et al.*, 1988). Basal expansion also plays a role in cell wedging in the chick neural tube (J. L. Smith and Schoenwolf, 1988). Cell adhesion molecules probably play a role in maintaining side-to-side adhesion of neurepithelial cells and thus resisting the shear forces generated in the neural tube during neurulation. For example, N-CAM is strongly expressed on the surface of cells of the neural plate and neural tube of *Xenopus* (Balak *et al.*, 1987; M. Jacobson, 1988) and the chick (Crossin *et al.*, 1985), as shown in Fig. 1.14.

During neural tube formation in the chick embryo, bundles of contractile microfilaments, which react specifically with antibodies to actin and myo-sin, coincide with the constricted apices of neurepithelial cells (Lee and Nageli, 1985; Nageli and Lee, 1987). This is most marked at the regions where the most acute bends in the neurepithelium occur, at the midline of the V-shaped early neural fold stage, and at the midlateral walls of the C-shaped midneural fold stage (Fig. 1.13). After closure of the neural tube, the apical microfilament bundles diminish in number and thickness.

Additional evidence supporting the concept of intrinsic cellular mechanisms of neurulation comes from the results of treating embryos with specific pharmacological agents. Cytochalasins, which block microfilament function, stop neurulation (Karfunkel, 1972; Morriss-Kay, 1983; but see Schoenwolf *et al.*, 1988). Neurulation is inhibited by treatment with colchicine or vinblastine, which prevents microtubule assembly (Karfunkel, 1971, 1972; O'Shea, 1982), and this evidence shows that microtubules are involved in maintaining the shape of neurectodermal cells (Waddington and Perry, 1966;

N-CAM   L-CAM

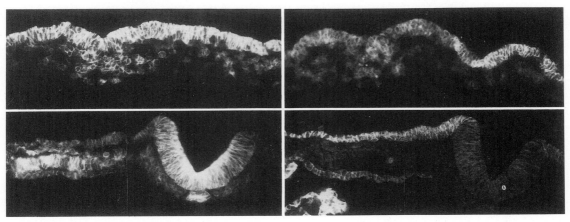

Figure 1.14. Expression of N-CAM and L-CAM (L-cadherin) during gastrulation and neurulation of the chick embryo. Both N-CAM and L-CAM are expressed by the epithelial cells of the blastoderm, but become down-regulated or masked in ingressing cells that will form the mesoderm (upper panels). At neurulation (lower panels), a striking border is formed between the N-CAM-rich neural ectoderm and the L-CAM-rich somatic ectoderm. Subsequently, N-CAM is expressed on all neural cells and L-CAM is completely lost from the nervous system though it continues to be expressed on epithelial cells derived from all three germ layers. From K. L. Crossin, C-M. Chuong, and G. M. Edelman, *Proc. Natl. Acad. Sci. USA* 82:6942-6946 (1985).

Burnside, 1971, Karfunkel, 1971). Papaverine inhibits neural tube closure in amphibian (Moran and Rice, 1970) and mouse embryos (O'Shea, 1982), probably by perturbing intracellular calcium which is required for the normal action of contractile microfilaments. Calcium ions are required for normal neurulation. In the absence of calcium ions the neural folds fail to fuse, and they collapse (Smedley and Stannisstreet, 1985). Restoration of calcium ions to the external medium results in rapid reelevation of the neural folds. Evidence that these effects are mediated by changes in the calcium ions inside the cells, rather than the effect on calcium-dependent cell adhesion molecules, is that papaverine prevents neurulation and the effect can be reversed by calcium ionophore A 23187, which increases calcium ion flux into cells.

Different lectins such as concanavalin A and wheat germ agglutinin bind specifically to sugar residues of cell membrane molecules, and several studies have shown changes in lectin binding during neurulation in frog and chick embryos (O'Dell *et al.*, 1974; Currie *et al.*, 1978, 1984; Takahashi *et al.*, 1979; Takahashi and Howes, 1986). Such developmentally regulated expression of sugar-containing molecules on the cell surface is probably related to

changes in cell–cell adhesion and interaction, but their mechanisms of action during neurulation remain to be discovered.

Much evidence showing that the forces for neurulation are intrinsic to the neurepithelium does not necessarily exclude a role of extrinsic factors, but the evidence for these is not compelling, and at most shows that the external structures have permissive and facilitatory roles. For example, the accumulation of extracellular matrix materials, especially nonsulfated glucosaminoglycans, at the site of neural fold elevation in the mouse suggests that increase of extracellular matrix components, especially hyaluronate, may be involved in neural tube formation (Morriss and Solursh, 1978a,b; Copp and Bernfield, 1988). In chick embryos, injection of hyaluronidase results in neural tube defects (Schoenwolf and Fisher, 1983). However, normal neurulation occurs in rat embryos cultured in hyaluronidase (Morriss-Kay *et al.*, 1986).

It has long been thought that neural tube formation can occur after isolation of the neural plate in amphibians (Glaser, 1914; Boerema, 1929; Holtfreter, 1939; Aufsess, 1941) and chicks (Roux 1895; for a review see Karfunkel, 1974). Other arguments against any necessary participation in neurulation by forces outside the neurectoderm itself are that the external structures vary along the length of the neural tube, and complete or partial removal of the notochord does not seriously affect neurulation or differentiation of nerve cells in the neural tube (Malacinski and Yoon, 1981). A midline specialization of the neurepithelium named the floor plate develops where the notochord is in contact with the neural plate, and this specialization has long been thought to have special functions in defining the basic plan of the brainstem and spinal cord (His, 1893; J. B. Johnston, 1902; Kingsbury, 1920, 1922, 1930). The floor plate is absent after removal of the notochord, but the mechanism by which the notochord may affect differentiation of floor plate cells is not known (Schoenwolf and Franks, 1984). A clue may be that a protein which binds to phospholipids and actin in the presence of Ca^{2+} is localized to the cells of the floor plate (McKanna and Cohen, 1989).

Grafting an additional notochord within 80 μm of the lateral wall of the neural tube in 2-day chick embryos stimulates differentiation of neurons and results in enlargement of the part of the neural tube nearest the notochord graft (van Straaten *et al.,* 1985). The evidence suggests that the notochord arranges the sclerenchymal cells, which then promote cell proliferation and differentiation in the neural tube (van Straaten *et al.,* 1989). This suggests that extrinsic forces help to shape the neural tube.

However, the extrinsic forces do not appear to be essential for the initiation of neurulation or for the complex series of changes in shapes of neurepithelial cells and in the maintenance of the cavity in the tube, which result in formation of a neural tube. The forces necessary for those changes are in the neurepithelial cells themselves.

The driving forces for neurulation are both extrinsic and intrinsic, but most investigators have concentrated on forces within the neurepithelium itself, particularly contractile microfilaments containing actin and myosin, mainly localized in the apical regions of the cells. In addition, the shape of the neurepithelial cells is regulated by intermediate filaments and microtubules (see Chapter 5). Cell-surface adhesion molecules and specialized membrane junctions maintain side-to-side contact between the neurepithelial cells. The net result of these cellular mechanisms in apical constriction and basal expansion, with the apex of the neurepithelial cells thrown into folds, so that the previously columnar cells become wedge shaped. To complicate the problem of how this is regulated, it should be remembered that neural tube bending and folding occur while the neurepithelial cells are actively proliferating, while interkinetic nuclear migration is occurring in those cells (see Section 2.2, Fig. 2.1) and at the same time as large changes occur in size and shape of tissues surrounding the neural tube.

2 The Germinal Cell, Histogenesis, and Lineages of Nerve Cells

For all those who are enchanted by the magic of the infinitely small, hidden in the bosom of the living being are millions of palpitating cells whose only demand for the surrender of their secret, and with it the halo of fame, is a lucid and tenacious intelligence to contemplate them, to admire and to understand them.

The final sentence of Ramón y Cajal's autobiography, *Recuerdos de mi vida: Historia de mi labor científica*, Tercera edición, 1923

2.1. Historical Orientation

A mind historically focussed will embody in its idea of what is "modern" and "contemporary" a far larger section of the past than a mind living in the myopia of the moment. "Contemporary civilization" in our sense, therefore, goes deep into the 19th century.

Johan Huizinga (1872–1945),
Homo Ludens, 1938

From its inception by Wilhelm His in 1887, the concept of subclasses of germinal cells that are the progenitors of corresponding classes of neurons and glial cells has been opposed by the concept of multipotential progenitors, put forward by Vignal (1888), Schaper (1894a,b), and Koelliker (1897). Both concepts have continued to exert powerful heuristic effects for more than a century.

Discovery of the germinal cells of the vertebrate nervous system, by Wilhelm His in 1887, can be fully understood only in historical context—it was only one of many interlocking pieces of research out of which a coherent picture of the behavior of cells during development was rapidly assembled in the second half of the 19th century (O. Hertwig,

1893–1896; E. B. Wilson, 1896). The contributions of His must also be viewed as part of the ongoing program to reconcile comparative anatomy and embryology with the gradual improvements in understanding cell structure and function (Koelliker 1852, 1854, 1879, 1896). That program gained momentum throughout the 19th century, and the investigation of the histogenesis of the nervous system was pushed forward rapidly by the advances made by cytologists and embryologists. In many ways it was a period like our own in which powerful new research techniques produced results that challenged the assumptions of the time. The cell theory put forward by Schwann in 1838 was radically modified during the next 50 years.[1]

[1]Schwann (1839) knew nothing of cell division: he conjectured that cells form by crystallization out of a fluid cytoblastema. Remak (1841) was the first to report formation of cells by division, which he observed in leukocytes of frog tadpoles, and to propose in 1852 that cells generally form in that way. Both Remak's and Schwann's theories were considered to be valid by Koelliker in the first edition of his *Handbuch der Gewebelehre* (1852). The stages of the mitotic cycle were described in the embryo of a flatworm by Schneider in 1873, and 2 years later Strassburger described mitosis in plants. A much more accurate description of the phases of the mitotic cycle was

41

Wilhelm His (1831–1904) towers over the field of research on histogenesis of the nervous system in the 19th century. He casts a long shadow into the 20th century through his pupils Franklin P. Mall, who brought the science of human embryology to the United States, and Friedrich Miescher, founder of the chemistry of nucleic acids and nucleoproteins. The new concepts of cell biology were transmitted to neuroembryology by His: He was the first to recognize the significance of cell migration in development of the central and peripheral nervous systems. He discovered the neural crest and showed that cranial and spinal ganglia are formed by cells which migrate from the neural crest (see Section 4.1 and Fig. 4.1). He was among the earliest to give evidence that the nerve fiber is an outgrowth of the nerve cell, the first to try to show when neuronal and glial cell lineages diverge, and he discovered that nerve cells originate by mitosis of stem cells near the ventricle of the neural tube. He showed that neurons originate from specific progenitor cells, which he called germinal cells (*Keimzellen*), recognizable by their mitotic figures lying close to the lumen of the neural tube (His, 1887a,b, 1888a,b, 1889a, 1890a,b).

It should be remembered that Walter Flemming's *Zellsubstanz, Kern und Zelltheilung* (1882) was hot off the press when His discovered the germinal cells in the neural tube of human embryos. Flemming's book provided the first clear demonstration of the transformation of the resting cell nucleus into the mitotic figure, and he showed that the essential event of mitosis is the duplication and division of the chromosomes. Flemming recognized that chromatin (which is the name he gave to the material in the nucleus which he stained with azo dyes) is probably the same as the nucleic acid which Miescher (1871) had purified from the nuclei of leukocytes and had called nuclein (reviewed by Hughes, 1952, 1959). By the mideighties, it had be-

come evident that chromatin, the material of the chromosomes (named by Waldeyer in 1888), is the basis of heredity. With those discoveries the links were forged between cytology, embryology, and evolution.

The great achievements of Wilhelm His are in no way diminished by the fact that he was misled by histological artifacts which were unavoidable at that time. Artifacts led him to conclude that there are two different classes of cells in the neural tube of the early vertebrate embryo: germinal cells that are visible as mitotic figures lining the lumen, which give rise to neurons, and spongioblasts that appear to form a syncytium, from which neuroglial cells originate (Fig. 2.1). These observations led His to formulate four separate theories: theory 1 was concerned with the different stem cells for neurons and glial cells; theory 2 was about the syncytium; theory 3 was about the significance of the large extracellular spaces and their contents; theory 4 was about guidance of migrating neuroblasts by radially aligned spongioblasts (M. Jacobson, in preparation).

His (1887a,b, 1888a, 1889) deduced that the germinal cell divides repeatedly: one daughter cell remains close to the lumen of the neural tube and reenters the mitotic cycle while the other daughter cell becomes a neuroblast. Then the neuroblast, which is incapable of further division, migrates away from the germinal layer and eventually develops into a neuron. Recognition of the asymmetrical division of the germinal cell was a significant conceptual advance that has become assimilated into modern theory (see Section 2.11).

The suffix "blast" derives from the Greek word *blastos,* which means a germ or a bud, and indicates that a cell is capable of further division.[2] However, neuroblasts in the vertebrates do not incorporate [³H]thymidine, which indicates that they have ceased DNA synthesis and mitosis, as we shall see in Section 2.2. Therefore, the cell called neuroblast by His is better referred to as an undifferentiated neuron or young neuron, and the term neuroblast is

---

given by Flemming (1882). He named the entire cycle "*karyomitosis*" and the individual nuclear changes "*mitoses.*" Before Flemming's work it was generally believed that the nucleus dissolves during cell division and reforms anew in each daughter cell. Virchow's dictum—*Omnis cellula e cellula*—was extended by Flemming with his "*Omnis nucleus e nucleo,*" which was finally completed by Watson and Crick with their "*Omnis DNA e DNA.*"

[2]Neuroblast (or archiblast) was a term invented by His (1868) to refer to the embryonic tissue that gives rise to the CNS in the chick embryo (which is now called epiblast) to differentiate it from the extraembryonic hemoblast (or parablast), which he believed to give rise to blood and mesenchyme. Only later did His (1889a) use the term neuroblast to refer to the cells rather than the entire tissue giving rise to neurons.

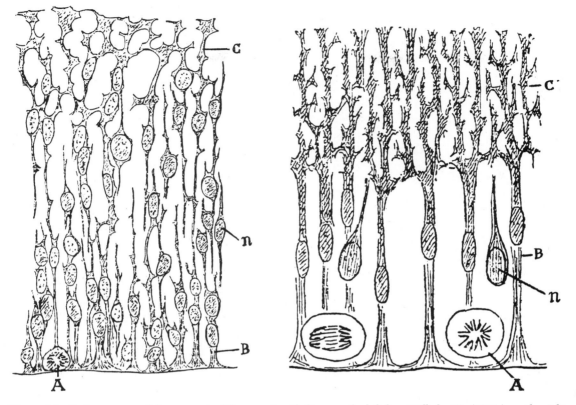

Figure 2.1. Early concepts of the structure of the neural epithelium, on the left from Wilhelm His (1887a), on the right from Ramón y Cajal (1894). The original drawing by His showing the germinal cell (A) undergoing mitosis near the ventricle, the spongioblasts (B) forming a syncytium, and neuroblasts (n) migrating from the ventricular germinal zone to marginal zone (C). Ramón y Cajal accepted the concept originated by His of separate populations of germinal cells, neuroblasts, and spongioblasts. Cajal did not believe that spongioblasts form a syncytium (see Section 5.1) but he did not have good counterevidence and that uncertainty is reflected in his drawing. Both His and Cajal knew of Flemming's description of the phases of mitosis, but His drew what he could see whereas Cajal drew idealized pictures of metaphase figures, two of which were most unlikely to be close together in the same section. Both thought that wide intercellular spaces are normally present in embryonic tissues, and that they provide pathways for cell migration. A fundamental difference between the two depictions of the same tissue is that His drew an accurate picture of a single histological section whereas Cajal combined many views in a single picture in his search for a synthetic principle by which to explain development of the neural epithelium.

best reserved for the progenitor of neurons in the invertebrates.

Another theory of neuronal and neuroglial histogenesis, in almost total disagreement with the theory of His, was proposed by Vignal (1888) and Schaper (1894a,b) and supported by Koelliker (1897). They based their theory on essentially the same histological observations as those of His, but they interpreted them in a different way. The observation that mitotic figures occur only in the cells lining the lumen of the early neural tube had been interpreted by His to mean that the mitotic

figures belong to germinal cells (*Keimzellen*), whereas he believed that the other cell nuclei of the neural tube belong to different classes of cells. He identified some as neuroblasts giving rise to neurons and others as spongioblasts giving rise to neuroglial cells. Alternative interpretations of the histological picture were given by Schaper (1897a,b). He suggested that *"the so-called 'Keim-zellen' of His lying near the central cavity of the neural tube, along the membrana limitans interna, are not to be considered as a special type of cell in contrast to the main epithelial cells in process of continuous proliferation"* (Schaper, 1897b). According to Schaper, the so-called germinal cells and spongioblasts are really cells of the same type which move to different levels in the neural tube during different phases of the mitotic cycle. The *"Keimzellen"* of His are merely cells that have rounded up close to the lumen in preparation for mitosis, after which the nuclei of the daughter cells move away from the lumen during interphase and return inward during prophase.

Schaper also showed that the young neuron, with a large, clear nucleus and abundant cytoplasm, can be distinguished from the neuroglial cell precursors. Some of the glial cell precursors have a small, round, densely chromatic nucleus and very scanty cytoplasm, but others may have different appearances (see Section 3.2). We would now call these cells *glioblasts*. Schaper showed that the young neurons and glioblasts migrate away from the lumen and form the mantle layer outside the germinal zone. Some of the cells in the mantle layer undergo mitosis. According to Schaper (1897a, p. 100), these are "indifferent cells," which he thought are capable of giving rise either to neurons or to neuroglial cells. These would now be called pluripotential progenitor cells.

Schaper's theory was premature (see footnote 1 in Chapter 1). On the authority of both His and Ramón y Cajal (1909, p. 637), Schaper's theory was consigned to oblivion. It was not accepted into a research program until 50 years later when new evidence in its favor was provided by F. C. Sauer (1935a,b). He confirmed that the neural epithelium, until the time of closure of the neural tube, consists of a single type of epithelial cell in various stages of the mitotic cycle. In addition, Sauer showed that the appearance of the cell changes and its nucleus moves to different positions in the cytoplasm during the different phases of the mitotic cycle.

2.2. Neurepithelial Germinal Cells during the Mitotic Cycle

The neural tube is initially formed of neurepithelial cells at different phases of the mitotic cycle (see Section 2.3). During the early stages of development of the neural tube, metaphase nuclei occur only close to the lumen or ventricle, whereas nuclei of different sizes and staining characteristics are seen at all levels between the ventricle and outer surface of the neural tube (Fig. 2.2). F. C. Sauer (1935a,b, 1936, 1937) identified telophase and early interphase nuclei as the smaller nuclei that form a series, gradually becoming larger and more basophilic as they are situated at increasing distances from the ventricle of the neural tube. He concluded that these nuclei are moving away from the ventricle following mitosis (Fig. 2.2). The late interphase and prophase nuclei form a series leading to mitosis as they approach the lumen. They are intensely basophilic and ovoid, with the sharper end pointing toward the lumen, and have 6–9 times the volume of the early postmitotic nuclei. Interphase is very short or nonexistent in rapidly dividing cells—the DNA synthesis recommences immediately after telophase. During interphase and prophase the neuroepithelial germinal cells are attached to the internal and external limiting membranes. During metaphase the cells lose their external attachment and round up toward the ventricle of the neural tube where cell division occurs. The daughter cells may both reenter the mitotic cycle or one or both may withdraw from the cycle. These postmitotic cells migrate out of the germinal zone to form a mantle layer near the external surface of the neural tube, where differentiation of various types of neurons and neuroglial cells occurs. Some of the neuroepithelial cells and neuroglial cells retain the ability to reenter the mitotic cycle if stimulated appropriately, whereas others leave the cycle temporarily (some neuroglial cells) or permanently (all neurons).

Thus, there are four possible proliferative states in the neural tube: proliferative germinal cells, both of whose daughter cells reenter the mitotic cycle; stem cells that contribute one daughter to the proliferative and one to the postmitotic population; temporarily nonmitotic cells capable of proliferation if stimulated; and permanently postmitotic cells. These populations may be anatomically segregated or may be mingled in the same region.

F. C. Sauer (1935a,b, 1936, 1937) correlated the size and histological appearance of nuclei with their distance from the lumen of the neural plate and neural tube of pig and chick embryos. He showed that the cells are separate, each bounded by a distinct plasma membrane, and that they do not form a

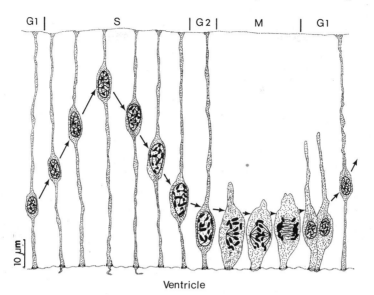

G1 | S | G2 | M | G1

10 μm

Ventricle

Figure 2.2. The cell nucleus moves to different levels of the neurepithelium during the mitotic cycle. A single neurepithelial germinal cell in the neural tube of the chick embryo is shown at approximately half-hour intervals at different phases of the mitotic cycle.

syncytium, as originally proposed by His and as was widely believed at that time, as shown in Fig. 2.1. Sauer observed that the cells of the neurepithelium are columnar, extend from the inner to the outer surface of the neural tube, and are joined to each other by terminal bars at the lumen. These observations have since been confirmed by electron microscopy (Duncan, 1957; Bellairs, 1959; Tennyson and Pappas, 1962; Brightman and Palay, 1963; H. Fujita and Fujita, 1963; E. Robbins and Gonatas, 1964a; S. Fujita, 1966; Wechsler, 1967; P. C. Baker and Schroeder, 1967; Fisher and Jacobson, 1970; Hinds and Ruffett, 1971).

In the neural plate and early neural tube the daughter cells reenter the mitotic cycle, but at later stages of development an increasing number of dividing neurepithelial germinal cells are seen with the plane of cleavage tangential, so that one daughter cell loses its basal attachment and does not reenter the mitotic cycle but migrates into the mantle layer (A. H. Martin and Langman, 1965; A. H. Martin, 1967).

It has been suggested that the orientation of the mitotic spindle may be important, not only in determining whether a daughter cell is released or remains attached to the luminal surface of the neu-

ral tube, but probably also in determining the spatial arrangement of cells. According to F. C. Sauer (1935a,b), during mitosis in the neural plate and tube the spindle axis is always tangential and the plane of cleavage is always radial so that the daughter cells lie side by side and retain their basal attachment at the lumen of the neural tube and both cells reenter the mitotic cycle. In the rat neurectoderm, mitotic spindles are preferentially oriented so that daughter cells are formed in the rostrocaudal axis (Tuckett and Morriss-Kay, 1985). In the ganglionic eminences of the newborn mouse over 90 percent of mitotic figures near the lateral ventricle cleave at right angles to the ventricular wall (Smart, 1976). The plane of cleavage is random in mitotic figures in the subventricular zone of the lateral ventricle (Smart, 1976).

The phenomena just described raise many unanswered questions about the mechanism of the to-and-fro movement of the nucleus and about the functions of such movement. It is possible that movement of the nucleus might allow regionally different cytoplasmic factors to enter the nucleus to promote differential gene activity. Interkinetic nuclear migration is not peculiar to neurepithelial germinal cells but is seen in a wide variety of embryonic

Table 2.1. Cell Cycle of Neurepithelial Germinal Cells[a]

Tissue	Species	Age	Cycle time	S	G_2	M	G_1	Reference
Neural tube	Chick	E1	5	—	—	—	—	Fujita (1962)
	Mouse	E10	8.5	4.6	0.6	1.3	2	Kauffman (1968)
	Mouse	E11	10.5	5.4	1.2	1.3	2.7	Same
	Mouse	E11	11	5.5	1	1	3.5	Atlas and Bond (1965)
Telencephalon	Mouse	E10	7	5.1	1	0.8	0.1	Hoshino et al. (1973)
	Mouse	E13	15.5	6.9	1	0.8	6.8	Same
	Mouse	E17	26	10.4	1	0.8	13.8	Same
Cerebral cortex	Mouse	E15	11	7.5	2	2	—	Langman and Welch (1967)
	Rat	E12	11	6–8	2	—	3.7	Waechter and Jaensch (1972)
	Rat	E18	19	6–8	2	—	11.2	Same
Cerebral subventricular zone	Rat	E18	19	6–7	—	—	10	Same
	Rat	P1	18.3	10	3.7	—	3.1	Same
	Rat	P6	17.2	10.8	2.5	—	2.5	Same
	Rat	P21	20.1	12.4	2.1	—	5.2	Lewis and Lai (1974)
Hippocampal dentate gyrus granule cells	Rat	P1–12	15.1–17.7	10.1–11.7	2.5–3.3	—	1.1–2.4	Lewis (1978)
Neural retina	Chick	E6	10	—	—	—	—	Fujita (1962)
	Mouse	P2	28	12.5	1.5	0.8	13	Denham (1967)
Optic tectum	Chick	E3	8	4	1.5	0.3	2.2	Wilson (1973, 1974)
	Chick	E4	9	5	1.5	0.4	2.1	Same
	Chick	E5	13	4	1.5	0.8	6.7	Same
	Chick	E6	15	5	1.5	1.4	7.1	Same
	Mouse	E10	8.5	5	1	1	1.5	Wilson (1974)
	Mouse	E11	11	6	0.9	1.2	2.9	Same
Rhombic lip	Rat	E14	12	—	—	—	—	Ellenberger et al. (1969)
Cerebellum external granule cells	Mouse	P1–10	21.5	7	2	0.6	11.9	Fujita et al. (1966)
	Mouse	P7–14	24	—	5	—	—	Miale and Sidman (1961)
	Mouse	P2–10	18	8.3	2	—	7.8	Mares et al. (1970)

[a] Time in hours.

tissues that are in the form of a pseudostratified epithelium (F. C. Sauer, 1936, 1937; Zwaan et al., 1969).

Changes in cell shape and the interkinetic nuclear movements that occur during the cell cycle probably involve dynamic changes in microtubules (Cassimeris et al., 1987, review) and require the action of contractile microfilaments (Citi and Kendrick-Jones, 1987, review), but the mechanisms have not been analyzed in neurepithelial cells (see Section 5.2). The involvement of microfilaments is suggested by the observation that cytochalasin B, a drug that inhibits the action of intracellular microfilaments, totally stops interkinetic nuclear migration in the neural tube of chick embryos (P. E. Messier and Auclair, 1974), but it does so by acting on apical microfilaments attached to terminal bars, thus breaking attachments between cells at the lumen of the neural tube.

It is not known how the duration of the cell cycle and the rate of proliferation of germinal cells are controlled. Sauer (1935b) pointed out that as the wall of the neural tube thickens during development, the distance the nuclei may have to travel is increased. This may be a cause of the progressive increase in intermitotic time that occurs during development (Table 2.1) if it is assumed that the rate of nuclear migration remains the same throughout development. The rate of nuclear migration in the neural tube of the 11-day mouse embryo is about 10 μm/hour (Atlas and Bond, 1965). How this compares with rates in other stages in the mouse or in other species is unknown. F. C. Sauer says that the movement of the nucleus away from the lumen occupies most of the intermitotic period and is much slower than the return movement in the premitotic period. According to Sauer (1935b), the volume of the nucleus doubles on the outward journey (from 98.7 to 127.5 μm^3 in chick) and doubles again on the inward journey (from 157.5 to 280 μm^3 pig; from 90 to 135 μm^3 in chick). Subsequent work has confirmed that nuclear size is related to nuclear DNA content (Szarski, 1976, review).

Additional evidence of intermitotic nuclear migration in the neural tube was obtained by Watterson (1965), who used colchicine to inhibit mitosis in the chick neural tube. Three hours after the chick embryo has been treated with colchicine, several layers of cells arrested in metaphase are seen close to the lumen of the neural tube. An increasing number of cells are affected, until almost all cells of the neural tube are arrested in metaphase, after about 7.5 hours of colchicine treatment. These observations of the effect of colchicine have been confirmed by Källén (1961, 1962) and by Langman *et al.* (1966), who used vincristine sulfate to inhibit mitosis. These experiments also show that cells at all levels in the neural epithelium, and not just the cells close to the lumen, can undergo mitosis. It is assumed, probably incorrectly, that colchicine blocks only cell division and that nuclear migration is unaffected, so that the nuclei are unable to reach the lumen because their migration is obstructed by layers of cells arrested in metaphase.

Intermitotic migration of the nuclei of neurepithelial germinal cells has also been confirmed independently by two methods: by cytophotometric measurements of the DNA content of nuclei at different depths in the neural epithelium (M. F. Sauer and Chittenden, 1959) and by observation of the position of labeled nuclei in the neural epithelium at progressively longer intervals after administration of a pulse of [3H]thymidine (M. E. Sauer and Walker, 1959; Sidman *et al.*, 1959; S. Fujita, 1962, 1963, 1965a, 1966; Atlas and Bond, 1965; A. H. Martin and Langman, 1965).

The amount of DNA in nuclei at various levels in the neural epithelium should provide a crucial test of whether nuclear migration occurs, since the DNA content of the telophase and early interphase nucleus is constant and characteristic of the species (Vendrely and Vendrely, 1956, review), and the DNA content of the nucleus is doubled during cell division before visible prophase (Alfert, 1950; Swift,

1950). Cytophotometrical measurements of the DNA content of the nuclei of the neural tube in the chick embryo neural tube stained for DNA by the Feulgen method (Feulgen and Rossenbeck, 1924; Hale, 1966) show that the DNA content of the nuclei is approximately proportional to their size (M. F. Sauer and Chittenden, 1959; Meek and Harbison, 1967). This is consistent with other observations showing that nuclear volume is a fairly reliable index of DNA content (Szarski, 1976, review), although some exceptions have been recorded (Billings and Swartz, 1969; C. J. Herman and Lapham, 1969). In the early neural tube the small nuclei close to the lumen contain more than the diploid value of DNA. This shows that the postmitotic gap (G_1) is very short, and DNA synthesis starts soon after mitosis while the nucleus is beginning its outward migration. Visible prophases are seen in the inner third of the neural epithelium, and the prophase nuclei contain the tetraploid amount of DNA, showing that they are in the postsynthetic (G_2) phase of the cell cycle. Therefore, while DNA replication is initiated during the outward migration of the nucleus, it continues during the movement of the nucleus toward the lumen (Fig. 2.3).

Additional evidence that DNA synthesis occurs mainly in nuclei in the outer half of the neural tube comes from the results of [3H]thymidine autoradiography. One hour after a single injection of tritiated thymidine, labeled nuclei appear only in the external half of the germinal cell layer of the cerebral vesicle of the 11-day mouse fetus (Sidman *et al.*, 1959), indicating that this is the site of DNA synthesis (Fig. 2.3). A single injection of [3H]thymidine is available for DNA synthesis for less than 1 hour in mammals, and only a single generation of cells takes up the label. These labeled nuclei migrate at approximately the same rate and divide synchronously (Sidman *et al.*, 1959; Atlas and Bond, 1965). Six hours after the injection, the labeled cells have arrived at the inner half of the germinal layer and numerous mitotic figures are labeled. Some of the labeled daughter nuclei migrate out into the mantle layer by 48 hours after the label has been given, and these cells remain labeled for their lifetime. Most labeled nuclei repeat the cycle of migration and mitosis in the germinal layer. With each cell division the radioactivity per daughter cell is halved. Similar results have been obtained after [3H]thymidine labeling of the nuclei of the neural groove,

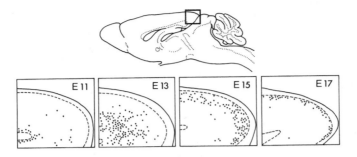

Figure 2.3. Inside-out sequence of time of origin of neurons in the cerebral isocortex of the mouse. Four different pregnant mice each received a single injection of [³H]thymidine on either the 11th, 13th, 15th, or 17th day of gestation. All the progeny were killed 10 days after birth, after the neurons of the cerebral isocortex have reached their final positions. Dots show the positions of labeled neurons in autoradiographs of sections of the occipital region of the cerebral cortex outlined in the rectangle. From J. B. Angevine, Jr., and R. J. Sidman, *Nature* 192:755–768 (1961).

neural tube, and spinal cord of the chick embryo (S. Fujita, 1962, 1963; H. Fujita and Fujita, 1964, Martin and Langman, 1965; Langman *et al.*, 1966). One hour after a single injection of [³H]thymidine, only nuclei in the outer half of the wall of the neural groove are labeled. Three hours later, labeled nuclei are seen mainly in the inner half of the wall, but 10 hours after injection of the label they have returned to the outer half of the wall (Martin and Langman, 1965), and the density of labeling is reduced to half that at the beginning. This shows that, within 13 hours, the labeled nuclei move from the outer to the inner margin of the neural tube, complete mitosis, and return to the outer half of the neural tube.

The rate of cell production is a function of the duration of the cell cycle and of the number of germinal cells. The duration of the cell cycle lengthens approximately linearly as development progresses (Fig. 2.4). The number of germinal cells first increases, then reaches a steady state, and finally declines as histogenesis ceases. Cumulative labeling experiments, in which repeated injections are given to make the [³H]thymidine continuously available for DNA synthesis, show that during the early phases of neurogenesis all the daughter cells reenter the mitotic cycle and thus the number of germinal cells increases. This period of symmetrical division of germinal cells (proliferative mode) in which the number of germinal cells increases logarithmically is followed by a period of asymmetrical division in which only one postmitotic daughter cell is produced at each

division of a germinal cell (stem cell mode), so that the population of germinal cells remains constant while the population of postmitotic cells increases arithmetically. Finally, some germinal cells enter their terminal cell cycle and produce two postmitotic cells. The rate of cell production gradually declines as the cell cycle increases in length

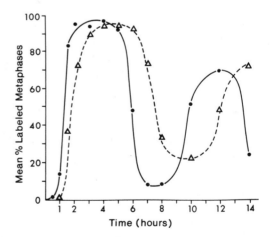

Figure 2.4. Progressive lengthening of the cell cycle occurs during development. Comparison of the duration of the mitotic cycle of neurepithelial cells of the mouse at E10 (solid line) and E 11 (dashed line). The mean percentage of labeled mitotic figures in the neural tube was determined after an injection of [³H]thymidine (1 μC/g) to pregnant mice. From S. L. Kauffman, *Exp. Cell Res.* 49:420–424 (1968).

and as germinal cells withdraw from the mitotic cycle.

2.3. Kinetics of the Cell Cycle of Neurepithelial Germinal Cells

In a proliferating cell population such as the neurepithelial germinal cells, the cells pass through a cycle of DNA synthesis and mitosis. The mitotic cycle has several phases—M, G_1, S, and G_2—as defined by A. Howard and Pelc (1953). They showed that S, the period of DNA synthesis (which can be recognized by observing the incorporation of tritiated thymidine into DNA), is separated from mitosis (M) by a period of several hours, which is called G_2; the period between the end of mitosis and the beginning of DNA synthesis is called G_1. Two main control points have been recognized; in G_1 controlling entry into the S phase, and in G_2 controlling entry into mitosis.

During mitosis (M phase), the maternal cell divides into two daughter cells, each with the diploid ($2n$) quantity of DNA. The duration of the M phase is usually 40–70 minutes (Table 2.1). Jelínek (1959) has shown that the M phase becomes progressively more prolonged during development of the chick embryo neural tube. At 3 days of incubation (E3), the M phase is 0.7 hour; at 4 days, 1.1 hours; and at 6 days, 2.5 hours. A similar increase in the duration of the M phase has been found in the chick optic tectum, the M phase increasing from 0.3 hour at E3 to 1.4 hours at E6 (D. B. Wilson, 1973, 1974). In the telencephalon of the mouse embryo, the duration of the M phase is constant at 0.8 hour from E10 to E17 (Hoshino *et al.*, 1973).

Following mitosis the cell enters the G_1 phase or postmitotic gap. Different cell populations show a wide range in the duration of G_1. It may be entirely absent in very rapidly proliferating cells, or it may last for hours, for days, or for the duration of the animal's life. There is a progressive increase in the duration of G_1 during development, and the gradual slowing of the cell cycle is largely due to lengthening of G_1 with each successive cycle. For example, in the telencephalon of the mouse, G_1 increases from 0.1 hour at E10 to 13.8 hours at E17 (Hoshino *et al.*, 1973). Most types of neurons are permanently arrested in the G_1 phase and are therefore diploid. Noncycling cells are said to be in G_0.

After mitosis the daughter cells may remain in the G_1 phase and commence cytodifferentiation, or one or both daughter cells may start DNA synthesis. In the early neural tube all the cells probably reenter the mitotic cycle; the cycle is short, G_1 is very short, and DNA synthesis starts immediately after mitosis during the initial stage of outward migration of the nucleus. Most neurons are permanently arrested in G_1, and glial cells may be temporarily suspended in G_1, waiting for the specific signals that promote their progress into a new round of DNA transcription.

The period of DNA synthesis is termed the S phase, which usually lasts for 6–8 hours and occupies about half of the total cell cycle in rapidly dividing cells. The rate of DNA synthesis is approximately constant during the S phase. Replication of the chromosomal DNA occurs during this time. DNA synthesis is usually completed before the onset of morphological prophase (Fig. 2.1).

The S phase is followed by a premitotic gap, or G_2 phase, which has a duration from 1 to 4 hours in various types of cells. The cell may be permanently arrested in the G_2 phase and retain the tetraploid amount of DNA. In neurons this occurs rarely, if at all. As a rule, the cell passes from G_2 into the M phase.

In neurepithelial germinal cells as well as glioblasts, the duration of mitosis is very short when compared with the duration of the cell cycle. This is reflected in the paucity of metaphase figures seen at all stages of development of the nervous system. Usually the total fraction of mitotic figures seen in histological preparations of the developing neural tube does not exceed 2–5 percent of nuclei.

There are several methods of determining the duration of the cell cycle that require counting the proportions of labeled and unlabeled mitotic figures in autoradiographs made after administration of [³H]thymidine. However, these methods are subject to large counting errors and to random variations in the distribution of mitoses because, in a rapidly proliferating population of cells, small changes in the duration of mitosis or in the intermitotic period may result in relatively large changes in the percentage of mitotic figures (Hughes, 1952; Saetersdal, 1958). Counts of mitotic figures should be interpreted very critically, regardless of the way in which they are expressed.

Three methods of expressing mitotic activity in terms of number of mitotic figures have been used:

1. The average number of mitotic figures per section (Hamburger and Keefe, 1944; Hamburger, 1948)
2. The number of mitotic figures per 100 cells capable of mitosis, i.e., the mitotic rate or mitotic index (Coghill, 1924, 1933; Derrick, 1937; Fujita, 1964, 1967)
3. The average number of mitoses per unit area, i.e., the mitotic density (Hamburger, 1948)

These expressions of mitotic activity are of very limited value unless the duration of the M phase in relation to the generation time is known and unless the fixation is adequate to preserve mitotic figures. Detection of mitotic figures in the CNS requires fixation by perfusion; immersion of the tissue does not result in sufficiently rapid penetration of the fixative, and significant loss of mitotic figures may occur as a result of slow fixation (Fleischauer, 1968; Cavanagh and Lewis, 1969). Duration of the phases of the mitotic cycle must also be taken into account, which seldom is the case. For example, the condition termed "neural overgrowth," which can be induced experimentally in chick embryos and which has been likened to neoplasia (Källén, 1962), is not due to increased proliferation, as was once thought; rather, the increased number of mitotic figures is due to lengthening of the M phase of the cell cycle (D. B. Wilson, 1972, 1974). The progressive lengthening of the duration of mitosis and particularly of the intermitotic period that generally occurs during development (Table 2.1) should always be taken into account when comparisons are made between mitotic activity measured at different stages of development.

The G_1 and G_2 phases are important control points in passage of cells through the mitotic cycle. Normally neurons are permanently arrested in G_1, and glial cells may be temporarily suspended in either G_1 or G_2. Many experimental conditions arrest cells in the G_1 or G_2 phases of the mitotic cycle, for example, radiation, excess thymidine, hydroxyurea, and mutual cell contact inhibition (Pardee *et al.*, 1978, review). Only the latter is of possible significance in normal development. Thus, proliferation of 3T3 fibroblasts in culture is inhibited by extracts of membranes from confluent cell cultures (Wittenberger *et al.*, 1978; Steck *et al.*, 1983). Cell surface glycopeptides extracted from mouse or bovine brain reversibly inhibit a variety of cell lines in the G_2 phase of the mitotic cycle (Kinders *et al.*, 1982; Charp *et al.*, 1983). This may be significant in view of the evidence summarized in the following section that the main control point of fission yeast and cleavage stage embryos is in G_2, that is, the control of entry into the M phase.

2.4. Mechanisms Controlling Cell Proliferation in the Neural Tube

Three experimental strategies have recently been used to investigate the mechanisms controlling entry of eukaryotic cells into and passage through the cell cycle: (1) genetic analysis of mutants, mainly yeast, that are defective in the cell division cycle (cdc mutants); (2) biochemical assays of protein kinases and other enzymes whose activities fluctuate during the cell cycle; (3) tests for inducers of mitosis in dividing cells, particularly cyclins and maturation promotion factor. The results of these experiments show that some of the mechanisms regulating the transition from G_2 to mitosis are similar in all eukaryotic cells.

The onset of mitosis coincides with phosphorylation of many intracellular proteins including lamin, vimentin, and histones. Protein kinases encoded by yeast genes cdc 28 and cdc 2 are required for transition from G_1 to S and from G_2 to mitosis (reviewed by Nurse, 1985; Hayles and Nurse, 1986; Lee and Nurse, 1988; Lohka, 1989). The fission yeast genes cdc 2^+ and its homologues in higher eukaryotes encodes a 34-kDa protein (p34cdc2) which contains a 16 amino acid sequence EGVPSTAIREISLLKE referred to as the PSTAIR sequence that is perfectly conserved in all cell cycle–controlling proteins but is not found in any other proteins. Antibodies against PSTAIR recognize p34cdc2 in cells of all eukaryotes from yeast to humans. The level of p34cdc2 is constant during the cell cycle, but p34cdc2 activity varies because it is a protein kinase which is complexed with a number of other proteins that regulate its kinase activity in an oscillatory pattern. Two of these proteins are products of fission yeast genes cdc 13 and cdc 25. The cdc 13 product is homologous with cyclin. The cdc 25 product is homologous with a protein that regulates mitosis in *Drosophila*, the product of the *string* gene (O'Farrell *et al.*, 1989). Periodic synthesis of cyclins controls mitosis in the blastula (Murray and Kirschner, 1989), but after early cleavage stages a transition occurs to control by periodic synthesis of the *string* gene product.

Cyclins are a family of proteins that control entry into mitosis in eukaryotic cells. Two types of cyclins, A and B, have been identified. Levels of cyclins increase as a result of synthesis during the cell cycle until metaphase, and then cyclins are rapidly degraded as the cell enters metaphase (Evans *et al.*, 1983). Resynthesis of cyclin then triggers another round of the cell cycle. Cyclin regulates the p34 kinase of maturation promotion factor, which in turn regulates Ca^{2+} release from intracellular stores. The increased intracellular Ca^{2+} triggers the start of metaphase.

Maturation promotion factor (MPF) (reviewed by Maller, 1985; Nurse, 1985; Cyert and Kirschner, 1988; Gautier *et al.*, 1988; Murray and Kirschner, 1989) is a mitotic protein kinase consisting of two subunits of 34 kDa and 45 kDa (catalytic and regulatory) encoded in higher eukaryotes by the homologues of yeast cell cycle control genes cdc 2^+ and cdc 13^+. Entry into and exit from the M phase are controlled by MPF. The p34 kinase subunit of MPF contains the PSTAIR sequence and probably acts by regulating intracellular Ca^{2+}. The 45-kDa subunit is cyclin which has to reach a certain level in order to activate the p34 kinase of MPF.

This mechanism of cell cycle regulation applies only to yeast, oocytes, and early stages of cleavage of the embryo. Other factors are involved in controlling the cell cycle at later stages of development (O'Farrell *et al.*, 1989). The natural factors that start and stop mitosis in the neurepithelium and that control the production of neurons and the neuroglia are not known, but factors that are functionally analogous to MPF are almost certain to be involved. Neuroglial cells are more convenient to study for this purpose than neurons because the neuroglia are easily grown in primary culture and continue to divide throughout life in the mammalian CNS. By contrast, neurons do not proliferate *in vitro* and are produced in mammals as a result of short bursts of intense mitotic activity in the neurepithelial germinal cells prenatally, or in granule cells in the neonatal period.

Polypeptide growth factors have been shown to stimulate cell proliferation in glial cells (see Section 3.4) and in a number of cultured cell lines, such as 3T3 fibroblasts (Rozengurt, 1986, review), in hematopoietic cells (Metcalf, 1985; Deuel, 1987, reviews), and in the immune system (Smith, 1988, review). Astrocytes are a source of growth factors and so are macrophages that enter the central nervous system during the late fetal and early postnatal periods and following injury (see Section 3.2). Growth factors that stimulate proliferation of neuroglial cells, known to be produced by brain macrophages, include interleukin I and tumor necrosis factor (Knighton, 1983; Merrill *et al.*, 1984; Giulian and Lachman, 1985; Giulian and Baker, 1985; Leibovich, 1987). Factors derived from astrocytes include glia maturation factor (Lim, 1985; Lim *et al.*, 1989a,b,c, 1990), platelet-derived growth factor and ciliary neurotrophic factor (Raff, 1989, review), and insulin-like growth factor (McMorris *et al.*, 1986). Because primary cultures of neuroglial cells can be made with ease, rapid progress has been made in identification of factors that stimulate glial cell proliferation and differentiation (see Section 3.3).

Chalones are substances which normally inhibit mitosis in various vertebrate tissues (Bullough, 1962; Iversen, 1976, 1981; Laurence and Thornley, 1976; Coomber and Scadding, 1983). They are water soluble and act locally, controlling repair of wounds (through dilution and thus disinhibition at the site of injury) and through the circulation. Chalones are tissue specific but not species specific.

The factors that control neurepithelial cell division during normal development are not known (in contrast with the trophic factors that support survival of young neurons; see Chapter 8). Progress in identifying neurepithelial cell mitogenic factors has been slow. This is not surprising when viewed in light of the history of discovery of the polypeptide hormones, the mitogenic lymphokines, that regulate T-lymphocyte proliferation (reviewed by K. Smith, 1988; Mizel, 1989). Almost 20 years elapsed after the initial report that plant lectins stimulate lymphocyte proliferation, to the demonstration, in 1965, of mitogenic effects of medium conditioned by cultured leukocytes. Another 10 years passed before a suitable assay system of cloned T lymphocytes was developed on which the effects of mitogenic lymphokines could be tested, which led directly to the isolation and biochemical characterization of interleukins. At first *"mitogenic lymphokines were thought to play a nutritional or supportive role, merely amplifying a process signalled entirely by antigen. No one thought it possible that lymphokines themselves could be responsible for stimulating cell division"* (K. Smith, 1988). Goethe said this long ago: *"Phrases often repeated finally become convictions and ossify the organs of intelligence"* (*On The Intermaxillary Bone*, Jena, dated 1786 but published 1836). The current concept is of cellular communication networks mediated by positive and negative signals from a variety of factors. These are discussed in this section as well as in Section 1.2 in connection with neural induction, Section 3.4 in relation to control of glial cell proliferation and differentiation, Chapter 7 in relation to hormones, and Chapter 8 in connection with various neurotrophic factors.

2.5. Summary of Methods of Cell Population Kinetic Analysis

Five experimental methods have been used to study cell population kinetics in the developing nervous system and other tissues.

1. Direct measurement of the time between mitoses may be obtained by the use of time-lapse cinephotomicrography, but this is applicable only to transparent organisms and to cells in tissue culture.
2. Colchicine or colcemid (or another stathmokinetic agent such as vinblastine, vincristine, or mitomycin C) is used to inhibit mitosis, and the numbers of cells blocked in metaphase are counted (Wright and Appleton, 1980, review).
3. Cell population kinetics can be analyzed by labeling a cohort of cells in the population and tracing the rate at which the labeled cohort moves from noncycling to cycling and from phase to phase in the cell cycle. Radioactive thymidine is used to label the DNA, and the numbers of labeled nuclei are assayed autoradiographically (Korr, 1980, review).
4. 5-Bromodeoxyuridine (BUdR, BrdU, or BrdUrd), which is incorporated into DNA instead of thymidine, is given as a pulse to label a single generation of cells in the S phase, and the labeled cells are detected at progressively later

times by means of an antibody to BrdU in tissue sections or by flow cytometry of dissociated cells (Grey *et al.*, 1986, review).
5. The quantity of DNA in every cell in the population, after disaggregation, can be measured directly by flow cytometry, and the distribution of cells at different phases of the cell cycle can be computed.

2.6. Cell Population Kinetics Studied with Agents That Inhibit Mitosis

Colchicine or colcemid inhibits mitosis by binding to tubulin, the subunit of the microtubules of the mitotic spindle, and so preventing their assembly (E. Robbins and Gonatas, 1964b; Borisy and Taylor, 1967b). Nocodazole has a similar action (De Brabander *et al.*, 1986). Colcemid, a derivative of colchicine, has a stronger affinity for tubulin but has a more rapidly reversible effect on mitosis (Kleinfeld and Sisken, 1966; Ray *et al.*, 1980). Colchicine has no effect on the rates of synthesis of DNA, RNA, or protein (E. W. Taylor, 1965; J. O. Karlsson *et al.*, 1971), or on the duration of the G_1, S, or G_2 phase (Puck and Steffen, 1963).

The minimal effective dose of colchicine that inhibits all mitoses is close to the toxic dose. Insufficient colchicine does not inhibit all the mitoses; but higher doses may be fatal and therefore the effective dose has to be determined by trial and error for every species. Colchicine also binds with high affinity to the tubulin of other types of cytoplasmic microtubules—for example, to neurotubules (Borisy and Taylor, 1967a; Wisniewski and Terry, 1968; Wisniewski *et al.*, 1968). Colchicine inhibits the elongation of axons and blocks the proximodistal transport of proteins in the axon (see Sections 5.4 and 5.9). The half-life of the colchicine–tubulin complex is 36 hours (Garland and Teller, 1973), and so the recovery from colchicine is slow. When administered in the correct dose, colchicine or colcemid arrests the cells in metaphase. The rate of entry of cells into the M phase, which is a measure of the rate of proliferation, can be obtained from the rate of increase of metaphase cells (Fig. 2.5).

Other drugs that block mitosis are more liable than colchicine to produce irreversible damage (L. Wilson *et al.*, 1974). Thus the vinca alkaloids, vinblastine sulfate and vincristine sulfate, bind to mi-

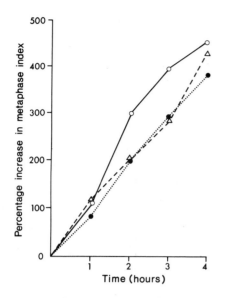

Figure 2.5. Measurement of the duration of the mitotic cycle from the percentage increase of metaphases after colcemid treatment. Metaphases were counted in the retina of the rat after administration of colcemid on postnatal day 2. The results of three experiments are shown. The duration of the mitotic cycle was approximately 1 hour. From S. Denham, *J. Embryol. Exp. Morphol.* 18:53–66 (1967).

crofilaments as well as to microtubules and also inhibit protein synthesis when given in doses sufficient to block mitosis (Creasey, 1968). The vinca alkaloids also have the disadvantage that they are insoluble in water. Mitomycin C, which is water soluble, inhibits mitosis by cross-linking the chromatids within the chromosomes. A dose of 20–40 μg/ml has been found to be effective in blocking mitosis (Kiehlman, 1966). Taxol binds tightly to tubulin in polymerized form, thus stabilizing microtubules (De Brabander *et al.,* 1986).

Other drugs have been used to inhibit cell proliferation in the developing nervous system. 5-Fluorodeoxyuridine (FUdR or FdUR) is not incorporated into DNA but stops mitosis by inhibiting thymidylate synthetase, resulting in a deficiency of thymidylic acid; DNA synthesis stops when thymidylic acid is no longer available, and this occurs rapidly, within hours of administration of FUdR. At low doses (10^{-8} to 10^{-6} M for ¼ hours) this is the only action of FUdR, and recovery can occur. The inhibitory effect of FUdR on mitosis can be reversed by thymidine in concentrations 100 times higher than

that of FUdR. At high doses FUdR results in chromosome breakage and cell death.

Cytotoxic agents which have a specific effect on cultured nonneuronal cells may have different effects on neurons or on neuronal stem cells *in vivo*. This is strikingly demonstrated by the drug 5-bromodeoxyuridine (BUdR, BrdU, or BrdUrd), an analogue of thymidine, which is incorporated into DNA instead of thymidine in cells that are engaged in DNA synthesis (Wilt and Anderson, 1972, review). BrdU is effective only if it is available during the S phase, and its effects may be prevented or reversed by equimolar concentrations of thymidine. BrdU has been reported to have little or no effect on cell viability or growth of mammalian or chick cells *in vitro*. However, the drug may cause chromosome breakage (Hsu and Somer, 1961) and may inhibit cell differentiation in chondrocytes *in vitro* (Abbott and Holtzer, 1968; Lasher and Cahn, 1969) and in myoblasts *in vitro* (Holtzer, 1972, review). Whether it can prevent or delay nerve cell differentiation *in vivo* remains to be shown.

There is good evidence that retinal ganglion cell precursor cells terminate their DNA synthesis shortly before differentiation of retinal ganglion cells occurs in the *Xenopus* embryo (M. Jacobson, 1968b; Beach and Jacobson, 1978a,b,c) and chick embryo (Kahn, 1973, 1974); and in Mauthner's neuron of *Xenopus* (Vargas-Lizardi and Lyser, 1974). Therefore, it seemed that the neural retina and Mauthner's neuron might be promising systems in which to use BrdU to inhibit cell differentiation without affecting cell viability. Initial reports suggested that it might be possible to achieve such a "chemical dissection" of the program of differentiation without affecting cell viability of retinal ganglion cells in *Xenopus* (Bergey *et al.,* 1973; R. K. Hunt *et al.,* 1977). In a more extensive study of the effects of BrdU injected in *Xenopus* embryos at different stages from gastrula to tailbud, at different doses ranging from ineffective to lethal, we found that at maximum doses that permit further development, the drug has little or no effect on the differentiation of the Mauthner neuron, and that it has a predominantly cytotoxic effect on the neural retina proportional to the dose, at all doses (Dribin and Jacobson, 1978). We were unable to see a specific effect on nerve cell differentiation *in vivo*.

BrdU is likely to be of use for analysis of cells *in vitro,* but its use *in vivo* in mammals is limited by its short metabolic half-life (Kriss and Revesz, 1961) and by its toxicity (Goz, 1978; Franz and Klienebrecht, 1982). The half-life of BrdU in amphibians is unknown, but it is most likely prolonged, as is the half-life of [3H]thymidine in amphibians (Beach and Jacobson, 1978c; Reyer, 1983).

Several monoclonal antibodies against BrdU have been used to stain small amounts of BrdU incorporated into cellular DNA (Gratzer, 1982; Raza et al., 1984; Gonchoroff et al., 1985). Because of its short half-life in vivo, BrdU can be used instead of [3H]thymidine to label only those cells that are actively synthesizing DNA immediately after the injection. The incorporated BrdU can be detected by means of the antibodies and the total DNA content of the cells can be measured simultaneously by means of flow cytometry (Dolbeare et al., 1983; Dean et al., 1984), as outlined in Section 2.8. The advantages and limitations of this technique are reviewed by Gray et al. (1986).

2.7. Autoradiographic Methods for Analysis of Cell Population Kinetics

Tritiated thymidine ([3H]TdR) becomes incorporated specifically into DNA during its synthesis, and, once incorporated, it remains permanently in the DNA, where it can be detected by means of autoradiography of tissue sections. The incorporation of thymidine into DNA proceeds by phosphorylation to its nucleotides: first to thymidine monophosphate, then to thymidine diphosphate, and finally to thymidine triphosphate, which is assembled, with other nucleoside triphosphates, into DNA (Cleaver, 1967). It should be noted that thymidine monophosphate is also synthesized from simple precursors such as aspartic acid. Thus the exogenously administered labeled thymidine is diluted by the endogenous pool of unlabeled thymidine monophosphate. Since the size of the pool cannot be known, it is not possible to calculate rates of DNA synthesis from the time course of incorporation of labeled thymidine. However, the endogenous pool of thymidine can be reduced by inhibiting endogenous synthesis of thymidine monophosphate by means of amethopterin (Siegers et al., 1974).

Because of the low energy of β-particles emitted from tritium (about one-fiftieth of the energy of

β-particles emitted from [14C]), an autoradiograph may be obtained with a resolution of 0.2–0.3 μm using light microscopy (Salpeter et al., 1974), that is, to within a single cell nucleus. By contrast the β-particles emitted from [14C] produce tracks extending for hundreds of μm in autoradiographs. By combining autoradiography with electron microscopy, a resolution as high as 6 nm may be achieved with tritium (Salpeter et al., 1969; Stevens, 1966) so that it is possible not only to identify the cell that has incorporated the [3H]thymidine into its DNA, but also to localize the site of DNA synthesis to the chromosomes, nucleolus, or mitochondria. Spurious results may be obtained as a result of the breakdown of [3H]thymidine (for example, due to self-radiolysis) and the incorporation of the radioactive breakdown products into macromolecules other than DNA (Wand et al., 1967).

Double-labeling with [3H]thymidine and [14C]thymidine is possible because of the different energies of their β-particles. In order to detect both labels in the same tissue, two layers of emulsion, separated by a layer of gelatin, are deposited on top of the histological sections. β-particles emitted from [3H] thymidine do not have sufficient energy to penetrate beyond the first emulsion layer, whereas the more energetic β-particles emitted from [14C]thymidine form tracks in the second emulsion layer. To detect both labels in the same tissue, the [3H] activity must be about 50 times greater than the [14C] activity (Schultze et al., 1976; Korr, 1980). Because of the relatively low resolution of [14C]-autoradiography, this method is not suitable for tissue in which the proliferating cells are closely packed, as in the neural tube and supependymal layer. Double-labeling autoradiography is best applied to tissues in which labeled cells are sparse, as in the adult brain, and is especially useful for studies of neuroglial cell proliferation (Korr et al., 1973, 1975).

The danger of radiation damage to the cells after incorporation of [3H]thymidine should be kept in mind (Samuels and Kisielski, 1963; Cleaver et al., 1972). There is less danger of chromosomal damage from [14C]thymidine than from [3H]thymidine because the greater energy of the β-particle emitted from [14C] is mainly absorbed outside the nucleus. For example, abnormalities of cell proliferation in the subependymal layer of the rat brain have been observed after the cells had incorporated [3H]thymidine and were attributed to endogenous irradiation of the cells by radioactive DNA (P. D. Lewis, 1968a). An excess of thymidine, whether radioactive or not, can inhibit DNA synthesis (Xeros, 1962; Blenkinsopp, 1967). A dose of 10 µCi/g body weight is usually used in mammals, and doses of [³H]thymidine larger than 20 µCi/g body weight cause radiation damage to various tissues (Cronkite *et al.*, 1962).

Labeled DNA can be detected by autoradiography in the developing nervous system within 5–10 minutes after injecting a single dose of tritiated thymidine directly into the embryo or injecting intraperitoneally or intravenously into the pregnant mammal. Injection of [³H]thymidine directly into the brain (Altman, 1962a) has the advantages of reducing the amount of thymidine used and of localizing the highest uptake of the label to a specific brain region or to the brain rather than other organs. Intracisternal injection of [³H]thymidine directly into the cerebrospinal fluid has very limited application because the nucleotide is unevenly distributed to the brain, with the result that labeling is capricious (Altman, 1963; Altman and Chorover, 1963). Another method, exposure of brain tissue to tritiated thymidine *in vitro*, is the only way in which human brain histogenesis can be studied autoradiographically. In this so-called *supravital labeling*, pieces of freshly excised human fetal brain are exposed to [³H]thymidine for 1 hour in a suitable culture medium, then fixed and processed for autoradiography (Rakic and Sidman, 1968, 1970). This method is also applicable to the study of cellular kinetics in excised brain tumors.

After a single injection the thymidine is available for DNA synthesis for only 30–60 minutes and is metabolized and excreted after 2 hours in mammals. Since the duration of labeling is short relative to the S phase, only cells of one generation, which are in the process of DNA synthesis while the [³H]thymidine is available, are labeled. This method is called *pulse labeling*. With each subsequent division, the label is halved, and this is measured by counting the number of silver grains over each cell in the autoradiograph. The labeled DNA is predominantly nuclear because the total quantity of mitochondrial DNA in the cell is only a small fraction of 1 percent of the nuclear DNA (Nass, 1969; Attardi *et al.*, 1982; Grivell, 1983; Borst *et al.*, 1984).

Interspecies differences in the availability of [³H]thymidine may have to be taken into account in planning experiments. For example, the clearance of the label from the plasma is about 10 times more rapid in monkeys than in rats (Nowakowski and Rakic, 1974). In monkeys a shorter pulse of label can be achieved, but to obtain the same level of labeling, the dose of [³H]thymidine has to be greater and the exposure time has to be longer for autoradiographs of monkeys than of rats. As the thymidine is cleared very slowly after injection into amphibians (D. H. Beach and Jacobson, 1979c) or after injection into the chorioallantois of chick embryos, it is not possible to label them with a short pulse. Pulse labeling can be achieved by injecting directly into the chick embryo when its size permits. In poikilothermic animals, the rate of DNA synthesis and the duration of the cell cycle are temperature dependent, so it is essential to record the temperature at which the experiments are done (Brugal, 1971).

Thymidine autoradiography after pulse labeling with a single injection of [³H]thymidine provides a relatively easy means of determining the duration of phases of the cell cycle. The time for the average grain count to decrease to half is approximately the generation time. The generation time can also be determined from the percentage of labeled mitosis (Quastler and Sherman, 1959; D. H. Beach and Jacobson, 1979a,b). The time taken for 100 percent of the mitotic figures to become labeled is approximately the duration of G_2 + M + ½ S. The percentage of labeled mitoses stays close to 100 for several hours and then decreases to almost zero. When the generation of labeled cells again enters the cell cycle, a new wave of labeled mitoses appears, each mitotic figure carrying half the label of the maternal cells; then the cycle repeats itself. The generation time can be obtained by measuring the time interval between two identical points (for example, the time at which the percentage of labeled mitoses reaches a maximum on two succeeding waves of labeled mitoses), as illustrated by Fig. 2.6. The duration of the S phase is approximately the time interval between the midpoints of the ascending and descending limbs of a wave of labeled mitoses. A useful discussion of the percent labeled mitosis curve is given by Shackney (1974). This method is practicable only when mitosis is frequent, as in the early neural tube and the subependymal layer of postnatal mammals, but is not suita-

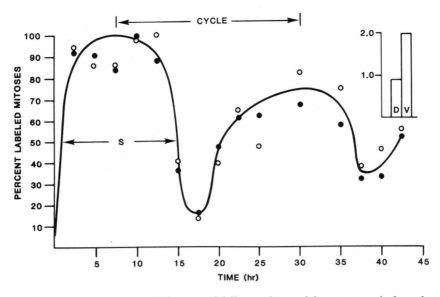

Figure 2.6. Measuring the cell cycle time and duration of different phases of the mitotic cycle from the percentage of labeled mitoses. Percentage of mitotic figures in the ventral (•) and dorsal (o) retinal margins labeled at different times after intraocular injection of 7.6 nl [³H]thymidine (1 μC/μl; Spec. Ac. 54.9 C/mmole) into the left eye of *Xenopus* embryos at Stages 57/58. Inset shows the average number of mitotic figures per vertical section in the right eye of the same animal. Although there were more than twice the number of mitotic figures in the ventral retina (V) than in the dorsal retina (D), the mitotic cycle was the same for both. The cycle time was ±20 hr; the S phase, ±13.5 hr. From D. H. Beach and M. Jacobson, *J. Comp. Neurol.* 183:615–624 (1979).

ble for regions of the nervous system where few mitoses occur.

The duration of the S phase and the generation time may also be obtained by cumulative labeling with [³H]thymidine. In this method, injections of [³H]thymidine are given at frequent intervals in order to make the nucleotide continuously available for DNA synthesis for hours or days. The following pattern of labeling is observed when [³H]thymidine is made available continuously to a population of proliferating cells at random phases of the cycle. The first cells to take up the label are those in the S phase, and therefore the percentage of cells labeled shortly after the injection will equal the percentage duration of the S phase relative to the generation time (G). If S = 50 percent of G, 50 percent of the cells start to incorporate the label immediately after it becomes available. Thereafter, the rate of labeling will be linear until 100 percent of the cells have become labeled in a period approximately equal to ½ S + G₂ + M + G₁ (that is, when the cells that have just completed DNA synthesis at the start of labeling have passed through G₂ + M + G₁ and entered the S phase). If,

instead of counting every cell that is lightly labeled, only heavily labeled cells are counted, a different result is obtained because the cell must complete a considerable part of its DNA synthesis in order to become heavily labeled. The time for 100 percent of the cells to become heavily labeled will be close to the generation time. In practice, an intermediate result is obtained. The cumulative labeling method is suitable for measuring cell cycle phases in the early neural tube but is impracticable in postnatal mammals because the time required to label all cells of a given type is too long.

Methods have also been devised for determining the durations of all phases of the cell cycle in a single experiment in which colchicine and [³H]thymidine are administered simultaneously at the start of the experiment and then by repeated injections in order to sustain their action for at least the time of the cell cycle. The durations of the phases of the cycle can be calculated from determinations of the percentages of labeled and unlabeled mitoses and interphase cells at progressive intervals after the beginning of the experiment (Puck and Steffen, 1963; Maekawa and Tsuchiya, 1968). In such an experiment the percentage of unlabeled interphase cells decreases linearly, in a time equal to G_1, to a minimum which represents the percentage of non-proliferating cells. The percentage of labeled metaphases increases linearly to a maximum in a time equal to the cell cycle. The percentage of metaphases that remain permanently unlabeled represents the percentage of the total cycle occupied by G_2. The ratio of unlabeled to labeled cells declines to a minimum in a time equal to S. The combination of colchicine and [3H]thymidine probably makes possible the analysis of the cell cycle with a higher degree of resolution than is obtainable by the use of either method alone (Wright and Appleton, 1980).

In summary, in mammals, a single injection of [3H]thymidine labels a single generation of cells that are in the S phase at the time of the injection. Analysis of the cell cycle kinetics can be done by counting the percentage of labeled mitotic figures, which is a measure of the time for the cohort of labeled cells to pass from one M phase to the next. The generation time is also given by the time taken for the number of autoradiographic silver grains to decrease to half.

Pulse labeling is useful for analysis of cell cycle kinetics only during the period of clonogenic cell proliferation, in regions where mitosis is frequent, and when all the cells reenter the mitotic cycle. Pulse labeling during nonclonogenic cell proliferation is a means of showing the time at which cells withdraw from the mitotic cycle (their "birthdates") because such cells, labeled in their terminal S phase, remain heavily labeled and can be identified after they have differentiated.

Repeated injections of [3H]thymidine (cumulative labeling) during the clonogenic period of cell proliferation will result in labeling of 100 percent of the cells in a time equal to the generation time. Cumulative labeling, started in the non-clonogenic period of cell proliferation, can distinguish the mitotically active cells from those that have withdrawn from mitosis before the beginning of labeling, and thus remain unlabeled. Cumulative labeling can also be used to label all the cells of a given type during their terminal S phase and thus can show the time during which a given cell type is generated. Cumulative labeling is very useful in submammalian vertebrates in which clearance of thymidine is slow, so that pulse labeling is not feasible. Cumulative labeling is impracticable in postnatal mammals because the time required to label all cells of a given type is too long. In practice an extended series of pulse labels is used for this purpose.

2.8. Flow Cytometric Methods for Analysis of Cell Population Kinetics

Flow cytometry (Gray *et al.*, 1986, review) has several advantages over radioactive thymidine methods of cell population kinetic analysis. Similar results have been obtained by both methods applied to intestinal epithelium (Cheng and Bjerknes, 1982). By means of flow cytometry the quantity of fluorescently stained DNA in every cell of the population can be measured directly. Since the quantity of DNA changes as the cell progresses through the cell cycle, it is possible to determine the distribution of cells through various phases of the cell cycle. Large numbers of cells can be studied rapidly with flow cytometry; measurements can be made at rates of thousands of cells per second and the total number of cells at each phase of the cycle can be counted directly (Crissman and Steinkamp, 1986, review).

In preparation for flow cytometry, the tissue is fixed and dissociated by gentle pipetting and by passing through a series of 20-μm nylon meshes. The dispersed cells are treated with RNase and stained with one or more fluorescent dyes before passing one at a time very rapidly through the cell sorter. The data are analyzed with a multi-Gaussian curve-fitting computer program (Fried and Mandel, 1979). This method has been applied most often in analysis of rapidly proliferating tissues such as malignant tumors. This technique promises to be very useful for studies of cell cycle kinetics in the nervous system, especially in rapidly proliferating tissue such as the neural tube, subependymal zone, and cerebellar external granular layer.

2.9. Summary of the Proliferation Kinetics of Neurons and Neuroglia

The data available in the literature on the proliferation kinetics of neuron and glial cell precursors have been assembled in Table 2.1. It can be seen that the evidence is as yet too fragmentary to show clearly whether there are consistent changes in the mean durations of the phases of the cell cycle of the precursors of neurons and glial cells. There is some indication that the cell cycle of germinal cells gradually becomes more prolonged during development of the chick neural tube (Jelínek, 1959; Fujita, 1962; Wilson, 1973, 1974) and neural tube of the mouse fetus (S. L. Kauffman, 1968; Hoshino *et al.*, 1973; Wilson, 1974). If the neurepithelial germinal cells behave like other dividing cells, their generation time would be expected to become progressively longer as development proceeds (Fig. 2.4). In mammalian cells this is due to progressive lengthening of the G_1 phase, whereas the S and G_2 phases remain relatively constant (Defendi and Manson, 1963; Cameron, 1964; Prescott, 1964; Wegener *et al.*, 1963, 1964). In amphibians all phases of the cycle increase progressively in duration from blastula to late tailbud stages (C. F. Graham and Morgan, 1966; Flickinger *et al.*, 1967). In the telencephalon of the mouse fetus the lengthening of the cell cycle is the result of an increase in the duration of G_1 and S phases, while the G_2 remains constant (D. B. Wilson, 1973, 1974).

The generation times of glial cell and neuronal progenitors are essentially the same, but significant differences between them with respect to other parameters of cell proliferation are summarized below and discussed in Section 2.10 (Korr, 1980). Reports that glial cell precursors have very long generation times, up to 50 days (Noetzel, 1962; S. Fujita, 1966; S. Fujita *et al.*, 1966), are probably based on incorrect assumptions about the labeling index (Korr, 1980). All types of neurons have similar cell cycle parameters during prenatal development in mammals, and there are only small variations between different mammalian species (Table 2.1). There appear to be significant differences between different vertebrate classes, but it should be noted that almost all studies of cell proliferation kinetics in the CNS have been done on rodents, and that very few data are available on submammalian species, with the exception of the chicken embryo.

Tritiated thymidine autoradiography has revealed great differences between neurons and glial cells in the programming of the final cell cycle: the neuron precursors enter their final cell cycle in a distinct germinal zone which contains proliferating cells and some postmitotic cells that are migrating out, whereas mitotically active glial cell precursors may be in any position and are usually extraventricular. The glial precursors may divide and migrate repeatedly (see Section 3.5). The result of these differences is that while neurons exposed to [³H]thymidine in their final cell cycle remain permanently and heavily labeled and can be easily identified in autoradiographs, glial cells that are labeled at the same time usually undergo further divisions which dilute the label to below detectable levels.

The most important concept that has emerged from the autoradiographic studies is that each distinct set of neurons originates in a fairly invariant timetable. Thus in any one neuronal set (which may contain several neuronal types) the entire population of each type of neuron completes the final cell cycle and becomes permanently postmitotic within a relatively short period, usually in less than 1 day in rodents. By contrast, glial cells in any region withdraw from the mitotic cycle over a much longer time than the neurons in the same region, or they may only withdraw from mitosis temporarily, waiting for the appropriate signals, especially growth factors, to stimulate their proliferation (see Section 3.4).

2.10. Time and Sequence of Origin of Neurons and Glial Cells in the Central Nervous System

Evidence of temporal and spatial regularities in the origin of neurons and glial cells in complex structures such as the cerebral cortex was extremely difficult to obtain before the advent in the 1960s of the technique of autoradiography following the administration of tritiated thymidine (e.g., Sidman *et al.*, 1959; Uzman, 1960; Angevine and Sidman, 1961; Miale and Sidman, 1961). Information about the times and places of origin of neurons in the developing nervous system is now obtained with relative ease by injecting pregnant mammals with tritiated thymidine (1–5 μCi/gram body weight) intravenously or into the amniotic fluid, killing the fetuses at various intervals after the injection, and examining their brains autoradiographically.

The nucleotide is available for less than an hour after injection in mammals. Therefore, the presence of the label in a cell is an indication that the cell must have been engaged in DNA synthesis during the hour following the injection. Thymidine is cleared more slowly in cold-blooded animals and may remain available for hours or even days after administration. The temporal resolution of the method is also poor in bird embryos when the nucleotide is injected into the extraembryonic regions of the egg rather than directly into the embryo.

Heavy labeling of cell nuclei is an indication that tritiated thymidine has been incorporated during the final period of DNA synthesis in preparation for the terminal mitosis of the heavily labeled cell. The label is then retained for the remainder of the life of the cell. Light labeling is an indication that the label has been diluted by several divisions of the cell after it has taken up the label. Absence of label is of little significance following a single injection of tritiated thymidine. However, cells that remain unlabeled after several injections of the nucleotide (cumulative labeling) may be regarded as postmitotic provided that there is no reason to suspect that the injected nucleotide was not able to enter the unlabeled cells.

There is great consistency in the pattern of labeling of cell nuclei with tritiated thymidine. According to Angevine (1965), *"plots made from littermates injected and processed in identical fashion could be superimposed to show remarkable similarity in number and placement of labelled neurons. The origin of neurons in the various regions [of the hippocampal formation of the mouse] follows a precise timetable; thus specimens injected at the same time yield identical patterns and specimens injected serially display an orderly succession of patterns."*

Spatial gradients of proliferative activity in the neurepithelial germinal zone are of great importance in programming the time of origin of neurons and number of neurons that are produced at any time. The spatiotemporal pattern of origin of neurons, revealed by [³H]thymidine labeling of cells during their terminal phase of DNA synthesis, shows that neurons assemble either by stacking in laminar structures or by packing into nuclear regions in regular spatiotemporal gradients. Such gradients are described as "inside-out" when the neurons that originate at successively later times migrate past those formed earlier and take up successively more external positions, that is, successively farther from the

ventricular germinal zone from which they originate. This "inside-out" pattern of assembly or stacking is generally characteristic of laminar structures, especially the cerebral cortex, optic tectum, and substantia nigra. There are some exceptions, such as the granular layer of the hippocampal dentate gyrus and the granular layer of the cerebellar cortex, but in such cases the granule cells arise from displaced germinal zones and not directly from the ventricular germinal zone. These cases of apparent "outside-in" assembly should be contrasted with those cases in which the neurons assemble in a true "outside-in" sequence, which is characteristic of nuclear regions such as the thalamus and hypothalamus (Fig. 2.7). Such lateral-to-medial gradients of time of origin of neurons have been reported in the isthmo-optic nucleus of the chick (P. G. H. Clarke *et al.*, 1976), the basal forebrain of the hamster (ten Donkelaar and Dederen, 1979), the hypothalamus of the mouse (Shimada and Nakamura, 1973) and rat (Ifft, 1972; Altman and Bayer, 1988a), the septal region of the rat (Bayer, 1979), the amygdala of the rat (Bayer, 1980), the rat thalamus (Altman and Bayer, 1979a,b,c, 1988a,b,c), the anterior thalamus of the rabbit (V. Fernandez, 1969), and the dorsal thalamus of the mouse (Angevine, 1970a,b), as shown in Fig. 2.7. By contrast, in the cerebellar cortex there are no simple gradients, but regional differences in time or origin and migration of Purkinje cells has been observed in the chick (Kanemitsu and Kobayashi, 1988) and rat (Altman and Bayer, 1985c).

A question that arises from the above is whether there are discretely different *histogenetic fields* in the germinal cell populations that give rise to cytoarchetectonically different regions of the CNS. The problem is why such discontinuities occur and why they are at regular positions, e.g., in the cerebral cortex. To what extent are they determined by extrinsic influences, e.g, from the thalamocortical afferents, and to what extent are they intrinsic to the cortical plate itself? The historical origin of this concept of parcellation of cerebral cortical areas is reviewed in Section 10.1 and the current evidence is discussed in Section 10.3.

Differences in the time of origin of different types of neurons are superimposed on the spatiotemporal gradients. It is a general rule, with few exceptions, that large neurons are produced before small ones in the same region of the nervous

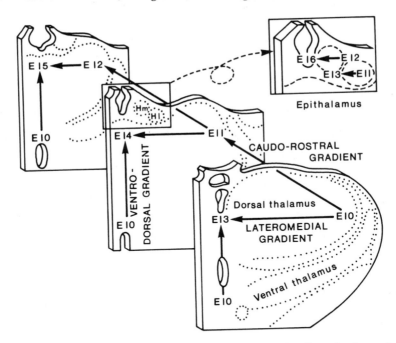

Figure 2.7. Gradients of time of origin of neurons determined autoradiographically in the diencephalon of the mouse embryo from E10 to E16. Hm and Hl are the medial and lateral habenular nuclei shown in the box. From J. B. Angevine, Jr. in *The Neuroscience: Second Study Program*, F. O. Schmitt (ed.), Rockefeller University Press, New York, 1970.

system, and the neurons produced last are small neurons such as granule cells or local circuit neurons.

Granule cell production continues after birth in all mammals that have been examined. Postnatal neurogenesis occurs in the following sites in the mouse:

1. In the main olfactory bulb and accessory olfactory bulb, granule cells originate from E1 to beyond P20 (Hinds, 1967, 1968 a,b; Hinds and McNelly, 1977). A similar timetable of granule cell production occurs in the rat in which granule cell production probably continues in the adult olfactory bulb (Kaplan and Hinds, 1977; Bayer, 1983).
2. In the hippocampus, granule cells of the dentate gyrus originate from E10 to P20 in the mouse (Angevine, 1965; Caviness, 1973; Vaughn *et al.*, 1977), as shown in Fig. 2.8. Postnatal generation of dentate granule cells also occurs in the rat (Altman, 1966b; Altman and Das, 1965b, 1967; Hine and Das, 1974; Schlessinger *et al.*, 1975, 1978; Kaplan and

Hinds, 1977; Bayer, 1980a), rabbit (Fernandez and Bravo, 1974), and rhesus monkey (Rakic and Nowakowski, 1981a).

3. In the brainstem nuclei, granule cells originate from the rhombic lip from E10 to P15 in the mouse (Taber Pierce, 1966, 1967a, 1973). For other species see the review by Altman and Bayer (1987).
4. Granule cells of the cerebellar cortex originate from E17 to P15 in the mouse (Miale and Sidman, 1961; S. Fujita *et al.*, 1966; S. Fujita, 1967; Mares *et al.*, 1970). References to other species are given in Section 10.13.

Large neurons, namely, the principal projection neurons, originate before the local-circuit neurons in mammals and submammalian vertebrates, for example, the olfactory bulb of the duck (Rebiere *et al.*, 1983). However, there are exceptions in submammalian vertebrates. An exception to the generalization that projection neurons originate early and local-circuit neurons originate late is found in songbirds, in which the majority of projection neurons from the "higher vocal centers" of the fore-

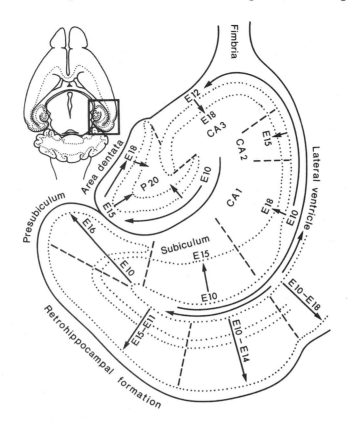

Figure 2.8. Gradients of time of neuron origin in the allocortex of the hippocampal formation of the mouse. Top left: A horizontal section of mouse brain, illustrating the position of the hippocampal region (rectangle), which is shown in greater detail below. A series of pregnant mice were each given a single injection of tritiated thymidine on different days of gestation (E10-E18), resulting in labeling of the fetuses. These were killed after birth, when the neurons had arrived at their final positions, and autoradiographs were made of their brains. Gradients of time of neuron origin are indicated by arrows. From J. B. Angevine, Jr., in *The Neurosciences: Second Study Program*, F. O. Schmitt (ed.), Rockefeller University Press, New York, 1970.

brain originate after P30 in the canary (Alvarez-Buylla *et al.*, 1988). However, in mammals there are many examples to support the generalization stated above. The retinal ganglion cells are formed first and differentiate before the receptors, bipolar cells, and amacrine cells in the same region of retina; although not necessarily before those cells in other parts of the retina that originated earlier (Sidman, 1961; S. Fujita and Horii, 1963; M. Jacobson, 1968b; Hollyfield, 1968; Kliot and Shatz, 1982; Walsch and Polley, 1985; Sengelaub *et al.*, 1986; Polley *et al.*, 1989). In the cerebellar cortex the Purkinje cells are formed first and then the Golgi Type II cells, followed by basket and stellate cells, and finally the granule cells. (Nineteenth-century work culminated in that of Ramón y Cajal, 1909–1911. Other refer-

ences are given in Section 10.11.) The large neurons are formed before the small neurons in the cerebellar roof nuclei (Miale and Sidman, 1961; Taber Pierce, 1967b). In the cerebral cortex the pyramidal cells are formed before the granule cells (Angevine, 1965; Hinds and Angevine, 1965; Bayer, 1980a) but the nonpyramidal cells of cortical preplate originate before the projection neurons (see Section 10.4). In the olfactory bulb the mitral cells are formed before the tufted cells and the granule cells are formed last (Hinds, 1968a,b; Creps, 1974a; Kaplan and Hinds, 1977; Bayer, 1983). The production of large neurons reaches a peak before production of small neurons in the spinal cord (H. Fujita and Fujita, 1963; Nornes and Carry, 1978; Sims and Vaughn, 1979; J. A. McConnell, 1981; Holley *et al.*, 1982; Altman and Bay-

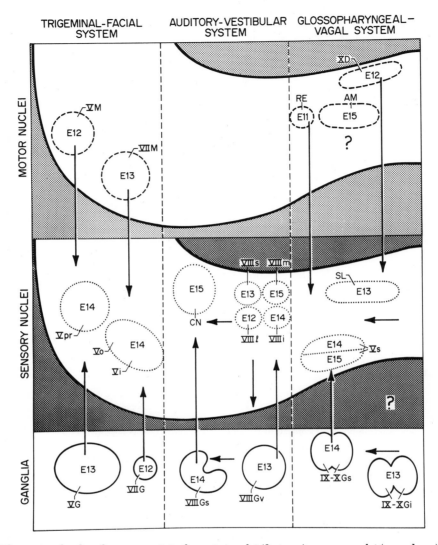

Figure 2.9. The temporal order of neurogenesis in the motor nuclei (first row), sensory nuclei (second row), and sensory ganglia (third row) in three related cranial nerve systems in the rat: the trigeminal facial (first column), the auditory-vestibular (second column; this system has no motor nuclei), and the glossopharyngealvagal (third column). Embryonic ages refer to days with peak neurogenesis. Vertical arrows refer to cytogenetic gradients (from earlier to later) in the motor nuclei and the sensory ganglia in relation to the sensory nuclei. Horizontal arrows indicate the matching cytogenetic gradients between the sensory ganglia and between the sensory nuclei in the auditory–vestibular and the glossopharyngeal-vagal systems. From J. Altman and S. A. Bayer, *Adv. Anat. Embryol. Cell Biol.* 74:1-90 (1982).

er, 1984, review), in the diencephalon (Angevine, 1968, 1970a), and in the cochlear nuclei (Taber Pierce, 1967a; but see Martin and Rickets, 1981).

There is also a tendency for motor nuclei to commence their histogenesis and complete their cell populations before the sensory nuclei at the same level of the neuraxis, and for the histogenesis of the motor systems to have a shorter duration

than that of the sensory systems. Studies of the brainstem, which has a similar plan in all vertebrates (Nieuwenhuys, 1974) substantiate those concepts particularly well, as shown in Fig. 2.9 (Taber Pierce, 1973; Nornes and Morita, 1979; Altman and Bayer, 1980a–d, 1982; Heaton and Moody, 1980; Shaw and Alley, 1982).

In some respects the ontogeny of the brain

appears to recapitulate its phylogeny. The "biogenetic law" that ontogeny recapitulates phylogeny should be regarded only as a parallelism, not as a necessary causal relationship, and always with the reservation that ontogenetic–phylogenetic parallelism may merely be the fortuitous result of the operation of circumstances and of principles of efficiency that are similar in evolution and in development. Bearing these reservations in mind, the parallels between ontogeny of the nervous system and its presumed phylogeny are often so striking as to demand explanations. It is the general rule that parts of the nervous system that may have appeared first in phylogeny have a tendency to appear early in ontogeny, and structures that may have arisen later in evolution also often arise late in ontogeny. For example, neurons in what is considered to be the phylogenetically older accessory olfactory bulb develop before their counterparts in the more recently evolved olfactory bulb (Hinds, 1968a; Bayer, 1983). The late origin of the hippocampal granule cells reflects the phylogenetic increase in granule cells in the hippocampus of placental mammals as compared with nonplacental mammals (Angevine, 1965). The early origin of the ventral thalamus in mammals reflects the early evolution of the homologous thalamic structures in submammalian vertebrates (Angevine, 1970a). The phylogenetically older accessory olive develops first ontogenetically (Harkmark, 1954; Ellenberger *et al.*, 1969).

In the cerebral isocortex, the neurons of the outer layers (except I) originate last and are the most recent to have appeared in evolution (see Section 10.6). Layers I and VI appear to have evolved first and are the first cortical layers to develop. In the cat, Marin-Padilla (1972) has shown that the first intracortical circuits are developed between layers I and VI; the Martinotti neurons of layer VI connecting with layer I and the horizontal neurons (Cajal–Retzius cells) of layer I projecting to layer VI (Fig. 2.10). These neurons, together with the pyramidal neurons of layer VI, are the first to form in the mammalian cortex, and initially form an organization that, according to Marin-Padilla (1972), resembles the reptilian neocortex. This precocious organization is completely transformed during late prenatal development, and its interconnections apparently disappear completely by the time of birth. This is an example of regressive differentiation of

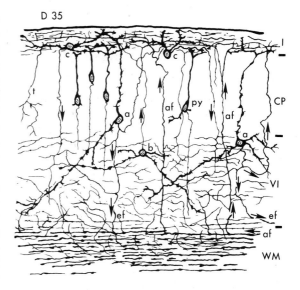

Figure 2.10. Organization of the cat neocortex at 35 days of gestation, illustrating its structure and basic neuronal types. During early gestation (E25–E45) the cortex is characterized by a superficial (layer 1) and a deep (layer VI) plexiform layer composed of ascending collaterals from the afferent fibers of the white matter and monoaminergic fibers from the brainstem. Three types of neurons are recognized in the neocortex of the cat during this gestational period: the horizontal neurons (c), with descending axons terminating in layer VI; the Martinotti neurons (b), with ascending axons terminating in layer I; and the pyramidal-like stellate neurons (a) with recurrent axonic collaterals to layer I and terminal efferent fibers. The cortical plate (CP) is composed of immature pyramidal neurons (py) at a bipolar stage of development. The dendrites of the three types of neurons of the primordial neocortical organization are covered by a few spinelike projections suggesting the presence of a postsynaptic apparatus. This, in addition to the obvious fiber and neuronal interactions between layers I and VI, supports the idea that the primordial neocortical organization of the cat is a functionally active structure. Layer I (superficial plexiform layer) has associative and projective characteristics. Analogies between the reptilian cortex (see Fig. 534 in Ramón y Cajal, 1911) and the primordial neocortical organization of the cat are suggested. Rapid Golgi method. Camera lucida drawing. From M. Marin-Padilla, *Z. Anat. Entwicklungsgesch.* 134:117-145 (1971).

cortical cytoarchitectonic fields, a concept introduced by Brodmann (1909, p. 226).

What is the purpose of preserving the genetic information and developmental processes for such transient structures that seem to have no nervous function in the embryo or fetus? Are such primitive structures truly vestiges of the state of organization reached by the ancestral forms? It has been suggested that transient vestigial structures in the embryo are necessary for the subsequent developmental events (de Beer, 1951). We should question whether such apparently vestigial neural circuits give a true indication of the neural circuitry of ancestral forms or whether they are so greatly modified and specialized that they cannot give more than a vague indication of the ancestral forms from which they might have evolved. Do the times of origin of neurons give a reliable indication of their phylogeny, or do the gradients of time of origin reflect a purely developmental adaptation to achieve an efficient assembly of complex structures? We shall consider this again in Section 10.2.

These examples show that the time of neuron origin depends on a complex set of factors, including the type of neuron, its position in the gradients of mitotic activity, and probably its phylogenetic status. It is important to recognize that the time of cell origin is not necessarily correlated simply with the time of any single aspect of cytodifferentiation, such as the formation of synapses. Cells may be "dormant" for relatively long times—months in the primate cerebral cortex—in their final positions, before they become connected in their definitive neural circuits. One cannot simply deduce the subsequent timetable of neuron differentiation from a knowledge of the time of neuron origin, one has to take other factors into consideration, such as the type of neuron, the region in which it is situated, and especially the time of arrival of the axons, usually from several sources, that are destined to synapse on the neuron in question.

To summarize: autoradiographic studies of the time of origin and migration of neurons and glial cells have revealed features that are common to many regions of the central nervous system, although there are some notable exceptions to these generalizations:

1. Spatial and temporal gradients of proliferation in the neurepithelial germinal zone
2. Separate origin of neighboring regions that are different cytoarchitectonically
3. An orderly sequence of production of large neurons first, then intermediate-sized neurons, and finally small neurons
4. Continuing production of glial cells after termination of production of neurons in any particular region of the brain

5. A predisposition for phylogenetically older parts of the brain to arise earlier in ontogenesis

2.11. Lineages of Neurons of Vertebrates and Invertebrates

Clonal analysis aims at a complete description of the growth of a clone (from the Greek word for a twig, meaning a cell population descended from a single progenitor cell): the number of descendants, their states of commitment, the amount of migration and cell mingling, their final positions, and states of terminal differentiation (reviewed by M. Jacobson, 1985a,b, 1990a). If the position of the labeled progenitor cell is known, fate maps can be deduced from the relationship between the positions of the progenitor cells and the positions and terminally differentiated types of their progeny.

The lineage of an identified ancestral cell may be either determinate or indeterminate with respect to the fates of the progeny. Determinate lineages result in stereotyped fates whereas indeterminate lineages result in variable fates during normal development of different individuals of the same species. Cell fates may be specified autonomously, without respect to conditions outside the cells in the lineage, or specification of cell fates may be contingent on cell interactions or other extrinsic conditions. Experimental tests of autonomy consist of observing any changes in fates of residual cells after cell ablation, or noting whether transplanted progenitor cells alter their fates after perturbations such as cell isolation, transplantation, fusion, or mitotic arrest, or whether fates of cells of a certain genotype are changed in chimeras or mosaics made of cells of two different genotypes. Cell lineages of vertebrates are always indeterminate and contingent on extrinsic conditions whereas lineages of invertebrates are, with few exceptions, determinate and autonomous. The concept of determinate and indeterminate cell lineages is considered in Section 1.3.

To trace cell lineages it is necessary to identify an individual progenitor cell and trace its progeny through successive cell divisions until they finally differentiate. This is called a prospective lineage analysis. It can be done by direct microscopic observation of embryos such as nematodes that are transparent and have small numbers of cells (Sulston and Horvitz, 1977; Kimble and Hirsch, 1979; Sulston *et al.*, 1983). It can also be done in embryos with large numbers of cells by using the techniques of injection of a heritable cell lineage tracer into an identified progenitor cell and then tracing the labeled progeny through successive cell generations (Jacobson and Hirose, 1978, 1981; Weisblat *et al.*, 1978).

When the position and identity of the initially labeled progenitor cell cannot be ascertained, the lineages of its progeny may be deduced retrospectively from analysis of their numbers, positions, and cellular phenotypes. This has to be done when tracing lineages after infection of a progenitor cell with a retroviral cell lineage tracer (Calof and Jessel, 1986; Turner and Cepko, 1987; Price *et al.*, 1987), and when analyzing aggregation chimeras (Mintz, 1971; Tettenborn *et al.*, 1971; McLaren, 1976), transplantation chimeras (reviewed by Harrison, 1935; Le Douarin, 1982), and genetic mosaics (reviewed by C. Stern, 1968; Gehring, 1978; Herman, 1989).

Several methods available for tracing a clone from a single progenitor cell will now be summarized and selected examples of their application will be given: (1) direct observation of lineages in the intact embryo; (2) analysis of animal chimeras and genetic mosaics; (3) tracing clones labeled with a retrovirus; (4) tracing clones originating from a single progenitor cell labeled with an intracellularly injected lineage tracer.

The entire lineage of the nematode, *Caenorhabditis elegans*, has been traced from the first cleavage of the egg through embryonic and postembryonic stages to the adult. This has been done by direct microscopic observation of living embryos and was feasible because the organism is transparent, and it rapidly undergoes an invariant pattern of cleavage to generate an invariant and small number of cells in the adult worm (Sulston and Horvitz, 1977; Kimble and Hirsch, 1979; Sulston *et al.*, 1983). Within the first hour after the first cleavage, five somatic founder cells and one primordial germ cell are generated by unequal cleavages (Fig. 2.11). This results in differential partitioning of cytoplasmic components that lead to lineage specific developmental fates of the blastomeres (Strome, 1989, review). During *C. elegans* hermaphrodite development, 1090 postmitotic somatic cell nuclei are generated but 131 cells undergo programmed cell death, including 20 percent of all presumptive neu-

ral cells. Only 959 cells form the adult worm of which 302 cells are in the nervous system. The nervous system of the adult worm consists of a cephalic part, a circumpharyngeal nerve ring, dorsal and ventral nerve cords, and their associated ganglia and sense organs.

One of the blastomeres AB, formed by the first division of the fertilized egg, is the founder cell that gives rise to 214 of the 222 neurons of the newly hatched first larval stage and all of the neurons formed during postembryonic stages (Fig. 2.11). Founder cell AB also gives rise to muscles, hypodermis, and other types of cells. Even at the terminal division, a cell can give rise to a nerve cell and a muscle cell. The animal does not have embryonic germ layers. The final population of neurons is formed by a series of highly invariant cell divisions, cell migrations, and cell deaths.

Because the cell lineages, migrations and cell positions are invariant in *C. elegans*, tracing lineage does not show whether cell fates are autonomous or contingent—perturbations are necessary for that: cell ablation, isolation, transplantation, fusion, or blockage of cleavage. Systematic ablation of single cells by means of a laser microbeam has been done with the aim of showing whether regulation of lineages can occur or whether lineages are cell autonomous (Sulston and White, 1980; Kimble, 1981; Sulston *et al.*, 1983). In most cases the surviving cells generated only those types of cells that they generated in unoperated embryos. No regulation occurs and the fates of cells are specified autonomously in most cases. In a few cases regulation occurs by a neighboring cell adopting the fate of the ablated cell. A group of cells capable of substituting for one another in that way is called an "equivalence group." Groups of cells similar to equivalence groups, in which one cell can substitute for the fate of another, have been found in the leech (Weisblat and Blair, 1984), the cockroach (Bate and Grunwald, 1981), and the frog, *Xenopus* (M. Jacobson, 1981b).

It is also possible to make genetic mosaics in *C. elegans* composed of cells of two different genotypes that can be recognized by phenotypic markers (Herman, 1984, 1989, review). Such mosaics can be used to show whether the phenotypes of identified cells depend only on their own genotypes (are cell autonomous) or whether they depend on interactions with other cells, which can be identified in the mosaics. Using mosaic analysis it has been possible to show that in worms with the *unc-3* mutation, which re-

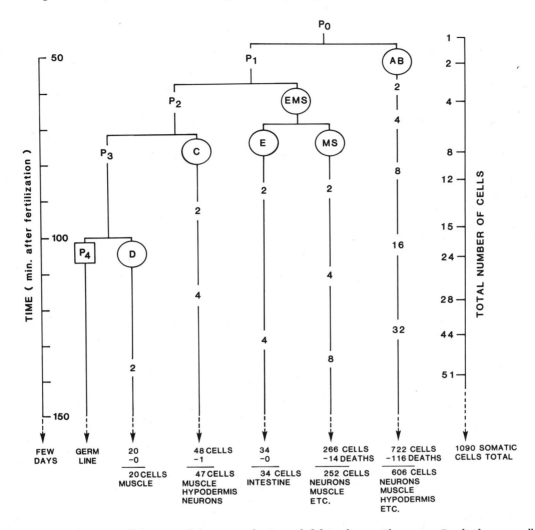

Figure 2.11. Embryonic cell lineages of the nematode *Caenorhabditis elegans.* The zygote, P$_0$, divides unequally to generate the first somatic founder cell, AB, and a germline cell, P$_1$. Further unequal division produce additional somatic founder cells (MS, E, C, and D) and the primodial germ cell, P$_4$. Each founder cell divides with a characteristic mitotic cycle time different from the others to generate a fixed number of progeny with different fates. Modified from data of J. E. Sulson, E. Schierenberg, J. G. White, and J. N. Thomson. *Dev. Biol.* **100**:64–119 (1983).

sults in severe incoordination of movements, the defect is localized in motoneurons derived from all four granddaughters of the founder cell ABp (Herman, 1989, review).

One of the advantages of *C. elegans* is that mutants can be selected which cause specific alterations in cell lineages without apparently causing general defects in cell functions (Sulston and Horvitz, 1981; Chalfie *et al.,* 1981; Greenwald *et al.,* 1983). Two of these are recessive mutations, *lin-4*

and *unc-86,* which cause various reiterations in postembryonic lineages, leading to increases in the numbers of cells. Another mutation, *lin-12,* causes one group of cells to adopt the fate normally reserved for another group, resulting in a homeotic transformation of one structure into another. Normally, *lin-12* appears to control alternative fates.

Recessive mutations in the genes *ced-3* and *ced-4* prevent almost all the programmed cell deaths that occur during development in *C. elegans* (Ellis and Horvitz, 1986; Avery and Horvitz, 1987). Using genetic mosaic analysis, Yuan and Horvitz (1990) show that *ced-3* and *ced-4* most likely act cell–autonomously to cause cell death in *C. elegans*. The surviving cells in those mutants, some of which differentiate as neurons, do not seem to have any affect on normal morphogenesis and function. In other words, the *ced-3* and *ced-4* mutations appear to be neutral, and it is not clear what purpose the cell death may serve during normal development. Horvitz *et al.* (1982) speculate that cells which are programmed to die are generated because it is easier to evolve a program to kill cells than to prevent their generation. Such an appeal to teleology is at best a weak form of reasoning, and carries no conviction in this case in which the death of cells seems to serve no useful purpose. It is significant that mutations in *ced–3* and *ced-4*, which prevent programmed cell death, have no effect on death of six sensory neurons, called the microtubule cells, caused by the mutation *mec-4 (e1611)* (Ellis and Horvitz, 1986). Death of the microtubule cells occurs because the mutation apparently makes the *mec-4* gene product cytotoxic. For additional discussion of cell death in invertebrates see Truman (1984) and Ellis and Horvitz (1986). Cell death in the vertebrate nervous system is dealt with in Chapter 8.

Cell lineages can be traced prospectively after injection of a heritable cell lineage tracer into a single progenitor cell, followed by identification of all labeled progeny at later stages of development. The tracer must be transferred at mitosis to the daughter cells and must be detectable in all the progeny. The tracer molecules must be nontoxic and of a size and charge that prevents their exit from the cells via gap junctions. These criteria are satisfied by horseradish peroxidase (M. Jacobson and Hirose, 1978; Hirose and Jacobson, 1979, 1981; M. Jacobson and Moody, 1984; Moody and Jacobson, 1983; Moody, 1987a,b); biotynilated HRP (M. Jacobson and Huang, 1984); and fluorescent- labeled dextran (Weisblat *et al.,* 1980b; Gimlich and Cooke, 1983; Sheard and Jacobson, 1987, 1990). Fluorescent tracers enable clones near the surface of the embryo to be monitored prospectively, and two or more clones can be labeled in the same embryo with different fluorescent tracers (Gimlich and Braun, 1985; Sheard and Jacobson, 1987, 1990).

Variants of this technique allow fates of labeled cells to be traced after transplantation to unlabeled

hosts. For example, by grafting labeled dorsal blastoporal lip to the ventral region of unlabeled *Xenopus* early gastrulae it was conclusively demonstrated that the induced nervous system originated mainly from the unlabeled host, and had thus changed their fates in response to the graft (Gimlich and Cooke, 1983; J. C. Smith and Slack, 1984; M. Jacobson, 1984a). Single cells labeled with horseradish peroxidase can be transplanted from a labeled donor to unlabeled host *Xenopus* embryos, where their fates can be noted. In that way it has been demonstrated that progeny of single transplanted progenitor cells change their fates after heterotopic transplantation, showing that their fates are contingent on position, not on origin from specified progenitors (M. Jacobson and Xu, 1989).

In vitro combination of embryonic cells of known lineages, labeled with cell lineage tracers, can be a good technique for investigation of the roles of cell interactions and cell lineages in embryonic pattern formation and in determination of different cell types. Cells labeled with HRP can also be excised and cultured *in vitro* in combination with unlabeled cells to observe the inductive interactions between labeled and unlabeled cells (M. Jacobson and Rutishauser, 1986) and to study cell migration and mingling (M. Jacobson and Klein, 1985; Klein and Jacobson, 1991).

One very significant finding of these cell lineage studies in the frog was that *"the relationship between an individual blastomere and any specific type of cell in the CNS was only probabilistic"* (M. Jacobson and Hirose, 1981). This conclusion applies to every type of cell and is vividly exemplified by the Mauthner neuron. *"Because one Mauthner's neuron normally differentiates on each side of the rhombencephalon, it can arise only from a single ancestral cell in each case, but the evidence is consistent with a probabilistic origin of Mauthner's neuron from more than one possible ancestral cell at the 64-cell stage"* (M. Jacobson and Hirose, 1981). In the zebrafish the origin of neurons from individually labeled ancestral cells also appears to be probabilistic (Kimmel and Warga, 1989).

In *Xenopus*, the small number of certain types of easily identified neurons (66 Rohon–Beard neurons and 82 primary motoneurons, mean total on each side of the spinal cord) makes it feasible to analyze their lineages quantitatively. This has been done by intracellular injection of HRP into single

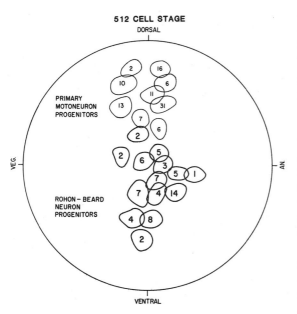

Figure 2.12. Probabilistic origins of Rohon–Beard neurons and primary motoneurons from two separate groups of progenitors in the 512-cell frog embryo. The embryo is shown in right lateral view (AN = animal pole; VEG = vegetal pole). Diameter of the embryo is about 1.3 mm. Single progenitor cells received an intracellular injection of horseradish peroxidase and the number of labeled Rohon–Beard neurons (RBN) or primary motoneurons (PMN) originating from each blastomere was counted at later stages, after the neurons had differentiated. Ancestral cells were labeled throughout the embryo, but only those which gave rise RBNs (thick outlines) or PMNs (thin outlines) are shown. The numbers denote the number of each type of neuron that originated from a single progenitor cell at the 512-cell stage. The mean total number of RBNs and PMNs on one side of the spinal cord in these embryos was 66 and 82 respectively. Thus, each progenitor produces an indeterminate, but small, fraction of the total. From M. Jacobson and S. A. Moody, *J. Neurosci.* 4:1361–1369 (1984).

progenitor cells in a series of embryos at successive cell generations, and later counting all the differentiated progeny of a single progenitor (M. Jacobson and Moody, 1984; Moody, 1989). Results of those experiments show that Rohon-Beard neurons and primary motoneurons originate from two different but neighboring groups of progenitors each composed of about 15 cells in the 512-cell *Xenopus* embryo. Each progenitor gives rise to a small and indeterminate fraction of the final population of descendants of a specific type (Fig. 2.12). Evidence

that individual progenitors are not predetermined to produce a certain number of a specific cell type is provided by the results of two different experiments. First, removal of the blastomere at the 16-cell stage from which most Rohon–Beard cells normally originate is followed by regulation resulting in development of the normal number of Rohon–Beard neurons (M. Jacobson, 1981a,b). Second, heterotopic transplantation of single blastomeres at the 512-cell stage is followed by complete regulation of their fates, including various types of neurons (M. Jacobson and Xu, 1989). Those results conclusively show that neuronal cell fates in *Xenopus* embryos are specified by local conditions, not by lineages from certain ancestral cells.

Fate maps can only be obtained if cell mingling is restricted after the time of initiation of a labeled clone. The fact that it is possible to obtain fate maps in amphibian embryos after labeling blastomeres in early cleavage stages shows that there must be restrictions of cell mingling. Paradoxically, very extensive cell mingling occurs in amphibian embryos, starting during gastrulation (Keller, 1978; M. Jacobson and Hirose, 1981; Nakatsuji and Johnson, 1982; M. Jacobson and Klein, 1985). Then how is it possible to obtain fate maps which show consistent relationships between the positions of individual blastomeres and the domains which all their progeny occupy at the completion of development (Fig. 2.13)? We have theorized that cell mingling is restricted across certain boundaries between morphological compartments but occurs relatively freely within such compartments, and that such compartments are established by groups of ancestral cells during cleavage stages, before the onset of cell mingling in *Xenopus* embryos (M. Jacobson, 1980, 1983, 1985a,b).

Evidence consistent with this compartment theory has been obtained by intracellular labeling of individual ancestral cells with a cell lineage tracer: clones initiated after the 512-cell stage are always confined to a single one of seven morphological compartments, whereas clones initiated at earlier stages frequently cross putative compartmental boundaries (M. Jacobson and Hirose, 1981; M. Jacobson, 1983). However, those results were not conclusive, mainly because the cells of a single clone initiated by labeling an ancestral at the 512-cell stage comprise only about 5 percent of the cells in a compartment, and thus do not clearly delineate the

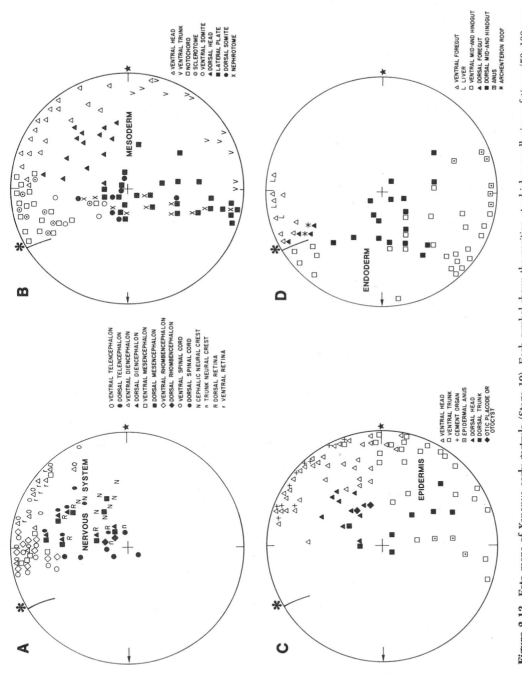

Figure 2.13. Fate maps of *Xenopus* early gastrula (Stage 10). Each symbol shows the position at which a small piece of tissue (50–100 μm diameter), consisting of cells labeled with horseradish peroxidase, was grafted from a totally labeled Stage 10 donor to the same position in an unlabeled Stage 10 host embryo. The asterisk shows the position of the dorsal blastoporal lip; the star is at the animal pole, the arrow is at the vegetal pole. After completion of gastrulation and neurulation, the hosts were processed histologically and the positions and histotypes of all labeled progeny were observed in the nervous system (A), mesodermal tissues (B), surface epidermis (C), and gut endoderm (D). All grafts giving rise to nerve cells also gave rise to at least one other histotype, and usually to several different histotypes. This is also observed when single labeled cells are grafted homotopically in *Xenopus* at Stage 10 (M. Jacobson and W.-L. Xu, *Dev. Biol. 131*:119–125, 1989), indicating that lineages have not diverged to give rise exclusively to nerve cells at the beginning of gastrulation. From M. Jacobson and W.-L. Xu, unpublished.

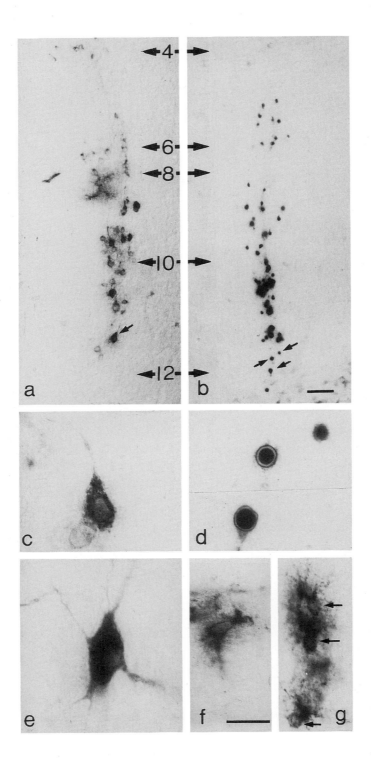

putative compartmental boundary. This limitation has been largely overcome by tracing the fates of two clones in the same embryo, each labeled with a different fluorescent tracer. Those experiments show that the two clones either approach one another without mingling, but do not cross boundaries at certain positions in all cases, or the clones mingle extensively on the same side of such boundaries (Sheard and Jacobson, 1987, 1990). A compartment is a purely morphological entity: *"The word compartment is used in the sense of a separate section of the overall structural pattern that has developed from a particular embryonic rudiment, the blastomere group. With respect to the fate map one may think of compartments as topological neighborhoods within the overall morphological pattern"* (M. Jacobson, 1983).

Another method for tracing cell lineages is to infect progenitor cells with a retrovirus carrying a reporter gene into the genome, and later to identify the infected progeny. Almost any gene can be inserted into a retrovirus vector but in order to qualify as a lineage tracer the reporter gene product must be nontoxic and easily detected histochemically, and the virus must be infective in the experimental animal but not in humans. Retrovirus vectors have been constructed for use in chick, mouse, and rat. Such vectors contain a suitable promoter, and as a reporter gene they contain the *Escherichia coli* β-galactosidase (β-gal) gene which is expressed at high levels in the infected cells and their progeny. The β-galactosidase activity can be detected histochemically. The retrovirus is injected extracellularly in a small volume containing a dose low enough to result in infection of very few, well separated cells, to ensure that isolated labeled clones are produced. Virus infects both mitotic and postmitotic cells but only integrates with the genome in cells in the S phase. Cells are infected at random, so that this method does not permit identification of the progenitor cell. Therefore, the lineages can only be deduced retrospectively and it may be difficult to rule out selective cell infection and selective survival of infected cells.

The main advantage of this technique is that small cells can be labeled close to or at their terminal cell division. Thus, it has been shown that a single progenitor in the vertebrate CNS can divide to produce a small clone or even only two progeny that are of different types—either different types of neurons (Calof and Jessel, 1986; Turner and Cepko, 1987; Price *et al.*, 1987; Gray *et al.*, 1988; Luskin *et al.*, 1988; Price and Thurlow, 1989; Sanes, 1989) or even neurons and glial cells (Galileo *et al.*, 1990), as shown in Fig. 2.14. This shows that there are multipotential progenitors in the vertebrate CNS but it does not show whether they are committed to produce only certain types of cells, although it is often inferred from the results summarized above that commitment in the nervous system is delayed until the terminal cell division. The main drawback of the retroviral tracer method is that it does not provide strong evidence regarding cell commitment or lineage autonomy.

Chimeric embryos formed by combining cells from different species or genera having cell autonomous markers have been of enormous value for studying cell migrations and interactions. The value of chimeras for the analysis of cell interactions during development was first grasped by Johann Friedrich Blumenbach (1752–1840), the Göttingen anatomist. In his *"Essay on Generation"* (1792) he describes how he made a chimera by fusing part of a green hydra with part of a brown hydra. He found that cells from both donors participated in restoration of a small but complete animal, by a process which he characterized as reconversion, or, as we would now say, regulation. This was a premature discovery, (M. Jacobson, in preparation). It was not until more than a century later that Gustav Born (1894, 1897) reinvented the method of combining tissues of two different amphibian embryos to form

Figure 2.14. Demonstration that different types of neurons and glial cells can originate from the same progenitor in the chick optic tectum. Chick embryos were infected with two different retroviruses, both of which insert the β-galactosidase gene into the genome of the infected cell, but one is localized in the cytoplasm, the other in the nucleus. Embryos injected with a mixture of both retroviruses contain clusters of labeled cells, either containing the cytoplasmic label (a) or nuclear label (b) but never both, showing that the clusters are clones. High-power pictures of cell marked with arrows in (a) and (b) show the cytoplasmic label (c) and nuclear label (d). Nuclear labelling allows additional cytoplasmic immunostaining to identify neurons shown in (e) (neurofilament +), or glial cell shown in (f) and (g). Arrows in (g) (GFAP + and glutamine synthetase +) show glial cell somata in a cluster. Magnification bar = 80 μm in (a) and (b) and 25 μm in (c)/ to (g). From D. S. Galileo, G. E. Gray, G. C. Owens, J. Majors, and J. R. Sanes, *Proc. Natl. Acad. Sci. USA* 87:458-462, 1990.

a mosaic or chimera in which further development involves interactions between the tissues of the two donors. He made combinations of dissimilar parts of two different species (heteroplastic combinations) or of different genera (xenoplastic combinations, a term coined by Geinitz, 1925). I should also mention that Gustav Born invented the technique of culturing frog embryonic tissues *in vitro* in a drop of frog lymph, and that, after Born's early death, both of those techniques were exploited by Ross Harrison (see footnote 4 in Chapter 5). In his elegant analysis of migration of epidermal cells and of the lateral line system in frogs, Harrison (1898, 1903) grafted the head of a darkly pigmented *Rana sylvatica* embryo to the body of the lightly pigmented *Rana palustris*. He could trace the dark lateral line organs migrating caudally into the lighter trunk and tail.

The term "animal chimera" was coined by Spemann (1921) to describe interspecific combinations. The use of xenoplastic transplantation by Spemann's students, Oscar Schotté and Fritz Baltzer, is described by Hamburger (1988). Spemann and Mangold (1924) made use of chimeras of two different species of urodeles in their experiments which proved that a grafted dorsal blastopore lip induces a nervous system in the tissues of the host (see Section 1.1). Interspecific amphibian chimeras were used often in the following decades to study tissue interactions and cell migrations, for example, from the neural crest (Lehman, 1927; Raven, 1931, 1936, 1937; Detwiler, 1937, 1938, review; G. Wagner, 1948; Thiebaud, 1983). Recently, interspecific avian chimeras formed of embryonic chick and quail tissues have been of immense value in studying migrations and fates of neural crest cells. We shall consider this at length in Chapter 4.

Retrospective clonal analysis can be made from mammalian chimeras formed by combining two early blastula stage embryos. Such chimeras have proved to be very useful for analysis of cell interactions, but for tracing cell lineages they have considerable limitations. Two eight-cell mouse embryos with different cellular markers can be combined, after removal of the zona pellucida, and they continue normal development after implantation in the uterus of a pseudopregnant mouse (Mintz, 1970, 1971; Tattenborn *et al.*, 1971; McLaren, 1972, 1976). The cells derived from the two donor embryos mingle extensively, so that it is impossible to determine the origin of any type of descendant from

any single progenitor. Conclusions about the number of descendant clones deduced from the distribution of the two types of descendants in the adult are also limited by lack of information about the amount of cell mingling, migration in and out of the tissue, and selective cell death (McLaren, 1976; West, 1978). The published number of clones at the time of foundation of a tissue ranges from 2 to 20 for different tissues (Mintz, 1970; Mintz and Sanyal, 1970; Sanyal and Zeilmaker, 1974, 1976, 1977; Wetts and Herrup, 1982).

Construction of composite embryos by combining two genetically distinct mouse embryos at about the eight-cell stage produces an aggregation mosaic animal. Cells of the adult are derived from one or other of the parents, and the distribution of cells will depend on the amount of mingling or of segregation of the two strains of cells at the time at which the presumptive fates of the cells had become established as a map. As J. H. Lewis *et al.* (1972) have pointed out, such experiments *"reveal only the relative size of the group of cells giving rise to a tissue, compared with the mosaic patch size, at the time when the presumptive fate of those progenitors first became definite. From this type of investigation the number of progenitors at the time of determination, that is, at the time of the first, decisive step of differentiation, cannot be deduced."* The difficulty of deriving the size of the stem cell pool from such experiments greatly reduces the usefulness of this technique. Indeed, the validity of some of the conclusions derived from studies of chimeric mice is questionable, for example, the conclusion that the retinal photoreceptors of the mouse are a clone originating from a group of 10 initiator cells near the center of the retina (Mintz and Sanyal, 1970). Because the cells from the two parents are able to mingle before the time of primary neural induction, the pattern of the mosaic in the neural plate is unpredictable and will tend to be fine grained, with the result that cells from both parents will contribute to all parts of the nervous system. Such mingling is seen in the cerebellum in which the Purkinje cells derived from each parent are randomly mixed, as shown in Fig. 2.15 (Dewey *et al.*, 1976; Mullen, 1977; Mullen and Herrup, 1979). Mullen estimated that coherent clones in the Purkinje cell layer average only 1.03 Purkinje cells. This number precludes any calculation of the number of clones from which the total population of Purkinje cells originated at the time they became committed. However, in some parts of the CNS of *Mus caroli*↔*Mus musculus* interspecific mouse chimeras, neurons and glial cells of the same genotype form large coherent clusters (Goldowitz, 1989). This is probably the result of preferential adhesion of like cells in such chimeras. From those results it is not possible to say whether the coherent clusters of cells are clones. In these mouse chimeras there are boundaries between regions populated by cells of one genotype and regions populated by the other which are reminiscent of the boundaries seen in the frog CNS.

In general, analysis of aggregation chimeras is a relatively weak method for tracing cell lineages, but it is a powerful method for determining whether cell fates are autonomous or are contingent on cell interactions and extrinsic factors. Intraspecific and interspecific chimeras have been used with great success in the analysis of cerebellar mutations (see Section 10.15) to show whether the gene action is confined to the affected cells or whether it involves cellular interactions (Mullen, 1977, 1978; Herrup and Mullen, 1979; Mullen and Herrup, 1979; Goldowitz and Mullen, 1982; Terashima *et al.*, 1986; Goldowitz, 1987, 1989a,b). This method does not have the certainty and precision provided by xenoplastic transplantation of genetically marked neural crest or neural plate cells, for example, transplantation between quail and chick embryos (see Section 4.3). This technique is especially useful for studying the paths of cell migration and for showing whether specification of cell fates is cell autonomous or contingent on conditions outside the cells (Fig. 2.16).

In *Drosophila* two types of genetic mosaics have been used to study cell lineage: gynandromorphs and X-ray-induced somatic crossing-over mosaics. Gynandromorphs are flies whose tissues are composed of a mosaic of male and female cells. They are produced through loss of an X chromosome at an early cleavage division, with the result that the animal is a mosaic of XO and XX cells (Sturtevant, 1929; Garcia-Bellido and Meriam, 1969; Hotta and Benzer, 1972; Janning, 1978). The X-ray-induced somatic recombination between homologous chromosomes can be initiated at later stages of development than gynandromorphy (C. Stern, 1968). The affected cell transmits its abnormality to its offspring, which form a clone. Because clonally related cells stay together during development of insects, the clones form large, compact groups of cells in the later stages of development or in the adult animal. In general, two tissues that share a stem cell pool should be correlated in mosaic composition provided that they did not diverge in development before the onset of mosaicism. Gynandromorphs have been used for determining the parts of the nervous system that are affected in behavioral mutants of *Drosophila* (Hotta and Benzer, 1970, 1972, 1973; Ikeda and Kaplan, 1970a,b; D. T. Suzuki *et al.*, 1971; Griglatti *et al.*, 1972). In these studies the mosaics consist of tissues which are heterozygous for a recessive behavior mutation located on the X chromosome and tissues which are hemizygous for the mutation. By testing many such mosaics, it can be determined which regions of the animal have to be hemizygous in order to produce the mutant behavior.

There have been several investigations of the genetic determinants of behavior in insects using genetic mosaics. P. W. Whiting (1932) made gynandromorphs of the parasitic wasp *Habrobracon*, in which the males and females have different behavior, and showed that the head controls sexual behavior in that species. Using genetic mosaics of *Drosophila*, it has been observed that specific behavioral or functional effects are associated with a mutant gene expressed in a specific tissue. Thus Ikeda and Kaplan (1970b) have shown that the hyperkinetic mutation, which causes shaking of the leg when the fly is etherized, is linked to the individual legs, while Hotta and Benzer (1970) have found that various abnormalities of visual behavior are due to defects within the compound eye. However, these studies are limited by the fact that the mosaicism of the nervous system has to be determined indirectly from the cuticular distribution of the mosaicism and by the construction of morphogenetic fate maps. Hotta and Benzer (1972) mapped the foci in the blastoderm from which the nervous structures arise that produce the mutant behavior: for example, the foci for the ether-induced leg shaking caused by the hyperkinetic[1] mutation were mapped to the thoracic ganglia. In fact, Ikeda and Kaplan (1970a,b) have shown, by electrophysiological recording, that the thoracic ganglion motoneurons are defective in the hyperkinetic[1] mutants. Combining the genetic mosaics with enzyme markers, Kankel and Hall (1976) have been able to derive fate maps for the nervous system by looking directly at the tissue dis-

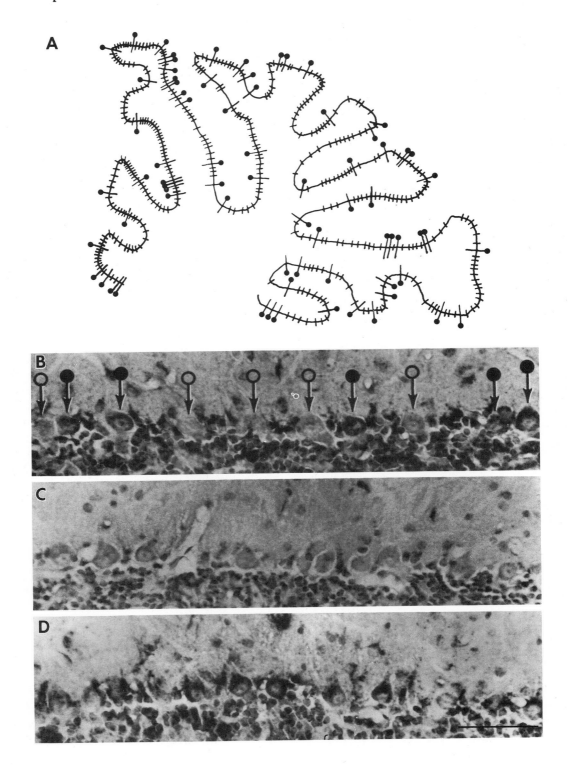

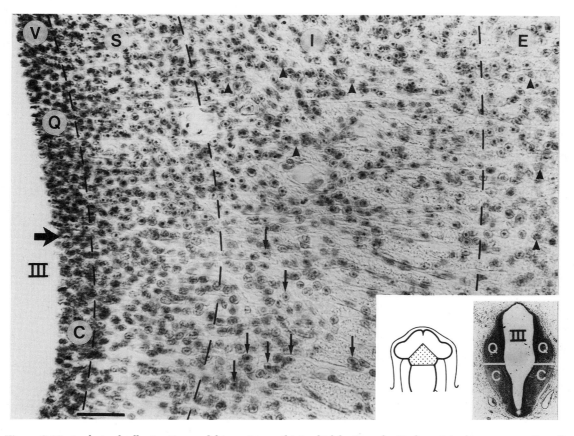

Figure 2.16. Analysis of cell migrations and fates using quail-into-chick brain grafts. Feulgen-stained transverse section of the diencephalon of a quail-into-chick chimera at E6. The transplant of the dorsal part of the diencephalon performed at E2 is shown diagrammatically in the inset (left). Donor and host cells are well separated in the subventricular layer (S). In contrast, the presence of isolated quail cells (small vertical arrows) in predominantly chicken regions and vice versa (arrowheads) in the intermediate zone (I) of the mantle layer indicates tangential movements in both directions. It is not known whether these are neurons or glial cells, probably the latter. In the external zone (E) of the mantle layer the presence of numerous host cells (arrowheads) in predominantly donor areas indicates the existence of large ventrodorsal cell movements at this level. White bars in the inset (right) show the virtual boundaries between host and donor tissues. III = 3rd ventricle; large arrow = ventricular boundary of the graft; bar = 25 μm; V = ventricular epithelium; Q = quail cells; c = chick cells. Modified from E. Balaban, M.-A. Teillet, and N. Le Douarin, *Science* 241:1339-1342 (1988).

Figure 2.15. Clonal analysis of cerebellar Purkinje cells of mosaic mice. (A) Location of Purkinje cells in a sagittal section of cerebellum of a $Gus^b/Gus^b \leftrightarrow Gus^h/Gus^h$ chimeric mouse. Positions of darkly stained Gus^b cells are shown by the dots, positions of unstained Gus^h cells are shown without dots. The distribution of Purkinje cells of the two genotypes is random. The average clone size is 1.7 cells. (B) Histochemical staining to show β-glucuronidase activity in Purkinje cells of a $Gus^b/Gus^b \leftrightarrow Gus^h/Gus^h$ chimera. Dark staining shows that the Purkinje cells are Gus^b/Gus^b (arrows with filled circles). Gus^h/Gus^h cells are unstained (arrows with open circles). (C) Cerebellar cortex of a Gus^h/Gus^h control. None of the Purkinje cells have β-glucuronidase activity. (D) Cerebellar cortex of a Gus^b/Gus^b control. All Purkinje cells have β-glucuronidase activity. Magnification bar = 50 μm. From R. J. Mullen (1977, 1978).

tribution of the X-linked enzyme activities. Their most significant finding is that only 3–10 blastoderm cells give rise to each major ganglion. Because a large population of neurons is derived from each stem cell in the blastoderm, they conclude that gynandromorphs with small clones in the nervous system cannot be obtained.

The method of somatic recombination has also been used to analyze the origins of cells forming an ommatidium in the compound eye of *Drosophila* (Hofbauer and Campos-Ortega, 1976; Ready *et al.*, 1976; Campos-Ortega and Hofbauer, 1977; Campos-Ortega *et al.*, 1978). The results show that the eight photoreceptors in a single ommatidium are not descendants of a single progenitor cell, and that cell commitment in the ommatidium is not determined by lineage. Such experiments offer the possibility of determining whether individual neuronal phenotypes are determined on the basis of lineage or position or both and also provide a possible means of understanding the genetic control of cell differentiation in the nervous system.

The main limitation of mosaics generated very early in development is that they cannot give the fine resolution required for lineage studies of individual neuronal phenotypes. Indeed, a fate map of the *Drosophila* brain has been achieved by direct embryological observation (Poulson, 1950) that equals and exceeds the resolution of fate maps so far derived from studies of genetic mosaics. The direct method of tracing lineages is possible because of the consistency with which neurons with particular functions and connections can be mapped to specific locations in the ganglia of some insects and because of the regular order in which the neurons originate from identifiable individual neuroblasts.

An important advance in understanding the relationship of cell differentiation to cell lineage and to cell position has come from studies by García Bellído *et al.* (1973) of the development of the mesothoracic disc in *Drosophila*. X-ray-induced somatic crossing-over is used to mark cells whose progeny form clones that are found to be confined to wing compartments. Each compartment has precisely defined borders and is made up exclusively of the surviving descendants of a small group of primordial cells; thus it is termed a *polyclone*. Genetic mosaics of homeotic mutants have shown that each compartment is controlled by a few genes called *selector genes*. An entire compartment is altered in

the homeotic mutant, which suggests that the compartment is the unit for genetic control of development of morphological patterns (see Section 1.2). By irradiating embryos at different stages of development, the progeny of marked cells can be followed in relation to compartment boundaries. Such experiments show that different structures, such as bristles and veins, within a compartment are not determined by a lineage mechanism but apparently by their position with respect to the compartment borders (García-Bellído, 1975).

The method for producing genetic mosaics by radiation-induced somatic cell mutations, first used for clonal analysis in *Drosophila*, has been adapted for use in zebrafish (Streisinger *et al.*, 1989). Zebrafish embryos heterozygous for the golden mutation are gamma-irradiated to produce homozygous labeled blastomeres. The progeny of those blastomeres have golden pigment instead of dark brown pigment found in the wild type in the pigmented retinal epithelial cells (Fig. 2.17). The frequency of induction of labeled clones varies with the dose of radiation and the stage of development—smaller clones are produced with lower doses at later stages. A single clone is produced at doses that produce mosaic eyes in less than 10% of embryos.

2.12. Control of Nerve Cell Number and Size

The number of neurons that reach maturity is the result of a balance between cell proliferation and cell death during neurogenesis. The limits to these parameters may be set by the genetic constitution, but the final size of the brain and the number of neurons and glial cells in the nervous system must be affected by many factors. These include genetic controls, hormones, growth factors, and nutrients within the developing system, as well as external factors such as nutrition and other environmental conditions. It is often necessary to make accurate counts of neurons and glial cells in order to determine precisely how and when such conditions may affect development of the nervous system. It is also important to obtain an accurate measure of the constancy and variability of the total number of neurons or the numbers in particular parts of the nervous system.

In mammals, the total number of neurons is

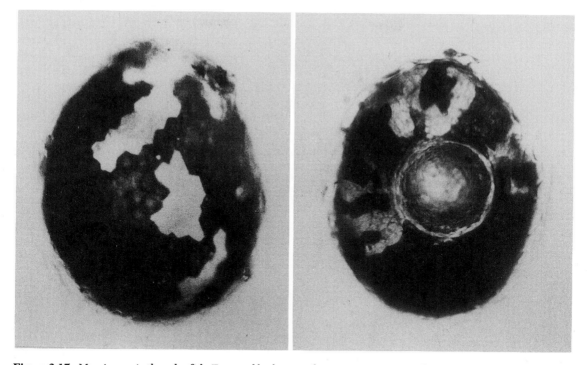

Figure 2.17. Mosaic eyes in the zebrafish. Front and back views of two eyes containing patches of golden (mutant) cells in the pigmented retina of a darkly pigmented (wild type) eye. These eyes are from 76 hours embryos heterozygous for a recessive mutation at the gol-1 locus, irradiated at the two-cell stage. The findings that each blastomere contributes to the pigmented retina, and yet the contribution of each progenitor is highly variable, indicate that extensive mixing occurs of the descendants of different blastomeres before the formation of the pigmented retina. From G. Streisinger, F. Coale, C. Taggart, C. Walker, and D. J. Grunwald, *Dev. Biol.* **131**:60-69 (1989), copyright Academic Press.

attained in the embryo or fetus, and postembryonic or postnatal increase in cells is largely or entirely due to addition of glial cells. Addition of neurons during a short period after birth in mammals is essentially limited to production of granule cells in a few restricted regions of the brain such as the olfactory bulb, hippocampal dentate gyrus, brain stem nuclei, and cerebellar cortex (see Section 2.10). These cases of restricted neurogenesis after birth in mammals are in sharp contrast to the cases of addition of neurons and glial cells to all parts of the nervous system throughout life in submammalian vertebrates and in some invertebrates. The addition of neurons throughout life poses the problem of how the newborn cells are integrated into the preexisting circuitry, and how the increase in neuron population affects behavior and memory. All the species in which continuous addition of cells occurs have complete repertoires of behavior in the young adult, and

any changes that occur as the animal grows must be very subtle. Such growth can occur by addition to the margins of the existing population or by interpolation into the existing population. Marginal histogenesis occurs in the retina and optic tectum of fish and amphibians continuously throughout life (see Sections 11.8 and 11.9). Interpolative histogenesis occurs in the mammalian brain, for example, the cerebellar cortex, where granule cells continue to be added to the existing circuitry for a relatively short period after birth (see Section 10.13).

There is a wealth of data on the constancy of numbers of neurons, but there are no explanations of how such constancy is controlled or achieved, or of why the number of neurons is constant. Apart from the concept that complex functions require a large number of neurons, we have no definite understanding of the relationship between a particular function of the nervous system and the number of neurons required to perform that function. Collecting data to show that a particular animal or part of its nervous system contains a constant number of neurons is far easier than reaching an understanding of the causes or of the functional significance of such constancy of cell content. In many invertebrates, the nervous system contains thousands or, at the most, tens of thousands of neurons. Counting the number of neurons by simple histological methods and mapping their locations and interconnections are within the realm of possibility in these invertebrates. The insect nervous system has a neuron count of about the same order of magnitude as that of the submammalian vertebrates, that is, between 10^6 and 10^7. The number is greater again by one or two orders of magnitude in mammals, and shows a regular phylogenetic increase until it culminates in humans with an estimated 10^{10} neurons.

Ogawa (1939) has counted and measured all the nerve cells and nerve fibers at various stages of development of an annelid worm and has found that the total number of nerve cells in the brain increases from 6000 to 10,000 from hatching to sexual maturity. Wiersma (1957) counted the neurons of the crayfish and found that the brain contains 70,000–80,000 neurons, while the total for the whole nervous system is about 95,000. This does not mean that the nervous system is simple in all invertebrates. The octopus has a brain of exceptional complexity, containing about 10^7 neurons in animals of 600–700 g body weight (J. Z. Young, 1963; Giuditta *et al.*, 1971); this is about the same as the number of neurons in the brains of some fish and amphibians—for example, 1.7×10^7 in the frog *Rana esculenta* (Kemali and Braitenberg, 1969). The numbers of cells in the octopus brain, neurons as well as glia, continue to increase with age allometrically with increase in body weight, reaching a total of 4×10^8 cells in octopus of 4.5 kg body weight (Packard and Albergoni, 1970; Giuditta *et al.*, 1971). The highest nervous centers of the octopus and some insects are more complex than many parts of the vertebrate brain (Ramón y Cajal and Sánchez, 1915; J. Z. Young, 1964). Reference to the work of Ramón y Cajal and Sánchez (1915) on the visual centers of insects is a chastening experience for anyone with a tendency to think of the invertebrate nervous system as simple. Cajal was quite explicit in this regard when he wrote: *"The complexity of the insect retina is something stupendous, discon-*

certing, and without precedent in other animals. . . .Compared with the retina of these apparently humble representatives of life (hymenoptera, lepidoptera, and neuroptera), the retina of the bird or the higher mammal appears as something coarse, rude, and deplorably elementary. The comparison of a rude wall clock with an exquisite and diminutive hunting-case watch fails to give an adequate idea of the contrast, for the hunting-case eye of the higher insect does not merely consist of more delicate wheels, but contains besides various highly complicated organs which are not represented in the vertebrates." A similar thought had been expressed by Robert Boyle (1627–1692) in his *"Disquisition about the Final Causes of Natural Things,"* in which he calls the eye of the fly a greater marvel than the sun.

Nevertheless, the simpler invertebrates have some advantages for studies of the factors that control the number of cells in the nervous system. In the near future the entire genome of the nematode (*Caenorhabditis elegans*) will be sequenced, and that knowledge will be related to the detailed program of development of the organism, including essentially complete knowledge of the genetic control of development of its nervous system (see Section 2.11). Many of those mechanisms are likely to operate in higher organisms. However, there will also be many mechanisms that are important in higher organisms but are not present in nematodes.

The small size of many neurons in insects is an advantage when studying them by electron microscope, but is a disadvantage for electrophysiological investigations. The large size of some neurons in certain invertebrates makes it relatively easy to inject tracers into them and to record their electrical actuality with intercellular microelectrodes. In many invertebrates the total number of neurons is quite constant, their positions are relatively invariant, and there is little variability in their connectivity patterns (Bullock and Horridge, 1965; M. J. Cohen and Jacklet, 1967; J. G. White *et al.*, 1976; Sulston, 1976; Sulston and Horvitz, 1977; Kimble and Hirsch, 1979; Sulston *et al.*, 1983). Even in arthropods, where the number and positions of neurons are remarkably constant, there are individual variations, particularly in the branching patterns of nerves, as Bullock and Horridge (1965) have emphasized. These are of great interest, particularly if the variations are determined genetically rather than as a result of developmental accidents. Variability of the position of the neuron soma not associated with the variability of the synaptic connections of the displaced neurons occurs in a snail (Benjamin, 1976). Such conservation of essentially normal connectivity in spite of gross malposition of nerve cell bodies has also been found in genetically determined developmental derangements of the mammalian nervous system (see Section 10.15).

The nervous system of insects consists of the brain located dorsally in the head connected to two bilaterally symmetrical, segmentally arranged chains of ventral ganglia, usually fused to form a single ventral chain of ganglia connected together by longitudinal nerves. During embryonic development each ganglion originates from a pair of neuromeres in each segment. After fertilization of the insect egg the zygotic nucleus undergoes many divisions without cell division to give rise to a syncytium containing thousands of nuclei. These migrate to the periphery, where each nucleus becomes enclosed in extensions of the egg cell membrane to give rise to the cellular blastoderm. In *Drosophila* the blastoderm-stage embryo is composed of about 6000 cells in a surface monolayer enclosing the yolk. Localized expression of segmentation and homeotic genes (see Section 1.2) results in development of segment primordia each of which forms a band around the embryo three to four cells wide at the anterior–posterior axis. The CNS is formed after gastrulation from a single layer of ventral ectoderm called the neurogenic region (Hartenstein and Campos-Ortega, 1988).

The ectodermal cells that give rise to the nervous system in insects are called the *neuroblast mother cells*, which undergo equal division to give rise to two neuroblasts, first so named by Wheeler (1891, 1893). The neuroblasts of insects are aptly named because they are true "blast" cells (Greek *blastos*, a germ or a bud) that divide to give rise to cells named *ganglion mother cells* by Bauer (1904), but which may be called second- or third-generation neuroblasts. The ganglion mother cells divide to form the *ganglion cells*, which are the postmitotic nerve cells (Fig. 2.18). In *Drosophila* as well as the grasshopper, each neuroblast generates an invariant lineage resulting in a stereotyped pattern of terminally differentiated neurons (Bate, 1976; Goodman, 1982; Doe and Goodman, 1985).

The first division of the neuroblasts tends to be unequal so that the ganglion mother cells are smaller than the neuroblasts, but later divisions become progressively more equal until, finally, an equal division gives rise to two ganglion mother cells. There are exceptions to this sequence; for example, in the optic lobes of the cockroach and stick insect, the divisions of neuroblasts are equal from the beginning (Malzacher, 1968). Moreover, there is evidence that in some insects the neuroblasts degenerate at the end of the larval stages (Wheeler, 1891; Bauer, 1904; Panov, 1960; Couin, 1965; Nordlander and Edwards, 1969; Starre-van der Molen, 1974; Bate, 1976). Neurogenesis proceeds in a rostral-to-caudal sequence, and the onset of degeneration of neuroblasts occurs in the same sequence in the locust (Bate, 1976). The same number of neuroblasts gives rise to the large and complex thoracic ganglia as to the small and relatively simple abdominal ganglia of the locust, and the number of neurons in a particular ganglion is controlled by selective cell death (Bate, 1976, 1982; Bate *et al.*, 1981).

As each ganglion mother cell is generated by division of the neuroblast, it displaces those generated earlier, so that a column of cells is formed, with the oldest cells at the head of the column farthest from the neuroblast. Experiments in which insect larvae and pupae have been fixed at progressive intervals after an injection of tritiated thymidine have shown that the age of any neuron can be determined by its distance from the proliferating center, since older cells are displaced by cells that are generated at later stages (Nordlander and Edwards, 1968a, 1969), as is shown in Fig. 2.18. The ganglion mother cells then divide once, with the spindle axis at right angles to the column of cells, each giving rise to two neurons (Bauer, 1904; Baden, 1936; Panov, 1960; Malzacher, 1968; Nordlander and Edwards, 1968b; Bate, 1976).

The maximum number of neuroblasts is rather small, about 110 in the stick insect and 140 in the cockroach (Malzacher, 1968; Bate, 1976; Bate and Grunewald, 1981). The number of neuroblasts diminishes during the late larval and pupal stages until they finally disappear in the pupa, either by degeneration or by final division into two mother cells.

The final number of neurons in insects is reached in the pupal stage, and no further production of neurons occurs later in development. During postembryonic nervous development in insects, only

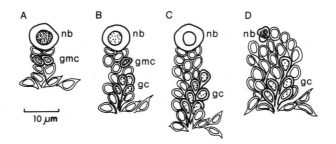

Figure 2.18. Neurogenesis in an insect. Position of labeled cells in a group of cells descended from one neuroblast (nb) in the brain of the monarch butterfly, fixed at successive intervals after an injection of tritiated thymidine at the beginning of the fourth instar. (A) The neuroblast and two ganglion mother cells (gmc) are labeled 2 hours after the injection. (B) At the beginning of the fifth instar, the neuroblast is less heavily labeled, another ganglion mother cell is labeled, and the original ganglion cells (gc) are lightly labeled. (C) Late in the fifth instar, label is not detectable in the neuroblast, indicating that it has been diluted by cell division. (D) Two days after pupation, the neuroblast is degenerating. Note that the density of labeling of ganglion cells does not diminish, indicating that the ganglion cells have not divided. From R. H. Nordlander and J. S. Edwards, *Arch. Entwicklungsmech. Organ.* **162**:197–217 (1969).

glial cells increase in number, although neurons as well as glial cells increase in size (Power, 1952; Panov, 1962; Gymer and Edwards, 1967; H. Korr, 1968; Malzacher, 1968). Neurons present in the larva may not be functionally connected, or the activity of neuronal circuits present in the larva or in the early instars may be suppressed by descending inhibition from the brain (Bentley and Hoy, 1970; Truman and Schwartz, 1982).

An alternative to histological methods of determining the total number of neurons plus glial cells is to measure the amount of DNA in the whole nervous system or parts of it (Santen and Agranoff, 1963; Winick and Noble, 1965; Oja, 1966; E. Howard, 1968; Nováková *et al.*, 1968; Stasny *et al.*, 1968; Margolis, 1969). The number of cells is obtained by dividing the total quantity of DNA in the nervous system by the quantity of DNA in a single euploid cell. The latter is a constant quantity for each species. For example, the DNA content of a single euploid brain cell is 6.4×10^{-12} g in the rat, 7.1×10^{-12} g in the cat, 6.5×10^{-12} g in the dog, and 7.1×10^{-12} g in humans (Heller and Elliott, 1954; Santen and Agranoff, 1963). The DNA content of a euploid cell of the chicken is 25×10^{-13} g, and from the total DNA content of the brain Margolis (1969) has calculated that the total number of cells in the chick brain at hatching is about 5×10^8. In the chick at hatching, the cerebellum, cerebrum, and optic lobes each contain about 16×10^7 cells, and the number of cells in these parts of the brain

changes in a systematic way during the postnatal period (Fig. 2.19).

The mean cell weight can be computed from the brain weight divided by the total brain DNA, with a correction for the weight of the extracellular fluid. The ratio of brain weight to DNA gives a rough-and-ready estimate of mean cell weight, but a measure of the variability of neuronal size and territory can be obtained only by much more tedious histological methods (Haddara, 1956; Sholl, 1956a, Mannen, 1966; Ware and Lopresti, 1975). The mean weight of the brain and the number of neurons are greater in male than in female mammals (Pearl, 1905; Blinkov and Glezer, 1968; Jerison, 1963; Calaresu and Henry, 1971; Ho *et al.*, 1980a,b). There are numerous anatomical differences between the brains of males and females (Arnold and Gorski, 1984; Toran-Allerand, 1984; Swaab and Hofman, 1984; see Section 7.9).

The size and complexity of the vertebrate brain make it very difficult to count the total number of neurons directly in histological sections, although direct counts have been made of neurons in small parts of the brain. For example, the total number of neurons in the ventral cochlear nucleus of humans is 48,010 (S.D. 4550), corrected for counting errors (Konigsmark and Murphy, 1970). The variability of cell size and number in the nervous system of vertebrates is not known because of serious limitations in the accuracy of methods of counting and measuring neurons and glial cells (Shariff, 1953; Nurnberger

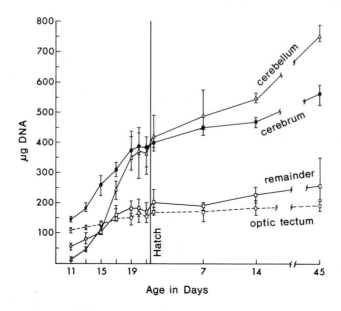

Figure 2.19. DNA content of parts of the brain of the chick at different ages before and after hatching. Each value, reported as micrograms of DNA per brain region (optic tectum, cerebrum, cerebellum, and remainder of the brain), is the average of at least six determinations. The vertical bars show the range of values obtained. From F. L. Margolis, *J. Neurochem.* 16:447–456 (1969), copyright Pergamon Press.

and Gordon, 1957; Haug, 1960, 1967b; Brizzee *et al.*, 1964). For example, the ratio of glial cells to neurons has to be determined by direct counts of cells in histological sections. Different glia-to-neuron ratios ranging from 10:1 to 1:1 have been obtained by different investigators using different counting methods and different methods of correcting for counting errors (Brizzee *et al.*, 1964). Counts of the total number of neurons in the cerebral cortex of humans vary widely and give an indication of the limitations of the methods that have been employed: The results have varied from 2.6×10^9 (Pakkenberg, 1967), to 5.5×10^9 (Burger, 1921), to 6.9×10^9 (Shariff, 1953), to 9.3×10^9 (Thompson, 1899), to 14×10^9 (von Economo and Koskinas, 1925). It is clear that more reliable cell counts, particularly in the mammalian brain, will have to be made before the real variability in the number of neurons and glial cells can be determined. Better stereological methods of counting neurons have been developed recently (Braendgaard and Gundersen, 1986; T. G. Beach and McGeer, 1987; Pakkenberg and Gundersen, 1988; Williams and Rakic, 1988, 1989; Nairn *et al.*, 1989; West and Gundersen, 1990). Such methods are essential for determining the individual

and intraspecies variations in the number of brain cells.

Variations between individuals at the same age of the same species may result from genetic, nutritional, hormonal, or other functional differences (Zamenhof, 1941, 1942, 1976; Kuhlenkampf, 1952; Altman and Das, 1964; Zamenhof *et al.*, 1964, 1966, 1968; E. Howard, 1965, 1968; E. Howard and Granoff, 1968; M. C. Diamond *et al.*, 1966). A large genetic variability in the number of neurons in the hippocampal formation of different strains of mice has been demonstrated by R. E. Wimer *et al.* (1976, 1978, 1980). The significance of such variability is discussed in Section 2.13.

Even the body temperature of the pregnant female has a marked influence on the number of cells that survive to birth in the fetus (M. J. Edwards, 1981, review). Increasing the body temperature of the pregnant female guinea pig by 3–4°C on the 18–25th days of gestation, for 1 hour, results in a 10 percent reduction in fetal brain weight (average gestation in the guinea pig is 68 days). Two heat stresses, each of 1 hour, produce a 13 percent decrease in brain weight, and a deficit of 26 percent in fetal brain weight follows eight periods of maternal heat stress, each lasting an hour (M. J. Edwards, 1969, 1971). The deficit in brain weight is due in large part to an irreversible reduction in the number of neurons and glial cells. The result is a brain with what appear to be normal proportions of neurons and glial cells but with fewer cells. Myelination is not affected. The effect of hyperthermia is to damage and destroy ventricular germinal cells of the telencephalon, and probably elsewhere in the brain, with resulting decrease in mitotic activity (M. J. Edwards et al., 1974, 1976, 1984; Wanner et al., 1976). The possible effects of hyperthermia on the human fetus should be kept in mind in cases of fever during early pregnancy. A connection between pyrexia during the first trimester of pregnancy and fetal brain damage or mental retardation in humans has been established (D. W. Smith et al., 1978; Pleet et al., 1981; Shiota, 1982; Spraggett and Fraser, 1982). An increase in number of neurons has been reported following hyperthermia and a decrease following hypothermia for a short period during incubation of the chick embryo (Zamenhof, 1976). In the chick, too, the period of neuron proliferation is especially sensitive to changes in temperature. Thus, raising the temperature from 37.5°C to 40.5°C on days 5–7 of incubation results in a 22 percent increase of the cerebellar cells that originate during those days (Purkinje cells, Golgi II cells, and neurons of the cerebellar roof nuclei). Embryos incubated at 35.3°C on E5-E7 have a 14.6 percent reduction in those neurons at hatching when compared with controls incubated at 37.5°C (Zamenhof, 1976).

The factors that control the number of glial cells are discussed in Sections 3.4 and 3.5. The concept that more highly evolved brains have a higher ratio of glial cells to neurons goes back to the nineteenth century and found its principal modern exponent in von Economo (1926). Friede (1954) reports that the mean number of glial cells per neuron (glia-to-neuron ratio) in all cellular layers of the mammalian cerebral cortex is 1.7 in humans, 1.2 in the horse, and 0.4 in the rabbit and mouse. These findings apparently support the concept of a phylogenetic increase in the glia-to-neuron ratio. However, in contradiction to this view, Hawkins and Olszewski (1957) show that the mean glia-to-neuron ratio is 4.5 in the whale, and they conclude that the increase in the number of glial cells per nerve cell is not correlated with phylogenetic status but with the size of the brain. The increase in glia-to-neuron ratio in

larger animals appears to be due to the fact that the size of the neurons is correlated with the size of the animal, so that large neurons may require more glial cells to support them, nourish them, or interact with them in ways that are not yet understood (Hawkins and Olszewski, 1957; Friede and van Houten, 1962; Friede, 1963). Methods of mechanically disaggregating the brain and separating neurons and glial cells have been devised (Raine et al., 1971; Sinha and Rose, 1971; Capps-Covey and McIlwain, 1975; K. D. McCarthy and Partlow, 1976a). These promise to clarify the factors that affect the number of cells in the brain and that alter the glia-to-neuron ratio.

The size and number of neurons are partly determined by the size of the animal. In the invertebrates as well as the vertebrates the size of the neurons is generally greater in larger species (Hanström, 1926; Goosen, 1949; Möller, 1950; Schulz, 1951; Nolte, 1953; Neder, 1959; Purves and Lichtman, 1985). The large neurons, such as the cerebral cortical pyramidal cells, have longer dendrites with more branches in large mammals than in small mammals (Shariff, 1953; Bok, 1959). However, among mammals, the body weight is more significantly related to the number of neurons than to neuron size; a 4-ton elephant is a million times larger than a 4-g shrew and the brain of the elephant (mean volume 4000 cm³) is more than 16,000 times larger than that of the shrew (Sorex, mean volume 0.24 cm³), yet the differences in the sizes of their neurons are only slight.

There is a good linear relation between the gestation time and the cube root of the brain weight at birth in all the mammalian orders: over a range of 16-655 days, the gestation time varies as the 0.334 power of the neonatal brain weight (Sacher and Staffeldt, 1974). In general, the rate of growth of the fetal brain varies little between mammalian species. The brain is the slowest-growing organ in the mammalian fetus, and it therefore sets important limits on the duration of gestation. To compensate for the longer gestation time, the smaller litter size, and hence the slower reproductive rate in large-brained species, the life span is directly proportional to the brain weight (Sacher, 1959).

The brain-to-body weight ratio decreases progressively during postnatal development in mammals (Pearl, 1905; Dubois, 1923; Donaldson, 1925; von Bonin, 1937; Brummelkamp, 1939; Hersh, 1941; Count, 1947; Sacher and Staffeldt, 1974; De-

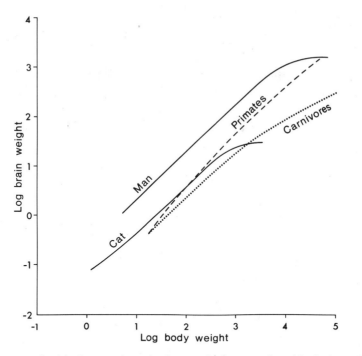

Figure 2.20. Allometric growth of the brain. Relationship between log brain weight and log body wieght during ontogeny in humans and the domestic cat (solid lines) and in a phylogenetic series of primates and carnivores (broken line). From E. W. Count, *Ann. N.Y. Acad. Sci.* 46:993–1122 (1947), copyright The New York Academy of Sciences, reprinted by permission.

kaban and Sadowsky, 1978; Ho *et al.*, 1980b). In humans the brain is about 18 percent of the body weight at 3 months gestation, 16 percent at 4 months, 14 percent at 5 months, and about 12 percent at birth. Thereafter, the brain weight diminishes to 10 percent of the body weight at 1 year of age and to about 2.5 percent at age 20. In the adult human, the brain consumes about 20 percent of the total oxygen consumption of the entire body (McIlwain, 1959). Epstein (1973) has suggested that the main limitation to the size of the human brain at birth is not the size of the maternal birth canal but the inability of the newborn to provide oxygen and glucose for a brain larger than 12 percent of the body weight. This problem does not arise in other mammals because their brain-to-body weight ratio is always less than that in humans. For example, at birth the brain-to-body weight ratio is 12 percent in humans, 8 percent in the chimpanzee, and only 5 percent in the cat. This difference between humans and other mammals persists throughout development (Fig. 2.20). According to Count (1947), *"a fetus of given body size always has a heavier brain than*

some extant relative of equal body size who is presumably less highly evolved." Statements such as this oversimplify the problem of the evolutionary tendency to increase brain-to-body weight ratio.

There are at least four factors that have to be taken into account when considering the significance of brain-to-body weight ratio differences: myelination, brain metabolism, differences of innervation of bone and soft tissues, and different ratios of principal neurons to local circuit neurons. The first is the fact that increase in brain weight after birth is largely due to myelin (see Section 3.11). The second is the limitation of size of the mammalian brain by the capacity of the body to supply it with energy. In poikilothermic animals, the limit may be set by the oxygen supply available to the embryo in the egg. In mammals, the placenta also sets a limit to brain size. Exchange between mother and fetus across the placenta is roughly proportional to the area of the placenta, and increases during gestation as the square of the placental diameter, but the nutritional requirements of the fetus increase as the cube of its linear dimensions. This sets a limit to the number of fetuses in large animals and limits the growth of the brain in multiple pregnancies. We can say that the Lilliputians in *Gulliver's Travels* could not have had the intellectual abilities they display in Swift's story; they are described as being scaled down to one-twelfth the size of a normal human, but with otherwise normal proportions. In fact, their body size could not have supported a brain larger than that of a dog, and their intellects would have had to be reduced accordingly. Similar misconceptions abound in the literature concerning giants and dwarfs. It occurs, more subtly, in the following proposition by Hans Reichenbach (1951, p. 132): *"Suppose that during the night all physical objects, including our bodies became ten times as large. On awakening this morning we should be in no condition to test this assumption, since our measuring rods and other instruments would have undergone congruent changes."* This statement ignores the fact that unless the fundamental laws of physics were also changed, a 10-fold increase in linear dimensions of the body would have to be attended by such great changes in *relative sizes* of the parts that the change in form would be noticed immediately. This is because increase in linear dimensions of the body results in increase of the body mass by the cube, but the cross-sectional area of the weight-bearing bones increases only as the square of the linear dimensions. In order to bear the additional weight of the soft tissues, the weight of the skeleton has to increase proportionately more than the increase in body weight. As a result, there is a smaller ratio of brain weight to body weight in large than in small animals (Goosen, 1949; Rensch, 1958).

This brings us to the third factor that is often not taken into account in considering the significance of brain-to-body weight ratio, namely, the fact that soft tissues have a much greater innervation than bone. Brain-to-body weight ratios should be calculated on the basis of soft tissue weight (preferably muscle mass, and making appropriate adjustments for the mass of viscera and blood) when comparing animals with very different skeletal mass (see, for example, Fig. 1 in Jerison, 1970, which does not take those factors into account in showing the relation of brain to body size in living and extinct animals). The allometric relationship between absolute brain size and body size is a crude one which fails to take functional differences into account. The problem of changes in physiological functions that are correlated with changes in body size has been well discussed by D'Arcy Thompson (1942), Adolph (1949), S. J. Gould (1966), Stahl (1970), Schmidt-Nielsen (1970, 1984), Pilbeam and Gould (1974), and Calder (1984). That brain size and the ratio of brain to body weight are not always reliable indices of "encephalization" is shown by the dolphins and whales, in which the brain is relatively large and the area of cerebral cortex is also relatively large, but the cortex is relatively thin (less than 2 mm) and relatively poor in local-circuit neurons in comparison with primates.

The fourth factor to take into account in considering the significance of brain size in relation to body size and to the evolution of the brain is the relative number of principal neurons and local-circuit neurons (see near the end of Section 1.6). Principal neurons form the main efferent and afferent pathways, and their axons form the peripheral nerves, whereas local-circuit neurons form the central integrating circuits. I have suggested that the number of principal neurons is correlated with the total body mass, whereas the number of local-circuit neurons can be more closely correlated with behavioral complexity than with the size of the animal (M. Jacobson, 1975a). Evidence that the numbers of principal neurons are matched with the sizes of the peripheral tissues they innervate is given in Chapter 8. From that evidence we can predict that there would be a better correlation between body size and size of brainstem and spinal cord than between body size and cerebral size. This has been confirmed by Hofman (1982). The body size might be expected to be closely correlated with the number of nerve fibers passing through the foramen magnum, and, in fact, Radinsky (1967) has shown that there is a coefficient of correlation of 0.976 between body weight and foramen magnum area in representatives of five orders of extant mammals. The increased number of principal neurons, such as spinal motoneurons and spinal sensory ganglion cells, in large animals is reflected in a linear relationship between the number of axons in peripheral nerves and the body weight (Schnepp and Schnepp, 1971; Schnepp *et al.*, 1971). This is the result of the afferent control of the number of principal neurons during ontogeny.

It is reasonable to expect the number of principal neurons to be closely related to body weight regardless of phylogenetic position, but the increase in the ratio of brain to body weight that occurs during phylogeny is probably due to an increase in local-circuit neurons. As an example, the ratio of granule cells to Purkinje cells in the cerebellar cortex is 1500:1 in humans, 950:1 in the rhesus monkey, 600:1 in the cat, 140:1 in the mouse, and 100:1 in the frog (Blinkov and Glezer, 1968). The stellate cells of the mammalian cerebral cortex increase from 31 percent of the total number of cortical neurons in the rabbit, to 35 percent in the cat, to 45 percent in the monkey (Mitra, 1955). These figures indicate a progressive evolutionary increase in the ratio of principal to local-circuit neurons. For several additional reasons dealt with elsewhere (M. Jacobson, 1974b; 1975a), the distinction between principal neurons and local circuit neurons will have to be made in the future when considering evolution of the brain and in making comparisons between brains of different species. This distinction is now beginning to be taken into consideration (e.g., Haug, 1981, 1987).

It has become conventional to recognize that the size of the cerebral hemispheres and of the cerebral cortex has increased disproportionately during mammalian evolution (Elias and Schwartz, 1971; Bauchot, 1978; Jerison, 1973, 1979; Hofman, 1982, 1985 a,b, 1988, 1989; Fox and Wilczynski, 1986; Haug, 1987). However, the various indices of encephalization do not take the complexity of cortical organization into account. Attempts to consider encephalization in ecological context (R. D. Martin, 1983) and in relation to evolution of intelligence (Passingham, 1975, 1981) are limited by lack of understanding of the principles of cerebral cortical organization and cortical mechanisms subserving behavior and intelligence.

Heterochrony is another important factor to be taken into consideration in the mechanisms that have led to evolution of greater brain complexity. Heterochrony is an evolutionary change in timing of developmental processes, and it can result in major changes in morphology (De Beer, 1951; Gould, 1977; Alberch et al., 1979; Alberch and Alberch, 1981). A small increase in the duration of cell proliferation can result in a disproportionately large increase in the number of nerve cells, and as local-circuit neurons are generally the last to be formed, they would be increased relative to the number of principal neurons.

The size of neurons may also be related to the lifespan and phylogenetic status of the animal. D'Arcy Thompson (1942) points out that *"such cells as continue to divide through life tend to uniformity of size in all mammals; those which do not do so, and in particular the ganglion cells, continue to grow, and their size becomes, therefore, a function of the duration of life."* However, it should be pointed out that the largest neurons are to be found in some invertebrates and that the largest neurons in the vertebrate nervous system are the first to be formed during development. Giant neurons are found only in the lower vertebrate orders—for example, Muller cells and other giant neurons in lampreys (H. P. Whiting, 1957; Rovainen, 1967a,b) and Rohon–Beard cells and Mauthner cells in fish and amphibians (Stefanelli, 1951; A. F. Hughes, 1957; Otsuka, 1962, 1964; Moulton et al., 1968; Kimmel and Eaton, 1976).

The size of the brain increases during postnatal life, owing primarily to an increase in cell size and myelination and only slightly to an increase in the number of cells. It has yet to be established that there is an increase in neuronal size as a result of learning and experience in mammals, although it is clear that neurons increase in size during normal maturation (Donaldson and Nagasaka, 1918; Kuhlenbeck, 1954; Brizzee and Jacobs, 1959; Schadé, 1959; Schadé and Groeningen, 1961; M. W. Fox et al., 1966; Ford and Cohan, 1968; Blinkov and Glezer, 1968).

The problem of neuron loss with aging is highly controversial—reports of stability of cell number are balanced by other reports of decline of the number of neurons. There is no doubt that in relatively healthy humans the weight of the brain declines gradually after age 30 and then diminishes rapidly after 80 years of age, but individual variability is very great (Ho et al., 1980a,b; Mani et al., 1986; Coleman and Flood, 1987; K. R. Brizzee, 1987; Scheff, 1987; Flood and Coleman, 1988). The question then is whether there is an inevitable physiological loss of neurons or glial cells or both, and whether the loss is due to a reduction in cell size or cell number or both. Pathological states—trauma, vascular insufficiency, nutritional deficiencies, toxins, and infective agents—must be taken into account. In the latter cases, the loss of neurons varies in different parts of the nervous system, so that counts made in one region may not correlate with counts made in another region. Even in one region, the different types of neurons may behave differently during aging or in response to infections, poisons, or insufficiency of oxygen or nutrients.

Until fairly recently, it was believed that the number of neurons inevitably declines with age and that brain weight declines linearly after middle age in humans (reviewed by Wright and Spink, 1959). That view has been challenged in more recent studies (Konigsmark and Murphy, 1970, 1972; E. Howard, 1973), and even in the earlier literature there are reports of failure to find neuron loss. Those reports deal mainly with the number of large, Type I neurons. For example, no change in the number of axons in the sciatic nerve is found in rats up to 850 days of age (Birren and Wall, 1956), nor is there a reduction in number of fibers in the ventral spinal roots of cats up to 50 weeks of age (Moyer and Kaliszewski, 1958). Large neurons, too, of the cat's spinal cord are undiminished until 50 weeks of age and are reduced in number only by 15 percent at 110 weeks (Wright and Spink, 1959). These reports of neuronal stability are supported by the observations that no reduction is found in the total number of neurons in the ventral cochlear nucleus counted in 23 human brains from birth to 90 years of age (Konigsmark and Murphy, 1972). Other brain stem nuclei have also been found to have a cell population that is not diminished in old age: the motor nucleus of the facial nerve (Van Buskirk, 1945), the dentate nucleus (Höpker, 1951), and the main nucleus of the inferior olive (Monagle and Brody, 1974).

By contrast, the cerebral cortex and cerebellar cortex seem to be more susceptible to loss of cells as a result of aging. Loss of neurons in the human cerebral cortex was reported by Brody (1955), and in the rat by Brizzee *et al.* (1968). Early reports of a gradual reduction in the number of cells in the rat cerebellum (Inukai, 1928) and the human cerebellum (Ellis, 1920; Harms, 1927) from birth to old age have not been confirmed by modern morphometric analysis, which shows that age is not correlated with the number of neurons in the human cerebral cortex (Haug, 1987). Accurate methods of assaying for the total number of cells by measuring the DNA content of the brain have shown that the DNA content of the cerebellum of the mouse remains constant from 60 to 470 days of age (Howard, 1973). As there is no cell production in the

cerebellum at that age, the results show that there is also negligible cell death. However, death of up to 3 percent of postmitotic cells occurs in the external granular layer of normal rats up to 21 days after birth (P. D. Lewis, 1975). In support of the concept of stability of the cerebellar cortical cells in the adult is the failure to find any electron microscopic evidence of degenerating cells in the cerebellar cortex of the adult rat, whereas in the same study, degenerating neurons were found in the lateral cerebellar nucleus (Chan-Palay, 1973).

The problems of individual variations and counting errors as well as the state of health have to be taken into consideration in assessing the meanings of these findings. In healthy laboratory animals there does not appear to be a decline in brain weight or brain DNA content with advanced age (E. Howard, 1973). The constancy of brain DNA content from maturity to very old age in the rat does not support the view that brain cell loss is inevitable. However, loss of neurons in restricted regions or replacement of neurons by glial cells cannot be detected by measuring total brain DNA content.

Increase in functional activity of the nervous system has been shown to produce an increased proliferation of glial cells which have the capacity to divide, even in adult mammals (see Section 3.5), but the evidence of increased neuronal proliferation due to functional activity is not compelling (see Section 6.12).

The size of the neurons is also related to their ploidy. However, reports that many large neurons, such as cerebellar Purkinje cells and hippocampal pyramidal neurons, continue DNA synthesis without cell division and attain a tetraploid quantity of DNA are now thought to be false (Mann and Yates, 1973a,b). The large neurons are capable of maintaining themselves with a diploid DNA content. In experimentally produced polyploid salamanders, newts, and frog, all the cells (including neurons and glia) are greatly enlarged, but the organs (including the brain) are normal in size and shape. Although the cells are increased in volume, there is a compensatory decrease in their numbers, as shown in Fig. 2.21 (Fankhauser, 1941, 1945a,b; Gurdon, 1959; Bradom, 1960; Pollack and Koves, 1977; Tompkins, 1978; M. Jacobson, 1978; M. Jacobson and Hirose, 1979; D. G. Sperry, 1988a,b). Brandon (1962) has shown that haploid salamanders also have brains of normal dimensions, since the cells, although small,

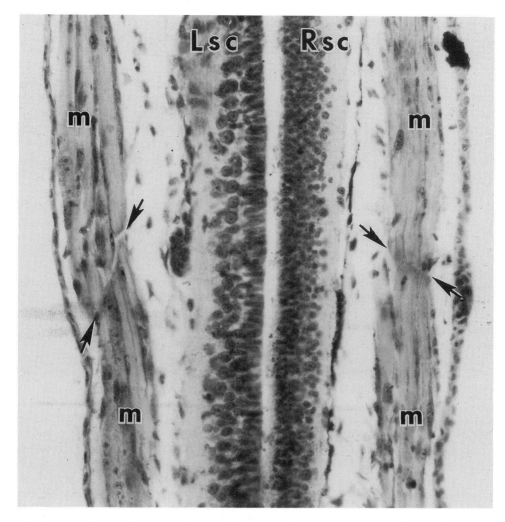

Figure 2.21. Size regulation in a *Xenopus* ploidy mosaic *Xenopus* embryos treated with a short heat shock just before the first cleavage of the zygote sometimes develop mosaicism as a result of one blastomere becoming polyploid (M. Jacobson and G. Hirose, *Science* 202:637–639, 1978). In this horizontal section through the spinal cord at a thoracic level, the left side is composed of polyploid cells, the cells are larger, and there are about half as many cells on the left side. However, bilateral symmetry and metamerism are essentially normal. For example, the positions of the spinal roots and the intermyotomal septa (arrows) are bilaterally symmetrical. Lsc = left side of spinal cord; Rsc = right side of spinal cord; m = somitic muscle. M. Jacobson, unpublished.

are increased in number (Fig. 2.22). Tetraploid mice at E14.5 and E16.5 days gestation are found to have about one-quarter as many cells as diploids of the same gestational age, but in the polyploids the nervous system contains many abnormalities (Snow, 1975). The total size of an animal may be set by the limits to protein synthesis, which in turn may be limited by the amount of ribosomal RNA. In fact, the number of ribosomal RNA cistrons per cell has

been shown to be twice as great in tetraploid as in diploid fish (Schmidtke *et al.*, 1975).

It is of considerable interest that the maze-learning ability of polyploid salamanders with a reduced number of very large brain cells is considerably worse than the learning ability of diploid salamanders (Fankhauser *et al.*, 1955). In this connection, Vernon and Butsch (1957) concluded that *"polyploidy, whether triploid or tetraploid,*

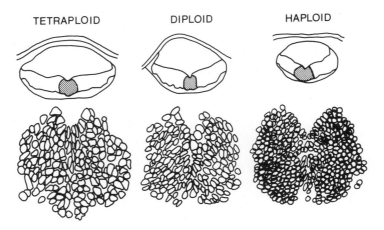

Figure 2.22. Size regulation of the brain in heteroploidy. Transverse sections through the medulla of tetraploid, diploid, and haploid newts. The nuclei in the shaded areas of the medulla are shown below in tetraploid, diploid, and haploid newts, to indicate the differences in size and number of the cells. From W. F. Bradom, *J. Exp. Zool.* 143:323:345 (1960) and *Biol. Bull.* 123:253-263 (1962).

brings about a decrease in maze-learning ability. It is not possible, however, to state whether such an effect is the result of the increase in cell size, the reduction in the number of cells, or the reduction in the number of neuronal connections that probably results from the reduced number of cells." Unfortunately, the learning ability of haploid salamanders, which have an increased number of neurons, has not been investigated. The relationship between brain size, number of neurons, and learning ability could also be studied very profitably in ants, in which the highest nervous centers, the corpora pedunculata, are very small in the males, larger in the females, and largest in the workers (Pandazis, 1930; Goll, 1967). "*The behavior of the three groups corresponds to their brain structure: the males may truly be called stupid, the females are far superior, and the highest faculties are those of the workers*" (Goetsch, 1957).

Growth of the nervous system, measured by changes in weight and size, has been found to correlate with the size of the species and with its ontogenetic stage and phylogenetic status. The difference in dimensions of the nervous system during development may be termed *ontogenetic relative growth*, whereas the difference in adult dimensions between related species may be termed *phylogenetic differential growth*. The same power function, y = bx^k, the allometric or relative growth function (Snell, 1892; J. S. Huxley, 1932), describes the rela-

tionships between homologous parts of a series of adult animals belonging to different species as well as the increase in size of any part of the brain during development of an individual (Hersh, 1941; Grenell and Scammon, 1943; Noback and Moss, 1956).

Written in straight-line logarithmic form, the allometric equation becomes $\log y = \log b + k \log x$, where b and k are constants and x and y represent variable parameters such as body weight, brain weight, the weight or the dimensions of different parts of the nervous system, or of the same part at different times during ontogeny, or in different animals that are closely related phylogenetically. If x and y conform to the relative growth equation and the constants do not change during ontogeny, a straight line with slope k is obtained on a double logarithmic plot, and $\log b$ is the y intercept (Fig. 2.20).

Depending on the values of b and k, the ontogenetic and phylogenetic relationship may be parallel, divergent, or convergent, or a combination of these three. An example of parallel allometry is given by Brummelkamp (1939), who showed that the brain weight to body weight relation in various groups of vertebrates (including fish, amphibians, and mammals) conforms to the allometric equation for each group, with $k = \frac{5}{9}$ for all groups; however, the value of b differs for each group. Jerison (1969) has plotted the brain and body weights for 198 vertebrate species (data from Crile and Quiring, 1940) showing that the data conform to the allometric equation with an exponent of $2/3$, close to the value obtained by Brummelkamp. Extending Brummelkamp's findings, Jerison (1969, 1974) shows that the value of the constant b is 10 times greater in the higher vertebrates (birds, mammals) than in the lower (fish, reptiles; see references in Platel and Delfini, 1986) and is clearly related to phylogenetic status of the group. The brain-to-body weight ratio is about twice as large in monkeys as in any other mammals, twice as large in the great apes as in monkeys, and twice as large in humans as in the great apes.

Unfortunately, the brain body weight ratio and relative growth curve do not differentiate between brain growth due to increase in cell size and growth due to increase in cell number and give no hint of the ratios of neurons to glial cells or of local-circuit neurons to principal neurons nor does it take differences in myelination into account. The allometric equation does not tell us anything about the mechanisms that control the growth of the nervous system and that determine its final size and shape and, most important, the mode of its organization. These limitations are generally acknowledged by morphologists. For example, E. S. Russell (1916, p. 312) states: *"Pure morphology is essentially a science of comparison which seeks to disentangle the unity hidden beneath the diversity of organic form. It is not immediately concerned with the cause of organic diversity."* There may be advantages, for purposes of comparative morphology, in the use of dimensionless numbers (see Stahl, 1962, 1970) and of nonmetric topological analysis (Kuhlenbeck, 1967; Thom, 1974). However, the most important advances in the past have come not from the application of this kind of "pure" morphology, but rather from the morphologists who make strong inductions regarding the functional significance of their morphological data.

2.13. Variations, Anomalies, and Errors of Neuronal Ontogeny and Their Significance

Variations are inherited differences between strains of the same species. Errors are unpredictable deviations from normal structure that are not determined genetically, except in the sense that everything in the organism is under some degree of genetic control. Distinction between true errors and variations is easily made in theory but is more difficult to make in practice. In practice, the distinction between variations and errors may be possible to make by showing that the former are inherited while the latter are not. The amount of variability has often been underestimated in what are generally considered to be extremely invariant neuronal structures.

Invariance of the structure of the nervous system is one of the primary phenomena that demand explanation. Another is the variation of brain structure between individuals or between different strains within a species. Variations are essential prerequisites for evolution by natural selection, but they have an evolutionary effect only when they result in selective advantages or disadvantages. As I have pointed out (M. Jacobson, 1970a,b, 1974b, 1975a), variability is largely but not exclusively found in the structures that develop last: in the local-circuit neurons and in the dendrites of principal neurons. These structures may be affected by mutations which may have no selective advantage and disadvantage, that is, they may be neutral. It is conjectured that such neutral mutations will accumulate because they are not eliminated by natural selection, and in time this accumulation will result in an increase in the polymorphism of the nervous system. As the polymorphism increases, certain structures may become advantageous or disadvantageous. The repository of neutral or nearly neutral mutations, which may provide the individual with negligible functional advantages under one set of environmental conditions, may become of significant advantage under different conditions. One may think of a pool of neurons waiting for opportunities to express latent functions. I call these *"opportunistic neurons."*

This theory of a mechanism of neural evolution is supported by several converging lines of evidence. First, it depends on the evidence of variability in the structure of the nervous system. Neuronal types and typical patterns of neuronal organization can be recognized because of their invariant features, but anyone who has had some experience of neuroanatomy and neurocytology is aware of the variability within cells of a given class and is struck by the frequency of anomalous patterns of neuronal organization in normal individuals in which such anomalies do not appear to result in abnormal functions. Secondly, it is supported by the evidence that some structural variations of the nervous system are genetically determined.

The nervous system of vertebrates consists of a very large number of types of cells, with each type showing a range of variations of structure and function. Many more cells of each type are produced during normal development than survive in the mature animal. Although the range of variability within each type of neuron in the large initial set and in the reduced final set has not been measured, it seems unlikely that all the cells in the initial set are identical. As is well known (Mayr, 1970, p. 82 *et seq.*), a range of variation may enhance the adaptability of a population: the greater the variation, the greater the *"efficiency of the exploration of the resources of the environment by the living matter"* (Dobzhansky, 1951). Therefore, such polymorphism is adaptive. The selection of the survivors that form the final set must be determined on the basis of some type of benefit, functional effectiveness, or what is termed "functional validation" (M. Jacobson, 1970b). We theorize that there is a competition between neurons which results in elimination of some neurons and the survival of others contingent on their fitness to survive (M. Jacobson, 1970b, p. 161, 334, 1974b; Hirsch and Jacobson, 1975). That a larger number of cells may survive if they are provided with additional peripheral targets shows that the death of cells is not inherently predetermined within the dying cells but is determined by factors in the postsynaptic target cells (see Section 8.2). The present understanding is that there is a quantitative disparity between the presynaptic set of elements and the postsynaptic targets on which they form synapses. It may also be assumed that there are qualitative differences between the elements of the presynaptic set and also between the elements of the postsynaptic set such that an element in one set will associate with an element in the other set, with a probability that varies as the range of different properties in each set of elements. Very slight differences between individual elements in each set may be sufficient to result in a struggle between the presynaptic elements for space on the postsynaptic cell or for a limited supply of some vital material produced by the target cells. Competition is keenest between individuals that are most similar and will finally result in one type completely displacing the other (Gause, 1932, 1934; Mayr, 1970; L. M. Cook, 1971).

Differences in brain structure which depend on the genotype have been described in many species, but such "neurological mutants" (see Section 10.15 for mutations affecting the cerebellum and Section 11.19 for anomalous visual pathways in albinos) are usually at such a large selective disadvantage that they could not have survived in natural conditions. However, there are striking variations in structure of the hippocampal formation in different strains of adult mice which are genetically determined (R. E. Wimer and Wimer, 1982) and which appear to have little or no selective value and may be neutral. Different strains of mice show a number of variations in the structure of the hippocampal formation: differences in the number of pyramidal neurons in specific hippocampal regions (R. E. Wimer *et al.*, 1976, 1978, 1980; Ingram and Corfman, 1980; R. E. Wimer and Wimer, 1982; Luzzatto *et al.*, 1988); differences in the distribution of mossy fibers (Barber *et al.*, 1974; Vaughn *et al.*, 1977; Fredens, 1981; Gozzo and Ammassari-Teule, 1983; Nowakowski, 1984). These variations that are inherited in inbred strains of mice appear to have no functional effects and to have neither selective advantage nor disadvantage. However, accumulation of such mutations may ultimately become advantageous or disadvantageous.

Such variations in structure should not be regarded as "errors" of development. Errors are chance deviations from the normal range, and any structure that occurs with a high probability in all individuals of the species cannot be called an error. Transient structures that appear only for a short period of development should not be termed "errors" if they occur predictably in all individuals. Such, for example, are the transient excesses of the number of synapses and neurons in many parts of the nervous system which are produced and then eliminated predictably at specific stages of development.

Whenever a careful search has been made, variability has been found even in the invertebrate nervous system, which has generally been regarded as very stereotyped. In the locust nervous system, two types of variability have been seen. Individual variations have been seen in the structure of identified neurons which conform to their type but show variability in the fine patterns of axonal and dendritic branching (Bullock and Horridge, 1965; Macagno *et al.*, 1973). Major variations occur in the brain of the locust, including cases in which axons project to lobes of the brain in which they are not normally found (C. Goodman, 1974). Duplication of cells has been seen as a rare anomaly in the ocellar interneurons of the locust (C. Goodman, 1974) and in the Mauthner neuron of amphibians (Stefanelli, 1951). Even in the projection of the retinula axons in the fly, which in most cases show great precision of their connections, some "erroneous" connections are occasionally found in "normal" animals (Meinertzhagen, 1972). In a leech that was found with more cells than usual in many of its ganglia, the supernumerary cells formed normal connections (D. P. Kuffler and Muller, 1974).

In newborn rats and newly hatched chicks, there is considerable individual variability in brain DNA content, which is an index of the total number of cells (neurons plus glial cells). For example, about 0.25 percent of chicks and 0.4 percent of rats have brain DNA content at birth or hatching that is well above the range of brain DNA content of individuals from the same litter or same batch of eggs (Zamenhof *et al.*, 1971c). It is not known whether these rare cases of high brain cell number result from increased cell proliferation or from diminished cell death nor is it known whether neurons or glial cells are affected. It is also not known whether the increased brain cell number results from a superior nutrient supply or whether it is caused by conditions within the embryo. No studies have been undertaken to determine whether the variability in brain DNA content is inherited.

Anyone who compares several brains will reach the conclusion that no two brains of individuals of the same species are exactly alike. There are always individual variations in all parameters, including brain weight (volume), neuronal packing density, mean size of specific types of cells, and number of neurons. In humans the degree of variability on such parameters is in the order of 15 percent (Haug, 1987). The range of variability in the human brain is large enough to have to be taken into consideration by neurosurgeons who probe the human brain stereotaxically, for example, to make lesions in the basal ganglia (Van Buren and Maccubin, 1962). Individual variability is most easily seen in the gyri and sulci of the human cerebral hemispheres (Bailey and von Bonin, 1951). The functional significance of individual variations of human brain structure is not known and neither are the genetic and developmental mechanisms that may give rise to individual variability in brain structure.

There are several species-specific, left–right asymmetries of brain structure and function in which individual variations of the dominant side occur, although one side is dominant in the majority of individuals. The evolutionary origins and genetic and developmental mechanisms of asymmetries and lateral dominance are not well understood (see footnote 6 in Chapter 1). Cerebral hemispheric functional dominance is present in birds and humans: passive-avoidance learning in chicks is a left-hemispheric function (Patel and Stewart, 1988), as is song learning in canaries (Nottebohm, 1971; Denenberg, 1981, review) and language learning in humans (Walker, 1980; Bradshaw and Nettleton, 1981, reviews). Asymmetry of cerebral cortical structures is known to be related to specific brain functions in humans, especially to the lateralization of language functions in the so-called Broca's and Wernicke's areas of the dominant cerebral hemisphere. This lateralization, which is probably genetically determined, is correlated with an increased size of the temporal planum and the frontal operculum—gyri related to cortical language functions, in the speech-dominant hemisphere (Geschwind and Levitsky, 1968; Geschwind, 1970, 1972; LeMay, 1976; Galaburda *et al.*, 1978; Galaburda, 1980; Falzi *et al.*, 1982). This asymmetry becomes measurable as early as the 29th week of gestation, and is well developed at birth (Witelson and Pallie, 1973; Wada *et al.*, 1975).

Hemispheric left–right asymmetries also occur in the great apes (LeMay and Geschwind, 1975; LeMay, 1976). In rats, there are left–right differences in thickness of the posterior regions of the cerebral cortex (M. C. Diamond *et al.*, 1981). The right hippocampal formation is larger than the left in the rat (M. C. Diamond *et al.*, 1983). Other asymmetries of brain structure also appear to be inherited, for example, the left–right asymmetry of the habenular nuclei in teleosts and amphibians (Braitenberg and Kemali, 1970). An additional habenular nucleus starts developing on the left side at the beginning of metamorphosis in frogs and attains full size about 2 months after metamorphosis (M. J. Morgan *et al.*, 1973). The same asymmetry—the presence of an accessory left habenular nucleus—is found in newts, but the asymmetry is reversed in newts with *situs inversus*, either produced by making lesions in the gastrula or present in natural populations in about 2 percent of individuals (von Woellwarth, 1950, 1969). Ludwig (1932) has reviewed the problem of the origins and functional effects of left–right asymmetry, but he was unable to arrive at any general explanations. The functional significance, developmental mechanisms, and evolutionary origins of left–right asymmetries in the nervous system remain largely unknown. They should not be thought of as "errors" of development.

Anomalous location of single neurons is fairly common, and even groups of ectopic neurons are found in a large percentage of adult human and primate brains when they are examined thoroughly (H. R. Schneider, 1968). This type of individual variability has been termed *heteromorphism* by Feremutsch (1952, 1960). Displaced and disoriented neurons are often found close to blood vessels which appear to have obstructed their migration. According to Ramón y Cajal (1929a), "*In all neural organs one occasionally sees atypical and accidental arrangements with regard to the path and orientation of axons. . . . All these aberrations are produced during fetal development and can be explained by obstacles which the neurons must surmount during their migration.*"

Ectopic neurons are found in the human brain in a number of pathological conditions and are occasionally seen in individuals with no neurological disease (see reviews by Ostertag, 1956; Crome and Stern, 1972; Norman, 1966). That some of these ectopias are the result of arrested migration is shown by the fact that the displaced neurons are situated in one of the migratory paths (Wiest and Hallervorden, 1958; Rakic, 1975a). Thus, ectopic olivary neurons, arrested in the medulla during migration from the rhombic lip via the pontobulbar body to the inferior olive, are seen in cases of pachygyria and of lissencephaly (A. E. Walker, 1942; Hanaway *et al.*, 1968). In almost all cases of human trisomy 18, ectopic neurons are seen arrested in the course of their migration along the corpus geniculothalamicum to the thalamus (Norman, 1966; Sumi, 1970; Terplan *et al.*, 1970). In the cerebellum, ectopic granule cells are often seen in the molecular layer in normal rabbits (Spacek *et al.*, 1973) and in normal humans (Brustowicz and Kernohan, 1952) as well as in a number of diseases of various etiologies. Although the mechanism of production of the ectopias is not known, the common factor in all these cases appears to be defective migration of the granule cells. In the reeler and weaver mutant mice, where the failure of migration of granule cells has been established with certainty, the underlying cellular defect is now known (see Section 10.15). Possible causes of the migration defect may be failure of development of some component of the mechanism of cell locomotion or failure to acquire the cell surface properties that are necessary for neurons to interact with cells along their paths of migration.

There are several ways in which "errors" of positioning, of orientation, or of the number of neurons may be corrected at later stages. The first means of eliminating malpositioned or disoriented cells is by cell death, yet the malpositioned cells survive in all the cases that have been cited above. In such cases, survival may be due to the formation of detailed axonal connections that provide sustenance to the malpositioned neurons. Other malpositioned cells die because their axons fail to find the correct synaptic targets. This form of "error correction" by elimination of redundant cells is what has been termed "natural selection" of nerve cells in the first edition of this book (M. Jacobson, 1970b, p. 161). This concept originated with Wilhelm Roux in his book *Der Kampf der Theile im Organismus* (1881), and of course I am in agreement with other authors who have followed me in accepting the concept of "natural selection" of neurons (Cowan, 1973; Prestige, 1974; Hollyday and Hamburger, 1976). They part company from me, however, when they adopt the view that death of redundant neurons in the spinal sensory ganglia or death of spinal motoneurons represents a mode of "error correction." It is undeniable that the excess production of neurons is in itself not an error. It is an invariant stage of development found in all individuals of the same species and is part of the normal developmental program, determined genetically in the first instance and performing a constructive function during development. This is a normal means of matching one set of neurons to another set, and the misconception that it is a form of "error" correction directs attention away from its significance as a mechanism of achieving optimum matching between pre- and postsynaptic elements.

Returning to the mechanisms of "error correction" in cases of malpositioning or misalignment of cells, there is considerable evidence that many such malpositioned neurons survive embryonic development and persist in the adult. An example of migration of up to 700 neurons beyond their usual assembly zone occurs in the isthmo-optic nucleus of the chick embryo (P. G. H. Clarke and Cowan, 1976; P. G. H. Clarke *et al.*, 1976). In this case, the majority of the misplaced neurons die, with the result that the anomaly is partly, but not entirely, corrrected. Subsequent experiments have shown that ectopic neurons are even more numerous than originally reported and that their loss is proportionately about the same as for the neurons within the isthmo-optic nucleus (Streit and Reubi, 1977; Hayes and Webster, 1981; O'Leary and Cowan, 1982, 1984). A considerable number of misplaced neurons of the chick embryo isthmo-optic nucleus survive beyond hatching, and in these cases one may regard such ectopias as a means of giving rise to a new form of neuronal organization. One may conceive of this as one way in which evolution of neuronal systems may occur.

In many cases, it seems that the ectopic neurons have formed essentially normal connections. For example, in the reeler mouse (see Section 10.15) the neurons of the cerebral cortex are malpositioned (Caviness and Rakic, 1978; Stanfield and Cowan, 1979), yet interhemispheric connections through the corpus callosum are normal, and it is probable that the correct connections are made within the cortex (Caviness, 1976; Caviness and Yorke, 1976,

1977; Dräger, 1981; Simmons *et al.,* 1982). In the cerebellum of the reeler mutant mouse, the malpositioned Purkinje cells appear to receive normal synaptic connections and do not form aberrant connections (Rakic and Sidman, 1972; Bliss and Chung, 1974), and in the weaver mutant mouse, the mossy fibers usually synapse normally on the ectopic granule cells (Rakic and Sidman, 1973b). The significance of aberrant synaptic connections which are formed in the cerebellum of the weaver mouse is discussed in Section 10.15.

Displaced cells persist either because they are integrated into the existing circuitry, as may occur even in some extreme cases of neuronal malpositioning, for example, the reeler mouse, or because they form novel functional systems or extend the functional capabilities of preexisting systems. If variations arise because of mutations whose effects are neutral, or are corrected at later stages of development, they will not be subject to natural selection but will tend to accumulate. Neuronal development need not be as invariant as is commonly supposed, provided that variants are either corrected or eliminated, or, if they persist, are either neutral or advantageous.

3 Neuroglial Ontogeny

On a perfectly translucent yellow field appear thin, smooth, black filaments, neatly arranged, or else thick and spiny, arising from triangular, stellate or fusiform black bodies! One might say they are like a Chinese ink drawing on transparent Japanese paper. The eye is disconcerted, so accustomed is it to the inextricable network stained with carmine and hematoxylin which always forces the mind to perform feats of critical interpretation. Here everything is simple, clear, without confusion. . . . The technique of dreams is now reality! The metallic impregnation has made such a fine dissection, exceeding all previous hopes. This is the method of Golgi.

Ramón y Cajal (1852–1934),
Histologie du système nerveux, Vol. 1, p. 29, 1909

3.1. History of Neuroglia

I have for this young researcher [Ramón y Cajal] the greatest regard, and as I have admired his great activity and initiative, I can appreciate the importance of his original observations. The small differences between his conclusions and my own cannot have an effect on my sentiments, as I am profoundly convinced that such divergence, by which one can push research forward, is always useful to science.

Camillo Golgi (1843–1926), *La rete nervosa diffusa degli organi centrali del sistema nervosa*, 1901

The original concept of neuroglia meaning "nerve glue" was based on Rudolf Virchow's assumption that there must be a mesodermal connective tissue element of the nervous system (Virchow, 1846, 1858, 1867). Even if neuroglial cells did not exist Virchow would have had to invent them as a requirement for his theory—as a bold conjecture thrown out for refutation. But techniques were inadequate to either corroborate or refute that conjecture. The mesodermal origin of neuroglial cells continued to receive corroboration (Andriezen, 1893; Weigert, 1895; W. Robertson, 1897, 1899, 1900a) in the face of strong counterevidence showing that both neurons and glial cells originate from embryonic ectoderm (His, 1889, 1901).

Virchow and his disciples were primarily interested in pathology and thus in neuroglial tumors and in the reaction of the neuroglia to disease and injury. Their theories guided practice in the direction of neuropathology, and away from normal development. Virchow's research program was aimed at showing that the causes of disease can be found in derangements of cells.

It is doubtful whether Virchow saw neuroglial cells in 1846 and there are no convincing pictures of them in Virchow's book, *Die Cellularpathologie* (1859), although he there discusses the theory of a neuroglial tissue. At that time the theory led and the facts followed. Progress was slow because techniques were inadequate in the 1840s and 1850s to provide reliable evidence. Virchow (1885) later described that period: *"The great upheavals that mi-*

croscopy, chemistry and pathological anatomy had brought about were at first accompanied by the most dismal consequences. People found themselves help-less . . . filled with exaggerated expectations they seized on any fragment which a bold speculator might chose to cast out."[1] Virchow's theory of the neuroglia consisted of two such bold speculations: first, that neuroglial cells form a connective tissue, and second, that neuroglia develop from mesoderm in the embryo. These conjectures were not Virchow's original creations. He derived the concept of tissues from Bichat (1801), who first proposed that tissues are where the functions of life and the dysfunctions of disease occur—Virchow extrapolated, saying that cells are where life and disease occur. Virchow obtained the concept of mesoderm from Remak to whom he is also indebted for the idea that all cells originate from other cells.[2]

The problem of the ectodermal or mesodermal origins of the neuroglial cells has a complex history. Wilhelm His (1889) corrected Virchow's misconception that the neuroglia form the connective tissue elements of the nervous system by showing that neuroglial cells as well as neurons originate from neurectoderm. This is considered at greater length in Section 2.1 in connection with the history of neurectodermal germinal cells. The problem was resolved in the last decade of the 19th century when numerous stains for connective tissue failed to stain neuroglial cells but only stained blood vessels in the

central nervous system: the Unna–Taenzer orcein method (Unna, 1890, 1891) and the Weigert (1898) resorcinol–fuchsin method for elastic fibers; the van Gieson (1889) acid fuchsin–picric acid stain for collagen; and the Mallory (1900) aniline blue stain for connective tissue. That so many different connective tissue stains failed to stain neuroglial cells could not conclusively falsify Virchow's theory because it could be maintained that glial cells are a special form of connective tissue that is not stained by any other method. That was the argument used by Andriezen (1893) and Weigert (1895). Contrariwise, the invention of specific neuroglial stains (Ramón y Cajal, 1913; Rio-Hortego, 1919, 1921a,b, 1932) was not considered to be conclusive refutation of Virchow's theory. Cajal could still maintain in 1920 that the glial cells belonging to his "third element" are of mesodermal origin. The most compelling evidence against it was that neuroglial cells in the embryo originate from the neurectoderm (His, 1889). However, the available evidence did not exclude the possibility of subsequent entry of mesodermal cells into the central nervous system. The gradual resolution of this problem is considered below, in connection with the history of the microglial cells.

His misidentified the progenitors of both the neurons and the neuroglial cells in the neural tube. He conjectured that neurons originate from germinal cells but the glial cells originate from a syncytial tissue named the *"myelospongium"* or *"neurospongium"* formed of spongioblasts (see Section 2.1). The theory that glial cells remain permanently anastomosed with one another continued to be corroborated by many authorities (Hardesty, 1904; Held, 1909; Streeter, 1912). In 1912, Streeter could confidently invert the truth by pronouncing that *"earlier conceptions of neuroglia cells were based on silver precipitation methods (Golgi) which failed to reveal the true wealth of their anastomosing branches, and there thus existed a false impression of neuroglia as consisting of scattered and independent cells."* At that time cells were believed to be naked protoplasmic bodies, lacking a membrane, and connected by protoplasmic and fibrous bridges (see Section 5.1 for a more extensive exposition of this preconception and the effects it had on evolution of the neuron theory).

The neurospongium theory was based entirely on artifacts (Fig. 2.2), and could not be refuted con-

---

[1]This state of affairs and of mind was not confined to science. In the mid-1850s Walter Bagehot in England was saying much the same thing about the social and political conditions in Europe. The period, he wrote, is an *"an age of confusion and tumult, when old habits are shaken, old views are overthrown, ancient assumptions rudely questioned, ancient inferences utterly denied. . . ." Physics and Politics* (1872; 1873 edition).

[2]In 1852 Remak stated that *"pathological cells and normal cells in general are. . . products or descendants of normal tissue cells."* In his book *Untersuchungen über die Entwickelung der Wirbelthiere* (1855, pp. 164–170), Remak developed the idea that all cells originate from other cells in the embryo, and not from a cytoblastema as Schwann had proposed. Virchow's celebrated pronouncement made in 1858 *Omnis cellula e cellula* (all cells from cells) is directly derived from Remak although Virchow failed to acknowledge this. Pagel (1945), Ackerknecht (1953), Kisch (1954), and Hall (1969) give Remak the priority for this correct version of the cell theory.

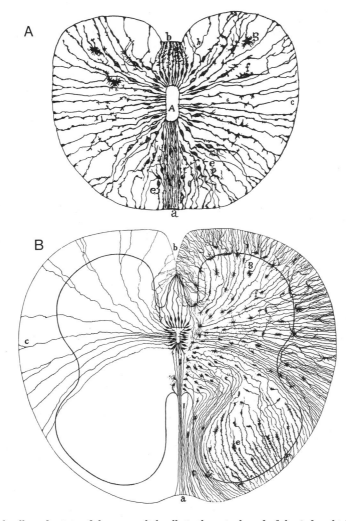

Figure 3.1. Epithelial cells and origin of the neuroglial cells in the spinal cord of the 9-day chick embryo (**A**) and 14-cm human embryo spinal cord (**B**). Golgi preparations. A = ependymal canal; a, b = epithelial cells of the posterior and anterior median sulci; these two types of cells maintain both peripheral and central attachments; c = ependymal cell; e = displaced epithelial cell migrating in the posterior horn; f = displaced epithelial cell migrating in the anterior horn; these two types of cells have entirely lost their central ends and conserved their peripheral ends terminating by conical boutons at the pia mater; g = epithelial cell about to become a neuroglial corpuscle; there remains no more than an outgrowth going to the pia mater. A from S. Ramón y Cajal, *Les nouvelles idées sur la structure du système nerveux*, 1894; B from M. von Lenhossék, *Der feinere Bau des Nervensystems*, 1893.

clusively until the 1950s when the electron microscope showed that all cells in the neurectoderm and neural tube are separated by narrow intercellular clefts from the beginning of development. In the 19th century the counterevidence to the neuroglial syncytium was already quite strong. Golgi staining of the neural tube always showed separate glial cells

forming a series of stages of development from the radially aligned spongioblasts to mature astrocytes, as shown in Fig. 3.1 (Koelliker, 1893; Lenhossék, 1893; Ramón y Cajal, 1894). As evidence against the neuroglial syncytium Alzheimer (1900) showed that one neuroglial cell may undergo pathological change while its neighbors remain normal. By the 1920s the neurospongium theory had been abandoned, not because it could be falsified conclusively, but because it failed to predict new observations predicted by the alternative theory that glial cells are always separate (Penfield, 1926, review).

The research program of His split into four separate research programs with different goals. The first dealt with the origins of neurons and glial cells from progenitors in the neural tube—His conjectured that neurons originate from germinal cells near the ventricle, and glial cells originate from spongioblasts which span the full thickness of the neural tube. The second theory dealt with the syncytial connections between cells in the neural tube. The third dealt with the enormous intercellular spaces which appeared as an artifact in sections of neural tube (Fig. 2.2). This space was supposed to contain a "central ground substance" in which the cells were embedded (Boeke, 1942; Bauer, 1953). A fourth theory dealt with the role of migration of neuroblasts in these spaces, guided by the radially aligned spongioblasts (Magini, 1888; His, 1889) (see M. Jacobson, in preparation). These theories illustrate Cajal's dictum that *"in biology theories are fragile and ephemeral constructions . . . while hypotheses pass by facts remain"* (Ramón y Cajal, 1928). He was also well aware that the facts were often indistinguishable from the artifacts.

The Golgi research program on neuroglia started in 1875 with Golgi's studies of glial cell tumors. Golgi's earliest papers on neuroglia were published in 1870 and 1871 using hematoxylin and carmine staining which was incapable of showing either neurons or glial cells completely. By 1873 Golgi had developed his potassium dichromate–silver technique, the first of his methods for metallic impregnation (see Section 6.2) which was capable of staining entire neurons and glial cells. In Golgi's 1875 paper on gliomas stained by means of his potassium dichromate–silver technique, he was able to give the first morphological definition of neuroglial cells as a class distinct from neurons. Golgi discovered the glial cell perivascular foot (see Fig. 5.1) and conjectured that the glial cell "protoplasmic process" mediates transfer of nutrients between the blood and brain (Golgi, 1895). This led ultimately to the modern theory of the blood–brain barrier (see Section 3.7). This is only one sign of the very progressive character of Golgi's research program, not only in terms of a great technical advance but also

because of its theoretical boldness.[3] By showing that the protoplasmic processes of neuroglial cells end on blood vessels and those of nerve cells end blindly, Golgi refuted Gerlach's theory that the protoplasmic processes (later called dendrites by His, 1890) end in a diffuse nerve net by which all nerve cells were believed to be interconnected. Having refuted Gerlach's theory, Golgi conjectured that the nerve net is really between afferent axons and the axon collaterals of efferent neurons. This reticular theory of nerve connections is discussed more fully in Section 6.1. Here it should be emphasized that it was a mature and progressive theory for its time, and that it became postmature and degenerative only near the very end of the 19th century. Guided by Golgi's conjectures about the relationship between neuroglial cells and blood vessels and about the active role of neuroglia in mediating exchange with the blood, progressive research programs have continued to the present time (see Section 3.18).

Golgi published his mercuric chloride method in 1879 but it went unnoticed until after he published his rapid method in 1887. The Golgi techniques were widely used after 1887 and were mainly responsible for the accelerated progress in neurocytology during the 1890s. One of the first advances was recognition of different types of glial cells. Astrocytes were named by Lenhossék (1891) who recognized them as a separate subclass although Golgi had identified them as early as 1873. Koelliker (1893) and Andriezen (1893a) subdivided them into fibrous and protoplasmic types according to the presence or absence of fibers in the cytoplasm. They noted that fibrous astrocytes predominate in white matter and protoplasmic astrocytes in gray matter.

There were two theories of astrocyte histogenesis. Schaper (1897) conjectured that the germi-

---

[3]A theory is mature when it is accepted in a research program where it operates to guide techniques to obtain new facts. A progressive theory is defined as one that leads the facts, a degenerative theory as one that falls behind the facts. A progressive theory stimulates research programs aimed at obtaining corroborative evidence or counterevidence. In a progressive research program many theories are proposed and tested. Their refutation and replacement is the basis of progress. A theory becomes degenerative when it fails to predict new facts and when the counterevidence becomes sufficient to falsify it.

nal cells of His, positioned close to the ventricle, divide to give rise to neuroblasts, spongioblasts, and "indifferent cells." He speculated that spongioblasts give rise to glial cells only in the embryo but indifferent cells persist in the postnatal period and give rise to both neurons and glial cells. A different theory was proposed by Koelliker (1890) and supported by Cajal (1909). They believed that spongioblasts persist into the postnatal period and are the only progenitors of all glial cells. Evidence for this was given by Lenhossék (1893), who showed a series of stages of astrocyte histogenesis, starting with detachment of radially aligned spongioblasts from the internal and external limiting membranes, followed by migration into the brain parenchyma where they continue to divide to give rise to astrocytes, as shown in Fig. 3.1. Transformation of radial glial cells into astrocytes in the spinal cord was confirmed by Ramón y Cajal (1896) in the chick embryo (Fig. 3.1). Almost a century later those premature discoveries (see footnote 1 in Chapter 1) were rediscovered; one might say they matured (Schmechel and Rakic, 1979a,b; Levitt and Rakic, 1980; Choi, 1981; Hajós and Bascó, 1984; Benjelloun-Touini *et al.*, 1985; Federoff, 1986; Munoz-Garcia and Ludwin, 1986a,b; M. Hirano and Goldman, 1988). Both Lenhossék and Cajal observed that the radial glial cells are the first glial cells to differentiate and this has also been confirmed with modern techniques (Rakic, 1972, 1981; Choi, 1981). Lenhossék and Cajal found that the peripheral expansions of some of the radial glial cells persist in the spinal cord to form the glia limitans exterior, and that too has recently been confirmed (Liuzzi and Miller, 1987).

Cajal's gold chloride–sublimate method stains astrocytes very well (see below), and this enabled him to confirm Lenhossék's theory of the origin of astrocytes from radial glial cells and to refute the theory that astrocytes originate from mesoderm (Cajal, 1913a, 1916). Cajal (1913b) also showed that astrocytes can divide in the normal brain and this too has recently been corroborated (see Section 3.3). Mitosis of astrocytes after brain injury was demonstrated by Penfield and Rio-Hortega (1926). When those theories of glial cell origins were originally proposed, they could neither be corroborated nor falsified by means of the histological evidence because no techniques for tracing cell lineages existed at that time. Those theories of glial cell lineages were bypassed for a century until more reliable techniques for tracing neuroglial cell lineages recently became available (see Section 3.3).

Oligodendroglial cells were discovered by W. Robertson (1899, 1900a) using his platinum stain. He did not understand their significance in myelination and he conjectured that they originate from mesoderm (he called them mesoglia, not to be confused with the mesoglia of Rio-Hortega, which are brain macrophages). They were rediscovered by Rio-Hortega (1919, 1921), who called them oligodendroglia because their processes are shorter and sparser than those of astrocytes. He made the distinction between perineuronal satellites in the gray matter, most of which he believed to be oligodendroglia, and interfascicular oligodendroglia situated in rows between the myelinated fibers of the white matter. From their anatomical position, and the fact that they appear only in late embryonic and early postnatal stages during the period of myelination, Rio-Hortega (1921b, 1922) conjectured that the oligodendroglia are involved in myelination in the central nervous system. Rio-Hortega (1921b) and Penfield (1924) also conjectured that a common precursor migrates into the white matter and then divides to produce astrocytes or oligodendroglia. This conjecture has only recently been possible to corroborate (see Section 3.3).

Before the introduction of good specific stains for glial cells (Ramón y Cajal, 1913; Rio-Hortega, 1919) it was not possible to differentiate, with any degree of certainty, between processes of neurons and those of neuroglia. Neuroglial cell processes were identified by a process of exclusion. Carl Weigert said that *"one recognized neuroglia as the structure that one could not or would not call neuronal"* (Rieder, 1906). Weigert understood that there was an urgent need for a specific neuroglial stain, and he spent 30 years trying to perfect one (Rieder, 1906). He pioneered the use of hematoxylin for staining nervous tissue, developed a very good stain for myelinated nerve fibers, and introduced aniline dye stains (with the help of his cousin Paul Ehrlich). Weigert (1895) was the first to invent a stain (fluorochrome–methylviolet) that was specific for glial cells, but it only stained glial fibers intensely, the remainder of the glial cell weakly, did not stain neurons, and failed to stain glia in embryonic tissue. It showed glial fibers apparently outside as well as inside the glial cells. Those findings misled Weigert to conclude that glial fibers form a connective tissue in the central nervous system analogous to collagen.

Nineteenth century theories of neuroglial functions in the adult nervous system reviewed by Soury (1899) include their nutritional and supportive functions, formation of myelin, formation of a glial barrier between the nervous system and the blood and cerebrospinal fluid, their role in limiting the spread of nervous activity, their proliferation and other changes in response to degeneration of neurons, and their involvement in conscious experience, learning, and memory. These theories of neuroglial functions were sustained more by clever arguments than by the available evidence; indeed, they continued to flourish because the means to test them experimentally were not available until recent times (see Table 3.1).

Soury (1899, pp. 1615-1639) gives a masterful critique of the theories of glial function that were being debated at the end of the 19th century. The theories were weakest in dealing with the origins and early development of glial cells and with their functions in the embryo. This is not surprising because the specific methods required for identifying embryonic glial cells were not invented until much later (the glia-specific histological stains of Ramón y Cajal, 1913, and Rio-Hortega, 1919; tissue culture of glial cells in the 1920s; identification of glial cells with the electron microscope after the 1950s; glial cell–specific antibodies after the 1970s). The concept that glial cells help to guide migrating neuroblasts and outgrowing axons, first proposed by His (1887, 1889) and Magini (1888), was not possible to test experimentally, for almost a century (Mugnaini and Forströnen, 1967; Rakic, 1971a,b). Their myelinating functions were suggested by a few but rejected by most authorities in the 19th century. It was thought that myelin in the CNS is produced as a secretion of the axon and in the peripheral nerves as a secretion by either the axon or the sheath of Schwann. This is considered in Section 3.6.

In 1913 Cajal introduced his gold chloride sublimate method for staining neuroglia. It stained astrocytes well but oligodendroglia were incompletely impregnated.[4] Cajal (1920) mistook the latter for a new type of neuroglial cell lacking dendrites, which he called the "third element." He thought that these *celulas adendriticas* (adendroglia, Andrew and Ashworth, 1945) are responsible for myelination of fibers in the CNS, and that they are of mesodermal origin. Rio-Hortega's ammoniacal silver carbonate method (1919), which clearly stains oligodendroglial and microglial cells, showed that these are the authentic "third element" and that Cajal's conclusions were based on incompletely stained cells. Cajal opposed this explanation, and although he reluctantly, and with reservations, acknowledged the authenticity of microglial cells, he continued to deny the existence of oligodendrocytes long after they were clearly demonstrated and their role in central myelination had been revealed (Rio-Hortega, 1919, 1924, 1928, 1932; Penfield, 1924). However, it is only fair to say that the definitive proof that oligodendrocytes are solely responsible for CNS myelination had to await the ultrastructural evidence (Farquhar and Hartman, 1957; R. L. Schultz *et al.*, 1957; Mugnaini and Walberg, 1964; R. L. Schultz, 1964).

As Penfield (1924) put it: *"Oligodendroglia has received no confirmation as yet though accepted by several writers. This is probably due to two causes; first, the difficulty of staining this element, and second, the fact that Cajal, repeating the work of his disciple, was unable to stain these cells, and, although he confirmed microglia as a group, he cast considerable doubt upon the validity of del Rio-Hortega's description of the remaining portion of the cells previously termed by Cajal 'the third element.'"* Then comes the critical thrust: *"As Cajal, the great master of neurohistology, has himself so often pointed out, it is extremely dangerous to assign value to negative results."* Wilder Penfield (1977), who worked with Rio-Hortega in Madrid in 1924, describes how the disagreement resulted in an estrangement between the two great Spanish neurocytologists and may have been a factor which precipitated the older man into a state of depression.

Even Ramón y Cajal did not escape being overtaken and corrected by his intellectual progeny. In

---

[4]Cajal's summary of his methods for staining the glial cells and his comments on the third element are given in the second volume of his autobiography, *Recuerdos de mi vida* (1917; 3rd ed. 1923), but these parts were omitted, together with most of Cajal's summaries of his methods, in the English translation of the 3rd Spanish edition by E. H. Craigie (*Recollections of My Life*, 1937, republished without correction, 1989). One of the central documents in the history of neuroscience deserves a better translation than this.

Table 3.1. Functions of Neuroglial Cells

Functions	Cell types	Selected references
1. Transport from blood to neurons	Astrocytes	Golgi, 1895; Wlassak, 1896; Abbott and Butt, 1986
2. Induction of vascular endothelial blood–brain barrier	Astrocytes	Stern and Peyrot, 1927; Joó, 1987
3. Myelination in CNS	Oligodendrocytes	Rio-Hortega, 1932; P. M. Wood and Bunge, 1984
4. Myelination in PNS	Schwann cells	Vignal, 1889; Geren, 1954; Robertson, 1955, 1987
5. Secretion of extracellular matrix	Schwann cells	Bunge and Bunge, 1981; Bunge et al., 1986
6. Axonal guidance	Astrocytes	His, 1898; Silver et al., 1982; Hankin and Silver, 1988
7. Stimulation of neurite outgrowth	Astrocytes	Nageotte, 1907; Tanaka and Obata, 1982; Gloor et al., 1986
8. Inhibition of neurite outgrowth	Oligodendrocytes	Schwab and Thoenen, 1985; Caroni and Schwab, 1989
9. Guidance of neuron migration	Radial glial cells	His, 1887; Magini, 1888; Mugnaini and Forströnen, 1967; Rakic, 1971a,b
10. Regulation of neuron morphogenesis	Astrocytes	Chamak et al., 1987; Barbin et al., 1988
11. Compartmentalization of neurons	Astrocytes	Steindler et al., 1988
12. Chromatolytic response to axotomy	Microglial cells	Graeber et al., 1988
13. Phagocytosis of cellular debris	Microglial cells	Rio-Hortega, 1932; Innocenti et al., 1983a,b
	Astrocytes	Wong-Riley, 1972; Ling et al., 1986
14. Transfer of proteins to axons	Invertebrate glial cells	Lasek et al., 1977; Gainer, 1978; Grossfeld et al., 1988
15. Initiation of Schwann cell mitosis	Microglial cells	Beuche and Friede, 1984; Lunn et al., 1989
16. Immune response	Microglial cells	Giulian, 1987; Streit et al., 1988
17. Uptake of neuroactive peptides	Oligodendrocytes, astrocytes	Reynolds and Herschkowitz, 1986
18. Production of interleukin I	Ameboid microglial cells	Giulian and Baker, 1985; Giulian et al., 1988
19. Production of PDGF and CNTF	Type I astrocytes; 0-2A glioblasts	Noble et al., 1988
20. Production of IGF	Astrocytes	McMorris et al., 1986; Balloti, 1987
21. Production of a and b FGF	Astrocytes	Gimenez Gallego et al., 1985; Pettman et al., 1985; Unsicker et al., 1987; Morrison, 1987
22. Production of GMF	Astrocytes	Lim, 1985
23. Production of NGF	Schwann cells	Rush, 1984; Finn et al., 1986; Korsching et al., 1986
24. Regulation of extracellular K^+	Astrocytes, Schwann cells	S. W. Kuffler, 1967; Newman, 1986; Chiu, 1987
25. Regulation of blood supply	Astrocytes	Paulson and Newman, 1987

historical perspective we see that what Cajal is to the neuron, Rio-Hortega is to the neuroglia (Diaz, 1972; Albarracín, 1982). Rio-Hortega was the first to deduce the origin and functions of oligodendrocytes and microglial cells correctly, the first to show their structural transformations in relation to their functions and to emphasize the dynamic state of these cells in normal and pathological conditions. His artistic talents equaled those of his mentor, but while Cajal's drawings have the nervous vitality and intensity of vision of a Velásquez, Rio-Hortega's figures display the deliberately perfected beauty of a Murillo.[5]

Two types of microglial cells in the mammalian CNS were first described by Rio-Hortega (1920, 1932): ameboid and ramified microglia. Ameboid microglia have short processes, appear to be motile and phagocytic, appear prenatally, and increase rapidly in the first few days after birth in the dog, cat, and rabbit. He concluded that these are macrophages originating from the blood, as Hatai (1902b) had observed earlier. Marinesco (1909) showed that brain macrophages ingest India ink and thus behave like macrophages elsewhere. Rio-Hortega and Asua (1921) showed that microglial cells are morphologically very similar to macrophages in other parts of the body. They conjectured that microglia and macrophages both originate from the reticuloendothelial system, which at that time was being vigorously discussed (Aschoff, 1924). The ameboid microglia appeared to Rio-Hortega (1921a) to originate in what he called "fountains" of ameboid cells at places where the pia mater contacts the white matter: beneath the pia of the cerebral peduncles, from the tela choroidea of the third ventricle, and from the dorsal and ventral sulci of the spinal cord. He identified another type, ramified microglia, with long processes, apparently sedentary and nonproliferative. These appear postnatally and persist in the adult. In his 1932 paper Rio-Hortega shows a series of transitional forms between ameboid and ramified microglia and concludes that these represent normal transformations between the two types of microglial cells, thus anticipating recent findings (Perry and Gordon, 1988). In the same paper Rio-Hortega shows that microglia migrate to sites of brain injury, where they proliferate and engulf cellular debris. These are the macrophages of the nervous system, whose roles in defense against infection and injury he was the first to recognize. Confirmation of most of Rio-Hortega's conclusions had to wait until the modern epoch, when the tools were forged that have made it possible to reveal the origins and functions of neuroglial cells.

The debate, started by Rio-Hortega (1932), about whether brain macrophages are derived

from the blood or from the brain has continued for 50 years (reviewed by Boya *et al.*, 1979, 1986; Adrian and Schelper, 1981; Schelper and Adrian, 1986). The presently available evidence shows that in adults both microglia and blood monocytes can contribute to brain macrophages, depending on whether the blood–brain barrier is intact or not. Present evidence shows that in the embryo the microglia originate from monocytes that enter the brain before development of the blood–brain barrier.

In modern times those who have concluded that brain macrophages are entirely hematogenous in origin include Konigsmark and Sidman (1965), S. Fujita and Kitamura (1975), Ling (1978; 1981), and Del Cerro and Mojun (1979). Those who have concluded that macrophages are derived from microglial cells include Maxwell and Kruger (1965), Mori and Leblond (1969), Vaughn and Pease (1970), Torvik and Skjörten (1971), Torvik (1975), and Boya (1976). The ultimate fate of the brain macrophages after repair of an injury is also controversial: they have been reported to degenerate (Fujita and Kitamura, 1976), return to the blood (Kreuzberg, 1968; McKeever and Balentine, 1978), or transform into microglial cells (Mori, 1972; Blakemore, 1975; Imamoto and Leblond, 1977; Ling, 1981; Kaur *et al.*, 1987), but the latter possibility is denied by Schelper and Adrian (1986). The same techniques, in the hands of skillful workers, have led to diametrically opposite conclusions. The brain macrophages may indeed originate from more than one source and have multiple fates, but the neurocytologist tends to select his facts according to prevailing prejudices—in this he is no different from other scientists and nonscientists. The main difference between them is that the scientist, more often than the nonscientist, submits his prejudices for refutation.

3.2. Identification of Developing Neuroglial Cells

Accurate methods for identifying different types of neuroglial cells are required to study their origins, lineages, and factors controlling their development. Improved standard transmission electron microscopy has provided better criteria by which to identify different types of glial cells and to correlate ultrastructure with developmental

---

[5]By comparison the majority of Golgi's published figures, redrawn by a draftsman, lack vivacity.

transformations and with functions (e.g., Peters *et al.*, 1976; Parnavelas *et al.*, 1983). Electron microscopic autoradiography has made it possible to identify the types of glial cells that are generated at different times and places (e.g., Skoff *et al.*, 1976)—matters that could not be finally resolved with light microscopic autoradiography. A number of enzyme markers have been used for cytochemical identification of neuroglial cell types (e.g., Kaur *et al.*, 1987). With a battery of glial and neuronal cell type–specific antibodies (e.g., Miller *et al.*, 1989), different types of neurons and glial cells can be identified during development, or in pathological states (e.g., Streit *et al.*, 1988), or in tissue culture, where their normal morphology is altered. These advances have, in turn, made it possible to use molecular biological technology to analyze the genetic and biochemical mechanisms of glial cell development, and to identify the cellular mechanisms, cell interactions, and molecular signals that control proliferation, migration, differentiation, and death of glial cells.

The structure and function of glial cells should be interpreted in dynamic terms. Even at very early embryonic stages, within the ventricular zone of the embryonic rat forebrain, the radial glial cells show heterogeneity in their expression of protooncogenes (J. G. Johnston and van der Kooy, 1989). Thus we expect to see morphological reflections of the varied functions of glial cells during development as well as in the mature nervous system. For example, we see differences between microglia at rest and during reaction to trauma (Graeber *et al.*, 1989), differences between astrocytes that reflect their interactions with neurons at different stages of development and in different functional states (Wilkin *et al.*, 1990), and differences between resting oligodendrocytes and those that are engaged in myelination. We have only to compile a list of functions that have been attributed to neuroglial cells (Table 3.1) to appreciate their diversity. In brief, we have to interpret the morphology of the neuroglial cells as well as of neurons in relation to the functional roles of the neurons or glial cells at the particular times and places at which they are observed and should expect the morphology to change under different conditions and at different stages of development. Such changes can vary from relatively slight ultrastructural alterations to complete transformation of the cell's morphology.

Such a transformation occurs in the radial neuroglial cells of the mammalian telencephalon. They are extremely elongated and span the full thickness of the brain and spinal cord at early stages while they function as guides for migrating neurons, but later, after neurogenesis has ceased, the radial neuroglia are transformed into astrocytes, as shown in Fig. 3.1 (Koelliker, 1893; Lenhossék, 1893; Ramón y Cajal, 1894, 1911, p. 847; Bignami and Dahl, 1974a,b; Rakic, 1975a; Choi and Lapham, 1978; Schmechel and Rakic, 1979; Voigt, 1989), and oligodendrocytes (Choi, 1981; Choi *et al.*, 1983; Choi and Kim, 1984; M. Hirano and Goldman, 1988). Using a monoclonal antibody that recognizes radial glial cells in light and electron micrographs, a series of transitional forms from the bipolar radial glial cell to the multipolar astrocyte can be identified (Misson *et al.*, 1988a,b). Transformation of cerebral cortical radial glial cells into astrocytes also occurs *in vitro* (Culican *et al.*, 1990).

Another dramatic transformation occurs when ameboid microglial cells of the fetal period differentiate postnatally into ramified microglial cells of the adult (Rio-Hortega, 1932; Murabe and Sano, 1962; Ling, 1981). This transformation can be mimicked *in vitro* by treating ameboid microglia with retinoic acid and dimethyl sulfoxide: the ameboid cells stop dividing, lose the ability to engulf latex beads, and grow long processes resembling those of ramified microglial cells (Giulian and Baker, 1986). A series of transitional forms between the ameboid and ramified microglial cells has been demonstrated in mouse brain, by using a monoclonal antibody specific for mouse monocytes to label the microglial cells, as shown in Fig. 3.2 (Perry *et al.*, 1985; Perry and Gordon, 1988).

Transmission electron microscopy has provided new criteria for identifying the astrocytes and oligodendrocytes (Farquhar and Hartmann, 1957; R. L. Schultz *et al.*, 1957; Luse, 1958, 1960; De Robertis and Gershenfeld, 1961; R. L. Schultz, 1964; Mugnaini and Walberg, 1964; Wendell-Smith *et al.*, 1966; Kruger and Maxwell, 1967; Vaughn and Peters, 1971; Peters *et al.*, 1976; Parnavelas *et al.*, 1983; Wood and Bunge, 1984) and for identifying the microglial cells (Mori and Leblond, 1969; Adrian and Williams, 1973; Adrian *et al.*, 1978; Blakemore, 1975; Ling *et al.*, 1986; LeVine and Goldman, 1988). The distinguishing electron microscopic features of the microglial cells are a small

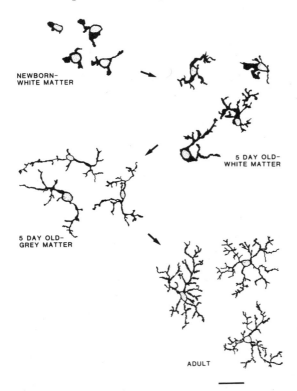

NEWBORN-
WHITE MATTER

5 DAY OLD-
WHITE MATTER

5 DAY OLD-
GREY MATTER

ADULT

Figure 3.2. Tranformations of macrophages which enter the developing CNS from the blood, pass through intermediate forms, and differentiate to become microglial cells of the adult. The cells are labeled immunocytochemically using the monoclonal antibody F4/80, which binds to antigen in the membrane and is specific for mouse macrophages. Scale bar = 25 μm. From Perry and Gordon, *Trends Neurosci.* 11:273–277 (1988).

nucleus containing dense chromatin clumps and light nucleoplasm, scant cytoplasm containing lipid inclusions, lysosomes, and abundant vesicles but sparse granular endoplasmic reticulum, scattered free ribosomes, and few or no microfilaments or microtubules (Peters *et al.*, 1976).

Microglial cells enter the CNS well before the onset of neuronal death (Ashwell, 1989). Nevertheless, microglial cells containing abundant electron-dense inclusion bodies and what seems to be phagocytosed debris, in the normal developing CNS, show that the microglial cells play a role as macrophages which remove the debris of cells that die during normal development and after injury to the CNS. These macrophages are especially numerous in those regions where massive neuronal death oc-

curs during development, for example, in the lateral motor column of the spinal cord of the chick embryo (see Section 8.6). Microglial cells proliferate around facial nerve neurons undergoing chromatolysis after transection of their axons (Graeber *et al.*, 1988; see Section 5.17). Macrophages are necessary for clearance of myelin and for initiating mitosis of Schwann cells during Wallerian degeneration, as discussed in Sections 3.9 and 5.17 (Beuche and Friede, 1984; Lunn *et al.*, 1989; Stoll *et al.*, 1989).

Brain macrophages can be recognized by their staining with silver carbonate (Stensaas and Reichert, 1971; Ling, 1976); by their uptake of horseradish peroxidase or carbon particles (Ivy and Killackey, 1978; McKenna, 1979; Leong *et al.*, 1983; Kaur *et al.*, 1986, 1987); and by cytochemical staining for nonspecific esterase (Ling *et al.*, 1982), thiamine pyrophosphatase (Murabe and Sano, 1982), aryl sulfatase (Ling, 1977), ATPase (Ling, 1977; Ferrer and Sarmiento, 1980), acid phosphatase (Ling, 1977); and 5'-nucleotidase (Kreutzberg and Barron, 1978; Kaur *et al.*, 1984, 1987). These enzymes are not specific for microglia, and also occur in macroglial cells (Vercelli-Retta *et al.*, 1976; Abe *et al.*, 1979; Zimmerman and Cammer, 1982). Immunocytochemical staining with a battery of available antibodies has been extremely useful for identifying microglial cells in various states of rest or activation (Streit *et al.*, 1988, review).

There is little difficulty in recognizing the two types of macroglial cells, namely, astrocytes and oligodendrocytes, when they are mature, although immature forms are more difficult to distinguish from one another. Immature astrocytes have more cytoplasmic organelles, granular endoplasmic reticulum, and microtubules than mature astrocytes. Mature Type 1 astrocytes have a lucent cytoplasm, sparse cytoplasmic organelles except for mitochondria which are prominent, and bundles of intermediate filaments 9 nm in diameter which stain with antibodies against vimentin as well as filaments which are stained with antibodies against their major subunit, the glial fibrillary acid protein (GFAP). In addition, they may contain lysosomes and glycogen granules and may be attached to a capillary. Type 1 astrocytes have finger-like or sheet-like processes which penetrate between the surrounding cells. Type 2 astrocytes have processes that associate with the internodes of myelinating axons.

Oligodendrocytes have fewer cytoplasmic processes than astrocytes, have abundant endoplasmic reticulum and ribosomes, have a high density of cytoplasmic organelles, and contain a prominent Golgi apparatus and vesicles and many cytoplasmic microtubules. Oligodendrocytes lack filaments that react with antibodies against vimentin or GFAP. The oligodendrocyte active in myelination has more extensive cytoplasmic processes, has more abundant cytoplasmic organelles, and therefore has a darker overall appearance than the mature, resting oligodendrocyte. Molecular markers of oligodendrocytes are the isoenzyme II of carbonic anhydrase (Ghandour *et al.*, 1980; Langley *et al.*, 1980; Cammer, 1984) and galactocerebroside (Raff *et al.*, 1979), which can be detected by immunostaining.

This summary of the characteristics of different types of glial cells barely does justice to the diversity of structures that are actually seen. This polymorphism is due to regional variations in cell structure and especially to differences that reflect various functional states. For those reasons, one has to be particularly critical of attempts to deduce glial cell lineage from electron microscopic pictures of small areas of fixed tissue. Schultz and Pease (1959) showed that it is almost impossible to differentiate among different types of ameboid microglial cells by their light or electron microscopic appearances. It is best to be skeptical of any interpretation such as that of Vaughn and Peters (1968) and Vaughn (1969) that *"small glioblasts, which resemble microglia very closely, are multipotential cells capable of producing macroglia as well as microglia."* Ideally, careful evaluation of cell types and transitional forms can provide circumstantial evidence of the lineage relationships between the forms. In practice, it is extremely difficult to deduce cell lineages from morphology. The fact that one type of cell can be recognized earlier in development than another is very poor evidence that the first gave rise to the second. Nevertheless, many authors have been victims of such *post hoc ergo propter hoc* reasoning.

3.3. Lineages of Macroglial Cells

The mechanisms by which different types of macroglial cells diversify may be cell lineage dependent and may also depend on cell interactions. This is one of the reasons for tracing cell lineages and for investigating the conditions that alter cell fates. Ideally, cell lineages are traced by marking an identified progenitor with a heritable cell lineage marker and tracing the labeled progeny. Recombinant retroviral tracers have shown that glial cells and neurons can originate from the same progenitor in the rat and chick embryo CNS (see Section 2.11).

Cell lineages cannot be deduced from purely descriptive morphological evidence or from the sequence of appearance of different cell types. Many such attempts have been made with inconclusive or conflicting results (Ramon-Moliner, 1958; Smart and Leblond, 1961; Vaughn, 1969; Skoff *et al.*, 1976a,b; Privat *et al.*, 1981). These early studies gave rise to a controversy over the identification of progenitors of various types of macroglial cells. Each of the logical alternatives has had its proponents: either the different glial cell types originate from different progenitors, or they originate from the same progenitor (simultaneously or successively), or one type transforms into another through intermediate forms (reviewed by Skoff, 1980; Wood and Bunge, 1984; Fedoroff, 1985).

Investigation of this problem has been greatly facilitated by the availability of cell type-specific antibodies that can be used to identify progenitors, possible intermediate forms, and terminally differentiated neuroglial cell types. Available cell type-specific markers include GD_3 ganglioside, a glycolipid marker of both neuronal and glial precursor cells in the cerebral subependymal zone and cerebellar external granular layer in young rats (Goldman *et al.*, 1984; Rosner *et al.*, 1984; M. Hirano and Goldman, 1988); carbonic anhydrase II, a marker of oligodendrocytes (Ghandour *et al.*, 1980; Kumpulainen *et al.*, 1983; Cammer, 1984); galactocerebroside, an oligodendrocyte marker (Raff *et al.*, 1979; Zalc *et al.*, 1981); vimentin, an intermediate filament marker of radial glial cells (Dahl *et al.*, 1981; Dupouey *et al.*, 1985; Traub, 1985, review; Hutchins and Casagrande, 1989); and glial fibrillary acidic protein, an intermediate filament marker of astrocytes (see Section 5.7; Eng *et al.*, 1971; Bignami *et al.*, 1972; Bignami and Dahl, 1974; Raff *et al.*, 1979; Raju *et al.*, 1981; Trimmer *et al.*, 1982). S100 protein (Moore, 1965) is detectable by immunocytochemistry in mature astrocytes (Matus and Mughal, 1975; Ghandour *et al.*, 1981a,b; Legrand *et al.*, 1981). It is expressed in mature astrocytes at a level at least 10 times that in other cell types. It is a dimer consisting of two 11-kDa subunits, alpha and beta, and is structurally related to the calcium-binding protein, calmodulin, and to intestinal vitamin D-dependent calcium binding protein (Kuwano *et al.*, 1984, 1986). S100 protein functions in calcium-dependent interactions with other proteins.

Glial cells can be identified unambiguously by their expression of certain combinations of these markers. Typically, oligodendrocytes are GC$^+$, CA$^+$, GFAP$^-$, whereas astrocytes are GFAP$^+$, GC$^-$, CA$^-$. Additional antibodies can be used to distinguish between types of astrocytes as discussed below. The "antigenic phenotypes" of differentiated glial cell types have been used to trace their origins from cells that appear earlier in development and express antigenic phenotypes of progenitor cells, for example, GD$_3$$^+$, which is a marker of glial progenitor cells in the postnatal brain. The appearance of "intermediate antigenic phenotypes" may be evidence for lineage relationships.

Simultaneous expression on one cell of markers that typically belong to two different glial cell types is one kind of evidence of development of transitional cell types. For example, expression of glial fibrillary acid protein (GFAP), an astrocyte marker, in oligodendrocytes in human fetal CNS has been interpreted to mean that both astrocytes and oligodendrocytes originate from the same progenitor and that transitional forms exist (Choi *et al.*, 1983; Choi and Kim, 1984, 1985). A similar conclusion may also be drawn from the evidence that carbonic anhydrase II, an oligodendrocyte marker, is also expressed in some developing astrocytes in the gray matter of adult rat CNS (Cammer and Tosney, 1988). GD$_3$ ganglioside, a marker of macroglial progenitor cells, is also expressed transiently in developing oligodendrocytes (Goldman *et al.*, 1984) but is lost from differentiated oligodendrocytes and astrocytes (Norton and Farooq, 1989). Cells with ultrastructural characteristics of oligodendrocytes also express GFAP (Choi *et al.*, 1983; Choi and Kim, 1984, 1985). It has been suggested that there is a lineage relationship between rat brain macrophages and oligodendrocytes on the evidence that cells with macrophage phenotype also express galactocerebroside, an oligodendrocyte marker (Mallat and Chamak, 1989). It should be recognized that those antigens may have distinct biological functions that are not directly related to cell lineages. Thus, vimentin is found in reactive microglial cells but not in quiescent microglia (Graeber *et al.*, 1988). The switch from vimentin to GFAP is related to the change from motile astrocytes with short processes to stationary astrocytes with long processes (Duffy *et al.*, 1982). The functional roles of intermediate filaments is considered at greater length in Section 5.7.

The analysis of glial cell lineages is facilitated by the ease with which glial cells from different regions of the CNS grow in primary cultures in which factors can be identified that alter cell proliferation and differentiation. Clonal culture of a single progenitor or observation of a single clone in a complex culture, and the use of cell type-specific antibodies can show the types of glial cells that originate from a single progenitor under different conditions, for example, in the presence or absence of growth factors or of specific blocking antibodies. Finally, the results of the tissue culture experiments have to be confirmed by observation *in vivo:* identification of the cells by means of light and electron microscopic immunohistology, and experimental alterations of cell proliferation, differentiation, and survival *in vivo,* after injections of growth factors, blocking antibodies, or cytotoxic agents, for example.

The power of such a program of experimental analysis is shown by recent studies of glial cell lineages in cultures of glial cell progenitor cells from the rat optic nerve (Raff, 1989; Wolwijk and Noble, 1989; Miller *et al.*, 1989, reviews) and from postnatal rat brain (Goldman *et al.*, 1984; LeVine and Goldman, 1988) or bovine brain (Norton and Farooq, 1989). This analysis depends on the fact that primary cultures of glial cells can be grown from optic nerve or brain from rats at various pre- and postnatal ages. The cells can be grown under different conditions (with or without fetal calf serum or growth factors) and the cultured cells can be identified by means of cell type-specific antibodies (Fig. 3.3).

The lineages of optic nerve glial cells have been analyzed by using a battery of cell type-specific monoclonal antibodies to characterize the types of glial cells that grow in cultures from optic nerves of rats at different embryonic and postnatal ages (Raff, 1989; Miller *et al.*, 1989, reviews). The 0-2A progenitors migrate into the optic stalk from the brain

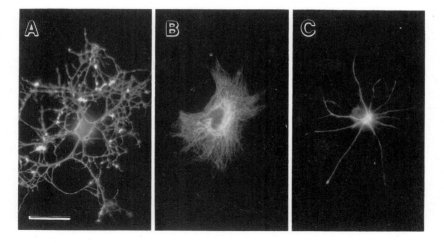

Figure 3.3. Three main types of macroglial cells in perinatal rat optic nerve. Immunofluorescence micrographs of cells in culture. (A) Oligodendrocyte labeled on its surface with monoclonal antibody against galactocerebroside. (B) Type 1 astrocyte labeled intracellularly with antiserum against GFAP. (C) Type 2 astrocyte labeled intracellularly with antiserum against GFAP. Magnification bar = 20 μm. Courtesy of Dr. M. C. Raff.

starting at E17 in rats (Miller *et al.*, 1989). They can be identified because they stain with A2B5 and NSP-4 antibodies and express vimentin. By contrast, the progenitor that gives rise to Type 1 astrocytes originates in the optic stalk itself, and it stains with anti-Ran-2 but not with antibody A2B5 (Raff *et al.*, 1984). Retinal astrocytes migrate from the optic nerve into the retina on E18–E22 in the rat (Watanabe and Raff, 1988; Ling *et al.*, 1989).

0-2A progenitor cells in adult rats have different characteristics from those in perinatal rats (Wolswijk and Nobel, 1989). The adult 0-2A cells express an antigen labeled with 04 monoclonal antibody (Sommer and Schachner, 1981) which is not expressed on perinatal 0-2A cells. Compared with the perinatal 0-2A cells, the adult 0-2A cells have a much longer cycle time (65 hours compared with 18 hours), a slower rate of migration (4 μm/hour compared with 21 μm/hour) and a longer time course of differentiation into oligodendrocytes *in vitro* (more than 5 days compared with less than 3 days). These differences appear to be functional modifications for different roles in the perinatal and adult periods: during the perinatal period rapid proliferation and fast migration are necessary, but those characteristics are not required in the adult.

Type 1 astrocytes appear first in the optic nerve of the rat fetus on E16, originating locally from the ventricular germinal cells of the optic stalk. They can be identified *in vitro* and *in vivo* by staining with antibodies to GFAP and a glycoprotein called Ran-2 but are not labeled with tetanus toxin or with A2B5 or NSP-4 antibodies. In culture without neurons they have a large cell body and lack long processes, but they change their morphology and form long processes when cocultured with neurons (Miller *et al.*, 1989). In the rat optic nerve, Type 1 astrocytes have long processes with endfeet surrounding blood vessels and others extending to the outer surface to form the glial external limiting membrane. Type 1 astrocytes react to injury by proliferating and forming a glial scar (Miller *et al.*, 1986).

Type 2 astrocytes appear in the rat optic nerve starting on P8–P10. They express NSP-4 antigen and surface glycoproteins stained by A2B5 antibodies. They are characterized specifically by 9-nm intermediate filaments containing GFAP and also stain positively for vimentin. Processes of Type 2 astrocytes enfold the nodes of Ranvier (ffrench-Constant *et al.*, 1986; ffrench-Constant and Raff, 1986).

Oligodendrocytes in the optic nerve appear first on the day of birth and continue to be formed until at least P14 in the rat. They express vimentin transiently but when fully differentiated they lack any kind of intermediate filaments. Oligodendrocytes can be stained specifically with antibodies against galactocerebroside, which is the major galac-

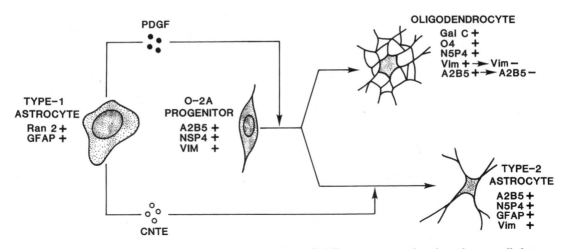

Figure 3.4. How the timing and direction of 0-2A progenitor cell differentiation are thought to be controlled. Type 1 astrocytes, the first glial cells to develop in the rat optic nerve, secrete PDGF, which stimulates 0-2A progenitor cells to proliferate until an intrinsic timing mechanism in the progenitor cell initiates the process that leads to oligodendrocyte differentiation. The first cells differentiate into oligodendrocytes on the day of birth. Beginning in the 2nd postnatal week a CNTF-like protein, which might also be made by Type 1 astrocytes, is produced in large amounts; it acts on residual proliferating progenitor cells to initiate their differentiation into Type 2 astrocytes. The cell morphologies are shown as they appear in culture of glial cells isolated from perinatal optic nerve (see Fig. 3.3). These glial cells can be identified unambiguously by their morphology and positive staining with antibodies. Modified from M. C. Raff, *Science* 243:1450–1455 (1989).

tolipid of myelin (Raff *et al.*, 1978; Ranscht *et al.*, 1982). Each oligodendrocyte extends processes to wrap around and myelinate about 10–20 axonal internodes.

The conclusions from those findings are that the two types of glial cells involved in formation of myelin at internodes and in formation of the nodes of Ranvier, namely, oligodendrocytes and Type 2 astrocytes, originate from the same progenitor called the 0-2A progenitor (Fig. 3.4). In the rat optic nerve the glial cells originate in a regular sequence: oligodendrocytes appearing at the time of birth and Type 2 astrocytes in the second postnatal week. The 0-2A progenitor cells are found throughout the CNS, wherever axons are myelinated (Goldman *et al.*, 1986; LeVine and Stallcup, 1987). Their characteristics change in the adult as they adapt for their role of slow replacement of macroglial cells (Wolswijk and Nobel, 1989).

Both 02A progenitors and Type 1 astrocytes probably originate by transformation from radial glial cells in the ventricular and subventricular zones and later migrate into white or gray matter. In the subventricular zone astrocytes develop by

transformation of radial glial cells (Choi and Lapham, 1978; Schmechel and Rakic, 1979; Levitt and Rakic, 1980; Dahl *et al.*, 1981; Schnitzer *et al.*, 1981; Bovolenta *et al.*, 1984; Pixley and DeVellis, 1984; Benjelloun-Touimi *et al.*, 1985; LeVine and Goldman, 1988; Misson *et al.*, 1988; Voigt, 1989). Oligodendrocytes in the spinal cord are derived from radial glial cells (Choi, 1981; Choi *et al.*, 1983; Choi and Kim, 1984; M. Hirano and Goldman, 1988).

It is significant that oligodendrocytes develop relatively late—always after completion of axonal outgrowth in the CNS. This is necessary because oligodendrocytes exert a strong inhibition on axonal growth and regeneration. This is caused by membrane-bound inhibitors on the surfaces of differentiated oligodendrocytes and CNS myelin of mammals, birds, and reptiles but not amphibians and fishes (Caroni and Schwab, 1988a,b, 1989; Schwab and Caroni, 1988). The inhibitory activity is not species specific. It is neutralized by monoclonal antibody IN-1, which binds to the isolated inhibitory molecules (35 kDa and 25 kDa) and to the surface of living oligodendrocytes. These inhibitory molecules develop only after the completion of axonal growth in the CNS but before my-elination (Caroni and Schwab, 1989). The differentiated oligodendrocytes are nonpermissive substrates for axonal growth in the CNS and *in vitro* (Schwab and Caroni, 1988). By contrast, astrocytes are either neutral or favorable substrates for axonal growth. Control of axonal growth is considered in Chapter 5.

3.4. Control of Glial Cell Development by Growth Factors

Whether 0-2A progenitor cells give rise to Type 2 astrocytes or to oligodendrocytes depends on growth factors, and there is good evidence that platelet-derived growth factor (PDGF) and ciliary neurotrophic factor (CNTF), produced by Type 1 astrocytes, control the production of oligodendrocytes and Type 2 astrocytes, respectively (Fig. 3.4).

0-2A progenitor cells dissociated *in vitro* from embryonic or newborn rat optic nerve stop dividing and differentiate within 2 days, either into oligodendrocytes (if cultured without serum) or into Type 2 astrocytes (if cultured in 10% fetal calf serum). There is good evidence that Type 1 astrocytes are the source of the factors that determine whether the 0-2A progenitor cells continue to divide and that determine the pathway of differentiation the 0-2A progenitor cells will enter. The evidence shows that Type 1 astrocytes secrete PDGF (Deuel, 1987, review), which stimulates proliferation of 0-2A progenitor cells. PDGF is a 32-kDa heterodimer consisting of two homologous polypeptide chains, A and B, that are disulfide linked. Each of them stimulates cell proliferation by binding to the same receptor, which is a 180-kDa membrane glycoprotein (Williams, 1989, review). Activation of the receptor by PDGF results in expression of many genes, including the *c-myc* and *c-fos* protooncogenes. The oncogene counterparts of these genes are associated with cell proliferation and transformation.

The mechanisms by which the cells stop dividing and differentiate to form oligodendrocytes appear to involve an intrinsic clock that counts the number of mitoses before the 0-2A cells withdraw from the mitotic cycle. Thus, PDGF would have only a permissive role in oligodendrocyte differentiation. By contrast, Type 2 astrocyte differentiation re-quires instructive factors, one of which is CNTF or a similar protein, released by Type 1 astrocytes (see Section 8.17). CNTF has a transient effect because the Type 2 astrocytes that it induces lose their GFAP after a few days and go on to become oligodendrocytes. By contrast, fetal calf serum contains factor(s) that promote permanent differentiation of Type 2 astrocytes and are therefore either different from CNTF or include additional factors.

In summary: the production of oligodendrocytes or Type 2 astrocytes from bipotential 0-2A progenitor cells is controlled by soluble growth factors. PDGF acts as a mitogen, stimulating division of 0-2A cells, which is a permissive condition for production of oligodendrocytes. CNTF is an instructive factor for Type 2 astrocyte differentiation. In addition to PDGF and CNTF, neuroglial cells secrete a number of other growth factors and also respond to factors that stimulate their proliferation. Three such factors have been well characterized, namely, glia maturation factor, insulin-like growth factor I, and colony-stimulating factors.

Glia maturation factor beta (GMF-beta) is a 17-kDa acidic protein that has been purified from bovine brain (Lim *et al.*, 1989a,b). Sequencing of GMF-beta shows no similarity to other known growth factors (Lim and Miller, 1988; Lim *et al.*, 1990). Using a monoclonal antibody against GMF-beta, Lim *et al.* (1987) showed that GMF-beta occurs in the CNS of all vertebrates from fish to primates, is maximal during development but persists throughout life, and is localized in astrocytes and in Schwann cells of growing and regenerating nerves but not in Schwann cells of intact adult nerves. However, GMF-beta is expressed 3 days after section of the sciatic nerve of the rat and continues to be expressed in Schwann cells associated with regenerating axons (Bosch *et al.*, 1989). GMF-beta stimulates proliferation and differentiation of astrocytes and Schwann cells in culture (Bosch *et al.*, 1984, 1989; Lim *et al.*, 1985, 1989a,b, 1990; Lim, 1985, review). GMF-beta may have an autocrine action on astrocytes, that is, secretion of the growth factor is not required. It also may have a paracrine action on neuroepithelial cells, involving short-range secretion. GMF inhibits proliferation and promotes differentiation of neuroblastoma cells *in vitro* (Lim *et al.*, 1988).

Insulin-like growth factors (IGF) I and II are

peptides that are structurally similar to proinsulin. IGF I is produced mainly in the liver in response to pituitary growth hormone and is bound to proteins in the blood. IGF I is also known as somatomedin C because it acts as an intermediate in the action of somatotrophin (growth hormone), which does not act directly on its target tissues (Froesch *et al.*, 1985, Nissley and Rechler, 1984; Baksin *et al.*, 1988, reviews). The IGF I receptor is an oligomer composed of a 130 kDa alpha subunit (115 kDa in the brain) containing the binding site, and a 90-kDa beta subunit with protein kinase activity, the phosphorylation of which is stimulated by the growth factor. Both IGF I and II and their receptors are found in fetal and adult mammalian CNS. The function of IGF II is not known. The IGF I gene is expressed in cultured astrocytes, indicating that IGF is produced by astrocytes, and addition of IGF I to cultured astrocytes stimulates their proliferation (Balloti *et al.*, 1987). IGF I increases the number of oligodendrocytes *in vitro* up to 60-fold, either by increasing proliferation or by promoting preferential differentiation from a bipotential precursor or both (McMorris *et al.*, 1986).

Colony-stimulating factors, which are glycoproteins that stimulate proliferation and differentiation of hematopoietic cells (Metcalf, 1985; Clark and Kamens, 1987), also promote the proliferation and inflammatory response of ameboid microglia *in vitro* or in the rat cerebral cortex (Giulian and Ingeman, 1988). Other immunomodulators including interleukin 1, interleukin 2, interferon gamma, and tumor necrosis factor have no effect on ameboid microglia *in vitro* (Giulian and Ingeman, 1988).

The concept that is supported by all these findings is that local cell interactions, mediated by polypeptide growth factors, exert positive and negative controls of glial cell proliferation and determine the entry of glial cells into alternative pathways of differentiation.

3.5. Glial Cell Production and Loss

Death and replacement of neuroglial cells in the adult human brain were first proposed long ago (F. Allen, 1912). This remained a premature theory until autoradiography enabled Smart and Leblond (1961) to confirm that macroglial cells are formed in the adult mouse brain.

Measurement of [^{3}H]thymidine uptake into macroglial cells shows that there is a continuous proliferation resulting in formation of about $150-240 \times 10^3$ new glial cells every day in the adult mouse (Smart and Leblond, 1961; Dalton *et al.*, 1968). Postnatal gliogenesis has since been repeatedly confirmed in mice and rats (Altman, 1962a, 1966a,b; Hommes and Leblond, 1967; Dalton *et al.*, 1968; P. D. Lewis, 1968a,b; Hinds, 1968a,b; Gilmore, 1971; H. Korr *et al.*, 1973; Smart, 1976, 1983; Sturrock, 1974a,b, 1979; Kaplan and Hinds, 1980; Korr, 1983; Parnavelas *et al.*, 1983; Debbage, 1986). Since the glial cell populations are in a steady state in healthy adult mammals, there must be loss of glial cells to balance their production. Pyknotic glial cells are evidence of glial cell death in the normal adult central nervous system (Korr, 1978b). The presence of glial cell progenitor cells in adult mammalian brains is proof that the potential for gliogenesis persists (see Section 3.3).

In adult rats the glial progenitor cell that gives rise to Type 2 astrocytes and oligodendrocytes in the optic nerve is fundamentally different from its counterpart in perinatal rats: the adult glial progenitor cell has a much longer cell cycle, slower rate of migration, different morphology, and different antigenic profile (Wolswijk and Noble, 1989). It is not known whether the 0-2A progenitor cells in the adult transform directly from the perinatal 0-2A cells or whether they have a different origin. Whereas almost all such evidence comes from mice and rats, there are some studies indicating that postnatal turnover of glial cells occurs in the rabbit (Robain, 1970; Sturrock, 1982), cat (Fleischauer, 1966, 1968; Haug, 1972), dog (Lord and Duncan, 1987), calf (Norton and Farooq, 1989), and monkey (Phillips, 1973).

From these studies it is clear that glial cells are produced and die throughout life in mice and rats, and probably in all mammals. After injection of tritiated thymidine followed by autoradiography, only macroglial cells are labeled, indicating that microglia do not proliferate in the healthy brains of postnatal mammals (Korr, 1980).

Differentiated astroglial and oligodendroglial cells are capable of proliferation but may remain temporarily arrested in the G_1 phase of the cell cycle. Mitotic oligodendrocytes comprise 21% of the mitotic population in the corpus callosum and hippocampal commissure of rats at P17. The rate of glial cell proliferation may be quite rapid: generation times between 19 and 20 hours were measured in the subependymal zone of the rat between E18 and P21, and these dividing subependymal cells are probably all glioblasts (Paterson *et al.*, 1973; P.D. Lewis and Lai, 1974; Sturrock and Smart, 1980). The earlier estimates of very long cell cycle times for glial cells (Noetzel, 1962; S. Fuji, 1966; S. Fujita *et al.*, 1966) were incorrect. Korr (1980b) found a cycle time of 20 hours for both oligodendrocytes and astrocytes. The durations of phases of the glial cell cycle remain the same from the end of the fetal period throughout postnatal life in the rodent brain (Korr, 1980).

In adult mammals no increase in total DNA content of the brain can be detected, so that cell production must be in equilibrium with cell loss. This turnover is mostly or entirely of glial cells: most authors agree that the only neurons formed postnatally in the mammalian brain are granule cells whose production is restricted to a relatively short postnatal period (Altman, 1963; Kaplan and Hinds, 1977; Kaplan, 1981; Altman and Bayer, 1987, review).

It is difficult to determine the time of prenatal onset of glial cell proliferation because the different types of immature glial cells are difficult to identify histologically, and because the label is diluted during the survival period of several weeks after a prenatal [³H]thymidine injection. However, the presence of labeled glial cells shows that their proliferation must have started before the time of injection of the tracer. Evidence of that kind reveals that glial cell proliferation starts during the period of neuron production, for example at E12 in the mouse olfactory bulb (Hinds, 1968), in the indusium griseum of the mouse at E11 (Sturrock, 1978b), and in the red nucleus of the rat at E11/12 (Korr, 1978a). These results are inconsistent with the concept that glial cell production starts only after neuron production has ceased in each region (Fujita, 1965, 1966). **The evidence shows that glial and neuronal cell production occur simultaneously in the mammalian CNS but that glial cell production continues after the cessation of neurogenesis.**

The neuroglial cells are formed by cells that have migrated away from the ventricular germinal zone at an earlier stage. Therefore, the precursors of glial cells, which are aptly termed *glioblasts* (Fujita, 1965a,b), must originate from the neurepithelial germinal cells at the same time as they give origin to neurons. Most glioblasts migrate into the intermediate or mantle zone and into fiber tract and commissures and continue proliferating in those extraventricular sites. Therefore, few mitotic figures are seen in the ventricular germinal zone during the period when glial cells are being produced in extraventricular sites—for example, after day 8 of embryonic development in the chick embryo hindbrain (Harkmark, 1954) or spinal cord (Bensted *et al.*, 1957; H. Fujita and Fujita, 1964; S. Fujita, 1965a,b).

Production of both types of macroglial cells starts prenatally, at the same time as neurons are produced. Neuronal and glial cell progenitors coexist in the cerebral ventricular zone of fetal monkeys (Levitt *et al.*, 1981). Further evidence of the early production of glial cells is that astrocytes are present in a laminated configuration preceding the final lineup of neurons in laminated structures such as the lateral geniculate nucleus (Hutchins and Casagrande, 1988, 1990) and cerebral cortex (Cooper and Steindler, 1980; Steindler *et al.*, 1988). Oligodendrocyte production starts somewhat later than astrocyte production in the same region. Monocytes enter the brain from the blood during the prenatal period and transform into microglial cells but this does not occur in adults (Ling, 1981; Streit *et al.*, 1988, review). Berry and Rogers (1966) found labeled astrocytes, oligodendrocytes, and microglial cells in the rat cerebral cortex after [³H]thymidine injection on E18. Labelled astrocytes were seen in the rat optic nerve after injection of [³H]thymidine on E15/16, but labeled oligodendrocytes were found only after postnatal injection (Skoff *et al.*, 1976b). **In all the regions mentioned, as well as in other regions (indusium griseum, olfactory bulb, and red nucleus), the onset of production of neurons and of glial cells occurs at about the same time. The apparent sequence of neurons first and glial cells afterward is due to the delayed differentiation of glial cells that are produced either before or at the same time as neurons, and to the difficulty of identifying immature glial cells in paraffin sections or even by means of electron microscopy.**

Glioblasts congregate in the subependymal zone (also named subventricular zone) in the lateral ventricles of the forebrain, starting at about E14 in the mouse (Langman and Welch, 1967; Sturrock and Smart, 1980; Sturrock, 1982). The subependymal glioblasts persist throughout life and give rise to all types of glial cells. The glial cells arising from the subependymal glioblasts migrate into and through the overlying white and gray matter. These glioblasts appear to be very susceptible to chemical carcinogens, whereas neurons and their stem cells are greatly resistant to the same agents. As a result, vulnerability of the nervous system to chemical carcinogens is minimal in the rat before 11 days of gestation, during the period of maximal production of neurons. The susceptibility to carcinogens increases after day 11 of gestation, reaches a peak toward the end of gestation, and declines to a low level after the first postnatal month. Virtually all tumors induced by carcinogens are gliomas (reviewed by Kleihues *et al.*, 1976; Russell and Rubinstein, 1977). Astrocytomas are the most frequent neoplasms of the human central nervous system. Several types of neoplasms (astrocytomas, schwannomas, meningiomas, neurofibromas) are associated with partial or complete loss of chromosome 22, and often with additional chromosome abnormalities. These abnormalities are also linked to loss of recessive tumor suppressive genes and expression of dominant oncogenes (Martuza *et al.*, 1988). The role of growth factors and extracellular matrix in proliferation of Schwann cell tumors is considered in Section 3.9.

Neurons affect proliferation and differentiation of glial cells. Mitotic inhibitory or excitatory signals pass from neurons to glial cells, depending on conditions. Thus, failure of production of glial cells occurs after death of the associated neurons. This has been observed in the superior colliculus of the newborn mouse after removal of an eye (DeLong and Sidman, 1962), in the optic tectum of the frog tadpole after eye removal (Cowan *et al.*, 1968), and in the spinal ganglia after removal of a limb (Carr, 1975, 1976). More direct evidence that neurons stimulate glial cell proliferation has been obtained in tissue culture. A pure culture of glial cells is nonproliferative, but addition of neurons stimulates mitosis in the glial cells (McCarthy and Partlow, 1976a,b; Hatten, 1985). In the absence of neurons, hippocampal astrocytes in culture proliferate rapidly, but addition of neurons rapidly inhibits glial cell mitosis and stimulates their differentiation (U. E. Gasser and Hatten, 1990).

Production of glial cells in the central nervous system of healthy adult mammals is well established (F. Allen, 1912; Smart, 1961; Smart and Leblond, 1961; Altman, 1962a, 1966a; Hommes and Leblond, 1967; Korr, 1978b; Sturrock and Smart, 1980; Sturrock, 1982). There is also a turnover of glial cells in various pathological conditions and states of increased function. Reactive hypertrophy without obvious hyperplasia of astrocytes occurs in many pathological conditions—for example, in slow loss of neurons in humans and in hypoglycemia—and has been most fully described and investigated in liver failure, so-called hepatocerebral disease (Cavanagh and Kyu, 1971; Cavanagh, 1974). In these conditions in which the astrocytes increase in size, the number of astrocytes of both fibrous and protoplasmic varieties may also increase, but such reactive hyperplasia is most often the result of acute or subacute loss of neurons (R. D. Adams and Foley, 1953).

The possibility, erroneous as it now seems, that in response to brain injury astrocytes might increase by "amitosis" or division of the nucleus without the formation of a mitotic figure has sometimes been proposed (Penfield, 1932; Hansson and Sourander, 1964; Hugosson *et al.*, 1968). However, in those studies the absence of mitotic figures was an artifact resulting from poor fixation (Cavanagh and Lewis, 1969). When perfusion fixation is used, glial cell mitoses are observed frequently. Lapham (1962) reported that reactive astrocytes may continue to synthesize nuclear DNA without undergoing mitosis and may thus become polyploid. Normal glial cells, however, are diploid, and with the exception of a report of tetraploidy in an unidentified type of glial cell in the human cerebellum (Lapham and Johnstone, 1963; Mann and Yates, 1973b), glial cells in several species have been shown to be diploid.

Several unrelated conditions are associated with an increase in the number of glial cells. An increase in the number of glial cells around motor neurons in the spinal cord of the mouse has been reported after greatly increased motor activity (Kuhlenkampf, 1952). Dehydration of rats results in an increase in the proliferation of glial cells in the hypothalamus (M. Murray, 1968). Autoradiography has also shown proliferation of glial cells in the brains of mice reared in an "enriched environment" (Altman and Das, 1964; Diamond *et al.*, 1964, 1966; see Section 6.12). The factors in these experiments that might have stimulated the production of glial cells are not known. Any of a variety of factors, such as increased sensory and motor activity, increased nutrition, or hormonal stimulation and metabolic changes, independently or in combination, might have stimulated proliferation of glial cells. These reports do not show whether the glial cells originate from stem cells or from fully differentiated neuroglial cells that remain quiescent under normal conditions. DNA synthesis can be reinitiated in fully differentiated glial cells in the adult mouse brain after injury (Ludwin, 1984).

Proliferation of glial cells has been observed around neurons undergoing chromatolysis after their axons have been cut (Cammermeyer, 1963, 1965a,b, 1970; J. Sjöstrand, 1965, 1966a,b; Chow and Dewson, 1966; Olsson and Sjöstrand, 1969; Vaughn and Pease, 1970; Vaughn et al., 1970; Young, 1977; Ling, 1978). In such cases, where peripheral nerves have been cut or crushed, there is no direct injury to the brain, and the labeled glial cells appear around the perikarya of the neurons far from the site of injury to the axons (see Section 5.16). The problem of the origin of these brain macrophages is controversial. Adrian and Smothermon (1970) concluded that the cells that enter the hypoglossal nucleus after injury to the hypoglossal nerve are mononuclear leukocytes. Others have concluded that the microglial cells that appear around axotomized neurons are produced by proliferation of intrinsic microglial cells (Vaughn et al., 1970; Sjöstrand, 1971; Stenwig, 1972; Berner et al., 1973; Torvik, 1975). There have been conflicting reports about the response of different types of glial cells to injury of the central nervous system. Cavanaugh (1970) reported astrocytic proliferation around a needle stab wound in the adult rat brain, whereas Murray and Walker (1973) found no evidence of glial cell proliferation following brain injury, but concluded that all the cells labeled with [³H]thymidine after brain injury are mononuclear leukocytes. One reason for the disagreement is that it is difficult to identify glial cells with the light microscope in autoradiographs because the heavy metal stains for glial cells are incompatible with autoradiography (Sidman, 1970). Electron microscopic evidence of tritiated thymidine labeling of mature oligodendrocytes, astrocytes, and microglia in the adult mouse brain after injury shows that all these types of glial cells respond to brain injury (Ludwin, 1984).

The classical view of Rio-Hortega (1919, 1932) was that microglial cells originate from the mesenchyme of the pia mater during the prenatal period and remain quiescent until activated and transformed into macrophages by trauma or infection. Later authors distinguished between the microglial cells that enter the brain from the blood and those that arise by mitosis of microglial cells in the brain (Maxwell and Kruger, 1965, 1966; Cammermeyer, 1965a–c; Sjöstrand, 1965, 1966a,b). Konigsmark and Sidman (1963a,b) found that after injection of [³H]thymidine into adult mice many labeled leukocytes appear in the blood but few labeled cells are found in the uninjured brain. However, after a stab wound has been made in the brain the previously labeled blood cells appear in the brain. They concluded that leukocytes are a major source of brain macrophages but left open the possibility that up to one-third of the labeled macrophages might originate in the brain. The same conclusion was reached by Adrian and Williams (1973a,b) and Matthews (1974). However, Schelter and Adrian (1986) strongly disagree with the conclusion that macrophages originate by transformation of microglial cells, although it is certain that transformation occurs in the opposite direction.

One of the difficulties in accepting the hematogenous origin of microglial cells in normal CNS was that they seem to enter the CNS much later than the vasculature (Jones, 1970; Mato and Ookawara, 1982), but this may be attributed to failure to identify the relatively few, small monocytes in the neural tube. For example, capillaries are present in chick embryo spinal cord at 4 days of incubation (Feeney and Watterson, 1946) whereas glial cells cannot be recognized until the 8th day (S. Fujita, 1965b). Finding a complete series of transitional forms leading to microglial cells either from the blood vessels or from other elements in the CNS, including the subventricular zone, would help to settle the origin of these cells. It has now been demonstrated by means of a monoclonal antibody specific for mouse macrophages that monocytes enter the central nervous system during embryonic stages and can be traced through a series of intermediate forms as they differentiate into microglia, as shown in Fig. 3.2 (Hume et al., 1983; Perry et al., 1985; Perry and Gordon, 1988). This resolves a major question that has been raised repeatedly throughout this chapter.

In summary, Type 1 astrocytes originate prenatally from neurepithelial cells in the ventricular germinal zone and subsequently migrate into the parenchyma of the CNS where they associate with blood vessels and contribute to formation of the blood–brain barrier (see Section 3.18). Type 1 astrocytes release mitogenic growth factors that promote proliferation and differentiation of oligodendrocytes and Type 2 astrocytes. They are also involved in formation of a glial scar after CNS injury. Type 2 astrocytes and oligodendrocytes originate from a common precursor, the 0-2A cell, that migrates postnatally into all regions of the CNS containing nerve fibers. Microglial cells originate from a specific population of mononuclear leukocytes which penetrate the blood brain barrier to enter the CNS during late fetal and early postnatal periods and transform into microglia.

The populations of astrocytes and oligodendrocytes are continuously renewed by a steady rate of cell proliferation and cell death in the healthy CNS throughout life. Short bursts of increased glial cell proliferation occur during normal development in response to neuron death, neurite outgrowth, synaptogenesis, and myelination, and in response to injury or diseases of the CNS. Macrophages that are mobilized at sites of injury originate both from endogenous microglial cells and from blood monocytes.

The mechanisms of normal turnover of neuroglial cell populations and of stimulation of increased proliferation are not well understood. Mitogenic growth factors are involved, secreted by brain macrophages and astrocytes, and possibly released from injured or dying neurons. Entry of glial cells into alternative pathways of differentiation is controlled by polypeptide growth factors. The action of these factors can be mediated by secretion and uptake through cell surface receptors, namely, paracrine action, or these factors may act internally during intracellular transport of the receptors and growth factors, resulting in autocrine stimulation of cell proliferation. Identification and characterization of these factors, their genes, sites of release and uptake, and the cellular mechanisms of their action are among the most important unfinished tasks.

3.6. A History of Schwann Cells and Myelination

Robert Remak (1837, 1838) discovered the differences between myelinated and unmyelinated nerve fibers, notably the presence of a medullary sheath and the greater diameter of the former. He also observed that unmyelinated fibers, which he called *"organic fibers,"* were characteristic of the sympathetic nervous system and could most easily be observed in the nerves to the spleen of ungulates. Remak (1838) described and illustrated the nuclei attached to the organic fibers before they were again observed by Schwann (1839) in the sheath which bears his name. Nonmedullated nerve fibers in peripheral nerves were first described by Remak (1838) in teased or dissociated peripheral nerves of the rabbit as elongated bands with an average diameter of 3–5 μm. These nonmedullated nerve fibers were henceforth called *"fibers or bands of Remak."*

The term *"myelin"* was introduced by Virchow (1859), to refer to the globules of fatty material, the so-called *"myelin-figures,"* that appear in association with degenerating nerve fibers or after placing fresh myelinated nerve in water. The myelin sheath of normal nerves was generally referred to in the German literature as *"Markscheide"* or *"Nervenmark,"* in the English literature as *"medullary sheath,"* and in French it is usually called *"myéline."* Ramón y Cajal took the term *"mielina"* and other terminology connected with the medullary sheath directly from Louis-Antoine Ranvier (1835–1922), who was one of the principal sources of Cajal's early knowledge of histology.

Summarizing what was then known about myelinated nerve fibers, Max Schultze (1870) states that *"the medullated fibres therefore consist essentially of two constituents, a cortex or sheath of medullary nerve substance, and an axial fibre or axis cylinder, which is either a primitive fibre or a bundle of fibrillae. The medullary sheath forms a more or less thick investment around the axis cylinder and consists of an oily substance containing protagon and capable of powerfully refracting light.*[6] *. . . The medullated fibres of the nerve centres are imbedded in an extremely delicate tenacious connective substance, the peculiar consistence of which preserves the fibres from injury. The medullated fibres of the peripheric nerves, . . . each possess in addition, and external to their medullary sheath, a special investment of connective tissue, constituting the so-called sheath of Schwann."* It is significant that Schultze does not mention the *"cell of Schwann"* in connection with the medullary sheath because at that time the nuclei that Remak (1838) had found along the nerve fiber, both medullated and unmedullated, were not called Schwann cells. Ranvier (1871, 1872) appears to have been the first to designate the cell of Schwann as a separate entity and to have discovered that a single Schwann cell occupies each internodal segment. Vignal (1889) dissected individual Schwann cells off the axon and showed that they ensheath the axon (Fig. 3.5).

In 1839 Schwann himself saw only the nuclei of the medullary sheath, and thus confirmed Remak's description of them. But Schwann supposed that those nuclei had originally belonged to a chain of cells which coalesced to form the nerve fiber. This "*cell-chain*" theory of development of the nerve fiber.continued to receive support for the following 60 years, even after His, Forel, Koelliker, and Cajal provided good evidence supporting the outgrowth theory of development of the axon (see Sections 5.1 and 6.1). The sheath of Schwann continued to be thought of as a syncytium containing many nuclei. As late as 1928 Cajal was willing to admit that the Schwann cells may coalesce to form a syncytium during nerve degeneration (Ramón y Cajal, 1928, p. 130).

Observations of myelination of nerve fibers growing in the tail fin of living frog tadpoles were started by Hensen (1864) and Koelliker (1886) and later their observations were extended by Harrison (1904) and Speidel (1932). Hensen noted that the nerves are at first unmyelinated but became myelinated initially by separate droplets of myelin which later coalesced. Koelliker observed that myelination starts in the neighborhood of the nuclei of the sheath of Schwann and that "*the myelinated regions are at first separated from one another by long unmyelinated stretches.*" Koelliker (1886) then concludes: "*I consider the primitive nerve fibers to be protoplasmic outgrowths of the central nerve cells, in which a central fiber separates from a thin protoplasmic mantle as the first rudiment of the axis cylinder. The nuclei of the sheath of Schwann possibly play a role, and under the influence of these nuclei the protoplasmic covering becomes transformed into real myelin by the deposition of fat. The myelinated fibers in the central nervous system show furthermore, that development of myelin can take place independently of external influences.*"

From the time of discovery of the myelin sheath by Remak there were two schools of thought about the origin of myelin, both of which had serious proponents until the 1950s: either it is a product of the sheath cells or it is formed by the axon itself (see M. Jacobson, in preparation for analysis of the competing research programs on myelination). Proponents of the latter theory pointed out that they could not recognize sheath cells in the central nervous system, and therefore the central myelin must originate as a secretion from the axons. This theory was defended by Koelliker (1896) and by Ramón y Cajal (1909, p. 618), who states that all authorities agree that myelin is "*a product of secretion of the axis cylinder.*" Some continued to hold this opinion as late as 1958 (see Windle, 1958, p. 74). There were also differences in opinion about whether myelin is intracellular or extracellular. Ranvier (1871, 1872) believed that myelin is produced by the sheath cells and is formed inside them, whereas many others thought of myelin as an extracellular material. For example, Ramón y Cajal (1928, p. 41) states that "*the nerve tube contains a thick oleaginous sheath which is placed between the cell of Schwann and the neurite, and which is interrupted, at intervals, to let in more freely the nutritive plasmas.*" By the beginning of the 20th century, the generally accepted concept of structure of the medullated nerve fiber, as described by Koelliker (1896) and Ramón y Cajal (1906), was that the myelin sheath is secreted by the axon and lies between it and the Schwann cells, which are surrounded by a clear "*membrane of Schwann.*" This is surprising when one considers the evidence, given below, that had been accumulating before 1900 indicating that myelin originates in nonneuronal cells supporting the axon. This is another example showing that mu-

---

[6]In 1864, Liebreich, a pupil of Hoppe-Seyler (1825–1895), one of the founders of biochemistry, proposed that protagon was the main chemical constituent of the brain, and that the other constituents, lecithin and cephalin, were its breakdown products. This was generally accepted for the next 30 years (reviewed by Wlassak, 1898), although in 1874 J. L. W. Thudichum (1829–1901) showed that protagon is not a chemical entity but a mixture of several chemicals, including phospholipids and cerebroside. In addition to discovering those chemicals, Thudichum also discovered and characterized brain glycolipids such as sphingomyelin. He is now justly regarded as the founder of neurochemistry, although in his time his findings were regarded as extremely controversial and were unjustly neglected (Rosenheim and Tebb, 1907; Drabkin, 1958; Tower, 1970).

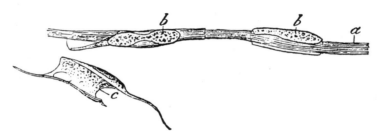

Figure 3.5. The earliest depiction of an individual Schwann cell (Vignal, 1889). The peripheral nerve (a) is shown ensheathed by two Schwann cells (b). One of these has a dumbbell-shaped nucleus, indicating that it may be ready to divide. Vignal dissected individual Schwann cells (c) off the axon, showing that they do not form a syncytium, as was then commonly believed.

tually contradictory theories have coexisted for long periods in the history of neuroscience.

Vignal (1889) first proposed that myelin is produced by Schwann cells and by the *"cellule de revêtement"* which surrounds the myelinated fibers in the CNS. Vignal states that the central myelinating cells *"originate from embryonic cells of the grey substance and have the same origin as the neuroglial cells."* This concept of myelin formation by supporting, nonneural cells is shown in drawings on pp. 27 and 33 of Vignal's book *Développement des éléments du système nerveux cérébro-spinal* (Paris, 1889), one of which is shown in Fig. 3.5. The origin of myelin from nonneural cells was also observed by Wlassak (1889), who showed that the first osmiophilic material appeared in the protoplasm of spongioblasts (i.e., the progenitors of neuroglial cells) in the CNS and in the protoplasm of the Schwann cells, and that these developed before the appearance of myelinated fibers. Wlassak (1898) concluded that *"the nervous supporting tissue at least in the embryonic organism does not merely have a mechanical but also a chemical function. It is a transport apparatus for certain materials which originate from the blood and are transferred to the nerve cells."* However, he was unable to show whether CNS myelin is made by the neuroglial cells or the nerve cells or both. This problem was not clarified further until the 1920s, when Rio-Hortega discovered the role of oligodendrocytes in formation of central myelin (see Section 3.1 and below). The origin of the myelin sheath could only be revealed conclusively with the aid of the electron microscope.

There were also wide divergences of opinion about the structure of the nodes. Remak (1838) and Koelliker (1852) had seen breaks in the medullary sheath but dismissed them as artifacts, and so they

were regarded until 1871. Ranvier (1871, 1872) was the first to demonstrate that each internodal segment is a separate unit associated with a single Schwann cell. In nerves of the mouse stained with silver nitrate he showed that the nodes interrupted all the layers of the myelin sheath and exposed the naked axon, in which there is a disc or ring of material, possibly forming a constriction in the axon itself. In his publications in Spanish, Ramón y Cajal also describes the nodes as *"interrupciones"* or *"estrangulaciones de Ranvier,"* terms which he borrowed from Ranvier, who used the terms *"anneaux constricteurs"* or *"étranglements annulaires"* for the nodes and *"segments interannulairs"* for the internodes. The nodes were termed *"Ranvierschen Schnürringe"* by Koelliker (1896) and other German writers. These terms show that the nodes were generally considered to be some form of constriction or interruption in the continuity of the axon, which were most easily seen in peripheral nerves. Bethe (1903) went so far as to propose that the nodes of Ranvier were septa completely interrupting the continuity of the axon except for the neurofibrils which penetrate the septa and which he thought are responsible for conduction of the nerve impulse. The presence of nodes interrupting the medullary sheath of nerve fibers in the CNS was first reported by Tourneux and Le Goff (1875) but denied by such authorities as Ranvier (1878) and Koelliker (1896). Only after Ramón y Cajal demonstrated nodes in the axons of neurons of the electric lobes of *Torpedo* in 1888 and in the granular layer of the cerebellum (1889) did Flechsig (1889) and Dogiel (1896) find nodes in other central myelinated fibers, using the methylene blue stain of Ehrlich (1885).

The incisures of Schmidt–Lanterman (Schmidt, 1874; Lanterman, 1876) were considered to be artifacts. Koelliker (1896, vol. 2, pp. 7–15) devotes eight pages to them and finally concludes that they are not present in normal living nerve fibers. An immense literature describing artifacts or debating the authenticity of structures in the axon and its medullary sheath was produced during the 19th century, and many terms had a transient currency. Consequently, the early descriptions of the myelin sheath are often impossible to reconcile with current knowledge. The most notorious of these fixation or precipitation artifacts are the cones of Golgi–Rezzonico, which were beautifully illustrated by Golgi (1880) as periodically repeating, cone-shaped spirals of a threadlike material (Golgi's original drawings are reproduced in Zanobio, 1975). Various perinodal apparatuses were minutely described and illustrated (Frommann's lines, spiny bracelets of Nageotte, Ranvier's crosses). These were probably due to selective penetration of stains into the axon at the nodes of Ranvier. Errors are universal, and they are noted here as the natural consequences of the limitations of the available techniques. Users are not to be condemned for the limitations of their methods, but the users themselves are made vulnerable by techniques.

The ectodermal origin of Schwann cells was first postulated by Nansen (1887).[7] This was supported by others (e.g., Froriep, 1907; Nageotte, 1905; Doinikow, 1911). Harrison (1906, 1924) proved the neurectodermal origin of Schwann cells by showing their absence after removal of the neural crest in amphibian embryos. Nageotte (1918) observed that several nonmedullated nerve fibers are enclosed within separate tunnels in a single sheath cell, but Ramón y Cajal (1933) claimed that each axon is individually enveloped by a special Schwann cell. Electron microscopy was to prove Nageotte in the right.

The history of this subject provides yet another example of a problem being hotly disputed by eminent neurohistologists for almost a century before it was finally resolved in a few years by the use of the electron microscope (Geren, 1954; I. D. Robertson, 1955). In retrospect it seems just as well that there were only a few investigators of myelin, because battalions of light microscopists armed with the best instruments and all the available techniques for staining myelin could never have resolved its structure and thus reached an understanding of its development. More progress was made in understanding myelin in the decade from 1954 to 1964 than had been achieved in the previous century. An excellent review of the early days of electron microscopy of myelin is given by J. D. Robertson (1987). The application of electron microscopy put an end to the debate and confusion that existed before 1953 by showing that in peripheral nerves the myelin sheath is a tongue of the Schwann cell wrapped around the

---

[7]Fridjhof Nansen (1861–1930) is well known for his Arctic explorations and his work of reconstruction after World War I, for which he was awarded the Nobel Prize for Peace in 1923. Here I wish to emphasize the point that he was able to entertain simultaneously parts of both the neuron theory and the reticular theory of nerve connections. Nansen learned the silver chromate technique directly from Golgi during a visit to Pavia in 1886. He had begun his investigations of the nervous system in 1882 and they were published in detail in 1886-1887 entitled *The Structure and Combination of the Histological Elements of the Central Nervous System*. He described the nerve cells and glial cells in the hagfish and marine annelids called myzostomes. Nansen adopted Golgi's classification of nerve cells into motor and sensory groups. He showed motor nerve cells with long axis cylinders emerging from the nerve centers, which bear collateral branches that ramify in the centers. The sensory nerve cells were shown with branched axons which connect with the collaterals of the motor nerve cells. Nansen did not see direct connections between these nerve fibers in the fibrillary plexuses as Golgi claimed to have found, and thus anticipated a part of what was to become the neuron theory. However, in agreement with Golgi, Nansen excluded the nerve cell body and dendrites from the conducting pathways. This is an important example

showing that significant parts of two opposing theories may be simultaneously tenable in the mind of a neuroscientist (see M. Jacobson, in preparation, for other examples). Nansen's work was published simultaneously with papers by Koelliker (1886), His (1886, 1887), and Forel (1887) which showed the individuality of nerve cells, outgrowth of the axon from the nerve cell body, and dependence of the axon's vitality on continuity with the cell body. That evidence established what came to be called the neuron theory as a rival to the already well-established reticular theory. From that time on the neuron theory continued to predict new findings while the reticular theory did not. Ramón y Cajal entered the field of neurocytology in 1888 and contributed his first really novel evidence supporting the neuron theory in 1890, namely, his description of migration of cerebellar granule cells and formation of their axons, the parallel fibers. Of course, His had already shown the independent migration of neurons from the neural crest in 1868 and in the neural tube in 1887.

axon like a scroll around a rod (Geren and Raskin, 1953; Geren, 1954; J. D. Robertson, 1955; A. Peters and Muir, 1959; A. Peters, 1960, 1964a,b). Ultrastructural evidence showing that myelination in the CNS is performed by oligodendrocytes wrapping cytoplasmic processes around axons was first provided by Farquhar and Hartman (1957), R. L. Schultz et al. (1957), and Mugnaini and Walberg (1964). This is discussed further in Section 3.11. If the truth about the mode of myelination had been revealed to Schwann he would have found it utterly unbelievable.[8]

The role of glial cells in myelination of axons in the CNS also remained an area of uncertainty and disputation until the 1960s. Several investigators had produced circumstantial evidence that interfascicular oligodendrocytes are involved in myelination. The rapid increase in oligodendrocytes in central tracts prior to their myelination and the invariable presence of oligodendrocytes during myelination in the CNS were very suggestive observations (Rio-Hortega, 1924, 1928; Penfield, 1924; Linell and Tom, 1931; Morrison, 1932). As the role of oligodendrocytes in myelination could not be proved, other hypotheses were entertained in which the role of myelin production was assigned to the axons themselves or to the astrocytes (Alpers and Haymaker, 1934; Scharf, 1951; Hild, 1957; Blunt et al., 1972). Finally, electron microscopy showed conclusively that there is continuity between the membrane of the oligodendrocyte and the myelin sheath and that the wrapping of the oligodendrocyte membrane around axons in the CNS is essentially the same as the process of myelination in peripheral nerves (Luse, 1956, 1960; Maturana, 1960; A. Peters, 1960, 1964a,b, 1966; M. B. Bunge et al., 1962; Kruger and Maxwell, 1966; Knobler and Stempak, 1973; C. Meier, 1976). Ironically, poor preparative procedures aided the initial studies of the layering of the myelin sheath: swelling resulted in slight separation of the layers and the scroll formation was easily

[8]History provides many examples of the ingenuities of biological adaptations, for example as described by Charles Darwin (1862) in "The Various Contrivances by which Orchids are Fertilized by Insects," which met with disbelief when they were first discovered. In a letter written in 1868, Darwin remarks "I carefully described to Huxley the shooting out of the Pollinia in Catasetum, and received for an answer, 'Do you really think I can believe all that?'"

seen. When better methods of intracardiac perfusion and fixation were used, the extracellular space between adjacent turns of the oligodendrocytes around axons in the CNS was absent and their interface was transformed into the intraperiod line (Peters, 1960; Maturana, 1960; Hirano et al., 1966; Hirano and Dembitzer, 1967; Hirano, 1968).

A powerful impetus to studies of development of myelinated fiber tracts was given by the discovery of degeneration (Wallerian degeneration) of the nerve distal to a transection, which was most easily traced in myelinated fibers (Waller, 1851; see Clarke and O'Malley, 1968; Denny-Brown, 1970). Although this showed that survival of the distal nerve segment and its myelin sheath depends on connection with the nerve cell body, it was also interpreted by many, including Cajal, to mean that myelin is produced by the nerve fiber. In 1885 Marchi and Algeri showed that a solution of osmic acid and potassium bichromate stains myelin sheaths of degenerating axons but not normal axons. This proved to be the most useful method of tracing myelinated fiber pathways in the CNS until the introduction of radioactive labeled tracers, horseradish peroxidase, and fluorescent tracers more than 80 years later.

Because myelinated fibers were most easily traced with the available histological techniques, the 19th century literature is dominated by studies of myelogeny. Flechsig (1876, 1920 review) was the first to recognize that myelination occurs at different times in different regions of the CNS, and to use this as a means of tracing fibers in the CNS. In 1876, Flechsig wrote: "During certain periods of fetal life, fibers can be distinguished from each other in a very striking manner, which in the adult are of uniform consistency and differ little from one another. This is because some of them already have a complete myelin sheath, whereas others still exhibit their naked axis cylinders. Thus we are in a position, especially in the compact white matter, to follow for a considerable distance fibers and fiber bundles that later on, owing to the uniformity of their components, become masked in their course." In this way he was able to demonstrate the course of the pyramidal tracts from the cerebral cortex to the spinal cord.

Numerous examples that support an evolutionary but not a revolutionary thesis of the nature of progress in neuroscience can be adduced from the history of myelin (M. Jacobson, Conceptual Foundations of Neuroscience, in preparation).

Concepts did not spring into existence fully formed like Athena from the head of Zeus, nor were the concepts that were most consistent with the evidence at the beginning necessarily the ones that finally turned out to be true. Completely contradictory ideas were held by well qualified people over many decades. For example, belief in the mesodermal origins of all glial cells was refuted very slowly, and the idea that myelin is a secretory product of the axons was held at the same time as the alternative theory that myelin is produced by nonneuronal cells. The contestants were either locked in a stalemate that could not be unlocked with the available techniques or they simply ignored their opponents. That is the main reason for persistence of the theory of axonal secretion of myelin even after the cumulative evidence was strongly, although not conclusively, against it. Crucial experiments that can solve a problem conclusively are very rare in the history of neuroscience, and that is one of the main reasons why conflicting theories can coexist for long periods. A theory that is ultimately accepted as true may languish unrecognized and unaccepted in the prevailing research programs: I call these premature theories.

3.7. How Schwann Cells Interact with Peripheral Nerve Fibers

Schwann cells enfold all axons in the peripheral nerves, including those that remain unmyelinated. Interactions with axons are involved in the following Schwann cell activities: mitosis (Wood and Bunge, 1975; McCarthy and Partlow, 1976; Salzer and Bunge, 1980; Salzer et al., 1980a,b; De Vries et al., 1982; Pleasure et al., 1985; Ratner et al., 1987); synthesis of basement membrane components (M. B. Bunge et al., 1982; Carey et al., 1983; Clark and Bunge, 1989); the expression of myelin components (Mirsky et al., 1980; Brocker et al., 1981; Politis et al., 1982; Poduslo et al., 1985; Brunden and Poduslo, 1987); expression of glia maturation factor (Lim, 1985; Bosch et al., 1989; see Section 3.4); uptake and release of nerve growth factor (Zimmerman and Sutter, 1983; Rohrer, 1985; Taniuchi et al., 1986; Heumann et al., 1987); and modulation of Schwann cell Na$^+$ and K$^+$ channels (Chiu, 1987;

Chiu and Wilson, 1989; Wilson and Chiu, 1990). Enteric neurons exert an inhibitory effect on Schwann cell and enteric glial cell DNA synthesis in culture (Eccleston et al., 1989). Thus inhibitory as well as excitatory signals pass from neurons to regulate mitosis and differentiation of Schwann cells.

The entire complex of Schwann cells and their ensheathed axons is surrounded by a basement membrane. Outside this is another covering of extracellular matrix which forms the endoneurium. Outside these are the epineurium and perineurium formed by fibroblasts. The extracellular matrix molecules surrounding the Schwann cells are secreted exclusively by the Schwann cells. They include laminin, entactin, haparan sulfate proteoglycan, and collagen Types I, III, IV, and V, which can be identified by means of specific antibodies (Bunge and Bunge, 1981; Bunge et al., 1986). Schwann cells secrete laminin in culture whether in contact with neurons or not (Cornbrooks et al., 1983). Although secretion of other extracellular matrix molecules by Schwann cells requires contact with neurons, metabolic labeling experiments show that the Schwann cells themselves secrete these molecules even when the neurons are removed before addition of the labeled precursors (Carey and Bunge, 1981; Carey et al., 1983). Ascorbic acid is required by Schwann cells in order to produce basement membrane (Eldridge et al., 1987). Ascorbic acid thus promotes myelination. Fibronectin, which is present in the extracellular matrix surrounding myelinated nerves, is probably produced by endoneurial fibroblasts and not by Schwann cells (Sanes, 1982; Sanes and Chiu, 1983). The endoneurial fibroblasts as well as the two external sheaths of peripheral nerves, the epineurium and perineurium, are of mesodermal origin (Haninec, 1988).

Schwann cells in culture have neuronal-type Na$^+$ and K$^+$ channels (Chiu and Ritchie, 1984; Gray and Ritchie, 1985). As Schwann cells change from the proliferative to myelinating mode they also lose voltage dependent potassium channels for both inward and outward K$^+$ flux (Chiu, 1987; Chiu and Wilson, 1989; Wilson and Chiu, 1990). CNS glial cells also express different ion channels depending on their differentiation (Barres et al., 1988; Cornell-Bell et al., 1990).

There has been some uncertainty about which lip of Schwann cell cytoplasm, inner or outer or both, moves during spiraling of the Schwann cell around the axon. Observations of Schwann cells ensheathing axons in tissue culture show that the Schwann cell nucleus revolves around the axon (Pomerat *et al.,* 1967; R. P. Bunge *et al.,* 1989). Recent observations *in vitro* correlated with electron microscopy show that the nuclear movement is in the direction of the advancing inner cytoplasmic tongue, while the outer cytoplasmic lip is anchored by extracellular matrix and macular adhering junctions, as shown in Fig. 3.6 (R. P. Bunge *et al.,* 1989).

Schwann cells, which are solely responsible for ensheathment and myelination of peripheral nerves, are derived from the neural crest and migrate into the peripheral nerves, where most of the Schwann cells originate by division. The mechanisms of their migration are dealt with in Section 4.3. The evidence that Schwann cells originate from the neural crest is that excision of the latter apparently resulted in total absence of Schwann cells in amphibian embryos (Harrison, 1924a; Detwiler and Kehoe, 1939; Hilber, 1943). In the chick embryo a small percentage of PNS cells originates from the ventral half of the neural tube, especially the Schwann cells of the ventral spinal roots and possibly some neurons of the sympathetic ganglia (Jones, 1939; Keynes, 1987; Lunn *et al.,* 1987; Loring *et al.,* 1988; Smith-Thomas and Fawcett, 1989).

The cells, known as satellite cells, which are responsible for myelination in the ganglia of the peripheral nervous system display different functional and structural characteristics in different locations: ganglia and nerves of the autonomic nervous system and of the enteric nervous system. In each of these regions the myelinating cells have unique characteristics. Schwann cells express a unique antigen (Schwann cell myelin protein, 75–80 kDa; Cameron-Curry *et al.,* 1989) *in vivo,* which is expressed by oligodendrocytes *in vitro* only, but not by satellite cells in peripheral ganglia or the gut. There are no Schwann cells in the gut but the enteric neurons are separated from nonneural cells by specialized cells that have some characteristics of astrocytes, including astrocytic intermediate filaments (Gabella, 1981; Jessen and Mirsky, 1983). Although the enteric glial cells originate from the neural crest, like Schwann cells, their differentiation is determined by local conditions in the gut. These differences may be determined partly by their origins from different subpopulations of neural crest

cells as well as by local conditions in the periphery, possibly along their routes of migration and in their final locations. After Schwann cells have differentiated at their peripheral locations a reduction occurs in their plasticity, as is shown by their failure to ensheath sympathetic neurons in culture (Roufa *et al.,* 1985). The problem of regional differentiation and plasticity of neural crest derivatives is discussed at length in Sections 4.5 and 4.6.

Commitment to Schwann cell differentiation may occur before they migrate out of the neural crest, but interaction between neurons and Schwann cells is required for their terminal differentiation. Rat neural crest cells explanted *in vitro* express early Schwann cell immunocytochemical markers and some of these cells differentiate into Schwann cells in culture (Smith-Thomas and Fawcett, 1989). This indicates that some neural crest cells may be predetermined to produce Schwann cells, and that migration and interactions along the route are not essential for Schwann cell differentiation. However, complete differentiation of Schwann cells requires interaction with neurons. For example, expression of S100 protein, an intracellular calcium-binding protein which is specific for mature glial cells including Schwann cells, requires neuronal stimulation (Holton and Weston, 1982a,b). Schwann cells produce galactocerebroside and myelin basic protein only when they are actively myelinating axons (Mirsky *et al.,* 1980; Jessen *et al.,* 1987).

After removal of the neural crest the peripheral nerves develop normally in the complete absence of Schwann cells. Nerve regeneration in the absence of Schwann cells also occurs in the unmyelinated nerve fibers of the cornea (Zander and Weddell, 1951). Myelination is not essential for the development and functioning of axons. Impulse conduction in axons commences, during development, before the formation of myelin sheaths (Ulett *et al.,* 1944; del Castillo and Vizoso, 1953; Carpenter and Bergland, 1957). Although myelination greatly increases the conduction velocity of the nervous impulse, normal impulse traffic occurs in unmyelinated axons.

Although peripheral axons can grow out and form functional connections in the absence of Schwann cells, an important role is played by Schwann cells in facilitating axonal growth and regeneration. The neurotrophic action of Schwann cells was considered to be their main function by the late 19th-century authorities, many of whom, like

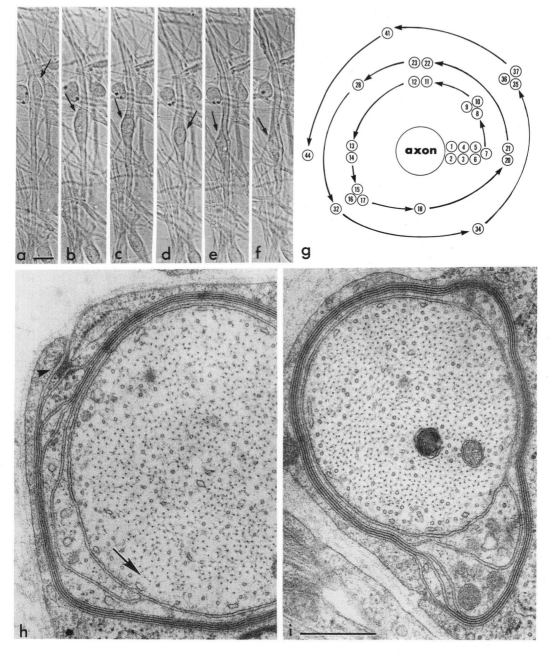

Figure 3.6. The direction of movement of the Schwann cell inner lip corresponds with the direction of movement of its nucleus. The direction of nuclear movement over a period of 44 hours *in vitro* is shown by arrows in (a)–(f). Myelin formed during that period. The nucleus moved in one direction 2.5 times round the axon as shown in (g). The axon at 44 hours is shown in (h) and it has three myelin-dense lines. The direction in which the inner Schwann cell cytoplasmic lip is pointing (arrow) corresponds with the direction of nuclear migration. (i) shows the internode about 100 μm distant from the section shown in (h). Magnification bars (a-f) = 10 μm; (h and i) = 0.5 μm. From R. P. Bunge, M. B. Bunge, and M. Bates, *J. Cell Biol.* **109**:273–284 (1989).

Cajal, denied that they played an essential part in myelination. Thus Ramón y Cajal (1905a, p. 205) states that *"growth, branching, and orientation of regenerated nerve fibers is governed by the attractive action of chemotactic substances produced by the cells of Schwann."* This is another example of a premature theory (see footnote 1 of Chapter 1). It was eclipsed by evidence showing that nerves grow normally in the absence of Schwann cells (Harrison, 1924a; Detwiler and Kehoe, 1939; Hilber, 1943). Only recently has the theory of Schwann cell neurotrophism become mature with the discovery that Schwann cells bind NGF and GMF, thus providing a neurotrophic substratum for growing and regenerating axons (Taniuchi *et al.*, 1988; Bosch *et al*, 1989).

Evidence for a neurotrophic action of Schwann cells is that optic nerve fibers will regenerate into a graft of peripheral nerve containing living Schwann cells but fail to grow into the same type of graft after the Schwann cells have been killed by repeated freezing and thawing (So and Aguayo, 1985; Berry *et al.*, 1988). The permissive conditions for such regeneration are production of extracellular matrix materials which are known to potentiate axonal growth and specific neurotrophic substances produced by Schwann cells. Schwann cells in adult nerves neither produce NGF nor do they express NGF receptors but they do both during normal outgrowth of axons and during axonal regeneration (Zimmerman and Sutter, 1983; Rohrer, 1985; Taniuchi *et al.*, 1986; Heumann *et al.*, 1987). Mechanisms of induction of NSF and NGF receptors in Schwann cells are not fully known. They include stimulation of Schwann cell mitosis by interleukin I secreted by macrophages (see Section 3.4) and by a factor produced by Schwann cells which is dependent on an extracellular matrix cofactor (Brockes *et al.*, 1986; Porter *et al.*, 1986, 1987), and glia maturation factor beta may also be involved (Lim, 1985, review; Bosch *et al.*, 1989).

3.8. Migration of Schwann Cells

Schwann cells migrate out proximodistally along the growing nerve fibers. This was first observed by Hensen (1864) and Koelliker (1886) in living nerve fibers visible through the skin of the frog tadpole's tail. The same preparation was later used by R. G. Harrison (1904) and Speidel (1932,

1933, 1935a,b, 1941, 1942, 1948, 1964, summary). Those findings have been confirmed using better microscopes (Webster and Billings, 1972; Billings-Gagliardi *et al*, 1974; Billings-Gagliardi, 1977). A short summary is given here of the main observation relevant to Schwann cell activities observed *in vivo*. Additional findings relevant to growth of axons are given in Chapter 5.

Schwann cells migrate at a maximum rate of 5 μm/minute in short spurts lasting a few minutes, and at an average rate of 40–90 μm/24 hours, in the tadpole's tail fin at about 20°C. They attach to an unmyelinated portion of the axon and never to a region that is myelinated. Myelination occurs in a proximodistal direction, although sometimes a gap is left between two myelinated internodes, which becomes filled in later. Myelination starts near the nucleus of the Schwann cell and spreads from there in both directions. The myelin close to the nodes is most unstable and breaks down under unfavorable conditions, leaving the remainder of the internode intact, closer to the Schwann cell nucleus.

The activities of Schwann cells can also be studied conveniently after cutting a nerve or after explanting a piece of peripheral nerve to tissue culture (summarized by Causey, 1960). After nerve section there is a delay of several days before Schwann cells begin migrating out of the cut ends of both stumps (Ramón y Cajal, 1928; J. Z. Young, 1942; Guth, 1956b). Rexed (1944) found that if an already degenerated nerve is cut again, there is no delay before migration of Schwann cells; thus their migration appears to be inhibited by the presence of normal nerve or accelerated by products of nerve degeneration. They migrate at a rate of about 0.3 mm/day out of the cut ends of mammalian peripheral nerves (Rexed, 1944). Eventually, the gap is bridged by the plasma clot, Schwann cells, and fibroblasts, which provide mechanical support and guidance for the axons growing out of the proximal nerve stump.

Schwann cell behavior in tissue culture has many similarities to that in real life. In tissue culture, practically no migration of Schwann cells occurs when the axons are intact, but the Schwann cells migrate away from the nerve when the axons degenerate (Abercrombie and Johnson, 1942, 1946; Abercrombie *et al.*, 1949). Some inhibition of movement of Schwann cells occurs when they come into contact with a regenerating axon *in vitro*. However, the Schwann cells still move about on the surface of the axon *in vitro*, as Speidel has observed in the living tissue. Full inhibition of movement of Schwann cells occurs only after they have formed a myelin sheath around an axon (Peterson *et al.*, 1958; Murray, 1959, 1965; Peterson and Murray, 1965; Pomerat *et al.*, 1967).

According to Lubinska (1961), the rate of migration of Schwann cells in tissue culture of mammalian nerves at 37°C is about 30 μm/hour, which is the same as the rate Rexed (1944) observed *in vivo*. A reduction in temperature diminishes the rate of migration to about 3 μm/hour at 20°C. which is the same as the rate reported in the tail fin of the tadpole. In tissue culture, the Schwann cells constantly change their shape. Their movement is intermittent. Schwann cells, like glial cells, pulsate in tissue culture (Russel and Bland, 1933; Lumsden and Pomerat, 1951; Ernyei and Young, 1966; Lumsden, 1968). Migration of Schwann cells ceases during mitosis in tissue culture and *in vivo*.

3.9. Schwann Cell Proliferation

Schwann cells continue dividing after migrating into peripheral nerves. Most of the Schwann cells are formed by mitosis in the peripheral nerves rather than by migration of postmitotic cells from the neural crest. Schwann cell proliferation is regulated by direct contact with the axon. Mitosis of Schwann cells is completed in about 1.5 hours from the time of rounding up to the time of separation of the daughter cells *in vitro* at 37°C (Lubinska, 1961). Proliferation of Schwann cells continues as long as the axon elongates and ceases after the axon stops growing. Axons stimulate proliferation of Schwann cells in culture (P. M. Wood and Bunge, 1975). One or more mitogens that stimulate Schwann cell proliferation are produced by neurons (Salzer *et al.*, 1980; Ratner *et al.*, 1984) and muscle (Murray and Robbins, 1982). The axon also controls the expression of myelin protein genes in Schwann cells (see Section 3.15).

Precisely the correct number of Schwann cells are formed to ensheath the axons, but if a peripheral nerve is repeatedly crushed the Schwann cells continue dividing, with a resulting overproduction of Schwann cells (P. K. Thomas, 1970). Schwann cells that have begun to form myelin no longer divide (A.

Peters and Muir, 1959; Asbury, 1967). In the adult, the mitotic activity of Schwann cells declines almost to zero, but they retain their ability to divide as they start proliferating in response to degeneration of the axon (Salzer and Bunge, 1980). The mitotic activity in Schwann cells reaches a maximum at 15–20 days after transection of a peripheral nerve in mammals, and the proliferation ceases after the axons have completed their regeneration (Abercrombie and Johnson, 1946; Abercrombie and Santler, 1957). The axis of the mitotic spindle in Schwann cells is always parallel to the long axis of the nerve (J. R. Martin and Webster, 1973).

Mobility and mitotic activity are characteristic of Schwann cells in the embryo and in certain pathological conditions in the adult. Inhibition of migration and proliferation of Schwann cells is controlled by the axon as well as by an autocrine mechanism of the Schwann cells which will be considered below. It is not due to the presence of myelin, because Schwann cells associated with unmyelinated axons are also sedentary and nonproliferative in the adult. However, in demyelinating diseases, the Schwann cells migrate and proliferate when the myelin breaks down, even though the axon appears to be intact. This abnormal proliferation may be associated with changes in the extracellular matrix. There is evidence that mitogenic response of Schwann cells to an autocrine glial growth factor is dependent on an extracellular matrix cofactor (Porter *et al.*, 1987). Neoplasms of Schwann cells occur as isolated schwannomas and as multiple neurofibromas (Russell and Rubinstein, 1977). The Schwann cells in these tumors secrete a glial growth factor which stimulates proliferation of normal Schwann cells (Brockes *et al.*, 1986). This appears to be an autocrine mechanism by which normal Schwann cells regulate their proliferation at a distance from nerve cells. Schwann cells can be stimulated to proliferate in culture by treatment with glial growth factor and forskolin (Porter *et al.*, 1986), and continuous treatment results in immortalization of Schwann cells (Langford *et al.*, 1988).

3.10. Determination of Internode Length

Schwann cells have some kind of territorial right to a particular length of axon. The initial length of all internodal segments in myelinated axons is about 200 μm (Friede *et al.*, 1981, review). During growth of the animal, the number of internodal segments does not change, but as the nerve elongates, the internodal segments become lengthened. Lengthening of the internodal segments during normal development may occur by passive stretching, which may also involve slippage of myelin layers (Vizoso, 1950; H. Webster, 1971; Friede, 1973a,b; Friede *et al.*, 1981, 1985), and by active remodeling of the myelin sheath. The time of stretching of the nerve in relation to the time of myelination varies and gives rise to considerable variation in the geometry of internodes in different nerves (Schäfer and Friede, 1988).

A few examples will show how variation in the length of myelinated segments can develop. The phrenic nerve elongates after the Schwann cells have started to form myelin, with the result that the number of internodes remains constant (140 in the rabbit) but the internodal length increases during growth of the animal (Friede *et al.*, 1985). By contrast, in the human laryngeal nerve, elongation occurs before myelination commences so that stretching of the internodal segments does not occur (O'Reilly and Fitzgerald, 1985). After regeneration of peripheral nerves in the adult rabbit, myelination of axons occurs without subsequent stretching, and all the internodes are about 300 μm long (Hiscoe, 1947; Vizoso and Young, 1948). However, stretching of nerves due to growth of the animal cannot be the only cause of elongation of the internodes because all nerve fibers in the same nerve are stretched equally, yet the internodes of large-caliber axons increase more than those of small-caliber axons in the same nerve, as was first reported by Key and Retzius in 1876.

During development the length of the internodal segment and the diameter of the axon increase proportionately so that in adult mammals there is a linear relationship between the two, as shown in Fig. 3.7 (Vizoso and Young, 1948; P. K. Thomas, 1955; Curtrecht and Dyck, 1970; Schlaepfer and Myers, 1973; Friede *et al.*, 1981, 1985). Unmyelinated nerve fibers do not show a proportionality between their diameters and the internuclear distances of their Schwann cells (Peyronnard *et al.*, 1975).

Internodal length and the final length of the axon do not increase proportionately. For example, in peripheral nerve and spinal roots of the cat, the increase in internodal length is up to twice the in-

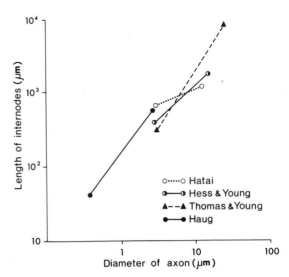

Figure 3.7. Diameter of myelinated axons and the length of their internodes. The measurements were made on adult animals and the data were abstracted from the following sources: S. Hatai, *J. Comp. Neurol.* 20:19–47 (1910), frog peripheral nerve; A. Hess and J. Z. Young, *Nature* 164:490 (1949), rabbit spinal cord; P. K. Thomas and J. Z. Young, *J. Anat.* 83:336-350 (1949), fish peripheral nerve; H. Haug, *Z. Zellforsch. Mikroskop. Anat. Abt. Histochem.* 83:265-278 (1967), cat cerebral cortex.

crease in total length of the axon, from the start of myelination to adulthood (Fried *et al.*, 1980; Berthold and Nilsson, 1987; Nilsson and Berthold, 1988). This indicates that active remodeling involving elimination of some internodes occurs in addition to stretching of the internodal segments (Berthold and Skoglund, 1968; Hildebrand *et al.*, 1985, 1986; Berthold and Nilsson, 1987).

The increase in diameter and internodal length of growing axons has important functional implications. The velocity of conduction of the nerve impulse in myelinated axons is directly proportional to the diameter of nerve fiber: For myelinated nerve fibers the ratio between conduction velocity and fiber diameter is 6.1 (Hursh, 1939; G. Schnepp *et al.*, 1971; Ritchie, 1984). For unmyelinated axons the conduction velocity is proportional to the square root of the diameter. Myelination thus greatly increases the efficiency of nerve conduction. Rushton (1951) concluded that, for axons less than 1 μm in diameter, conduction is faster without myelin, but Waxman and Bennett (1972) have shown that even for axons of 0.2 μm, which is about the smallest diameter at which axons in the CNS are myelinated, the conduction velocity is faster with myelin than without it. During evolution of the nervous system there has been a tradeoff between the optimal conduction velocity in nerve fibers and their packing in minimum space.

Propagation of the action potential in myelinated axons is saltatory, from node to node (A. F. Huxley and Stämpfli, 1949), and this is another reason why the conduction velocity increases with lengthening of the internodal segments during growth of the axon (Sanders and Whitteridge, 1946; Ridge, 1967). As a result, the time taken for the action potential to traverse the peripheral nerve fiber tends to remain constant as the animal grows. Presumably, the increase in conduction velocity in myelinated axons in the CNS also compensates for lengthening of the axons. The conduction time in axons tends to remain constant during growth of the nervous system in spite of the great increases in distances that the nerve impulses must traverse (Scherrer et al., 1968). For an excellent review of increase in conduction velocities during development, see Hildebrand and Skoglund (1971).

3.11. Development of the Myelin Sheath

Electron microscopy enabled Geren (1954) to discover all stages in the ensheathment and myelination of axons in the sciatic nerve of the chick and thus to solve a problem that had defied the powers of the most skillful light microscopists for a century. The initial stage of ensheathment consists of enfolding of the axon by the Schwann cell, leaving a channel (the mesaxon) open to the extracellular space (Gasser, 1958). Then a tongue of cytoplasm extends from the Schwann cell as a spiral around the axon, ensheathing the latter in many turns of Schwann cell cytoplasm and membranes. Finally, compaction of the Schwann cell membranes occurs as the cytoplasm is squeezed out of the internodal portion and remains only as an inner collar close to the axon, as perinodal loops of cytoplasm near the nodes of Ranvier, as an outer collar containing the nucleus of the Schwann cell, and as the bridges of cytoplasm forming the Schmidt–Lanterman clefts (Figs. 3.8 and 3.9).

At first the Schwann cells surround bundles of many axons, but as the Schwann cells proliferate they each associate with fewer axons. If the axons remain unmyelinated, they are merely enfolded by cytoplasmic processes of Schwann cells, each of which also enfolds several other axons. But axons destined to be myelinated establish a one-to-one relationship with Schwann cells, which stop dividing and start wrapping around the axon (A. Peters and Muir, 1959; A. Peters and Vaughn, 1967; H. Webster, 1971; H. Webster et al., 1973). Myelin continues to be formed while peripheral nerves elongate and increase in caliber during growth of the body. A single peripheral nerve axon may finally have up to 100 layers of myelin.

In the CNS myelination is accomplished by oligodendrocytes. The morphological processes of central myelination have been well reviewed by P. M. Wood and Bunge (1984). Significant differences between peripheral and central myelination will be discussed where relevant in the following sections. Oligodendrocytes cultured in the absence of neurons or other cell types can express the main glycolipids and proteins of the myelin sheath (Lemke, 1988), and they do so in a defined medium without requiring unknown growth factors (Gard and Pfeiffer, 1989). This is quite different from the Schwann cells, which require contact with neurons or treatment with specific mitogens in order to initiate myelination (P. M. Wood, 1976; Salzer and Bunge, 1980; Salzer et al., 1980; S. Porter et al., 1987).

The point of exit of the cranial nerves and spinal roots is a boundary at which a transition between central and peripheral myelin occurs. We do not know when and how this transition develops, and little attention has been given to this problem. The transition' is not hard and fast, because Schwann cells can invade the CNS in order to myelinate axons that have been demyelinated, for example, by diphtheria toxin (Hildebrand, 1989), or to myelinate regenerating central axons, for example, after spinal cord compression or in demyelinating diseases such as multiple sclerosis (McDonald, 1974; Prineas, 1985, reviews). The myelin formed by Schwann cells in the spinal cord expresses peripheral nerve antigens (Ghatak et al., 1973; Itoyama et al., 1983).

Before the formation of myelin lamellae there is a period of greatly increased lipid synthesis in the Schwann cells and interfascicular oligodendrocytes that can be detected histochemically and bio-

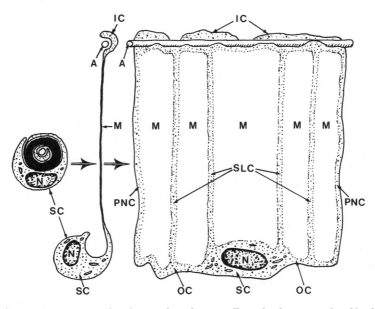

Figure 3.8. Myelination of axons in peripheral nerves by Schwann cells. Left: The axon enclosed by the Schwann cell, before the development of myelin. Right: The cytoplasmic process of the Schwann cells wrapped around the axon and formation of lamellae of compact myelin. A = axon; EMA = external mesaxon; IMA = internal mesaxon; IPL = intraperiod line; MDL = major dense line; SC = Schwann cell.

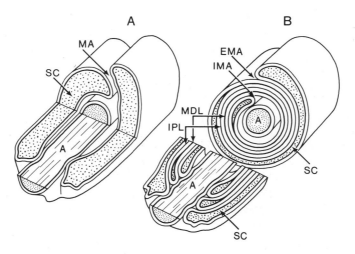

Figure 3.9. "Unrolled" Schwann cell and myelin sheath. A = axon; M = myelin, IC = inner collar of Schwann cell cytoplasm; N = nucleus of Schwann cell; PNC = perinodal cytoplasm of Schwann cell; OC = outer collar of Schwann cell cytoplasm; SC = Schwann cell; SLC = Schmidt–Lanterman cleft. Modified from H. deF. Webster, *J. Cell Biol.* **48**:348–367 (1971).

chemically. The intense synthetic activities of oligodendrocytes during the period of maximum myelination result in a 1500 percent increase in the total quantity of myelin in the brain of the rat during the period from 15 days to 6 months after birth. During this period the increase in brain weight is largely due to the accumulation of myelin. A biochemical index of the degree of myelination in any part of the nervous system can be obtained from the phospholipid content at any stage of development relative to the phospholipid content of the same region in the adult. Although phospholipids are not restricted to myelin, they are most abundant there, and phospholipids continue to increase while myelin is forming. Therefore, the incorporation of ^{32}P into brain lipids can be used as a rough index of the rate of myelination during development. In the brain of the rat, accumulation of cholesterol and phospholipid increases dramatically 7–10 days after birth. The accumulation of cerebroside, the most characteristic lipid in myelin, is a useful index of the development of compact myelin. Increase of cerebroside occurs only during the period when myelin layers first appear, that is, from the 10th to the 20th day after birth (Cuzner and Davison, 1968).

Metabolic turnover of myelin, lipids, and proteins varies during development: there is a high rate of synthesis in early development which gradually changes to a state of metabolic stability in adults (reviewed by Benjamins *et al.*, 1984; Benjamins and Smith, 1984). Some myelin lipids such as cerebroside, sulfatide, and cholesterol turn over very slowly. There is efficient reutilization of components of myelin lipids. Regarding the structural proteins of myelin, MBP and PLP have half-lives of the order of 2–3 weeks during early development but in the adults their turnover is too slow to be measured accurately. A large number of enzymes involved in synthesis and transport of components of myelin have recently been identified but consideration of them is beyond our scope (for reviews see Lees and Sapirstein, 1983; Norton and Cammer, 1984).

Before the onset of myelination there is a period of intense proliferation of interfascicular oligodendrocytes in the central nervous system and of Schwann cells in peripheral nerves. During this period these myelinating cells are most sensitive to irradiation. X-irradiation of neonatal rats and mice results in defects in myelination and changes in the compostion of myelin (Diller *et al.*, 1964; Schjeide

et al., 1968). The intense proliferation of oligodendrocytes in central fiber tracts prior to myelination has been called myelination gliosis by Roback and Scherrer (1935). This proliferation ceases at the onset of myelination (Dekaban, 1956; Majno and Karnofsky, 1958; Friede, 1961). Myelination in each region of the brain is always preceded by an increase in vascularization (Craigie, 1925, 1938; Dunning and Wolff, 1937; J. F. Feeney and Watterson, 1946; Sakla, 1965; R. M. Barlow, 1969; Otto and Lierse, 1970; Sturrock, 1981, 1982b).

The emphasis on myelination as an indication of functional maturation of the brain (Flechsig, 1920; F. Tilney and Casamajor, 1924; Langworthy, 1928b, 1930, 1933; F. Tilney, 1933; Windle *et al.*, 1934) was once popular, but should now be regarded as an oversimplification. Correlation of myelination and development of function in the pyramidal tracts is discussed by Huttenlocher (1970). Although it is obvious that the behavioral capacities of newborn animals increase during the period of myelination, there is no reason to regard the former as a direct consequence of the latter. Obviously, myelination cannot be taken as an index of maturity of the unmyelinated fibers, which are merely enfolded by satellite cells without developing a sheath of compact myelin. Impulse traffic starts in axons during development, before they develop myelin sheaths (Ulett *et al.*, 1944; J. del Castillo and Vizoso, 1953; F. G. Carpenter and Bergland, 1957; Naka, 1964; Kelerth *et al.*, 1971; Fulton *et al.*, 1980; Fulton and Walton, 1986; Shibata and Moore, 1987; Ziskind-Conhaim, 1988). Precocious motor activities develop in the newborn opossum before myelination commences (Langworthy, 1928a). Nevertheless deficits in myelination or abnormal myelination are also associated with significant functional neurological derangements (see Section 3.17).

In rats, rabbits, and mice, myelination begins only 2 days after birth in the ventral roots and in ventral and lateral tracts of the spinal cord, and then extends in a rostrocaudal direction, with the first myelin appearing in the brain in the internal capsule and posterior commissure at 10 days and starting last in the corpus callosum and association areas of the cerebral cortex at 15–21 days of age (J. B. Watson, 1903; F. Tilney, 1933; S. Jacobson, 1963; A. N. Davison *et al.*, 1966). The sequence of myelination is similar in the opossum (Langworthy, 1928a), cat (F. Tilney and Casamajor, 1924; Langworthy,

1928b), sheep (Romanes, 1947; R. M. Barlow, 1969), and human (Flechsig, 1920; Keene and Hewer, 1931, 1933; Langworthy, 1930, 1933; Conel, 1939–1963; Yakovlev and Lecours, 1967), although the time scale differs in different species.

Myelination not only starts late, when cellular proliferation and migration in the nervous system have virtually ceased, but also continues until at least 16 weeks of age in the rat and until well into the first decade in the life of humans. As a first approximation, the sequence of myelination of neurons occurs in the same order as their time of origin and differentiation. Phylogenetically older regions of the nervous system tend to be myelinated before those that have arisen more recently in phylogeny, and in each region the large neurons with long axons are myelinated before small neurons with short axons. However, this orderly sequence becomes obscured with time because the duration of myelination occupies a fairly large fraction of the neonatal period.

3.12. Axonal Induction of Schwann Cell Functions

Whether the Schwann cell does or does not form a myelin sheath is determined by the type of axon with which it associates. All the evidence shows that the axon stimulates the Schwann cells to form myelin. This capacity of the axon depends on its continuity with the perikaryon, for the Schwann cells disassociate from the axon if it is disconnected from the perikaryon (Ramón y Cajal, 1928, and many later authors). This may indicate that the Schwann cell requires one or more substances that are made in the neuron cell body and transported down the axon. Evidence that the expression of the genes for the major structural proteins of peripheral myelin is regulated by contact of the Schwann cell with the axon is given in Section 3.15. Other evidence of an effect of the axon on Schwann cells is that after nerve transection NGF receptors are expressed in all the Schwann cells distal but not proximal to the transection (Taniuchi *et al.*, 1986). NGF receptors of the low-affinity type are found on mature Schwann cells cultured without contact with axons (Distefano and Johnson, 1988). One may think of the Schwann cells as a low-affinity,

high-capacity reservoir of NGF for use by growing and regenerating axons.

Experiments in which myelinated and unmyelinated nerves are cross-united show that Schwann cells are able to associate as easily with axons that become myelinated as with those that remain unmyelinated. The myelination of regenerated axons depends on the type of neuron and not on the type of Schwann cell. Only myelinated nerves become remyelinated, regardless of the nature of the peripheral nerve stump into which they grow. Although all Schwann cells have the potential to produce myelin, they do so only when in contact with the appropriate peripheral nerves (Langley, 1898; Langley and Anderson, 1904a,b; Simpson and Young, 1945; Weinberg and Spencer, 1975; Aguayo *et al.*, 1976a,b; Bray *et al.*, 1981, review). Evidence supporting this conclusion was obtained by joining the proximal stump of a myelinated nerve to the distal end of an unmyelinated nerve, in which the Schwann cells in either the proximal or distal stump had been prelabeled with [³H]thymidine (Weinberg and Spencer, 1976). In that situation the labeled Schwann cells do not migrate from the proximal to the distal stump, and axons regenerating into the distal stump are myelinated by the Schwann cells of the unmyelinated nerve.

The formation of a myelin sheath and the number of layers of myelin are also determined by the diameter of the axon; myelination does not start until the axon reaches a certain minimum diameter and continues as long as the axon grows (Duncan, 1934a,b; Friede, 1973a,b). Myelin-associated glycoprotein (MAG) appears to be responsible for the myelination of large diameter axons rather than small-caliber axons in the peripheral nervous system (Owens and Bunge, 1989). In mammalian peripheral nerves, axons smaller than about 1 μm are unmyelinated, and in myelinated nerves, the number of layers of myelin is porportional to the diameter of the axon (Sanders, 1948; M. A. Matthews, 1968; Friede and Samorajski, 1968; Friede, 1972, 1973a,b). By contrast, in the CNS axons as thin as 0.2 μm in diameter may be myelinated, although it is uncommon to find central myelinated axons less than 0.4 μm in diameter (M. A. Matthews, 1968; Waxman and Pappas, 1971; Franson and Hildebrand, 1975). This is another example of the difference between central and peripheral myelination which will be enlarged upon in the following section. These observations indicate either that small axons do not stimulate the Schwann cell to myelinate them or that Schwann cells are incapable of forming a myelin sheath around small axons. It is not definitely known whether Schwann cells can ensheath artificial fibers. Ernyei and Young (1966) have reported the formation of myelin sheath by Schwann cells around fibers of glass, nylon, rayon, and tungsten, 5–30 μm in diameter, in cultures of sympathetic and dorsal root ganglia of mice. However, Field *et al.* (1968b) failed to confirm this.

One of the most promising experimental strategies for studying interactions between Schwann cells and axons has been to graft a segment of one type of nerve into a gap in another type (Aguayo *et al.*, 1982, 1983, reviews). The Schwann cells originate locally in such peripheral nerve grafts and do not enter the graft with the regenerating axons from the proximal stump or migrate into the graft from the distal nerve stump. Such experiments have proved that the neuropathy in trembler mice (see Section 3.16) is due to a primary disorder of Schwann cells and is not due to a disorder of the axons, as is shown in Fig. 3.10 (Aguayo *et al.*, 1976c, 1977). Similar experiments, in which segments are grafted between myelinated and unmyelinated nerves, have shown that myelin production is determined by the axon with which the Schwann cell interacts. Thus Schwann cells from unmyelinated cervical sympathetic nerves will produce myelin when in contact with regenerating axons of the sural nerve (Aguayo *et al.*, 1976a,b).

The influence of the Schwann cell on the caliber of its associated segment of the axon has been demonstrated by grafting a segment of sciatic nerve reciprocally between a normal mouse and a trembler mouse (Aguayo *et al.*, 1976c). The trembler is a dominant mutant in which a defect of Schwann cells causes widespread deficiency of myelination and reduction of axon caliber (see Section 3.16). Transfer of normal Schwann cells to a segment of sciatic nerve of the trembler mouse results in normal myelination of that segment and in an increase of the caliber of the trembler axons in the myelinated segment. Conversely, the segment of normal sciatic nerve populated by trembler Schwann cells has a deficit of myelination and a local reduction of axonal caliber. This shows that axon caliber is controlled to a considerable degree by the local influence of the Schwann cell. The mechanism of this influence is not known. It may be due to a local change in the axon resulting in local increase in neurofilaments or neurotubules.

3.13. Structure of the Myelin Sheath

Electron micrographs of fixed and stained myelin show a periodicity consisting of two electron-dense bands, the major dense line and the intraperiod line, separated by a lucent zone. The electron-dense lines are due to proteins, while the lucent regions are due to lipids (Raine, 1984, review). The *major dense line* is formed by apposition of the two inner layers of the plasma membrane of the Schwann cell in peripheral nerve, or oligodendrocyte in the CNS, with the cytoplasm squeezed out. Pockets of Schwann cell cytoplasm remain where the membranes have not fused, namely, at the incisures of Schmidt–Lanterman and at the paranodal region (Figs. 3.8 and 3.9). The *intraperiod line* is formed by apposition of the two outer layers of plasma membrane, with the extracellular space obliterated. A potential extracellular space remains, because the extracellular marker, lanthanum, may penetrate between the myelin layers. Schmidt–Lanterman incisures are found in peripheral but not in central myelin.

The structures of central and peripheral myelin sheaths are slightly different, reflecting their formation by different types of cells (Raine, 1984, review). In peripheral axons, the Schwann cell cytoplasm consists of a broad tongue forming an outer collar containing the cell nucleus and an inner collar adjacent to the axon, as shown in Fig. 3.9. In central axons the cytoplasm of the oligodendrocyte is connected to the sheath by a process that is prominent early in development (Figs. 3.11 and 3.12) and during remyelination (Fig. 3.13) but which later becomes very slender and may be as long as 10 μm. Unlike the Schwann cell, which is attached to one axon, a single oligodendrocyte myelinates several axons, and the glial cell body may not be adjacent to its myelin sheath. The main difference at the nodes of Ranvier is the presence of processes of Schwann cell cytoplasm covering the nodes in peripheral axons, whereas processes of Type 2 astrocytes enfold the

PROXIMAL GRAFT DISTAL

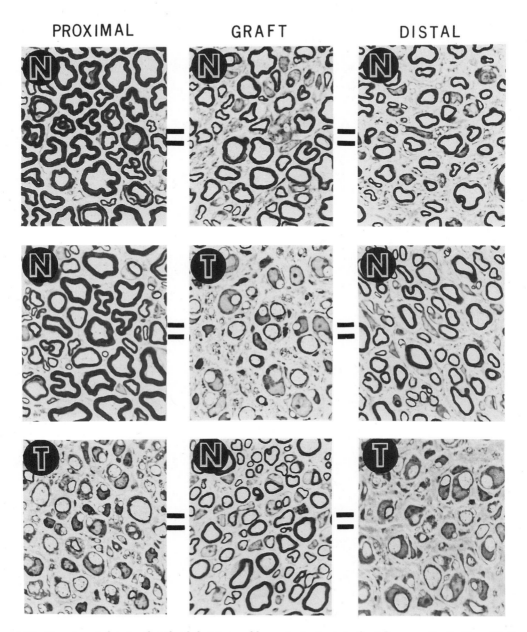

Figure 3.10. Experiment showing that the defect in trembler mutant mice is in the Schwann cells. Grafting of Schwann cells between segments of the sciatic nerve of normal (N) and trembler (T) mice. Two months after grafting, cross-sections were made of sciatic nerves 3 mm proximal to the graft, in the middle of the graft, and 3 mm distal to the graft. Phase micrographs show myelinated and unmyelinated axons: normal-to-normal graft (top row), trembler-to-normal graft (middle row), and normal-to-trembler graft (bottom row). Normal-grafted Schwann cells myelinate trembler host axons growing through the graft, but trembler-grafted Schwann cells fail to myelinate normal axons. From A. J. Aguayo, M. Attiwell, J. Trecarten, S. Perkins, and G. M. Bray, *Nature* **265**:73–75 (1977).

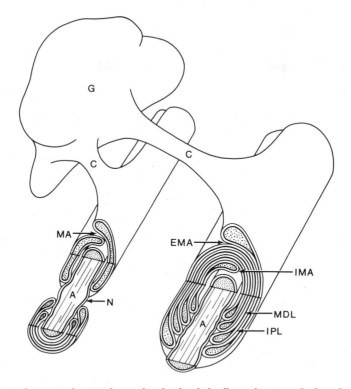

Figure 3.11. Myelination of axons in the CNS by an oligodendroglial cell. Myelination is farther advanced on the axon at the right than on the axon at the left. A = axon; C = cytoplasmic process of oligodendrocyte; EMA = external mesaxon; IMA = internal mesaxon; IPL = intraperiod line; MA = mesaxon; MDL = major dense line; N = node; G = oligodendroglial cell.

axon at the nodes of central axons (ffrench-Constant *et al.*, 1986; ffrench-Constant and Raff, 1986).

3.14. Developmental Changes in the Lipid Composition of Myelin

The major lipid constituents of myelin are phospholipids, glycolipids, and sterols (Smith, 1983; Lees and Brostoff, 1984; Norton and Cammer, 1984). In mammals, the phospholipids, chiefly phosphatidyl ethanolamine and lecithin, constitute 26–44 percent of the dry weight; glycolipids, including sphingomyelin, cerebroside, and ganglioside, constitute 12–22 percent of the dry weight; sterols, mainly cholesterol, range from 11 to 22 percent of the dry weight in different mammals. The structural proteins that are specific for myelin are reviewed in Section 3.15. They constitute about 20 percent of the dry weight of myelin.

There are differences between the lipid and protein compositions of central and peripheral myelin, as is to be expected because they are formed by different types of cells, the Schwann cells in peripheral nerves and the oligodendrocytes in the CNS (reviewed by Benjamin and Smith, 1985; Raine, 1984; for myelin proteins see Section 3.15). Peripheral myelin has double the sphingomyelin content of central myelin; the ratio of cerebroside to sphingomyelin is about 1 in peripheral myelin but about 2 in central myelin. As a result of these differences the myelin period is about 10 percent less in central than in peripheral myelin of the same animal.

The composition of myelin changes considerably during development (Norton and Poduslo, 1973; Norton and Cammer, 1984, review). In the rat, the myelin galactolipids increase by about 50 percent and lecithin decreases by a similar amount from birth to about 2 months of age. At the same time,

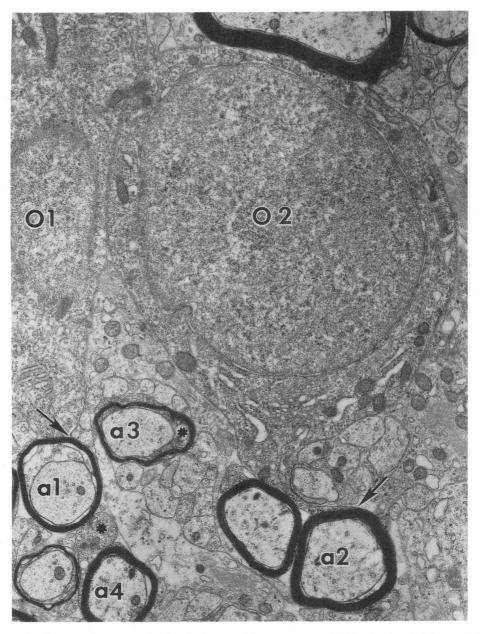

Figure 3.12. Myelination of CNS axons by oligodendrocytes. Electron micrograph of the spinal cord of the cat at P5 showing two oligodendrocytes, O1 and O2, attached to axons a1 and a2. Arrows show points of continuity between the cell body and mylin sheath. Cell cytoplasm associated with the sheaths of axons a3 and a4 is marked by an asterisk. At this magnification the connection to the perikaryon cannot be seen. The cytoplasm of the sheath associated with a4 appears as a large loop. Mag. ×10,800. Electron micrograph kindly provided by M. B. Bunge.

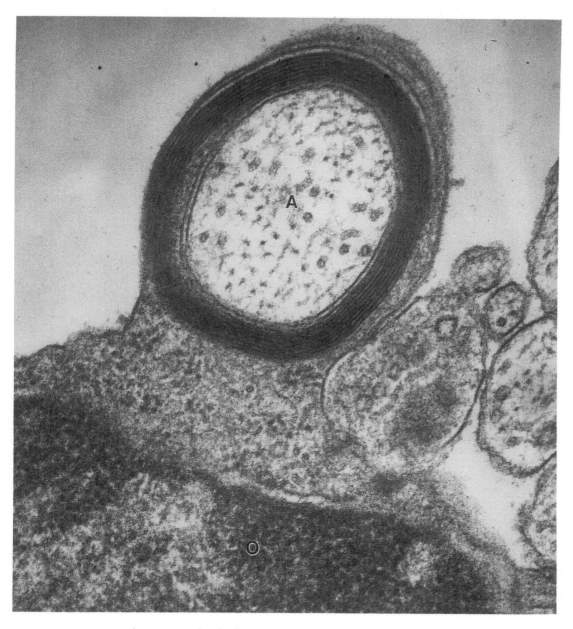

Figure 3.13. Connection between an oligodendrocyte (0) and the myelin sheath around an axon (A). This electron micrograph was taken of part of the cerebral white matter 3 days after demyelination produced by intracerebral implantation of Ariethyltin acetate. From A. Hirano, *Dev. Neurosci.* 11:112–117 (1989), copyright S. Karger AG, Basel.

the polysialogangliosides decrease and the mono-sialoganglioside, G_{M1}, increases to become the main ganglioside of adult myelin. In the rat these changes are not completed until 2 months of age. Similar changes occur in humans.

3.15. Myelin Structural Proteins and Their Genetic Control

The main structural proteins of myelin are proteolipid protein (PLP), which is confined essentially to central myelin; P_o protein, which is found only in peripheral myelin; myelin basic protein (MBP); 2′,3′-cyclic nucleotide 3′-phosphohydrolase (CNP); and myelin-associated glycoprotein (MAG). The latter three are present in both central and peripheral myelin.

Let us first consider the four structural proteins of central myelin. PLP is the main structural protein of CNS myelin, comprising 50 percent of the total protein (Lees and Brostoff, 1984, review). PLP is synthesized on rough endoplasmic reticulum of oligodendroglial cells. It is acylated, very hydrophobic, and spans the myelin membrane. PLP is involved in myelin compaction and maintenance of the intraperiod line of central myelin (Duncan et al., 1987). In the jimpy mutant mouse, synthesis of defective PLP occurs because of a defect in splicing of its mRNA (Duncan et al., 1987; Sutcliffe, 1988, review; see Section 3.16).

MBP accounts for about 30 percent of the total myelin protein in both the central and peripheral nervous systems (Omlin et al., 1982). It is involved in myelin compaction and in maintenance of the major dense line. In the shiverer mutant mouse, MBP is lacking and so is the major dense line (see Section 3.16). MBP is synthesized on free ribosomes in oligodendrocytes and Schwann cells (Coleman et al., 1982; Griffiths et al., 1989). There are at least four isoforms of MBP (21.5, 18.5, 17, and 14 kDa in the ratios of 1:10:3.5:35) in the rat and mouse and a fifth has been found in the mouse (Lees and Brostoff, 1984; Newman et al., 1987). They are translated from RNAs derived from alternative splicing of the primary transcript from a single gene.

CNP is a specific myelin-associated enzyme. It comprises about 5 percent of total protein in central and peripheral myelin (Norton and Cammer, 1984, review).

MAG comprises about 1 percent of total CNS myelin protein. It belongs to the immunoglobulin family of molecules and has similarities to other cell adhesion molecules, L1 and NCAM (Martini and Schachner, 1986; Salzer et al., 1987). It mediates adhesion of oligodendrocyte and Schwann cell processes to axons, but it is finally excluded from compact myelin, as shown in Fig. 3.14 (Trapp and Quarles, 1984; Quarles, 1985). The deficit in Quaking mutant mice is an inability to remove MAG during the process of myelin compaction (see Section 3.16). There are two isoforms of MAG, large (MAG-L) and small (MAG-S), which differ by 10 amino acids at the carboxyl terminal which forms the cytoplasmic domain (Salzer et al., 1987). Both forms are found in central and peripheral myelin. MAG-S is more abundant during development whereas MAG-L predominates in the adult.

These four myelin proteins can be detected by immunocytochemistry in oligodendrocytes shortly before the start of myelination (Sternberger et al., 1979; Roussel and Nussbaum, 1981; Hartman et al., 1982; Monge et al., 1986) and their mRNA's can be detected by in situ hybridization (Zeller et al, 1984; Kristensson et al., 1986; Trapp et al., 1987; Jordan et al., 1989). Their expression occurs in oligodendrocytes grown in vitro independently of neurons (Zeller et al., 1985; Dubois-Dalcq et al., 1986).

The genes for the four central myelin proteins and for the peripheral myelin protein, P_o, have been cloned and sequenced; their isoforms are produced by alternative splicing, and the mRNAs encoding the isoforms have been identified (Zeller et al., 1984; de Ferra et al., 1985; Naismith et al., 1987; Takahashi et al., 1985; Diehl et al., 1986; Arquint et al., 1987; Bernier et al., 1987; Lai et al., 1987; Sutcliffe, 1988, review).

MBP and PLP mRNAs can be detected by in situ hybridization in mouse brain at 6 hours after birth, before the histological appearance of myelin (Verity and Campagnoni, 1988). Expression of mRNAs for the major structural proteins of CNS myelin reaches a peak at 20 days of age. PLP mRNA remains associated with oligodendrocyte cell bodies, associated with rough endoplasmic reticulum. By contrast, MBP mRNAs are associated with free ribosomes and move from the cell body to the oligodendrocyte processes. MBP and PLP increase in the CNS during maturation, whereas MAG decreases (Trapp and Quarles, 1984).

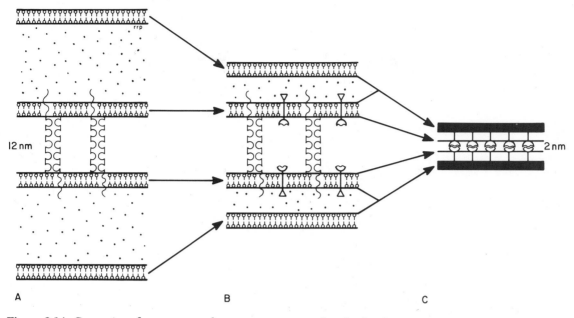

Figure 3.14. Conversion of mesaxon membranes to compact myelin The distribution and membrane orientation of P_o protein and MAG are shown only in the inner two membrane bilayers. (A) Initial mesaxon wraps contain MAG but little P_o protein. The extracellular space, 12–14 nm wide, between juxtaposed mesaxon membranes contains MAG shown in a homphilic MAG-to-MAG association. (B) P_o protein is inserted as the mesaxon membranes increase in length. The cytoplasmic domains of MAG molecules prevent fusion of cytoplasmic leaflets of these mesaxon membranes. (C) MAG is removed and compaction of myelin occurs. The extracellular space (2 nm) is set by homophilic binding between P_o molecules or by heterophilic interaction between P_o and acidic lipids. From B. D. Trapp, *J. Cell Biol.* **107**:675–685 (1988). Copyright Rockefeller University Press.

We shall consider the main structural proteins of peripheral myelin. The major structural protein of compact peripheral myelin is P_o, which is not found in central myelin. This is an integral membrane glycoprotein of molecular weight 28–30 kDa, which comprises about 50 percent of the total protein of peripheral myelin (Lees and Brostoff, 1984). It is involved in compaction of peripheral myelin (Lemke and Axel, 1985). Expression of P_o and MBP mRNAs in Schwann cells is regulated by contact with axons of the appropriate type and caliber (Trapp *et al.*, 1988).

In peripheral nerves MAG is an integral membrane glycoprotein of molecular weight 98–100 kDa which functions as a cell adhesion molecule during the attachment of Schwann cells to axons. Immunocytochemical studies have shown that MAG is the major structural protein of the mesaxon membranes of Schwann cells, whereas P_o protein is the major structural protein of compact peripheral myelin (Trapp, 1988). During myelin compaction, P_o protein replaces MAG in the mesaxon membrane (Fig.

3.14). MAG is excluded from compact peripheral myelin but persists at Schmidt–Lanterman incisures, paranodal myelin loops, and mesaxon membranes of peripheral myelinated axons (Trapp and Quarles, 1982; Martini and Schachner, 1986).

The 18.5 kDa isoform of MBP, termed P1 in peripheral myelin, and another basic protein, P2, are localized on the cytoplasmic side of the plasmalemma at the major dense line and are involved in compaction at the major dense line.

The distribution of mRNA species encoding peripheral myelin proteins has been shown by *in situ* hybridization (Trapp *et al.*, 1987; Griffiths *et al.*, 1989). P_o and MAG transcripts are concentrated at the perinuclear region of Schwann cells, presumably on the rough endoplasmic reticulum, which is the site of synthesis of these glycoproteins. During myelin compaction the P_o protein is inserted into the mesaxon membrane while MAG is removed (Fig. 3.14). In quaking mice there is a failure of removal of MAG from the compacting myelin (Trapp, 1988). Phospholipid protein mRNA and the protein have both been detected in Schwann cell cytoplasm but the protein is evidently degraded as it does not enter into compact myelin of peripheral nerves (Pucket *et al.*, 1987; Griffiths *et al.*, 1989).

MBP and P_o accumulate rapidly in Schwann cells that are actively myelinating (Wood and Engel, 1976; Lemke and Axel, 1985; Willison *et al.*, 1987), whereas only small quantities of these proteins appear in Schwann cells that are not forming myelin (Brockes *et al.*, 1979; Trapp *et al.*, 1981, 1987; Willison *et al.*, 1988). Production of MBP and P_o is reduced rapidly in the distal, degenerating segment of the nerve after axotomy (Mirsky *et al.*, 1980; Politis *et al.*, 1982; Poduslo *et al.*, 1984; Willison *et al.*, 1988; Trapp *et al.*, 1988). MBP mRNA and P_o mRNA levels decrease in the distal segment rapidly after nerve transection, showing that axonal regulation of MBP and P_o gene expression occurs primarily at the level of mRNA synthesis (Trapp *et al.*, 1988).

3.16. Genetic Mutations Causing Defective Myelination

Mutations causing abnormalities of myelination in mice include quaking (Sidman *et al.*, 1964), jimpy (Phillips, 1954; Sidman *et al.*, 1964), trembler (Falconer, 1951; Henry and Sidman, 1988), and shiverer (Privat *et al.*, 1979).

Quaking is an autosomal recessive mutation which results in greatly reduced development of central and peripheral myelin. The deficit in the quaking mutant is a failure of myelin compaction resulting from inability to remove MAG from the mesaxon membrane (Trapp, 1988; Fig. 3.14). Northern blot analysis of RNA from quaking mouse brain shows that the transcripts are qualitatively normal but PLP and MBP transcripts are both considerably reduced in quantity, whereas the MAG transcripts are significantly increased in quantity (Konat *et al.*, 1988). This increase in MAG transcripts may be either a compensatory response or a sign of dysregulation. Homozygous quaking mice also have hyperplasia and abnormal vacuolation of oligodendroglial cells (Samorajski *et al.*, 1970; Freidrich, 1975). In spite of severe neurological dysfunction, including paresis and seizures, the homozygous quaking mice survive for a year or more (Hogan and Greenfield, 1984).

Jimpy is a sex-linked recessive mutation that results in severe reduction of central myelination of hemizygous male mice (Phillips, 1954; Sidman *et al.*, 1964). Oligodendrocytes are reduced in number (Kraus-Ruppert *et al.*, 1973; Meier and Bischoff, 1975). Peripheral myelin is not affected. Jimpy hemizygous males have weakness and seizures starting shortly after birth and they die between 25 and 35 days of age. Female carriers are mosaics due to random X-inactivation; therefore, about half the oligodendrocytes are affected and half are normal. The female carriers show about 30 percent reduction of central myelination at birth, but recovery occurs as the result of compensatory proliferation of oligodendrocytes that carry the normal gene (Bartlett and Skoff, 1989). The primary defect in splicing of PLP transcripts results in synthesis of dysfunctional PLP which is shorter than normal and has an altered carboxyl end (Nave *et al.*, 1986; Sutcliffe, 1988, review). Cultures of oligodendrocytes from jimpy mice also express the jimpy phenotype. However, jimpy oligodendrocytes appear nearly normal when grown in medium conditioned by normal glial cells (90% astrocytes), indicating that the jimpy cells lack a factor provided by astrocytes (Bartlett *et al.*, 1988). Other evidence that extrinsic factors can rescue jimpy oligodendrocytes is that they are capable of producing MBP and myelin when transplanted into shiverer mouse brain in which MBP is totally absent (Gumpel *et al.*, 1987).

There are two forms of trembler mutations, an autosomal dominant and a semidominant-J mutant (Henry and Sidman, 1988). The central myelin appears normal but there is a virtual absence of peripheral myelin in both forms of trembler mutation, in either the homozygous or heterozygous condition. The difference between them is that the semidominant-J mutant mice die before 1 month of age whereas the dominant form survives for a year or more. The basis for this difference is not known, but Henry and Sidman (1988) suggest that the absence of peripheral myelin is in itself not sufficient to result in total disablement and death because it is compatible with survival in the dominant form.

Mice with the recessive autosomal mutation *dystrophic* (Michelson *et al.*, 1985) have progressive wasting of limb muscles. They show a failure of ensheathment of axons by Schwann cells, defects in Schwann cell basal lamina, and defective myelination of peripheral nerves, especially of the spinal nerve roots in the homozygous mice (Bradley and Jenkinson, 1973; Madrid *et al.*, 1975; Okada *et al.*, 1976; Bradley *et al.*, 1977; Jaros and Bradley, 1979). The primary defect is not known. However, the defect is corrected in chimeras of dystrophic and shiverer mice (deficiency of myelin basic protein serves to label the shiverer Schwann cells). In such chimeric mice the dystrophic Schwann cells do not show any functional or structural defects (Peterson and Bray, 1984).

Shiverer is an autosomal recessive mutation which in the homozygous conditions results in almost total lack of myelin in the CNS, and in total lack of all four types of MBP. The defect is a deletion of the gene for MBP (Campagnoni *et al.*, 1984; Roth *et al.*, 1985; Kimura *et al.*, 1985, 1989). From 2 weeks of age the affected mice start shivering and convulsions occur at a later age, resulting in death. In the heterozygous condition, the shiverer mutation does not cause abnormal behavior but results in reduction of MBP to about 50 percent of normal. Complete rescue from the mutant phenotype occurs in transgenic shiverer mice into whose genome a recombinant gene for the most abundant (14 kDa) form of MBP has been inserted (Kimura *et al.*, 1989), as shown in Fig. 3.15.

3.17. Abnormalities of Myelination

Because the myelination involves a sequence of proliferative and synthetic activities of myelinating cells and also requires the cooperative activity of the axon, abnormalities of myelin development might result from a variety of disturbances in proliferation and motility of myelinating cells, or from defects in ensheathment of axons by myelinating cells, or from deficiencies in enzymes or substrates required for the synthesis of myelin.

During the time of myelination the CNS is especially vulnerable to undernutrition (Dobbing, 1963; Culley and Mertz, 1965; Benton *et al.*, 1966; A. N. Davison and Dobbing, 1966; H. P. Chase *et al.*, 1967; Clos and Legrand, 1969, 1970; Sima and Sourander, 1978; Lai and Lewis, 1980a,b; Wiggins, 1982, review; see Section 7.2). Insufficient nutrition during that period results in a delay in myelination and a deficiency in the total quantity of myelin. The effect is on synthesis rather than degradation of my-

elin. It is also probable, although not fully demonstrated, that undernutrition results in reduced proliferation of oligodendrocytes as well as in a reduction in the quantity of myelin that they synthesize (Lai *et al.*, 1980; Lai and Lewis, 1980; Clos *et al.*, 1982a,b). During the peak period of myelination in the rat, it is established that each oligodendrocyte synthesizes 3 times its own weight of myelin daily (Norton, 1976). It is also evident that the oligodendrocytes require a large supply of precursors necessary for myelin synthesis. As expected, the development of blood vessels in the brain is correlated with myelination (Sturrock, 1981, 1982a,b). Although malnutrition results in reduced synthesis of CNS myelin, the composition of myelin is normal in experimentally undernourished rats and in undernourished humans (J. H. Fox *et al.*, 1972; Krigman and Hogan, 1976). Recovery of myelination is not complete in rats fed freely after 20 days of postnatal undernutrition (Wiggins *et al.*, 1976). Malnutrition results in 20–30% reduction in the total number of oligodendrocytes in the white matter of the rat cerebellum, an effect which is not reversible (Lai *et al.*,1980; Lai and Lewis, 1980; Clos *et al.*, 1982a,b). Myelination is retarded and reduced in the cortical white matter (Bass *et al.*, 1970a,b) and corpus callosum (Robain and Ponsot, 1978; Lai *et al.*, 1980) in malnourished rats. The effects of malnutrition on the developing nervous system are protean and are considered at greater length in Sections 7.1 and 7.2.

After CNS demyelination due to diphtheria toxin or multiple sclerosis, remyelination occurs by a process that is similar to normal but is incomplete (Bunge *et al.*, 1961; A. Hirano *et al.*, 1969; Ghotak *et al.*, 1973; Itoyama *et al.*, 1983; A. Hirano, 1989, review). In such cases the myelin sheath has fewer layers and shorter internodal length than normal in proportion to the caliber of the axon (Prineas, 1985; Hildebrand, 1989).

Abnormal behavior and mental retardation occur in several metabolic diseases in which deficiencies in the formation of myelin have been reported in humans, for example, in phenylketonuria (Crome *et al.*, 1962) and inherited disorders of amino acid metabolism (Prensky *et al.*, 1968). In those cases, it is not known whether the myelin deficiency and the behavioral impairment are causally related or merely coincidentally associated. Thyroidectomy of rats at birth results in 30 percent reduction in the dry weight of myelin obtained from the whole brain at

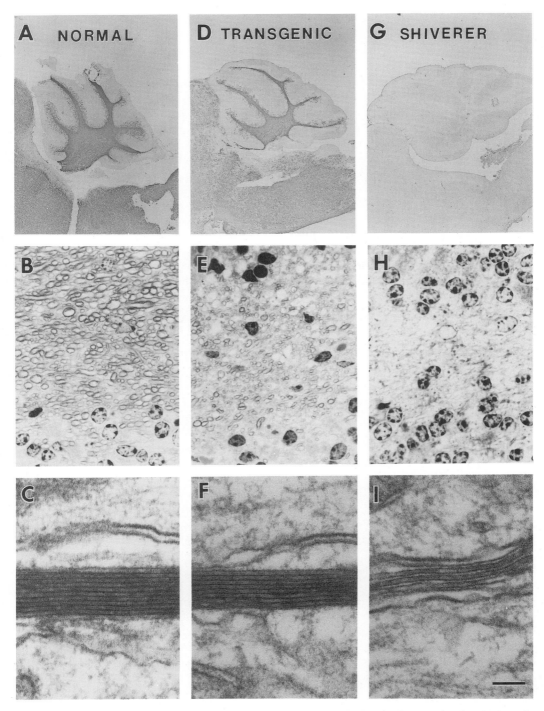

Figure 3.15. Gene therapy of transgenic shiverer mice. A recombinant gene coding for the most abundant (14 kDa) form of myelin basic protein (MBP), including the native promoter, was injected into homozygous shiverer zygotes to produce transgenic shiverer mice. The transgenic animals recovered from shivering and had essentially normal myelination as illustrated here. Panels A–C are from a normal control; D–F from a transgenic shiverer; G–I from a homozygous (*shi/shi*) mouse. The upper three panels show a sagittal section of the cerebellum immunostained for MBP. The middle three panels show toluidine blue-stained sections of the white matter near the granular layer. The lower three panels show electron micrographs of myelin in the white matter. Magnification bar = 50 nm. From M. Kimura, M. Sato, A. Akatsuka, S. Nozawa-Kimura, R. Takahashi, M. Yokoyama, T. Nomura, and M. Katsuki, *Proc. Natl. Acad. Sci. USA* 86:5661–5665 (1989).

43 days of age, but there is no change in the time course of myelination or the composition of myelin as compared with normal rats (Balázs *et al.*, 1969; Clos *et al.*, 1982a,b). The effects of thyroid hormone on CNS development are considered in detail in Section 7.4.

3.18. Vascularization of the CNS

It is appropriate to consider this topic in relationship to glial cells because in mammals and most other vertebrates the astrocytes induce and maintain the functions of the vascular endothelial cells which form the blood–brain barrier, a term first used by Stern and Peyrot (1927). The blood vessels in the CNS form a distinct anatomical compartment, separated completely from cells of neurectodermal origin by a basement membrane, which is the combined product of the endothelial cells and the perivascular glial cells (Caley and Maxwell, 1970; Phelps, 1972; Bär and Wolff, 1972; Povlishok *et al.*, 1977; Marin-Padilla, 1988). Glial cells participate in the immune response in the CNS: the perivascular glial cells can present antigen to T cells (Fontana *et al.*, 1984, 1987), a function which they share with the capillary endothelial cells and choroid plexus.

In elasmobranch fish the blood–brain barrier is not formed by the endothelial cells but by the perivascular glial cells themselves, which are connected by tight junctions and which have selective carrier mechanisms for transporting water-soluble molecules to the neurons (Cserr and Bundegaard, 1984; Gotow and Hashimoto, 1984; Abbott and Butt, 1986).

The neural plate and early neural tube are avascular. Blood vessels grow in the meninges before penetrating into the CNS from the pial surface. This vascular penetration starts at the level of the medulla and progresses rostrally in the brain (Streeter, 1918; Padget, 1948, 1957; Allsopp and Gamble, 1979) and caudally in the spinal cord (Gillilan, 1858; Strong, 1961; Sturrock, 1981, 1982). Vascular endothelial cells proliferate rapidly. Their mitosis is stimulated by basic fibroblast growth factor which they themselves secrete (Schweigerer *et al.*, 1987). By using quail-chick chimeras to trace the origins of the brain vascular endothelial cells, Stewart and Wiley (1981) showed that the endothelial

cells originate from outside the nervous system. The endothelial cells are actively motile. Their filopodia perforate the basement membrane and penetrate between the glial endfeet which form the glial external limiting membrane and the endothelial cells migrate between the brain cells (Nousek-Goebl and Press, 1986; Marin-Padilla, 1988, review).

Brain vascular morphogenesis occurs by sprouting of existing blood vessels rather than by aggregation of migrating endothelial cells, such as that which occurs during early development of the cardiovascular system. In the brain, the sprouts of endothelial cells form compact masses initially, but a lumen is formed as the result of secretion of extracellular matrix materials by the endothelial cells (Nabeshima *et al.*, 1975; Krahn, 1982; Furcht, 1983). The sprouts coalesce to form anastomotic capillary loops.

Angiogenesis is controlled by angiogenic factors that have been identified in tumors (Folkman, 1985) and brain (Klagsbrun and Shing, 1985; Risau, 1986). Angiogenesis is inhibited by protamine, a 5.4-kDa basic protein (Taylor and Folkman, 1982). Angiogenesis is adaptive, so that formation as well as regression of brain capillaries is correlated with the developmental state of the CNS. This regression of capillaries occurs during the period of disappearance of germinal zones such as the cerebellar external granular layer, the cerebral subventricular layer, and the ventricular germinal layer. The mechanisms controlling regression of capillaries are not known. Angiogenesis in the nervous system (Jones, 1970; Bär and Wolff, 1972, 1975; Gamble, 1975; Hauw *et al.*, 1975; Wolff *et al.*, 1975; Marin-Padilla, 1985, 1988) is similar to that in healing wounds (Cliff, 1963; Schoefl, 1964; McKinney and Panner, 1972) and neoplasms (Folkman, 1982).

Brain capillary endothelial cells differ from those in other organs in several important respects (Joó, 1987, review). Brain capillary endothelial cells form continuous tight junctions that prevent molecules from passing between the endothelial cells and thus form a blood–brain barrier. This barrier develops in all vertebrates (Cserr and Bundegaard, 1984) and some invertebrates (Abbott *et al.*, 1986). Materials either have to diffuse through the endothelial cells, and this is limited to fat-soluble molecules, or water-soluble molecules have to be specifically and very selectively transported across the brain capillary endothelial cells

(Davson *et al.*, 1987; Pardridge, 1983, reviews). Evidence, to be given later, shows that these specialized functions of brain capillary endothelial cells develop under control of astrocytes.

Capillary endothelial cells in organs outside the CNS lack special transport mechanisms, and therefore, macromolecules have to pass out of the blood through fenestrations in the capillary walls. Such fenestrations are also found in capillaries in the circumventricular organs in the dorsal midline of the third and fourth ventricles (Weindel, 1973; Pickel *et al.*, 1986), the pineal gland (Wislocki and Leduc, 1985), the hypothalamus, and the pituitary gland, where their function is to permit peptides to cross the capillary endothelium (Voitkevich and Dedov, 1972; Eurenius, 1977).

That the blood–brain barrier in mammals is formed by the CNS capillary endothelial cells is shown by the fact that horseradish peroxidase (HRP), injected intravenously, does not enter the CNS. Conversely, HRP injected into the brain ventricle is not prevented from entering the brain by the astrocytes but is stopped by the endothelial cells from entering the blood (Reese and Karnovsky, 1967; Brightman and Reese, 1969). The tight junctions between brain capillary endothelial cells in mammals or between perivascular glial cells in elasmobranch fish can be temporarily loosened by injection of a hypertonic solution of a water-soluble nonelectrolyte such as urea or mannitol into the carotid circulation, thus opening the blood–brain barrier (Rapoport, 1970; Rapoport *et al.*, 1981; Mackie *et al.*, 1986).

There is considerable evidence that astrocytes induce the functional development of brain capillary endothelial cells, as originally suggested by the observations on the origin of brain blood vessels in chick-quail chimeras (Stewart and Wiley, 1981). Endothelial cells *in vitro* only express the functional characteristics required for their functioning as the blood–brain barrier when cocultured with astrocytes. These characteristics include induction of enzymes (De Bault and Cancilla, 1980; Beck *et al.*, 1986) and increased development of tight junctions (Tao-Cheng *et al.*, 1986). Type I astrocytes grafted to the eye induce permeability changes in the nonneural capillary endothelial cells of the iris (Janzer and Raff, 1987).

Developmental changes in the density of the brain microvasculature have been studied by several methods. The stages during which vascularization of the CNS has been reported is probably biased by the methods used for detecting newly formed blood vessels. Perfusion with fixatives gives an overestimate of the time of vascularization whereas injection with India ink and gelatin (Strong, 1961; Koppel, *et al.*, 1982) gives an underestimate because the injected material is more viscous than blood and fails to enter many capillaries (Sturrock, 1981, 1982). This may be the reason for the finding that the cerebellar external granular layer in the rat is virtually devoid of capillaries throughout its development (Koppel *et al.*, 1982). Staining for microvascular alkaline phosphatase (Bell and Scarrow, 1984; Norman and O'Kusky, 1986) is a better method of quantitating the density of brain blood vessels than injection with India ink. However, alkaline phosphatase only becomes cytochemically detectable in the luminal plasma membrane of the endothelial cells at P12–P24 in the mouse brain (Vorbradt *et al.*, 1986), so the early stages of angiogenesis are not detected by this method. At earlier stages of development, angiogenesis can be studied with monoclonal antibodies that stain vascular endothelial cells (Pardanaud *et al.*, 1987; Coffin and Poole, 1988).

Brain angiogenesis and functioning of the blood–brain barrier start very early in the CNS (Saunders and Mollgard, 1984), but the period of maximal sprouting of brain capillaries is delayed until more advanced stages of CNS development corresponding with the period of dendritic growth and glial cell proliferation (Dunning and Wolff, 1937; Sakla, 1965; Otto and Lierse, 1970). These events occur during the 2nd and 3rd postnatal weeks in the rat cerebral cortex (Bär and Wolff, 1973; Bär, 1978) and during the 2nd–7th postnatal weeks in the cat cerebral cortex (Ben Hamida *et al.*, 1983). A direct relationship between angiogenesis and myelination has been reported in the mouse brain (Sturrock, 1981, 1982a,b) but was not found in the cat cerebral cortex (Ben Hamida *et al.*, 1983). Increased proliferation of brain capillary endothelial cells occurs in association with proliferation of oligodendroglial cells in female carriers of the jimpy mutation in mice (Bartlett and Skoff, 1989; see Section 3.16). The ventricular germinal zone and subependymal zone are also sites of very active angiogenesis and these are also the most common sites of brain hemorrhage in premature infants (Leech and Kohnen, 1974).

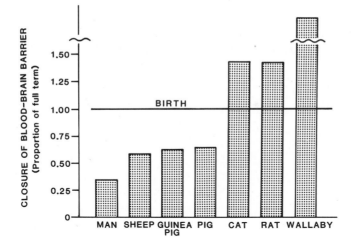

Figure 3.16. Time of closure of the blood–brain barrier may occur either before or after birth in different mammals. In humans it occurs in gestation and in the cat and rat during the neonatal period, in the Tammar wallaby, which is born after only 27 days of gestation, the closure occurs near the end of the period of 250 days while the young wallaby is in the mother's pouch. Modified from C. E. Johanson (1989).

There is conflicting evidence regarding the time of development of a functional blood–brain barrier (Mollgard and Saunders, 1986, review). Complete impermeability to macromolecules has been reported from the earliest stages of development (Saunders and Mollgard, 1984; Mollgard and Saunders, 1986). This is correlated with the presence of tight junctions very early in development as shown by electron microscopy and freeze fracture (Mollgard and Saunders, 1975). However, variable results have been obtained when the permeability of the developing blood–brain barrier has been tested by means of markers such as HRP. For example, Mollgard and Saunders (1986) found the barrier to be closed to proteins from early fetal stages whereas Stewart and Hayakawa (1987) found a gradual closure with age, only becoming completely closed postnatally in the rat (Ferguson and Woodbury, 1969; Bradbury, 1979; Lossinsky et al., 1986; Johanson, 1989, review). As shown in Fig. 3.16, the time of closure occurs at different times in different species: in humans and other primates, sheep, guinea pig, and pig, closure occurs in the first half of gestation, in the cat, rat, and mouse, closure occurs about the 3rd postnatal week; and in the wallaby, it is delayed for months after entry into the mother's pouch. In this context, it is of considerable practical significance to know the status of the vascular supply to grafts of fetal brain tissue to the adult brain. Al-

lografts of fetal brain to the mammalian cerebral cortex are rapidly invaded by blood vessels and a blood–brain barrier develops after grafting in the brain parenchyma (Broadwell et al., 1987; Dusart et al., 1987; Krum and Rosenstein, 1989), but not when grafts are placed in the ventricle (Rosenstein, 1987).

Development of the nerves supplying the brain arterioles probably occurs over the same extended period as the growth of the brain vascular system. There are at least three separate sources of innervation of the blood vessels supplying the CNS: the arteries on the surface are innervated by nerves of peripheral autonomic origin (Nelson et al., 1970); central serotonergic nerves from the raphe nuclei supply arterioles that penetrate from the pia into the brain parenchyma (Edvinsson et al., 1983), whereas the small arterioles throughout the brain are innervated by fibers of noradrenergic neurons in the locus coeruleus (Rennels and Nelson, 1975). There is considerable evidence that nerve growth factor regulates the sprouting of nerve fibers innervating the brain vasculature (Menesini-Chen et al., 1978; Stenevi and Björklund, 1978; Crutcher et al., 1979, 1981). These nerve fibers are in a highly plastic state, and their density is probably continuously changing as a result of terminal sprouting to adapt to functional requirements.

Development of the choroid plexus and secretion of cerebrospinal fluid by the choroid plexus starts early during mammalian embryonic development, coinciding with the phases of mitotic activity in the ventricular germinal layer and subependymal layer (Kappers, 1958; Tennyson and Pappas, 1968; Chamberlain, 1973; Sturrock, 1979). Correlation of glycogen in the choroid plexus cells with brain metabolic activity suggests that the CSF may supply nutrients to the developing brain (Kappers, 1958; Sturrock, 1979).

In summary: the blood vessels that grow into the CNS form a distinct anatomical compartment, separated from the neurectodermal cells by a basement membrane. The brain capillary endothelial cells are joined by tight junctions, so that all exchange between blood and brain occurs by transport through the endothelial cells, particularly by pinocytosis. This exchange is highly selective, so that many toxins, drugs, and even ions are excluded from the brain whereas others, glucose and amino acids, are selectively transported across the blood–brain barrier. The barrier functions of the endothelial cells are induced and maintained by the astrocytes that form a glial cell layer between the capillaries and the neurons. Development of the brain microvascular system adapts to the functional requirements of the brain and is maximal during periods of increased neuronal and glial cell proliferation, growth and differentiation of dendrites, synaptogenesis, and myelination. The functional state of the brain microvasculature is also controlled by monoaminergic nerve fibers originating from neurons in the brain stem. These neurons supplying the brain arterioles are among the most plastic in the CNS, and probably continue growth and sprouting throughout life under the influence of nerve growth factors, including those produced by glial cells, as a form of adaptation to changing functional requirements. Ontogenetic interactions between astrocytes, brain capillary endothelial cells, and nerves innervating the brain blood vessels are a major problem for future research to resolve.

4   The Neural Crest
and Its Derivatives

. . . a physiological system . . . is not a sum of elements to be distinguished from each other and analyzed discretely, but a pattern, that is to say a form, a structure; the element's existence does not precede the existence of the whole, it comes neither before nor after it, for the parts do not determine the pattern, but the pattern determines the parts: knowledge of the pattern and of its laws, of the set and its structure, could not possibly be derived from discrete knowledge of the elements that compose it.

Georges Perec (1936–1982), "La vie,
mode d'emploi" (1978)

4.1. Historical Perspective

The principle, whereby the germinal discs of organ rudiments are represented in a planar pattern, and conversely, every single point of the germinal disc reappears in an organ, I name the principle of organ-forming germinal regions.

Wilhelm His (1831–1904),
Unsere Körperform, p. 19, 1874

In 1868 Wilhelm His discovered the neural crest and he traced the origin of spinal and cranial ganglia from the neural crest (Fig. 4.1). These discoveries raised several theoretical problems—the origin and boundaries of the neural crest, the modes of cell migration, and the fates of cells of neural crest origin. For the past century these problems—origin, migration, and fate—have been the main conceptual platforms from which research programs on neural crest development have been launched.

The first of those research programs was aimed at finding the origins and morphological boundaries of the neural crest in the brain as well as the spinal cord. Wilhelm His thought that the neural crest originates from the *Zwischenstrang* (meaning "intermediate cord") situated between the cutaneous ectoderm and the neural plate, and he regarded it as distinct from the neural tube and the lateral ectoderm, both anatomically and with respect to the structures to which it gives rise. A priority dispute arose when Balfour (1875, 1878) announced the "discovery" of the neural ridge, part of the neural tube, as the origin of the spinal ganglia in elasmobranch fish. Wilhelm His (1879) then asserted his claim to priority of discovery of the origin of the cranial and spinal ganglia from a distinct organ-forming zone, the neural crest. Wilhelm His (1874) identified the neural crest as one of the organ-forming germinal zones as defined in the epigraph to this section, and he conjectured that it contained subsets of cells with restricted fates. During the following century that conjecture was subjected to numerous weak refutations and partial corroborations, and it has recently received further corroboration (Maxwell *et al.*, 1988; Fontaine-Perus *et al.*, 1988; Baroffio *et al.*, 1988; Smith-Thomas and Fawcett, 1989).

143

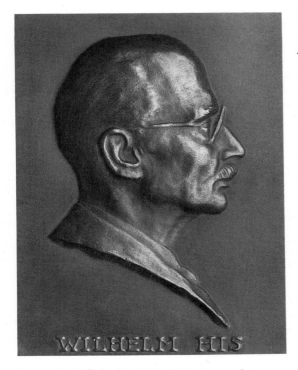

Figure 4.1. Wilhelm His (1831–1904): *Vir praeclarissimus.* Discoverer of the neural crest and of the origin of the peripheral nervous system (1868); discoverer of cell migration in the vertebrate central and peripheral nervous systems (1868, 1889); discoverer of outgrowths of nerve fibers from nerve cells in chick and human embryos (1887, 1888a); discoverer of the origin of neurons by mitosis of ventricular germinal cells (1887). He showed that neuroglial cells originate from neurectoderm and not from mesoderm as was previously believed (His, 1889). He greatly advanced the science of human embryology (His, 1880, 1882, 1904). One of his minor achievements was to have identified the skull of J. S. Bach by showing that clay reconstruction of the face made on Bach's skull closely resembled an oil painting of the elderly Bach (His, 1895). This portrait harmonizes with the classical style of his scientific research and writing—the style is formal; it is not lacking in expression but the expression is in the force of the logic and the wit rather than in the sentiment. He was a product of the Swiss enlightenment: pursuit of self interest was tempered by liberal values, moral high-mindedness, and public service.

The problem of migration of neural crest cells was conceived by His as part of the general problem of cell migration and cell assembly during morphogenesis, in purely mechanistic terms of mechanical guidance either of coherent masses of cells or of individual cells. This mechanistic theory was greatly influenced by Carl Ludwig, professor of physiology at Leipzig, to whom His dedicated *Unsere Körperform* (1874), as a kind of mechanistic embryological manifesto. The aim of his manifesto was to refute theories which held that nonmaterial vital forces were at work during development, for example, Ernst Haeckel's "morphogenetic forces" ("*formbildende Kräfte*") and Justus Liebig's "life forces" ("*lebens Kräfte*") (see Section 11.1). Mechanistic materialism of the kind upheld by His, Moleschott, Ludwig, and others was unable to refute vitalistic theories because there always remained some phenomena which could not be given a completely mechanistic explanation. Vitalists were unwilling or unable to disclose the conditions for refutation of their theories, and by placing them virtually beyond refutation they also place them outside the empirical sciences (see footnote 1 in Chapter 11).

The history of research on the neural crest can be divided into three overlapping research programs. The first program started with the discovery of the neural crest by Wilhelm His in 1868 and lasted until about 1900. Its primary objectives were to describe development of the neural crest in terms of cellular activities and to fit the observations into comparative morphological and evolutionary theories (summarized in Neumayer, 1906). To achieve those objectives it was necessary to improve microscopic and histological techniques. His made important contributions to those technical advances, such as the invention in 1866 of the first microtome to have a micrometer advance (His, 1870).

This epoch may also be dated from the publication of the first significant treatise on comparative embryology (Balfour, 1880, 1881, Vol. 2 deals with the vertebrates). Twenty-six years later the achievements of this research program were collected in the magisterial compendium edited by O. Hertwig (1906, over 5000 pages dealing with all the classes of vertebrates, with chapters by such luminaries as O. and R. Hertwig, W. Waldeyer, F. Keibel, K. von Kupffer, H. Braus, E. Gaupp, W. Flemming, and F. Hochstetter, to note only the most famous). There has been no other period of 26 years in the history of embryology in which so much has been done by so few.

Wilhelm His made the distinction between two periods of development in general, and nerve cells in particular: the period of cell proliferation or "numerical growth," as he called it, and the period of "trophic growth," which is characterized by nerve cell differentiation and by outgrowth of nerve fibers (His, 1868, p. 187). He was also the first to give convincing histological evidence that the nerve fibers are outgrowths from the nerve cells, although the concept that nerve fibers are protoplasmic outgrowths of the nerve cell had been proposed earlier by Bidder and Kupffer, Remak, and Koelliker (see Sections 5.1 and 6.1). The observation, first made by His, that nerve fibers grow out only after neural crest cells migrate to the sites at which ganglia are formed was critical evidence that rendered dubious the theory, then considered to be certain, that all neurons are connected by delicate fibers from the start of their migration.

One of the most significant advances during this epoch was the report by Julia Platt (1893) that she could follow "mesectoderm" from the neural crest to cartilages of the head in *Necturus*. This was the first experimental evidence challenging the dogma of origin of cartilage from mesoderm, and thus a refutation of the germ layer theory. Her findings were confirmed by von Kupffer in cyclostomes (1895), Dohrn (1902) in selachians, and Brauer (1904) in the limbless amphibian *Gymnophiona*. These findings raised fundamental questions about the origins of mesodermal segmentation of the head. The segmental pattern of the head and the relationships of the cranial nerves had been worked out by methods of comparative anatomy (Van Wijhe, 1883; O. Strong, 1895; J. B. Johnston, 1898; C. J. Herrick, 1899). The question arose about how the primary mesodermal segmentation of the head could be related to origin of cartilage cells from the apparently unsegmental cranial neural crest. The answer emerged as a result of the transplantation experiments that were the vogue during the next epoch. It was that the segmental pattern must develop primarily in the mesenchyme of the head that is not of neural crest origin; later the neural crest cells, which are not themselves segmentally determined, migrate into the predetermined metameric pattern of the mesenchyme (Landacre, 1910, 1914, 1921; Stone, 1922, 1929; Celestino da Costa, 1931; Starck, 1937; Ortmann, 1943).

The first research program terminated gradually after about 1900 with the decline of interest in comparative anatomy and with the reciprocal rise of the research program of experimental embryol- ogy. These two research programs, which overlapped in time, correspond with what Merz (1904) calls the morphological and genetic concepts of nature. The first tries to explain development in terms of rules that underlie invariant or universal patterns of morphological organization such as segmentation, polarity, and symmetry, or more generally in terms of body plans. It attempts to define homologous forms that show how morphological patterns have been conserved during development and evolution. The second tries to explain the genetic rules by which the patterns are expressed and change during development and evolution. These views are not mutually exclusive, of course, and both views were held by many workers. However, after 1900 the genetic view gained ascendancy.

The second research program can be called the Program of Experimental Embryology. It may be dated from 1888 with publication of a report by Wilhelm Roux showing that destruction of one of the first two blastomeres of the frog embryo results in development of only one-half of the embryo from which partial regeneration of the other half appears to occur. Roux's experimental method of analysis set an example for the entire research program. However, his interpretation that the egg is a self-differentiating mosaic, and even the reproducibility of his results, were later challenged by Oscar Hertwig (1894, Vol. 2 is a critique of Roux). The crucial counterexample to Roux's result was the discovery by Hans Driesch that separation of the first two blastomeres of the sea urchin embryo results in development of two complete larvae. It has been said that while Roux pointed the way to the methodology of experimental embryology, the fundamental problem of development, namely, embryonic regulation, was raised by Driesch, and that the heir to both traditions was Spemann (Horder and Weindling, 1985). Certainly, with regard to the history of the neural crest, the relative role of self-differentiation and of regulation of crest cells has been an important issue.

This program was defined by Wilhelm Roux in 1894 with his manifesto, the celebrated *"Einleitung,"* published in the first issue of his journal *Archiv für Entwickelungsmechanik*. The opening sentence states that *"Developmental mechanics or causal morphology of organisms, which this Archiv is dedicated to serve, is the **Doctrine of the causes of organic form**, consequently the doctrine of the* *causes of the origin, maintenance, and involution of these forms.*" The experiment is the method of causal analysis, Roux declared. The comparative embryologists and anatomists have arrived where the new science of Entwickelungsmechanik is starting, Roux states, and he refers in a single sentence to the work of Wilhelm His. It is also strange that the name of His does not appear in the long list of those who gave their support to the new *Archiv*.

Manifestos proclaiming new theses always exaggerate their importance and originality, and Roux's was no exception. The three distinctive features of Roux's contribution were all derivative. His preformationism was derived from a long tradition and most directly from Weismann and His, albeit with modification. Roux's mechanistic materialism also had a venerable tradition, but for the present purposes it is only necessary to say that Roux's outlook was less rigorously and uncompromisingly materialistic than that of His. Roux's claim that he had introduced a totally new causal–analytic experimental method was true only in that the experimental method became increasingly used in embryology after Roux. Experimental perturbation of development had been used to analyze development long before—we have seen in Section 2.11 how Friedrich Blumenbach (1752–1840) made animal chimeras of differently colored hydra to show that the whole animal can be reconstituted by regulation of the different parts and not by regeneration of each part separately (Blumenbach, 1792). Experimental analysis of artificial fertilization of frog eggs, performed by Lazzaro Spallanzani (1789), is another early example of the causal analysis of development prior to the era of *Entwickelungsmechanik*.

Two important experimental techniques were invented at the start of this research program, namely, tissue culture and analysis of chimeras. Tissue culture was invented by Wilhelm Roux (1893) and Gustav Born (1895) but was first used for studying neurite outgrowth by Ross Harrison (1910, 1912, see footnote 4 in Chapter 5). Surprisingly fast, a spate of publications appeared in which nervous tissue was studied *in vitro* (Lewis and Lewis, 1911, 1912a,b; Herlitzka, 1911; Marinesco and Minea, 1912) and the technique has remained indispensable to the present time. The second important technical advance made at that time was the analysis of amphibian chimeras by Gustav Born (1876) and Ross Harrison (1903) (see Section 2.11). The technique of interspecific and intergeneric grafting was very useful in the early studies of neural crest migration in urodeles (Lehman, 1927; Raven, 1931, 1936, 1937; Detwiler, 1937). In frogs, chimeras made up of cells from two species with different cellular markers have also been used quite often since the early experiments of Born and Harrison (G. Wagner, 1948; Thiébaud, 1983; Sadaghiani and Thiébaud, 1987; Krotoski *et al.*, 1988). Analysis of neural crest development has been greatly advanced by using the quail/chick chimera introduced by Le Douarin in 1969 (Le Douarin, 1973; Le Douarin and Teillet, 1973).

Another advance made during this period was clarification of the contribution of ectodermal placodes to cranial ganglia. This was first done by Landacre (1910, 1912, 1916) in the fishes *Ameiurus* and *Lepidosteus* and the dogfish *Squalus*. Later he was able to trace the fates of neural crest cells in the head because of their characteristic pigmentation and yolk granules in the urodele *Plethodon* (Landacre, 1921). The placodal contributions to cranial ganglia were further defined by Knouff (1927, 1935) in the frog. The vital staining method of Vogt (1925, 1929) was used to trace the fates of cranial neural crest in urodeles by Detwiler (1937a), Yntema (1943), and Hörstadius and Sellman (1946).

Studies on mammalian neural crest development were limited to descriptive observations, and the advances that were made by the methods of experimental embryology, using amphibian embryos, could not be applied at that time to mammalian embryos. The first description of neural crest in a mammal was given by Chiarugi (1894) in the guinea pig. This was followed by the extensive series of guinea pig embryos studied during the 1920s by Celestino da Costa (1931) and Adelmann's (1925) classical study of cranial neural crest development in more than 200 rat embryos. Those descriptive studies are unlikely to be repeated and are still valuable sources of information.

Perhaps the most significant achievement of the 2nd research program on neural crest development was the demonstration that neural crest cells are pluripotent and that they can give rise to a wide range of cell types in all three classical germ layers (reviewed by Raven, 1931–1933, 1936; Starck, 1937; Hörstadius, 1950). The ablation and grafting experiments of the earlier part of this epoch have been repeated more recently using better techniques and have been extended to include avian and mammalian embryos. That program also remained incomplete, so that the mechanisms of cell migration, inductive cellular interactions, and cell determination remained to be elucidated by molecular biological methods.

In the Developmental Neurobiology Research Program, from the 1960s, the search for molecular mechanisms has dominated the field. The thrust of the new research program was articulated by Joshua Lederberg in the introduction to the first volume of *Current Topics in Developmental Biology* (1966): *"The field has had enough fancy; more recently its methodology has been under enormous pressure to accommodate the inspirations of molecular biology and the models of development that can be read into microbial genetic systems. But now, as this volume amply shows, it is responding."*

4.2. Introductory Overview

Mountains of material about neural crest have grown up since its discovery, and since then, at regular intervals, extensive reviews have been written about it. It now seems to have become like Venice, about which Henry James could write, in 1909, that *"there is notoriously nothing more to be said about it,"* but he went on to write a lot about it nevertheless.

Like the neural plate, the neural crest is derived from embryonic ectoderm. It is located in the angle between the dorsolateral part of the neural tube and the overlying ectoderm, extending from the diencephalon to the tail. A great variety of cell types originate from the neural crest (Table 4.1), including all neurons and glial cells of the peripheral nervous system, except those neurons of the cranial sensory ganglia that originate from cranial ectodermal placodes. Neurons in the central nervous system that originate from the neural crest include the mesencephalic nucleus of the 5th cranial nerve and possibly the Rohon–Beard neurons in the dorsal spinal cord.

The neural crest can first be seen histologically as a separate population of cells at the lateral margins of the neural folds, and later as cells that separate from the neural folds as the latter fuse dorsally to complete the closure of the neural tube. Neural crest cells begin emigrating before closure of the neural tube, commencing at the level of the mesencephalon and progressing in a rostrocaudal sequence. Maturation of the extracellular matrix surrounding the neural crest is one of the conditions necessary for initiation of emigration of cells from the crest (Löfberg *et al.*, 1985, 1989). Emigration from the crest occurs both as coherent populations as well as individual cells. Newly emigrating cranial neural crest cells preferentially enter a lateral pathway under the surface ectoderm, whereas the majority of trunk neural crest cells enter a ventral pathway between neural tube and somites (Weston, 1963; Le Douarin, 1973), as shown in Fig. 4.2.

Characteristic migration patterns of neural crest cells are determined by the local environment, especially by oriented extracellular matrix molecules along the migration pathways (Löfberg *et al.*, 1980; Brauer and Markwald, 1988; Newgreen, 1989). Cells continue to emerge from the neural crest and migrate along well-defined routes to occupy specific sites in the periphery. They divide and mingle locally as they migrate. The basic patterns of neural crest origin, migration, and formation of various peripheral structures are similar in embryos of all vertebrate classes (Reviewed by Neumayer, 1906; Holmdahl, 1928; Raven, 1936; Harrison, 1938; Hörstadius, 1950; Bartelmez, 1962; Weston, 1970; Le Douarin, 1982, 1986).

How are the neural crest cells set apart, in the first instance, from the neural plate and the lateral ectoderm? What are the developmental potentials of individual neural crest cells at different positions and stages of development and how are they realized? What factors are involved in release of cells from the neural crest? What are the mechanisms of their migration and what conditions stimulate or inhibit migration? How are neural crest cells entrapped or arrested at specific peripheral sites? What controls their proliferation and their final numbers at different peripheral locations? What factors control differentiation of various types of cells of neural crest origin? Neural crest derivatives occupy all the classical germ layers (Table 4.1), and this poses yet another set of questions about the validity of the germ layer theory (see Section 1.1).

Research methods that have been used to find answers to these questions include surgical removal or grafting, tissue culture, fate mapping, and cell lineage tracing using a variety of techniques for la-

Table 4.1. The Derivatives of the Neural Crest[a]

1. Peripheral nervous system (PNS)
   (a) **Neurons**
       (i) Cranial sensory ganglia V, VII, IX, X (proximal parts) — Yntema, 1943; D'Amico-Martel and Noden, 1983; Tan and Morriss Kay, 1986
       (ii) Spinal sensory ganglia — Teillet *et al.*, 1987
       (iii) Sympathetic ganglia and plexuses — Kirby and Gilmore, 1987
       (iv) Parasympathetic ganglia and enteric plexuses — Le Douarin and Teillet, 1974; Gershon, 1981; Kirby and Stewart, 1983
       (v) Mesencephalic nucleus of V — Narayanan and Narayanan, 1978
       (vi) Rohon–Beard neurons — Du Shane, 1938; Chibon, 1966
   (b) **Neuroglial cells of entire PNS** — Teillet, 1971
   (c) **Schwann cells** — Weston, 1970; Noden, 1978
2. Endocrine and paraendocrine cells
   (a) **Adrenal medulla** — Teillet and Le Douarin, 1974
   (b) **Calcitonin-secreting cells** — Polak *et al.*, 1974
   (c) **Carotid body Type 1 cells** — Pearse *et al.*, 1973
3. Pigment cells — Du Shane, 1938; Newth, 1956; Teillet, 1971; Epperlein and Löfberg, 1984; Tucker and Erickson, 1986
4. Mesectodermal derivatives
   (a) **Meninges**: pia-arachnoid of prosencephalon and part of mesencephalon. — Harvey and Burr, 1926; Le Lièvre, 1976
   (b) **Visceral skeleton and anterior ventral skull bones** — Chibon, 1966, 1967; Noden, 1986
   (c) **Connective tissue**
       (i) Corneal endothelium and stroma — Johnston *et al.*, 1979
       (ii) Tooth papillae — Chibon, 1970; Kirby *et al.*, 1983; Bockman *et al.*, 1987
       (iii) Dermis, smooth muscle, and adipose tissue of skin of head and ventral part of neck — Raven, 1936
       (iv) Connective tissue of glands (salivary, lacrymal, thymus, thyroid, pituitary) — Le Douarin and Jotereau, 1975
       (v) Connective tissue and smooth muscle of arteries of aortic arch origin — Le Lièvre and Le Douarin, 1975; Kirby *et al.*, 1983, Sumida *et al.*, 1989
       (vi) Mesenchyme of dorsal tail fin — Du Shane, 1935

[a]Selected references are provided to aid further access to the literature, and do not indicate priority.

beling neural crest cells. Each method has limitations as well as certain advantages. Removal of small parts of neural crest to observe the resulting defects has been the classical method of elucidating the fates of neural crest cells. To study their migrations and subsequent fates, homotopic grafts of labeled crest cells or injection of a cell lineage tracer into a single neural crest progenitor has been carried out. Heterotopic transplantation of labeled neural crest cells can show whether their fates were determined at their original or at their final positions. Clonal culture can show how many types of cells originate from a single neural crest cell under various conditions.

The roles of specific molecules in different phases of development of neural crest cells can be studied immunocytochemically by observing when certain antigenic molecules are expressed and by showing that antibodies which recognize those molecules also perturb neural crest development in specific ways *in vivo* and *in vitro*. The putative roles of such molecules can be tested in tissue culture or *in*

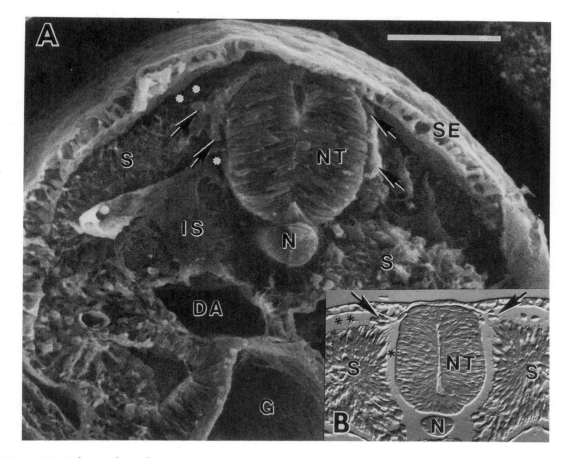

Figure 4.2. Pathways of neural crest migration in the trunk of the 2-day chick embryo. (A) Scanning electron micrograph of a transverse slice through the trunk showing the neural crest (arrowheads) migrating into the dorsolateral pathway (two asterisks) and mediolateral pathway (one asterisk). (B) Transverse plastic section at about the same level as (A) viewed with differential interference contrast optics. DA = dorsal aorta; G = gut; IS = intersegmental artery between two somites; N = notochord; NT = neural tube; S = somite; SE = surface epithelium. Magnification bar ± 100 μm. Micrographs kindly provided by G. C. Schoenwolf.

vivo by either increasing (by local injection) or reducing (by means of antibodies or enzymes) those molecules in the neural crest, the migration pathways, or the peripheral destinations of neural crest cells. Messenger RNA extracted from subpopulations of neural crest cells can be used to construct cDNA libraries that can be screened with antibodies or oligonucleotide probes to clone genes that are involved in neural crest development. *In situ* hybridization and Northern blot analysis can be used for identification of neural crest specific mRNA.

Although many important problems remain incompletely resolved, the main features of development of neural crest cells can now be summarized. Neural crest cell lineages diverge from CNS cell lineages at an early stage, during gastrulation. The mechanisms of initial determination of cell types within the neural crest remain unknown. When transplanted from one segmental level to another in the trunk, they can give rise to the full range of terminally differentiated cell types, indicating that multipotential precursors are present. However, trunk and head neural crest cells are not fully interconvertible, showing that some restriction of fates occurs in the neural crest itself. Heterogeneity has also been defined by differences in the immunoreactivity of subpopulations of cells in the neural crest.

Restrictions of potentialities of some neural crest cells start before their emigration but determination of various cell types is completed by conditions in their peripheral environments. Such factors include materials in the extracellular matrix onto which neural crest cells can adhere preferentially, and which determine the routes of migration to various peripheral destinations; factors which stimulate cell differentiation, for example, outgrowth of neurites; and trophic factors, which promote survival of differentiated cell types.

Behavior of neural crest cells is also modulated by changes in their surface receptors for extracellular molecules and by changes in cell adhesion molecules at the cell surface. These changes at the cell surface determine whether crest cells adhere more strongly to one another or to extracellular matrix materials, and thus migrate either as a coherent multicellular tissue or as independent cells, and whether they cease migration and cohere to form ganglia.

Some neural crest derivatives retain considerable developmental plasticity and thus resemble some other populations of embryonic cells that migrate and mingle on the way to their final positions. Commitment to programs of terminal differentiation is delayed in such cells, and they retain the ability to undergo transdifferentiation without cell divisions, even after they are fully differentiated, in response to changes of environmental conditions. Such plasticity apparently has the advantages of neither requiring tight control of pathways of cell migration to predetermined destinations nor requiring regulation of the final population size by means of cell death.

4.3. Migration and Fate of Neural Crest Cells

Various experimental methods have been used for tracing the origins, migrations, and fates of neural crest cells. They are, first, histological recognition of neural crest cells in normal embryos; second, ablation of the crest or neural folds; third, grafting crest to other sites or explantation into culture systems; fourth, grafting marked crest cells from one level to the same or another level in the neural axis; and, fifth, labeling individual cells in the neural crest with a heritable cell lineage tracer.

Identification of neural crest cells by visible characteristics such as size and pigmentation enabled the early investigators to map their migration routes and fates with remarkable accuracy (Landacre, 1921). Recently introduced methods of clonal analysis by means of heritable cell lineage tracers (see Section 2.11), especially when combined with monoclonal antibodies that recognize neural crest cells, will eventually make it unnecessary to use transplantation for studying neural crest migration.

Ablation and grafting are still indispensable methods for studying the role of cell interactions and extrinsic factors in specification of cell fates and cell determination. Some of the disadvantages of deducing cell fates from defects resulting from ablation of parts of the crest are that small ablations are often repaired from the neighboring parts of the crest, while large ablations may include adjacent central nervous tissue and may disrupt normal development. Ablation and grafting of relatively large populations of neural crest cells have the disadvantage that they may fail to show *all* the derivatives of the crest: because the operations may have been performed after migration of some crest cells had occurred, because selective death and survival of different subpopulations of the grafts may occur, and because specific tissue interactions required for differentiation of some or all crest derivatives may not be possible at the graft site.

Vital staining of neural crest cells has also been used to trace the fate of the cells (Detwiler, 1937a; Yntema, 1943), but this technique is now mainly of historical interest. Another strategy for marking the neural crest cells has been to graft to an unlabeled host the neural crest from an embryo labeled with tritiated thymidine. The labeled cells can subsequently be identified by means of autoradiography in amphibians, birds, and mammals (Weston, 1963; Weston and Butler, 1966; Johnston, 1966; Chibon, 1967; Noden, 1975; Tan and Morriss-Kay, 1986; Morriss-Kay and Tan, 1987). It is not possible to trace cells into late stages of development with this method because dilution of the label to undetectable levels occurs in rapidly dividing cells such as those of neural crest origin. This limitation also applies to labeled lectins, such as wheat germ agglutinin–gold conjugate (Smits van Prooije *et al.*, 1987; Chan and Tam, 1988). Injection of labeled lectin into the amniotic sac of the mouse embryo results in total labeling of the embryo from which labeled cells can be grafted to unlabeled embryos.

The use of a natural cell marker which is stable and can be seen in all the cells that originate from a transplant has great advantages over artificially introduced markers which are diluted as a result of cell division. Raven (1937) grafted neural crest between two genera of amphibians with different sizes of nuclei (xenoplastic grafting) and was able to identify the cells that originated from the graft. More recently, some elegant studies have been done by grafting of neural tube and crest between quail and chick (Le Douarin, 1973). Identification of the cells derived from chick or quail grafts is possible because of characteristic differences between the interphase nuclei stained with the Feulgen technique; the nucleolar-associated chromatin is dispersed in the chick but forms large clumps of heterochromatin in the quail (Fig. 1.9).

A nuclear marker is available for the frog, *Xenopus,* in which quinicrine staining results in punctate fluorescence of nuclei of cells of *Xenopus borealis,* which are used for grafting to *Xenopus laevis* embryos, in which uniform nuclear fluorescence occurs (Thiébaud, 1983). The fates of cephalic neural crest in *Xenopus* have been mapped in this way, by orthotopic grafts of *Xenopus borealis* neural crest to *Xenopus laevis* hosts at the open neural plate stage (Sadaghiani and Thiébaud, 1987; Krotoski *et al.*, 1988). Such experiments have been done only at relatively late stages of development when the neural crest can be identified and excised and grafted to new positions. The grafts can be exchanged between the same or different levels of the neuraxis (homotopic or heterotopic grafting) or between the same or different stages of development (isochronic or heterochronic grafting), and the types of cells derived from the grafts, their migration routes, and their final positions can be demonstrated (reviewed by Le Douarin, 1982, 1986). The results of such grafting experiments are considered in Section 4.6.

Grafting as a means of tracing migration patterns of neural crest cells (although not as a means of assaying their states of determination) may eventually be rendered obsolete by the use of special histological staining of neural crest cells (Nichols, 1986) and by the use of a panel of monoclonal antibodies that can be used to identify all the different phenotypes at all stages of development. The use of antibodies that specifically stain subpopulations of neural crest cells before migration (Marusich *et al.*, 1986a,b; Barald, 1988a,b), during migration (Vincent *et al.*, 1983; Vincent and Thiery, 1984; Tucker *et al.*, 1984; Rickmann *et al.*, 1985), and after arrival in the periphery (Barald, 1982; Dodd *et al.*, 1985; Regan *et al.*, 1986; Sieber-Blum, 1989) show that the terminally differentiated phenotypes of neural crest cells may appear at different stages, before, during, or after their migration.

4.4. Factors Regulating Migration and Differentiation of Crest Cells

The effects of extracellular matrix molecules on neural crest cell motility and morphology have been studied by explanting crest cells on glass or plastic coated with extracellular matrix molecules, or into three-dimensional collagen gels. Extracellular matrix materials have been shown to regulate neural crest migration and differentiation. These include fibronectin (Newgreen and Thiery, 1980; Mayer *et al.*, 1981; Thiery *et al.*, 1982; Duband and Thiery, 1982; Hynes and Yamada, 1982; Duband *et al.*, 1986; Perris *et al.*, 1989), laminin (Newgreen and Erickson, 1986; Duband and Thiery, 1987; Perris *et al.*, 1989), tenascin (Mackie *et al.*, 1988; Epperlein *et al.*, 1988; Halfter *et al.*, 1989), collagen Type I and IV (Frederickson and Low, 1971; von der Mark *et al.*, 1976; Newgreen *et al.*, 1982; Duband and Thiery, 1987), and hyaluronic acid and chondroitin sulfate, which may be in the form of either glycosaminoglycan or the proteoglycan (Derby, 1978; Pintar, 1978; Brauer *et al.*, 1985). Crest cells adhere strongly to laminin, which is specifically localized as the major component of basement membranes of epithelia bounding the pathways of migration of neural crest cells (Newgreen, 1984; Sternberg and Kimber, 1986; Erickson, 1987; Halfter *et al.*, 1989; see Section 5.11 for details of laminin structure and its function during neurite elongation).

Basement membranes contain four macromolecules as their major components: Type IV collagen, laminin, entactin, and proteoheparan sulfate (reviewed by Timpl and Dziadek, 1986; Furthmayr, 1988). Cytotactin (also called tenascin, brachionectin, J1) is a large extracellular proteoglycan found in basement membranes of the neural tube, in the migration pathways of neural crest cells, and in the mature vertebrate CNS. It functions as a cell–cell and cell-substratum adhesion molecule (Erickson and Bourdon, 1989; Chiquet-Ehrismann, 1990, reviews).

It should be noted that the term "basement membrane" is used to refer to the material deposited on the epithelial cell surface as seen with light microscopy. Basement membrane consists of basal lamina plus additional material (Bluemink et al., 1984; G. R. Martin and Timpl, 1987; Leblond and Inoue, 1989). Standard transmission electron micrographs show only the electron-dense middle layer, the lamina densa, and not the inner lamina rara (also called lamina lucida) or the outer pars fibroreticularis, which connects the basement membrane to connective tissue (LeBlond and Inoue, 1989). I prefer to use the term "basal lamina" only when referring to electron micrographs.

Migration of neural crest cells occurs by a combination of passive displacement of coherent populations and active migration of individual cells. Active migration can be seen in tissue culture, and that it can also occur in vivo is shown by the fact that neural crest cells transplanted in ventral positions can migrate dorsally in the opposite direction to normal (Hörstadius and Sellman, 1946; Weston, 1963; Erickson et al., 1980).

The classical cases of migration of individual neural crest derivatives are pigment cells and Schwann cells, which can easily be seen through the transparent epidermis of the tail fin of the frog tadpole (Harrison, 1904, 1924a,b; Speidel, 1964; Billings-Gagliardi, 1977). This is discussed in Section 3.8. Adequate intercellular spaces must be present, and the crest cells start their migration as spaces appear between somites and neural tube and between neural tube and ectoderm (Fig. 4.2). These are the two pathways entered by the newly emigrating crest cells, the dorsal or dorsolateral pathway being favored by the majority of cephalic neural crest cells, whereas the majority of trunk crest cells enter the ventral pathway (Pratt et al., 1975; Thiery et al., 1982; Newgreen et al., 1982; Brauer et al., 1985; Brauer and Markwald, 1987). Using the fluorescent dye DiI (Honig and Hume, 1989) to label the neural tube and crest in chick embryos, Serbedzija et al. (1989) have demonstrated that in the chick embryo crest cells enter the ventral pathway first and the dorsal pathway last.

The importance of intercellular space is shown in the patch mutant mouse in which a space opens prematurely between ectoderm and somites, and neural crest cells invade that space 2 days before their normal time (Erickson and Weston, 1983). The crest cells enter spaces between compact tissues and do not penetrate through basement membranes of the epidermal ectoderm, neural tube, somites, or blood vessels. By contrast, growing nerve fibers have no such difficulty in penetrating basement membranes, and this may be correlated with the evidence showing that domains of the laminin molecule, and cell receptors, involved in promoting nerve fiber extension are different from those involved in cell adhesion on laminin substrates (Edgar et al., 1984; Lander et al., 1985a,b).

The roles of extracellular matrix molecules in release of neural crest cells from the neural folds and in migration and trapping of neural crest cells have been studied by several methods. Specific histological stains and antibodies show that the pathways of neural cell migration are correlated with characteristic distributions of extracellular matrix molecules.

The extracellular matrix is not homogeneous, and different subpopulations of neural crest cells associate preferentially with specific components of the extracellular matrix (Brauer et al., 1985). The composition of the extracellular matrix changes during development. Some of the matrix is produced by the neural crest cells themselves, so that the initial wave of neural crest cells modifies the extracellular matrix encountered by neural crest cells migrating later. The spatial arrangement of extracellular matrix components may be as important as the composition of the extracellular matrix (Oldberg and Ruoslahti, 1982; Brauer et al., 1985; Schittny et al., 1988). Therefore, the behavior of neural crest cells on a flat surface coated with purified extracellular matrix components is probably a very inadequate model of conditions in real life. This limitation also applies to in vitro observations of growth cone activity and morphology, which have many features in common with migrating neural crest cells. (See Section 5.11.)

Fibronectin and laminin are the preferred substrates for neural crest migration *in vivo* (Newgreen and Thiery, 1980; Mayer *et al.*, 1981; Krotoski *et al.*, 1986; Duband and Thiery, 1987) and *in vitro* (Tucker and Erickson, 1984). Neural crest migration is maximal on relatively low concentrations of purified laminin and is reduced at higher concentrations, and migration is increased when laminin is associated with nidogen (Perris *et al.*, 1989). Fibronectin and laminin contain the sequence Arg-Gly-Asp-Ser (RGDS) as part of the cell attachment domain, and this sequence is recognized by cell membrane receptors belonging to the integrin family (Buck and Horwitz, 1987; Hynes, 1987; Ruoslahti and Pierschbacher, 1987; Ruoslahti, 1988, review). Neural crest cells migrate in synthetic basement membrane matrices containing laminin, fibronectin, and collagen, but their migration is inhibited by a synthetic peptide Gly-Tyr-Ile-Gly-Ser-Arg (YIGSR) which blocks the RGDS sites in the cell binding domain of laminin and fibronectin (Bilozur and Hay, 1987). Neural crest cells modulate their levels of vinculin and talin, which link the cytoskeleton to integrin and thus to cell membrane adhesive sites for extracellular matrix molecules (Duband and Thiery, 1990).

Evidence that fibronectins are involved in migration of neural crest cells is that their migration is partially blocked by antibodies against fibronectin (Rovasio *et al.*, 1983) or the fibronectin receptor (Bronner-Fraser, 1986) or by a peptide containing the cell-binding domain of fibronectin (Boucaut *et al.*, 1984). Fibronectins are already present in the migration pathways before emigration begins. Therefore, either the crest cells lack fibronectin receptors prior to their migration or fibronectin is not the only stimulus for initial migration from the neural crest. Grafts of extracellular matrix components attached to membrane filters stimulate initial emigration of neural crest cells in the Axolotl embryo (Löfberg *et al.*, 1985). This shows that the premigratory neural crest cells have the ability to migrate, but their initial migration is triggered by extracellular matrix components.

Cell migration requires a delicate balance between the strengths of cell–cell adhesion and cell–substratum adhesion. Migration occurs when the cells have sufficient adhesion for traction but not sufficiently strong adhesion to one another or to the substratum to be immobilized. Neural crest cells

migrate into regions of moderate fibronectin concentrations *in vivo* (Thiery *et al.*, 1982) and *in vitro* (Yamada and Kennedy, 1984). Neural crest cells have high binding affinity for fibronectin during their migration, but this diminishes as the cells aggregate to form ganglia (Rovasio *et al.*, 1983). Fibronectin present in the migration pathways is replaced by laminin at the sites of neural crest cell aggregation (Rogers *et al.*, 1986; Kimber, 1986; Duband and Thiery, 1987).

Changes also occur in adhesive properties of neural crest cells: NCAM (Thiery *et al.*, 1984; Duband *et al.*, 1985) and N-cadherin (Hatta *et al.*, 1987; Duband *et al.*, 1988) are expressed on all neurepithelial and neural crest cells prior to migration but disappear from migrating neural crest cells and reappear on the surface of cells when they aggregate to form ganglia (Fig. 4.3). As they emigrate, neural crest cells lose their adhesion mediated by N-cadherin and reduce their adhesion due to NCAM. They regain those cell-adhesion molecules when they reaggregate to form ganglia (Duband *et al.*, 1985, 1988). At the same time fibronectin present in the migration pathway is replaced by laminin at the sites of neural crest cell aggregation (Rogers *et al.*, 1986; Sternberg and Kimber, 1986; Duband and Thiery, 1987).

Tenascin (cytotactin; Chiquet-Ehrismann *et al.*, 1986) is another glycoprotein of the extracellular matrix that is found in the migratory pathways of neural crest cells in amphibian, avian, and mammalian embryos (Mackie *et al.*, 1988; Epperlein *et al.*, 1988). Its distribution is much more restricted than that of fibronectin, being localized to the anterior half of each somite in the chick embryo, which is also one of the pathways for migration of neural crest cells (Mackie *et al.*, 1988). Tenascin on the substratum promotes quail neural crest cell migration, probably by facilitating attachment (Halfter *et al.*, 1989).

The role of collagens in neural crest migration is uncertain. There are at least 10 different kinds of collagen (Martin *et al.*, 1985) but only Types I, III, and IV are common. They provide mechanical strength to connective tissues and may form oriented pathways for cell migration. Types I and III form banded fibers whereas Type IV is nonfibrillar and is specifically localized in basement membranes. Type I collagen is associated with fibronectins in the extracellular migratory pathways of neural

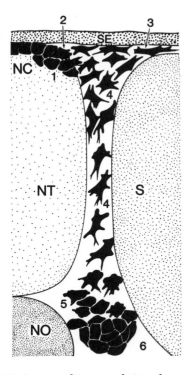

Figure 4.3. Some conditions regulating release, migration, aggregation, and differentiation of neural crest cells. (1) Cell adhesion molecules, N-CAM, and N-cadherin maintain adhesion of neural crest cells to one another. (2) Cells at the surface of the neural crest are exposed to extracellular matrix components, especially fibronectin, laminin, and tenascin, which stimulate cell migration out of the crest. Cells migrating in the dorsolateral migration pathway (3) and the ventromedial migration pathway (4) are subjected to different extracellular conditions which determine their fates. Cell adhesion molecules (CAMs) are down-regulated on the surfaces of migrating neural crest cells. Extracellular conditions which do not support cell migration result in rounding up of cells (5) and expression of CAMs on the cell surfaces results in cell aggregation (6). Components of extracellular matrix play a role in determining the fates of neural crest cells in different locations. NC = neural crest; NO = notochord; NT = neural tube; S = somite; SE = surface ectoderm.

crest cells, but Type III collagen is not observed in those pathways. Type IV collagen is associated with laminin and entactin (Carlin *et al.*, 1981) in basement membranes that form boundaries to the routes of migration of neural crest cells (Duband and Thiery, 1987).

Hyaluronic acid and chondroitin sulfate are present in the migration pathways of neural crest cells. Hyaluronic acid is synthesized by the neural crest cells, ectoderm, somites, and neural tube cells. Crest cells do not adhere to hyaluronic acid (Fisher and Solursh, 1979). The role of hyaluronic acid appears to be to expand the extracellular spaces and so facilitate migration of neural crest cells (Derby, 1978; Pintar, 1978). High, but not low, concentrations of hyaluronic acid inhibit migration of neural crest cells in culture, possibly by reducing adhesivity of the substrate (Tucker and Erickson, 1984). Therefore, it is possible that high concentrations of hyaluronic acid may be one of the factors that stop migration of neural crest cells at sites of ganglion formation. Chondroitin sulfate reduces crest cell adhesion to fibronectin or to collagen *in vitro* and may act in this way *in vivo* (Morris, 1979).

In summary, neural crest cell migration is controlled by complex factors, including cell adhesion molecules and extracellular matrix molecules. Extracellular conditions, especially their affinity for fibronectin and laminin, determine their paths of migration. There may be differences between populations of crest cells in their preferences for various extracellular conditions. Release of cells from the neural crest seems to depend on the balance between the strength of their adhesion to one another by means of cell surface adhesion molecules and their adhesion to extracellular matrix molecules, especially fibronectin and laminin, in the peripheral pathways. The adhesion molecules and their receptors provide neural crest cells with anchorage, traction for migration, and possibly signals for growth and differentiation. Cell migration is facilitated by hyaluronic acid which expands the extracellular spaces. Neural crest cells adhere much more strongly to fibronectin and laminin than to collagen, chondroitin sulfate, or hyaluronate, so that the relative abundance of these extracellular matrix molecules may determine the routes of migration and the preferences for subpopulations of crest cells to enter those routes. Extracellular matrix conditions which do not favor cell motility, combined with relatively greater adhesion between the neural crest cells themselves than between cells and substratum, result in reaggregation of the crest cells and formation of peripheral ganglia.

The conditions that result in determination of the large variety of cellular phenotypes of neural crest origin and their terminal differentiation in the peripheral tissues are considered in the following sections. Local conditions in the periphery are critical for terminal differentiation, and in some cases the involvement of neurotrophic molecules has been demonstrated. The problems of nerve cell maintenance, survival, or death and the roles of neurotrophic molecules are dealt with at greater length in Chapter 8.

4.5. Diversification of Neural Crest Cells

A variety of cell types distributed throughout the animal are derived from the neural crest (Table 4.1). Therefore, we have to ask how the neural crest cells migrate to their final positions and how they differentiate appropriately at many different sites.

The neural crest gives rise to neurons and glial cells in cranial and spinal sensory and autonomic ganglia, enteric ganglion cells of the entire digestive tract, Schwann cells of peripheral nerves, pigment cells in all tissue except the retina, chromaffin cells of the adrenal medulla, several types of endocrine and paraendocrine cells, and a variety of types of connective tissue. Only those crest derivatives of relevance to the nervous system are considered here. Development of Schwann cells is discussed at length in Sections 3.7–3.12. Development of sensory and autonomic ganglia is dealt with in Sections 8.10 and 8.14.

The leptomeninges (pia and arachnoid mater) of part of the mesencephalon and the entire diencephalon and telencephalon (i.e., prosencephalon) originate from neural crest. The leptomeninges of part of the mesencephalon, rhombencephalon, and spinal cord as well as the entire dura mater are of mesodermal origin. These two origins of leptomeninges have been demonstrated in amphibians (Harvey and Burr, 1926; Harvey et al., 1933) and birds (Van Campenhout, 1937; Ayer-Le Lièvre and Le Douarin, 1982). Thus, if the telencephalic region of the neural tube is transplanted to another part of the body in larval *Ambystoma*, the transplanted brain develops without pia-arachnoid, whereas the leptomeninges develop with the brain if neural crest is transplanted with neural tube.

Cranial sensory ganglion neurons originate from neural crest as well as from the cranial ectodermal placodes, but the neuroglial (satellite cells)

of these ganglia are entirely derived from the neural crest (D'Amico-Martel and Noden, 1983). The neurons of the proximal parts of ganglia of the IXth and Xth cranial nerves originate from neural crest, whereas the placodes are the sole source of neurons of the distal parts of those ganglia (petrosal and nodose ganglia, respectively) and neurons of the vestibuloacoustic (VIIIth) ganglion (Halley, 1955; Batten, 1958). The trigeminal ganglion of the Vth cranial nerve and the geniculate ganglion of the VIIth nerve contain neurons of crest and placode origin. These conclusions are derived from the classical histological observation on bird and mammalian embryos (reviewed by Hörstadius, 1950; Nichols, 1986) and from tracing grafted, labeled cells in chick embryos (Narayanan and Narayanan, 1980; Ayer-LeLièvre and Le Douarin, 1982; D'Amico-Martel and Noden, 1983) and in rat embryos (Tan and Morriss-Kay, 1986; Chan and Tam, 1988). All the primary sensory neurons in the spinal ganglia are of neural crest origin, and so are all the glial cells (satellite cells) in the cranial and spinal ganglia.

There are important histological and functional differences between crest- and placode-derived primary sensory neurons. The neuropeptide excitatory synaptic transmitter, substance P, is present in all cranial sensory ganglionic neurons of crest origin but very rarely in those of placodal origin (Fontaine-Perus et al., 1985). Those of neural crest origin are small, occupy the proximal part of the ganglion, and require nerve growth factor (NGF) for their survival (see Sections 8.10 and 8.14). By contrast, the neurons of placode origin are large, occupy the distal part of the ganglion, and are not dependent on NGF. Both types of primary sensory neurons require brain-derived neurotrophic factor (BDNF, Barde et al., 1982; see Section 8.17) for survival and for promoting nerve fiber outgrowth (Lindsay et al., 1985).

BDNF supports survival of placode-derived and neural crest-derived sensory neurons (Barde et al., 1982; Thoenen et al., 1987; Davies et al., 1987; Ernsberger and Rohrer, 1988; Hofer and Barde, 1988; Rodrigeuz-Tébar and Barde, 1988). Evidence that migrating dorsal root ganglion (DRG) neurons require trophic support from the neural tube is that implantation of a silastic membrane between the neural tube and the migration pathway from neural crest to the DRG results in death of all the DRG neurons. These neurons can be rescued by impregnation of the silastic membrane with BDNF or neural tube extract before implantation (Kalcheim and Le Douarin, 1986; Kalcheim *et al.*, 1987).

The spinal sensory ganglia originate entirely from the neural crest, as is shown by their absence after adequate extirpation of the neural crest at an early stage of development (Harrison, 1924a; Detwiler, 1937a). Quail–chick chimeras show that neurons and neuroglial cells of dorsal root ganglia are entirely of neural crest origin (Teillet, 1971). Detwiler (1934, 1937a) concluded that the neurons of the sensory ganglia form compact aggregates under the influence of the somites. Removing somites results in loss of the corresponding ganglia, whereas additional ganglia develop in juxtaposition to supernumerary somites. Weston (1963) also showed an enhanced rate and duration of migration of neural crest cells in somite mesenchyme and an attenuation of migration between the somites. Neural crest cells migrate ventrally, from the dorsal aspect of the neural tube, through the lateral part of the sclerotome, but only through that part of the sclerotome which is in the rostral part of each somite (Rickmann *et al.*, 1985). This may be a factor that results in segmental aggregation of cells to form spinal ganglia. Further development of the spinal dorsal root ganglia of the chick embryo is described in Section 8.10.

The postganglionic neurons of the autonomic nervous system are all derived from cells that migrate out of the neural crest (W. His, Jr., 1897; Van Campenhout, 1930b, 1931; Detwiler, 1937a; Detwiler and Kehoe, 1939; E. Müller and Ingvar, 1923; Yntema and Hammond, 1947; Nawar, 1956). The sympathetic neurons migrate from the neural crest to form a primary sympathetic chain along the dorsolateral surface of the aorta. Many of the sympathetic neurons reach their prevertebral positions considerably before the aggregation of neurons to form the spinal ganglia (Detwiler, 1937a). Some neurons of the primary sympathetic chain persist as the prevertebral sympathetic ganglia, but the majority migrate laterally, using the segmental branches of the aorta as routes of migration, to form the secondary chain of paravertebral sympathetic ganglia (Tello, 1925; Van Campenhout, 1931).

Van Campenhout (1930b, 1931) first showed that the postganglionic parasympathetic neurons in the walls of the thoracic and abdominal viscera migrate into the viscera from the neural crest and do not differentiate from mesodermal or endodermal cells, and this has been repeatedly confirmed (Le Douarin and Teillet, 1974; Le Douarin, 1982, review). The debate as to whether any neurons of the autonomic nervous system differentiate locally from mesodermal or endodermal cells or whether they are all derived from the neural crest was carried on for 80 years after the discovery of the neural crest (reviewed by Yntema and Hammond, 1947) and is now of historical interest only. A neural crest origin for all neurons and associated glial cells of the autonomic nervous system has been conclusively demonstrated in quail–chick chimeras (reviewed by Le Douarin, 1982).

Schwann cell originate from the neural crest, apparently from all cephalic as well as trunk levels. The Schwann cells move out of the neural crest along the nearest outgrowing peripheral nerves, dividing as they migrate. Local ablation of neural crest results in total absence of Schwann cells from the peripheral nerves in the region (Harrison, 1924a; Detwiler and Kehoe, 1939; Hilber, 1943). Their modes of migration, the major extracellular matrix components with which they come into contact, and the cellular interactions between neurons and Schwann cells are dealt with at length in Sections 3.7–3.12.

Rohon–Beard neurons are of interest because, like the neural crest itself, they have a transient existence (Rohon, 1884; Beard, 1895). It has never been conclusively shown whether they originate from the neural crest or from the neighboring neural tube. Beard (1895) first described their apparent migration from the neural crest as well as their initial axon outgrowth and later degeneration and pointed out that other cells looking like Rohon–Beard neurons migrate into the mesenchymal tissue dorsal to the neural tube and myotomes, to become extramedullary neurons in an elasmobranch fish, the skate *Raja batis*. Chibon (1967) claimed to have demonstrated the origin of Rohon-Beard cells from neural crest in the amphibian *Pleurodeles*, but this is doubtful because his method of surgical removal and transplantation of neural crest could not avoid inclusion of the neighboring neural fold. Clonal analysis, using intracellularly injected horseradish peroxidase or fluorescent molecules as heritable cell lineage tracers, shows that Rohon–Beard neurons and trunk neural crest originate from separate, although adjacent, groups of ancestral cells in the *Xenopus* embryo as early as the 512-cell blastula stage (M.

Jacobson and Moody, 1984; M. Jacobson and Sheard, 1989). Other indications that Rohon–Beard neurons are different from any other neural crest derivatives and are probably not of neural crest origin is that they originate and are determined very early during gastrulation (Lamborghini, 1980; M. Jacobson and Moody, 1984), and they differentiate and form connections before any other neural crest derivatives (M. Jacobson and Huang, 1985).

The origin of trigeminal mesencephalic neurons from cranial neural crest is controversial. The other alternative sources of their origin are the neural tube and the mesencephalic ectodermal placodes. Uncertainties have arisen because the conclusions drawn from grafting or ablation of embryonic rudiments are notoriously liable to errors. Many rudiments are close together, as is the cranial neural crest and ectodermal placodes. In frogs, Piatt (1945) reported that trigeminal mesencephalic neurons originate from the mesencephalic ectodermal placode. Kollross and McMurray (1955) concluded that trigeminal mesencephalic neurons originate from neural crest, whereas Lewis and Straznicky (1979) claimed that they originate from the alar plate of the mesencephalic neural tube.

In chick embryos, the trigeminal mesencephalic neurons originate from neural crest (Narayanan and Narayanan, 1978). Nevertheless, trigeminal mesencephalic neurons fail to respond to NGF either when injected into the chick embryo at E6–E14, or when excised at E16 and cultured in the presence of NGF (Straznicky and Rush, 1985). This and other examples of neurons derived from neural crest which apparently lack NGF receptors and which fail to respond to NGF or to anti-NGF antibodies are discussed in Sections 8.9 and 8.15.

The ganglion cells and associated neuroglial cells of the gut are derived exclusively from neural crest (Andrew, 1971). The factors and conditions that result in differentiation of several functional classes of enteric neurons are not known. That these conditions are likely to be complex is shown by the fact that in the adult there are cholinergic and several types of peptidergic enteric neurons, and there are also enteric neurons that transiently express catecholamines in the embryo (Gershon, 1981; Gershon *et al.*, 1984). It is likely that the different enteric neuronal phenotypes are determined by local differences in the tissue microenvironment and by cellular interactions (Patterson, 1978; Gershon,

1981). The differences are not determined by the origins of cells from different levels of the neural crest, because neural crest from trunk levels that normally do not contribute to enteric ganglia can do so after transplantation of trunk neural crest to the vagal level, and in co-cultures of neural crest with gut. The interactions required for differential expression of enteric ganglion cell phenotypes may be very complex. A possible indication of this is the prolonged time between their entry into the gut and the first overt signs of their differentiation: 12 hours in the chick embryo (Allen and Newgreen, 1980) and 5 days in the mouse embryo (Rothman and Gershon, 1982).

The origin of the ganglion cells in the gut and the associated glial cells has been analyzed by using the technique of transplanting quail neural tube into chick, and this method of analysis has also contributed to solving the problems of the prospective potency of neural crest cells, the selectivity of their migration routes, and the factors involved in control of their differentiation. Le Douarin and Teillet (1973) showed that the ganglion cells in the intestinal wall in the plexuses of Auerbach and Meissner arise from two different levels of the neural crest. In the chick embryo, ganglion cells for the entire length of the digestive tract are derived from neural crest of the caudal rhombencephalon at the level of somites 1–7, whereas lumbosacral neural crest caudal to somite 28 gives rise to some enteric ganglion cells of the intestine below the umbilicus and is the main source of neurons of the ganglion of Remak (Fig. 4.4). These two sources of origin thus correspond to the vagal and lumbosacral divisions of the parasympathetic nervous system, whereas the sympathetic ganglia develop from an entirely different region of trunk neural crest at the level of somites 8–28. The chromaffin cells of the adrenal medulla originate only from neural crest at somites 18–24.

The neural crest cells migrate into the gut via the branchial arches and dorsal mesentery, and they divide as they migrate. They colonize the gut in a single wave, in a rostrocaudal direction, as far as the caudal hindgut. The most caudal part of the hindgut is colonized separately from the sacral neural crest (Gershon, 1981; Le Douarin, 1982, reviews). These events occur from E3 to E8 in the chick (Yntema and Hammond, 1954; Le Douarin and Teillet, 1973) and from embryonic days 11 to 16 in the mouse (Rothman and Gershon, 1982, 1984; Payette *et al.*,

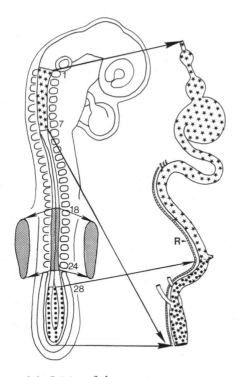

Figure 4.4. Origins of the enteric nervous system from different levels of the neural crest. Anterior and posterior levels of the embryonic neural axis from which the enteric ganglion cells originate as demonstrated by isotopic and isochronic transplantations of quail neural tube into chick embryo (Le Douarin and Teillet, 1973). The neurons arising from the anterior level (between the levels of somites 1 and 7) colonize the whole gut. Those which come from the posterior level located behind somite 28 contribute only to the formation of the ganglia of the postumbilical gut. The neural crest of the cervical and dorsal region (from somites 8 to 28) does not participate in the formation of enteric ganglia but gives rise to adrenergic orthosympathetic neurons and to adrenomedullary cells which come from the precise level of somites 18–24. R = nerve of Remak originating from the lumbosacral level of the neural axis (behind somite 28). From N. M. Le Douarin and M.-A. M. Teillet, *Dev. Biol.* 41:162–184 (1974), copyright Academic Press, Inc.

1984). The myenteric plexus is formed first and the precursors later migrate from the myenteric ganglia, through the circular muscle layer, to the submucosa (Gershon *et al.*, 1980). The extrinsic nerves and accompanying Schwann cells (also of neural crest origin) enter the gut later (Rothman *et al*, 1986).

Factors in the gut that support growth of peripheral nerves and Schwann cells are different from those that promote migration of enteric ganglion cell precursors. This is shown by the observation that in *lethal spotted* (*ls/ls*) mutant mice there is total failure of colonization of the terminal hindgut by enteric ganglion cell precursors but the ingrowth of peripheral nerves and Schwann cells occurs normally (Rothman *et al.*, 1986; Payette *et al.*, 1988). The *lethal spotted* mutant is an animal model for congenital megacolon, also known as Hirschsprung's disease in humans. Defects in extracellular matrix material, especially excess basement membrane components, occur in the terminal hindgut of *lethal spotted* (*ls/ls*) mice, before, during, and after invasion of the hindgut by neural crest cells (Rothman *et al.*, 1986), as shown in Fig. 4.5. Payette *et al.* (1988) propose that the aganglionosis in these mice may be due to an excess of the signal that normally stops neural crest cell migration in the gut.

4.6. Determination of Neural Crest Cell Fates

There is a regional origin of different derivatives of the neural crest, and the question arises whether the neural crest cells from each region are homogeneous or heterogeneous in their prospective potency. There is abundant evidence that some cells from each level retain the potency to differentiate into the cell types normally originating from other levels, but those observations of the behavior of multicellular grafts could not exclude the possibility of selective death or survival of subpopulations of cells with different prospective potencies. This difficulty was not adequately taken into account in drawing conclusions from the results of grafting quail neural tube to different levels of the neural axis in chick embryos (Le Douarin and Teillet, 1974; Le Douarin, 1982, 1986). In all cases the neural crest cells migrate along the usual routes from the graft to the appropriate tissues, showing that there are constraints on the route of migration which lead the cells to the proper terminal sites at each level. On the other hand, the neural crest cells differentiate according to the sites in which they settle, regardless of their origin, showing that the grafts contain some cells which are pluripotent, that they are not fully determined at the beginning of their migration, and that their terminal differentiation is controlled by local factors along the route and at the end of their migration. These

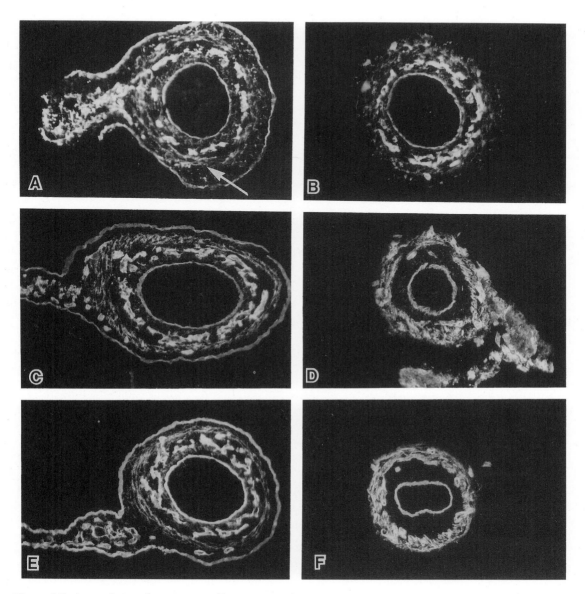

Figure 4.5. Accumulation of components of basement membranes associated with failure of neural crest cells to colonize the distal hindgut in the lethal spotted mutant mouse. Comparison of collagen Type IV and laminin immunofluorescence in the proximal and distal colon of mice at E14. Collagen Type IV immunoreactivity in the proximal colon (A) and distal colon (B) of normal controls is compared with proximal colon (C) and distal colon (D) of *ls/ls* mice. The basement membranes of the mucosa, serosa (absent in distal colon), and blood vessels are brightly stained. The position of the developing circular smooth muscle layer is shown by the arrow pointing to thin strands of immunoreactive material in the intercellular spaces between the myoblasts. Laminin staining in the proximal colon (E) and distal colon (F), both in *ls/ls* mice, has the same pattern as collagen Type IV staining. Note the accumulation of collagen Type IV and laminin in the outer portion of the gut wall of *ls/ls* mice. Magnification X177. From R. F. Payette, V. M. Tennyson, H. D. Pomeranz, T. D. Pham, T. P. Rothman, and M. D. Gershon, *Dev. Biol. 125*:341–360 (1988), copyright Academic Press, Inc.

experiments do not exclude the possibility that cells that are already committed to certain fates while in the crest fail to migrate or fail to survive. Early diversification of cells in the crest itself is shown by evidence that different subpopulations of neural crest cells express specific differentiation antigens prior to their emigration (Ciment and Weston, 1982; Barald, 1982; Payette *et al.*, 1984). The nonneural mesenchymal derivatives of the cephalic neural crest have been shown to be fully committed early as they differentiate into connective tissue regardless of their final location, after transplantation in the intact embryo (Noden, 1978; Le Douarin, 1982). However, periocular mesenchyme cells, which normally form cartilage in avian embryos, can give rise to enteric ganglion cells after they invade the gut in cocultures of gut and neural crest (Smith-Thomas *et al.*, 1986).

In principle, the problem of heterogenity of the neural crest should be possible to resolve by clonal culture of single cells removed from the crest from different segmental levels and at different stages of development (A. M. Cohen and Konigsberg, 1975; Sieber-Blum and Cohen, 1980; Sieber-Blum and Sieber, 1984; Baroffio *et al.*, 1988). However, the results of such experiments have been equivocal. Clonal culture of quail trunk neural crest cells results in clones consisting entirely of melanocytes, or clones containing only adrenergic neurons, or clones containing both (Sieber-Blum and Cohen, 1980). Either these three types of clones originate from the same progenitor that fails to express its full developmental potential in some cases, or they are the progeny of three different progenitor cells. There is evidence in favor of the latter, but falling short of proof (Sieber-Blum and Sieber, 1984). Clonal culture of quail cranial neural crest shows heterogeneity of the cells with respect to their differentiative capabilities—some clones originate from pluripotent cells, others from partially or fully determined cells (Baroffio *et al.*, 1988).

The time of initial determination of the neural crest is at the early gastrula stage in the *Urodele* amphibian embryo, as shown by the earliest time after which cells fated to become neural crest will autonomously differentiate as such after heterotopic transplantation (Raven, 1935). However, there is no direct evidence on this point in other vertebrate classes. During the relatively extended period between gastrulation and the initial emigration of neu-

ral crest cells, there would be ample time for subsets of crest cells to undergo separate paths of determination. Ablation or transplantation of relatively large populations of cells or labelling the entire neural crest with fluorescent tracers (Serbedzija *et al.*, 1989) are useful methods but are incapable of showing conclusively when and how separate subpopulations of ectodermal cells become committed to form the various derivatives of the neural crest. To discover when the fates of crest cells diverge from one another it is necessary to perform a clonal analysis, starting at a specific stage of development, labeling a single neural crest precursor at a selected position with a heritable cell lineage tracer and later tracing the migration pathways, final positions, and phenotypes of the labeled descendants. A number of exogenous cell markers are available, including intracellularly injected macromolecules and retroviral tracers (M. Jacobson, 1986, 1990, reviews; see Section 2.11). Orthotopic and heterotopic grafting of single cells labeled with one of these heritable cell lineage tracers can show whether the labeled descendants have changed fates in their new locations (M. Jacobson and Xu, 1988).

The prospective potency of neural crest cells, that is, the number of alternative differentiation pathways that they are capable of entering under various experimental conditions, has been assayed by transplantation or culture of crest cells. Transplantation and culture experiments are ultimately limited by the accuracy of identification of the terminally differentiated descendants of neural crest precursors. Therefore, an important part of the program of investigation of cell fates has been the invention and refinement of techniques for accurate identification of specific cell types. Methods of immunocytochemistry, using cell type–specific antibodies have been extremely useful for identification of differentiated cells of neural crest origin (Barald, 1982; Ciment and Weston, 1982; McKay and Hockfield, 1982; Schachner, 1982; Vincent *et al.*, 1983; Vincent and Thiery, 1984; Dodd *et al.*, 1985; Regan *et al.*, 1986; Sieber-Blum, 1989). *In situ* nucleic acid hybridization and Northern blot analysis can be used for cellular and tissue localization of neural crest-specific messenger RNA molecules at different stages of development (Anderson and Axel, 1985).

The results of transplantation and culture experiments at first led to the conclusion that neural crest cells are pluripotent and that the neural crest cell population is relatively homogeneous (Le Douarin *et al.*, 1978; Teillet *et al.*, 1978; Sieber-Blum and Cohen, 1980; Loring *et al.*, 1981). Other experiments showed that the neural crest contains pluripotent stem cells but that they are heterogeneous with respect to their fates before migration (A. M. Cohen and Koenigsberg, 1975; Le Douarin *et al.*, 1978; Sieber-Blum and Cohen, 1980; Schweitzer *et al.*, 1983; Anderson *et al.*, 1985; Sieber-Blum and Sie-

ber, 1985; Xue *et al.*, 1985; Anderson and Axel, 1986; Le Douarin, 1986; Baroffio *et al.*, 1988). The concept of homogeneity and pluripotentiality was challenged when antibodies showed that certain antigens typical of differentiated cells of neural crest origin were first detectable in subpopulations of cells in the neural crest before and during their early migration (Barald, 1982, 1988a,b; Barald and Wessels, 1984; Ciment and Weston, 1982; Vincent *et al.*, 1983; Marusich *et al.*, 1986a,b; Barbu *et al.*,

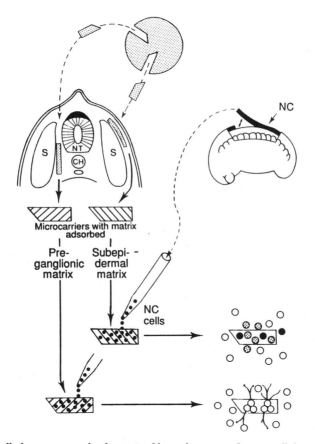

Figure 4.6. Neural crest cell phenotypes can be determined by pathway-specific extracellular matrix molecules. Microcarriers, approximately 0.15 by 0.4 mm, are implanted into the trunk region of stage 25 Mexican axolotl embryos (*Ambystoma mexicanum*) either subepidermally or in the presumptive region of the dorsal root ganglia. Implanted microcarriers are left in the embryo for adsorbance of matrix material for 10–12 hours. Just before the onset of local neural crest cell migration, they are removed from the embryo and transferred to plastic dishes for cell culture or further processed for characterization of the adsorbed matrix material. Pure populations of premigratory neural crest cells are obtained from the neural crest. Explanted neural crest cells can be deposited site specifically onto the matrix-covered microcarriers, or within the same culture dish, onto the plastic surface beside the carriers and incubated for up to 5 days at 20°–22° C in a serum-free medium. Open circles = undifferentiated cells; filled circles = melanocytes; dotted circles = xanthophores; and circles with projections = neurons. From R. Perris, Y. von Boxberg, and J. Löfberg, *Science* 241:86–89 (1988), copyright American Association for the Advancement of Science.

1986; Ziller *et al.*, 1987; Weston *et al.*, 1988). However it should be noted that staining with antibodies indicates the prospective significance of neural crest cells, that is, their differentiation if left undisturbed, which is not the same as all the possible fates that they may have after transplantation or tissue culture (Patterson, 1978; Hawrot, 1980).

The sympathoadrenal precursor cells are perhaps the best-studied case of determination of neural crest derivatives by environmental factors. Both the chromaffin cells of the adrenal medulla and the noradrenergic neurons of the paravertebral sympathetic ganglia originate from the midtrunk level of the neural crest (corresponding with somites 18–24). Normal chromaffin cells develop when the midtrunk level of the neural crest in chick embryos is removed and replaced by quail neural crest from other trunk levels that do not normally give rise to chromaffin cells (Le Douarin, 1982). Fully differentiated chromaffin cells are converted into neurons, without dividing, when treated with NGF *in vitro* (Unsicker *et al.*, 1978; Ogawa *et al.*, 1984; Doupe *et al.*, 1985a,b). Evidence of conversion of chromaffin cells to nerve cells includes outgrowth of nerve fibers, formation of synapses (Ogawa *et al.*, 1984), and expression of neuron specific messenger RNA (Anderson and Axel, 1985). This transdifferentiation is blocked by glucocorticoids, which suggests that secretion of glucocorticoids by the adrenal cortical cells is one of the factors that determines differentiation of chromaffin cells in the adrenal gland. These observations support the hypothesis that adrenal chromaffin cells and sympathetic noradrenergic neurons originate from the same precursor cells in the neural crest (Landis and Patterson, 1981).

The importance of inductive cell interactions along the route of migration is shown by the work of A. M. Cohen (1972) and Norr (1973). The differentiation of sympathetic neurons containing norepinephrine depends on an inductive action of the somitic mesenchyme on the neural crest cells during their migration (A. M. Cohen, 1972). The somitic mesenchyme has this inductive action only if it has previously been in contact with ventral neural tube and notochord (Norr, 1973). When neural crest cells are excised and cultured clonally before any contact with somitic mesenchyme has occurred, only melanocytes but no neural cells differentiate (A. M. Cohen and Konigsberg, 1975). It is not known whether these inductions require direct cell-to-cell contact or whether they may be mediated by diffusible molecules or by components of the extracellular matrix (Bissell *et al.*, 1982).

Determination of region-specific cell types can result from differences in the conditions along the alternative migration pathways. Perris *et al.* (1988) show that premigratory neural crest cells grown on nitrocellulose coated with extracellular matrix components from the dorsolateral migration pathway ("subepidermal matrix") differentiate into pigment cells (Fig. 4.6). The same population of neural crest cells differentiate into neurons when grown on nitrocellulose conditioned with extracellular matrix from the ventral migration pathway ("preganglionic matrix").

5   Axonal Development

*If there exists any surface or separation at the nexus between neurone and neurone,
much of what is characteristic of the conduction exhibited by the reflex-arc might be
more easily explainable. . . . The characters distinguishing reflex-arc conduction
from nerve-trunk conduction may therefore be largely due to intercellular barriers,
delicate transverse membranes, in the former.*

*In view, therefore, of the probable importance physiologically of this mode of
nexus between neurone and neurone, it is convenient to have a term for it. The term
introduced has been synapse.*

Charles Scott Sherrington (1857–1952), *The Integrative Action of the
Nervous System*, 1906

5.1. Historical Perspective

*When you are criticizing the philosophy of
an epoch, do not chiefly direct your attention to those intellectual positions which its
exponents feel it necessary explicitly to defend. There will be some fundamental assumptions which adherents of all the variant systems within the epoch unconsciously
presuppose. Such assumptions appear so
obvious that people do not know what they
are assuming because no other way of put-
ting things has ever occurred to them.*

Alfred North Whitehead (1861–1947),
Science and the Modern World, p.
71, 1925

The history of ideas about the forms and
functions of neurons shows that the conditions
which permit different scientists to uphold totally
opposed hypotheses are, firstly, that the evidence
is contradictory and inconclusive and, secondly,
that one or both hypotheses are based on erroneous assumptions. One of the major assumptions of the late 19th century was that animal cells
lack a cell membrane. The cell surface was be-

lieved to be a transition between two phases, without special structure. Therefore, it was assumed
that protoplasmic bridges between cells could
freely appear and disappear. To recognize the significance of this fundamental assumption is to gain
an entirely fresh view of the history of rival theories of formation of nerve connections. Proponents of the *neuron theory* believed that nerve
cells only come into close contact and are never in
direct protoplasmic continuity, whereas proponents of the *reticular theory* believed that nerve
cells are directly connected by protoplasmic
bridges or networks. The reticular theory is consistent with the fundamental assumption that cells
lack membranes; the neuron theory is in conflict
with that assumption.

The concept of the cell without a surface
membrane is as old as the cell theory itself. Schwann (1839, p. 177) wrote: *"Many cells do not seem
to exhibit any appearance of the formation of a cell
membrane, but seem to be solid, and all that can be
remarked is that the external portion of the layer is
somewhat more compact."* No special structures or
functions were attributed to the cell surface, but the
"physical basis of life" that was so much discussed by

19th-century biologists was assumed to reside in minute particles and fibers in "the protoplasm" (reviewed by Hall, 1969). For example, Max Schultze (1861) defined cells as *"membraneless little lumps of protoplasm with a nucleus."* The concept that the cell lacks a membrane was supported by Carl Gegenbauer in his influential essay on the evolution of the egg, published in 1861. Sedgwick (1895) regarded the embryo as a giant protoplasmic mass in which numerous cell nuclei are embedded. In discussing the structure of nerve cells, Koelliker (1896, Vol. 2, p. 45) believed that the *"central cells lack a definite membrane and possess as boundaries only the tissues of the grey substance, which consists in varied proportions of nerve fibers, glial cells and blood vessels."* In the 1st edition of E. B. Wilson's very influential book *The Cell in Development and Inheritance* (1896, p. 38), I came across the statement that *"the cell-membrane or intercellular substance is of relatively minor importance, since it is not of constant occurrence, belongs to the lifeless products of the cell, and hence plays no direct part in the active cell-life."* Wilson maintains the same opinion in the 2nd edition (1902, p. 53), but in the 3rd edition (1925, p. 54) he provides some evidence for the existence of a plasma membrane.

The intellectual climate before about 1920 nurtured the concept of protoplasmic connections between neurons. When the inadequate histological methods of those times failed to resolve membranes between cells, it was quite reasonable to assume that the cells are connected to form a syncytium. This flawed assumption, as much as the histological artifacts, formed the basis for reticular theories of connections between neurons.

All the reticular theories of neuronal connectivity claimed that neurons are in direct protoplasmic continuity, and form various types of networks (Gerlach, 1858, 1872; Golgi, 1882–1883, 1891; Apáthy, 1897). The outlines of these theories have so often been reviewed that they do not require repetition insofar as they narrate the sequences of events and their main ideas (Stieda, 1899; Soury, 1899; Barker, 1901; Ramón y Cajal, 1932; Van der Loos, 1967; Clarke and O'Malley, 1968). However, none of those authors seem to have recognized that the unstated assumption beneath all the variant theories was that cells normally lack a cell membrane. We can now understand more adequately how the minds of the proponents of different theories of neuronal organization were conditioned by the prevalent assumptions about cellular organization, and how far their theoretical speculations exceeded what they could have seen in their histological preparations.

The idea that nerve cells are directly interconnected through a network of fine fibers is usually attributed to Camillo Golgi (1843–1926). However, that notion was originally the brainchild of Joseph von Gerlach (1820–1896). In sections of the spinal cord stained with carmine or gold chloride, Gerlach (1872) saw a fine feltwork of fibers in the gray matter. He interpreted this to be a genuine network formed by anastomosis between branches of the dendrites, which were at that time called protoplasmic processes. Remak (1854) and Deiters (1865) had shown that the branched protoplasmic processes are different from the single, unbranched axis cylinder, but they had not been able to show how they end or form connections in either the central or peripheral nervous systems (see Sections 6.1 and 7.1). Gerlach (1872) depicted the sensory fibers of the dorsal roots originating indirectly by branching from a diffuse nerve network formed by interconnected branches of the protoplasmic processes. Gerlach's concept was accepted by all neuroanatomists at that time because it was consistent with the prevailing belief in protoplasmic bridges connecting cells in general.

Gerlach's construct was eventually demolished by Golgi (1882–1883), using his method of impregnation with potassium bichromate and silver nitrate, which revealed the entire neuron for the first time. Golgi (1882–1883) showed that, contrary to Gerlach's construct, the protoplasmic processes end freely, without any interconnecting network, and appear to make contact only with blood vessels and glial cells (Fig. 5.1). Therefore, he thought that they must have nutritive functions, and he looked elsewhere for the conducting pathways between nerve cells. He believed that he had found them in the axon collaterals, which he discovered. Golgi then made the distinction between two main types of neurons: type I with a long axon and type II with a short axon. He suggested that the axon collaterals of type I neurons are connected directly by a diffuse nerve network (*"reticola nervosa diffusa"*) to branches of the axons of type II neurons, thus excluding the dendrites from the conducting pathways (Fig. 5.1). Golgi at first treated this as a speculative hypothesis, and the diffuse nerve network is merely

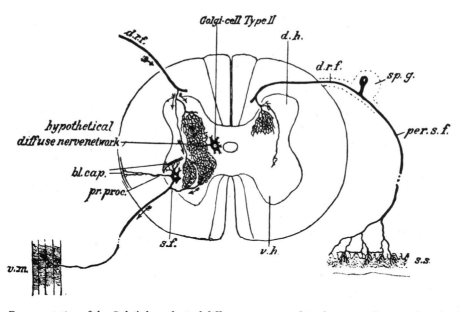

Figure 5.1. Representation of the Golgi's hypothetical diffuse nerve network in the mammalian spinal cord. The network was supposed to be formed by anastomosis between collaterals of incoming dorsal root fibers (d.r.f.), the much branched axons of Golgi type II cells, and collaterals (s.f.) of Golgi Type I cells (the motor neuron). The direction of impulse traffic is shown by the arrows. The cell body and dendrites were supposed to be excluded from the conduction pathways, and the dendrites were supposed to connect with blood capillaries (bl. cap.) and to be purely nutritive in function. From L. Barker, *The Nervous System and its Constituent Neurones* (1901).

discussed but never shown in any of the numerous figures in his 1882-1883 papers or in his long polemical paper of 1891 which deals specifically with the question of the functional significance of the nerve net.[1] Pictures of the *"reticola nervosa diffusa"* are shown for the first time in two figures in a communication from Golgi which appears in the *Trattato di fisiologia* of Luigi Luciani (1901), and the same figures are reproduced in Golgi's *Opera Omnia* (1903, Figs. 41 and 42) and his Nobel lecture (1907). One figure shows a network formed by axon collaterals of granule cells of the hippocampal dentate gyrus, the other depicts a network in the granular layer of the cerebellar cortex formed by axonal branches of the basket cells. Neither of these curious illustrations shows the 2nd type of cell participating in the network, as the theory requires. On this point the text also reveals Golgi's reluctance to commit himself to specific details, saying that these figures only *"give an idea of the network"* (Golgi, 1907, p. 15; see also Section 6.1 for Golgi's statement that he regarded the network as a hypothesis, not a proven fact).

The reticular theory, increasingly destitute of empirical and intellectual support, found its final refuge in structures of incredible subtlety, at the limits of resolution of light microscopy.[2] These are aptly described by Golgi (1901) as *"di organizza-*

---

[1]Golgi was quick to understand that his theory precludes strict functional localization in the central nervous system (CNS). This theoretical issue is a significant component of Golgi's thinking about structure–function correlation in the CNS which merits far more attention than can be given to it here. One can merely comment that the reticularists were unanimously opposed to the concept of strict functional localization while the neuronists generally supported the idea of localization of functions in the CNS. Reticularists also underestimated the significance of specificity of neuronal connections and therefore overestimated the role of plasticity in development and in recovery from injury of the CNS (e.g., Bethe and Fischer, 1932a,b). This is considered further near the end of this section and in Section 11.1.

[2]The diffuse nerve net and all the other incredibly fine interneuronal fibrils and networks were hypostatized entities that existed only as mental constructs. It is virtually impossible to refute a theory supported by hypostatized entities because those entities can be reinvented as required to save the theory. That strategy saved the reticular theory for over 80 years until the electron microscopic evidence refuted it.

zione di meravigliosa finezza." These structures took the form of tenuous fibrillar networks that were depicted as direct extensions of intracellular neurofibrils (Apáthy, 1897; Bethe, 1900, 1903, 1904; Held, 1905). Such fancies had to be abandoned when it was shown that neurons are separated at some large synapses by a membrane which is not crossed by neurofibrils and that the neurofibrils do not enter all synaptic terminals (Bartelmez and Hoerr, 1933; Hoer, 1936; Bodian, 1937, 1942). The neurofibrils that are stained with silver in light microscopic preparations of mammalian central nervous tissue were eventually shown to be clumps of neurofilaments when examined with the electron microscope (Peters, 1959; Gray and Guillery, 1961).

Evidence showing a discontinuity from neuron to neuron came from four quarters: embryology, histology, physiology, and pathological anatomy.[3] The first embryological evidence of the individuality of neurons was reported by Wilhelm His (1886, 1887, 1889). He demonstrated that neuroblasts originate and migrate as separate cells and that nerve fibers grow out of individual neuroblasts and have free endings before they form connections. In 1887 His described with remarkable accuracy the outgrowth of the nerve fiber: *"The fibers which grow out from the nerve cells advance by growing into existing interstitial spaces between other tissue elements. In the spinal cord and in the brain, the medullary stroma already formed, provides pathways for expansion and its structure undoubtedly determines the course of the process of extension. . . ."* These observations were later confirmed by Ramón y Cajal (1888, 1890a,b,c, 1907, 1908). This evidence showing free outgrowth of axons did not shake the faith of the reticularists because they could point out that it did not exclude the later development of protoplasmic continuity between neurons after they had made contact (Nissl, 1903; Bethe, 1904; Held, 1905). Of course, the fact that axons and dendrites develop as independent extensions of the neuron did not prove that the entire neuron remains an independent cell, but evidence for that gradually accumulated. Ramón y Cajal (1888, 1890a,b,c, 1907) showed that neurons stained by means of the Golgi technique were always completely isolated from others, and he followed Golgi in assuming that they were revealed in

[3]To maintain a logical flow of concepts in this section, I have discussed theories of outgrowth of fibers from nerve cells in greater detail in Section 6.1.

their entirety. This assumption could not be tested before the advent of the electron microscope.

During the 19th century there were three main theories of development of the axon: the cell-chain theory, the plasmodesm theory, and the outgrowth theory. According to the cell-chain theory, originated by Schwann and supported by F. M. Balfour among other excellent embryologists, the axon is formed by fusion of the cells that form the neurilemmal sheath. This theory of development was an extrapolation from interpretations of regeneration of peripheral nerves, in which Schwann cells and fibroblasts were mistaken for the precursors of the regenerating axons. Ramón y Cajal (1928, pp. 7–16) heaps scorn and derision on this theory and on its proponents who are *"little acquainted with the severity and rigour of micrographic observations, and with the secrets of histological interpretation,"* but his rhetoric cannot conceal the fact that histological observations alone, without experimental evidence, were insufficient to disprove the cell-chain theory. It is fair to say that Cajal tended to use such rhetorical flourishes to conceal weaknesses in his arguments. The cell-chain theory was finally refuted by the elegant experiments of Harrison (1904, 1906, 1924a), when he showed that removal of the neural crest, from which the Schwann cells originate, results in the development of normal nerve fibers in the absence of Schwann cells. He also demonstrated that removal of the neural tube, which contains the developing neurons, prevents the formation of nerves, although the Schwann cells are left intact.

The plasmodesm or syncytial theory originated with Viktor Hensen (1835–1924) and was supported by Hans Held (1866–1942). According to this theory, the nerve fiber differentiates from preestablished filaments that connect all the cells of the nervous system. This theory was founded on the fundamental assumption, which has been discussed above, that cells originate as a syncytium in the embryo and retain protoplasmic bridges throughout life. This theory was consistent with much of the evidence available at that time and was widely supported. For example, as late as 1925 in the 3rd edition of *The Cell in Development and Inheritance,* E. B. Wilson was still defining plasmodesms as *"the cytoplasmic filaments or bridges by which in many tissues adjoining cells are connected."* The plasmodesm theory provided explanations for sever-

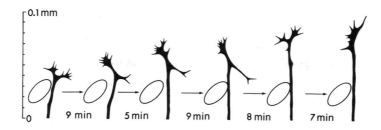

Figure 5.2. Six successive views of the end of a growing nerve fiber, showing its change of shape and rate of growth. The sketches were made with the aid of a camera lucida at the time intervals indicated. The red blood corpuscle, shown in outline, marks a fixed point. The average rate of elongation of the nerve was about 1 μm/minute. The total length of the nerve fiber was 800 μm. The observations were made on a preparation of frog embryo ectoderm, isolated in lymph, 4 days after isolation. Adapted from R. G. Harrison, *J. Exp. Zool.* 9:787-846 (1910).

al observations that were supposed to support the contact theory of the synapse; for example, reflex delay was ascribed to slowing of conduction during passage of the nerve impulse across extremely thin plasmodesms.

The outgrowth of nerve fibers was eventually demonstrated in tissue culture by Ross Harrison (1907b, 1910).[4] Harrison excised pieces of neural tube from early tailbud frog embryos, at a stage before any nerve fibers are present, and explanted the tissue into a drop of frog lymph suspended from a coverslip. Nerve fibers grew out of the explant, in some cases from single isolated cells, for distances up to 1.15 mm at rates ranging from 15.6 to 56 μm/hour (Fig. 5.2). Harrison's observations were very rapidly confirmed by other reports of outgrowth or regeneration of axons in tissue culture of nervous tissue of amphibians (Hertwig,

---

[4]Harrison is usually credited with having invented tissue culture but he had several forebearers. Nevertheless he deserves the credit for having seized the opportunity to use a new technique to solve an old problem. The earliest report of culture of fragments of chick embryo medullary plate in warm saline was made by Wilhelm Roux in 1893, and the following year Gustav Born was the first to culture fragments of amphibian embryos (reviewed by Loeb, 1923; Oppenheimer, 1971). After 1910, Harrison abandoned tissue culture in favor of surgical alteration of whole embryos because he recognized the limitations of tissue culture for answering questions about specification of structures in relation to position in the embryo. For Harrison's contributions to experimental embryology see Oppenheimer (1966). I should call Harrison a scientists' scientist because he often succeeded in devising an experiment that cut through the knottiest problem with a single stroke, which is what we would all like to do.

1911–1912; Legendre, 1912; Oppel, 1913), chick (Burrows, 1911; Lewis and Lewis, 1911, 1912; Ingebrigtsen, 1913a,b) and mammals (Marinesco and Minea, 1912 a–d).

The locomotion and growth of epithelial cells, young neurons, and nerve fibers in tissue culture were shown to occur only when they are in contact with a surface such as fibrin fibers in a fluid medium, or are at the interface between the solid substratum and liquid medium, or are at the liquid–air interface (Loeb, 1902; Harrison, 1910, 1912; W. H. Lewis and Lewis, 1912). This phenomenon was called *stereotropism* by Loeb (1902) and Harrison (1911, 1912), *contact sensibility* by Dustin (1910), and *tactile adhesion* by Ramón y Cajal (1910, 1928). Wilhelm His was the first to recognize the importance of mechanical factors in embryonic development. This and many other important contributions of Wilhelm His to developmental neurobiology are reviewed by Picken (1956). His clearly understood and described cases of axonal guidance by the tissue substratum and his 1894 review of the mechanical basis of animal morphogenesis contain numerous aperçus of the concepts and mechanism of nerve growth later promoted by Ross Harrison and by Paul Weiss.

These results were the final confirmation of the theory of the outgrowth of nerve fibers from young neurons first stated tentatively by Koelliker in 1844: *"The fine fibers arise in the ganglia . . . as simple continuations of the processes of the ganglion-globules. In other words, the processes of the ganglion-globules are the beginnings of these fibers."* Only 13 years later Bidder and Kupffer could assert *"with the greatest degree of certainty, that . . . every fiber must . . . be conceived merely as a colossal 'outgrowth' of the nerve cell"* (see Section 6.1). In 1886 Koelliker could state quite definitely that *"I consider the primitive nerve fibers to be protoplasmic outgrowths of the central nerve cells"* (Koelliker, 1886). This was only one of five cardinal theories and several auxiliary theories which ultimately united around the end of the 19th century to construct a theory of organization of the nervous system. The others were that the nerve cell and fibers are parts of the same unit; that dendrites are fundamentally different from axons; that nerve cells connect by surface contact and not by cytoplasmic continuity; that the contact area between neurons acts as a one-way valve for conduction of nervous activity; that the contact regions are the principal sites of functional integration and modifiability; and that nerve cells and their connections are initially formed in excess, and the redundancy is eliminated during later development. Construction of the general theory ("the neuron theory") from these components is considered in Section 6.1.

Harrison (1910) observed the growth of the axons from the Rohon–Beard cells, which are the primary sensory cells and which can be seen in the dorsal part of the neural tube just beneath the epidermis in living frog embryos. Beard (1896), in his original description of the development of Rohon–Beard neurons, had accurately depicted the outgrowth of the axon from the cell body, but he failed to draw the general conclusion. Harrison observed that as the axon grows out of the Rohon–Beard cell into the subepidermal tissue, it slowly increases in length and gives rise to many branches. The growth of the axons of Rohon–Beard cells occurs in the same way as the growth of axons in tissue culture. The tip of the initial outgrowth, as well as the end of each branch, consists of an enlargement from which ameboid terminal filaments are constantly emitted and retracted. These were the first observations of the activities of the growth cone during normal development in a living animal. They fully confirmed Cajal's descriptions of growth cones in fixed specimens, and they provided a standard by which to assess whether growth cones in histological preparations are normal or artifactual. The fact that Harrison's observations on the growth of living nerve fibers agreed with descriptions of the growth of axons in histological preparations of the developing nervous system at one stroke established the validity of histological observations of Koelliker (1886), His (1886, 1887, 1889), and Cajal (1888, 1890a–c), which were far more detailed and diverse than any that could be obtained *in vitro* at that time. Harrison's experiments had, in his own estimation, taken the mode of formation of the axon *"out of the realm of inference and placed it upon the secure foundation of direct observation."*

Harrison coined the term "exploratory fibers" for the nerve fiber that precedes the rest in the development of a fiber pathway. Cajal gives many vivid descriptions of these pathfinders. For instance, during the outgrowth of the dorsal spinal root from the spinal sensory ganglia, he says, *"a bundle of precocious bipolar cells strikes with its cones, like battering-rams, on the posterior basal membrane and opens a narrow breach in it. Other sensory fibers, differentiating later, make use of this opening, and assault the interior of the spinal cord along its dorsal portion."*

Cajal was the most vigorous advocate of the neuron theory, and it is significant that he never doubted the objective reality of the cell membrane. The sources of his conviction are difficult to trace because he does not discuss the evidence or defend his belief in the existence of the cell membrane. Already in the 1st edition of *Elementos de Histologia Normal* (1895, p. 303) he defines a *"fundamental membrane"* which is *"a living organ of the cell which is a continuation of the protoplasm."* In the 4th edition of his *Manual de Histologia Normal* (1909, pp. 150, 154) he says: *"All the cells of the central nervous system and sensory organs as well as the sympathetic possess a membrane of extreme thinness, a fundamental membrane. . . . This membrane is not a peculiarity of certain neurons, it is a general property without exceptions."* This statement is made *ex cathedra*, without supporting evidence, as if it were a self-evident truth, at a time when most authorities, even some who supported the neuron doctrine, held the opposite opinion, namely, that the cell membrane is either a histological artifact or a lifeless structure without significant function.

I have been unable to determine whether Cajal's belief in the existence of a cell membrane preceded or followed his adoption of the neuron theory. The two beliefs are now seen to be so obviously interdependent that it is not easy to understand how, at that time, it was possible to affirm the one while denying the other. Yet none of the other supporters of the neuron theory shared Cajal's deep conviction, not Koelliker, not Lenhossék, not van Gehuchten. Nor can one find any discussion of the authenticity of the nerve cell membrane in the 19 massive volumes of *Biologische Untersuchungen* (1881–1921) of Gustaf Retzius, a consistent proponent of the neuron theory. The matter was ignored, either because they did not understand the importance of the cell membrane or because they denied its very existence. For example, Koelliker (1896, Vol. 2, p. 48) states that *"with reference to the envelope of the nerve cell, it can be shown with certainty that the latter apparently at all times lacks a cell membrane."* Another defender of the neuron theory, Mathias Duval in his *Précis d'Histologie* (1897, p. 774) says of the nerve cell that *"formerly one described it as having an envelope, by reason of artifacts produced by coagulating reagents; nowadays it is recognized that it is a naked protoplasmic body."*[5] All those who opposed the neuron doctrine were at least logically consistent in also denying the existence of a nerve cell membrane. Thus, after reviewing the evidence, Sterzi (1914, p. 19) concludes that *"a cellular membrane does not exist. . . . The nervous cytoplasm is in direct relationship, through fine reticular fibrils that constitute the interstitial part of the nervous tissue."* Cajal's convictions were not dogmatic—he was too shrewd not to be willing to acknowledge that exceptions to the neuron theory may exist. He admits that perineural connective tissue cells but not the neurons are sometimes connected by protoplasmic bridges. He says that *"these mesodermic cells form a net with meshes of variable size,"* and he shows axons *"growing through the plasmatic interstices [of the] anastomozed fibroblasts"* (1928, p. 183 and Fig. 101D). Cajal treats reports of protoplasmic connections between Schwann cells with skepticism (1928, p. 83) but finally agrees that in degenerating nerves the Schwann cells form a syncytium (1928, p. 130 and Fig. 23).

In his final statement on the evidence for the neuron theory, Cajal (1933) still finds it necessary to ask: *"Do the terminal nerve arborizations actually touch the nude protoplasm of the cell or do limiting membranes exist between the two synaptic factors?"* Then comes the prescient conclusion: *"I definitely favor this latter opinion, although with the reservation that the limiting films are occasionally so extremely thin that their thickness escapes the resolution power of the strongest apochromatic objectives."*[6] He then admits that *"neuronal discontinuity, extremely evident in innumerable examples, could sustain exceptions . . . for example those existing in the glands, vessels and intestines."*

The achievements of Cajal may be seen as signals rising far above the intellectual noise. But it is not always possible to see how they were generated in Cajal's mind, or even how he found the empirical stimuli for his creativity. His autobiographical account of his creative processes, *Recuerdos de mi vida* (1st ed. 1917, 3rd ed. 1923), deserves to be treated with as much skepticism as respect. His *Reglas y consejos para investigación cientifica* (1923) shows how difficult it must have been for him to discipline his unrepentent romanticism.[7] In Cajal the genius of the artist and scientist were combined to a unique degree. He had the gift, usually granted only to the artist, of incorporating vague and chaotic elements of experiences into an orderly synthesis. The artist is more or less free to adopt, modify, or invent a language to represent and express his experience. The scientist is not so free and usually lacks the originality and courage that are necessary to liberate himself from the assumptions of his times.

[5]*"The power of holding two contradictory beliefs in one's mind simultaneously, and accepting both of them"* is how George Orwell defined "doublethink" (*Nineteen Eighty-Four*, Part 2, Chapter 9). Lack of insight is associated with doublethink in the benign form exercised by Koelliker and the others in this case. The malignant form, described in Orwell's novel, occurs when both beliefs are held in full consciousness of the contradiction.

[6]The cell membrane was one of those hypostatized entities like "the synapse" which were given a name before they could be identified physically. Cajal's reservations show that even by 1933 the cell membrane remained a hypothetical construct rather than a physically identified structure.
[7]Cajal's much admired literary style evidently was influenced by the 19th century writers whose works are catalogued in his library, among them the Valencian novelist Blasco Ibañez, and the philosopher Ortega y Gasset. Cajal corresponded with Ortega y Gasset and agreed with the elitist philosophy expressed in Ortega's *Revolt of the Masses*. Cajal's bitter complaints about his disadvantages as a Spaniard on the periphery of European affairs is even more forcefully stated in Ortega's *Invertebrate Spain*. For further reflections on Cajal's style see M. Jacobson, *Conceptual Foundations of Neuroscience*, in preparation.

Cajal's methods of drawing from the microscope can be inferred from his own testimony and other evidence. There is a solitary reference to his use of a camera lucida (Ramón y Cajal, 1891, legend to Fig. 1), but to suggest that he used such a drawing aid habitually (De Felipe and Jones, 1988) is like saying that a life preserver is needed by a powerful swimmer within reach of the shore.[8] Cajal describes different models of camera lucida in his *Manual de Histologia Normal*, but he also describes other instruments such as the microspectroscope and the polarizing microscope, which he probably never used. Further evidence against his habitual use of the camera lucida is that the latter is neither mentioned in Cajal's autobiography nor visible in the photographs showing him at his worktable.[9] Cajal's line drawings of Golgi or silver preparations were evidently made with a metal pen or a goose quill, with which the width of the line can be delicately shaped by varying pressure on the point. Penfield (1954) saw Cajal writing with a goose quill (but not drawing with one or wiping it on his bedsheets, as stated by De Felipe and Jones, 1988). For halftone figures, he used pencils, crayon, and fine paintbrushes (Penfield, 1977, p. 104). Cajal was well aware also of the special artistic effects obtainable with paper of different grades and textures (cf. Ramón y Cajal, 1905, p. 36). I believe that he could have used the camera lucida for laying out the picture at low magnification, but that the details were drawn freehand, keeping one eye and hand on the microscope while using the other hand and eye for drawing. This was the way in which students were trained to use the monocular microscope for making histological drawings, and it was also the principal method recommended by Cajal. He notes in his *Manual de Histologia Normal* (p. 36, 4th ed., 1905) that this method *"requires a facility for copying from nature as well as artistic taste which, alas, does not always coexist in the dedicatees of the natural*

sciences." Cajal would undoubtedly have found this direct method no less accurate and much less cumbersome than using a camera lucida attached to his microscope, especially when a very strong source of light is required for viewing the image of a Golgi preparation 100 μm thick. From his own evidence it is certain that his preferred method of freehand drawing would have been inhibited and frustrated by the use of a camera lucida.

Cajal's unique gift was his ability to grasp in a novel synthesis the relationships between neurons that were seldom if ever seen in a single view through the microscope. Justifying this method, he wrote: *"A histological drawing is never an impersonal copy of everything present in the preparation. If that were true our figures would be far too complicated and almost incomprehensible. By virtue of an incontestable right, the scientific artist, for the purpose of clarity and simplicity, omits many useless details. . . . In order to decrease the number of figures artists are sometimes forced to combine objects which are scattered in two or three successive sections"* (Ramón y Cajal, 1929a).

Cajal had definite presuppositions regarding the functional significance of the living structure he observed in dead, fixed specimens and was not averse to making bold inferences that went beyond anything that he could have seen. For example, in his drawings the conspicuous arrows pointing in the assumed direction of flow of nerve activity were meant to show an intrinsic property of the neuron to conduct in one direction only, a *"dynamic polarization"* of the cell (Fig. 5.3). His vivid description of activity of the growth cone, which he saw only as a fixed and stained structure, is also typical of the strong inductive vein in his mode of thought. Cajal's procedure was akin to that of the method of Chinese painting called *xie-yi hua*, literally "writing the meaning painting," which I have described as a combination of uninhibited fluency with deep insight (M. Jacobson, 1985).

The most compelling pathological–anatomical evidence of discontinuity between one neuron and the others comes from the experiments of von Gudden (1870, 1874, 1881) and Forel (1887). They observed that when axons are cut degeneration is confined to the corresponding neurons. Reactive changes occur in neighboring glial cells (Weigert, 1894; Nissl, 1894), but the neighboring, uninjured neurons remain unaffected (see Section

[8]It is possible that the editors of the journal *La Cellule* required more information than Cajal was in the habit of giving in his unrefereed publications in which there is no mention of the camera lucida (e.g., Ramón y Cajal, 1892).
[9]De Felipe and Jones (1988, p. 5) also err in stating that their Fig. 1 shows *"one of Cajal's favorite Zeiss microscopes, purchased after 1885."* That microscope was actually a gift made to Cajal in 1885 from the Provincial Council of Zaragoza (cf. *Recuerdos de mi vida: Historia de mi labor científica*, Chapter 1). The microscope in question is correctly identified in Albarracín, 1982, p. 97.

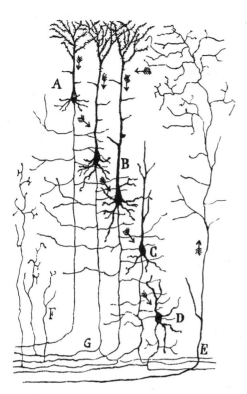

Figure 5.3. Schematic illustation of the probable currents and the nervosoprotoplasmic connections between the cells of the cerebral cortex. A = small pyramidal cell; B = large pyramidal cell; C and D = polymorphic cells; E = fiber terminal coming from other centers; F = collaterals of the white matter; G = axis cylinder bifurcating in the white matter. From S. Ramón y Cajal, *Les nouvelles idées sur la structure du système nerveux chez l'homme et chez les vertébrés*, Reinwald, Paris, 1894.

6.1). After the discovery of specialized nerve terminals called "endkolben" (terminal knobs) or "endfüsse" (endfeet) (Held, 1897; Auerbach, 1878; Ramón y Cajal, 1903; Wolff, 1905), it became apparent that these endings are not in direct continuity with the neurons they contact. This could be deduced from the fact that injury to a neuron results in rapid degeneration of its nerve terminal structures but not of the neurons that they contact (Hoff, 1932; Foerster *et al.*, 1933). Conversely, after nerve injury resulting in retrograde degeneration there is not an immediate effect on the nerve endings in contact with the degenerating neurons (Barr, 1940; Schadewald, 1941, 1942). That the acute degenerative changes are confined to the injured neuron was much later

confirmed with the electron microscope (de Robertis, 1956; reviewed by Gray and Guillery, 1966).

Physiological experiments showed that conduction in nerve fibers is bidirectional whereas conduction in reflex pathways is unidirectional. Sherrington (1900, p. 798) proposed that one-way conduction in the reflex arc is due to a valve-like property of the junction between neurons, which he named the synapse in 1897. Thus the unidirectional conduction in the central nervous system was conceived by Sherrington to be a function of one-way conduction at the synapse and not due to the "dynamic polarization" of the entire neuron from dendrites to axon, as conceived by van Gehuchten (1891) and Ramón y Cajal (1895). Additional physiological evidence supporting the concept of the synapse was provided by measurements of the reflex conduction time, which showed a delay of 1–2 msec more than could be accounted for by the conduction time in the nerve fibers (Sherrington, 1906, p. 22; Jolly, 1911; Hoffmann, 1922; Lorente de Nó, 1935, 1938).

The question of whether transmission of excitation from neuron to muscle is electrical or chemical was first discussed by du Bois-Reymond (1877, p. 700 *et seq.*), who concluded in favor of chemical transmission, largely on the basis of the effects of curare. The accumulation of evidence in favor of chemical transmission at the vagus endings in the heart (Loewi, 1921, 1933), at the neuromuscular junction (Dale, 1935, 1938), and in autonomic ganglia (Feldberg and Gaddum, 1934; Dale, 1935) dealt directly only with transmission at synapses in the peripheral nervous system. Both Adrian (1933) and Eccles (1938) argued that the rapid speed of conduction across central synapses precludes chemical transmission. This objection was removed after it was shown that cholinesterase can act within milliseconds on the amounts of acetylcholine released at the neuromuscular junction and probably also at central synapses (Nachmansohn, 1940).

The advent of the electron microscope and of intracellular microelectrode recording finally proved the identity of synapses in both central and peripheral nervous systems. Until the invention of glass knives for cutting ultrathin sections (Latta and Hartmann, 1950), the electron microscope revealed little more than the light microscope, namely, that there was what appeared to be a single membrane separating the neurons at the synapse (reviewed by Robertson, 1987). Later electron microscopic observations of synapses made with tissues fixed in osmium tetroxide, embedded in methacrylate, and sectioned with glass knives showed the presynaptic and postsynaptic membranes separated by a synaptic cleft about 20 nm wide (Robertson, 1952; Palade and Palay, 1954). Synaptic vesicles, which characterize presynaptic nerve endings (Palade and Palay, 1954; de Robertis and Bennett, 1955), were immediately recognized as possible storage sites of chemical transmitters (del Castillo and Katz, 1956). After the introduction of epoxy embedding (Glauert *et al.*, 1956, 1958) and potassium permanganate fixation (Luft, 1956), it became possible to see the structure of the presynaptic and postsynaptic membranes and to obtain more accurate measurements of the width of the synaptic clefts. Even before glutaraldehyde fixation (Sabatini *et al.*, 1963) provided reliable pictures of cytoplasmic structure, the first attempts were made to find ultrastructural differences between excitatory and inhibitory synapses (Gray, 1959; Anderson *et al.*, 1963; reviewed by Eccles, 1964).

The crucial physiological evidence proving the existence of chemical synaptic transmission was obtained by means of intracellular microelectrode recording at the neuromuscular junction (Fatt and Katz, 1951; Fatt, 1954), in the vertebrate spinal cord (Brock *et al.*, 1952), and in the abdominal ganglion of *Aplysia* (Tauc, 1955). Intracellular microelectrode recording showed that the excitatory postsynaptic potential is thousands of times greater than can be accounted for by electrotonic transmission from neuron to neuron, thus making it certain that the observed amplification is mediated by chemical synaptic transmission. This evidence settled the long-standing controversy between electrical and chemical theories of synaptic transmission (reviewed by Eccles, 1959, 1964, who reversed his early position in support of electrical transmission to finally accept the general validity of chemical transmission at central synapses). It is ironic that no sooner had the dispute been resolved in favor of chemical synaptic transmission than the first report appeared of an authentic case of electrical transmission in the crayfish giant fiber to motor fiber synapses (Furshpan and Potter, 1957). When potassium permanganate fixation allowed membrane structure to be resolved with the electron mi-

croscope, it became evident that the presynaptic and postsynaptic membranes are in close apposition at electrically coupled synapses, whereas a synaptic cleft is characteristic of chemical synapses (Robertson, 1963; 1965; Pappas and Bennett, 1966).

In addition to the preconceived ideas about the absence of cell membranes, the other main reason for the slow acceptance of the neuron theory was that the evidence in its favor arrived in bits and pieces from several different disciplines, over a period of more than 50 years.[10] The neuron theory was built up gradually, by a process of conjecture and refutation. Such theoretical constructs can include approximations, need only have sufficient internal consistency to work, and can be continually adjusted to fit the data.

The theory of scientific revolutions, as expounded by Kuhn (1962, 1970, 1974), does not provide a satisfactory explanation of how the neuron theory ultimately replaced the reticular theory, both of which are components of different paradigms. The neuron theory replaced the reticular theory because it was a more consistent predictor of discoveries and ultimately because the electron microscopy evidence falsified the reticular theory. It is said by Kuhn (1970) that scientific paradigms are created under the influence of the *Zeitgeist* (a term invented by Goethe for events that occur *"neither by agreement nor by fiat, but self-determined under the multiplicity of climates of opinion"*). Yet the history of the neuron and reticular theories shows that both existed in the same *Zeitgeist* and people continued to believe in the reticular theory long after the passing of the *Zeitgeist* in which the theory had grown up. There were also some central figures who remained indifferent to either theory, which shows that the climate of opinion did not affect them crucially. As an example of this indifference it is instructive to quote Wilhelm Wundt (1904), the founder of physiological psychology: *"Whether the definition of the neurone in general, and whether in particular the views of the interconnexion of the neurones pro-*

---

[10]Formulation of the neuron theory occurred so gradually that when it was announced publicly by Waldeyer in 1891, Cajal was taken by surprise and complained that *"all Waldeyer did was to publish in a weekly newspaper a resumé of my research and to invent the term neuron."* Sherrington (1949) notes that Waldeyer's paper was published *"without consulting Cajal"* and *"somewhat to Cajal's surprise."*

mulgated especially by Ramón y Cajal will be tenable in all cases, cannot now be decided. Even at the present day, the theory does not want for opponents. Fortunately, the settlement of these controversies among the morphologists is not of decisive importance for a physiological understanding of nervous functions." Wundt was wrong but he had enormous influence (see Titchener, 1921; Boring, 1950). Wundt's reactionary view of the neuron theory is consistent with his archaic exposition of neuroanatomy which occupies the 1st volume of his very influential textbook *Principles of Physiological Psychology* (5th ed., English transl., 1904) in which the important advances in neuroanatomy and neurocytology of the previous decades are completely ignored.

The physiological psychologists, more than any other group of neuroscientists, continued to support the last vestiges of the reticular theory or variants of it. Karl Lashley (1929) was still upholding a theory of equipotentiality of different regions of the cerebral cortex 50 years after Golgi had proposed a similar theory (see footnote 1 in Chapter 5 and Section 11.1). According to Lashley (1929, 1937), learning and memory depend on the quantity of cortex, not on the specific cortical region. After destruction of large regions of cortex, the *engram* (Lashley's term for the form in which memory is stored) moves to another place without losing its essential form, as in the *"harmonious equipotential system"* proposed by Driesch (1908) to account for embryological regulation in his vitalistic view (see Section 11.1). Sperry's chemoaffinity theory of formation of specific nerve connections (Sperry, 1963) was a reaction to theories of equipotential or random neural networks and to theories of development of functional specificity from an initially diffuse neural network. This is considered at greater length in Section 11.1.

The synapse was conceived as a theoretical necessity by Sherrington in 1897, more than 50 years before it was conclusively shown to exist and function as a physical entity. None of the 19th-century proponents of the different theories of connections between neurons lived to witness the final solution of their problem. Ironically, neither the intracellular microelectrode technique nor electron microscopy owed anything to the rival theories of nerve connections—the stimuli for their invention came from other sources and those techniques were first applied to other problems

before being put to use in solving the problem of neuronal connections. The problems were resolved by opportunistic application of any techniques that seemed likely to work, and finally by means of microelectrode recording and electron microscopy, not merely as a result of wrangling about different theories.

This understanding of the history of neuronal connections and of the neuron theory is different from the generally prevalent view. I see the neuron theory reaching its canonical form, as we finally understand it, only gradually as a result of convergence and coalescence of several theoretical positions and research programs rather than as a revolutionary overthrow of one theory by another.

In Section 6.1 we shall examine the theoretical positions as parts of several research programs, in which different techniques and different values were favored by their protagonists. The techniques that were favored by the neuronists, especially the Golgi methods, corroborated their position by showing free nerve endings. The reticularists favored techniques, for example, the gold technique of Apáthy, and neurofibrillar stains, which apparently revealed fine fibrils directly connecting nerve cells. The neuronists conceived of strict localization of function in the nervous system, whereas the reticularists conceived of diffusely distributed functions. These differences were, in general, also related to different values, for example, as reflected in the mechanism-versus-vitalism and in the nature-versus-nurture debates.[11] The importance of values in neuroscience research programs is discussed further in my *Conceptual Foundations of Neuroscience* (M. Jacobson, in preparation).

It is true that the adversarial theoretical positions occupied by the neuronists and the reticular-

---

[11]As late as 1923 Emil Rohde proposed that all cells, including neurons, originate from a multinucleated syncytium rather than by cell division. I mention this aberration mainly to point out that it was seized upon by E. S. Russell (1930, p. 221) as evidence for a vitalistic theory of the organism. The affinity of vitalists for the reticular theory of nervous organization is related to their need for some empirical evidence for the "wholeness" of the organism, as they understood it (see Russell, 1930, 1946). For additional discussion of relationships between vitalism and theories of nervous development see Sections 3.1 and 11.1.

ists had a powerful heuristic effect, driving them on to seek evidence to corroborate their own position and to refute that of their adversaries. The research program progressed by means of a dialectical process of conjecture and refutation. Because refutation always lags behind conjecture, and because each side held tenaciously to its own theoretical position for as long as possible in the face of counter–evidence, both theories continued to be contested long after the reticular theory became impossible to defend. The reticular research program, with its untenable theory, selective techniques, and special world view, became a degenerating program in the sense that it was supported by artifacts and refuted by the facts.

History provides many examples to show that to gain a scientific reputation it is sufficient to apply a new technique to resolve an old problem, but it is neither necessary to be a profound thinker nor to support the correct theory. As Schopenhauer remarks in a celebrated footnote in *The Art of Controversy* (Parerga and Paralipomena, 1851), in order to win a dispute *"unquestionably, the safest plan is to be right to begin with; but this in itself is not enough in the existing disposition of mankind, and, on the other hand, with the weakness of the human intellect, it is not altogether necessary."*

5.2. General Overview

This chapter and Chapter 6 are concerned mainly with development and maintenance of neuronal form and polarity. Neurons are highly polarized structurally and functionally as individual cells and as elements in neural circuitry. The "dynamic polarization" of the nerve cell was discovered by Van Gehuchten in 1891 and was made a centerpiece in Cajal's conception of neuronal circuits (Ramón y Cajal, 1895). The polarity is reflected in the initial directions of outgrowth of axons and dendrites, in structural and functional differences, particularly in the organization of the cytoskeleton and the presence of ribosomes and Golgi elements in dendrites and their absence from axons. Polarity is manifested by the direction of release and uptake of materials and selective intracellular transport of different materials. The polarity is also expressed by the distribution of presynaptic and postsynaptic membrane spe-

cializations, which determines the direction of impulse traffic in neuronal circuits.

How do the various components develop which ensure the polarity of the neuron? To what extent is polarity intrinsic and to what extent and by what means is polarity determined by external conditions? The same questions may be asked about the differentiation of neuronal types: to what extent is diversification of neuronal types determined by cell lineage and to what extent by cell interactions and extrinsic factors? The role of lineages in determination of cellular phenotypes has been considered in Section 2.11. The main consideration in this chapter is the origin and maintenance of neuronal polarity and form as expressed in differentiation of the axon. Development of dendrites and synapses is discussed in Chapter 6.

In this chapter evidence will be given to show that the differential distribution of cytoplasmic molecules and organelles in dendrites and axons results from the configuration of the neuronal cytoskeleton and selective transport of molecules from the cell body into the axon and dendrites. The microtubules, because of their intrinsic polarity and their selective association with certain proteins that function as transport motors, determine the polarity of the entire neuron. Polarity of microtubules is a consequence of the intrinsic polarity of tubulin molecules which give the microtubules plus and minus ends. Microtubules in the axon are all aligned with their plus ends pointing to the axonal growth cone whereas microtubules in dendrites point in either direction.

There are three microtubule-associated proteins (MAPs), which are mechanicochemical nucleotide triphosphatases that function as motors involved in axonal transport: kinesin, dynein, and dynamin. Kinesin functions as the retrograde motor, dynein as the anterograde motor, and dynamin mediates sliding between microtubules. Organelles and molecules are specifically linked to one of these motors and thus transported preferentially toward one end of the microtubule. For example, ribosomes and Golgi elements are specifically transported to the minus end of microtubules and can therefore enter dendrites but not axons.

In addition to transporting molecules selectively, the cytoskeleton determines neuronal shape, motility, and growth, especially the plasticity of growth cones. The polarized organization of the cytoskeleton, by selectively transporting enzymes, plasma membrane molecules, and receptors, determines the functional repertoires that are specifically localized to different parts of the nerve cell.

Charles Bonnet (1720–1793) was indeed prophetic when he described the organism as *"a marvellous assemblage of an almost infinite number of tubes differently figured, calibrated and twisted"* in his *Contemplation de la Nature*, first published in 1764. Bonnet derived this idea from Albrecht von Haller (1708–1777), who recognized that the organism is formed of fibers which are composed of elementary subunits held together by a cohesive substance. In his very influential *Prima linea physiologiae* (English ed. 1754, Chapter 1, p. 2) von Haller states that *"the primary simple fibre, such as we rather comprehend from reason than from sense, is composed of earthy particles adhering longitudinally, and connected by intervening and cohesive gluten."* These men had embarked on a research program whose aim was to find a purely mechanistic view of the organism. Molecular neurobiology is a culmination of this program to achieve what I term *"the mechanization of the brain picture."*

5.3. The Cytoskeleton

The structural components of the neuron may be observed in living nerve cells or extruded cytoplasm or axoplasm by means of new techniques of light microscopy (Allen and Allen, 1983; Allen et al., 1983). At a higher resolution the cytoskeleton has been studied by standard transmission electron microscopy (Wuerker and Palay, 1969; Le Beux, 1973; Metuzals and Tasaki, 1978; Metuzals et al., 1981) or better in unfixed material treated by rapid freezing and by immunocytochemical techniques (Hirokawa, 1982; Schnapp and Reese, 1982). The main structural components of the axon are the plasma membrane, on the cytoplasmic surface of which is a network of actin and actin-like microfilaments 6–8 nm in diameter (Metuzals and Tasaki, 1978; Hirokawa, 1982); longitudinally arrayed microtubules 24 nm in diameter; and 8- to 11-nm-diameter neurofilaments, suspended in a granular matrix (Wuerker and Palay 1969; Le Beux, 1973;

Metuzals et al., 1981; Schnapp and Reese, 1982). Cross-bridges (4–6 nm in diameter, 20–50 nm in length) connect neurofilaments, microtubules, and membrane-bound organelles (D. S. Smith, 1971; D. S. Smith et al., 1977; Shelanski et al., 1981; Hirokawa, 1982, 1988a,b, 1989a,b; Schnapp and Reese, 1982). Microtubule-associated proteins MAP1A, MAP2, and tau proteins are known to be components of the cross-bridges between microtubules and between microtubules and neurofilaments (see Section 5.5). Neurofilament 145-kDa and 200-kDa proteins form components of cross-bridges between neurofilaments (Hirokawa et al., 1984; Hisanaga and Hirokawa, 1988). MAP1C and kinesin are microtubule-associated ATPases which form dynamic links between microtubules and membrane-bound organelles (Valee et al., 1989, review).

The axon also contains membrane-bound organelles, including axoplasmic reticulum, lysosomes, microvesicles, and mitochondria. Axons differ from dendrites in their cytoplasmic organelles: ribosomes and Golgi elements are present in dendrites but absent from axons. The main consequence of this difference is that synthesis of proteins and glycoproteins occurs in dendrites but materials required for axonal growth, maintenance, and repair are synthesized in the cell body and transported into the axon.

The network of protein microfilaments and microtubules in the cell is termed the cytoskeleton. These include actin filaments (Pollard and Cooper, 1986, review), intermediate filaments, mainly neurofilaments (Steinert and Roop, 1988, review), and microtubules (Dustin, 1984; Allen, 1987, reviews), distributed in longitudinal arrays and bundles in specific configurations in the cytoplasm. The polymerized cytoskeletal proteins are in dynamic equilibrium with pools of unpolymerized subunits (Okabe and Hirokawa, 1990). These cytoskeletal proteins are linked together by a variety of associated proteins (Matus, 1988, review) whose interaction with the cytoskeleton results in changes in cell shape, cell movements, endocytosis, exocytosis, movements of organelles, and intracellular transport of materials.

The term "cytoskeleton" is not entirely satisfactory because these proteins not only form structural supports, but are also responsible for movements of cells and movements of materials in cells. Changes in shape of the cell require interaction between the cytoskeleton and the plasma membrane (Weatherbee, 1981; Pollard and Cooper, 1986, review) and movements of cytoplasmic organelles result from interactions between the microtubules and associated proteins that act as motors for transport in either the cellulofugal (anterograde) or cellulopetal (retrograde) direction (reviews by Hilfer and Searls, 1985; Schliwa, 1986; Sheetz, 1987; Bershadsky and Vasiliev, 1988; Obar et al., 1990). Intracellular transport is considered at greater length in Section 5.8.

5.4. Microtubules

Microtubules are very abundant in neurons and glial cells. They have two main functions: to provide mechanical stability and to provide the conduits along which membrane-bound organelles are transported. In addition, microtubules are found in the mitotic spindle and in cilia which are present in all neurons.

Microtubules are built up of protofilaments of tubulin dimers to form a cylindrical polymer of indefinite length, with an external diameter of 24 nm, a wall 5 nm thick, and a hollow core 14 nm in diameter. Cytoplasmic microtubules typically have 13 protofilaments coiled helically. The tubulin dimer is a 100-kDa complex of two nearly identical proteins called alpha- and beta-tubulin. The dimers are all oriented in the same direction in the microtubule, giving it an intrinsic structural polarity, with plus and minus ends. In mammalian brain, tubulin comprises about 20 percent of the total soluble protein. Tubulin is conveyed anterogradely in the axon by slow transport and is added to elongating microtubules at their plus ends.

Microtubules are in a condition of dynamic instability, undergoing phases of elongation and rapid shortening (Kirschner and Mitchison, 1986a,b; Schulze and Kirschner, 1986, 1987). They are stabilized by an energy-dependent mechanism involving hydrolysis of GTP and by microtubule-associated proteins (MAP) (Cassimeris et al., 1987, review).

The spatial configuration of microtubule polymerization in the cell is organized by centrosomes and by the kinetochores of the mitotic spindle. Polymerization of microtubules requires hydrolysis of GTP and the dynamic equilibrium between the tubulin pool and microtubules is affected by many factors, especially the concentration of Ca^{2+} in the presence of calmodulin (Kotani et al., 1985). Calmodulin binds Ca^{2+} and then interacts with MAP2 and tau protein which stabilize microtubules by forming cross-bridges between them (see Section 5.5). Assembly of tubulin into microtubules in cells occurs in head-to-tail order (Bergen and Borisy, 1980), with the minus end of the filament anchored in a microtubule organizing center, where polymerization is suppressed, and addition of tubulin subunits to the filament occurring exclusively at the free, plus end (Kirschner, 1980). The polarity of microtubules in the cell can be revealed in electron microscopic sections. Tubulin added to cross-sections adopts a configuration which appears as hooks on the microtubules with their direction indicating the orientation of the microtubule: clockwise hooks indicate that the plus end of the microtubule points to the observer; counterclockwise hooks indicate the opposite (Heidemann and McIntosh, 1980; Enteneuer and McIntosh, 1981).

The microtubules in the axon are all oriented the same way, with the plus end pointed in the direction of the growth cone and the minus end anchored in a microtubule-organizing center located in the cell body (Burton and Paige, 1981; Heidemann, 1981). Microtubule-organizing centers are present in dendrites from which microtubules extend with their plus ends either toward or away from the cell body, except in the distal dendritic arborizations, within about 15 μm of the growth cones, where all microtubules are oriented the same way with the plus end pointing to the growth cone (Baas et al., 1988).

Microtubules are associated with the membranes of neurons, notably at the membrane densities of pre- and postsynaptic junctions (Bird, 1976; Gray 1975; Westrum and Gray, 1971, 1977; Kelly and Cotman, 1978). Microtubules are also connected by means of filamentous bridges with membrane-bound organelles in neurons (Yamada et al., 1971; Gray, 1978; Hirokawa, 1982, 1988a,b, 1989a,b; Schnapp and Reese, 1982). These bridges are composed of protein ATPases which act as the motors for transporting organelles. MAP1C acts as the retrograde motor and kinesin functions as the anterograde motor (see Sections 5.5 and 5.8).

The number of microtubules in inversely proportional to the caliber of the axon. In the cat there are 11 microtubules/μm^2 in 10-μm myelinated axons and over 100 microtubules/μm^2 in unmyelinated fibers with caliber less than 0.1 μm^2 (Fadic *et al.*, 1986). The ratios are similar in sensory, motor, and sympathetic axons at all ages in rats (Banks *et al.*, 1975; Alvarez *et al.*, 1982; Alvarez and Zarour, 1983; Fadic *et al.*, 1986; Foúndez and Alvarez, 1986; Saitua and Alvarez, 1988). Therefore, there may be a limit to the number of microtubules that can be formed as the axon increases in caliber.

5.5. Microtubule-Associated Proteins (MAPs)

These are polypeptides that are associated with microtubules in neurons and glial cells where they form molecular cross-bridges that play important roles in the assembly and stabilization of microtubules (reviewed by Nunez, 1986; Olmsted, 1986; Matus, 1988). Large MAPs and smaller tau proteins are very important because they regulate the assembly of microtubules which are essential for development, stability, and plasticity of the long cytoplasmic processes that characterize neurons and astrocytes. A significant difference between cells that have such long processes and those that do not have them is that the former have MAPs whereas the latter lack MAPs.

MAPs can be classified into a very-high-molecular-weight group ($\sim$320–350 kDa), consisting mainly of MAP1A and of less abundant MAP1B and MAP1C and MAP5; a group with intermediate molecular weights ($\sim$70–280 kDa), of which MAP2 is the most abundant in adult neurons and MAP3 and MAP4 are more abundant in astrocytes; and a lower-molecular-weight group, of which the tau proteins (55–62 kDa) are most abundant in axons. Antibodies prepared against the different forms of MAPs have shown that they are compartmentalized intracellularly, are distributed specifically in neurons or glial cells, and are developmentally regulated.

Intracellular compartmentalization of MAPs in different regions of the same cell probably results from association of MAPs with components other than the microtubules. This is suggested by evidence that MAPs bind to neurofilaments (Letterier *et al.*, 1982; Heimann *et al.*, 1985; Hirokawa, *et al.*,

1988a) and actin filaments. Binding to actin is regulated by phosphorylation of MAPs (Nishida *et al.*, 1981; Seldon and Pollard, 1983; Sattilaro, 1986). Phosphorylation increases the binding of MAPs to actin and neurofilament protein but reduces assembly of microtubules (Murphy and Flavin, 1983).

MAP1A and MAP1B are related in subunit composition but are expressed in different times and places in the developing rat nervous system (Schoenfeld *et al.*, 1989). MAP1B is abundant in the newborn rat brain and decreases whereas MAP1A increases during postnatal development. MAP1B is abundant in growing axons. MAP1B persists in the adult olfactory nerve and hippocampal mossy fibers, indicating that these fibers continue to grow in the adult rat. MAP1A is abundantly expressed in growing and mature dendrites. In addition, MAP1A and MAP1B are expressed in glial cells (Bloom *et al.*, 1984, 1985; Calvert and Anderton, 1985).

MAP2 exists in high-molecular-weight ($\sim$280 kDa) and low-molecular-wieght ($\sim$70 kDa) forms whose relative abundance changes during development. Both forms of MAP2 appear to be encoded by the same gene (Garner and Matus, 1988). The high-molecular-weight MAP2 is found mainly in developing dendrites *in vivo* (Bernhardt and Matus, 1984; Burgoyne and Cummings, 1984; De Camilli *et al.*, 1984; Tucker *et al.*, 1988a–c), as well as *in vitro* (Kosick and Finch, 1987), showing that the dendrite localization is not specified by external conditions (Caceras *et al.*, 1984). MAP2 is found in the developing cerebellar Purkinje cell dendrites but disappears from mature dendrites (Tucker *et al.*, 1988c). MAP2 is also expressed in spinal motoneuron axons (Papasozomenos *et al.*, 1985), in mouse brain astrocytes (Couchie *et al.*, 1985), and in astrocytes of the optic nerve, but not in astrocytes of the optic tract (Papasozomenos and Binder, 1986). High-molecular-weight MAP2 (280 kDa) is found only in neurons and is the most abundant MAP in adult mammalian brain. Low-molecular-weight MAP2 (70 kDa) is relatively more abundant in embryonic brain, where it exists in glial cells and in developing neurons before the high-molecular-weight form is expressed (Tucker *et al.*, 1988c).

Abundant expression of MAP3 (180 kDa) occurs in astrocytes but not in neurons (Huber *et al.*, 1985). MAP4 ($\sim$210 kDa) is also specifically localized in astrocytes but not in neurons (Parysek *et al.*, 1984; Olmsted *et al.*, 1986). MAP5 ($\sim$320 kDa)

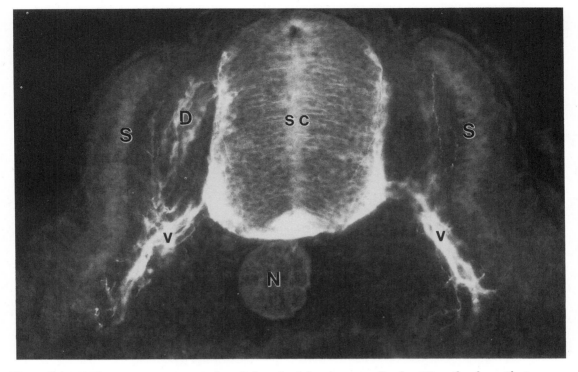

Figure 5.4. MAP5 in outgrowing axons in the spinal cord and dorsal root ganglia of an E3 quail embryo. The transverse section has been stained with fluorescent anti-MAP5 monoclonal antibody. D = dorsal root ganglion; N = notochord; S = somite; SC = spinal cord. Photograph kindly provided by R. P. Tucker.

has been found exclusively in neurons, cell bodies, dendrites, and axons, and is 10 times more abundant in newborn rat brain than in the adult (Calvert and Anderton, 1985; Bloom *et al.*, 1985; Riederer *et al.*, 1986; Tucker, 1988a; Garner *et al.*, 1989). MAP2 appears to be a component of cross-bridges between microtubules and neurofilaments (Hirokawa *et al.*, 1988).

Expression of different MAPs varies systematically during development: MAPs 2C, 3A, 3B, 5, and juvenile tau (~48 kDa) are abundant during embryonic and early postnatal stages in the rat brain and are greatly reduced after postnatal day 20. The specific functions of some of these embryonically expressed MAPs are not known, but others have been correlated with early stages of brain development. For example, MAP3 is found in radial glial cells and MAP5 is the only MAP now known to be expressed in neurons during their migration, before their terminal stages of differentiation. MAP5 is the only neuronal MAP that is abundant in growing ax-

ons in the 3 day quail spinal cord (Tucker *et al.*, 1988a,b), as shown in Fig. 5.4. This should be compared with Cajal's depiction of the 3-day chick embryo spinal cord in which he discovered the growth cones in 1890 (Fig. 5.5). In the quail spinal cord MAP2C first appears in motoneuron cell bodies on E3 and in axons and glial cells at later stages and becomes less abundant on E5–E7. Tau protein is expressed in outgrowing axons, starting on E3 (Tucker *et al.*, 1988).

Expression of MAP1A (Riederer and Matus, 1985; Bernhardt *et al.*, 1985; Schoenfeld *et al.*, 1989) and MAP2A (Burgoyne and Cumming, 1984; Binder *et al.*, 1984) occurs postnatally during the period of most extensive outgrowth of dendrites. Phosphorylated MAP1B is concentrated in axons and is most abundant in developing axons, whereas unphosphorylated MAP1B is localized in the cell body and dendrites (Sato-Yoshitake *et al.*, 1989). MAP1A and MAP2 are components of cross-bridges between microtubules (Hirokawa, 1987a,b), and

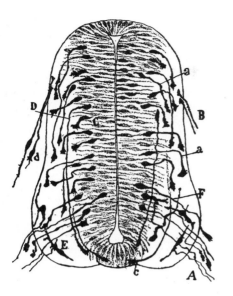

Figure 5.5. Growth cones in the spinal cord of the 3-day chick embryo. A = ventral spinal nerve fibers; a = axon; B = dorsal root fibers; C = growth cone on a very short axon; c = growth cone on a commissural fiber; D = commissural fiber; d = dorsal root ganglion cell; E = ventral horn motor nerve cell; F = fiber of lateral motor nerve cell. From S. Ramón y Cajal, *Anat. Anz.* 5:609–613 (1890).

MAP2 also cross-links neurofilaments and microtubules (Hirokawa *et al.*, 1988a). Whereas MAP1B is a long molecule forming long cross-brdiges between microtubules, tau proteins are short, rod-like molecules, forming short cross-bridges (Hirokawa *et al.*, 1988b).

Tau protein is found only in neurons (Drubin *et al.*, 1986; Papasozomenos and Binder, 1987) and is localized mainly to the axon in association with microtubules (Cleveland *et al.*, 1977a,b; Binder *et al.*, 1985; Peng *et al.*, 1986; Kosik and Finch, 1987; Hirokawa *et al.*, 1988b). Tau promotes polymerization of tubulin. It exists in at least four forms which result from posttranslational modification (Goedert *et al.*, 1989; Kanai *et al.*, 1989). The change from the juvenile form of tau protein to the adult tau protein is correlated with stabilization of the adult form of the neuron (Mareck *et al.*, 1980; Couchie and Nunez, 1985; Nunez, 1986; Hirokawa *et al.*, 1988). The highly phosphorylated form of tau is a major component of the paired helical filaments in neurons in Alzheimer's disease (Wischik *et al.*, 1985; J. G. Wood *et al.*, 1986).

Dynein (MAP1C), kinesin, and dynamin are microtubule associated ATPases that perform the functions of motors that move materials on microtubules (Fig. 5.6). Dynamin is a polypeptide which mediates microtubule bundling and sliding between microtubules in an ATP-dependent manner (Obar *et al.*, 1990); that is, it mediates movements between microtubules rather than between microtubules and vesicles. MAP1C is a form of dynein and causes movement of materials, vesicles, and organelles from plus to minus along microtubules, whereas kinesin transports materials in the opposite direction (Vale *et al.*, 1985c, 1986; Paschal *et al.*, 1987; Sheetz, 1987, review; Valee *et al.*, 1989, review). Because microtubules in the axon are oriented with their plus ends pointing toward the growth cone (Burton and Paige, 1981), MAP1C is the retrograde motor and kinesin is the anterograde motor (Hirokawa *et al.*, 1989b). When kinesin-coated latex beads are applied to purified microtubules in the presence of ATP they move at a rate of 0.3–0.4 μm/second along the microtubules in a minus-to-plus direction, which is analogous to anterograde axonal tranport (Vale *et al.*, 1985c, 1986). Similarly, when microtubules and ATP are applied to a glass coverslip coated with MAP1C, the microtubules glide rapidly along the surface of the MAP1C layer at 1.25 μm/second at room temperature, which is in the range for retrograde transport of particles (Paschal *et al.*, 1987; Vallee *et al.*, 1989).

5.6. Microfilaments

Actin microfilaments, 6–8 nm in diameter, are ubiquitous cytoskeletal components of neurepithelial cells, glial cells, and neurons. They function with other cytoskeletal elements to determine cell shape and cell movement. Globular actin (G-actin) subunits form a cytoplasmic pool which is in dynamic equilibrium with actin polymers which form double helical filaments (F-actin). These filaments are organized into bundles and networks by means of cross-linking proteins, the most abundant of which is filamin (Pollard and Cooper, 1986, review). The resulting complex has the viscoelastic properties of a gel, especially its property of recoiling rapidly in response to a large transiently applied force but of deforming gradually in response to a small, but steadily applied, force. However, rapid change of shape, accompanied by change from

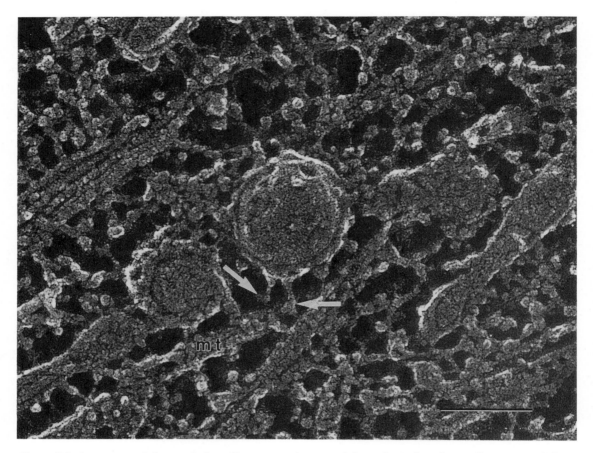

Figure 5.6. Structures with the morphology of kinesin appear to cross-link membrane-bound organelles to microtubules in the neurite. A rat spinal cord was processed for quick-freeze, deep-etch electron microscopy, and neurite regions rich in membrane-bound organelles and microtubules were examined. Numerous rod-shaped structures were observed to span the space between organelles and microtubules, and many of these apparent cross-bridges are reminiscent of kinesin involved in cross-linking synthetic microspheres to microtubules. Magnification bar = 100 nm. From N. Hirokawa, K. K. Pfister, H. Yorifuji, M. C. Wagner, S. T. Brady, and G. S. Bloom, *Cell* **56:**867-878 (1989).

gel to sol physical state, can be accomplished by the action of the enzyme gelsolin, in the presence of increased free Ca^{2+}, which cuts actin filaments (Yin, 1987, review). Such gels underlie the plasma membrane, forming the membrane skeleton, and surround synaptic vesicles (Inestrosa *et al.,* 1976; Hirokawa *et al.,* 1989a). Actin depolymerization is necessary for release of transmitter from synaptic vesicles (Bernstein and Bamburg, 1989).

Actin filaments are held together in the form of bundles or actin cables by means of special bundling and cross-linking proteins. These actin cables can pull on the plasma membrane at focal contact sites, where the actin filaments are attached by at least four different attachment proteins (including talin and vinculin on the cytoplasmic side of the focal contact) to transmembrane linker proteins, which bind to components of the extracellular matrix (fibronectin and vitronectin). The fibronectin receptor is an important linker protein belonging to the integrin family, which serves as a link between cytoplasmic microfilaments and extracellular fibronectin. Focal contacts are the sites of the tightest adhesion between cells and substrate surfaces, there being only 10–15 nm separating the plasma membrane from the substratum at those sites.

Fibronectin has been shown to promote growth of axons *in vitro* as well as *in vivo* (see Section 5.11).

Neural crest cells migrate preferentially on fibronectin substrates (Newgreen and Thiery, 1980; Mayer *et al.*, 1981; Thiery *et al.*, 1982; Duband and Thiery, 1982; Hynes and Yamada, 1982; Tucker and Erickson, 1984; Duband *et al.*, 1986; Perris *et al.*, 1989). This was considered in more detail in Section 4.4.

Actin filaments have polarity: they grow by addition of actin monomers at the plus end, and when they are in dynamic equilibrium there is an equal loss of monomers from the negative end, a process known as *treadmilling*, which is driven by energy derived from hydrolysis of ATP (Tilney *et al.*, 1981; Bonder *et al.*, 1983; Wang, 1985; Korn *et al.*, 1987). Rapid treadmilling occurs in filopodia and lamellipodia of the growth cone: the actin monomers are added at the plus end of the microfilaments near the growing tip and removed from the minus end of the microfilaments inside the growth cone (Wang, 1985). The concept of treadmilling was first defined more than 300 years ago by René Descartes (1596–1650), as a theoretical model of the movement of animal spirits, in particle form, along nerve fibers (see Section 11.1): *"As fast as any particle is detached at the extremity of each fibril, another is attached at its root"* (*La description du corps humain*, first published in 1664).

Many different proteins are known that bind to actin filaments and specifically regulate the form of the actin filament network (Pollard and Cooper, 1986, review). Some actin-binding proteins can control the polymerization or breakdown of actin filaments, others attach actin filaments to the plasma membrane. Neurons and glial cells have a network of actin filaments beneath the plasma membrane, forming a cortical layer known as the membrane skeleton (Bray *et al.*, 1986; Hirokawa *et al.*, 1989a). Bundles of actin filaments complexed with myosin are attached to the plasma membrane, and their contraction is involved in changes in cell shape and in cell locomotion. The contractions necessary to produce movements of the cytoplasm are caused by nonmuscle myosin molecules interacting with ATP and with bundles of actin filaments which are attached to the plasma membrane (Clarke and Spudich, 1977; Citi and Kendrick-Jones, 1987, review; Korn and Hammer, 1988, review). Phosphorylation of the light and heavy myosin chains enables their assembly into filaments and thus enables the interaction between nonmuscle myosin

and actin filaments (Craig *et al.*, 1983; Citi and Kendrick-Jones, 1986; Barylko *et al.*, 1986). Contractile movements of axons, which can be seen in tissue culture (Pomerat, 1961; Weiss *et al.*, 1962; Burdwood, 1965; Weiss, 1972), are probably mediated by actin and myosin. The functions of such movements are not known, but have been said to be involved in transport of materials (Weiss, 1963, 1964, 1972).

Cytochalasin and phalloidin are drugs that affect actin function by changing actin polymerization. Cytochalasins inhibit cell locomotion, changes of cell shape, phagocytosis and cytokinesis, production of microspikes, and formation and motility of lamellipoda (Cooper, 1987). Cytochalasins bind to the growing ends of actin filaments (their membrane-associated ends; Tilney *et al.*, 1981), thus preventing addition of actin subunits. Phalloidin binds specifically to actin filaments and prevents their depolymerization. It does not cross the plasma membrane and must be injected into the cell. Fluorescent-labeled phalloidin can be used to display actin filaments in cells.

Spectrin is a cytoskeletal protein localized mainly on the cytoplasmic side of the nerve cell membrane (Levine and Willard, 1981), where it is bound to intermediate filaments and actin to form the so-called membrane skeleton (Goodman and Zagon, 1984, review). The spectrin is a long, thin rod about 100 nm in length. It is formed of two large polypeptide chains, alpha-spectrin (240 kDa) and beta-spectrin (235 kDa). These heterodimers link head-to-head to form 200-nm-long tetramers. The tail ends of several tetramers are joined together by actin and an 82-kDa protein to form a network underlying the cytoplasmic surface of the plasma membrane (Marchesi, 1985). Another protein, ankyrin (210 kDa) links the beta-spectrin to the cytoplasmic domain of a transmembrane protein (100 kDa) called band 3. This membrane infrastructure allows the cell to withstand stresses and enables it to return to its original shape after deformation. There are two forms of brain spectrin, only one of which cross-reacts with antibodies to erythrocyte spectrin. Spectrin (240/235) is abundant in axons and presynaptic terminals, is less abundant in the nerve cell body, and is absent from glial cells. By contrast, brain spectrin (240/235E) is present in some glial cell types and in neuronal cell bodies and dendrites, but is absent from axons. Spectrin is transported in the axon with the slow component (see Section 5.9).

Clathrin is a 170-kDa protein that is involved in receptor-mediated endocytosis and is the main constituent of coated vesicles (Pearse, 1975, 1976; Goldstein *et al.*, 1979; Salisbury *et al.*, 1983). Brain clathrin polymerizes together with clathrin-associated proteins (30–36 kDa) to form baskets or filaments (Schook *et al.*, 1979; Heuser and Evans, 1980; Listani *et al.*, 1982; Pearse *et al.*, 1982). Clathrin and clathrin-associated proteins are transported anterogradely in soluble form in the axon with the slow component b (SCb), as discussed in Section 5.9 (Garner and Lasek, 1981; Gower and Tytell, 1987).

5.7. Intermediate Filaments

Intermediate filaments have a diameter of 8–10 nm and are composed of protein subunits (40–200 kDa) (reviewed by Fuchs and Hanukoglu, 1983; Steinert *et al.*, 1985; Traub *et al.*, 1985; Steinert and Roop, 1988). Intermediate filaments are encoded by a large multigene family with specific patterns of expression in different tissues: neurofilaments (neurons), glial filaments (astrocytes), vimentin (mainly cells of mesodermal origin, but also immature astrocytes, reactive microglial cells, and dividing neuroepithelial cells), desmin (muscle), and keratins (epithelial cells). With the exception of keratins, all other types of intermediate filaments have substantial similarities in their amino acid sequences.

Monoclonal antibodies have been produced that react with many or all types of intermediate filaments. There are specific intermediate filaments in different types of cells, as can be demonstrated with monoclonal antibodies that exclusively stain only one type of intermediate filament (Lin *et al.*, 1984, review). The antigenic diversity has been put to good use in detecting the developmental expression of different intermediate filaments by means of panels of antibodies.

No method has contributed more to studies of expression of different gene products during cell differentiation than the use of antibodies (Valentino *et al.*, 1985, review). Antibody staining of Western blots can be used to detect extremely small amounts of specific polypeptides and to show their changes during development. Tissue sections stained with antibodies and examined with light or electron microscopy can reveal the cellular distribution of specific antigens. It should be remembered that different antibodies can be raised against epitopes on the same molecule, and that varying staining patterns may result because posttranslational modification of the antigenic molecule may make epitopes inaccessible or may give rise to new epitopes. Immunocytochemical methods tend to show the regions of highest concentration of antigen. The quantity of antigen present in such small regions of high concentration may represent a tiny fraction of the total quantity in the tissue. In other parts of the tissue the antigen may be below the threshold of detectibility or may be hidden by background staining, especially when immunofluorescence methods are used. In spite of such limitations, which may complicate interpretation of the data, the use of cell type–specific antibodies and of antibodies against specific molecules has revolutionized research on nerve cell differentiation.

Neurofilaments are intermediate filaments which are uniquely found in neurons. They are distributed in the dendrites, cell body, and axon in characteristic longitudinal arrays of single neurofilaments or of neurofilament bundles linked by cross-bridges (Schnapp and Reese, 1982; Hirokawa, 1982; Lazarides, 1982; Hirokawa *et al.*, 1984; Hisanaga and Hirokawa, 1988). Neurofilaments are present as polymeric structures and there is little neurofilament protein in monomeric form in the axon (Morris and Lasek, 1984) except at the synapses where neurofilaments are specifically degraded (Roots, 1983). The specific histological staining of neurons with silver salts is due to the affinity of some part of the neurofilaments for silver (Peters, 1959; Gray and Guillery, 1961; Phillips *et al.*, 1983). Neurofilaments are found in all vertebrate neurons but are said to be absent from arthropods (Lasek *et al.*, 1985).

Mammalian neurofilaments are composed of three different protein subunits with different molecular weights (73 kDa, 145 kDa, 200 kDa) designated, light, medium, and heavy (L, M, H) (Liem *et al.*, 1978; Schlaepfer and Freeman, 1978; Willard and Simon, 1981; Sharp *et al.*, 1982). Electron microscopy shows that the L subunits form a core filament around which two filaments, formed by the M and H, are coiled, with the M and H subunits exposed at the surface forming cross-bridges linking neurofilaments (Willard and Simon, 1981; Sharp et al., 1982; Hirokawa, et al., 1984; Hisenaga and Hirokawa, 1988). Neurofilaments are unique among intermediate filaments in forming such cross-bridges (Wuerker and Palay, 1969; Wuerker, 1970; Hirokawa, 1982). The cell body and dendrites of mature neurons contain mostly L and M, while the H subunit is characteristic of axons (Hirokawa et al., 1984).

Each of the three neurofilament subunits is the product of translation of a different mRNA (Czosnek et al., 1980), and the genes encoding them have been cloned (Lewis and Cowan, 1985, 1986; Myers et al., 1987). Expression of the different subunits is regulated independently in different types of neurons and at different stages of development.

Although all three neurofilament subunit types have been reported to appear simultaneously in neurons in the peripheral nervous system (PNS) (Cochard and Paulin, 1984), there is considerable evidence that the heavy subunit appears gradually after the others in the central nervous system (CNS) as well as the PNS (Shaw and Weber, 1982; Pachter and Liem, 1984; Glicksman and Willard, 1985; Foster et al., 1987; Carden et al., 1987; Lee et al., 1987; Figlewicz et al., 1988). The appearance of the cross-linking H polypeptide characterizes the change from rapid axonal growth to a steady-state condition and it also correlates with a marked reduction in the velocity of axonal transport (Willard and Simon, 1983). It has been suggested that gradual development of the H form is related to stabilization of the axon (Carden et al., 1987) or to stabilization of the neuron with respect to its degree of developmental plasticity (Figlewicz et al., 1988). The physical basis of such a stabilization appears to be the formation of cross-bridges between the H subunits of neighboring neurofilaments.

All three forms of neurofilament proteins undergo extensive posttranslational modifications which result in the addition of amino acid sequences and in phosphorylation at the COOH terminal (Julien and Mushynski, 1982; Glicksman and Willard, 1985). One of the results of posttranslational modification is antigenic variety, allowing the different forms of the neurofilament protein to be detected by means of antibodies (e.g., Sternberger and Sternberger, 1983; Carden et al., 1985; Shaw et al., 1986). Such studies have shown that posttranslation-

al modifications of the medium and heavy forms occur during transport of the neurofilament protein down the axon (Nixon et al., 1982; Bennett and Di-Lullo, 1985). Neurofilament polypeptides are conveyed anterogradely in the axon by slow flow (Hoffman and Lasek, 1975; Lasek and Hoffman, 1976). Antibodies to phosphorylated forms of neurofilament protein specifically stain axons in mammals (Sternberger and Sternberger, 1983, 1984), birds (Bennett, 1987), frog (Szaro and Gainer, 1988), and some invertebrates (Cohen et al., 1987; Eagles et al., 1988).

Neurofilament proteins can first be detected in postmitotic neurons and are absent from dividing neuroepithelial cells, in which vimentin is the predominant intermediate filament protein. Vimentin is a 57-kDa protein subunit of intermediate filaments expressed in many types of cells, including immature glial cells (Dahl et al., 1981; Bignami et al., 1982; Dupouey et al., 1985; Traub, 1985; Hutchins and Casagrande, 1989), and together with GFAP in developing and mature astrocytes (Schnitzer et al., 1981; Tapscott et al., 1981b; Trimmer et al., 1982). Vimentin immunoreactivity is found in ependymal cells (Schnitzer et al., 1981) and radial glial cells (Dent et al., 1989). Vimentin is expressed in neuroepithelial cells but gradually disappears from postmitotic neurons as the neurofilament proteins are expressed (Tapscott et al., 1981a; Jacobs et al., 1982; Bennet, 1987). For further consideration of vimentin expression in neuroglial cells see Section 3.3.

Separation of microtubules and neurofilaments results from treatment with the neurotoxin iminodiproprionitrile (IDPN; Griffin et al., 1978, 1982, 1983). Following IDPN treatment the neurofilaments aggregate at the axonal perimeter and the microtubules are clustered at the center of the axon (Papazomenos et al., 1981). Transport of neurofilaments can be blocked with IDPN without significantly affecting transport of tubulin, and thus neurofilaments accumulate at the axon hillock (Griffin et al., 1978, 1982). This shows that transport of neurofilaments is normally linked to the microtubules, but not the reverse. The role of neurofilaments in axonal transport is apparently not an essential one. They are also said to be unnecessary on the evidence that neurofilaments are sparse or absent from axons of some arthropods such as the cockroach and crayfish (Lasek et al., 1985).

Glial fibrillary acid protein (GFAP) is a 51-kDa protein of 10-nm glial intermediate filaments found in astrocytes characteristically (Eng *et al.*, 1971; Bignami *et al.*, 1972; Bignami and Dahl, 1974; Raff *et al.*, 1979; Raju *et al.*, 1981; Trimmer *et al.*, 1982). GFAP is also expressed in radial glial cells of the urodele spinal cord (Zamora and Mutin, 1988) and in goldfish retina Müller cells (Bignami, 1984). Oligodendrocytes and Schwann cells express GFAP transiently during development (Borit and McIntosh, 1981; Barber and Lindsay, 1982; Dahl *et al.*, 1982).

As astrocytes mature they switch from vimentin to GFAP production (Dahl, 1981; Dahl *et al.*, 1981; Schnitzer *et al.*, 1981; Bovolenta *et al*, 1982, 1987; Pixley and de Vellis, 1984; Hutchins and Casagrande, 1989). In the corpus callosum and corticospinal tract the switch from vimentin to GFAP expression occurs only after astroctyes contact nerve fibers (Valentino *et al.*, 1983). Contact with axons is also required for expression of GFAP in astrocytes of cerebellar white matter (Bovolenta *et al.*, 1984) and optic nerve and tract (Bovolenta *et al.*, 1987). In mouse cerebellum the expression of GFAP mRNA is correlated with the time course of expression of GFAP protein (Lewis and Cowan, 1985). The switch from vimentin to GFAP is correlated with a reduction of astrocyte motility and differentiation of long astrocyte processes (Duffy *et al.*, 1982). Differentiation of glial cells and the use of intermediate filament antibodies as glial cell markers are discussed further in Section 3.3.

5.8. Transport of Materials in Nerve Cells: Overview

Neurons must produce very large quantities of protein because all proteins required for growth, maintenance, and function of the axon are synthesized in the cell body and then transported to the axonal terminals, and because the volume of the axon is thousands of times greater than the volume of the nerve cell body. This dependence of the axon on the cell body starts with the initial outgrowth of the axon and continues throughout life.

Even at the fastest rate of anterograde axonal transport (50–400 mm/day), materials produced in the cell body may be *en route* for weeks before

arriving at the presynaptic terminals. Materials such as nerve growth factor, transported in a retrograde direction at about 200 mm/day, may journey for days or weeks from the peripheral nerve terminals to the cell body. These delays set severe limits on participation of the cell body in regulation of the activities of growth cones and axonal presynaptic endings. Similar constraints operate in the control by the cell body of dendritic growth cones and dendritic postsynaptic specializations such as spines.

Transport of materials probably also occurs in both directions in dendrites. However, the distances are shorter than in axons and the delays are also shorter. Moreover, local synthesis of proteins takes place in dendrites close to postsynaptic structures such as dendritic spines where the machinery of synthesis is well placed to respond rapidly to synaptic activity.

Transport of materials within the neuron has a fourfold significance in relation to development of the nervous system. First, transport from the cell body to the axonal and dendritic endings is a way of providing materials for growth and renewal of components which have a shorter lifespan than that of the neuron as a whole. Second, it provides materials for the formation, maintenance, and functions of the synapses. Third, transport of materials to the cell body from the axon terminal allows recirculation of axonal components. Fourth, trophic molecules and other signals are transported retrogradely from the extracellular environment at the tips of the axon and from the axon's postsynaptic targets.

There are four different classes of evidence showing transport of materials in axons:

1. Light microscopic cinematography, and video-enhanced differential interference microscopy show movements of membrane-bound organelles in both directions in the intact axon or in isolated axoplasm (Kirckpatrick *et al.*, 1972; Cooper and Smith, 1974; Breuer *et al.*, 1975; Allen and Allen, 1983; Allen *et al.*, 1983; Schnapp *et al.*, 1985; Valee *et al.*, 1985).

2. A ligature tied around a peripheral nerve results in accumulation of materials in the axons mainly proximal to the ligature, and release of the constriction is followed by anterograde movement of the materials accumulated above

Table 5.1. Axonal Transport

Component (rate, mm/day)	Composition	Selected references
Fast anterograde (50–400)	Membrane-associated materials; GAPs; Na$^+$-K$^+$ ATPase; transmitter-associated proteins; catecholamines; mitochondrial membrane components	Taxi and Sotelo, 1973; Courand and DiGiamberardino, 1980; DiGiamberardino, 1980
Fast retrograde (200)	Materials entering axon by endocytosis; lysosomal hydrolases; NGF; viruses; tetanus toxin; HRP and other tracers	Stoeckel et al., 1975; Kristensson et al., 1978; Thoenen and Barde, 1980; Mesulam, 1982; Ugolini et al., 1989
Slow anterograde (0.2–8)	Cytoskeletal proteins and associated proteins	Hoffman and Lasek, 1975
SCa (0.2–1)	Tubulin; neurofilament protein; MAPs; tau protein; spectrin	Black and Lasek, 1980; Okabe and Hirokawa, 1990
SCb (1–2)	Actin; clathrin; clathrin-associated proteins; myosin-like proteins; spectrin; soluble enzymes; calmodulin	Garner and Lasek, 1981; Lasek et al., 1984; Gower and Tytell, 1986

the ligature, as first shown by Weiss and Hiscoe (1948) and subsequently reported by many others (Bisby, 1982a, review). Accumulation of membrane-bound organelles and vesicles in the axon proximal and distal to a ligature has been observed with the electron microscope (R. S. Smith, 1980; Tsukita and Ishikawa, 1980).

3. Retrograde axonal transport has been demonstrated of viruses (Bodian and Howe, 1940, 1941a,b; Kristensson et al., 1974, 1978; Tsiang, 1979; Kucera et al., 1985; Gillet et al., 1986; Lycke and Tsiang, 1987; Ugolini et al., 1987, 1989); horseradish peroxidase (Kristensson and Olsson, 1971, 1973; Kristensson, 1975, 1978, review; LaVail, 1975, review; Mesulam, 1982, review); tetanus toxin (Stoeckel et al., 1975; Harrison et al., 1984); and nerve growth factor (Hendry et al., 1974a,b; Paravicini et al., 1975; Stoeckel and Thoenen, 1975; Stoeckel et al., 1975; Thoenen and Barde, 1980, review; see Section 8.18).

4. The kinetics of axonal transport have been studied by injecting a radioactive precursor such as [^{35}S]-methionine in the vicinity of the nerve cell bodies where the amino acids are rapidly incorporated into proteins which are transported from the cell body into the axon. At intervals after such a pulse of labeled amino acids, the nerve containing the labeled axons is removed and cut into 1- to 3-mm segments, and the labeled proteins are measured bio-

chemically or autoradiographically. Because these methods give averages for different axons and various proteins, their limit of resolution of the rate of axonal transport is no better than about 0.1 mm/day.

These methods reveal two main rate components of axonal transport, called fast and slow, each of which includes several subcomponents (Table 5.1). Slow transport includes all proteins of the cytoskeleton and associated proteins of the axoplasmic matrix (Liem et al., 1978; Griffin et al., 1978; Black and Lasek, 1980; Garner and Lasek, 1981, 1982; Brady and Lasek, 1982; Gozes, 1982; Lasek, 1982; Lasek et al., 1984; Gower and Tytell, 1986). By contrast, fast transport includes plasma membrane proteins such as Na$^+$ and K$^+$ ATPase, acetylcholinesterase, components of mitochondria, membranous organelles, and vesicles as well as neurotropic viruses. Fast transport at rates of 50–400 mm/day occurs in both directions in the axon: fast anterograde transport of proteins and organelles toward the axon terminals, and fast retrograde transport of materials that enter the axon terminals by endocytosis.

Slow transport is anterograde exclusively. The molecules composing the slow component show two main peak velocities, which are termed slow components a and b (SCa, 0.2–1 mm/day; SCb, 1–2 mm/day). SCa consists mainly of tubulin and neurofilament protein, and also includes MAPs tau protein and brain spectrin (Hoffman and

Lasek, 1975; Black and Lasek, 1980; Okabe and Hirokawa, 1980). SCb consists of actin, myosin, clathrin, spectrin, and various enzymes (Garner and Lasek, 1981, 1982; Lasek *et al.*, 1984; Gower and Tytell, 1986). SCa is uniformly distributed throughout the axon whereas SCb is concentrated near the plasma membrane. These materials may be in transit for weeks or months, and it is thus essential to maintain their stability for such long periods. The total quantity of materials transported in the slow components is about five times the quantity transported in the fast components (J. J. Bray and Austin, 1969; Sjöstrand and Karlsson, 1969).

5.9. Transport of Materials in the Axon

The concept of the nerve fiber as a hollow tube for conducting vital materials to and from the CNS was the prevailing doctrine during the 17th and 18th centuries (E. Clarke, 1968). The concept was not entirely without experimental evidence to support it. Thus Alexander Monro *primus* (1732) inferred that animal spirits were blocked from entering the diaphragm when a ligature was tightened around the phrenic nerve, and he noted that a few contractions of the diaphragm could be elicited by squeezing the nerve distal to the ligature. The historical literature describing the effects of ligating peripheral nerves is voluminous but those experiments did not result in the discovery of axoplasmic flow because swelling of the nerve proximal to the compression was seen as a form of edema, and because it was believed that the axon receives nutrition from local sources and from Schwann cells in peripheral nerves. Ramón y Cajal (1928, pp. 290–304) describes the result of ligating the sciatic nerve of the rabbit and very plainly shows ballooning of the axons above the ligature and thinning of axons below, but he too drew the wrong conclusions. He thought that the pressure stimulates axonal growth above the constriction and that the thin fibers below the constriction show that *"the trophic influence exercised by the central neurones is of a dynamic and not of a material nature. . . . assimilation and growth of the axons are purely local processes. . . . they are not influenced by materials or chemical reserves of the soma or nucleus of the neurones . . ."* (Ramón y Cajal, 1928, p. 302). Cajal's experiment, in principle, was

capable of demonstrating axonal flow, but he interpreted the evidence in terms of false concepts. This is another example to show that concepts have an existence which is almost independent of the validity of the evidence that goes to support them.

It was not a significant advance in experimental design, but a different theoretical position, that allowed the first modern demonstration of proximodistal flow of axoplasm by Weiss and Hiscoe in 1948. They started with the concept of bulk flow of the axoplasm and showed that the swelling and distortion of axons that arise proximal to a ligature tied on a peripheral nerve moves distally at a rate of about 1 mm/day after the ligature is removed. The results were dominated by the slow component of anterograde axonal transport, which constitutes more than 80 percent of the mass of transported materials, and Weiss and Hiscoe did not recognize the significance of retrograde transport. Their work bypassed the earlier discovery by Bodian and Howe (1940, 1941a,b) of retrograde axonal tranport of poliovirus at a rate of 30 mm/day. That phenomenon was viewed as unique to viruses and the chance to generalize it was lost. Consequently, the use of viruses and other exogenous molecules as tracers of axonal transport was delayed for 30 years. The use of the herpes simplex virus I as a retrograde transneuronal tracer has only recently been introduced (Kristensson *et al.*, 1978; Ugolini *et al.*, 1987, 1989).

Hundreds of research papers on transport of materials in the axon have appeared in the past decade and the importance of the subject is also reflected in the frequency of reviews (Lubinska, 1964; Lasek, 1970, 1982; Ochs, 1972a,b, 1981; Jeffrey and Austin, 1973; Grafstein, 1975; Heslop, 1975; Lasek and Hoffman, 1976; Grafstein and Forman, 1980; Baitinger *et al.*, 1982). Axonal transport of labeled molecules provides a nondestructive means of tracing axonal pathways using anterograde and retrograde tracers, and there is a vast literature dealing with those tracing techniques using horseradish peroxidase (Mesulam, 1982, review) and fluorescent tracers (Swanson, 1983, review).

Direct evidence that axoplasmic transport involves microtubules is that particles can be seen moving along microtubules *in vitro*: latex microspheres coated with kinesin or MAP1C can be seen moving on microtubules applied to glass coverslips (Vale *et al.*, 1985c, 1986). Axoplasmic transport is inhibited by colchicine and related drugs that bind to microtubules (Wuerker and Kirkpatrick, 1972; L. Wilson *et al.*, 1974, reviews). Reversible inhibition of outgrowth and elongation of nerve fibers in cultures of chick dorsal root ganglia is produced by colchicine in low concentrations (2.4×10^{-8} M to 1.2×10^{-7} M), and retraction of axons occurs within 30 minutes at high colchicine concentration (1.2×10^{-7} M to 2.4×10^{-6} M; K. M. Yamada *et al.*, 1970; M. P. Daniels, 1972). Recovery from colchicine occurs in about 12 hours after cessation of treatment. Colcemid has the same effect as colchicine, but recovery occurs within a few hours. Treatment with high concentrations of colchicine, resulting in retraction of the nerve fiber, also results in a reduction in the number of microtubules per unit cross-sectional area (Chang, 1972; M. P. Daniels, 1975). Local injection of colchicine into the sciatic nerve of the rat inhibits the rapid transport of amine storage granules in the adrenergic nerve fibers (Dahlström, 1968). Injection of colchicine into the hypoglossal or vagus nerves completely blocks both slow and fast transport of protein (Sjöstrand *et al.*, 1970). Colchicine has also been found to inhibit slow transport of protein in the crayfish nerve cord (H. L. Fernandez *et al.*, 1970), and to inhibit fast transport of neurosecretory material in the supraoptic neurons of the rat (Norström *et al.*, 1971). Fast transport is more sensitive than slow transport, but both are inhibited by colchicine.

The concentration of colchicine that is required to totally inhibit slow axonal transport is large enough to have numerous other toxic effects. These include inhibition of nucleoside transport (Mizel and Wilson, 1972) and a variety of abnormalities seen with the electron microscope in glial cells as well as in neurons: infolding of the nuclear membrane and alterations of the appearance of the endoplasmic reticulum, Golgi apparatus, and mitochondria (J. O. Karlsson *et al.*, 1971; Hansson and Sjöstrand, 1971). The fact that lumicolchicine, which has some of the toxic effects of colchicine but does not bind to tubulin, does not block axonal transport (M. T. Price, 1974) is also evidence that inhibition of axonal transport by colchicine is not due to indirect toxic effects but to a direct effect on microtubules.

There are several lines of evidence which are inconsistent with models of bulk axonal flow as originally conceived by Paul Weiss (1963). Firstly, the rates of axonal transport of cytoskeletal proteins are unrelated to the diameter of the axon. The rate of bulk flow of any kind of non-Newtonian fluid would be a function of axon diameter. Secondly, soluble proteins move slowly but organelles move much faster. The opposite would be predicted from a bulk flow model. Other evidence that is not consistent with bulk flow is that the total number of microtubules in all the branches of one axon is about 10 times the number in the main axonal stem (Zenker and Hohberg, 1973). Moreover, individual microtubules extend only part of the length of the axon (Bray and Bunge, 1981), and because their elongation occurs only at the plus end of each microtubule, they must be in dynamic equilibrium with a pool of tubulin throughout the length of the axon. Although the greatest concentration of plus ends is at the axon terminals or growth cones, the total number of plus ends of microtubules in the entire axon far exceeds the number concentrated at the axon terminals.

Components that are related structurally and functionally are transported together at slow velocities (Lasek *et al.*, 1984). For example, neurofilaments, microtubules, and MAPs (especially tau proteins, which are abundant in axons) all move together at the same rate in the SCa component, whereas actin and associated proteins move at a different rate in the SCb component and in a separate compartment of the axon. According to one model, most of the neurofilament and microtubule protein is transported in the form of stable, insoluble aggregates and polymers whereas most of the transported actin is in the form of soluble monomers (Morris and Lasek, 1982). According to a different model, there is a continual exchange between stationary polymerized cytoskeleton and soluble subunits: accordingly, soluble subunits produced by disassembly of stationary polymers would be transported for a short distance and then be added to the stationary polymerized cytoskeleton (Okabe and Hirokawa, 1990). This model is based on recent evidence showing a continuous exchange between the cytoskeleton and a soluble pool of subunits (Lim *et al.*, 1989; Okabe and Hirokawa, 1990).

The observation that soluble tubulin and neurofilament subunits are present in very small quantities in the axon was thought to signify that the SCa represents a bulk movement of the assembled cytoskeleton and that little interchange occurs between the assembled cytoskeleton and the pools of subunits (Lasek, 1986; McQuarrie, *et al.*, 1986).

However, Okabe and Hirokawa (1990) have shown that the polymerized axonal cytoskeleton is stationary but its components undergo continual turnover involving local disassembly and replacement with soluble free subunits which are transported down the axon. A region of axon labeled with fluorescent tubulin or actin was photobleached just proximal to the advancing growth cone. After bleaching, the growth cone continues to advance but the bleached zone remains stationary, although there is considerable elongation of the fluorescent axon distal to the bleached zone. This shows that translocation of microtubules and actin filaments does not occur during axon elongation. However, transport of tubulin and actin molecules to the growth cone is necessary for axon elongation. Analysis of recovery, after bleaching of a short zone of fluorescently labeled axon, led Okabe and Hirokawa (1990) to propose a model in which the polymerized cytoskeleton is stationary, but tubulin and actin turn over with half-times of about 45–90 minutes for tubulin and 15–30 minutes for actin and are continuously replaced by tubulin and actin subunits transported down the axon.

Saltatory movements of particles in both directions in living axons can be seen with light microscope cinematography (Burdwood, 1965; Berlinrood et al., 1972; Kirkpatrick et al., 1972; Cooper and Smith, 1974; Breuer et al., 1975; Forman et al., 1977). Movement of single organelles in the living axon can be seen with video-enhanced differential interference contrast microscopy (Allen and Allen, 1983; Allen et al., 1983; Burmeister et al., 1988). Movement of latex beads and of isolated axoplasmic organelles occurs along purified microtubules (Vale et al., 1985c; 1986; Paschal et al., 1987; Vallee et al., 1989) and occurs in both directions along single microtubules dissociated from squid axons (Schnapp et al., 1985). Individual particles move smoothly on purified microtubules, which indicates that the oscillatory and saltatory movements of organelles seen in vivo are due to encounters within the axon. Nevertheless, the net transport is in one direction and the rates correlate well with rates of fast axonal transport determined by metabolic labeling.

It has been suggested that the smooth endoplasmic reticulum (ER) might extend from the cell body continuously in the axon to the presynaptic terminals and thus serve as a channel for flow of materials (Palay, 1958b; A. Peters et al., 1970; Droz et al., 1975; Rambourg and Droz, 1980). Materials transported rapidly in the axon, either to or from the cell body, are localized within tubules and cisternae of the smooth ER. Herpes simplex virus, transported from the nerve endings to the perikaryon, is localized within the ER, and its localization can be made without ambiguity (Kristensson et al., 1974). Likewise, horseradish peroxidase, ferritin, or thorium dioxide is taken up by pinocytosis into vesicles which form multivesticular bodies that apparently coalesce to form cisternae in the preterminal part of the axon (Holtzman, 1971; Birks et al., 1972). Horseradish peroxidase is always surrounded by smooth ER and is localized within tubules and cisternae of ER as it flows in the axon (Sotelo and Riche, 1974). Catecholamine granules, transported from the cell body in the fast phase of axonal flow, are also confined within the smooth ER (Taxi and Sotelo, 1973). The smooth ER forms a continuous system of channels from the perikaryon to the axonal terminals (Droz et al., 1975; Rambourg and Droz, 1980). Tubules of smooth ER, 60–120 nm in diameter, apparently provide channels for fast flow in both directions in the axon. These ER tubules come into close apposition with the plasma membrane of the axon, indicating that an exchange of materials may occur at such points of contact. In the preterminal region the smooth ER forms a network of fine tubules, 20–30 nm in diameter, from which synaptic vesicles appear to bud. Radioactive labeled proteins, conveyed by fast axonal flow from the cell body, are difficult to localize unambiguously to the smooth ER because such localization is almost at the limits of resolution of electron microscopic autoradiography. However, by compressing the axon to impede axonal flow temporarily, Droz et al. (1975) have shown by means of high-resolution autoradiography that radioactive labeled proteins, conveyed by fast axonal flow, are localized to regions containing accumulations of smooth ER (Fig. 5.7). The evidence, taken as a whole, shows that the smooth ER probably provides channels for rapid transport of a diversity of materials from the axonal terminals to the cell body, as well as from the sites of their synthesis in the cell body to the axon and presynaptic terminals.

The fate of the transported material is diverse: some material is utilized for renewal of axonal structures, some is metabolized, some is recirculated by retrograde axonal flow, while other material is re-

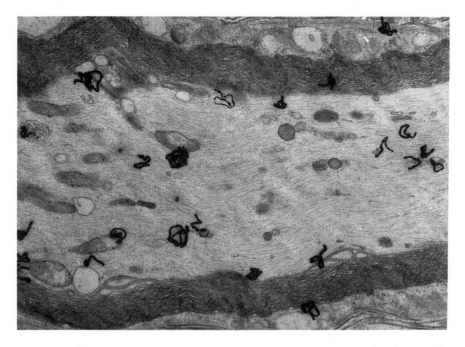

Figure 5.7. High-resolution autoradiograph of a postganglionic axon excised 3 mm from the ciliary ganglion of a chicken injected with tritiated leucine 24 hours before. The silver grains are associated with neurofilaments, mitochondria, and multivesicular bodies in the axoplasm. By courtesy of B. Droz.

leased at the terminals. A significant fraction of the transported material is offloaded or deposited along the length of the axon (Gross and Beidler, 1975; Ochs, 1975; Muñoz-Martinez *et al.*, 1981; Snyder, 1986, 1989). Proteins or peptides released from nerve terminals may be taken up by postsynaptic cells (Korr *et al.*, 1967; Alvarez and Püschel, 1972; Grafstein and Laureno, 1973; Droz *et al.*, 1973) or transferred directly from pre- to postsynaptic cell after inhibition of protein synthesis.

Subcellular localization of various materials that flow in axons has been studied, either by autoradiography, using light and electron microscopy (Fig. 5.7), or by fractionation of homogenates of brain or nerve after the administration of radioactive materials that are incorporated into identifiable components of the nerve cell. Electron microscopic autoradiographs made after injection of radioactive amino acids have shown that the fast-moving proteins in the axon on the way to the nerve endings are located in the plasma membrane, smooth ER, and amine storage granules. The mitochondria as a whole move with the slow flow, but components of

mitochondrial membranes are conveyed with the fast flow, and virtually all glycoproteins move directly to the nerve endings (J. O. Karlsson and Sjöstrand, 1971a–c; G. Bennett *et al.*, 1973; Droz *et al.*, 1973). By contrast, the bulk of the fast-moving protein is deposited in the axon *en route* (Concalon and Beidler, 1975). In the nerve endings, the fast-moving proteins and glycoproteins are located principally in synaptic vesicles and the presynaptic plasma membrane (Fig. 5.8).

The slow-flowing proteins have been localized, in electron microscopic autoradiographs, to bundles of neurofilaments, neurotubules, mitochondria, and plasma membrane. In contrast to the fast-flowing materials, which largely arrive at the nerve endings, most of the slowly flowing protein is deposited along the entire length of the axon, and probably less than 5 percent enters the nerve endings (Droz *et al.*, 1973).

In homogenates of brain and nerves, the fast-flowing proteins and glycoproteins are associated with "particulate" fractions thought to contain plasma membranes, synaptic vesicles, and other parti-

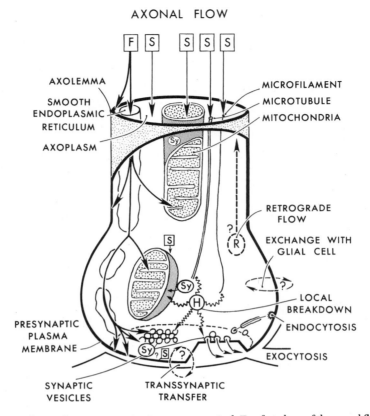

AXONAL FLOW

Figure 5.8. Dynamic condition of synaptic proteins in an axon terminal. F = fast phase of the axonal flow; S = slow phase of the axonal flow; Sy = sites of local protein synthesis or of local incorporation of labeled amino acids; H = hydrolytic enzymes such as proteinases and peptide hydrolases; R = retrograde flow. From B. Droz, *Brain Res.* **62**:383-394 (1973).

cles, whereas the slow-flowing proteins are found in the "soluble" fraction (which does not indicate that they are soluble *in vivo*) consisting of nonparticulate components of axoplasm and microtubule and microfilament proteins (Cuénod and Schönbach, 1971; J. O. Karlsson and Sjöstrand, 1971a–c; DiGiamberardino *et al.*, 1973). The neurotubule and neurofilament proteins compose more than 75 percent of the slow component of axonal flow in mammals (P. N. Hoffman and Lasek, 1975; Lasek and Hoffman, 1976).

In studies that set a standard of excellence in this field, Droz *et al.* (1973), G. Bennett *et al.* (1973), and DiGiamberardino *et al.* (1973) characterized the axonal transport of protein and glycoprotein from the preganglionic cell bodies in the third nerve nucleus to the giant calyciform terminals in the ciliary ganglion. They found that fast-flowing

proteins, moving at a rate of about 288 mm/day, are mainly used for renewal of various membranes (synaptic vesicles, mitochondria, endoplasmic reticulum, and plasma membrane, particularly the presynaptic membrane). They observed a wave of slowly flowing protein moving down the axon at a rate of 1.5–10 mm per day, most of which is deposited in the axoplasm along the entire length of the axon, with less than 5 percent arriving at the nerve endings. These proteins are deposited in regions of axoplasm devoid of synaptic vesicles and mitochondria.

The lifespan of materials in the neuron has been studied by determining the rate of disappearance of material pulse-labeled with radioactive precursors (reviewed by Dunlop, 1983; Shahbazian *et al.*, 1989). Kinetic studies, using high-resolution autoradiography and cell fractionation techniques, have shown that various components of the neuron are continually replaced, and that the proteins and glycoproteins of the nerve endings turn over at various rates and are replaced by material transported from the cell body. Renewal of synaptic proteins has been reviewed by Droz (1973). Not surprisingly, in view of the heterogeneity of materials that flow in nerve fibers, their turnover times range from hours to months. Proteins conveyed by slow transport turn over slowly, with half-lives of about 3 weeks in the axon and 10–18 days in the presynaptic region (J. O. Karlsson and Sjöstrand, 1971a; Droz *et al.*, 1973; H. L. Koenig *et al.*, 1973; Droz, 1973). Rapidly transported proteins turn over at varying rates in nerve endings; one fraction turns over in less than 1 day (Cuénod and Schönbach, 1971; J. O. Karlsson and Sjöstrand, 1971c), another fraction containing fucosyl glycoproteins turns over in about 10 days (Marko and Cuénod, 1973; G. Bennett *et al.*, 1973), while another component appears to have a turnover time of several months (Elam and Agranoff, 1971).

Whether there are changes in the rate of axonal flow during development is quite controversial. We have to ask whether the reported changes in rate of flow are due to maturation and aging or whether they are due to differences in temperature (particularly as a result of cooling of embryos and newborn animals), changes in dimensions of the nerves (rate of change in length and in diameter may be independent variables), or other variables that are usually uncontrolled or not even considered. The addition of new axons to the developing nerve and the elongation of axons that occur during the experimental period have to be taken into account when studying slow axonal flow in growing nerves. When these factors are taken into account, no change in rate of transport of AChE is found in the phrenic nerve of rats at different ages (Inestrosa and Alvarez, 1988).

Many reports of changes in rate of slow flow do not take all these factors into consideration. For example, in one of the more carefully controlled studies of changes in rate of fast axonal flow during maturation, Hendrickson and Cowan (1971) reported an increase in rate of fast flow of protein in optic nerve fibers of the rabbit. They determined the earliest time of appearance of labeled protein in the superior colliculus after injection of [^{3}H]leucine into one eye. In 6-day-old rabbits, they found a rate of flow of 120 mm/day, increasing to 150 mm/day by the end of the 3rd week postnatally, and attaining the adult level of about 200 mm/day at the end of the 4th week. This is almost twice the value obtained by essentially the same method by J. O. Karlsson and Sjöstrand (1968) in adult rabbits. The rate of slow flow, reported by Hendrickson. and Cowan (1971), diminished from 5 mm/day at the end of the 1st week to 2 mm/day in rabbits greater than 4 weeks of age. Increase in the rate of fast flow of protein was also found in the chick embryo, where no fast flow of protein could be detected at 7 days of incubation (Marchisio and Sjöstrand, 1972), and the rate almost doubled between 10 and 18 days of incubation (Marchisio *et al.*, 1973). On the other hand, Ochs (1973), in a careful study, found that the rate of fast flow in sciatic nerve remained remarkably uniform in cats 2 weeks of age (389 + 29 mm/day) and 6 weeks of age (426 + 34 mm/day) compared with adult cats (430 + 27 mm/day) and adult dogs (439 + 34 mm/day). Ochs (1972a,b) reported similar rates, about 410 mm/day, for fast flow in peripheral motor and sensory nerves as well as in central tracts of a variety of mammalian species.

In experiments on chick embryos and newborn mammals, the rate of fast axoplasmic flow is likely to be reduced significantly by cooling the animals even slightly. Fast axonal flow has a Q_{10} of 2–2.6 (Ochs and Smith, 1971, 1975), which means that a change of temperature of only 0.5°C will change the rate of fast flow by 15 mm/day. This seems to be the main or only reason for the slower rates of rapid axonal flow found in cold-blooded as compared with warm-blooded animals. In cold-blooded animals, increased temperature accelerates the rate of slow axonal transport (Grafstein and Forman, 1980, review; Cancalon, 1983b) and increases the rate of peripheral nerve regeneration (Lubinska and Olekiewicz, 1950; Cancalon, 1983a; Kleinebeckel and Schulte, 1988). Neither the species, type of nerve, nor caliber of the axons appears to affect the rate of fast axonal flow, if allowance is made for temperature differences. In the light of the evidence now available, the changes in rate of fast flow that have been reported during development may well be due to lowering of the body temperature of embryos or newborn animals during the experiment. The reported changes in rate of slow flow also need to be corrected for changes in the number and dimensions of the axons during development. In brief, inadequate controls of the varying parameters of the developing nerve make it impossible to draw reliable conclusions about changes of rate from many of the published reports on flow rates in developing nerves.

Transport of protein and organelles in dendrites is a controversial and unresolved problem (Thoenen and Kreutzberg, 1981; Sasaki *et al.*, 1983). It has been difficult to obtain good evidence of transport of proteins in dendrites. Ribosomes in dendrites are responsible for local synthesis of proteins in dendrites (Stewart and Levy, 1982; Steward and Falk, 1986), and flow is difficult to detect against a background of local synthesis. In one study, dendritic transport of protein at a velocity of 50–200 μm/minute, which is too fast to be accounted for by diffusion alone, was inferred from observations of dendritic labeling after a brief survival period after intracellular injection of radioactive amino acids (Schubert *et al.*, 1971). This transport is blocked by colchicine, which indicates that microtubules are involved (Schubert *et al.*, 1972).

Transport of RNA in dendrites of hippocampal neurons in culture has been observed: after giving a pulse of [³H]-uridine the label is at first restricted to the cell nucleus and recently synthesized RNA is transported selectively into dendrites (Davis *et al.*, 1987). The rate of RNA transport in dendrites (0.26–0.5 mm/day; Davis *et al.*, 1990) is similar to the rate of Veg 1 mRNA transport in *Xenopus* oocytes, which has been shown to require microtubules and microfilaments (Yisraeli *et al.*, 1990). One of the abundant mRNAs in dendrites has been found by *in situ* hybridization to code for the alpha subunit of calcium/calmodulin-dependent protein kinase (Burgin *et al.*, 1990). The role of Ca^{2+} and kinases in modulating assembly of the cytoskeleton, especially in growth cones, is discussed in Section 5.11.

5.10. Retrograde Axonal Transport

Many different molecules are taken up at axonal endings and transported back to the nerve cell body (Kristensson, 1978, review; Bisby, 1982, review). The mechanism of retrograde axonal transport involves linkage between membrane-bound organelles and microtubules by MAP1C, as described in Section 5.5. The rate of retrograde transport is fast, about 200 mm/day. Materials are transported retrogradely only if packaged in membranes or endocytotic vesicles. This is shown by the observation that carboxylated microbeads are retrogradely transported after entering the axon by endocytosis (L. C. Katz *et al.*, 1984; Cornwall and Phillipson, 1988), but are only transported anterogradely following injection directly into the axon (Adams and Bray, 1983).

Retrograde axonal transport is specifically inhibited by the drug EHNA, an adenosine analogue, without affecting anterograde transport (Vallee *et al.*, 1989, review). Vanadate and drugs such as colchicine which bind to tubulin inhibit both anterograde and retrograde axonal transport. Foreign materials such as horseradish peroxidase (HRP) (Mesulam, 1982), fluorescent-labeled molecules (Swanson, 1983), and fluorescent latex microspheres (Cornwall and Phillipson, 1988) have been used for experimental observations of retrograde axonal transport. Axons also serve as a route for retrograde transfer of physiologically significant materials such as nerve growth factor (see Section 8.18).

Although a considerable time has elapsed since W. H. Lewis (1931) first used the term *pinocytosis* for ingestion of extracellular fluid by macrophages, the study of protein uptake by cells from the extracellular fluid was neglected for a long time (Ryser, 1968; Steinman *et al.*, 1973; Willingham and Paston, 1984, review; Goldstein *et al.*, 1985, review). There are three kinds of evidence for pinocytosis by nerve endings. First, pinocytosis has been observed in neurons in tissue culture (A. F. Hughes, 1953; Nakai, 1956; Klatzko and Miquel, 1960; Burdwood, 1965). Second, indentations of the surface membranes of nerve terminals have been seen by electron microscopy, and these are considered to be evidence of pinocytosis (K. H. Andres, 1964, K. H. Andres and Von Düring, 1966; Waxman and Pappas, 1969; Holtzman and Peterson, 1969; Moor *et al.*, 1969; Akert *et al.*, 1972). Third, uptake of electron-opaque tracers from the extracellular space into axons can be seen with the electron microscope (Birks, 1966; Holtzman and Peterson, 1969; Birks *et al.*, 1972; Zacks and Saito, 1969; Malmgren *et al.*, 1978; Anderson *et al.*, 1981; Mesulam, 1982). This is discussed later in connection with retrograde transport of HRP. These observations show that the neuron is capable of taking up material from the extracellular space by means of pinocytosis and that transfer of materials between glial cells and neurons, or between neurons, may occur in that way.

Probably the first report of retrograde movement of materials in nerve fibers was made by Matsumoto (1920), who observed the movement of material stained with neutral red in sympathetic nerve fibers in tissue culture. Both anterograde and retrograde axonal transport are demonstrated by materials dammed up at both sides of a constriction on a nerve (Lubinska, 1964, review; R. S. Smith, 1980; Tsukita and Ishikawa, 1980). Since then, there have been several reports of particles moving visibly in both directions in living nerve fibers (Burdwood, 1965; Pomerat, 1961; Berlinrood et al., 1972; P. D. Cooper and Smith, 1974; D. S. Forman et al., 1977; R. S. Smith and Cooper, 1980; Koles et al., 1982). Such observations have been greatly improved by video-enhanced contrast microscopy and digital image enhancement (Allen et al., 1981, 1983; Allen and Allen, 1983).

Retrograde movement of poliomyelitis virus in nerves had been shown as early as 1940 by Bodian and Howe. They demonstrated that movement of poliomyelitis virus is blocked by freezing and then thawing a short segment of the nerve, which disrupts the axons without affecting the periaxonal space, indicating that the virus moves within the axons rather than between them (Bodian and Howe, 1941a,b). Certain viruses are specific for nerve or glial cells or both. Poliomyelitis and rabies viruses are selective for neurons and are transported retrogradely from the site of infection to the CNS, but in the CNS they are transported both anterogradely and retrogradely (Tsiang, 1979; Kucera et al., 1985; Gillet et al., 1986; Lycke and Tsiang, 1987). Transport of rabies virus is blocked by colchicine (Bijlenga and Heaney, 1978). Herpes simplex virus (types 1 and 2) infects both neurons and glial cells. The virus can enter peripheral axons and travel in the axon at a rate of 30 mm/day to the cell body, where it may remain latent but can be reactivated by damaging the peripheral nerve (Walz et al., 1974). The virus is localized within cisternae of the smooth ER (Kristensson et al., 1974; Lycke et al., 1984). There is evidence that other neurotropic viruses use the smooth ER as channels for their transmission within the neuron. Neurotropic viruses replicate after entering the neuron and are subsequently transferred retrogradely from cell to cell and may thus be used as retrograde transneuronal tracers

(Kristensson et al., 1978; Ugolini et al., 1987, 1989).

Tetanus toxin is taken up by nerve fibers, apparently nonselectively because it accumulates in motor, sensory, as well as sympathetic nerves, and is transported retrogradely to the cell body at a rate of about 7.5 mm/hour (Stoeckel et al., 1975). Prior administration of neuraminidase abolishes the uptake of tetanus toxin, indicating that the toxin binds to gangliosides of the axonal membrane. Tetanus toxin B-IIb fragment has been used as a retrograde transneuronal tracer (Buettner-Ennerver et al., 1981).

Radioactive amino acids injected into the tongue muscles appears in the nerve cell bodies of the hypoglossal nucleus (W. E. Watson, 1968). Kristensson and Olsson (1971, 1973) showed that Evans blue-labeled albumin and HRP appear in the hypoglossal neurons or spinal cord motoneurons after those protein tracers are injected into tongue muscles or gastrocnemius muscle, respectively. The rate of transport of these exogenous proteins is 120 mm/day.

HRP, a 44-kDa protein, has been used to show that retrograde axonal flow occurs in peripheral nerves as well as in axons in the CNS. Only basic isoenzymes of HRP are endocytosed and retrogradely transported. Uptake of HRP is most likely by weak electrostatic interaction between the positively charged HRP molecules and negatively charged groups on the cell surface, leading to weak adsorptive endocytosis (Key and Giorgi, 1987). HRP conjugated to wheat germ agglutinin (WGA) is also taken up by weak adsorptive endocytosis but the WGA has a higher affinity for neuronal membranes than basic HRP (Gonatas et al., 1979). Electrical stimulation of nerves increased uptake of HRP into their endings at the neuromuscular junction (Holtzman et al., 1971; Heuser and Reese, 1973; Heuser et al., 1974). HRP is transported inside cysternae of smooth endoplasmic reticulum in the axon (Sotelo and Riche, 1974). Retrograde flow of HRP has thus become a useful neuroanatomical technique for tracing pathways (Kristensson, 1975, 1978, review; LaVail, 1975, review; Kristensson and Olsson, 1977; Malmgren et al., 1978; Mesulam, 1982, review). HRP can also be used as a retrograde transneuronal tracer of nerve pathways (Harrison et al., 1984).

Retrograde transport of normally occurring materials in the axon has been studied by tying one or two ligatures on peripheral nerves and measuring the accumulation of material distal to the ligature. In this way, retrograde transport of acetylcholinesterase has been found at a rate of about 134 mm/day in dog peroneal nerve (Lubinska and Niemierko, 1971) and 70–120 mm/day in rabbit vagus nerve (Sjöstrand and Frizell, 1975). Retrograde transport of choline acetyltransferase in the rabbit hypoglossal nerve occurs at a rate of 50–60 mm/day (Sjöstrand and Frizell, 1975).

Nerve growth factor (NGF) is taken up by receptor-mediated endocytosis at the nerve ending and is transported back to the cell body in adrenergic sympathetic neurons and spinal sensory neurons (Hendry et al., 1974a,b; Paravicini et al., 1975; Stoeckel and Thoenen, 1975; Stoeckel et al., 1975; Thoenen and Barde, 1980, review), and surprisingly, also in motoneurons (Yan et al., 1988; Wayne and Heaton, 1988). This transport is blocked by colchicine. The rate of retrograde transport of NGF in sensory neurons is about 13 mm/hour, while in adrenergic sympathetic neurons it is about 2.5 mm/hour. The concept of uptake and retrograde axonal transport of materials with a trophic action on the neuron, or carrying a signal to the perikaryon from the target organs, has been well established by evidence obtained over a period of several decades (see Section 8.16).

Some foreign substances that enter the axon and are transported to the cell body can be toxic. The signal that initiates chromatolysis after axotomy may be of this kind (see Section 5.16). Ricin communis agglutinin (RCA), when injected into a nerve, is rapidly taken up by axons, is transported retrogradely and results in cell death—so called "suicide transport" (Wiley et al., 1982; Yamamoto et al., 1983, 1984; L. R. Johnson et al., 1985, R. G. Wiley and Oeltman, 1986; Ling and Leong, 1987, 1988; Ling et al., 1989). RCA has become a useful reagent for tracing the central projections of primary afferents from peripheral nerves (Yamamoto et al.,1983; Leong and Tan, 1987; Ling and Leong, 1987).

5.11. The Growth Cone

Elongation of neurites occurs exclusively at their growth cones, which are the actively growing tips of all branches of axons and dendrites. Growth of the plasma membrane occurs by insertion of membrane components at the growth cone. Growth of the axonal cytoskeleton also occurs by assembly in the growth cone. These components are delivered from the cell body to the axonal growth cone by axonal transport. Delivery of cytoskeletal and associated proteins by slow axonal transport sets a limit to the rate of axonal elongation and regeneration. Growth cone movements, produced by actin filaments, determine the direction of growth of axons and probably also of dendrites. Dendritic growth is considered at length in Chapter 6, and what follows in this section relates to axonal growth cones.

The axonal growth cone's functions are ultimately under control of the cell body which is the source of all the components of the growth cone except those obtained by endocytosis from the environment. Delays in arrival of molecules transported retrogradely from the growth cones to the cell body and in their transport out to the growth cone, set limits to the role of the cell body in regulation of growth cone activities. Therefore, the activities of growth cones are regulated by local conditions. The direction of elongation of the growth cone can be influenced by mechanical guidance by the substratum, extracellular matrix molecules, diffusible extracellular growth factors, and by electric fields (reviewed by Kater and Letourneau, 1985; Lander, 1987; Bray and Hollenbeck, 1988; Van Hoof et al., 1989).

In 1890 Ramón y Cajal discovered the axonal growth cone.[12] In his autobiography (1917, Chapter 8) he writes: *"I had the good fortune to see for the first time that fantastic ending of the growing axon. In my sections of the spinal cord of the three day chick embryo, this ending was displayed as a protoplasmic conglomeration of conical form, endowed with ameboid movements. It could be compared with a living battering ram, soft and pliable, which advances, mechanically thrusting the obstacles encountered in its path, until it reaches the region of its peripheral termination. This curious terminal club*

---

[12]Cajal admits in his autobiography that both he and Lenhossék independently discovered the growth cone in 1890, but he claims priority because his publication was first. At about the same time, Koelliker (1890), van Gehuchten (1891), and Retzius (1893, 1894) also clearly showed growth cones (*Wachstumskeule; cones d'accroissement*).

was baptised by me: the cone of growth" (Fig. 5.5).[13]

The question of where elongation occurs in the developing axon was thoroughly discussed by Ramón y Cajal in his inimitable manner in *Degeneration and Regeneration of the Nervous System* (1928, p. 362 *et seq.*). He concluded that *"longitudinal growth of nerve fibres is especially localized to their free ends, where the cone of growth is situated"* and *"the cone of growth possesses two important functions: to lengthen the conductor (longitudinal growth), and to create new nerve paths."* However, *"the increase of calibre of the axon is a function of the entire fibre."* In the previously cited work (p. 370) Cajal states: *"The act of axonic growth and emission of branches imply complex processes of organization of the membrane, the neuroplasma, and the neurofibrillar network.—The neuroplasma must be conceived, not as an inert liquid, but as a complex protoplasmic organ, full of special invisible units."* This is a pure conjecture for which Cajal received the inspiration from the micromechanical models of living organisms constructed in the 17th and 18th Centuries (see Section 1.1; reviewed by Hall, 1979).

That the axon does not elongate like a growing hair from its proximal region or at all points along its length was evident from Harrison's (1910) observations of the relationship of the growth cone to fixed external markers (Fig. 5.2), and also was evident from observations by Speidel (1942) on the elongation of axons in the tail fin of the frog tadpole, showing that axonal extension occurs only at the growth cone. Growing nerves can be seen easily through the transparent epidermis of the tail fin of frog tadpoles. Koelliker (1886, 1905) and R. G. Harrison (1904, 1924a,b) observed the migration of Schwann cells along these nerves. Speidel described their growth, the movements of their endings, and their myelination (Speidel, 1932, 1933, 1935a,b, 1941, 1942, 1964). Because the growth cones at the tips of the cutaneous nerve fibers behaved like those in tissue culture, extrapolation from the culture system to the

living tissue could be made with more confidence than is usually possible. Branching of the axon actually occurs at the end, although collateral branches may occur along its length. During myelination, branches that are not at a node of Ranvier are eliminated.

During normal growth of cutaneous axons of the tadpole, Speidel observed extension, retraction, branching, and elimination of branches by autotomy, all occurring continuously (Figs. 5.9 and 5.10). One can clearly see in Speidel's figures that the lengths of the proximal segments between branching points remain constant as the axon extends distally, thus confirming earlier observations showing that extension occurs at or close to the growth cones (Ramón y Cajal, 1928, pp. 362–370). This has been confirmed by D. Bray (1970, 1973b), as shown in Fig. 5.11. Speidel observed that retraction of a growing axon may occur spontaneously or may be induced by mechanical obstruction, injury, or noxious chemicals such as alcohol. During retraction of the axon the axoplasm can be seen flowing proximally, and the axon terminal is transformed into a lanceolate retraction club. The rate of retraction is usually the same as that of extension, about 40 μm/hour.

Advances in microscopy and imaging used to observe growing axons labeled with fluorescent dyes that are transported to the growth cone have made it possible to extend Speidel's original observations on the behavior of living growth cones (W. A. Harris *et al.*, 1987). Retinal axons growing to the optic tectum in *Xenopus* embryos bear growth cones that are relatively small but very actively motile and are similar in morphology and behavior to those growing on nonadhesive surfaces in tissue culture. As they approach their targets they slow down and become larger and more elaborate. Similar changes in morphology of growth cones have also been seen in growth cones of *Xenopus* retinal ganglion cells labeled with lucifer yellow—the growth cone morphology changes in relation to different conditions along the optic nerve pathway (Holt, 1989). Similarly, in histological preparations of the developing optic nerve fibers of the mouse, the growth cones increase in size and number of filopodia as they enter the optic chiasm (Bovolenta and Mason, 1987).

Growth cones are structurally and functionally different from the rest of the neuron. Most of the interactions of the neuron with its

[13]In Craigie's English translation of Cajal's autobiography the words *"of the spinal cord"* are omitted from the second sentence of this quotation on p. 369. I have found many other significant omissions and errors in that translation. Therefore, I have verified all quotations for this edition and, where required, have made fresh translations of all excerpts from Cajal's writings as well as new translations from the works of other authors.

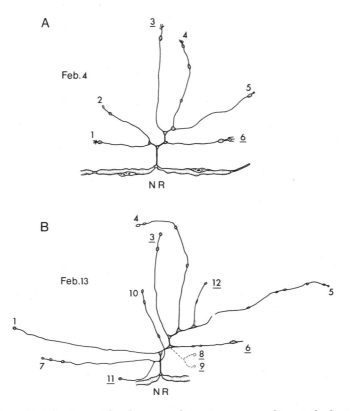

Figure 5.9. Remodeling of developing peripheral nerve endings. A young axonal terminal arborization seen through the transparent tail fin of a living frog tadpole, showing its growth from February 4 (A) to February 13 (B). The endings are numbered to show the changes in their positions and lengths during the period of observation. An underlined number signifies a branch located deeply, away from the skin. Growth cones were present on endings 1, 3, 4, and 6 on February 13. Endings 2, 8, and 9 were eliminated. Six new endings (7–12) developed during the period of observation. From C. C. Speidel, *J. Comp. Neurol.* **76**:57-69 (1942).

environment take place at the growth cone. Only the growth cone moves—as the axon or dendrite elongates, the cell body and proximal segments of the axon or dendrite are, in most cases, attached and stationary. There are exceptions in which the cell body itself migrates, as in the case of the cerebellar granule cells. However, the addition of new material during the elongation of the axon, and probably also of dendrites, occurs at the growth cone, which is solely responsible for the choice of direction, for selecting a pathway, and finally, for selecting a suitable target at which to stop elongating.

The external morphology of growth cones varies from a relatively simple pointed, paint-brush-like ending with a single thin, finger-like extension called a filopodium, to an elaborate fan-like expansion bearing a profusion of filopodia and broad and flat extensions called lamellipodia. The appearance of the growth cone is similar in different species, both invertebrate and vertebrate. Growth cones have been observed in the Rohon–Beard cells of living frog embyros (Harrison, 1910), the out-growing axons in the tail fin of the intact, living frog tadpole (Speidel, 1933, 1941), and the peripheral nerves (Roberts and Taylor, 1982) and spinal cord neurons of frog embryos (M. Jacobson and Huang, 1986). Growth cones of grasshopper neurons *in vivo* (Goodman *et al.*, 1982; Bastiani *et al.*, 1985), of axons growing in tissue culture of *Aplysia* neurons (Burmeister *et al.*, 1988; Goldberg and Burmeister, 1988), and of the snail *Helisoma* (Haydon *et al.*, 1985; Kater and Mattson, 1988; Kater *et al.*, 1988) resemble growth cones of vertebrate neurons *in*

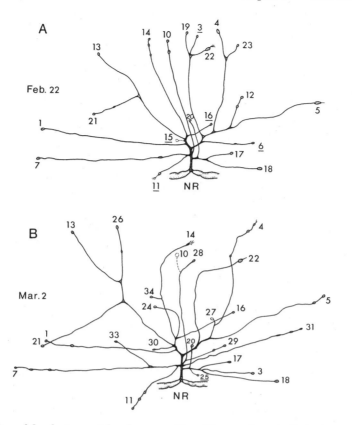

Figure 5.10. **Remodeling of developing peripheral nerve endings.** The axonal terminal arborization shown in Fig. 5.9 was observed from February 22 (A) to March 2 (B). Eleven new endings had appeared by February 22, and 11 more by March 2. Some endings were eliminated, others retracted, others extended, and some showed no changes. Note that these observations show that the lengths of the proximal segments of the branches remain constant but growth occurs only at the growth cones. From C. C. Speidel, *J. Comp. Neurol.* **76**:57-69 (1942).

vitro from amphibians (Harrison, 1907a,b, 1910, 1912, 1914), chick embryos (W. H. Lewis and Lewis, 1912; A. F. Hughes, 1953; Nakai, 1956, 1960; D. Bray, 1970, 1979, 1982; K. M. Yamada *et al.*, 1970, 1971; Wessells *et al.*, 1971a,b; Letourneau, 1982; Connolly *et al.*, 1985), rat (Argiro *et al.*, 1985), and human fetuses (Nakai and Kawasaki, 1959), to give only selected references.

Ultrastructure of the growth cone is correlated with its functional activities: elongation and growth; motility and active exploration; uptake of materials; secretion of enzymes, neurotransmitters, and trophic agents. Fixation with aldehyde and standard methods of staining for electron microscopy show that the growth cones of axons contain a core of the usual cytoplasmic organelles, including microtubules, 10 nm-neurofilaments and 7-nm mi-

crofilaments, and many mitochondria, vesicles, and cisternae of smooth ER and a network of microfilaments in the cortical cytoplasm associated with the plasma membrane (del Cerro and Snider, 1968; Tennyson, 1970; K. M. Yamada *et al.*, 1971; D. Bray and Bunge, 1973; Skoff and Hamburger, 1974; del Cerro, 1974; G. G. Fox *et al.*, 1976; Tsui *et al.*, 1983). Growth cones of glial cells have essentially similar appearances to those of neurons (del Cerro, 1974).

Tissue frozen very rapidly provides a different electron microscopic image from that produced by aldehyde fixation (Cheng and Reese, 1985, 1987, 1988). After quick freezing, the growth cones lack the abundant smooth ER and vesicles seen in aldehyde-fixed tissue, but have flattened membrane saccules resembling the Golgi apparatus, and the membrane-bound organelles are arranged in a spe-

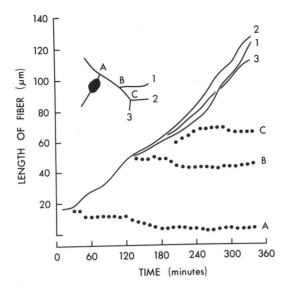

Figure 5.11. Axonal growth occurs only at the growth cone. Lengths of outgrowing axonal branches of a single sympathetic ganglion neuron in culture were measured from time-lapse photomicrographs. Lengths were measured from the cell body to the growth cones and branch points. The cell is shown as it appeared at 300 minutes after the start of the observations. From D. Bray *J. Cell Biol.* 56:702–712 (1973).

cific order in the long axis of the growth cone. Using the quick-freezing technique, Cheng and Reese (1987) studied growth cones in the chick embryo optic tectum, after exposure to ferritin for varying times. They observed that the ferritin appeared first in coated pits near the base of the growth cone, and at successively later times in coated vesicles, smooth vesicles, individual membrane saccules near the base of the growth cone, and finally in the stacked saccules progressively nearer the tip of the growth cone. These observations show that the membranes are recycled by endocytosis at the base of the growth cone and enter the flattened saccules which represent a pool of membrane materials available for addition to outgrowing filopodia.

The growth cone extends, spinning out the neurite behind it. Observations of growing axons, initially with conventional light microscopy and recently with video-enhanced contrast differential interference microscopy (Burmeister *et al.*, 1988), show that as the leading edge of the growth cone advances, the base of the growth cone becomes transformed into the neurite. The direction taken by the leading edge is determined by both stimulation

and inhibition of growth cone motility resulting from contact with the extracellular matrix and with the surfaces of other cells and neurites, as well as by diffusible growth-promoting molecules, of which NGF has been most fully characterized.

Advance of the growth cone starts with the formation of thin veils extending between thin finger-like processes called filopodia or microspikes. Vesicles, and then other organelles, enter the veil from the proximal core of the growth cone, which consists of a mass of actin microfilaments in which axonal neurofilaments and microtubules end. The veil becomes like the proximal core region of the growth cone whose structure has meanwhile become transformed into that of the axon. The filopodia are motile extensions of the growth cone, with a length of up to 10–20 μm and a diameter of about 0.3 μm. There may be from 1 to 30 filopodia on a single growth cone. They contain a central bundle of actin filaments which extend from the layer of actin filaments adjacent to the plasma membrane of the growth cone (Reese and Reese, 1981; Letourneau, 1983). Filopodial extension most probably results from addition of actin monomers at the distal ends of the parallel microfilaments (Argiro *et al.*, 1985) by mechanisms similar to extension of the acrosomal process of the sperm (Tilney and Inoue, 1982). The filopodia extend and retract rapidly at a rate of about 6–10 μm/minute, and they are in constant motion. They adhere to other cells or foreign bodies that they touch. The adhesion of filopodia to other cells is mediated not by NCAM, but by proteoglycans called adherons (Schubert *et al.*, 1985a,b, 1986) which form filaments extending from the filopodial tip (Tsui *et al.*, 1985, 1988). Filopodia are very active, extending, retracting, and moving laterally, when neurons are cultured on nonadhesive surfaces such as glass or plastic, but the growth cone activity decreases when the glass or plastic is coated with adhesive molecules such as polylysine. Growth cones of embryonic neurons are larger and more active than those of adults (Argiro *et al.*, 1985).

As the growth cone extends, lamellipodia and filopodia move away from its leading edge in a movement known as "*ruffling*" (Abercrombie, 1980; Bray and Chapman, 1985; Hollenbeck, 1988). This movement of the growth cone is inhibited by agents that alter actin polymerization, e.g., cytochalasins and phalloidin (Cooper, 1987). The mechanism of extension at the growth cone is quite similar to that observed during the extension phase of movement of many types of cells. This movement is driven by the network of actin filaments adjacent to the plasma membrane (Stossel *et al.*, 1982, review). Change of the cortical actin from a gel to a sol which can flow into the center of the growth cone probably occurs in a way analagous to that which occurs during elongation of the pseudopod of the amoeba (Taylor and Condeelis, 1979). The contraction phase of the filopodia probably serves to pull the growth cone bodily forward and to change the direction of growth (Bray and Chapman, 1985).

The principal cause of axonal extension is insertion of new material into the growth cone. New plasma membrane is added mainly at the base of the growth cone (Bray, 1970; Griffin *et al.* 1981; Pfenninger and Malié-Pfenninger, 1981). Plasma membrane components are delivered by fast axonal transport, whereas the cytoskeletal proteins are supplied by slow axonal transport, and this limits the rate of axonal elongation and regeneration (Wujek and Lasek, 1983). Assembly of microtubules occurs at the growth cone (Letourneau and Ressler, 1984; Bamburg *et al.*, 1986). The growth cone interacts with its environment and determines the direction of axon elongation (Letourneau, 1979; Taghert *et al.*, 1982; Candy and Bentley, 1986).

Selective inhibition of growth cone motility occurs when growth cones of one type of neuron contact a neuron of a different type (Kapfhammer *et al.*, 1986; Kapfhammer and Raper, 1987; Moorman and Hume, 1990) or when neuronal growth cones contact oligodendrocytes (Caroni and Schwab, 1988a,b, 1989; Schwab and Caroni, 1988; Chiquet, 1989, review; see Section 3.3). Such behavior of growth cones could serve to restrict axonal growth to specific pathways and may also be involved in inhibition of growth of axons when they meet specific targets. Inhibition of growth cone motility and of axonal extension by contact with oligodendrocytes may be a basis for the failure of axon regeneration in the mammalian central nervous system.

Factors that can modify the morphology of growth cones are intrinsic, namely, the type of neuron, stage of development, and functional state; and extrinsic, especially contact with different molecules in the substratum and local environment, for example, nerve growth factor, laminin, and fibronectin, which promote axon elongation. The effects of local environment in tissue culture

have been most frequently studied and reviewed (Cotman and Banker, 1974; Johnston and Wessells, 1980; Landis, 1983; Letourneau, 1983; Kater and Letourneau, 1985; Lockerbie, 1987; Bray and Hollenbeck, 1988). Rapidly growing axons have growth cones with simpler morphology than slowly growing axons, and the most complex growth cones are seen close to targets or at points of decision such as the optic chiasm (Bray and Hollenbeck, 1988, review; Holt, 1989). It is not known exactly how the extracellular conditions are transduced to result in changes in growth cone motility and elongation but there is considerable evidence that intracellular free calcium ions are involved.

Growth cone morphology and motility can be regulated by the level of intracellular free Ca^{2+} ions. There are three different ways in which calcium can modulate microtubule assembly and thus influence axonal elongation: the first is via Ca^{2+}-dependent kinases that can phosphorylate cytoskeletal proteins; the second is by a direct effect of Ca^{2+} on tubulin; the third is via the calcium-binding protein calmodulin, which interacts with tau proteins and MAP2 which stabilize microtubules by forming cross-bridges between them. In addition, rapid changes in growth cone shape and motility can result from changes in actin microfilament polymerization, which is influenced by Ca^{2+} (see Section 5.6).

The relationship between intracellular Ca^{2+} and growth cone activity has been studied by Kater and collaborators in the large growth cones of the snail, *Helisoma*, growing in culture, using calcium-binding fluorescent dyes such as fura-2 (Grynkiewicz *et al.*, 1985) to indicate changes in intracellular calcium (Cohan and Kater, 1986; Cohan *et al.*, 1987; Mattson and Kater, 1987; Kater *et al.*, 1988, review). Some neurons of Helisoma extend axons actively while others are stationary, and the level of intracellular free Ca^{2+} in motile growth cones is 2–3 times higher than in nonmotile growth cones (Cohan *et al.*, 1987). Serotonin applied to individual growth cones causes them to stop moving and to round up (Haydon *et al.*, 1987). Electrical stimulation has the same effect (Cohan and Kater, 1986). Those treatments causes an increase in intracellular free Ca^{2+} from 125 to 330 nM (Cohan *et al.*, 1987). Those effects and the effects of calcium ionophore and calcium channel blockers (Mattson and Kater, 1987) show that there is an optimal level of about 100–150

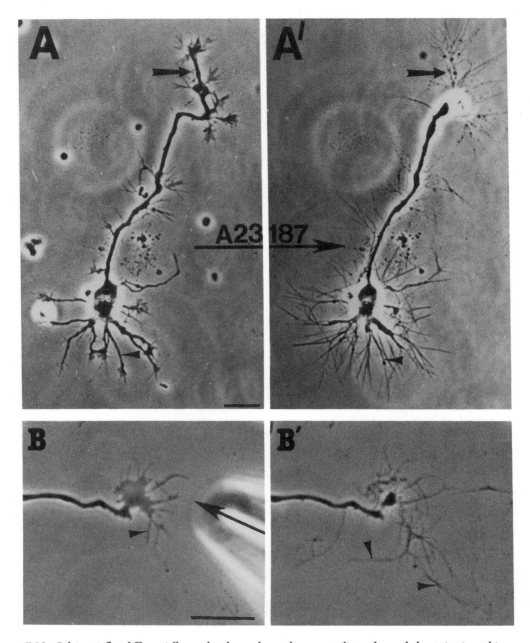

Figure 5.12. Calcium influx differentially regulated axonal growth cone motility and axonal elongation in rat hippocampal pyramidal cells in culture. An isolated pyramidal neuron is shown before (A) and 20 minutes after (A') application of 1 μm calcium ionophore A23187. The arrow points to the axon, the arrowhead to the dendrites. After treatment with calcium ionophore filopodial microspikes extend from axon and dendrites, and the shafts of both axon and dendrites retract. Formation of microspikes results from actin polymerization to form microfilaments, while retraction of the neurite shafts results from calcium-induced depolymerization of microtubules. (B, B') The effect of focal application of A23187. Arrow in (B) shows the flow of A23187 from the micropipette. (B') shows retraction of the axonal shaft and formation of microspikes. Differential sensitivity of microfilaments and microtubules to Ca^{2+} is believed to be a mechanism for regulation of growth cone motility and neurite elongation in response to neurotransmitters and growth factors. Magnification bar = 10 μm. Kindly provided by Mark P. Mattson.

nM Ca^{+2} at which growth cones are motile, and either much higher or much lower calcium levels result in retraction of filopodia and cessation of growth cone extension (Fig. 5.12).

The activities of the growth cone involve making and breaking adhesive contacts with components of the extracellular matrix. For this purpose migrating neurons and growth cones secrete proteases and plasminogen activators which result in activation of proteolytic enzymes which break down components of the extracellular matrix (Krystosek and Seeds, 1981; Pittman, 1985; Monard, 1988, review; Pittman and Buettner, 1989). The rate of axonal growth is also modified by protease inhibitors secreted by glial cells and fibroblasts.

In the past few years various lines of evidence have indicated that glial cells may produce factors which stimulate outgrowth of axons from PNS and CNS neurons (see Sections 3.7 and 8.19). Nageotte (1907) was the first to report that in transplanted sensory ganglia the satellite cells appear to exert a strong attraction on the regenerating axonal sprouts. This is what Cajal meant when he referred to *the nutritive and tutorial functions of the glial cells.* The glia-derived neurite promoting factor (GdNPF or GDN) is a potent serine protease inhibitor, similar to the protease nexin-I which is released from fibroblasts (Guenther *et al.*, 1985; Gloor *et al.*, 1986; Monard, 1988, review). It is a polypeptide of 43 kDa released from cultured glial and glioma cells. It is similar to GDN in normal brain, especially in the adult primary olfactory system where it is likely to be involved in continual renewal of neurons (Reinhard *et al.*, 1988). GDN promotes axon outgrowth from cultured sympathetic neurons but does not support their survival, and GDN also potentiates the growth-promoting efforts of NGF on sympathetic neurons (Zurn *et al.* 1988).

The current theory of the combined effects of proteases and protease inhibitors, which have opposing actions, is as follows. By degrading components of the extracellular matrix, proteases may facilitate the motility of the filopodia on the growth cones, but reduce their adhesive contacts. Protease inhibitors have the opposite effects: by forming complexes with proteases they may stabilize growth cone adhesion and thus potentiate axon extension (Monard, 1988). In theory, excessively strong adhesion would result in inhibition of the motility of the

growth cones; therefore, there must be a balance between the activities of proteases and protease inhibitors. Failure to achieve this balance may be one of the reasons for lack of successful regeneration in the CNS. Other causes of failure of regeneration in the CNS of higher vertebrates may be lack of trophic factors, nonpermissive conditions such as lack of laminin and fibronectin in the adult mammalian CNS and active inhibition of axon extension by oligodendrocytes.

Growth cone motility, shape, and direction of growth are directly regulated by NGF in tissue culture (see Section 8.16 for the mechanism of action of NGF). Axons can respond to NGF in solution and to NGF bound to the substratum (Gundersen, 1985).

Growth of rat sympathetic axons is stimulated directly by NGF (Campenot, 1977, 1979). The direction of growth of chick embryo dorsal root ganglion axons can be altered by application of NGF (Gundersen and Barrett, 1979, 1980). Sudden increase in NGF level results in rapid retraction of growth cones (Griffin and Letourneau, 1980), while addition of NGF is followed by spreading of growth cones on axons growing from chick DRG neurons in culture (Connolly *et al.*, 1985). Removal of NGF causes a loss of ruffles and rounding up of growth cones of chick sympathetic axons, and addition of NGF results, in less than 30 seconds, in reinitiation of ruffling (Connolly *et al.*, 1985). These effects are the result of direct action of NGF on the growth cone and they occur in growth cones on axons severed from the cell body. The direct effect of NGF on growth cone motility is probably mediated by *ras* proteins which are abundant in axons of NGF-sensitive neurons such as dorsal root ganglion neurons (Furth *et al.*, 1987; Sudol, 1988). Introduction of *ras* proteins into PC12 cells or freshly dissociated chick embryo neurons from dorsal root, ciliary, or nodose ganglia results in promotion of neurite outgrowth (see Section 8.16).

Laminin, a glycoprotein molecule of the extracellular matrix, is a potent promoter of neurite outgrowth in tissue culture. It acts on all types of PNS neurons and many types of CNS neurons. However, laminin is only transiently present in the embryonic vertebrate CNS and is not found in the adult mammalian CNS. Neurons respond to laminin only when it is bound to the substratum. Laminin has a powerful growth-promoting effect but does not promote neuron survival (reviewed by Lander, 1987; G. R. Martin, 1987; Sephel *et al.*, 1989).

In adult animals laminin is limited to basement membranes of which it forms the most abundant component (Martin and Timpl, 1987; Leblond and Inoue, 1989; Yurchenco and Schittny, 1990). Laminin is a very large glycoprotein (850 kDa) consisting of an A chain (~400 kDa) and two B chains (each ~210 kDa) disulfide-linked to each other, in the shape of a cross with three short and one long arm. The neurite-outgrowth fragment is at the end of the long arm. Laminin binds to other molecules of the basement membrane and to epithelial and muscle cells that are in contact with basement membranes *in vivo*. Laminin also interacts with itself, with cell surface proteoglycans, and with integrin receptors. In tissue culture, laminin has neurite-promoting activity at concentrations of 10–100 ng/ml.

Peripheral nerve axons can interact with laminin in basement membranes, in epithelia and muscles (Sanes *et al.*, 1986). Outside the CNS, at the regions of outgrowth of cranial and spinal nerves and along the peripheral nerve pathways, laminin may promote the outgrowth of those nerves (Rogers *et al.*, 1986; Krotoski *et al.*, 1986; Riggott and Moody, 1987). The role of laminin in guidance of migrating neural crest cells is discussed in Section 4.4.

Laminin is absent from the adult vertebrate CNS (Alitalo *et al.*, 1982), but it appears to be present transiently and in low abundance in the embryonic vertebrate CNS (Liesi, 1985a; Madsen *et al.*, 1986; McLoon *et al.*, 1986; J. Cohen *et al.*, 1987; Letourneau *et al.*, 1988). Retinal ganglion cells *in vitro* respond to the neurite-promoting effect of laminin during the period of normal axonal outgrowth (J. Cohen *et al.*, 1986; Hall *et al.*, 1986; Halfter *et al.*, 1987), and during the time when laminin-like immunoreactivity is present in the optic axon pathway (Liesi *et al.*, 1985b; McLoon *et al.*, 1986; J. Cohen *et al.*, 1987).

It has been suggested that in the absence of laminin, the Thy-1 protein supports neurite outgrowth in the CNS (R. Morris, 1986; Bolin and Rouse, 1986; R. J. Greenspan and O'Brien, 1989). Antibodies to Thy-1 protein can serve as a substrate capable of promoting outgrowth of neurites from rat retinal ganglion cells (Leifer *et al.*, 1984) and enhance survival of mouse Purkinje cells *in vitro* (Mes-

ser *et al.*, 1984). Thy-1 protein has an interesting form of attachment to the outside of the plasma membrane: its terminal cysteine is covalently bonded to a membrane glycolipid containing phosphatidyl inositol (Tse *et al.*, 1985). This type of attachment is involved in signal transduction across cell membranes, mediated by second messengers (Hokin, 1985). This suggests that Thy-1 located in elongating axons, for example on cerebellar climbing fibers (Morris *et al.*, 1985), may be involved in signal transduction.

Fibronectin is a glycoprotein which is widely distributed, but its role in promoting axon growth in the PNS is related to its localization in basement membranes and interstitial matrices. Fibronectin does not exist in the adult vertebrate CNS but is transiently present in the CNS during embryonic development (reviewed by Yamada, 1983; Furcht, 1983; Hynes, 1985; Lander, 1987; Dufour *et al.*, 1988). Fibronectin is composed of two disulfide-linked polypeptides (each ~220 kDa) both encoded by the same gene. A variety of isoforms of fibronectin subunits are produced as a result of differential gene splicing and posttranslational modification and these probably have different functions. Fibronectin is a relatively weak promoter of neurite outgrowth compared with laminin, when they are bound to the tissue culture substratum. Fibronectin stimulates growth of a wide variety of PNS neurons (Baron-van Evercooren *et al.*, 1982; Rogers *et al.*, 1983; Manthorpe *et al.*, 1983; Gundersen, 1987), but CNS neurons do not respond to fibronectin (Rogers *et al.*, 1983). Fibronectin has not been found in the adult CNS but transient fibronectin immunoreactivity in the CNS occurs during development (Pearlman *et al.*, 1986; Chun *et al.*, 1986). Fibronectin is widely distributed in peripheral tissues (Furcht, 1983; Krotoski *et al.*, 1986; Sanes *et al.*, 1986) where it may play a role in stimulating peripheral axonal growth.

Antibodies have been produced which completely block the neurite-promoting effects of laminin and fibronectin in culture (Bozyczko and Horwitz, 1986; Hall *et al.*, 1987; Letourneau *et al.*, 1988). These antibodies react with integrins which are cell surface receptors for laminin and fibronectin (Ruoslahti and Pierschbacher, 1986, 1987; Hynes, 1987). The effect is mediated by cell surface receptors of the integrin family located on the growth cone surface which recognize RGDS (Arg-Gly-Asp-Ser) sequences in the laminin and fibronectin molecules. The membrane receptors interact with actin microfilaments on the cytoplasmic side of the membrane of the growth cone and filopodia (Buck and Horwitz, 1987; Ruoslahti and Pierschbacher, 1987). Evidence that migration of neural crest cells involves interaction between integrin receptors and extracellular matrix molecules is given in Section 4.4.

These adhesive interactions between growth cones and the extracellular matrix can be modulated during development in several ways. Changing the distribution and number of integrin receptors and cell adhesion molecules can alter the strength of adhesion. Posttranslational modifications, especially phosphorylation, can provide another means of regulating integrins. Developmentally regulated expression of extracellular matrix molecules can alter their abundance and localization.

An example of developmental regulation of responsiveness to laminin is seen in chick retinal ganglion cells (Cohen et al., 1986, 1987; Hall et al., 1987). Retinal neurons from E6 chick embryos are stimulated to extend neurites on either laminin or type 1 astrocytes, whereas E11 retinal neurons fail to grow neurites on laminin but do so on astrocytes (Cohen et al., 1986). This is correlated with a loss of integrin receptors by the retinal cells between E6 and E11 (Hall et al., 1987) and they preferentially adhere to one another and to other cells that express cell adhesion molecules. After E11, retinal cells still continue to express N-cadherin and NCAM (Neugebauer et al., 1987). Similarly, the neurite outgrowth response of embryonic chick ciliary ganglion neurons to laminin is developmentally regulated: laminin receptors are gradually lost between E8 and E14 whereas the ability to extend neurites in response to Schwann cells persists, probably because of persistence of N-cadherin and L1 cell adhesion molecules (Tomaselli and Reichardt, 1988). The cell adhesion molecules N-cadherin and L1 (NgCAM) are produced by Schwann cells in outgrowing and regenerating peripheral nerves. Schwann cells also produce NGF and secrete laminin into the endoneural basal lamina (Cornbrooks et al., 1983; Palm and Furcht, 1983). Interactions between growing nerve fibers and Schwann cells are discussed at length in Section 3.7.

Growth cones can take up proteins (ferritin, 500 kDa; HRP, 44 kDa) and carboxylated mi-crobeads by pinocytosis from the extracellular space (Holtzman, 1971; Birks et al., 1972; M. B. Bunge, 1973a; del Cerro, 1974; Mesulam, 1982; L. C. Katz et al., 1984; Cheng and Reese, 1987; Cornwall and Phillipson, 1988). This capacity for pinocytosis persists at the presynaptic and postsynaptic membranes in the adult neuron (U. Smith, 1971). Some of the particles taken into the growing neuron are rapidly transported toward the cell body enclosed within membrane vesicles, as described in Section 5.10 (Sotelo and Riche, 1974; Droz et al., 1975; L. C. Katz et al., 1984; Cornwall and Phillipson, 1988).

Changes from the actively growing to the stable, and relatively stationary, state of the growth cone and its transformation to presynaptic endings are related to changes in cytoskeletal components. Evidence in support of this hypothesis is that treatment of neurons in culture with taxol, which increases polymerization of tubulin to form microtubules, results in loss of motility of growth cones (Letourneau and Ressler, 1984) and also inhibits formation of branches (Letourneau et al., 1986). Taxol treatment of neurites *in vitro* also stabilizes them and overcomes their inability to grow without solid support (Letourneau et al., 1987). Conversely, when cultured neurons are treated with microtubule-depolymerizing drugs, neurites retract and motile filopodia extend from them (Bray et al., 1978). The growth cone contains a network of actin filaments, which are one of the main components of the ruffling membrane and filopodia. The addition of cytochalasin B to cultures of actively extending neurites results in immediate inhibition of movement of the growth cones and stops elongation of the neurites (Wessells et al. 1971b; Cooper, 1987). These observations show that polymerized microtubules characterize the stable growth cone whereas actin filaments and neurofilaments characterize the actively extending growth cone. It has been suggested that this change is due to MAPs, specifically with a change from the types of MAPs that associate with microtubules and neurofilaments in actively elongating axons, for example, MAP5 (Fig. 5.4), to the types of MAPs, especially the tau proteins, that associate preferentially with stable microtubules (see Section 5.5).

The growth-associated protein GAP-43 is found in large amounts specifically in outgrowing axons during normal development and its synthesis and axonal transport are increased during nerve regeneration (Skene and Willard, 1981a; Kalil and Skene, 1986; Benowitz and Routtenberg, 1987, review; Gordon-Weeks, 1989, review). GAP-43 is a 24-kDa membrane-associated phosphorylated protein. Neurons with high-affinity NGF receptors also have high levels of GAP-43 mRNA (Verge et al., 1990). It is present in axonal growth cones but not in dendritic growth cones (Goslin et al., 1988). GAP-43 is also expressed during neurite outgrowth of PC12 cells (Skene and Willard, 1981b). By contrast, axons in the mammalian CNS which do not regenerate effectively do not contain GAP-43 (Skene and Willard, 1981a). Other evidence that it performs a function in axonal growth is that axonal growth cones contain relatively larger amounts of GAP-43 than other parts of the axon (Meiri et al., 1986, 1988; Skene et al., 1986). GAP-43 has been localized to the membrane skeleton subcellular fraction (Meiri and Gordon-Weeks, 1990). This observation is consistent with electron microscopic immunocytochemical localization of GAP-43 to the region adjacent to the plasma membrane (van Lookeren Campagne et al., 1989). There it probably plays a role in regulation of changes in the sol–gel state of the plasma membrane-associated actin filaments which result in rapid changes in cell shape (Stossel et al., 1981) and growth cone motility (Bray and Chapman, 1985). Presumably GAP-43 is also involved in changes in shape of the growth cone. GAP-43 is expressed throughout the entire population of olfactory receptor neurons in adult rats (Verhaagen et al., 1989). These neurons are continuously replaced throughout adult life in all vertebrates (Graziadei and Monti Graziadei, 1978). The persistence of GAP-43 in the hippocampal formation of the adult CNS suggests that it may be involved in memory and learning.

It has been suggested that plasticity of the adult nervous system concerned with memory and learning may employ mechanisms that function in developing growth cones (Greenough, 1984; Routtenberg, 1985, 1986). Changes in the structure and function of synapses and possibly sprouting of axon terminals and formation of new synapses may occur as a result of long-term potentiation (Bliss and Lomo, 1973). There is increasing evidence that activity of protein kinase C in growth cones and synapses is positively correlated with long-term potentiation (Akers and Routtenberg, 1985; Lovinger et al., 1987; Nelson et al., 1989), and that neurite out-growth is promoted by phorbol esters which stimulate protein kinases in growth cones (Hsu et al., 1984; Natyzak and Laskin, 1984). Therefore, it is a very plausible theory that neuronal activity results in changes in growth cones and in formation of synaptic connections, mediated by protein phosphorylation. For additional information regarding the role of neuronal activity on synaptogenesis see Sections 11.15 and 11.20.

5.12. Outgrowth of the Axon

The single major feature that distinguishes nerve cell differentiation and growth from that of all other types of cells is outgrowth of the axon from the nerve cell body in a specific direction, along a specific pathway, to form synaptic connections with specific targets. The proper functioning of the nervous system absolutely depends on the outgrowth of axons to make connections with the correct postsynaptic targets within the CNS as well as between the central neurons and peripheral receptor and effector organs. The invariance of the direction of initial outgrowth of the axon, its trajectory, and its targeting on postsynaptic sites are the essential features of axonal development.

The final pattern of neuronal connections may be regarded as the result of five distinct processes, which are expressed in a coordinated program: (1) outgrowth of axons and selection of pathways to their appropriate destination; (2) dendritic outgrowth and formation of specific dendritic morphology; (3) selection of specific targets by axons; (4) elimination of incorrect and redundant synapses, axonal and dendritic branches, and of mismatched neurons; (5) functional refinement of the final pattern of synaptic connections. The first of these processes in considered in this chapter. The others are considered in Chapter 6.

Growth of axons to their appropriate targets is accomplished by an intrinsic tendency for outgrowth of axons from young neurons and by interactions between the growth cones and their environment. These include:

1. Passive guidance by oriented structures in the pathways, such as collagen, cartilage, blood vessels

2. Local conditions which permit, enhance, or inhibit axonal elongation, including electrical fields, extracellular matrix molecules, cell adhesion molecules, and integrins
3. Active modification of the extracellular matrix by enzymes released by the growth cone
4. Growth factors released by cells in the axonal pathways and by axonal targets
5. Inhibition of axonal growth and stabilization by conditions at the targets
6. Modification of axons and dendrites in response to nerve activity

Sprouting of axons in the young neurons is not random. The initial outgrowth of the axon normally occurs in the direction it must take to reach its correct destination. For example, all young ganglion cells of the retina of vertebrates send their axons radially inward toward the optic stalk. This cannot be due entirely to mechanical forces within the retina, which would predispose an equal number of optic axons to grow radially outward. This is rarely seen, and when it happens the optic axons that initially take an aberrant course usually double back to grow in the right direction (Ramón y Cajal, 1910, 1929a). Neurons that have a single axon when mature can put out more than one axon during development, for example, in the cardiac ganglion of *Xenopus* (Heathcote and Sargent, 1985) and retinal ganglion cells of *Xenopus* (Holt, 1989).

In each region of the CNS, the axons grow out in a characteristic and consistent direction, with only slight variations of their direction and course of growth (Szentágothai and Székely, 1956a, Lyser, 1966; M. Jacobson and Huang, 1985). Axonal outgrowth always precedes dendritic outgrowth, as can be seen in Cajal's figure of the 3-day chick embryo spinal cord (Fig. 5.5). The earliest outgrowth of axons can be seen in neurons labeled from the time of their origin from ancestral cells labeled with HRP (Fig. 5.13): the axon always emerges on the side facing the target and grows directly to the target along stereotypic pathways (M. Jacobson and Huang, 1985). That this is not due to an intrinsic polarity of the pathway in the CNS is shown by the behavior of axons growing out of and into a segment of spinal cord inverted rostrocaudally before initial outgrowth of axons: axons originating in the normal orientation grow through the disoriented segment of spinal cord without deviation, and axons originating

in the inverted segment grow in the wrong direction into the normal CNS (Huang and Jacobson, 1986). This shows that external conditions are only permissive but do not provide instructions about direction of elongation. The evidence to be given later shows that polarization of the neuron is inherent but can be modified by polarizing influences in the cellular environment.

Axons are quite different from dendrites and those differences appear from the earliest stages of their development. There is an intrinsic polarity and a strong tendency for neurons to express a specific phenotype during normal development and in tissue culture. Mattson *et al.* (1989) found that hippocampal pyramidal neurons which both originated as sister cells from the same progenitor are similar in morphology and were always either both sensitive or both resistant to glutamate. By contrast, nonsister neurons located close together were not similar in their morphology or glutamate sensitivity. These findings show that morphology and glutamate sensitivity are determined by cell lineage rather than by the environment. Sister neuroblastoma cells that originate from the same maternal cell have similar patterns of neurite outgrowth (Solomon, 1979, 1981). When the neurites are made to retract and regrow they recapitulate their previous neurite morphology (Solomon, 1980). During normal development interconversion between axons and dendrites is not seen but such interconversion can occur in rat hippocampal cells in culture. Cutting the growing axon of a cultured hippocampal neuron close to the cell body causes it to regrow as a dendrite (Dotti and Banker, 1987). The shorter the length of the proximal stump in relation to the other processes, the higher the probability of regrowth of a dendrite (Goslin and Banker, 1989). The mechanism of this response to injury involves entry of calcium into the injured neurite and a direct effect of Ca^{2+} on the cytoskeleton (Mattson *et al.*, 1988b,d, 1990, review).

During normal development initiation of axonal and dendritic growth are influenced by nonuniform extrinsic conditions—adhesion molecules, extracellular matrix molecules, growth factors produced by glial cells and by axonal targets. There is good evidence for a role of astrocytes in determining neuron polarity. Rat sympathetic neurons in culture do not develop dendrites in the absence of satellite cells or serum, but extend axons under all other culture conditions that were tested

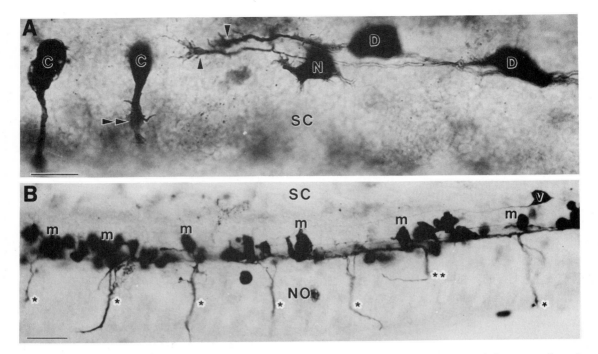

Figure 5.13. Initial neurite outgrowth from spinal cord neurons in *Xenopus* embryos. Neurons in whole mounts of spinal cord are labeled with HRP injected into their ancestral cells 24 hours earlier at the 32-cell stage. These neurons are at Stage 24. Their neurites started growing out 2–3 hours earlier, and they elongated at rates of 31–73 µm/hour, growing directly to their targets, and rarely making errors. (A) shows the dorsal half of the spinal cord, (B) the ventral half. C = commissural neurons; double arrowheads indicate the axonal growth cone bearing filopodia. Filopodia also emerge from the neuron soma. D = dorsal longitudinal neuron; filopodia emerge from the neurite shafts and the growth cones (arrowheads). N = neuron at the stage of initial neurite outgrowth with filopodia on the cell body. (B) Motoneurons (m) with axons emerging from the ventral spinal roots (asterisks). The double asterisk shows a rare case of an aberrant axon. SC = spinal cord. NO = notochord. V = ventral longitudinal neuron. Magnification bars are 50 µm. Modified from M. Jacobson and S. Huang, *Dev. Biol.* **110**:102–113 (1985), copyright Academic Press, Inc.

(Bruckenstein and Higgins, 1988a,b). Only axons grow out of neurons that are cocultured with astrocytes derived from a different brain region, but dendritic growth is stimulated by coculturing neurons and astrocytes from the same brain region (homotopic cocultures) (Denis-Donini *et al.*, 1984; Chamak *et al.*, 1987; Autillo-Touati *et al.*, 1988). The dendrites growing in homotopic cocultures express the dendritic marker, MAP2 (Chamak *et al.*, 1987). Mesencephalic neurons grow much larger dendrites when grown in medium conditioned with mesencephalic astrocytes than with striatal astrocytes (Rousselet *et al.*, 1988). The primary effect of the astrocyte-conditioned medium is to modify adhesion of neurons to the substratum—axons elongate under low-adhesion conditions and dendrites develop when the neuron adheres strongly to the substratum

(Rousselet *et al.*, 1990). Experiments in which neurons are cultured in the presence of different extracellular matrix molecules also show that decreased adhesion of the cell body to the substratum results in inhibition of dendritic growth but not of axonal growth, as shown in Fig. 5.14 (Chamak and Prochiantz, 1989a,b).

As a rule, the axon emerges from the pole of the neuron nearest the external surface of the neural tube. Mall (1893) first suggested that where this rule does not hold, the young neuron has rotated from its original axis: some observations are consistent with his suggestion. A small percentage of cortical pyramidal neurons either fail to rotate completely or become misaligned (Fig. 5.15), and such neurons may be found in any degree of disorientation. Regardless of the orientation of the neuron, the axon often emerges from the basal pole of the neuron and the main dendrite from its apex, indicating that the initial outgrowth of the axon and dendrite is determined by factors within the neuron and not in the surrounding tissue. The direction of outgrowth of the apical dendrite continues to conform to the axis of the neuron, even when the neuron is inverted (Van der Loos, 1965; Stensaas, 1967b; A. Globus and Scheibel, 1967c; Valverde *et al.,* 1989). The axon arises occasionally from an anomalous position on the cell body or a dendrite and grows in its usual direction; or, after having grown a short distance in the direction that had been predetermined in the neuron, it makes a hairpin bend to grow toward its correct destination (Fig. 5.15). Ramón y Cajal (1929a, p. 90) described inverted young neurons in the medulla of the chick embryo which have a hairpin bend on the axon which runs in the correct direction regardless of the direction of the initial outgrowth. These observations indicate that the initial direction of outgrowth of the axon is predetermined in the neuron but that the direction of further elongation is determined by factors in the tissue through which the axon grows.

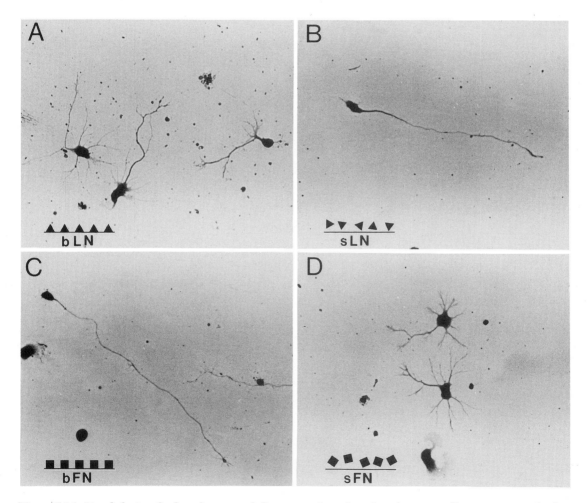

Figure 5.14. Morphologies of cultured mesencephalic neurons depend on the substratum: adhesion promotes dendritic growth but axons develop under low-adhesion conditions. Mesencephalic neurons were cultured for 48 hours in a defined serum-free medium on different substrata: (A) bound laminin, bLN; (B) soluble laminin, sLN; (C) bound fibronectin, bFN; (D) soluble fibronectin sFN. The mean surface area of the cells was similar under all conditions. Modified from B. Chamak and A. Prochiantz, *Development* 106:483–491 (1989).

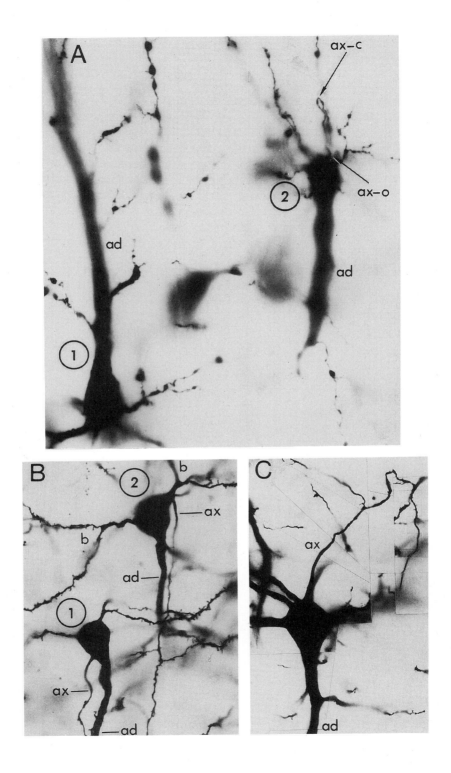

Experiments aimed at defining factors that determine the polarity of the Mauthner neuron have given results that are consistent with those described earlier. Rostrocaudal inversion of the presumptive Mauthner cell in the amphibian gastrula or neurula results in the development of an inverted Mauthner neuron (Stefanelli, 1950, 1951; C. O. Jacobson, 1964; Hibbard, 1965a). In many cases the axons continue growing in the wrong direction and end in the head rather than the tail, but in some cases the axon grows out for a short distance toward the head and then bends back, decussates normally, and grows down the spinal cord in the usual manner (Fig. 5.16). By contrast, the dendrites do not adjust their orientation but grow out in conformity with the original polarity of the cell body (Stefanelli, 1950).

From these observations one can draw the following conclusions about the factors that determine the polarity of the neuron: The polarity of the neuron is reflected in differences between the morphology of axon and dendrites, especially in the organization of the cytoskeleton and membrane specializations, and in the absence of protein synthesis in the axon. The axon and dendrites grow out in a predetermined manner during normal development, axonal outgrowth generally preceding dendritic outgrowth. Extrinsic conditions may be permissive—weak adhesion of the neuron to the substratum favors axonal outgrowth whereas strong adhesion favors dendritic outgrowth. In some cases cues in the environment may provide instructions about the direction of axonal outgrowth.

Studies of inverted neurons show that their axons grow out in a direction related to the intrinsic polarity of the neuron but the axon may either continue growing in that direction regardless of orientation with respect to substratum or reorientation may occur with respect to the substratum.

Dendrites of inverted or malpositioned neurons do not reorient but conform to the orientation of the cell body. These findings show that conditions for axonal outgrowth are different from those favoring dendritic outgrowth and suggest ways for discovering the molecular mechanisms.

There is a great deal of anatomical and physiological evidence of specific connectivity within the CNS, discussed in Chapter 11. Nerve fibers grow relatively long distances, bypassing many other neurons on the way, to connect with a specific group of cells. In some cases, the connection is made with a specific neuron or even with a specific part: axon, soma, or dendrite. Peripheral nerves grow to make contact with specific muscles or with specific sense organs, as discussed at length in Chapter 9.

Some nerves in the adult run a long and tortuous course from origin to termination. This might lead one to suspect that, in the embryo, potent forces must have guided the nerves to their destination. However, the first nerve fibers in the PNS as well as the CNS have to grow very short distances in a straight line to reach their targets (M. Jacobson and Huang, 1985). For example, the first motor nerves grow directly from the spinal cord into the myotomes, which move away from the cord only later. In the limb bud of the chick embryo, the motor axons have to grow less than 1 mm to reach the limb muscles, and development occurs rapidly, so that the first nerve fibers penetrate the limb bud on the 4th day of incubation and the gross pattern of limb innervation has developed by E7 (Fouvet, 1973; Landmesser, 1978; Lance-Jones, 1979; Pettigrew *et al.*, 1979; see Sections 9.4 and 11.3). Such peripheral nerves as the facial or the recurrent laryngeal branch of the vagus are obvious examples in which the course of the nerve has been distorted by the growth of other structures. In the case of the facial nerve, in addition to deformation of the path-

---

Figure 5.15. Inverted pyramidal cells in the rabbit cerebral cortex have inverted dendrites but correctly oriented axons. (A) Two pyramidal cells in the cortex of a 5-day-old rabbit. Cell 1 is correctly oriented; cell 2 is inverted. In cell 2 the axon origin (ax-o) is at the usual site, the pyramid base. After growing initially toward the pia, the axon makes a hairpin curve (ax-c) to grow in the correct direction. The orientation of the apical dendritic shaft (ad) conforms with the orientation of the cell body. (B) Two inverted pyramidal cells in the deeper half of the occipital cortex of an adult rabbit. The axon (ax) in cell 1 originates from the region between the cell body and the apical dendrite (ad). The axon in cell 2 originates from the base of the apical dendrite. The axon occurs in the correct direction, but the apical dendritic shaft is incorrectly oriented in both cells. (C) Pyramidal cell from the cerebral cortex of an adult rabbit showing the axon (ax) growing in the wrong direction initially and then turning to grow in the correct direction. The apical dendritic shaft (ad) is incorrectly oriented. From H. Van der Loos., *Bull. Johns Hopkins Hosp.* 117:228–250 (1965).

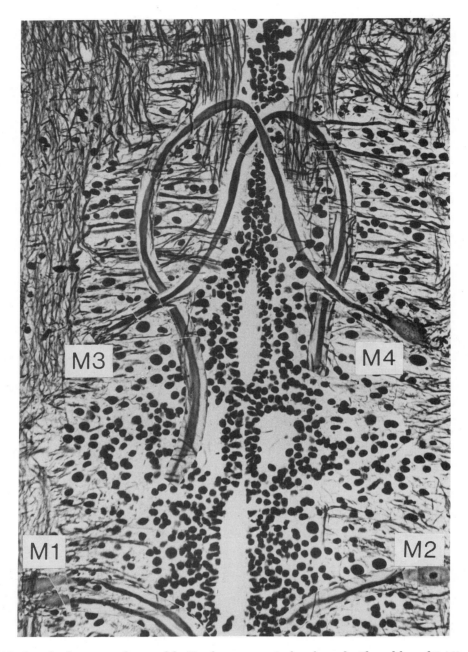

Figure 5.16. Growth adjustments of axons of the Mauthner neurons in the salamander *Pleurodeles waltii*. M1 and M2 are the normal Mauthner's neurons of the host (duplicated on the left side). M3 and M4 are Mauthner's neurons in a segment of medulla grafted with anteroposterior axis reversed. The axons of the grafted Mauthner's neurons decussate, curve back, and grow in the correct direction. Composite photograph, × 130. From E. Hibbard, *Exp. Neurol.* 13:289–301 (1965), copyright Academic Press, Inc.

way of the peripheral nerve, the nerve cell bodies become displaced after they have formed connections with the periphery.

These examples show that the pathways taken by fully developed nerve fibers may give a misleading impression of the courses taken by the first fibers to reach their targets. The final course of peripheral nerves, as well as central tracts, is the result of stretching and passive displacement of the nerves due to growth and movement of the tissues through which they run. This has been called "passive stretching" by R. G. Harrison (1935) and "towing" by Weiss (1941a). An extreme case of passive stretching is that of the lateral line nerve, which innervates the lateral line sensory placode while it is in the head and is then towed as the placode migrates into the tail (R. G. Harrison, 1903). Another remarkable case occurs in the teleost fish *Gadus*, in which the pelvic fins are displaced to a jugal position, rostral to the pectoral fins, but the origin of the peripheral nerves from lumbosacral levels of the spinal cord shows the original segmental level of the jugal fins that they innervate.

The earliest axons to grow out were called *pioneer fibers* by Harrison (1910). He thought of them as mechanical guides for secondary fibers that grow out later, forming bundles or fascicles (Weiss, 1941). The concept of pioneer fibers has been supported by evidence that the first axon to grow out almost always reaches its target by the shortest route and without error. This has been observed in *Xenopus embryos* (M. Jacobson and Huang, 1985) and insect embryos (Bate, 1978; Bentley and Kishishian, 1982; J. S. Edwards, 1982; Goodman *et al.*, 1982). That the primary fibers are not fundamentally different from the secondary fibers in insects is shown by the observation that the secondary fibers can successfully navigate a virgin pathway after destruction of the pioneer fibers (Bentley and Kishishian, 1982).

What guides the pioneer fibers to their targets? Preformed extracellular tunnels between neurepithelial cells or glial cells may guide outgrowing axons, as Wilhelm His (1886, 1887, 1904) proposed originally (Singer *et al.*, 1979; Nordlander and Singer, 1978). Preformed glial pathways may act as guides for axons in the corpus callosum (J. Silver *et al.*, 1982). Neural cell adhesion molecules on glial cells along the pathways (Rutishauser, 1983) and on the outgrowing axons (Balak *et al.*, 1987) play a role in promoting side-to-side adhesion between axons

(Rutishauser *et al.*, 1978; Rutishauser and Edelman, 1980). Axon outgrowth and fasciculation can be perturbed by antibodies to NCAM *in vitro* (Rutishauser *et al.*, 1978; Buskirk *et al.*, 1980) and *in vivo* (Thanos *et al.*, 1984; J. Silver and Rutishauser, 1984). Extracellular matrix molecules along the pathways promote axonal growth, as described in Section 5.11.

It should be emphasized that the initial pathways over which pioneer neurons grow to reach their targets are rarely more than 100 μm in length, and the outgrowing axons elongate rapidly and reach their targets within hours. For example, in *Xenopus* embryos the pioneer fibers in the CNS elongate at rates of 41–75 μm/hour and contact their targets 1–3.5 hours after their initial outgrowth from the young neurons in the CNS (M. Jacobson and Huang, 1965). Those dimensions and times would be sufficient for development of gradients of diffusible neurotrophic molecules, released from the axonal targets (see Section 5.16), as well as for electric fields to be generated which could promote growth of pioneer axons (see Section 5.13).

The problem of selective connectivity is discussed at greater length in Chapters 9 and 11. At this point, we are trying to account for the mechanisms of axonal guidance which might be at work in determining that axons grow along the appropriate pathway and arrive at the correct destination. There may be intermediate destinations, so-called "guideposts," to which the axon grows on the way to its final destination (Bate, 1976; Ho and Goodman, 1982; Goodman *et al.*, 1982; Bentley and Kishishian, 1982; Taghert *et al.*, 1982). This, of course, does not solve the problem of axonal guidance but only introduces another level of complexity involving specification of intermediate targets as well as the final targets. In principle, axons may reach their targets by a random search process, or by specific guidance by electric fields, by the substratum or by diffusible neurotropic molecules released by their targets, or by a combination of these mechanisms. We should make clear distinctions between at least four components of this process; first, choice of the initial direction of outgrowth from the nerve cell body; second, selection of a pathway; third, selection of branching points and of pathways for collateral branches; fourth, selection of one or more targets. Because different mechanisms are likely to subserve guidance of axons over short and long distances. We should also make distinctions between short-range guidance, acting only by direct contact of over a distance no greater than a few tens of micrometers, and long-range guidance, acting over distances of hundreds of micrometers.

The main factors that may affect the direction of growth of nerve fiber are electric fields, chemical difference in the environment, and the nature of the substrate, which includes molecules on the surfaces of other neurons and glial cells in the axonal pathways, and diffusible growth-promoting factors. It seems likely that all of these factors may play some part. We may conceive of the axon navigating through an *"epigenetic landscape"* filled with some molecules that are stably attached, others that are transiently present, as well as diffusible ions and molecules. Some of these are permissive, others instructive, and yet others may be inhibitory. Unfortunately, the proponents of special theories of nerve growth have each emphasized one parameter to the exclusion of all others. A single parameter, such as cell adhesion (Edelman, 1988b), can be regarded as the most potent and universal only by taking a peculiarly shortsighted view which excludes other equally significant parameters from proper consideration. Here I concur with Mencius (Meng Tzu, 7 A.26): *"What I dislike in these 'unique positions' is that they make a travesty of the Way. They make one point and overlook a hundred others."*

5.13. Role of Electric Currents in Nerve Growth

There is now good evidence that extracellular electric fields can guide the growth and orientation of neurites in tissue culture, and the fact that the magnitude of the experimentally applied currents is in the range of currents measured *in vivo* make it plausible that electric fields have roles in normal development (reviews by Jaffe and Nuccitelli, 1977; Robinson, 1985; Faber and Korn, 1989).

The theory that electrical fields are involved in the growth and specific orientation of axons and dendrites forms the basis of the theory of neurobiotaxis proposed by Ariëns Kappers (1907, 1917, 1921, 1932). This theory underwent changes in the course of time. It started as a theory of polarization of the neuron as a result of growth of axons and

dendrites in different directions in response to electric fields, and later included the concept that *"simultaneousness of excitations or their successive occurrence is the leading factor"* in formation of axodendritic connections (Ariëns Kappers *et al.,* 1936). Both parts of the theory were premature and remained for many decades unsupported by any direct evidence. The theory of neurobiotaxis had considerable heuristic value and stimulated many experimental tests. Early attempts to test the theory (S. Ingvar, 1920; Peterfi and Williams, 1933; Karssen and Sager, 1934; Weiss, 1934; Marsh and Beams, 1946; D. Ingvar, 1947) were hampered by primitive stimulating and recording equipment, contamination of the culture medium by the electrodes, and by the use of relatively large pieces of nervous tissue rather than isolated cells (Jaffe and Nuccitelli, 1977, review). This is one of the most interesting cases to consider if we want to establish the criteria necessary to refute a theory. It shows that neither weak corroboration nor weak refutation is sufficient to determine the survival of a strongly heuristic theory. In any event, both parts of Ariëns Kappers' theory have received increasing corroboration in recent years. The evidence in support of the role of correlated nerve activity in neural development is given in Sections 11.15 and 11.20. Here we discuss the growth effects of electric fields.

Resolution of the problem of the growth effects of electric fields has been made possible by invention of a linearly vibrating electrode (Jaffe and Nuccitelli, 1974) and a circularly vibrating microelectrode (Freeman *et al.,* 1985) capable of accurate measurement of current densities near the theoretical limit. Jaffe and Poo (1979) showed that neurites extending out of explanted pieces of chick dorsal root ganglia grow faster in a weak electric field toward the cathode. Neurites growing from dissociated neurons of *Xenopus* embryos change direction to grow in the direction of the cathode (Hinckle *et al.,* 1981; Patel and Poo, 1982). Changes in the rate and direction of growth cone extension result from focal electric current pulses applied by means of a micropipette to neurites growing in culture: slowing of the rate of growth cone extension occurs in response to positive current and increase in the growth rate occurs in response to application of negative current in front of the growth cone. Application of a negative focal current at an angle with respect to the direction of growth results in turning of the growth cone toward the electrode (Patel *et al.*, 1984, 1985; Freeman *et al.*, 1985). The magnitude of current required to produce the effects is in the order of a few pA per square micrometer which is in the range of current density produced by biological potentials such as miniature end-plate potentials (Patel *et al.*, 1985). Currents measured from growth cones of goldfish retinal ganglion cells *in vitro* are in the range of 10–100 nA/cm^2 and appear to flow into the filopodial tip and out at its base (Freeman *et al.*, 1985). Ion substitution experiments show that most of this current is carried by Ca^{2+} ions which probably enter through activated voltage-sensitive Ca^{2+} channels on the filopodial tips (Freeman *et al.*, 1985). We have already reviewed the evidence showing that growth cone motility is regulated by the level of intracellular Ca^{2+} (Section 5.11). The calcium current is also associated with spontaneous release of transmitter from the growth cone (Young and Poo, 1983).

Migration of neural crest cells is influenced by applied electric fields. *Xenopus* neural crest cells (Stump and Robinson, 1983; Cooper and Keller, 1984) and quail neural crest cells migrate in a weak electric field toward the cathode (Erickson and Nuccitelli, 1982).

There appear to be several mechanisms by which weak electric currents alter nerve growth. Firstly, the effects appear to be mediated by influx of Ca^{2+} ions which can alter polymerization of microfilaments, act directly on tubulin, or act via calmodulin on MAPs and tau proteins which stabilize microtubules by linking them together by crossbridges. In addition, Ca^{2+}-dependent kinases can phosphorylate cytoskeletal proteins. It has also been conjectured that the electric field might result in lateral redistribution of charged, mobile molecules in the plasma membrane (Jaffe, 1977). Evidence to support this conjecture is that binding of concanavalin A to the plasma membrane abolishes the effects of electric current without affecting neurite elongation (Patel and Poo, 1982).

5.14. Chemotropism

The response of growth cones to chemoattractants was first proposed as a hypothesis by Ramón y Cajal (1898) who provided a wealth of circumstantial evidence, but no proof of the neurotropism hypothesis. The experiments of Forssman (1898, 1900), Lugaro (1906), Marinesco (1907), Dustin (1910), as well as his own (Ramón y Cajal, 1910, 1919), summarized by Cajal (1928, pp. 328–392), are well worth repeating, using modern techniques to tap this rich source. Numerous observations on the regeneration of peripheral nerves indicate that the nerve fibers from the proximal stump of the nerve show a preference for entering the peripheral stump (Ramón y Cajal, 1928). Forssman (1898, 1900) coined the term *neurotropism* to describe the attractive influence of the distal stump. Ramón y Cajal (1910, 1928) thought that the regenerating nerve fibers might be attracted by chemicals released from the degenerating nerve or from Schwann cells.

Many attempts to determine whether the "powerful alluring substances" postulated by Ramón y Cajal (1928, p. 278) are released from degenerating nerve have given negative results, and it is only in the past few years that convincing evidence has been obtained of stimulation of nerve fiber outgrowth by target tissues acting at a distance of up to 1 mm *in vitro*. Nerve fibers in tissue culture are not deflected by a piece of degenerating peripheral nerve (Weiss, 1934). This experiment is obviously merely a preliminary to many more refined investigations of the effects of various tissues, tissue extracts, and chemicals on the growth of axons in tissue culture which are now being attempted.

Negative results were obtained by Weiss and Taylor (1944), who performed experiments to determine the effect of the peripheral nerve stump on the outgrowth of nerve fibers from the proximal stump. After transecting the sciatic or tibial nerve of the rat, they used a Y-shaped arterial cuff to join the cut ends. The nerve fibers were given a choice between growing into a branch containing the distal nerve stump or into a branch containing a blood clot or tendon. Abundant regeneration occurred into both branches, irrespective of whether the "neurotropic lure" was present or not, or whether the branch was open or closed (Fig. 5.17). We now know that macrophages and reactive Schwann cells at the site of nerve section are sufficient to stimulate regeneration (see Section 5.15). However, by focusing exclusively on the conditions in the distal segment, Weiss and Taylor failed to look for factors at the site of section.

Under the rubric of *chemotropism* we lump

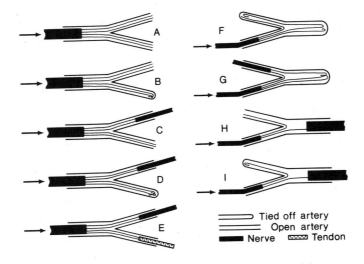

Figure 5.17. Nonselective axonal regeneration in the rat from the proximal cut end of the sciatic nerve or its tibial branch (arrow) into a Y-shaped arterial cuff with one arm containing degenerating nerve and the other arm tied off, left open, or containing tendon. The entire cuff was filled with blood clot. Nerve fibers regenerated nonselectively into both arms of the arterial cuff. From P. Weiss and A. C. Taylor, *J. Exp. Zool.* 95:233–257 (1944).

together many phenomena that seem to show that nerve fibers grow up a concentration gradient toward the source of some diffusible substance—that is, they exhibit positive chemotaxis. There is little evidence that nerve fibers might exhibit negative chemotaxis. Chemotaxis involves action at a distance and should therefore be distinguished from chemoaffinity, which involves contact between cells. Demonstration of stimulation of growth cones by diffusible molecules requires that the molecules form a gradient extending to the outgrowing axons with a peak at the site of release from the targets, that the growth cones possess receptors for those molecules, and that they stimulate axonal elongation and change in direction of growth.

The distance of 1 mm is the maximum over which a concentration gradient can be set up within a few hours in developing tissues (Crick, 1970, 1971; Munro and Crick 1971). Coughlin (1975) has shown that growth of parasympathetic nerve fibers is specifically stimulated by their normal target organ, the submandibular gland. The submandibular ganglion of the fetal mouse shows little axonal outgrowth when grown alone *in vitro*, but vigorous outgrowth occurs toward a piece of submandibular gland epithelium when the ganglion and epithelium are sepa-

rated by up to 0.5 mm. This stimulation occurs through a filter with 0.1-µm pores. The stimulation of axonal growth is not potentiated by NGF and is not inhibited by NGF antiserum. Considerable but not absolute specificity is shown; stimulation of axonal outgrowth is greatest toward the normal target organ, the submaxillary gland, but less outgrowth occurs toward the preputial gland and no outgrowth is seen toward a variety of other embryonic mouse tissues. Neither in this nor in any of the other demonstrations of stimulation of axonal outgrowth has the chemotropic agent been identified. However, the history of discovery of the nerve growth factor and other neurotrophic factors (see Chapter 8) should remind us that such agents may be present in such low concentrations in normal embryonic tissues that it may be virtually impossible to extract them without some prior information about their chemical nature, and that the neurotropic agents may be found in high concentration in totally unexpected places. More than 80 years ago the man who was the first to use the method of tissue culture to study growth of nerve fibers wrote: *If it could be shown in tissue culture that there is an attraction between growing nerve fibers taken from a certain part of the nervous system and a particular kind of peripheral cell, and between another type of central neuroblast and a different peripheral cell, then we should have direct evidence for the existence of those more subtle [sic] factors which seem to be necessary to account for the definitive establishment of particular nervous connections. The few experiments which I have directed to this end have given negative results, which is not surprising when the crudities of the method are borne in mind, but since it is possible to introduce many refinements into these methods, an ultimate solution of the problem in this way does not seem to be beyond hope of attainment* (Harrison, 1910).

Experiments of the kind imagined by Harrison have recently been done and have provided evidence for chemotropism in the CNS and PNS. Axons grow toward various tissues, over a distance of 0.5–1 mm in tissue culture (Chamley *et al.*, 1973; Ebendal, 1976a,b; Ebendal and C. O. Jacobson, 1976). In such experiments, sympathetic ganglion or another nervous tissue from chick embryos is confronted by one or more target tissues separated by about 1 mm from one another in the same culture medium, and the outgrowth to different target tissues is observed. Ebendal and C. O. Jacobson (1976) found that fibers grow out of spinal, trigeminal, sympathetic, and Remak's (colon) ganglia preferentially toward the following tissues, listed in diminishing order of their stimulatory effect: heart, kidney, colon, liver, skin, skeletal muscle, spinal cord. That the colon has the strongest stimulating effect on Remak's ganglion may indicate a specific chemotaxis. These results indicate that a substance or substances emanating from the target tissues stimulate growth of axons toward the targets.

Some more evidence for chemotropism is that neurites of commissural neurons of the rat embryo spinal cord are attracted at a distance by the ventral floor plate cells *in vitro* (Tessier-Lavigne *et al.*, 1988). Those commissural axons normally grow toward the floor plate in order to cross to the opposite side, but having crossed the midline they grow away from the floor plate. Another case of chemotaxis *in vitro* is the attraction of trigeminal ganglion neurites by epithelial cells of the head, mediated by an unidentified factor, not NGF (Lumsden and Davies, 1983, 1984, 1986; Davies *et al.*, 1987).

The possibility of chemotaxis of nerve fibers is strengthened by the fact that some other kinds of cells have been shown to move up a concentration gradient toward the source of some diffusible sub-stance. Chemotaxis of bacteria (see Adler, 1966; Adler and Tso, 1974) and of leukocytes toward bacterial products (McCutcheon, 1946; H. Harris, 1954; Grimes and Barnes, 1973; S. H. Zigmond, 1974) was well known at the end of the 19th century, and examples are cited by Ramón y Cajal (1909–1911, Vol. 1, p. 658) in support of his theory of neurotropism. Other examples of chemotaxis are provided by the ameboid forms of the cellular slime molds which move up a concentration gradient of cyclic AMP (Bonner, 1947; 1959; Konijn *et al.*, 1968; M. H. Cohen and Robertson, 1971; Gerisch *et al.*, 1975), by the chemotaxis of spermatozoa to female gonophores in some hydroids (Miller, 1966; Miller and Brokaw, 1970), and by the attraction of the miracidia of *Schistosoma* by amino acids released from snails (MacInnis *et al.*, 1974). The chemotactic response of neutrophil leukocytes to bacteria has been elucidated at the molecular level and appears to be analogous in many respects to the behavior of growth cones. Neutrophils can respond to extremely low concentrations, in the order of 10^{-10} M of bacterial chemoattractant peptides to which they have specific receptors, and they migrate up the attractant gradient by detecting a difference in concentration of about 1 percent between the leading and trailing edge of the cell (Devreotes and Zigmond, 1988). It is almost certain that growth cones respond to chemoattractants, and that the mechanisms of such neurotropism will prove to be similar to those in other types of cells.

5.15. Effects of Separating the Axon from the Cell Body: Nerve Degeneration and Chromatolysis

Cutting the axon results in a train of events that extend in both directions from the cut and may also extend across the synapses in both directions. The term "trophic" was first used by Waller (1851) to describe the influence of the cell body on its axon and target tissues. The anterograde effects of separating the cell body from the axon are, first, degeneration of the distal axonal segment (direct Wallerian degeneration), which is deprived of vital materials necessarily supplied by axonal flow from the cell body; second, transneuronal anterograde effects on the end-organ (see Chapter 9) and target neurons which may re-

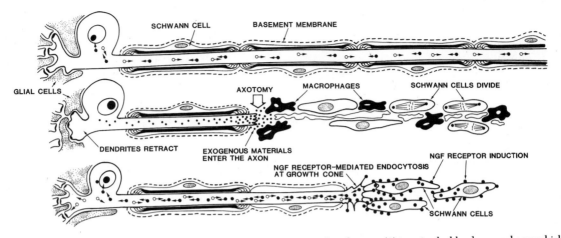

Figure 5.18. Wallerian degeneration in the distal stump of a cut peripheral nerve: (1) invasion by blood macrophages which destroy myelin and initiate mitosis of Schwann cells (Beuche and Friede, 1984; Lunn *et al.*, 1989); (2) entry of Ca²⁺ and protease activation results in autolysis of the distal axonal stump (Schlaepfer, 1974); (3) induction of NGF receptors on Schwann cells and secretion of NGF by Schwann cells, followed by receptor-mediated uptake of NGF by the proximal axonal stump, and retrograde transport of NGF, leads to axonal regeneration (Taniuchi *et al.*, 1988).

sult in their death, as described in Section 8.2. Indirect Wallerian degeneration of the proximal stump of the axon may occur.

The retrograde effects may result from entry of cytotoxic materials into the axon at the site of injury. They are also the result of separating the cell body from its target tissues which are sources of trophic factors, and the same effects occur after removal of the target tissue before the axons arrive. Killing the target cells after the axons have connected with them may result in transneuronal retrograde degeneration. The retrograde effects in the cell body are known as chromatolysis: increased RNA and protein synthesis in the cell body, manifested as a dispersal of Nissl granules, swelling of the neuron, displacement of the nucleus to an eccentric position, dendritic retraction associated with stripping of some or all of the boutons from the injured neuron. Glial cells proliferate and their processes grow around the injured neuron, effectively isolating it from presynaptic input. These changes may lead either to cell death or to regeneration of the axon. Macrophages, which enter the site of injury, release interleukin I, which stimulates Schwann cell mitosis. Newly formed Schwann cells express NGF receptors and produce NGF, which promotes axon regeneration (Fig. 5.18). Very young neurons die rapidly after

cutting their axon but they become less sensitive to axotomy as they grow older. There is evidence that older peripheral nerves are protected by a store of ciliary neurotrophic factor, probably produced by Schwann cells (Sendtner *et al.*, 1990; see Section 8.17).

Chromatolysis is a term coined by Marinesco (1909) for a characteristic sequence of changes that occur in the nerve cell body after its axon has been cut. Experiments have been limited to the type of neuron whose axon is long enough to cut surgically. Chromatolysis occurs in motor and sensory nerves in both vertebrates and invertebrates. After an axon has been cut, chromatolysis may occur without any changes being visible in the proximal segment of the axon except for a short length of axon close to the site of injury. Young neurons are much more sensitive to axotomy and die rapidly after their axons are cut, but they become less sensitive as they grow older (Vulpian, 1868; Gudden, 1870; LaVelle and LaVelle, 1984, review). Nissl (1892, 1894) first described changes in basophilic granules in the nerve cell body after severing its axon, and these have since been called *Nissl granules*. An excellent review of the literature on Nissl granules and an account of the changes in Nissl granules during development of the neuron have been given by LaVelle (1951, 1956). The lucid and thorough reviews by Lieberman (1971, 1974) make additional comments largely redundant here, and only a brief description of chromatolysis and its relevance to development will be given.

Chromatolysis is not a lysis but a change of the protein synthesis of the neuron. The arrays of parallel cisternae of rough ER in the normal, mature neurons of vertebrates are an indication that the cell body is synthesizing protein for export into the axon, some of which forms the packaging for synaptic transmitters that are secreted at the axon terminals. This may be called the *secreting* mode of synthesis. By contrast, the cell body of the growing neuron, or the neuron that is regenerating an axon and is synthesizing enzymes and proteins for growth, has few parallel long cisternae of rough ER but has an abundance of free polyribosomes. This may be called the *growing* mode of synthesis. Chromatolysis is an indication of change from the secreting to the growing mode.

Degeneration of the distal or peripheral section of the axon severed from its cell body was first described by Waller (1851) after cutting the glossopharyngeal and hypoglossal nerve of the frog and is called *anterograde degeneration* or *Wallerian degeneration*. This invariably occurs rapidly, within days to weeks, in all vertebrates and insects (J. S. Edwards and Palka, 1973; D. Young, 1973), but occurs very slowly, over a period of months, in central neurons of crustaceans (Wine, 1973). It shows that the survival of the axon depends on its continuity with the perikaryon of the neuron. But in the giant axons of annelids, which are septate, with cell bodies at intervals, fusion of the cut ends can occur (Yolton, 1923; Stough, 1930; Birse and Bittner, 1976). In some axons of the crayfish (Hoy *et al.*, 1967; Hoy, 1973; Bittner, 1973) and leech (Van Essen and Jansen, 1977), the distal part of the axon, when isolated from its cell body, can survive for a long time, and the cut ends of the axon can heal together. Restoration of function may occur after regeneration of the axon to form connections with its target cells as well as after axonal fusion.

Wallerian degeneration of axons of vertebrates can first be seen histologically close to the site of axotomy. By conventional histological methods axons are seen to start fragmenting by the 3rd or 4th day after axotomy, but observations of living fibers have revealed changes occurring within minutes of the injury, up to several millimeters distal to a crush (Williams and Hall, 1971). Degeneration then progresses in a centrifugal direction in the distal segment of the axon and the loss of axons is complete in 3 or 4 weeks. The large-diameter axons degenerate more rapidly than the finer axons. The cellular debris is removed by macrophages which invade the degenerating nerve from the blood and are usually seen in large numbers approximately 5–7 days after axotomy (Olsson and Sjöstrand, 1969). Proliferation of Schwann cells in the degenerating nerve occurs within a few days of axotomy (Ramón y Cajal, 1928; Abercrombie and Johnson, 1946; J. Joseph, 1948; G. A. Thomas, 1948). Nerves undergoing Wallerian degeneration maintain essentially normal conduction velocity until late in the process, whereas the conduction velocity is diminished relatively early as a result of degeneration due to disease (Erlanger and Schoepfle, 1946; Gilliatt, 1961).

Changes in the proximal stump of the axon are called *retrograde degeneration* and are not evident until 10–20 days after axotomy in adult animals, although they can occur earlier in newborn animals (Ranson, 1906, 1912; Brodal, 1940a; Torvik, 1956; Cole, 1968). The intensity of retrograde degeneration of the axon decreases centrally and usually does not extend more than a few centimeters proximal to the lesion (Ranson, 1906, 1912; Ramón y Cajal, 1928). Except for this short segment, the central end of the axon does not degenerate unless degeneration of the cell body occurs. Degeneration of the entire proximal axonal stump occurs and is called indirect Wallerian degeneration (van Gehuchten, 1903; Grant, 1970; Aldskogius, 1974). The large-caliber axons are affected before the fibers of smaller diameter in both Wallerian and retrograde degeneration.

The most characteristic change that occurs during chromatolysis of vertebrate neurons is a dissolution of the Nissl granules. Evidence that the Nissl granules contain nucleic acid was obtained as long ago as 1895 by Hans Held from their staining properties and high phosphorus content. Ribonucleic acid was finally demonstrated in the Nissl granules and in the nucleolus by means of ultraviolet microspectrophotometry (Caspersson, 1940, 1950; H. Landström *et al.*, 1941). Electron microscopy revealed that Nissl granules consist of arrays of flattened cisternae of ER with attached ribosomes (Palay and Palade, 1955; Deitch and Murray, 1956; A. Peters *et al.*, 1970). During chromatolysis in neu-

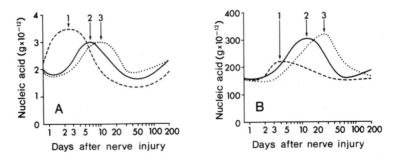

Figure 5.19. Changes in neuronal RNA during chromatolysis. Changes in nucleolar RNA (A) and in total cell-body RNA (B) in neurons of the hypoglossal nucleus of the rat after crushing of the hypoglossal nerve at different distances from the hypoglossal nucleus. The different levels at which the nerve was crushed were as follows: at the base of the skull (curve 1), at the carotid bifurcation (curve 2), and distally in the tongue (curve 3). The closer to the nerve cell body that the axon was injured, the earlier the onset and decline of the increase in RNA. From W. E. Watson, *J. Physiol. (London)* **196**:655–676 (1968).

rons of vertebrates, the long parallel cisternae of ER disperse and are replaced by randomly oriented small cisternae which are displaced toward the periphery of the cell. An increase in the number of free ribosomes occurs at the same time as an increase in volume of the nucleolus (Barr and Bertram, 1951; H. A. Lindsay and Barr, 1955; Haggar, 1957; Porter and Bowers, 1963). Haggar (1957) observed a 31 percent increase in volume of the nucleolus 7 days after axotomy and a return to normal by 41 days. Increase in RNA synthesis in the nucleolus and increased ribosomal synthesis also occur (Hydén, 1943, 1960; Brattgard *et al.*, 1957; Eckholm and Hydén, 1965). The uptake of tritiated uridine into RNA first increases in the nucleus and nucleolus and then in the cytoplasm (Porter and Bowers, 1963; W. E. Watson, 1968). The closer the site of axotomy is to the cell body, the sooner the onset of chromatolysis (Geist, 1933; Bodian, 1947). The nucleolar RNA content of hypoglossal neurons reaches a maximum about 3 days after crushing of the hypoglossal nerve as it emerges from skull, 5 days after crushing it at the level of the carotid bifurcation, and about 9 days after crushing it in the tongue (Fig. 5.19). This indicates that the latent period increases by about 1 day/millimeter distance between the cell nucleus and site of axotomy (W. E. Watson, 1968).

In addition to changes in the quantities, distribution, and activities of ER and ribosomes during chromatolysis, many other changes have been observed. An increase in the volume of the cell body

usually occurs during chromatolysis. For example, 3–12 days after cutting the hypoglossal nerve, Brattgard *et al.* (1957) observed an increase of almost threefold in the volume of hypoglossal neurons. The nucleus is usually displaced from the center of the cell body toward the base of one of the dendrites (Ramón y Cajal, 1928). The Golgi apparatus may undergo displacement to the periphery of the cell, and dispersion of the Golgi apparatus has been reported by investigators using classical methods of impregnation (Penfield, 1920; Ramón y Cajal, 1928, Fig. 204; Moussa, 1955–1956) or histochemical methods of detecting enzymes in the Golgi apparatus (Barron and Tuncbay, 1962, 1964; Söderholm, 1965; Watanabe, 1965). However, as seen with the electron microscope, the changes in the Golgi apparatus during chromatolysis are minimal, at most consisting of dilatation of the cisternae (Lieberman, 1969). In guinea pig vagal motoneurons the plasma membrane becomes irregular, forming invaginations and protrusions some of which have the appearance of growth cones (Engel and Kreuzberg, 1988). However, such changes of the surface membrane have not been noted in other species (Lieberman, 1971, review). The marked species differences in severity of chromatolysis are not understood. For example, facial nerve crush results in severe chromatolysis in adult rabbits, mild chromatolysis in adult mice, and no reaction in adult rats (Torvik, 1976).

Changes in the enzymes of neurons undergoing chromatolysis and during recovery, as well as in the associated glial cells, have been shown by means of histochemical techniques. The increase in acid phosphatase, an enzyme characteristic of lysosomes (Bodian and Mellow, 1945; Cerf and Chacko, 1958; Barron and Tuncbay, 1964; Holtzman et al., 1967), as well as in various forms of lysosomes (Barron and Tuncbay, 1964; Holtzman *et al.*, 1967; M. R. Matthews and Raisman, 1972) is an indication of increased intracellular catabolism in neurons undergoing chromatolysis.

Glial cells associated with chromatolyzed neurons undergo proliferation within a few days after axotomy (Brodal, 1940a; Torvik, 1956; Cammermeyer, 1965a, 1970, review). Using the light microscope, these glial cells have been variously identified as oligodendrocytes (W. E. Watson, 1965) or microglial cells (Sjöstrand, 1965, 1966a,b; 1971; Kreutzberg, 1966). With the electron microscope, these proliferating cells have been classified as multipotential glial cells (Vaughn and Peters, 1968, 1971; Vaughn *et al.*, 1970). The term "multipotential glia" is meant to refer to a cell type that can develop into either astrocytes or oligodendrocytes. The existence of such cells was first postulated by Schaper (1897a,b) and has since been amply confirmed (see Section 3.3) but whether they are the glial cells which react to chromatolysis is doubtful.

There is no doubt that microglial proliferation occurs in response to neuronal injury (see Section 3.4.). The proliferation of microglial cells around axotomized neurons has been observed with the electron microscope after sciatic nerve transection in adult rats (Kerns and Hinsman, 1973b), after hypoglossal nerve section in adult rats and rabbits (Fernando, 1971; Hamberger *et al.*, 1970b; Sumner and Sutherland, 1973), after facial nerve section in adult mice (Blinzinger and Kreutzberg, 1968; Torvik and Skjörten, 1971b) or newborn rabbits (Torvik, 1972), and after spinal nerve transection in frogs (D. L. Price, 1972). The glial reaction is prevented by injection of actinomycin D before axotomy, but as the drug also prevents chromatolysis, it is not known whether the effect on glia is direct or indirect (Torvik and Heding, 1969; Torvik and Skjörten, 1974). In all these studies, there is no visible response of the oligodendrocytes, and the reaction in the astrocytes is limited to changes in ultrastructure and increase in glial fibrillary acidic protein, without evidence of mitosis (Aldskogius, 1982; Reisert et al.,

1984; Graeber and Kreuzberg, 1986). The proliferating cells, which will be simply termed *microglial cells* in the absence of more definitive identification, do not appear to arise from pericytes (Kerns and Hinsman, 1973a). There is considerable evidence that they are not derived from the blood (W. E. Watson, 1974b,c, reviews). They do not act as macrophages unless chromatolysis results in neuronal death. They surround the injured neurons, become inserted into the synaptic clefts, and only rarely are seen to have engulfed the displaced boutons (Blinzinger and Kreutzberg, 1968; Hamberger *et al.*, 1970b; Sumner and Sutherland, 1973; Sumner, 1975).

The glial response starts a few days after axotomy and reaches a maximum during the second week. It is accompanied by dendritic retraction (Grant, 1965; Grant and Westman, 1968; Sumner and Watson, 1971) and by stripping of some presynaptic terminals from the dendrites and soma. This was discovered prematurely by Ruth Barnard in 1940, then forgotten and rediscovered later (Grant, 1965; Blinzinger and Kreuzberg, 1968). The degree of presynaptic disconnection apparently depends on age; the boutons are almost completely lost in newborn rabbits (Torvik and Söreide, 1972) but are reduced to about 50 percent in adult rats (Cull, 1974; Sumner, 1975). There is evidence that excitatory synapses only are disconnected (Sumner, 1975). The disconnected presynaptic terminals withdraw a short distance but are not destroyed. They can reconnect after the injured axon has restored its contact with its end-organ (Sumner and Watson, 1971; W. E. Watson, 1974c), but the boutons remain disconnected if nerve regeneration is delayed (Sumner, 1976).

The changes summarized here occur in the neurons of vertebrates during chromatolysis. Different changes are seen in the neuron of invertebrates, where the cytoplasm has a uniform basophilia due to the uniform distribution of free ribosomes and the paucity of ER (Mathotra, 1960; Trujillo-Cenóz, 1962; Rosenbluth, 1963; Coggeshall, 1967). The response of invertebrate neurons to axotomy consists of aggregation of ribosomes onto ER in the perinuclear region to form arrays of rough ER that look rather like Nissl granules in neurons of vertebrates. This aggregation is maximal about 3 days after axotomy in the cockroach, then begins to disperse and disappears after about 2 weeks (M. J. Cohen and Jacklet, 1965, 1967; M. J. Cohen, 1967; Jacklet and M. J. Cohen, 1967b). Chromatolysis in the neurons of cephalopod molluscs seems to be similar to that in vertebrate neurons (J. Z. Young, 1932).

The severity of chromatolysis, the latency of onset after axotomy, and the delay before recovery vary according to the severity of the injury as well as the distance of the axotomy from the cell body. Chromatolysis occurs more rapidly, is severer, and has a longer duration and slower recovery the nearer the site of axotomy to the nerve cell body. The type of neuron, morphological characteristics of the affected neurons, and the age and species of the animal also play a part in determining the severity of chromatolysis. Von Gudden (1870b) discovered that retrograde degeneration of the proximal stump of an axon and chromatolysis are much more rapid and severe in newborn animals. This is the basis of the Gudden method of mapping the distribution of degenerating neuron perikarya after cutting their axons (for examples, see Brodal, 1940a; Romanes, 1946; Torvik, 1956).

The effect of age on the time course and severity of chromatolysis is a reflection of the state of maturity of the neuron, of its state of synthesis at different ages, and of differences in availability of trophic factors at different ages.

If the peripheral nerve axon is cut during the period when synthesis is directed to dendritic growth and synaptogenesis, little or no chromatolysis is seen because the neuron is already in a state of maximal protein synthesis. At a later age, when synthesis is largely directed at production of materials to be transported to the axonal endings, cutting the axon results in a change of protein synthesis from a secreting to a growing mode of synthesis. In a sense, that is a reversion to a mode of synthesis found at an earlier stage of development. That may be why young neurons show less marked chromatolysis, and very young neurons may show none of the classical changes after their axons are cut during the period of maximal dendritic growth: they are already in the growing mode at the time of axotomy.

Why young neurons are more likely than old neurons to die after axotomy is an old problem that has recently been solved with the discovery that ciliary neurotrophic factor (CNTF) applied to the end of the cut facial nerve in young rats can prevent chromatolysis (Sendtner *et al.*, 1990). Apparently young neurons lack CNTF and that is why young neurons have a greater susceptibility than older neurons to injury, toxins, anoxia, and transsynaptic degeneration, both retrograde and anterograde (see Section 8.17). The literature shows that the change in vulnerability to axotomy occurs rapidly as the neuron matures. Thus Romanes (1946) found that axotomy produces rapid and almost total loss of motoneurons supplying the hindlimb in the newborn mouse, but by 1 week of age the motoneurons recover completely after axotomy. The transition to greater resistance to axonal section is seen in a single animal in relation to the time of origin of the motoneurons supplying the hindlimb—those that supply the more proximal muscles are situated most ventrally in the ventral horn of the spinal cord, are the first in the field, and are more resistant to axotomy than those that are born later and supply distal leg muscles (Romanes, 1946). A similar reduction in vulnerability to axotomy of hypoglossal neurons is seen in the cat: dendritic degeneration of hypoglossal neurons can be seen with silver impregnation only when axotomy is performed in kittens less than 11 days old but not in kittens at 20 days of age or in adult cats (G. Grant, 1970).

LaVelle (1973, review) has shown that the strength of the chromatolytic reaction at different stages of development is related to the maturity of the nucleolus. In the facial nucleus of the hamster, the nucleoli have not developed fully before birth, and facial nerve section results in death of the facial neurons with little or no chromatolysis. After birth, as the nucleoli mature, the strength of chromatolysis increases. The survival of axotomized facial neurons also increases from complete degeneration of all the facial neurons within 6 days after axotomy at birth to nearly 90 percent survival 30 days after axotomy at 15 days of age (LaVelle and LaVelle, 1958). The evidence also shows that the increasing ability with age of neurons to survive is correlated with the maturation of their capacity for RNA and protein synthesis (McLoon and LaVelle, 1981).

Chromatolysis is a complex of changes representing repair activities rather than the direct response to injury. Chromatolysis is a consequence of disconnecting the cell body from the terminal connections of the axon, be they sense organs or muscles, rather than the result of injury *per se*. However, it is also likely that toxic materials can enter the neuron at the site of injury and after retrograde transport to the cell body can induce chromatolysis (Kristensson and Olsson, 1975, 1976; Kristensson, 1984).

Chromatolysis can be produced by a variety of means without cutting or crushing the axon. Chromatolysis develops after infection of motoneurons with poliovirus (Bodian, 1948). Blocking axonal flow with colchicine produces chromatolysis without either blocking impulse conduction or overtly damaging the neuron (Pilar and Landmesser, 1972). Chromatolysis occurs in peripheral adrenergic neurons after treatment with 6-hydroxydopamine, which is selectively taken up at adrenergic nerve endings, and results in their degeneration (Angeletti and Levi-Montalcini, 1970). Additional evidence that chromatolysis can occur without axotomy is that botulinum toxin injected into the tongue muscle results in chromatolysis of the hypoglossal neurons without interrupting them (W. E. Watson, 1969). This may be caused either by botulinum toxin blocking uptake of trophic factors by the nerve endings or by damage to the nerve endings allowing extracellular materials to enter the axon.

Chromatolysis occurs rapidly in primary sensory neurons of all sizes in cranial and spinal sensory ganglia of mammals after their peripherally directed axons have been cut, but it does not occur, even after years, following section of their centrally directed axons (Hinsey et al., 1937; Tower, 1937a; Hare and Hinsey, 1940; Lassek and Perry, 1944; Lieberman, 1968; Carmel and Stein, 1969). This is indirect evidence that chromatolysis is caused by disconnection of the cell body from the peripheral supplies of trophic factors rather than by injury itself. The ganglion cells survive because they are sustained by two sources of trophic stimulation—from the CNS and from the periphery (see Section 8.7).

Neurons in the mammalian CNS can survive after axotomy at some distance from the cell body but die rapidly after axotomy close to the cell body. This has long been thought to be due to the presence of intact axonal branches proximal to the point of axon section. This has come to be known as the theory of the *sustaining collaterals*, initially propounded by Ramón y Cajal (1928). Evidence consistent with of this theory was obtained by Fry and Cowan (1972). They studied the response to cutting the axons of neurons in the lateral mammillary nucleus, which has axons running in one tract connected to the thalamus (mammillothalamic

tract) and axons running in another tract connected to the tegmentum (mammillotegmental tract). A slight loss of cells in the mammillary nucleus occurs when the former tract is cut, and no cell loss results from section of the latter tract, but after cutting of both tracts 60 percent of the cells of the nucleus die and the remainder are shrunken. The authors concluded that at least 60 percent of the neurons have axonal branches in both tracts, and that cutting one branch is insufficient to cause the cells to die. As a general rule, after section of axons in the CNS, retrograde degeneration usually stops at the axon collaterals that are nearest the lesion (Powell and Cowan, 1964; Cole, 1968; Grant, 1970; Wolff et al., 1981).

The theory of sustaining collaterals applies also to the severity of chromatolysis after axotomy in fully developed neurons, showing that the neuron's dependence on the postsynaptic target cells persists throughout life. The type of neuron that has axonal branches arising relatively close to the cell body shows little chromatolysis and does not usually die after one of its axonal branches is cut, presumably because it is sustained by the trophic factors obtained from the intact axonal branches. By contrast, some types of neuron such as retinal ganglion cells that have single long axons that branch close to their targets are very vulnerable: section of the main axonal trunk results in marked chromatolysis and leads to neuronal death if axonal regeneration does not occur. However, the species differences in the regenerative capacity of CNS axons should be taken into account. After optic nerve section the retinal ganglion cells undergo chromatolysis in all vertebrates but in mammals they all rapidly shrink and die, whereas in goldfish they swell and all regenerate and in frogs some die and some regenerate. In goldfish and frogs the retinal ganglion cells behave like mammalian peripheral neurons.

An intriguing and unsolved problem is the nature of the signal that initiates the changes in the nerve cell body after axonal transection located at a relatively great distance from the perikaryon (Cragg, 1970). The stimulus that initiates chromatolysis must be transmitted to the cell body from the point of axonal injury. The signal must be associated with the injured neurons because the chromatolysis is confined to them and does not affect adjacent, uninjured neurons. Therefore, the signal cannot be some product of injury that is released into the extracellular fluids, but must travel retrogradely in the axon. The message that starts chromatolysis is also unlikely to be electrical. Antidromically conducted action potentials arising from injury currents might have some effect on motoneurons but not on sensory neurons, in which the impulse traffic is normally in the direction of the cell body.

The possibility that chromatolysis is started by material that enters the axons at the site of the lesion and is transported to the cell body is rendered more plausible since the demonstration that HRP, applied to the cut or crushed region of the facial nerve of mice, is transported in 6 hours to the perikarya in the facial nucleus (Kristensson and Olsson, 1974). Chromatolysis is seen in those neurons 12 hours after axotomy. HRP can enter intact presynaptic endings by pinocytosis, as discussed in Section 5.10. The hypothetical signal could then flow in the axon to the cell body where it could regulate the synthesis of materials required for growth and maintenance of the axon. Another route which the signal for chromatolysis might take is the plasma membrane, in or on which materials have been shown to be transported at a rate of a few millimeters per day from the nerve ending to the cell body (Koda and Partlow, 1976). Transport of a signal in the axon is consistent with the observation that the duration of the latent period before onset of chromatolysis is related to the distance of axotomy from the cell body—the longer the axonal stump, the greater the reservoir of the material. In the goldfish Mauthner neuron the onset of chromatolysis occurs at 10, 20, and 40 days after cutting the axon at 5, 10.5, and 20 mm from the cell body, indicating retrograde transport of the signal at an average rat of 0.5 mm/day at

15.6°C (Zottoli *et al.*, 1984). Observations in mammals imply that the signal for chromatolysis travels up the axon at a rate of about 4–5 mm/day (Cragg, 1970). A rate of 65 mm/day has been reported for the transport of the signal for chromatolysis in the red nucleus of the rat (Egan *et al.*, 1977a,b).

Another possible mechanism for initiation of chromatolysis involves cutting off a supply of trophic molecules from the periphery. The latter model is not consistent with evidence that chromatolysis occurs in embryonic neurons in culture after their axons, which lack connections with end-organs, have been cut (Levi and Meyer, 1945). The hypothesis that loss of a substance transported from the target organ initiates chromatolysis is also not consistent with the evidence that RNA synthesis is further increased by a second axotomy proximal to the first or by repeated crushing of the axon (W. E. Watson, 1968). However, these latter observations are consistent with the hypothesis that material entering the axon at the site of injury starts chromatolysis (Kristensson and Olsson, 1974, 1975, 1976; Kristensson, 1984). This mechanism is discussed in Section 5.10.

The signal(s) that start chromatolysis have not been identified. The evidence indicates that different signals may be effective and that the severity of chromatolysis may depend on complex conditions including species, age, type of neuron, distance of the lesion from the cell body, and severity of the lesion. At least two conditions acting separately or together may start chromatolysis: entrance of materials at the site of injury which are retrogradely transported to the cell body; and blockade of retrograde axonal transport of factors which maintain the resting state or which inhibit the growing state of RNA and protein synthesis.

6 Formation of Dendrites and Development of Synaptic Connections

I find the fundamental features of a theory of the central ganglion cells in the observation of Remak, that every cell makes connection exclusively with only one motor nerve cell root, and that this is a fiber chemically and physiologically different from all other central processes. . . . The body of the cell is continuous, without interruption, with a more or less large number of processes which branch frequently. . . . These processes which . . . must not be considered as the source of axis cylinders, or as having a nerve fiber growing from them . . . will hereafter be called protoplasmic processes.

Otto Friedrich Karl Deiters (1834–1863),
*Untersuchungen über Gehirn und
Rückenmark des Menschen und
der Saugethiere,* 1865

6.1. Historical and Theoretical Perspective

*So long as one only substitutes one theory
for another, in the absence of direct proof,
science gains nothing; one old theory deserves another.*

Claude Bernard (1813–1878),
*Leçons sur la physiologie et la
pathologie du système nerveux,*
Vol. 1, p. 4, 1858

Five cardinal theories of the organization of nervous systems originated in the second half of the 19th century and formed the basis of the neuron theory on which modern neuroscience research programs are constructed. The most important advance in our understanding of the historical development of the neuron theory is that it did not originate in the 1880s and 1890s as a single theory but was constructed over a much longer period, starting in the 1840s, by convergence of at least five different cardinal theories and several other auxiliary theories. Those cardinal theories were, firstly, that the nerve cell and its fibers are parts of the same unit (Wagner, 1847; Koelliker, 1850; Remak, 1853, 1855); secondly, that nerve fibers are protoplasmic outgrowths of nerve cells (Bidder and Kupffer, 1857; His, 1886); thirdly, that dendrites and axons are fundamentally different types of nerve fibers (Wagner, 1851; Remak, 1854; Deiters, 1865; Golgi, 1873, 1882–1885); fourthly, that nerve conduction occurs in only one direction—from dendrites to axons in the same nerve cell, and from axons to dendrites between different nerve cells (van Gehuchten, 1891; Lenhossék, 1893; Ramón y Cajal, 1895); fifthly, that nerve cells are connected by surface contact and not by cytoplasmic continuity (Koelliker, 1879, 1883, 1886; His, 1886; Forel, 1887). In addition to those five cardinal theories, a number of additional auxiliary theories also entered into construction of the neuron theory, especially the theory that the contact regions, named synapses by Sherrington (1897, 1906), are the principal sites of functional integration and modification. One of the consequences of understanding the historical development of the neuron theory in these terms is that priority for its discovery cannot be fairly attributed to a single individual, least of all to Ramón y Cajal, who only appeared on the scene in 1888 after the theory had been largely constructed by others.

A revolutionary advance in understanding the cellular organization of the CNS occurred in the decades before those cardinal theories were promulgated. It was necessary to advance from the elementary level of understanding that the brain is composed of separate globules and fibers suspended in a fluid or ground substance (Ehrenberg, 1833, 1836; Purkinje, 1837; Valentin, 1836, 1838, among many others), to the higher level of understanding that the globule and fiber belong to the same cell. This advance was mainly accomplished by Rudolph Wagner (1847), Albert Koelliker (1850), and Robert Remak (1853, 1855). The theory of the unity of nerve cells and fibers was advanced further by the conjecture that nerve fibers grow out of nerve cells (Bidder and Kupffer, 1857; His, 1886).

The discovery of the difference between dendrites and axons (Wagner, 1851; Remak, 1853; Deiters, 1865) intensified efforts to discover how nerve cells are connected together. The earliest theories were based on the assumption that there is a special tissue consisting of fine fibrils forming the link between neurons. Joseph Gerlach (1872) thought this linkage was made by fine fibrils connecting dendrites of different neurons. Camillo Golgi (1882–1885) thought that the linkage was formed by a fiber network interposed between afferent axons and collaterals of efferent axons.

Albert Koelliker (1879, 1883, 1886) was the first to conjecture that nerve cells are connected by contact and not by continuity. It is significant that the first good evidence in support of the contact theory was experimental and not merely histological, because histological methods were at that time not capable of resolving the problem—

August Forel (1887) showed that, after eye enucleation or lesions of the visual cortex, degeneration was confined to the injured neurons and did not extend to those in contact with them.

It should be emphasized that all these theories, including those which were eventually refuted, were at first progressive, in the sense that they were ahead of the facts (there were few facts on which to base any theory). They were also mature, in the sense that they could be accepted immediately into the construction of research programs and could guide research within the constraints of available techniques. Only in the late 1880s and early 1890s were the facts accumulated to unify and consolidate the five cardinal theories into the neuron theory.

Let us start by considering the level of conceptualization that had been reached in the first half of the 19th century. The concept that the nervous system consists of separate globules and fibers prevailed until the 1840s. It was believed that globules and fibers originate separately and that when they join, which occurs only rarely, it was a secondary and perhaps an impermanent union. The early microscopic observations of nervous globules were probably artifacts created by chromatic aberration. Joseph Lister (1830), who developed the achromatic objective, concluded that virtually all previous microscopic observations of histological structure were invalid because of the gross optical aberrations produced by the available lenses. The poor methods of fixation, sectioning, and staining also set severe limitations on the accuracy of histological observations. Construction of the research program concerning nerve cells and fibers and their connections was closely linked to the progress of microscopic and histological techniques (see Section 6.2).

The theory that the nerve fiber is an outgrowth of the nerve cell was originally proposed by Bidder and Kupffer (1857, p. 116): *"It can be stated with the greatest degree of certainty, that the nerve cell is endowed with the conditions for allowing the fiber to grow as a direct extension out of itself. . . . every fiber must thereafter until its peripheral termination, regarded morphologically, be conceived merely as a colossal 'outgrowth' of the nerve cell."* This theory was based on very flimsy evidence, but it was a mature theory in the sense that it could be accepted into a research program. Its heuristic power was tremendous, and it has continued to guide research until now. It was also a progressive theory in that it was ahead of the facts. It continued to lead the facts for the following 50 years or more, as they were slowly accumulated, culminating in Harrison's (1910) demonstration of nerve fibers growing in tissue culture.

Here we have an interesting exercise in assigning priorities. Priority of discovery of the unity of the nerve cell and fiber could be awarded to Remak for having shown the unity between fibers and sympathetic ganglion cells (1838); to Helmholtz (1842) for showing it in an invertebrate; to Koelliker (1844) for generalizing that concept to all nerve cells. Priority of discovery of outgrowth of fibers from nerve cells could be claimed by Bidder and Kupffer (1857), who first advanced the idea; by His (1886) for histological demonstration of fiber outgrowth from cells in chick and human embryos; by Cajal for discovery of the axonal growth cone, in 1890(c); and by Harrison (1910) for showing nerve fiber outgrowth in tissue culture. Is priority established by the one who pronounced the original theory, or who gave the first but inconclusive evidence, or who finally proved the theory? Or should priority be given to those who invented the techniques that made it possible to obtain the facts? No doubt they all did well and all deserve praise, but I think that priority belongs principally to the one who planted the tree of knowledge, less to those who tended it and pruned it, and least to those who marketed the fruit.

Wilhelm His was the first to obtain histological evidence showing that the axon grows out of the nerve cells in the spinal cord of the chick embryo. In 1886 His made this pregnant statement: *"As a firm principle I advocate the following law: that every nerve fiber extends as an outgrowth of a single cell. That is its genetic, its nutritive and its functional center; all other connections of the fiber are either merely collaterals or are formed secondarily."* From the deduction of Forel that nerve fibers end by contacting other nerve cells in the nerve centers, and those of His that the fiber is an outgrowth of the nerve cell, the neuron theory began to be constructed. His could not see the full extent of outgrowing nerve fibers in his preparations stained with carmine, gold, or hematoxylin, and he did not have the advantage of apochromatic lenses or of the Golgi technique, both of which became generally available after 1886. For example, His was unable to see the growth cones and could not at that time deal ex-

plicitly with the question of how one neuron connects with another. It is not sufficiently appreciated that in 1856 His had obtained the earliest evidence that nerve fibers end freely in preparations of cornea stained with silver nitrate and blackened by exposure to light. His suggested that nerve fibers in the centers might also end freely but could not obtain evidence with the techniques at his command.

An indirect approach to this problem was taken by August Forel in 1887 which led him to obtain the first experimental evidence showing that nerve cells connect by contact and not by continuity. Forel's work was based on the discovery by Bernard von Gudden (1870, 1874) that removal of the eye of the newborn rabbit results, after a short survival period, in atrophy of the visual centers. He thus provided the first method for tracing pathways in the CNS. He extended this method in 1881 to show that lesions in the cerebral cortex result in degeneration in the corresponding subcortical structures. It was clear that acute degeneration is confined to the injured nerve cells, but von Gudden did not understand the general significance of his results. That was accomplished by Forel, who in 1887 showed that removal of one eye of a rabbit results in degeneration restricted to the optic nerve fibers without extending to nerve cells of the lateral geniculate nucleus, whereas removal of the visual cortex results in loss of the lateral geniculate neurons without apparently affecting the optic nerve fibers. From this Forel made the brilliant deduction that there are two separate neurons linking the retina to the cerebral cortex and that they make contact but do not form direct connections in the lateral geniculate nucleus. In his autobiography (published posthumously in 1935) Forel states: *"I considered the findings of Gudden's atrophy method, and above all the fact that total atrophy is always confined to the processes of the same group of ganglion-cells, and does not extend to the remoter elements merely functionally connected with them. . . . All the data convinced me ever more clearly of simple contact. . . . I decided to write a paper on the subject and risk advancing a new theory . . . and sent it immediately to the Archiv für Psychiatrie in Berlin. However, this periodical was then appearing at long intervals, so my paper did not appear until January 1887. . . . Without my knowledge Professor His of Leipzig had arrived at similar results, and had published them in a periodical which was issued more promptly, in October 1886, so that formally speaking the priority was his."*

Cajal, in Chapter 5 of his autobiography, deals with the contributions of His and Forel in the following manner: *"Two main hypotheses disputed the battlefield of science: that of the network, defended by nearly all histologists; and that of free endings, which had been timidly suggested by two lone workers, His and Forel, without rousing any echo in the schools. . . . My work consisted just in providing an objective basis for the brilliant but vague suggestions of His and Forel."* Their statements were certainly neither timid nor vague. Perhaps Cajal's perception of the contributions of His and Forel reflects his lack of understanding of their classical or Apollonian style in contrast to his own romantic or Dionysian style (M. Jacobson, in preparation).[1]

Let us now consider the history of concepts of dendritic form and function and the origins of the cardinal theory that dendrites are fundamentally different from axons. In 1851 Rudolph Wagner described the large nerve cells in the electric lobe of the brain of *Torpedo* and noted that usually only one of its several processes is continuous with the nerve fiber (Wagner, 1851, Vol. 3, p. 377). Before that time nerve cells had been described as ganglionic globules, notably by Christian Gottfried Ehrenberg (1833, 1836), Gustav Gabriel Valentin (1836, 1839), and Jan Evangelista Purkinje (1837a,b), but the relationship of globules to nerve fibers was incorrectly understood, and the dendrites had not been identified. For example, Valentin (1836, 1838) thought that the fibers approach the ganglionic globules and even loop around them without making contact. In 1837 Purkinje described the ganglionic globules (they were called cells only after 1839) that now bear his name in the cerebellar cortex and showed the cell body and proximal part of the dendrites without identifying the latter. In the 1st edition of

Koelliker's *Mikroskopische Anatomie* (1850–1852) the dendrites are not identified as such.

Wagner's identification of two different types of nerve cell processes was confirmed in the multipolar nerve cells of the spinal cord of the ox by Robert Remak (1854), who also clearly showed that the axon is in direct continuity with the nerve cell body. Those observations were made by Remak on tissue sections sent to him by Stilling, who was the master of the freehand technique for cutting thin frozen sections. The relationship of the cell body to the two types of processes was described more clearly by Otto Deiters, who dissected single motor neurons from the spinal cord of the ox, after macerating the cord in a weak solution of potassium dichromate. He showed that the dendrites, which he named protoplasmic processes, are different from the axon, and he generously gave priority to Remak for discovery of two different nerve cell processes (see the epigraph to this chapter). Deiters also described a separate system of fine fibers originating from the dendrites, which he believed to run into the ground substance in which he thought nerve cells are embedded. This was the source of the idea that there are two systems of fibers connecting neurons. Deiters, and later Gerlach, thought that axons connect with one another to form one system but a separate system is formed by the connections between dendrites of different nerve cells. Deiters' observations, which were published posthumously in 1865 by Max Schultze, elevated the difference between axon and dendrites to a general theory of nerve cell morphology. This theory was characterized by Henle (1871, p. 26) in his historical review of the progress of anatomy, as the single most important advance made up to that time in understanding the nervous system. Only the proximal segments of large dendrites could be seen until Golgi, in several works published between 1873 and 1886, showed the complete dendritic trees of neurons in the spinal cord, olfactory bulb, and cerebral and cerebellar cortex. However, it was only in 1890 that they were named dendrites by His. Another important distinction was made by Nissl (1894), who showed that the basophilic granules which now bear his name extend from the cell body into dendrites but never into axons.[2]

---

[1]The contributions of Koelliker, His, and many others to the construction of the neuron theory continue to be undervalued and those of Cajal to be exaggerated. The following statement by a distinguished neuroanatomist is typical: *"During the last decade of the century neuroanatomy advanced more rapidly than any of the other disciplines. The phenomenal growth was due almost entirely to the work of one man, Santiago Ramón y Cajal, who from 1888 to 1911 almost single-handedly created modern neuroanatomy"* (Nature 341:493, 1989). If some people wish to set up Cajal as a household idol, that is an aberration of historical perspective and personal faith which is not worthy of dispute.

[2]We owe to Ramón y Cajal (1889) the suggestion that the peripheral fibers of sensory ganglion cells are dendrites. It is one of his less fortunate conjectures, and was soon

By 1860 a major unresolved problem was recognized to be the way in which nerve cells are connected together in the CNS. Koelliker was able to state in 1863 (p. 313): *"The case is related undoubtedly to the connections of the nerve cells to one another. Many describe anastomoses and see such where others find nothing definite. I could name many well known researchers who have shown me such variations with which I could not agree."* Gerlach (1872, p. 353) claimed to have discovered the necessary link in the form of a very fine feltwork of fibrils between nerve cells in the spinal cord stained with carmine and ammonia or with gold. Gerlach conceived of the feltwork arising from the tips of the fine branches of the protoplasmic processes forming one system of connections between nerve cells and conceived of a separate system of connections between axons.[3] I have been able to

find only two reports claiming to corroborate Gerlach's theory. One of these is by Boll (1874), and it is of interest because it shows fine fibers linking the protoplasmic processes (dendrites) of Purkinje cells. That might possibly have been a premature discovery of the parallel fibers.

Adequate counterevidence to Gerlach's theory could not be obtained with the existing techniques and was delayed until invention of the Golgi technique and publication of Camillo Golgi's major work. Golgi showed protoplasmic processes (dendrites), fully stained for the first time, in the spinal cord, cerebellar cortex, cerebral cortex, and olfactory bulb (Fig. 6.1). He showed that the protoplasmic processes end blindly, without any connections to one another, and thus totally demolished Gerlach's theoretical construct. We should recognize the significance of Golgi's discoveries in relation to his progress ahead of his predecessors and contemporaries and not only in relation to the later advances made by his followers. Golgi's view of the cellular structure of the CNS was as far in advance of those of his predecessors as the views of Cajal were in advance of those of Golgi. Cajal could see farther not only because he had sharp vision, but because he stood on Golgi's shoulders.

Golgi proposed that dendrites end on or close to blood vessels, and he believed that they have nutritional functions and are not in the main conducting pathways.[4] Golgi rejected the authenticity of Gerlach's fibrillar feltwork, but he proposed that the link between nerve cells is a network of fibrils which form connections between afferent axons and the collaterals of efferent axons. Golgi did not show a picture of his conjectured network or reticulum but in 1886 he described it in very guarded terms: *"Out of all these branchings of the different nerve processes there arises, of course, an extremely complicated texture which extends throughout the whole grey substance. It is very probable that out of the innumerable further subdivisions there arises a net-*

---

corrected by Retzius (1891b), although the mistake was subsequently repeated by many others until the electron microscope resolved the problem. Retzius (1891b) showed that in *Amphioxus*, which lacks spinal ganglia, the sensory neurons have dendrites which branch in the spinal cord and axons which run in the dorsal roots to the periphery. He also pointed out that analogous conditions exist in annelids and crustaceans (Retzius, 1890, 1891b).

[3]Gerlach (1872, p. 353) says: *"The cells of the grey substance provided with nerve and protoplasmic processes are therefore doubly connected with the nerve-fiber elements of the spinal cord, on the one hand by means of the nerve process which becomes the axis-fiber of the tubules of the anterior roots, and secondly through the finest branches of the protoplasmic processes which constitute a part of the fine plexus of nerve-fibers of the grey substance."* The functional consequences of such a system did not seem to have occurred to Gerlach. Gerlach's well-known figure showing the dendritic terminal branches of two nerve cells connected by a fiber with a lateral branch does not indicate the direction of flow of nerve activity, and Gerlach simply did not think in such terms. He failed to understand the Bell–Magendie Law when he wrote (1872, p. 354): *"Jacubowitsch (1857) . . . transferred the law of Bell, which had been applied more or less successfully to the white columns of the spinal cord, to the grey substance, and maintained that the larger cells of the anterior cornua were motor, and the smaller cells of the posterior horns the sensory elements, notwithstanding that every tyro was aware that neither the conditions requisite for voluntary movements, nor those for sensation, are present in the spinal cord . . ."* While Gerlach was venting his scorn on Jacubowitsch's essentially correct concept he was unable to see the defects in his own theory.

[4]Golgi's concept has recently been revived by the finding of close contacts between blood vessels and developing dendrites of spinal motoneurons in juvenile and adult cats (Ulfhake and Cullheim, 1986, 1988). *"It remains to be shown that the contacts between motoneuron dendrites and fine blood vessels have a functional significance, but it is tempting to speculate on the possibility of a more direct communication between the humoral system and central neurons . . ."* (Ulfhake and Cullheim, 1988).

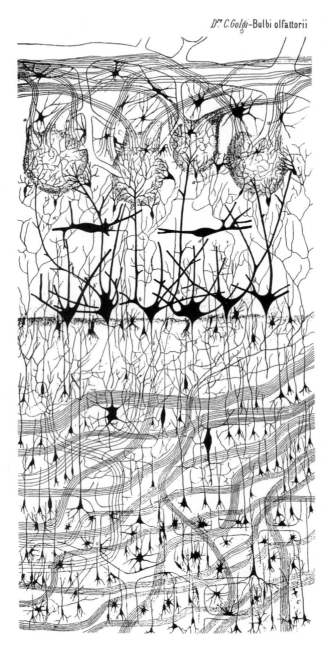

D. C. Golgi - Bulbi olfattorii

Figure 6.1. Structure of the olfactory bulb of a dog revealed by means of Golgi's newly invented technique of metallic impregnation of nerve cells, using potassium dichromate and silver nitrate. In the original figure the nerve cells and processes are shown in black and blue and the glial cells in red. Golgi states that although this figure is semischematic, it is an accurate depiction made with the aid of a *camera chiara* (same as a *camera lucida*). Golgi discovered the astrocyte perivascular endfeet (seen at the top left). At the time of publication of this figure Golgi was uncertain about the modes of connection of nerve cells, and he shows the axons as well as dendrites ending blindly. The figure was made with an achromatic objective at a total magnification of 250× and was the best that could be obtained until apochromatic objectives became available in 1886 and enabled others to build on Golgi's work using his staining methods. From C. Golgi, *Riv. sper. freniat. Reggio-Emilia* 1:405-425 (1875).

work, by means of complicated anastomoses, and not merely a feltwork; indeed one would be inclined to believe in it from some of my preparations, but the extraordinary complexity of the texture does not permit this to be stated for certain."

There followed the well-known dispute between the supporters of Golgi's reticular theory (notably Apáthy, Bethe, Held, Nissl) and the supporters of the alternative theory of neuronal connections by contact (Koelliker, 1879, 1883, 1886, 1887; Forel, 1887; His, 1886, 1889; Ramón y Cajal, 1890, 1891; Lenhossék, 1890, 1892; Retzius, 1892; Van Gehuchten, 1892; Vignal, 1893). This polemic is discussed in some detail in Section 5.1. None of the supporters of the neuron theory actually saw the synaptic contact zone, only the free nerve endings. It should be noted that all these proponents of the theory of neuronal contact at first also admitted that there were some neurons linked by protoplasmic anastomoses. The difference between the opposing factions was that while one side asserted that contact between nerve cells is the rule and anastomoses are the exception, the reverse was asserted by the other side. This is most clearly seen in Koelliker's theoretical position, which shifted progressively from the reticular to the neuron theory. The confrontation between these opposing theories, unpleasant as it often was, had great heuristic value, resulting in efforts to obtain corroborative and refutative evidence.

Evidence showing that dendrites are in the direct conducting pathway accumulated rapidly to refute Golgi's theory that dendrites only have nutritive functions. Firstly, many bipolar neurons had been described, for example, in the spinal ganglia and cranial ganglia of fish (Wagner, 1847) and in the cochlear and vestibular ganglia. In those neurons the dendrites had to be in the conducting pathway. Max Schultze (1870, p. 174) said, *"It is obvious that such a ganglion cell is only a nucleated swelling of the axis cylinder."* Secondly, many neurons were found in which the axon comes off a dendrite rather than the cell body, for example, in cerebellar granule cells (Ramón y Cajal, 1888, 1890). In the invertebrate nervous system, where the cell body is outside the line of conduction, the beautiful methylene blue and Golgi preparations of Retzius (1890, 1891, 1892a) clearly showed dendrites as a necessary part of the conduction pathways and failed to show any signs of Golgi's conjectured network.

Let us now consider how concepts of the organization of specific regions of the CNS evolved historically. A number of regions were selected by Golgi for study with his metallic impregnation techniques—the spinal cord, cerebellar cortex, hippocampal formation, and cerebral neocortex, and these became the principal battlefields on which different theories of organization of nervous connections were fought (M. Jacobson, in preparation). Briefly, I confine the discussion to the history of concepts of organization of the olfactory bulb.

The direct connection of olfactory nerve fibers to dendrites of mitral cells in the glomeruli of the olfactory bulb was discovered by Owsjannikow (1860) and Walter (1861). Their discovery that the olfactory nerve fibers connect directly with protoplasmic processes (dendrites) was contrary to all concepts at that time. Their findings were disputed by Golgi (1875), who pointed out that the olfactory nerve fibers often stain when the mitral cell dendrites fail to stain, and *vice versa,* and that he could find no connection between them. Instead, Golgi claimed to have found fiber-to-fiber connections between the olfactory nerve endings and fine nerve fibers entering the olfactory glomeruli. Golgi's depiction of cellular relationships in the olfactory bulb was correct in many aspects, was a significant advance over earlier concepts, and formed the basis for all subsequent studies. For example, Golgi discovered the astrocytic perivascular endfoot (shown clearly at the top left of Fig. 6.1), and he correctly recognized the relationship between astrocytes and brain capillaries (see Section 3.1). Golgi (1875, 1882) gave the first modern description of the olfactory mitral cells and their relationship to the glomeruli as shown in Fig. 6.1, but he failed to trace the mitral cell axons out of the olfactory bulb. He correctly showed mitral cell dendrites entering the glomeruli, but instead of contacting the olfactory afferents he showed the dendrites contacting blood vessels. Golgi did not fail to see the irregularities on the surface of dendrites but he regarded them as artifacts caused by metallic precipitates. The dendrites are depicted with perfectly smooth surfaces in Golgi's figures of olfactory bulb, spinal cord, cerebellar cortex, and cerebral cortex. He also depicted many mitral cell dendrites ending blindly in the external plexiform layer. Golgi's observations led him to the wrong conclusion that all dendrites end blindly in association with blood vessels and are not nervous conducting elements. Golgi thought that the olfactory nerve fibers connect with fine nerve fibers which enter the glomeruli from the olfactory tract (Fig. 6.1). As we know now, the only fibers from the olfactory tract which end near the glomeruli, but do not enter them, are the centrifugal fibers originating from the nucleus of the horizontal limb of the diagonal band, and it is probable that Golgi erroneously traced those into the glomeruli. He correctly showed some of those fibers ending in the external plexiform layer and also correctly showed other fibers ending in the granule cell layer (these are now known to originate from the anterior olfactory nuclei of both sides). We should remember that he had then only recently invented his method of metallic impregnation of nerve cells, which he gradually improved over the following decade. Also, his observations were made before the invention of apochromatic microscope objectives in 1886. Golgi's advance over his predecessors was at least as great as the further advances that were made by Koelliker, Lenhossék, van Gehuchten, Retzius, and Cajal. To deny Golgi the full credit due to the original discoverer, because he failed to see as far as his successors, is like denying the credit to Columbus for discovering America, because he did not land at New York and failed to explore the entire continent.

Golgi's error regarding the blind ending of the mitral cell dendrites and the fiber-to-fiber connections in the olfactory glomeruli persisted until 1890. The problem could then be resolved with apochromatic objectives, which Golgi did not have when he did his pioneering neurocytological investigations. Ramón y Cajal (1891), van Gehuchten and Martin (1891), Retzius (1892b), and Koelliker (1892), using Golgi's technique, showed that the olfactory nerve fibers end by contacting mitral cell dendrites, and that the mitral cell axons extend into the olfactory tract. Axodendritic contacts were also demonstrated between climbing fibers and cerebellar Purkinje cell dendrites (Ramón y Cajal, 1888, 1890; Retzius, 1892) and between optic nerve terminals and dendrites of neurons in the optic tectum of the chick embryo (Ramón y Cajal, 1891; van Gehuchten, 1892).[5]

The original demonstration of a specialized presynaptic ending at an identified synapse was made by Held (1897a), who showed that during development of the giant presynaptic terminals (the calyces of Held) on the cells of the trapezoid nucleus there is a clear line of demarcation between the axon and the dendrite on which it ends. However, Held incorrectly concluded that the two neurons fuse later in development. The axon terminal expansions were named "Endfüsse" (endfeet) and "Endkolben" (Held, 1897; Auerbach, 1898). Ramón y Cajal (1897) immediately understood the significance of these specializations as a means of increasing the contact area, and he was also the first to show that presynaptic terminal expansions occur as a rule and to demonstrate them clearly by means of his reduced silver stain. In 1903 Cajal refers to these axon endings as "mozas," "anillos," "varicosidades," "bulbos," and "botones" (knobs, rings, varicosities, bulbs, and buttons). They were called "boutons terminaux" by van Gehuchten (1902). The terminology was simplified when Sherrington (1897) introduced the term "synapse," and it became conventional to refer to presynaptic and postsynaptic structures and functions.

Confrontation between the reticular theory and neuron theory did not end with these advances—the reticular theory merely changed from a progressive to a retrogressive theory, meaning that it was overtaken by the facts and continued to be supported only by histological artifacts. For example, in support of the reticular theory, there were several reports which claimed that fine filaments cross between neurons at the synapse and that those filaments persist even after degeneration of the presynaptic terminals (Tiegs, 1927; Boeke, 1932; Stöhr, 1935). In support of the neuron theory it was shown that the end bulbs of degenerating axons swell and disappear completely within 6 days after axotomy, without apparently affecting the cell on which they terminated (Hoff, 1932). This became an effective method of tracing fibers to their terminations, and it generated a vast literature from the 1930s to the 1950s. The reticular theory was by then only a historical relic. It was finally refuted when the synapse

---

[5]Priority for discovery of synaptic spines and for correctly conjecturing their function belongs to Cajal (1891, 1892), although the demonstration that spines are involved in formation of synapses was not possible to make without the electron microscope (Gray, 1959), and further conjectures and subsidiary theories of spine function have since been made by many others (Rall, 1974; Swindale, 1981; Crick, 1982; Gray, 1982). See M. Jacobson, *Conceptual Foundations of Neuroscience*, in preparation, for the historical dynamics of discovery of dendritic spines.

could be studied with the electron microscope (Palade and Palay, 1954).

Many examples of axo-somatic junctions were also compelling evidence that a fine network does not form the link between neurons. For example, Ramón y Cajal showed the contacts between cerebellar basket cell axonal terminals and Purkinje cell bodies in 1888, the contacts between centrifugal optic nerve fibers retinal cells in birds in 1889 and 1892, and the terminations of cochlear nerve fibers on cell bodies in the ventral cochlear nucleus of mammals in 1896. The evidence conclusively refuted Golgi's theory, but Golgi continued to adhere to it despite the counterevidence—an outstanding case of tenacity (see footnote 1 in Chapter 11).

A theory of synaptic receptors was first proposed by Langley (1906) from his experiments on the effects of nicotine on neuromuscular transmission in the chicken. Langley (1906) stated that the *"receptive substance . . . combines with nicotine and curari [sic] and is not identical with the substance which contracts."* This theory was included in a research program that had started with the simultaneous discovery by Claude Bernard and Albert Koelliker, about 1844, that curare blocks transmission at the neuromuscular junction (Bernard, 1878, pp. 237–315), and it culminated in purification of the nicotinic acetylcholine receptor, its molecular cloning, and elucidation of its primary structure (reviewed by Changeux *et al.*, 1984; Schuetze and Role, 1987). Additional information on the history of theories of synaptic transmission is given in Section 5.1.

The theory that dendrites change shape and retract or extend in response to functional demands was widely held at the end of the 19th century. The theory of ameboid movements of the dendrites was proposed by Rabl-Rückhard (1890) and Duval (1895). At first Cajal (1895) supported the theory and added to it the possibility that neuroglial cells penetrate into the space left by retraction of dendrites during sleep or anesthesia. Later Cajal (1909–1911) argued that the theory was unsupported by any evidence showing the required anatomical changes at synapses, but, as we know, lack of evidence is not a good reason for abandoning a theory—for that there must be well-corroborated counterevidence. Some counterevidence was obtained by Sherrington (1906, p. 24), who pointed out that the reflex delay ("latent period") is longer on the second occasion when a reflex is produced in

two stages than when a single full-strength reflex is produced: *"This argues against an amoeboid movement of the protoplasm of the cell being the step which determines its conductive communication with the next."* That was a fine argument at the time, but subsequent research has shown changes in synaptic size and shape as a result of stimulation (Sotelo and Palay, 1971; Baily and Chen, 1983, 1988; Lnenicka *et al.*, 1986; Wernig and Herrara, 1986), and the molecular mechanism for rapid changes in size and shape of dendritic spines has been discovered (Coss, 1985; Fifková, 1985a,b).

We should now consider the theory that synapses initially develop in excess and are later eliminated selectively. The concept of competition and selection on the basis of "fitness," "adaptiveness," and "competitiveness" derives from Charles Darwin. Once the selectionist idea was grasped it could be extrapolated to deal with populations of molecules, cells, nerve fibers, synapses, or any other parts of the organism. The first to do so was Wilhelm Roux in 1881 in his book *Der Kampf der Theile in Organismus* ("Struggle between the Parts of the Organism"). Charles Darwin considered this *"the most important book on Evolution which has appeared for some time"* and noted that its theme is *"that there is a struggle going on within every organism between the organic molecules, the cells and the organs. I think that his basis is, that every cell which best performs its functions is, in consequence, at the same time best nourished and best propagates its kind"* (Darwin, 1888, Vol. 3, p. 244). As Roux recognized, competition is keenest between individuals that are similar and will finally result in one type completely displacing the other. In his 1881 book, Roux introduced two other principles of biological modifiability and plasticity: *trophische Reizung* ("trophic stimulation") and *funktionelle Anpassung* ("functional adaptation"). In his autobiography Roux (1923) noted that he had shown that these are *"also applicable as a partial elucidation of adaptation during learning in the spinal cord and brain"* (1881, p. 196; 1883, p. 156; 1895, Vol. 1, pp. 357, 567).

In a single theoretical construct, Roux included competition, trophic interactions, and functional adaptation as causes of plasticity. This was a premature theory in the sense that it was too far in advance of the facts to be of immediate use in constructing research programs (see footnote 1 in Chapter 1).

Starting in the 1960s, the technical methods were devised that could be used to test this theory and include it in a research program. The theory of competition and selection was then reinvented in more modern terms. This was done without acknowledging Roux's priority in spite of attention having been drawn to his contribution in both previous editions of this book. By contrast, the significance of Roux's theoretical construct was well known to his contemporaries, but it was difficult to test the theory with techniques available during the 19th century.

Ramón y Cajal was aware of Roux's theory of cellular competition and selection. Cajal showed that overproduction of axonal and dendritic branches represents a normal phase of development in which excessive components are eliminated. He tells us: *"We must therefore acknowledge that during neurogenesis there is a kind of competitive struggle among the outgrowths (and perhaps even among nerve cells) for space and nutrition. . . . However, it is important not to exaggerate, as do certain embryologists, the extent and importance of the cellular competition to the point of likening it to the Darwinian struggle . . ."* (Ramón y Cajal, 1929). The last sentence indicates the influence of Roux's theoretical position, which is the origin of so-called neural Darwinism (Edelman, 1987). Cajal (1892, 1910) also adopted Roux's idea of trophic agents in the mechanism of competitive interaction, survival of the fittest, and elimination of the unfit nerve terminals, synapses, and even entire nerve cells. Since then selectionist mechanisms have been proposed for development of functionally validated synaptic connections (Hirsch and Jacobson, 1974; Changeux and Danchin, 1976), for development of connections between sets of neurons by various forms of competitive interaction between nerve terminals, and for development of behavior and learning (Jerne, 1967; Changeux *et al.*, 1984; Edelman, 1987).

The first evidence of specificity of formation of synaptic connections was obtained by J. N. Langley (1895, 1897), who showed that, after cutting of the preganglionic fibers of the superior cervical ganglion, selective regeneration of presynaptic fibers occurs from different spinal cord levels to the correct postganglionic neurons. Thus, stimulation of spinal nerve T1 dilates the pupil but does not affect blood vessels of the ear whereas the opposite effect is produced by stimulation of T4; T2 and T3 have both effects, but to different degrees. Langley (1895) proposed the theory that preganglionic fibers recognized postganglionic cells by a chemotactic mechanism. Guth and Bernstein (1961) concluded that this selection was made on the basis of competition between the presynaptic terminals.

Experimental tests of competition between cells or cellular elements are very difficult to do. When one structure supplants another during development, the deduction is often made that one has been eliminated as a result of competition. However, there are cases in which one structure is replaced by another without any competition, for example, the pronephros by the mesonephros and the latter by the metanephros. In that case there is not even a causal relationship between the three kidneys that develop in succession. In general, mere succession is not evidence of causal relationship and is thus not evidence of mechanism, competitive or otherwise (M. Bunge, 1959; Mayr, 1965; Nagel, 1965). An experimental test of neuronal competition was first done by Steindler (1916) by implanting the cut ends of the normal and foreign motor nerves into a denervated muscle. Steindler found no selective advantage of the normal nerve. When two different nerves neurotize a muscle, the resulting pattern is a mosaic in which individual muscle fibers are innervated at random by one nerve or the other. Steindler's observations have been repeatedly corroborated (Weiss and Hoag, 1946; Bernstein and Guth, 1961; Miledi and Stefani, 1969). Similarly, when two optic nerves are forced to connect with one optic tectum, their terminals segregate to form stripes and patches in the optic tectum of the goldfish (Levine and Jacobson, 1975) and the frog (Constantine-Paton and Law, 1978).

Several theories of the possible mechanisms of competitive exclusion and elimination of synapses have been proposed. The oldest of these is the theory of formation of selective connections between neurons that have correlated activities. This is an extension of the psychological theory of association of ideas. That theory, deriving from the epistemology of John Locke and David Hume, was first given a neurological explanation by David Hartley. In his *Observations on Man* (first published in 1749), Hartley proposed that mental associations form as a result of corresponding vibrations in nerves (an idea that Newton had thrown out in the last paragraph of his *Principia*). The step from a psychological to a neurophysiological theory of association appears to have been made before the mid-19th century, as evidenced by Herbert Spencer's statement: *"As every student of the nervous system knows, the combination of any set of impressions, or motions, or both, implies a ganglion in which the various nerve-fibres concerned are put into connection"* (*Principles of Psychology*, 1855). The hypothesis that synapses form or become altered between neurons whose electrical activities coincide has become widely accepted in approximately the way in which it was formulated by Ariëns Kappers *et al.* (1936): *"The relationships which determine connections are synchronic or immediately successive functional activities."*

The general idea that learning is predicated by selective strengthening of synapses (Ramón y Cajal, 1895) has been accepted and elaborated in various forms (Hebb, 1949, 1966; J. Z. Young, 1951; Eccles, 1964; Konorski, 1967; Beritoff, 1969; Anokhin, 1968; Stent, 1973). Neurophysiological theories of strengthening of synapses between neurons that have synchronous functional activities imply that linkages initially are extensive but become more restricted, functionally and anatomically, as a result of functional activity. In this view, the final arrangement is the result of cooperative interactions between neurons. This view has been extended to include competitive functional interactions between neurons—neurons with equal activities being able to maintain connections with a shared postsynaptic target, while functional imbalance results in the more active neuron excluding the less active neuron from a share of the postsynaptic space (Guillery, 1972a; Sherman *et al.*, 1974; Sherman and Wilson, 1975; C. Blakemore *et al.*, 1975; Edelman, 1987).

Theories of competitive elimination of synapses are based on the assumption that presynaptic terminals compete with one another for necessary molecules in limited supply such as trophic factors (Ramón y Cajal, 1919, 1928; Changeux and Danchin, 1976; M. R. Bennett, 1983); or that synapse elimination occurs as a result of secretion of inhibitory or toxic factors (Marinesco, 1919; Aguilar *et al.*, 1973; O'Brien *et al.*, 1984; Connold *et al.*, 1986). In 1919 Cajal noted that these factors could be produced by and act upon presynaptic or postsynaptic elements, or both, and that neurotrophic factors could also be secreted by glial cells. It was also recognized that the nerve cell body has a trophic influence on the axon and on the peripheral structures with which it con-

nects (Goldscheider, 1898; Parker, 1932). It was also conjectured that a retrograde trophic stimulus travels from peripheral structures to neurons. The observation that dendrites of spinal motor neurons sprout only after their axons have grown into the muscles led to the theory that a neuron's dendritic growth is dependent on its axonal connections (Ramón y Cajal, 1909–1911, p. 611; Barron, 1943, 1946; Hamburger and Keefe, 1944). Related to this is the "modulation theory" of Paul Weiss (1936, 1947, 1952), according to which the motoneuron modulates its central synaptic connections to match the muscle with which its axon connects. That theory is discussed in Section 11.4.

6.2. Technical Goals and Technical Constraints

To appreciate the achievements of the early neurocytologists it is necessary to recognize the difficulties under which they labored. A summary of the technical methods they had to work with will show that after 1830 when the achromatic compound microscope became available, and apochromats after 1886, the limits to what could be observed were set by methods of tissue processing, more than by the resolving power of available microscopes. Alcohol was the only means of fixation until Adolph Hannover started using chromic acid for fixation in 1840. Until formalin was used as a fixative (Ferdinand Blum, 1895), it was not possible to fix large pieces of nervous tissue without producing gross artifacts. Frozen serial sectioning, done freehand, was introduced by Benedikt Stilling in 1842. Stilling's magnificent atlas of low-power (~10×) serial sections published in 1859 *"laid the foundations for the modern anatomical study of the spinal cord"* (Clarke and O'Malley, 1968). Freehand sectioning was required until several models of freezing microtome were invented during the 1870s and 1880s. Embedding in paraffin wax was introduced in 1869 and in celloidin in 1882. However, a microtome capable of cutting serial section ribbons was not invented until 1884 (Threlfall, 1930; Bracegirdle, 1978).

The complexity of interlacing of fibers in the CNS led to attempts to loosen the tissue by various methods of maceration. Nerve cells teased out of macerated tissue were the first animal cells to be seen in isolation. The well-known illustration of a single motor neuron dissected by Otto Deiters (1865) from the macerated spinal cord is a good example of what could be accomplished by a very skilful operator. Partial separation of cells was more often used in tissue sections, for example, by Max Schultze in his studies of the nerve endings and structure of the inner ear (1858), olfactory organ (1862), and retina (1866). Schultze fixed the tissues in osmic acid and mounted them, with light compression, in iodinated serum, which caused slight separation of individual cells and tissue layers.

Little progress in staining was made until the 1860s. Carmine was first applied to animal tissues by Joseph Gerlach in 1858, but it stained nerve fibers faintly, and this led to errors in tracing nerve fibers to their terminations. Peripheral nerve fibers could be stained with silver (Wilhelm His, 1858) or with gold (Julius Cohnheim, 1866), but those stains produced serious artifacts when applied to the CNS. The gold stain, much improved by Apáthy (1897), led him to see neurofilaments crossing the synaptic junctions and extending without interruption through several neurons.

Golgi made significant advances in understanding the morphology of dendrites, starting with his 1873 paper in which he introduced the technique of metallic impregnation of nerve cells, using potassium dichromate and silver nitrate. In that paper Golgi gave the first essentially correct description of the morphology of the major classes of cells in the cerebellar cortex. It was not surpassed, except by Golgi's paper of 1886, until the early work on the cerebellar cortex by Ramón y Cajal (1888, 1892) and Koelliker (1890), both of whom relied on the Golgi technique.

Golgi published his mercuric chloride method of impregnation in 1879 and his rapid method in 1886, and he was also the first to use the method of injection of fixative directly into an artery (Golgi, 1886, p. 30). Why did these revolutionary technical advances go unheeded until they were rediscovered by Koelliker in 1887? There are several reasons that are worth considering because they illustrate some of the peculiarities of communication of scientific information at that time. Publication of his 1873 and 1879 papers in local Italian journals consigned Golgi's results to virtual oblivion for a decade until he published his 1886 paper in a journal that had a wide circulation for its time. Cajal contended with

similar difficulties of very limited circulation of his papers published before 1889. The German-speaking states of central Europe were then the centers of research on microscopic anatomy in general, and especially on neurocytology. Until the mid-1880s there were more neuroscientists working in those central European lands than in all other countries. Communication of new ideas and techniques was fastest within the central countries, slower from the central to the peripheral countries, and very much slower in the other direction.

Koelliker made several visits to Golgi at Pavia (Fig. 6.2), the first in 1887, and after that he started using the Golgi technique. He was largely responsible for renewing interest in the Golgi technique after its long neglect (Koelliker, 1887). In the same year Cajal first learned of the Golgi technique and used it so effectively that he was able to demonstrate his Golgi preparations, showing evidence in support of the neuron theory, at the congress of the German Anatomical Society, at Berlin in 1889. There, Cajal first met Koelliker, His, Lenhossék, Retzius, and van Gehuchten, all of whom had already made significant contributions to advance the five cardinal theories which together formed the neuron theory.

Techniques, theories, and values meshed together effectively by about 1885 to construct what we can now call the neuron research program. Before that time neither the techniques nor the theories were mature. We have already indicated how the techniques were developed from about 1830 to 1885, and how the five cardinal theories together formed the neuron theory. Values too had changed during that period. The positivist conviction that science has the power to explain the structure and functions of the nervous system and to apply that knowledge for the benefit of mankind gave added value to research on the nervous system. The conviction that the human brain is a product of organic evolution gave added value to research on animal brains. The mechanical materialistic conception of nature gave added value to reductionist methods for studying the nervous system. During the period from 1830 to 1885 the change occurred from gross anatomical studies to microscopic, biophysical, and chemical investigations of the structure and functions of the nervous system. As new facts emerged the neuroscientists' image of the brain changed.

The Golgi techniques were mainly responsible for the rapid advances made in neurocytology after

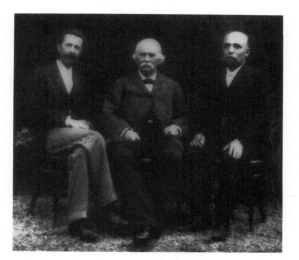

Figure 6.2. A group portrait taken at Pavia, about 1900. From right to left: Camillo Golgi (1842–1926), Albert Koelliker (1817–1905), and Giulio Bizzozero (1846–1901). The latter was an important hematologist, especially noted for his discovery of the reticulocyte and for his research, in collaboration with Golgi, on the hematogenous phases of the malaria parasite. Koelliker was one of the principal founders of neurocytology and one of the originators of the neuron theory. He was a frequent visitor to Pavia, where he learned at first hand of Golgi's metallic impregnation techniques in 1887.

1887, and in the resulting change in the image of the brain. Before Golgi the cellular composition of the brain was half-hidden and the globular cells were seen floating in an amorphous ground substance which occupied more than 50 percent of the volume of the gray matter. The Golgi techniques revealed the dendrites fully for the first time and gave an image of cellular diversity that could not have been imagined before. The picture of the brain that was revealed by the Golgi technique provoked urgent questions about how to reduce the multiplicity of neuronal types to some unifying principle and how to give functional meanings to the diversity of neuronal structures. Another question was whether neurons are connected together diffusely or in circuits. And, if they formed circuits, what their operational principles were. Those questions could not have been asked before the Golgi era. Their answers now appear self-evident but we should remember that they only became so because of the adventurous minds of our 19th-century predecessors.

Other techniques served different purposes, for example, the myelin stain of Weigert (1882) and the methods of anterograde and retrograde tracing fiber pathways which have already been mentioned (Gudden, 1870, 1874; Marchi, 1885; Forel, 1887; Nissl, 1894). In 1904 Max Bielschowsky published

his silver impregnation method which stains both myelinated and unmyelinated nerve fibers, and this was supplemented by the pyridine silver technique of Ranson (1911) and the silver protargol method of Bodian (1936), which stained unmyelinated fibers better than any previous methods. Ranson (1911, 1912a, 1915) first showed that the majority of unmyelinated fibers in peripheral nerves are afferents and traced them to the small neurons of the dorsal root ganglia. This is discussed further in Section 9.1. Selective silver staining of degenerating nerve fibers and nerve terminals was greatly improved by the methods of Nauta (1950, 1957) and of Fink and Heimer (1967).

An important technical advance was Ehrlich's discovery in 1885 that methylene blue injected intravenously in living animals could stain their nerves. The principal advantage of this technique was as a complement to the Golgi technique. By showing that dendritic spines have identical appearances when stained with methylene blue and with his double-impregnation modification of the Golgi method, Ramón y Cajal (1891, 1896) proved that dendritic spines are not artifacts caused by metallic precipitation, as Golgi, Koelliker, and others at first suggested.

With the aid of the Golgi technique and

Ehrlich's methylene blue technique, very rapid progress was made in recognizing that the pattern of dendritic branching is characteristic of different types of nerve cells. Many investigators contributed to this understanding, notably Golgi (1882–1885, 1886, spinal cord, cerebellar cortex, cerebral cortex, olfactory bulb); Koelliker (1887, 1890, spinal cord, cerebellar cortex, cerebral cortex); Dogiel (1888, 1891, retina); Ramón y Cajal (1889, 1890, 1891, retina, spinal cord, cerebellar cortex, cerebral cortex, olfactory bulb); Martinotti (1890, cerebral cortex); Van Gehuchten (1891, 1892, spinal cord, cerebellar cortex, cerebral cortex, symphathetic ganglia); Lenhossék (1890, spinal cord); and Retzius (1892, olfactory bulb, cerebellar cortex; 1890, 1892, morphology of neurons of crustaceans and annelids).

In the century after the invention of the Golgi technique, the study of dendritic growth and form had barely advanced to the stage that the plant and animal taxonomists had surpassed two centuries earlier. Classification of the forms of dendritic trees was based on the concept of the neurophenotype and on the conviction that the form of each neuron, especially the form of its dendritic tree, is a characteristic and invariant feature of a distinct neuronal type. Individual neurons belonging to the same type may exhibit a limited variability, but they are assumed to share certain invariant features that make it possible to assign that cell to its proper type. Such a system of classification of neurons can easily become an artifice, based merely on differences or on similarities of form that are useful as an aid to identification but that have no other functional or developmental significance. The danger of dwelling on externals alone is well shown in the history of taxonomy (Goerke, 1973, pp. 89–105). The danger is greatest when the classification is based on a single technique such as the Golgi method. This has resulted in classifications of dendritic branching patterns which are reminiscent of the efforts of the taxonomists before Linnaeus to classify plants into trees, bushes, and herbs (Ramón Moliner, 1962, 1968; Percheron, 1979a,b). More advanced methods of topological analysis of dendritic branching patterns have been introduced (Uylings *et al.*, 1975, 1983; Berry and Bradley, 1976; Berry and Flinn, 1984; Van Pelt and Verwer, 1982, 1984; Verwer and Van Pelt, 1983).

Investigation of the growth of dendrites would be impossible without the Golgi methods of metallic impregnation of neurons, and a brief summary of the advantages and limitations of two of the most frequently used of these methods may be of assistance in assessing the value of the results obtained with Golgi methods (reviewed by Hill, 1896; Kallius, 1926; Polyak, 1941; Ramón-Moliner, 1957, 1970; Morest and Morest, 1966; Scheibel and Scheibel, 1970, 1978; Valverde, 1970; Schierhorn and Nagel, 1977; Millhouse, 1981; Morest, 1981; Braak and Braak, 1985).

The Golgi–Cox method consists of the precipitation of metallic mercury in the neuron after fixation in potassium dichromate and mercuric chloride. This method impregnates the cell body fully, impregnates the dendrites for most of their length but not into their terminal branches, and shows only the initial portion of the axon. The metallic precipitate rarely penetrates into the fine dendritic branches or into dendritic spines or filopodia on growing dendrites. The advantage is that the background is clear and unimpregnated cells can easily be counterstained. Less than 5 percent of the neurons are impregnated by the Golgi–Cox method, apparently at random without any selectivity (Smit and Colon, 1959; Ramon-Moliner, 1970; Pasternak and Woolsey, 1975). Therefore, the method is useful for obtaining the frequency of different types of neurons and for quantitative studies (Sholl, 1956a,b).

The rapid Golgi method involves precipitation of silver chromate within the neurons after fixation in a solution of osmium tetroxide and potassium dichromate. Numerous methods of the rapid Golgi technique using aldehyde fixation have been invented but the quality of the preparations rarely approaches that of the classical technique (Braak and Braak, 1985, review). The rapid Golgi method generally impregnates the entire neuron, but it is more capricious and results in more unusable sections than the Golgi–Cox method. Less than 5 percent of neurons are impregnated (Scheibel and Scheibel, 1970). Impregnation depends on whether a cell process extends into a crystal of silver chromate which forms a nucleation center. The metallic precipitate spreads from the nucleation center to fill the entire cell (Spacek, 1989). The rapid Golgi method cannot be used for counting the frequency of different types of neurons, but its great advantage is that it usually impregnates the entire cell. This has been confirmed by high-voltage electron microscopy (Chan-Palay and Palay, 1972; Chan-Palay, 1973). Dendritic spines, growth cones, and filopodia are made visible by this method. Entire dendritic and axonal trees are often impregnated down to the finest branches so that they can be traced to their synaptic terminals.

For more than a century the Golgi method has continued to give more information about the growth and form of neurons than any other technique, and it remains the main method for studying dendritic morphogenesis in the human brain (Conel, 1939–1963; Braak, 1976). Only quite recently have other techniques been invented for filling neurons with opaque or fluorescent materials such as horseradish peroxidase (HRP) (Cullheim and Kellerth, 1976, 1978; Snow et al., 1976; Adams, 1977; Keefer, 1978; Rose, 1982; Ulfhake and Kellerth, 1981, 1983; Egger and Egger, 1982; Cameron et al., 1983, 1985; Cullheim et al., 1983, 1987a,b; M. Jacobson and Huang, 1985); fluorescent dyes such as Procion yellow or Lucifer yellow (Stretton and Kravitz, 1968; Milburn and Bentley, 1971; Tauchi and Maslund, 1984); or filling neurons with cobalt chloride, which can be precipitated intracellularly as cobalt sulfide (Pitman et al., 1972; Scalia and Fite, 1974; Székely and Gallyas, 1975; Görcs et al., 1979; Urbán and Székely, 1983; Antal, 1984). These intracellular markers can be introduced into the living nerve cell by injection or iontophoresis through a micropipette or may enter the neuron to a more limited extent by diffusion through the cut end of the axon (Iles and Mulloney, 1971; Kater et al., 1973). Intracellular injection of a cell lineage tracer such as HRP into the neuronal stem cell results in labeling of the progeny and shows the neurites labeled from the beginning of their outgrowth (M. Jacobson and Huang, 1985). Other methods for studying dendritic morphogenesis are immunocytochemistry and electron microscope serial section reconstruction. For example, high-molecular-weight MAP2 (see Section 5.5) is expressed mainly in developing dendrites (Bernhardt and Matus, 1984; Burgoyne and Cummings, 1984; De Camilli et al., 1984; Tucker et al., 1988a–c). Antibodies to MAP2 can be used to identify dendrites and to distinguish them from axons.

The Golgi technique and other methods of filling the entire neuron have brought us within reach of attaining the goal set by Descartes of geometrizing the brain, which has proved too laborious, if possible at all, without their aid. Now that the three-dimensional geometry of the neuron can be derived with the aid of the computer from reconstructions of serial sections (a method pioneered by Levinthal and Ware, 1972; D. R. Reddy et al., 1973; Rakic et al., 1974; Antal, 1984), it is possible to correlate the form of the neuron with its ontogeny and with its function in ways that were extremely difficult in the past (Hollingworth and Berry, 1975; Berry et al., 1978, 1980). Computers are useful, but they are neither indispensable nor sufficient: a keen eye for recognizing patterns in nature and for accurately identifying different types of cells and the knack of interpreting structure in functional terms cannot, at the present time, be supplanted by the computer, but creative interactions with a computer can greatly extend our ability to deal with complex, developing systems.

6.3. Regularities of Dendritic Development

Outgrowth of dendrites generally occurs after the outgrowth of the axon. In most cases it is fairly certain that the axon has formed connections before the differentiation of dendrites commences (Ramón y Cajal, 1909, p. 611; Barron, 1943, 1946). After the neurons have migrated to their final positions, there is often a long delay before full differentiation of the dendrites occurs. The young neuron has relatively short and thick dendritic processes, but these develop a complex system of branches which resemble the branching of multiaxiate plants. It is not certain whether branching occurs only at the tips of existing dendrites or whether branches also or only emerge preterminally. Branching results in a great increase in the surface area of the dendrites, which form more than 90 percent of the postsynaptic surface of the neuron (Sholl, 1955; Schadé and Baxter, 1960; Mannen, 1965, 1966; Mungai, 1967). The size, shape, and pattern of dendritic branching seen in neurons impregnated by the Golgi method are characteristic for each type of neuron. There are differences in proportion and structure of different types of neurons, and particularly in the pattern of dendritic branching, on which a system of classification may be based.

A century after the characteristic differences between axons and dendrites were established by light microscopy (see Section 6.1), distinctive fine structural characteristics were revealed by electron microscopy. But this also showed many variations of these characteristics (Peters *et al.*, 1976). For example, large axons contain a high ratio of microfilaments to microtubules, whereas dendrites of the same caliber have the reverse, but this does not always apply to fine axons and fine dendritic branches. Microtubules in axons are all oriented with their plus ends pointing away from the cell body whereas they are found in either plus or minus orientation in dendrites. Microtubule-associated proteins (MAPs) are compartmentalized in the neuron, with some much more abundant in dendrites (see Section 5.5). MAP1A occurs in growing and mature dendrites, where it is a component of cross-bridges between microtubules. High-molecular-weight MAP2 is found mainly in outgrowing dendrites, where it is a component of cross-bridges between microtubules and neurofilaments. Dendrites contain ribosomes, rough and smooth endoplasmic reticulum, and Golgi apparatus, whereas axons do not contain any of those structures. Axons may be myelinated, but dendrites very rarely have a myelin sheath. Axons usually have presynaptic specializations, whereas dendrites usually have postsynaptic specializations, but this rule is broken by relatively infrequent dendrodendritic, axoaxonal, and reciprocal axodendritic synapses.

Striking spatial and temporal regularities in the development of dendrites have been observed. There are differences between the developmental chronology of neurons with long axons (Golgi type I, or principal neurons) and those with short axons (Golgi type II, or local circuit neurons). The development of large neurons, in general, occurs earlier than the development of small neurons in any particular region of the nervous system (see Sections 2.10 and 10.2). It is important when making comparisons of different developmental stages to restrict the comparison to corresponding regions of the nervous system. In any region of the brain, the dendrites of local-circuit neurons, with short axons (Golgi type II), differentiate later than dendrites of the principal neurons, which have long axons. For example, in the dorsal nucleus of the lateral geniculate body the principal neurons that send their axons to the visual cortex mature before the local-circuit neurons, which have short axons that end within the lateral geniculate nucleus. In the lateral geniculate nucleus of the cat the principal neurons have almost completed their development by the end of the 2nd postnatal week when differentiation of dendrites of local-circuit neurons begins (Morest, 1969b).

Maturation of dendrites tends to occur in ventrodorsal or inside-out sequence; dendrites of neurons in the ventral lateral geniculate nucleus mature before those in the dorsal lateral geniculate nucleus; the dendrites of the cortex of the brain mature later than the dendrites of the central nuclei projecting to the cortex; and within the cortex the dendrites of deeper layers tend to develop before those in more superficial layers (Schadé *et al.*, 1962; Morest, 1969b).

In general, the motor neurons develop before the sensory neurons in the same region of the nervous system (see Section 2.10). Within ascending sensory systems (auditory, somatosensory, visual, and olfactory) the neurons mature in ascending order, beginning with those nearest the peripheral receptors and terminating with the neurons at the highest level of the neuraxis.

Dendrites of superior cervical ganglion cells grow in proportion to body size throughout life (Purves *et al.*, 1986a; Voyvodic, 1987). The size of the dendrites is related to the size of the target, the submandibular gland in the rat (Voyvodic, 1989). The complexity of primary dendritic branches of superior cervical sympathetic neurons is directly proportional to body size in small mammals (Purves and Lichtman, 1985). The superior cervical ganglion is an interesting choice for studies of this kind because there are large age-related changes in the morphology of the superior cervical ganglion cells and other sympathetic ganglion cells (De Castro, 1932). These changes may have misled Ramón y Cajal (1919) when he classified sympathetic neurons on the basis of the length of their processes into those with short dendrites only, those with long dendrites only, and a 3rd class with both long and short dendrites. Amprino (1938) showed that the morphology of the dendrites of superior cervical ganglion cells changes during development: in humans at birth all the ganglion cells have long dendrites, and they shorten later in life. Nevertheless, comparative studies of the superior cervical ganglion cells in mammals show that there are species differences related to differences of body size (Purves *et al.*, 1986, 1988; Snider, 1987; Ivanov and Purves, 1989).

The shapes of dendritic trees may give an indication of their evolutionary history, but it is in the nature of such hypotheses about the evolution of structures which have left no fossil record that inferences about evolution can be made only tentatively from the evidence of comparative and devel-

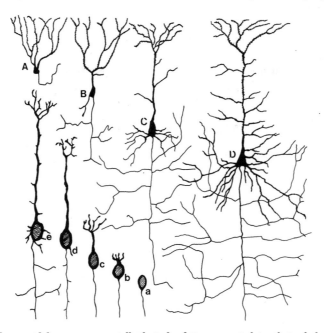

Figure 6.3. Ontogeny of pyramidal neurons especially their dendrites, recapitulates their phylogeny, according to Ramón y Cajal (1894). Pyramidal cells of various vertebrates: (A) frog; (B) lizard; (C) rat; (D) human. Progressive stages of development of a pyramidal neuron are shown in (a)–(e).

opmental studies. The well-known figure drawn by Ramón y Cajal (Fig. 6.3) is an early attempt to show a relationship between the development of the dendrites of pyramidal neurons of the mouse and a phylogenetic series of pyramidal cells from the frog, lizard, mouse, and human. The concept of dendritic ontogeny recapitulating its phylogeny has been implicitly accepted since Ramón y Cajal's time (Noback and Purpura, 1961; Poliakov, 1965; Stensaas, 1967a; Sanides, 1969). In particular, the notion has gained general acceptance that the forms of dendritic trees have become increasingly elaborate during evolution, and that, for pyramidal cells, there has been a general evolutionary tendency for the basal dendrites to expand more than the apical dendrites.

6.4. Dendritic Outgrowth and Branching

Ramón y Cajal (1909–1911) observed that the dendrites of spinal motor neurons and cerebellar Purkinje and granule cells undergo regressive changes, analogous to pruning of a tree. He distinguished an initial phase of outgrowth of an excessive number of dendritic branches followed by a phase of regulation and resorption of the redun-

dant dendrites. He proposed that a selection among the dendritic outgrowths takes place during development, presumably on a functional basis. That is, those dendritic branches that play an essential part in the functions of the dendrites persist, while those that are functionally inappropriate disappear. Ramón y Cajal's description in his autobiography is more picturesque: *"I noticed that every outgrowth, dendritic or axonic, in the course of formation, passes through a chaotic period, so to speak, a period of trials, during which there are sent out at random experimental conductors most of which are destined to disappear. . . . What mysterious forces precede the appearance of the processes, promote their growth and branching . . . and finally establish those protoplasmic kisses, the intercellular articulations, which seem to constitute the final ecstasy of an epic love story?"*

Many of Cajal's conclusions regarding the growth of dendrites have received support from later investigations. The pruning of the shaggy, spine-like branchlets from cerebellar Purkinje cells is described in Section 10.12. A similar process occurs in the dendrites of neurons of the brainstem reticular formation of cats: at birth the dendrites as well as the cell bodies are covered with spines which are

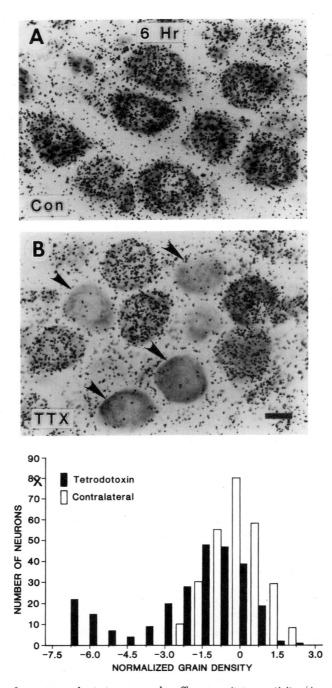

Figure 6.4. Regulation of protein synthesis in neurons by afferent excitatory activity. (A and B) Photomicrographs of neurons from nucleus magnocellularis (the cochlear nucleus) of the chick (magnification bar = 10 μm). These autoradiographs are taken from two sides of the same tissue section. The right inner ear of this animal was infused with tetrodotoxin for 6 hours, which blocked all action potentials in the cochlear nerve. One-half hour before the animal was killed it was given an injection of tritiated leucine. The tissue was then prepared for autoradiography to reveal the amount of leucine incorporated into proteins. On the side of the brain receiving input from the normal ear (A) the neurons are all heavily labeled. However on the side of the brain connected with the silent cochlear nerve, two effects are evident. First, there is a population of neurons (arrowheads) that

almost entirely lost by the 3rd postnatal month (M. E. Scheibel *et al.*, 1973). Retinal ganglion cells in the cat undergo a phase of exuberant growth followed by elimination of excessive intraretinal axonal branches and collaterals as well as dendritic branches and spines (Dann *et al.*, 1987, 1988; Ramoa *et al.*, 1988). The ganglion cells in the cat retina at E35–E37 are very small and simple with dendrites aligned radially, but by E50 the three main classes (alpha, beta, gamma) of adult ganglion cells can first be recognized (see Section 11.17). From E50 to P7 the dendrites increase very rapidly in size and complexity and develop excessive branches and spines. These are rapidly reshaped to reach adult configurations at the end of the 1st postnatal month although growth of the neurons continues to adulthood (Ramoa *et al.*, 1988). Evidence that these excessive dendritic branches and spines may be eliminated as a result of competition for afferents is discussed later. It is not known what happens to the synapses on the dendritic spines which disappear. It seems very likely that in such cases there are temporary synaptic connections which later disappear or are displaced to other parts of the neuron. This has been shown to occur for the transient climbing fiber connections which are initially made with the spines on the Purkinje cell body but which later move to the dendrites when the spines disappear from the cell body (see Section 10.12).

Dendrites differentiate in conjunction with the specific axonal terminals with which they form synaptic connections. This suggests that the afferent axonal terminals might stimulate the development of dendrites. There is a large body of evidence showing that removal of afferents or blockade of afferent excitatory synaptic activity results in functional and structural changes in dendrites of the postsynaptic neurons. Deafferentation results in rapid changes in the metabolism of postsynaptic neurons (Kupfer and Downer, 1967;

Lippe *et al.*, 1980; Durham and Woolsey, 1984; M. R. Meyer and Edwards, 1982; Steward and Rubel, 1985; Born and Rubel, 1988). For example, after cochlea removal in the newly hatched chick, protein synthesis in the nucleus magnocellularis (the avian cochlear nucleus) is reduced by 50 percent within 0.5 hour, and after 6 hours the protein synthesis ceases in one-quarter of the neurons (Steward and Rubel, 1985). Comparable reduction in protein synthesis in nucleus magnocellularis neurons occurs after tetrodotoxin blockade of action potentials in the auditory nerve, as shown in Fig. 6.4 (Born and Rubel, 1988).

Deafferentation results in structural changes which can lead to atrophy and death of the postsynaptic neurons (Jones and Thomas, 1962; Gentschev and Sotelo, 1973; Guillery, 1974; A. Globus, 1975; Murphey *et al.*, 1975; Benes *et al.*, 1977; Gulley *et al.*, 1977; Parks, 1979, 1981; Rubel *et al.*, 1981; Caceres and Steward, 1983; Deitch and Rubel, 1984). Partial removal of excitatory afferents can result in rapid and selective atrophy of the deafferented dendritic branches with little or no effects on the remaining dendritic branches, as shown in Fig. 6.5 (Deitch and Rubel, 1984).

The number of afferents is an important factor which determines the size and complexity of dendritic trees. In some places dendrites may compete for the available afferents and that appears to be one of the ways in which the sizes of dendritic trees are adjusted to fit into the available space. For example, in the retina, if a region is surgically depleted of retinal ganglion cells there is considerable enlargement of ganglion cells and their dendrites in the cell-poor region in cats (Leventhal *et al.*, 1988b) and monkeys (Leventhal *et al.*, 1989). This effect has been considered to be the result of dendritic competition for afferents (Perry and Maffei, 1988) or for trophic factors (Eysel *et al.*, 1985). The sensitive period for dendritic plasticity in the retina ends between P40 and P60 in the cat

---

are devoid of label, indicating little or no protein synthesis. These cells will undergo cell death if the blockade of their afferent activity continues. Second, the remaining neurons are labeled, but generally less heavily than on the normal side of the brain; these neurons will atrophy, but not die. The graph at the bottom shows data (grain densities from six animals) treated in the same way. For each animal the grain densities are normalized on the basis of the mean and S.D. found on the normal (contralateral) side of that brain.

Note that on the side ipsilateral to tetrodotoxin blockade (TTX = filled bars) most of the neurons show a modest (~25 percent) decrease in grain density. About one-third of the cells show grain densities more than 3 z-scores below the normal side; these correspond to the unlabeled cells in (B). From D. E. Born and E. W. Rubel, *J. Neurosci.* 8:901–919 (1988), copyright Society for Neuroscience.

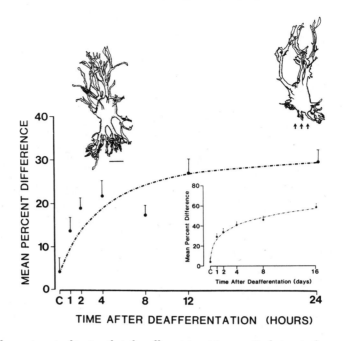

Figure 6.5. Results of experiments showing that the afferent input to a particular part of a neuron regulates that part independently of the other parts. A normal cell from nucleus laminaris of the chickbrain stem is shown at the top left. Its bipolar, symmetrical dendrites get separate, but matched, input. When the excitatory input to the ventral dendrite is eliminated by cutting the afferent axons, the ventral dendrites atrophy (arrows at top right cell) but the dorsal dendrites remain unchanged. This cell is from an animal 8 days after cutting of the axons to the ventral dendrites. The graphs show the rapid atrophy of the ventral dendrite. By 2 hours after cutting of the afferent axons the ventral dendrite is about 20 percent smaller than the dorsal dendrite. By 12 hours, which is before any degeneration of axons can be seen, it is about 25 percent atrophied. From J. S. Deitch and E. W. Rubel, *J. Comp. Neurol.* **229**:66–79 (1984).

(Eysel *et al.*, 1985). Leventhal *et al.* (1989) showed that the cell bodies and dendritic fields of ganglion cells in the cell-poor region were about 10 times larger than normal in cats and primates, but they still retained the morphological characteristics of their classes (Fig. 6.6). The enlarged dendrites of retinal ganglion cells at the edge of a cell-poor region are turned away from the cell-rich region in rats, cats, and in the peripheral retina of monkeys (Perry and Linden, 1982; Eysel *et al.*, 1985; Leventhal *et al.*, 1988b, 1989). However, in the central area of the monkey retina the dendrites are always directed toward the fovea regardless of their relationship to the cell-poor region (Leventhal *et al.*, 1989). This may occur because of the greater number of afferents converging on retinal ganglion cells in the region of the fovea in primates.

Dendritic growth cones have been recognized in Golgi preparations and with the electron microscope. The initial contacts between dendritic and axonal growth cones result in formation of immature synaptic junctions (Bodian, 1966; Del Cerro and Snider, 1968; Morest, 1969a,b; Tennyson, 1970; Kawana *et al.*, 1971; Hinds and Hinds, 1972, 1976b; Hayes and Roberts, 1973; Skoff and Hamburger, 1974; Vaughn *et al.*, 1974; Mason, 1985; Vaugh, 1989). This is considered in relation to formation of axodendritic synapses in Section 6.5. Dendritic growth cones are enlargements of some, but not all, growing tips of the dendrites. Dendritic growth cones possess one to four filopodia. They resemble axonal growth cones (see Section 5.11) except that dendritic growth cones lack the undulating membrane seen on some axonal growth cones. Axonal growth cones contain GAP-43, a protein with growth regulatory functions (Mein *et al.*, 1986; Skene *et al.*, 1986; Benowitz and Routtenberg, 1987, review; Gordon-Weeks, 1989, review), which is absent from dendritic growth cones (Goslin *et al.*, 1988; see Section 5.11). The ultrastructure of den-

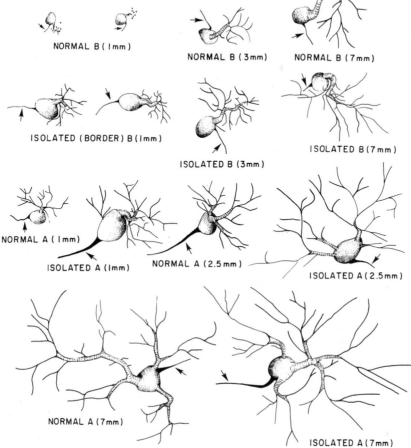

Figure 6.6. A- and B-type ganglion cells in normal and cell-poor regions of the squirrel monkey (*Saimiri sciureus*) retina. The cell-poor regions resulted from three small lesions made close to the optic disc in this monkey's retina at 1 day of age; the animal received HRP injections into one LGNd at about 3 years of age. Notice that the cell bodies and dendritic fields of isolated central A and B cells are much larger than those of their normal counterparts. Also notice that even though the cell bodies of isolated central cells are similar in size to those of isolated peripheral cells, their dendritic fields are smaller. Isolated A and B cells in paracentral regions of monkey retina (2–5 mm from the fovea) are only slightly larger than their normal counterparts. Isolated cells in peripheral regions (more than 5 mm from the fovea) are not obviously larger than normal. Magnification bar = 80 μm. Arrows point to axons. From A. G. Leventhal, S. J. Ault, D. J. Vitek, and T. Shou, *J. Comp. Neurol.* **286**:170–189 (1989).

dritic and axonal growth cones is similar. They contain a network of 5-nm microfilaments and a variable number of vesicles and cisternae of smooth endoplasmic reticulum. They contain few or no ribosomes, mitochondria, or microtubules. The main identifying features of dendritic growth cones are their continuity with a dendrite and the presence of microfilaments, one or more filopodia, and axondendritic synapses. It should be noted that all these features are apparently also seen in dendritic retraction bulbs. Dendritic branches are retracted (Sumner and Watson, 1971; L. A. Goldstein *et al.*, 1990) as well as extended, and the problem arises of the fate of the synapses that are present on the dendritic growth cones. It seems probable that during the period of "trial and error" some transient synapses are eventually eliminated. It is in the nature of such evanescent structures to be elusive.

Barron (1943) suggested that development of the dendrites of some neurons is delayed until their axons have reached their targets, and that a retrograde signal transmitted from the axon terminals to the cell body is required for the initiation of dendritic growth. This theory is consistent with the following evidence. Firstly, the evidence that dendrites retract after axotomy and extend after axonal regeneration (Sumner and Watson, 1971; Purves, 1975; Yawo, 1987) can be interpreted to mean that dendritic growth is maintained by a trophic factor transported retrogradely from the axonal targets. Secondly, there is good evidence that NGF is transported retrogradely in sensory and sympathetic axons (Hendrey *et al.*, 1974; Stöckel *et al.*, 1975; Korsching and Thoenen, 1983), and in cholinergic neurons of the basal forebrain (Seiler and Schwab, 1984). Thirdly, treatment with NGF results in dendritic growth enhancement of NGF-responsive neurons (Snider, 1988).

There are several types of neurons in which the axons form synaptic connections before or at the same time as their dendrites form synaptic connections. The mitral cells of the mouse olfactory bulb make axonal connections on the same day, E15, as synapses form on their dendrites (Hinds and Hinds, 1976a). The axons of association neurons of the rat spinal cord make connections 1 day earlier than synapses form on their dendrites (Vaughn *et al.*, 1974). The dendrites of the principal neurons of the lateral geniculate nucleus differentiate at the time of arrival of the optic axons in the lateral geniculate nucleus. The afferent optic axons in the dorsal lateral geniculate nucleus have growth cones and filopodia that are in contact with growth cones and filopodia of the dendrites of local-circuit neurons (Morest, 1969b). The filopodia and growth cones diminish in number as the dendrites mature, but they can still be seen on many mature dendrites. Dendrites of motoneurons in the spinal bulbocavernosus nucleus extend and retract their dendrites in response to changes in testosterone levels in male rats throughout life (L. A. Goldstein *et al.*, 1990; see Section 7.10). Those findings suggest that some growth adjustments are still occurring, even in mature dendrites. They have obvious implications for theories of neuronal plasticity and of learning. The dendrites of local circuit neurons of the medial geniculate body of the adult cat have growth cones (Morest, 1971). In adult canaries the dendrites of neurons in the brain centers subserving singing are stimulated to grow by gonadal hormones (De Voogd and Nottebohm, 1981). The evidence that local-circuit neurons continue to grow in adult mammals supports Cajal's conjecture that these cells play a role in the higher nervous activities of humans (Ramón y Cajal, 1901).

Development of the dendrites occurs at the same time as the development of axodendritic and dendrodendritic synapses, and it will have become clear from the previous discussion that synaptogenesis and dendritic growth are interdependent processes. As a general rule, axodendritic synapses tend to start developing before axosomatic synapses on pyramidal cells of the cerebral neocortex and on cerebellar Purkinje cells, although in the latter case there are transient connections of climbing fibers on somatic spines before dendritic synapses develop (Pappas and Purpura, 1961; Voeller *et al.*, 1963; Purpura *et al.*, 1964; Marty and Scherrer, 1964; Meller *et al.*, 1968a,b; Molliver and Van der Loos, 1970; Crepel *et al.*, 1976). Moreover, axodendritic synapses are formed over an extended period during postnatal growth of dendrites in the mammalian cerebral cortex and cerebellar cortex.

The proper functioning of the dendrites depends on their coming into the proper relationship with axons that are destined to form synapses on them. Dendritic spines are the main postsynaptic sites on most neurons (Gray, 1959; Spacek and Hartmann, 1983; Spacek, 1985; Coss, 1985, review), and because inhibitory and excitatory inputs are often spatially segregated on different regions of the dendrites, spines are important for integration of synaptic inputs (Feldman, 1984, review). How the spines develop in the correct positions, in the correct numbers, and how they are maintained and modified are important questions to answer. To what degrees are spine development and modification determined by afferents, by the spine itself, and by the postsynaptic neuron?

The normal stages of development of dendritic spines are not well understood in terms of cellular and molecular mechanisms. It is not clear why synaptic junctions form early during development of dendritic spines in some types of neurons while in others the spines form first and synaptic junctions form later. Development of dendritic spines usually occurs after the formation of axodendritic synapses, but the spines can develop and persist in the absence of synapses on them. There is ample evidence that spines can develop in the absence of presynaptic terminals after experimental removal of the afferents, in some mutations, as well as during normal development.

Serial thin sections of developing Purkinje cell dendrites reveal many spine-like structures which do not possess synapses. However, postjunctional specializations always form together with presynaptic endings on Purkinje cell spines during normal development (Landis, 1987). Synapses form first and the spines develop later in the hippocampal dentate gyrus of the rat (Cotman et al., 1973a). The same sequence is seen on the gemmules (which is another name first given to spines by Berkley, 1897) of granule cells in the olfactory bulb of the mouse embryo (Hinds and Hinds, 1976b).

Transient synaptic junctions are formed between parallel fibers and the dendritic shafts of Purkinje cells during normal postnatal development (Mugnaini, 1969; Altman, 1971, 1972), but in normal adults the parallel fibers synapse exclusively on dendritic spines of Purkinje cells (Landis and Reese, 1974; Palay and Chan-Palay, 1974; Hanna et al., 1976). The shaft and spine junctions are similar in thin-sectioned electron microscopic preparations, but in freeze-fractured preparations the shaft junctions lack the particles aggregated on the extracellular side of the postsynaptic membrane that are characteristic of mature synapses on dendritic spines (Landis, 1987). These particles represent transmembrane proteins which are lacking in the synapses on dendritic shafts. There is evidence in cerebellar mutant mice that development of synapses on shafts is independent of formation of spine synapses and that dendritic spines can develop in the absence of presynaptic input (see Section 10.15 for an account of mutations affecting development of the cerebellum). For example in the staggerer mutant mouse the Purkinje cell dendritic spines fail to develop and parallel fibers make transient synaptic junctions with dendritic shafts and with glial cells before most of the granule cells die (Sotelo, 1973, 1975; Landis and Sidman, 1978). Formation of presynaptic specializations on Purkinje cells shows a certain degree of autonomy of the development of the presynaptic endings. In the weaver mutant

mouse there are few parallel fibers yet the Purkinje cells form numerous dendritic spines complete with postsynaptic specializations (Rakic and Sidman, 1973a,b; Hirano and Dembitzer, 1973, 1975; Sotelo, 1973, 1975a,b; Hanna et al., 1976; Landis and Reese, 1977). Postsynaptic specializations also develop on dendritic spines of Purkinje cells devoid of presynaptic junctions in reeler mice (Rakic, 1976; Mariani et al., 1977; Landis and Landis, 1978). Purkinje cell dendritic spines also develop in the absence of parallel fibers after experimental destruction of granule cells (Phemister et al., 1969; Herndon et al., 1971; Altman and Anderson, 1972; Hirano et al., 1972; Hirano and Dembitzer, 1975; Herndon and Oster-Granite, 1975). Deafferentation of Purkinje cell dendritic spines results in elongation, narrowing, and often branching of spines (Sotelo, 1973, 1975a,b; Herndon and Oster-Granite, 1975; Hirano and Dembitzer, 1975; Landis and Reese, 1977; Chen and Hillman, 1982a,b, 1985).

There is increasing evidence showing that changes in size and shape of dendritic spines and of their postsynaptic specializations play significant functional roles during development and in the mature nervous system. Developmental changes in size and shape of dendritic spines can be seen in Golgi preparations—the spines appear to be thinner and longer initially (Schüz, 1981). Quantitative analysis of Golgi preparations shows constancy of proportions of the head and stalk of dendritic spines during development but the diameter of the spines increases by 21–29% from birth to maturity in the guinea pig cerebral cortex (Schüz, 1986).

Dendritic spines contain high concentrations of actin and myosin, as shown by light and electron microscopic immunocytochemistry (Matus et al., 1982; Caceres et al., 1983; Markham and Fifková, 1986; Morales and Fifková, 1989). These are supposed to be responsible for changes in shape of dendritic spines in response to synaptic stimulation, specifically that the neck shortens and increases in diameter (Chang, 1952; Globus and Scheibel, 1967; van Harreveld and Fifková, 1975; Moshkov et al., 1977, 1980; Lee et al., 1980; Fifková and Anderson, 1981; Brandon and Coss, 1982; Rausch and Scheich, 1982; Burgess and Coss, 1983; Coss, 1985, review; Fifková, 1985a,b, reviews; Wentzel et al., 1985; Petukhov and Popov, 1986).

Because it is not possible to record directly from individual dendritic spines, biophysical models

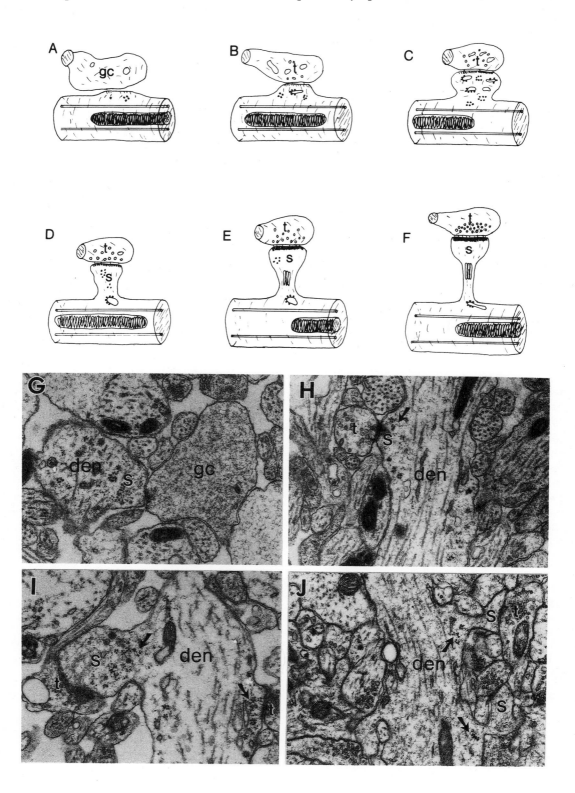

have been constructed to test the effects that changing spine dimensions might have on synaptic efficiency. Chang (1952) first conjectured that changes in the length and width of the spine neck could modulate synaptic efficiency: lengthening would reduce transmission and shortening would result in enhanced transmission of synaptic current from the spine head to the dendrite (Diamond *et al.*, 1970; Rall, 1970, 1974, 1978; Koch and Poggio, 1983; Perkel and Perkel, 1985; Rall and Seger, 1988). Another theory is that changes in spine dimensions could alter diffusion of proteins and ions in and out of the spine (Shepherd, 1979, p. 364; Gamble and Koch, 1987; Brown *et al.*, 1988; Harris and Stevens, 1988, 1989). For further discussion of the effects of activity on dendritic spines see Section 6.11.

The theory that changes in dendritic size and shape are structural bases for learning, initially proposed as a premature theory a century ago (Rabl-Rückhard, 1890; Duval, 1895; Ramón y Cajal, 1895), has recently attained maturity (Petit, 1988; Markus and Petit, 1989, review). Changes in synaptic size and shape appear to account for changes in synaptic efficiency at the neuromuscular junction (Wernig and Herrara, 1986, review) and during learning in *Aplysia* (Baily and Chen, 1983, 1988). Changes in morphology of synaptic terminals have also been reported in phasic motoneurons subjected to tonic stimulation (Lnenicka *et al.*, 1986), and in the lateral vestibular nucleus of the rat (Sotelo and Palay, 1971). Long-term potentiation results in an increased proportion of synapses, with presynaptic density pushing into the postsynaptic element in the hippocampal dentate gyrus and area CA1 (Desmond and Levy, 1983, 1986a,b; Markus and Petit, 1989). The protein synthesis and posttranslational

modification of proteins required for spine growth and modification are carried out by polyribosomes associated with membranous cysternae at the base of the dendritic spine (Steward *et al.*, 1988). Polyribosome clusters associated with membranous cysternae are located at the base of many dendritic spines (Steward and Levy, 1982; Steward, 1983b) as well as at the subsynaptic region of many other types of synapses (Steward and Ribak, 1986). Polyribosome clusters are sites of protein synthesis, and almost all polyribosomes in dendrites are associated with dendritic spines. The specific requirement of many different synapses on the same neuron located far from the protein-synthesizing machinery in the cell body has to be supplied by transport of RNA from the cell nucleus (see Section 5.4) and by local protein synthesis. The location of polyribosome clusters close to the base of each dendritic spine enables protein synthesis to be regulated by activity at individual synapses (Steward and Levy, 1982; Steward, 1983b), as shown in Fig. 6.7.

During synaptogenesis there is a considerable increase in the number of dendritic spines with underlying polyribosomes (Steward and Falk, 1985, 1986). During reinnervation of the hippocampal dentate gyrus there is an increase in polyribosomes associated with reinnervated dendritic spines (Steward, 1983a) and a corresponding increase in protein synthesis (Fass and Steward, 1983; Steward and Fass, 1983). These findings suggest that polyribosomes and membranous cysternae associated with synapses are involved in synthesis and posttranslational modification of classes of proteins that are specifically required by synapses, and that are needed quickly and therefore cannot be supplied efficiently by transport from the cell body (Steward *et al.*, 1988).

Figure 6.7. A possible sequence of synaptic maturation indicating the relationship between polyribosomes and synapses at various stages of synapse maturation. This is based upon studies of synaptogenesis in the dentate gyrus and hippocampus. Polyribosomes are most prominent during the time that primitive contacts differentiate into mature synapses with prominent postsynaptic membrane specializations. (G)–(J) Sample electron micrographs of synaptic contacts in the developing dentate gyrus. (G) A primitive contact from the molecular layer of the dentate gyrus of the 4-day-old rat. In this photomicrograph, a presumed growth cone (gc) is apposed to a dendrite with polyribosomes. A few vesicles are present at this contact site, and the postsynaptic membrane specialization is barely evident. This profile is the type represented by (A). (H) A somewhat more mature synapse from the dentate gyrus of a 4-day-old rat. Note the more prominent postsynaptic membrane specialization and the selective localization of the polyribosomes near the contact site. This profile is the type represented in diagram (B). (I) Two synapses from the dentate gyrus of a 7-day-old rat, during the phase when polyribosomes are most prominent. These profiles are the type illustrated in diagram (C). (J) Two synapses from the dentate gyrus of 20-day-old animals. At this age, synapses appear more mature, although polyribosomes are still more prominent than in mature animals. (A–E) are from O. Steward, L. Davis, C. Dotti, L. L. Phillips, A. Rao, and G. Banker, *Mol. Neurobiol.* 2:227–261 (1988). (G–I) are from O. Steward and P. M. Falk, *J. Neurosci.* 6:412–423 (1986).

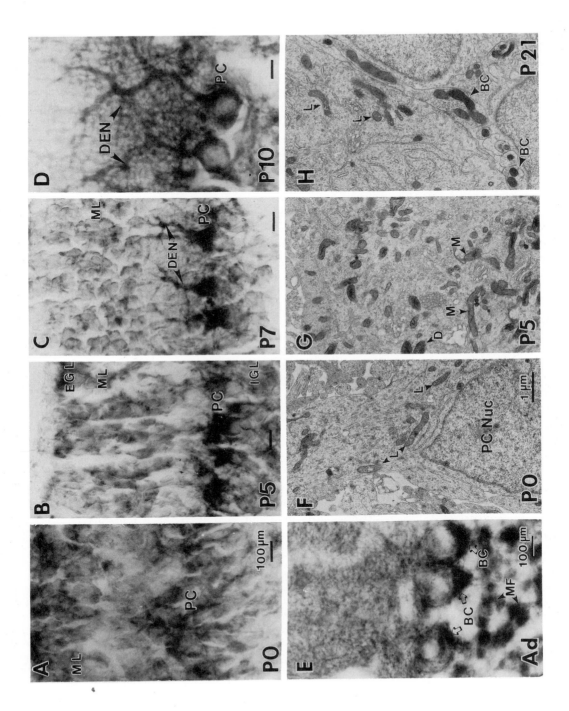

Very long-lasting changes can occur after synaptic activity, and such long-term potentiation (Bliss and Lomo, 1973) is localized to individual activated synapses and does not spread to other synapses on the same neuron (Andersen et al., 1977; McNaughton et al., 1978). This is evidence that the modification is effected at individual synapses as a result of functional activity. There is considerable evidence that protein synthesis is required for synaptic modification (Duffy et al., 1981; Fifkova et al., 1982; Stanton and Sarvey, 1983; Deadwyler et al., 1987).

Dendrites are sites of the highest oxidative energy metabolism in the nerve cell (Creuzfeldt, 1975). This is shown by the high density of mitochondria and high level of cytochrome oxidase activity, which peaks during the period of synaptogenesis (Wong-Riley, 1989, review). The level of cytochrome oxidase activity is closely correlated with the type of synaptic input: increased synaptic activity results in enhanced cytochrome oxidase activity in postsynaptic neurons, whereas inhibitory inputs result in lowering of cytochrome oxidase activity (Kageyama and Wong-Riley, 1982). Deafferentation or pharmacological blockade results in reduction of the level of cytochrome oxidase activity in the postsynaptic neurons. This has been observed in the cortical barrels of adult mice after removal of vibrissae (Wong-Riley and Welt, 1980), and in the visual system of the cat after eye enucleation, monocular visual deprivation, or blockade of action potentials (Wong-Riley, 1979; Wong-Riley and Riley, 1983; Kageyama and Wong-Riley, 1986). Development of synapses on rat cerebellar Purkinje cells is closely correlated with cytochrome oxidase activity and with density of mitochondria (Mjaatvedt and Wong-Riley, 1988), as shown in Fig. 6.8. The Purkinje cell somatic spines receive input, presumably excitatory, from climbing

fibers starting at P3 and these are replaced by inhibitory basket cell synapses beginning at P10, while the climbing fibers shift their excitatory synapses to the Purkinje cell dendrites. Thus, in the mature Purkinje cell the soma receives inhibitory input and the dendrites excitatory input (see Section 10.12). The cytochrome oxidase activity in mitochondria is higher in the soma during the period of somatic spine synapses with climbing fibers and lower after they are replaced by inhibitory basket cell terminals. The cytochrome oxidase activity in the Purkinje cell dendrites is correlated with the amount of excitatory axodendritic synaptic activity.

Many conditions influence ontogeny of dendrites and synapses, for example, the levels of nutrition, thyroid hormone, and sex hormones (Lauder, 1983, review). These are discussed in Chapter 7. Neurotransmitters also affect development of dendrites and synapses. Evidence that catecholamines (dopamine, serotonin) alter growth cone motility in tissue culture may indicate an effect on synaptogenesis (Haydon et al., 1987; Lankford et al., 1988; Mattson, 1988, review). Norepinephrine secreted by early arriving axons in the cerebral cortex appears to inhibit synaptogenesis (Felton et al., 1982; Parnavelas and Blue, 1982). Norepinephrine is involved in the plasticity of the visual cortex (Kasamatsu et al., 1984; Gordon et al., 1988, reviews; see Section 11.21). Continuous blockade of opioid receptors significantly increases dendritic growth and spine density in the cerebral cortex and cerebellar cortex of neonatal rats, which suggests that endogenous opioids inhibit development of dendrites and dendritic spines (Hauser et al., 1989).

The growth of dendrites and the formation of axodendritic synapses in the cerebral cortex have been correlated with changes in the electroen-

Figure 6.8. Cytochrome oxidase activity in the developing rat cerebellar cortex. High levels of cytochrome oxidase activity occur in dendrites, which receive excitatory input during development. At birth (PO) the Purkinje cells have very low levels of cytochrome oxidase histochemical reaction product as seen with light microscopy and electron microscopy. Lightly reactive mitochondria (L) predominate (F). Increasing numbers of moderately (M) and darkly (D) reactive mitochondria are seen with the EM at P5 (G), and the quantity of cytochrome oxidase reaction product increases in the dendrites as they receive more excitatory input on P5–P10 (B–D). As the excitatory input from climbing fibers is replaced by inhibitory input from basket cells, from P10 to adulthood, the quantity of cytochrome oxidase in the dendrites diminishes and lightly reactive mitochondria predominate at P21 (H). Note the basket cell terminals (BC), with their darkly reactive mitochondria, synapsing directly on the Purkinje cell soma (H). In the adult this can be seen with light microscopy (E). DEN = dendrite; EGL = external granule cell layer; IGL = internal granule cell layer; ML = molecular layer; PC Nuc = Purkinje cell nucleus; magnification bar = 100 μm (A–E); 1 μm (F–H). Adapted from A. E. Mjaatvedt and M. T. T. Wong-Riley, *J. Comp. Neurol.* 277:155–182 (1988).

cephalogram and in evoked cortical electrical responses (Ellingson and Wilcott, 1960; Huttenlocher, 1966, 1967; Myslivecek, 1968; G. H. Rose and Lindsley, 1968; Molliver and Van der Loos, 1970). Little is known about the development of dendrodendritic synapses, which are numerous, especially in the mammalian brain, and which are thought to have important functions (Shepherd, 1972; Schmitt *et al.*, 1976).

6.5. General Comments on Development of Synapses

Structure and function of mature synapses provide the points of departure from which progressively earlier stages of development have been studied (E. G. Jones, 1983; Vaughn, 1989, reviews). Ultrastructural features by which developing synaptic junctions may be recognized are: parallel, opposed plasma membranes belonging to presynaptic and postsynaptic elements; a cleft between them which contains denser material than is ordinarily found in extracellular spaces; synaptic vesicles near to or in contact with the presynaptic membrane; and some structural specializations associated with the cytoplasmic surfaces of presynaptic and postsynaptic membranes, generally starting in the postsynaptic elements and developing later in the presynaptic elements.

Functions of developing synapses may be inferred from their ultrastructural resemblance to mature synapses and from the presence of transmitters determined by biochemical and immunocytochemical methods. Synaptic vesicles in contact with the presynaptic membrane implies release of transmitter, and this may be corroborated by electrophysiological detection of synaptic potentials. Causal–analytical developmental studies aim to discover the mechanisms by which the presynaptic and postsynaptic elements come together. These mechanisms include cooperative cell interactions (guidance, growth control, temporal coincidence, cell recognition, functional validation) and competitive cell interactions involving selective affinity, exclusion, elimination, or survival.

Development of synapses is certainly one of the central problems in developmental neurobiology. Before discussing the present knowledge in detail it may be useful to make some general comments. Synaptogenesis may be controlled directly by the cell body as well as indirectly by the environment of the developing dendrites and axonal terminals. Because many neurons have axonal branches that terminate in a variety of ways it is unlikely that the cell body exerts a direct control of all the synapses made by its axonal terminals. For example, the auditory nerve fibers branch to form several different types of endings in different parts of the cochlear nucleus (Lorente de Nó, 1933a; M. L. Feldman and Harrison, 1969). It seems unlikely that different instructions can be issued by the cell body to different branches of the same axon. The local conditions at the axonal terminals, and especially the nature of the postsynaptic neuron, must play an important part in controlling the formation and differentiation of the synapse. There is good evidence that presynaptic and postsynaptic elements both determine the form of the synapse (Parks *et al.*, 1990).

The development of the synapse involves an interaction between the presynaptic and postsynaptic elements. It would not be correct to attribute the primary or determinative role to either component. It is also unlikely that the specificity of synaptic connections depends only on a single factor such as the biochemical compatibility or affinity between presynaptic and postsynaptic elements, as Sperry (1963) has proposed. This is not to deny that specific affinities and disaffinities between presynaptic and postsynaptic elements are necessary for the formation of some or even all synaptic connections, but such affinities may not be sufficient. The two elements must first come into close proximity or even into contact, and the time at which the nexus is made may also have to be specific. Functional activity may be necessary to ensure full maturation and permanent stability of the synapses. A number of factors, each of which is necessary but not sufficient, may have to act in combination to result in the functional development of the synapse. The preestablished harmony of normal development ensures that all the components are present in the right places at the right times. Thus it is best to observe the processes of synaptogenesis under normal conditions, using probes that perturb normal development as little as possible. Observations can now be made on essentially unperturbed developing synapses over periods of days or weeks using fluorescent dyes that label either postsynaptic structures (Purves *et al.*, 1986; Wigston, 1989) presynaptic endings (Yoshikami and Okun, 1984; Lichtman *et al.*, 1985; Magrassi *et al.*, 1987; Purves *et al.*, 1987; Robbins and Polak, 1987; Lichtman *et al.*, 1987; Purves and Voyvodic, 1987), or extracellular matrix components of the synapse (Sanes and Cheney, 1982; Kelley *et al.*, 1985; Ko, 1987; Scott *et al.*, 1988).

Inferences made from observations of normal development tend to be weak because they can show only whether events are correlated in time and space, and not whether they are causally related. To show causal relationships the effects of breaking the causal chain must be analyzed, and recovery after restoration of the causal chain must be demonstrated, as Wilhelm Roux was among the first to emphasize (see Section 4.1). The disadvantage of this strategy is that experimental intervention may result in changes that are not part of normal development. Extreme caution should be exercised in trying to interpret such results in terms of normal developmental processes. Even "gentle" interference may alter normal development, while heroic manipulations of the developing nervous system, such as exposure to chemical toxins, irradiation, virus infection, or surgery, may inhibit normal developmental processes as well as create ones that do not exist under normal conditions. Some examples of this sort are the formation of anomalous synaptic connections by retinal axons after destruction of the superior colliculus in newborn mammals (Schneider, 1981; Campbell and Frost, 1988) and anomalous synaptic connections of cochlear nuclei which develop after ablation of the otocyst in chick embryos (Jackson and Parks, 1988).

There are some good experiments involving formation of aberrant connections which shed light on problems of normal development, such as whether the form of the synapse is determined predominantly by the presynaptic or postsynaptic element. Parks *et al.* (1990) have shown that both elements influence the form of synaptic junctions in the auditory relay nuclei of the chick embryo. In birds the cochlear axons form large calyciform endings on neurons of the nucleus magnocellularis (NM), the primary auditory nucleus. By contrast, the NM neurons form small presynaptic boutons on neurons of the nucleus laminaris, the secondary auditory relay nucleus (Rubel and Parks, 1988). Ablation of the

cochlea in the chick embryo results in formation of anomalous projections from the normal NM to the deafferented NM. However, the anomalous NM–NM nerve fibers form neither large calyciform endings nor the typical small boutons but take on an intermediate form (Parks *et al.*, 1990). This shows that pre- and postsynaptic elements both play roles in determining the form of the synapse.

In addition to physicochemical compatibility of the presynaptic and postsynaptic elements, the correct timing of the connection may be important. If the axon and dendrite fail to make contact at the right time, their subsequent development may be abnormal. A principle of competitive exclusion may operate to ensure specificity of synaptogenesis: termination of different types of axons on specific regions of the postsynaptic membrane may occur as a result of the restricted availability of synaptic sites during the time of arrival of axonal terminals at the postsynaptic membrane. As each fresh contingent of axons arrives at the postsynaptic membrane, it may be excluded from the synaptic sites that have been occupied and may be constrained to occupy synaptic sites that remain vacant on the most recently developed dendritic branches. This is one of the ways in which a topographically organized projection may develop.

Spatial patterning of synaptogenesis which may be due to the time of arrival of different presynaptic endings is seen in the formation of axodendritic synapses on granule cells of the hippocampal dentate gyrus. D. I. Gottlieb and Cowan (1972) found that the ratio of crossed to uncrossed inputs to the hippocampal granule cells correlates with the time of origin of the granule cells; the earlier their origin, the greater the proportion of uncrossed inputs. Thus at the time the first formed granule cells are ready to receive synapses on the proximal portions of their dendrites, the only afferents present are those from the same side of the hippocampus, whereas the fibers from the opposite side do not approach the dentate gyrus until some days later. From such evidence it has been inferred that recognition between the specific afferents and the dentate granule cells is unnecessary; all that seems to be required is that the axons arrive at a time when the granule cell dendrites are ready to receive them.

Precise coordination of the development of presynaptic and postsynaptic elements may be necessary in some cases, but microprecise timing is not required if the growth of dendrites occurs in response to the arrival of the appropriate axonal terminals. One may imagine a situation in which the ingrowing axons stimulate the growth of dendrites on which they are destined to terminate or stimulate a mutual interaction between axons and dendrites. Situations in which one type of migrating neuron moves through the dendritic field of another type with which it is destined to synapse also invite speculations about possible interactions between the two neurons. For example, the cerebellar granule cells migrate through the dendritic field of the Purkinje cells with which the granule cell axons (the parallel fibers) are destined to synapse (Ramón y Cajal, 1909–1911), as discussed in Sections 10.12 and 10.13.

If there are rules that apply to synaptogenesis, they remain elusive, and it is likely that they will not be revealed by studying synaptogenesis with the electron microscope alone. Biochemical, histochemical, and immunocytochemical studies of synaptogenesis *in vivo* and *in vitro* are required before further progress can be made in identifying the components of developing synapses. Electrophysiological recording from identified synapses during their development is required in order to determine their functional development and to correlate their function with structure as revealed with the electron microscope. All such studies have been severely limited by sampling problems, the heterogeneity of the cell population, and the asynchrony of development of cells in the same population. The changes in a single synapse may be very rapid, occurring in hours, while the sequence of events is, at best, inferred from observations of large numbers of synapses made at intervals of days.

The obvious truth that both the pre- and postsynaptic components of any synapse must be present at the same time in the same place before they can form a synapse does not necessarily mean that the temporal coincidence is the cause of the formation of the synapse. The observations are equally consistent with a neuronal recognition mechanism, and for that mechanism to be effective it is also necessary for the components to come together and be ready to interact at the right time in development. I have labored this point only because the relationship between cause and effect is often hard to define clearly in the analysis of the development of complex systems such as

the nervous system (M. Bunge, 1959; Mayr, 1965; Nagel, 1965). Setting aside the niceties of philosophical arguments about causality, I am taking the common-sense view that a cause should be a necessary and sufficient condition that invariably precedes an event—in this case, the formation of a synapse. In most cases, nerve cells come together during development without forming synapses. That the proper components are present at a certain time and place is a necessary but not sufficient condition for the formation of a synapse. It seems as if there must be some degree of mutual affinity between the neurons, or neuronal recognition, before the "correct" synaptic associations can develop. Neuronal recognition, therefore, as a mechanism of achieving association between the "correct" neurons, requires that the neurons be prelabeled before they form any association. This introduces the problem of the origin of the labels and their spatial deployment in sets of neurons and their expression during neuronal recognition in the formation of synaptic connections. Neurons, usually at some considerable distance apart initially, grow toward each other to form a synaptic connection; this raises the problem of the mechanisms of targeting of presynaptic on postsynaptic elements in the development of neuronal connections and the precision of such neuronal targeting. This theme is taken up more amply in Section 5.12 and Chapter 11.

6.6. Timetables of Synaptogenesis

The onset of synaptogenesis occurs according to a remarkably invariant timetable. In each region of the mammalian nervous system there is usually a difference of less than 1 day between individuals of the same species in the appearance of the first synapses on any particular type of neuron. Synapses appear suddenly and increase very rapidly in numbers thereafter. Excessive production of synapses, followed by elimination of redundant synapses, occurs in many regions.

Recently it has become possible to obtain a measure of synaptogenesis from the quantities of proteins associated specifically with synaptic vesicles (Knaus *et al.*, 1986; Moore and Bernstein, 1989), as discussed in Section 6.7. In the past, the increase in connectivity in the developing cerebral cortex has

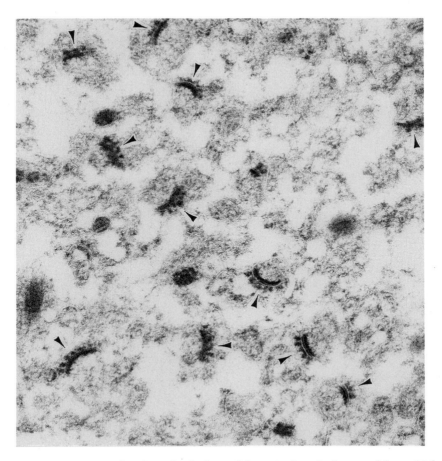

Figure 6.9. Synaptic junctions stained in the molecular layer of the parietal cerebral cortex of the rat 26 days after birth. Ethanolic phosphotungstic acid stain. Arrowheads point to synaptic junctions that are much more deeply stained than the background. 24,000×. By courtesy of F. E. Bloom.

been obtained from the cell-to-gray coefficient (von Economo, 1926; V. B. Peters and Flexner, 1950; Shariff, 1953; Sholl, 1953). The cell-to-gray coefficient was introduced by von Economo (1926) as an index of connectivity or functional capacity of the cerebral cortex, the rationale being that more neuronal interconnections might be present when the cell bodies are widely spaced. The value of the cell-to-gray coefficient for comparative studies is limited by its variability, owing to slight technical differences in the hands of different investigators (Haug, 1956; Eayrs and Goodhead, 1959). Estimates of neuronal connectivity may also be obtained from counts of the frequency of synaptic profiles seen with the electron microscope. Counts of synaptic boutons are limited because if boutons are cut in a plane of section that does not include the pre- and postsynaptic membrane specializations, they can only be identified by the presence of synaptic vesicles which are not uniformly distributed. Moreover, individual boutons may form different numbers of synaptic contacts so that the number of boutons may remain constant or may even diminish while the number of synaptic contacts increases (Beaulieu and Collonnier, 1988). Counts of synaptic contacts have been obtained in electron microscopic sections stained with ethanolic phosphotungstic acid, which selectively stains synaptic junctions, as Fig. 6.9 shows (Bloom, 1972; D. G. Jones, 1973, D. G. Jones *et al.*, 1974).

Most quantitative studies of synaptogenesis use synaptic density as an index of changes in numbers

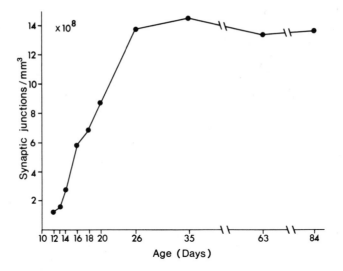

Figure 6.10. Rapid increase in the number of synapses in the cerebral cortex of the rat from birth to P26. The number of synapses in the molecular layer of the parietal cortex was counted with the electron microscope in thin sections stained with ethanolic phosphotungstic acid. From G. K. Aghajanian and F. E. Bloom, *Brain Res.* 6:716–727 (1967).

of synapses, but this requires correction for the rapid increase in volume which occurs at the same time (de Groot and Bierman, 1986, review). This is important to consider when studying synapse elimination. Synaptic density may decrease although the number of synapses increases, if the volume increases relatively more than the absolute number of synapses in a certain region, as shown by Hinds and Hinds (1976a) in mouse olfactory bulb. This may be an explanation for the reports of apparent postnatal decrease in number of synapses in some regions of the spinal cord (Conradi and Ronnevi, 1975; Weber and Stelzner, 1980). Rapid increase of the number of synapses has been reported in many regions of the mammalian CNS during the early postnatal period (Aghajanian and Bloom, 1967; Lund and Lund, 1972; Vaughn and Grieshaber, 1973; Vaughn *et al.*, 1975; Cragg, 1975; Oppenheim *et al.*, 1975; Hinds and Hinds, 1976a; Dyson and Jones, 1980; Brand and Rakic, 1984; Blue and Parnavelas, 1983).

Dramatic increase in the connectivity of the mammalian cerebral cortex occurs during the early postnatal period of development. Eayrs and Goodhead (1959) estimated that a 10-fold increase in connectivity occurs between days 12 and 30 after birth in the cerebral cortex of the rat. Aghajanian and Bloom (1967) calculated a sevenfold increase amounting to 12×10^6 synapses per cubic millime-

ter, in the molecular layer of rat parietal cortex from the 12th to the 26th day after birth (Fig. 6.10). In the molecular layer of the hippocampal dentate gyrus of the rat, less than 1 percent of the adult number of synapses are present at 4 days after birth, but the number doubles every day until it attains more than 90 percent of the adult value at 30 days after birth (B. Crain *et al.*, 1973). In the olfactory bulb of the mouse, the total number of synapses increases more than 1000 times during the 16-day period from E14, when the first synapses appear, to P10 (Hinds and Hinds, 1976a). Even more rapid postnatal increases of the number of synapses have been reported in the cat visual cortex (Cragg, 1972b) and the rat cerebellar cortex (Woodward *et al.*, 1971; Cragg, 1972a). These observations show that synapses must form rapidly, but they do not allow any estimate to be made of the time of formation of a single synapse. They show that there is a net increase of synapses but do not show whether individual synapses persist or are lost.

The theory of neuronal modification by selective depletion (M. Jacobson, 1973) was proposed at a time when synaptogenesis was viewed as an entirely constructive process. According to Hebb (1949), learning results in the formation of more synapses. Regressive events during development of the nervous system were viewed as mechanisms of error elimination (Cowan, 1973). Since then the

evidence has grown to show that overproduction of synapses occurs in widespread regions of the central and peripheral nervous system, and that elimination of synapses occurs universally in the central and peripheral nervous system. The theory of *"neuronal modification by selective depletion"* states that overproduction of synapses is genetically programmed and that the final configuration occurs by elimination of synapses on the basis of cell interactions and functional validation: *"The effect of these interactions is to reduce the initial redundancy, to selectively promote the development of neuronal structures that can coexist because they are mutually compatible or mutually interdependent. . . . The reduction of structures, including synapses, which this theory predicts, results in increased matching of the functions of the nervous system with the conditions of the world in which the creature lives. As Herbert Spencer put it, it is a process which brings the inner and outer relations of the organism into closer correspondence"* (M. Jacobson, 1973). This theory predicts that synaptic overproduction is genetically predetermined and is not affected by experience but that experience acts by eliminating and stabilizing synapses that have already formed; a process termed *functional validation.* Other theories also predict that activity stabilizes synapses but do not state explicitly that there is an initial overproduction of synapses (Stent, 1973; Changeux and Danchin, 1976). The ratio of inhibitory to excitatory synapses per neuron should also be taken into account as an important variable that might be affected by synapse elimination, but it rarely is considered in reports of the total number of synapses.

There are numerous reports.of synapse overproduction followed by synapse elimination during normal development. For example, in the cerebral cortex of the rhesus monkey (*Macaca mulatta*), synaptic density increases during the last 2 prenatal months, reaches a peak about 2 months after birth and then decreases gradually to reach adult levels of synaptic density by about 3 years of age (Rakic *et al.,* 1986). Premature delivery of the rhesus monkey 3 weeks before term does not alter the rate of synaptogenesis or synapse overproduction but can modify existing synapses (Bourgeois *et al.,* 1989). Synaptogenesis in the human striate cortex peaks at 2–4 months after birth. This is followed by elimination of about 40 percent of synapses between ages 8 months to 11 years (Huttenlocher and de Courten,

1987). Overproduction of synapses occurs in the visual cortex of the cat (Cragg, 1975; Winfield, 1981). The transient synapses on the somatic spines of cerebellar Purkinje cells are described in Section 10.12. The spinal motoneurons of the newborn kitten have synapses on the initial segment of the axon, but no synapses are found on this region in the adult cat. These synapses are removed and phagocytosed by glial cells during the 2nd week after birth. (Ronnevi and Conradi, 1974). Removal of other synapses on the cell body and dendrites of spinal motoneurons also may occur in the kitten during the 2nd postnatal week (Conradi and Ronnevi, 1975). Synapse elimination in the ciliary ganglion (Landmesser and Pilar, 1972) is discussed later.

The majority of synapses observed during the early stage of synaptogenesis in the embryonic mouse spinal cord are axodendritic synapses on dendritic growth cones and filopodia (Vaughn *et al.,* 1974; Vaughn and Sims, 1978; Vaughn, 1989, review). In the lateral marginal zone of the mouse spinal cord at E12–E13, approximately 65–75 percent of axodendritic synapses are located on dendritic growth cones or filopodia, as shown in Fig. 6.11. The percentage of synapses located on dendritic growth cones diminishes to about 30 percent on E16 and at the same time synapses on differentiated dendrites increase to about 70 percent of axodendritic synapses (Vaughn *et al.,* 1974; Vaughn and Sims, 1978). This has been interpreted to mean that the majority of axons initially form synaptic junctions on dendritic growth cones and filopodia, and as the dendrites continue to grow the synapses are left behind on the progressively more differentiated dendrites, as illustrated in Fig. 6.12. The spatiotemporal sequence in which dendrites encounter axons may be significant in determining the pattern of dendritic branching—this has been called the synaptotropic hypothesis (Vaughn *et al.,* 1974; Vaughn, 1980) or the synaptogenic filopodial theory (Berry and Bradley, 1976a,b).

The temporal sequence of formation of synaptic connections between different neurons is correlated with the times of neuronal origin and differentiation (reviewed by Altman and Bayer, 1987; Vaughn, 1989; see Section 3.10). This correlation has been found in the olfactory bulb (Hinds and Hinds, 1976a), cerebral cortex (Molliver and van der Loos, 1970; Cragg, 1972; Krisst and Molliver, 1976; Krisst, 1978), cerebellar cortex (Larramendi, 1969;

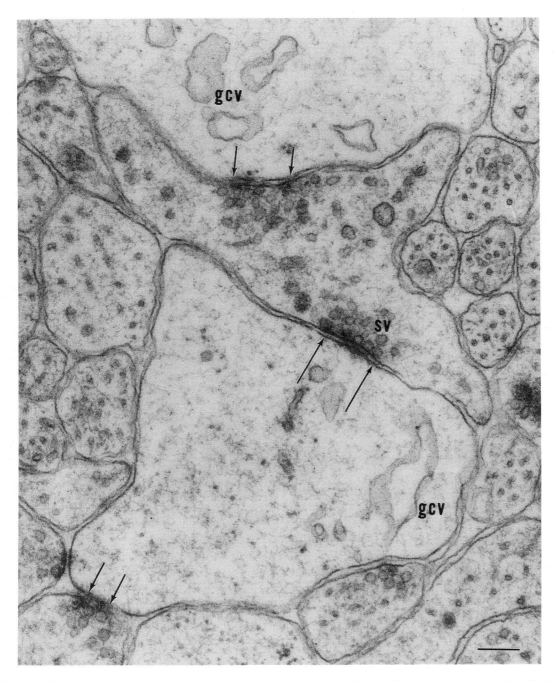

Figure 6.11. Synaptic contacts on the growth cones of motoneuron dendrites in developing mouse spinal cord. The postsynaptic elements contain vacuoles and vesicles (gcv) typical of growth cones on dendrites. The presynaptic elements contain synaptic vesicles (sv) aggregated near the synaptic contact zones (shown by arrows). The presynaptic element in the upper part of the figure appears to be a filopodial extension of an axonal growth cone, whereas the one in the lower left corner is a main axonal shaft. Magnification bar = 0.2 μm. Electron micrograph provided by James E. Vaughn.

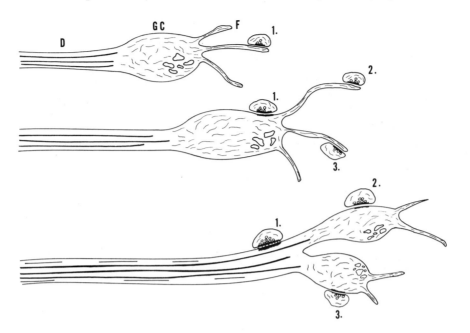

Figure 6.12. A graphic representation of the synaptotropic hypothesis of dendritic branching. In the upper drawing, a differentiated dendrite (D) expands into a growth cone (GC) that, in turn, gives rise to several filopodia (F). One of these filopodia receives a synaptic contact (1), and it becomes a new growth cone in the middle drawing. Synapse 1 thus becomes located on the growth cone without having changed its absolute position in the neuropil. New filopodia extend from the new growth cone, and two of them simultaneously receive synaptic contacts (2 and 3). As shown in the 3rd drawing, this results in the formation of two growth cones from the synaptically contacted filopodia (2 and 3) and, consequently, in dendritic branching. From J. E. Vaughn, C. K. Henrikson, and J. A. Grieshaber, *J. Cell Biol.* **60**:664-672 (1974), with permission of The Rockefeller University Press.

Altman, 1972; Kornguth and Scott, 1972; Foelix and Oppenheim, 1974; Shimono *et al.*, 1976), and spinal cord (Vaughn and Grieshaber, 1973; Vaughn *et al.*, 1975).

Synaptogenesis starts before neurogenesis is completed. Thus newborn neurons migrate to their definitive levels in the cortex, bypassing cortical neurons upon which synapses have already formed or are in the process of formation. However, synaptogenesis may be delayed in some cases. The presynaptic endings and their postsynaptic targets may be juxtaposed for days before they form synaptic connections. For example, in the cerebellum of the mouse, the stellate cells lie closely surrounded by parallel fibers before they connect together. This is not due to some inability of the parallel fibers, because they connect with Purkinje cell dendrites while delaying the formation of synapses with stellate cells (Larramendi, 1969). In the olfactory bulb of the mouse there is a delay during which both the presynaptic and postsynaptic elements are close together before the olfactory axons synapse on the mitral cells (Hinds and Hinds, 1976a). A similar delay in formation of synapses between optic axons and neurons in the tectum of the chick embryo has been reported (Crossland *et al.*, 1974a).

Although granule cells are formed postnatally in the olfactory bulb, all types of synapses are already present in the mouse olfactory bulb at birth, which is a sign of the precocity of the olfactory system. This should be compared with the delayed, postnatal synaptogenesis in the neocortex (Molliver and Van der Loos, 1970; Cragg, 1975a,c). The majority of the synapses in the mouse olfactory bulb are axodendritic, but dendrodendritic synapses are also present at birth (Hinds and Hinds, 1976a,b).

The fact that synapses are commonly seen on dendritic as well as on axonal growth cones shows that neither need be completely mature to enable synaptogenesis to commence. There may be cases, however, in which the onset of synaptogenesis is delayed until some essential components of the pre- or postsynaptic membranes are synthesized or take up their positions in the synaptic membranes.

Correlation between structure and function of developing synapses shows the general rule that function precedes development of specialized synaptic structures. An indication of the precocity of synaptic function relative to synaptic structure is that immature cerebellar Purkinje cells of the rat respond to several putative synaptic transmitters on the 1st and 2nd days after birth, whereas synapses can first be seen on the 3rd day postnatally (Woodward et al., 1971). The chick ciliary ganglion is another example in which synaptic transmission begins at embryonic Stage 26.5 (E4.5) but few synapses can be seen with the electron microscope at Stage 33.5 (E7.5) when all ganglion cells show synaptic potentials (Landmesser and Pilar, 1972). In the ciliary ganglion there are two classes of cells, choroid and ciliary, with different preganglionic inputs, which can be distinguished functionally and morphologically. The preganglionic axons selectively connect with the proper postganglionic cells, indicating that their functional specificity is expressed from the start of synaptogenesis. The morphology of the synapses in the ciliary ganglion undergoes marked changes during development. Synaptic connections are initially made by fine terminal branches of presynaptic axons and at those stages (Stages 26.5–33, E4.5–E7.9) synaptic transmission is chemical. These axonal terminals appear to retract and from Stage 36 (E10) are displaced by calyces, so that by Stage 40 (E14) all ciliary cells have calyces. At the same time there is an increase in electrical transmission until, at 2 days after hatching, 80 percent of synapses are electrically transmitting. The calyces are temporary structures which disappear by 2 weeks after hatching and break up into a cluster of boutons. This morphological transformation does not impair electrical transmission.

6.7. Ultrastructural Differentiation of Synapses

Considering the astronomical number of synapses developing at any one time—and the period of synaptogenesis is relatively long relative to the time of development of a single synapse—it is in-

evitable that all stages are present except at the very beginning and end of the period. There is no general rule about the order of development of the presynaptic and postsynaptic structures, but in each case the order is apparently invariant. Thus, in the spinal cord of the amphibian embryo, increased density of the presynaptic membrane is seen before the postsynaptic specializations are visible (Hayes and Roberts, 1973, 1974). Synthesis of transmitter in the presynaptic neuron and, presumably, its release at the presynaptic terminals occur independently of development of the postsynaptic specialization during normal development of the chick spinal cord (Zukin et al., 1975) and mouse cerebellum (McLaughlin et al., 1975). Clustering of synaptic vesicles at the presynaptic membrane can be induced in tissue culture by latex beads coated with polycations (Burry et al., 1980, 1984; Peng et al., 1987, 1988).

Development of postsynaptic structures is sometimes seen before the arrival of the presynaptic terminals, and development of the postsynaptic membrane specializations is often seen before presynaptic specializations can be seen with the electron microscope. For example, in the olfactory bulb of the mouse, Hinds and Hinds (1976a,b) verified in serial sections that postsynaptic specializations develop before presynaptic membrane thickenings are apparent, but the presynaptic endings are, nevertheless, close to the developing postsynaptic structures. Rees et al. (1976) have obtained good evidence that postsynaptic structures can develop before presynaptic membrane thickening occurs in the isolated superior cervical ganglion and spinal cord of the rat fetus (Fig. 6.13). They found a series of stages in the formation of synapses after the spinal cord axons arrive in the ganglion. Soon after the initial contact between axonal growth cones and ganglion cells, the latter show an increase in the size of the Golgi complex and an increase in the number of coated vesicles adjoining the postsynaptic membrane. This is followed by thickening of the postsynaptic membrane, and only later is the specialization of the presynaptic membrane shown by the appearance of presynaptic dense projections and synaptic vesicles.

Dense material develops in association with the cytoplasmic surfaces of presynaptic and postsynaptic membranes, usually starting first in the latter (Adinolfi, 1972a,b; Blue and Parnavelas, 1983b;

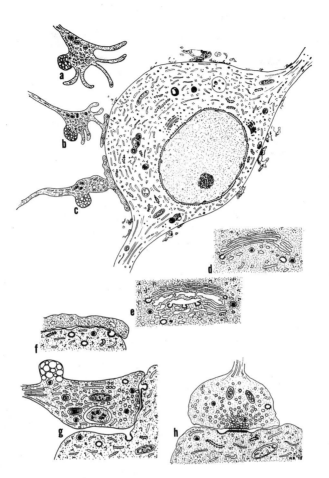

Figure 6.13. Stages of synaptogenesis on the soma of an isolated superior cervical ganglion neuron in culture. The superior cervical ganglion cell as it appears after 2–3 days in culture. Some cellular debris resulting from the mechanical dissociation process clings to the plasmalemma. The nucleus is eccentric, and the cytoplasm is characterized mainly by polysomes, smooth and rough endoplasmic reticulum, Golgi apparatus, mitochondria, multivesicular bodies, and other lysosomal structures. At (a), the soma is approached by a growth cone of a neurite growing out of the spinal cord exhibiting filopodia, a mound area, branched membranous reticulum, and several large lysosomes. At (b), a single filopodium of this growth cone is shown contacting the neuronal surface. Other filopodia are withdrawing. At (c), only the highly flattened, contacting process remains, and its surface membrane has developed many close contacts with the somal plasmalemma. Inset (d) shows the typical Golgi apparatus of a cultured superior cervical ganglion neuron before contact. A few coated vesicles are in continuity with cisternae or present in the adjacent cytoplasm together with an occasional large dense-cored vesicle. Changes occurring in the Golgi complex of a contacted neuron are shown in (e). A greater number of coated vesicles are present, some being continuous with the region of the maturing face of the Golgi complex. These coated vesicles migrate to the neuronal surface in the area of filopodial contact and there fuse with the plasmalemma (as at f), thereby contributing membrane with undercoating (postsynaptic density). This is considered to be the first definitive sign of synaptic specialization. A more advanced stage of synaptogenesis is diagrammed in (g). On the presynaptic side, synaptic vesicles and large dense-cored vesicles appear among the growth cone organelles and cluster at that part of the membrane apposed to the postsynaptic density. In (h), the large amount of membranous reticulum, lysosomes, and mound area typical of the growth cone is no longer present. A few mitochondria, some reticulum, occasional large dense-cored vesicles, and numerous synaptic vesicles now characterize the ending. Presynaptic dense material gradually appears, some cleft material is seen, and the cleft widens. Postsynaptic membrane density increases in length as the addition of large coated vesicles continues. From R. P. Rees, M. B. Bunge, and R. P. Bunge, *J. Cell Biol.* 68:240–263 (1976).

Krisst and Molliver, 1976) and later developing in association with both presynaptic and postsynaptic membranes (Lund and Lund, 1972; Foelix and Oppenheim, 1975; Vaughn et al., 1975; Brand and Rakic, 1984). Synapses with more dense material in the postsynaptic elements are more frequent on dendrites whereas symmetrical synapses develop more commonly on the cell body, although synapses of both types occur at both locations, and the appearance may also depend on the plane of section. These membrane densities include amorphous dense cytoplasmic material, microtubules, microfilaments, and intramembranous particles (McGraw et al., 1980; Nagy and Witkowsky, 1981; Landis et al., 1983; Westrum et al., 1983). Particles in the postsynaptic membrane of the neuromuscular junction are probably acetylcholine receptors (Heuser et al., 1974; Rash and Ellman, 1974; Heuser and Salpeter, 1979). The thickness and density of membrane specializations increase with synaptic maturation (Jones, 1983, review).

Dendritic spines contain polyribosomes, especially in large spines, a network of microfilaments, intermediate filaments, and smooth endoplasmic reticulum (Landis and Reese, 1983; Spacek, 1985), as well as actin and microtubule-associated protein MAP2 (Caceras et al., 1983). Coated vesicles and coated pits are seen in both elements of developing synapses (Vaughn and Sims, 1978; McGraw and McLaughlin, 1980). These are evidence of membrane expansion and recycling and intake of materials from the extracellular space.

Asymmetrical axodendritic synapses seem to go through an intermediate stage of development in which the pre- and postsynaptic membrane thickenings are equally dense. Hinds and Hinds (1976b) found that, early in development of the mouse olfactory bulb, there are more symmetrical axodendritic synapses on growth cones, and later in development the number of asymmetrical synapses increases. This sequence has also been found in the mammalian cerebral neocortex (R. Johnson and Armstrong-James, 1970; Adinolfi, 1972a,b; Cragg, 1972b,c), in the cerebellar cortex of the chick (Foelix and Oppenheim, 1974), and in the spinal cord of the rat fetus (M. K. May and Biscoe, 1973). The size of the synaptic contact zone rapidly reaches adult size and does not change significantly during synaptic maturation in different species and locations (Vaughn, 1989, review). This is in contrast with neu-

romuscular synapses, which increase considerably in size during postnatal maturation (Herera and Banner, 1987; Lichtman et al., 1987).

The first synaptic vesicles to form are round and clear, whereas markedly flattened vesicles develop later (Bodian, 1966a,b, 1968; Adinolfi, 1972; Lund and Lund, 1972; Krisst and Molliver, 1976). Synaptic vesicles appear to bud off the smooth endoplasmic reticulum (Teichberg and Holtzman, 1973). The increasing number of synaptic vesicles is a good index of synaptic maturation (Dyson and Jones, 1980; Blue and Parnavelas, 1983b; Jones, 1983, review). A number of proteins have been identified that are associated with synaptic vesicles (Trimble and Scheller, 1988, review). Antibodies to these proteins have been used as sensitive assays of synaptogenesis (Knaus et al., 1986; Moore and Bernstein, 1989). Synaptophysin (Navone et al., 1986) is a 38-kDa integral membrane glycoprotein present in the membrane of classical clear synaptic vesicles. Synaptophysin has a cytoplasmic domain containing a Ca^{2+} binding site which is involved in exocytosis of the synaptic vesicles. The level of synaptophysin during development is closely correlated with the time course of synaptogenesis (Knaus et al., 1986). Synapsin I and III are phosphoproteins found on the cytoplasmic surface of synaptic vesicles (De Camilli et al., 1983). The synaptic vesicles are immobilized and localized at the presynaptic membrane by a cytoskeletal lattice (Hirokawa, 1983; Peng, 1983). This process is regulated by phosphorylation of synapsin 1 in the walls of the vesicles (Bahler and Greengard, 1987). Levels of synapsin 1 are precisely correlated with synaptogenesis in the rat suprachiasmatic nucleus (Moore and Bernstein, 1989).

Whether glial cells play any role in synaptogenesis is not known but it is tacitly assumed that they are not essential. This is based on negative evidence—synapses form in tissue culture in the absence of glial cells. Synaptic junctions develop transiently between axons and radial glial cells or astroglial cells, apparently as a phase of normal development (Henrikson and Vaughn, 1974; Oppenheim et al., 1978; McGraw and McLaughlin, 1980), and some more durable axoglial synapses may also develop (Ebner and Colonnier, 1975). Their possible functions are not known. Glial cells participate in eliminating synapses and in the disconnection of synapses that occurs after neuronal injury. After axotomy and anterograde axonal degeneration, the degenerating presynaptic boutons are pinocytosed by the dendrites (Walberg, 1963).

6.8. Topographical Specificity of Synaptic Connections

Specificity of connections to a restricted part of the neuron is well established by anatomical and physiological methods. In the pyramidal cells of the cerebral cortex, the excitatory synapses are mainly restricted to specialized postsynaptic structures, the dendritic spines, whereas inhibitory synapses occur on dendritic shafts and on the cell body (Anderson *et al.*, 1963, 1966; Blackstad and Flood, 1963). In these pyramidal neurons the cell body accounts for only 4 percent of the surface area, the dendrites comprise 96 percent, and the dendritic spines alone account for up to 43 percent of the total surface of the neuron (Mungai, 1967). In stellate neurons of the cerebral cortex, the dendrites, which have bulbous dilations but no spines, occupy up to 87 percent of the surface area (Mungai, 1967).

Topographical specificity of presynaptic terminals on the dendrites and cell body seems to be universal. For example, the central three-fifths of the apical shafts of pyramidal cells in the striate cortex receive geniculostriate afferents, and oblique branches of the apical dendrites and the basal dendrites receive intracortical afferents from Golgi type II neurons and axons that cross in the corpus callosum (A. Globus and Scheibel, 1966). Ultrastructural differences between presynaptic terminals on different parts of the neurons in the cat visual cortex have been demonstrated by Colonnier (1968). He found that the dendritic spines of the pyramidal cells in the visual cortex receive only presynaptic terminals containing round synaptic vesicles, which are presumed to contain excitatory synaptic transmitter (Uchizono, 1965, 1966).

Probably the best-documented example of topographic specificity of synaptic connections is provided by the pyramidal cells of CA1 and CA3 of the mammalian hippocampus (Blackstad 1956; Andersen *et al.*, 1966; D. I. Gottlieb and Cowan, 1973). The distribution of afferent connections is very strikingly segregated on different parts of the hippocampal pyramidal cells. Commissural and septal afferents synapse on the basal dendrites. Intrahippocampal inputs from the basket cells synapse on

the cell bodies of the pyramidal cells. These two inputs are probably inhibitory, as indicated by the markedly flattened synaptic vesicles. The inputs to the apical dendrites of the pyramidal cells are excitatory, as evidenced by their round and clear synaptic vesicles. On the pyramidal cell apical dendrites, the inputs are also segregated as follows: entorhinal afferents synapse on the tips of the dendrites; commissural and septal afferents are confined to the central parts of the dendrites; and the proximal parts of the apical dendrites receive dentate afferents (Fig. 6.14).

6.9. Synaptic Stability and Lability

The problem of continuous turnover of synapses in the adult has received very little attention. Massive elimination of synapses in the developing mammalian CNS should alert one to the possibility that some synapses in the adult, which are generally considered permanent, are continually degraded and completely replaced. However, it would be extremely difficult to obtain evidence of slow turnover of synapses. The best evidence at present available shows that neuromuscular synapses are stable for at least several months (Lichtman *et al.*, 1987).

Activation of synapses which are normally functionally ineffective can occur following injury to the CNS. These synapses are normally ineffective in activating the postsynaptic cell but they become functionally effective after injury to neighboring pathways. In this way latent pathways have been demonstrated in the spinal cord (Basbaum and Wall, 1976; Guth, 1976; Goshgarian and Guth, 1977; Wall, 1977; Devor and Wall, 1978, 1981a,b; Devor, 1983; Seltzer and Devor, 1984). Unmasking of ineffective synapses has been demonstrated in the somatosensory cortex (Wall and Egger, 1971; Frank, 1980), trigeminal nuclear complex (Dostrovsky *et al.*, 1982), and dorsal column nuclei (Merrill and Wall, 1972; Dostrovsky *et al.*, 1976; Millar *et al.*, 1976). This is considered at greater length in Section 11.7. The mechanism of unmasking of functionally ineffective synapses is not known but several conjectures have been made: release of the postsynaptic neuron from chronic inhibition or development of hypersensitivity (Cragg and McLachlan, 1978; Devor *et al.*, 1986), or retraction of glial cell processes resulting in elevated extracellular po-

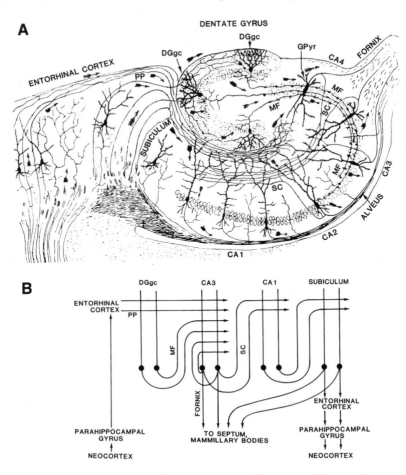

Figure 6.14. Specificity of synaptic connections in the hippocampal formation of the rat. The organization of the main afferents, efferents, and principal neurons of the hippocampal formation is shown in (A), after Ramón y Cajal (1911), and schematically in (B). The giant pyramidal cells (GPyr) in area CA3 project association fibers to the midzone of the dentate granule cell dendritic field, project Schaffer collaterals (SC) to the midzone of dendrites of CA1 pyramidal cells, project to other CA3 pyramidal cells, and send commissural fibers via the fornix to synapse on the midzone of dendrites of dentate granule cells (DGgc) in the contralateral hippocampus. Granule cells in the dentate gyrus (DGgc) project mossy fibers to synapse on the inner zone of dendrites of CA3 pyramidal cells. Fibers originating in the entorhinal cortex project via the perforant path (PP) to synapse on the outer zone of dendrites of pyramidal cells in all parts of the hippocampus. CA1 pyramidal cell axons project mainly to the subiculum. The commissural inputs and the interneurons of the hippocampus are not illustrated.

tassium (Hatten, 1985, 1986). Goshgarian *et al.* (1989) report electron microscopic evidence of astrocytic retraction from between phrenic motoneurons as early as 4 hours after their axons are cut.

Presynaptic terminals disconnect from neurons undergoing chromatolysis. Boutons are disconnected from the dendrites and cell body of the motoneuron after its axon has been cut (Barnard, 1940; Blinzinger and Kreutzberg, 1968; Hamberger *et al.*, 1970b; Kerns and Hinsman, 1973b) and from

autonomic postganglionic neurons undergoing chromatolysis (M. R. Matthews and Nelson, 1975). The disconnection of boutons occurs as the dendrites of the injured neuron retract (Grant, 1965; Grant and Westman, 1968; Sumner and Watson, 1971) so that the numerical density of boutons may be only slightly diminished, although their total numbers may be reduced to about 50 percent in adult rat hypoglossal neurons (Cull, 1974), or to almost zero in facial neurons of newborn rabbits (Torvik and Soreide, 1972). In the adult rat these changes occur during the 2nd–5th week after the hypoglossal nerve is cut. The changes occur more rapidly in the adult rabbit hypoglossal neurons, beginning within 4 days and increasing to a maximum in the 2nd week (Hamberger *et al.*, 1970b). The boutons do not retract far, but they are separated from their postsynaptic sites by glial cell processes that grow into the widened synaptic clefts. The boutons reconnect with the postsynaptic membrane after regeneration of the injured axon has restored contact with its target cells (Sumner and Watson, 1971). This is the only known case of formation of synapses in the adult mammalian CNS.

The disconnection and reconnection of boutons are correlated with changes in synaptic transmission to the injured neuron. This has been observed in the ciliary ganglion after section of the ciliary nerves (Pilar and Landmesser, 1972). Depression of the synaptic transmission through other sympathetic ganglia after section of the postganglionic nerve (G. L. Brown and Pascoe, 1954; Acheson and Remolina, 1955; C. C. Hunt and Riker, 1966; Pilar and Landmesser, 1972) indicates that disconnection of some presynaptic terminals occurs after section of the postsynaptic nerve. A similar interpretation can be made of the altered presynaptic input to spinal motoneurons undergoing chromatolysis (Eccles *et al.*, 1958b; Kuno and Llinás, 1970; Kuno *et al.*, 1974a,b; Mendel *et al.*, 1974).

Marked astrocytic reaction and microglial proliferation are always seen in the vicinity of the chromatolytic nerve cell (Aldskogius, 1982; Graeber and Kreutzberg, 1986). This is discussed at greater length in Section 5.15. Because neuroglial cell reaction and proliferation are not seen around normal neurons, it is unlikely that normal synapses undergo periodic disconnection and reconnection, as Sotelo and Palay (1971) have suggested. Synaptic turnover, if it occurs, must either be very slow or it must not provoke a glial cell response. There is, at present, no evidence of loss or gain of synapses in the healthy adult mammalian brain.

6.10. Comments on Neuronal Plasticity

The term "plasticity" is used to refer to certain types of adjustments of the developing nervous system to changes in the internal or external milieu. For the present purposes, the term is limited mainly to the adjustments that are adaptive, that is, that tend to return the system to its former state or enable the system to function and the organism to survive under the changed conditions. Some derangements of the normal organization, produced by injury, are considered because they may reveal developmental processes that are more difficult to investigate during normal development. An example is the reconstitution of the external granular layer of the cerebellum after its partial destruction by X-rays (Section 10.14). Another good example is the rerouting of embryonic axonal projections to anomalous targets after their definitive targets have been removed during early development. This may occur because specific projections develop from initially widespread projections as a result of retraction of axons from temporary targets (see Section 10.9). Therefore, removal of the definitive targets may leave the axons permanently in possession of their embryonic targets. One of the mechanisms of such plasticity may be that the axons depend on their targets for trophic support, and after removal of the definitive source of trophic support the axon is forced to depend on alternative sources. This discussion is mainly concerned with structural changes such as the growth of new axonal and dendritic branches and the formation of new synaptic connections. Changes in function of preexisting synapses or changes in behavior without recognizable structural changes are not included here.

The diverse phenomena that go by the name of plasticity are unlikely to be the result of one mechanism. There are particular cases of abnormal development resulting in dysfunction when the use of the term is exasperatingly inappropriate. Changes in response to injury that are nonfunctional or malfunctional may have the same relationship to adaptive or constructive plasticity as pathological processes in general have to normal functions. History shows that in the many cases in which the study of deranged function has advanced the knowledge of physiological processes there has been no doubt about which processes were deranged and which were normal. The distinction, which needs to be sharply defined, is frequently blurred in the literature on plasticity in the developing nervous system. The term plasticity is often applied equally to destructive and maladaptive as well as to constructive and adaptive changes in the nervous system. In such cases, unless the term is used with proper qualifications, it loses much of its heuristic value. Whenever the term *"plasticity"* appears in the literature, the reader is called upon to exercise his discernment to the maximum to give a meaning to the term that is appropriate to the context in which it appears.

6.11. Plasticity and Rigidity of Developing Dendrites

One of the main problems of development of dendrites is to understand the processes that give the dendritic tree its characteristic shape in each type of neuron. Since each cell has the same genotype, how does this become expressed as a variety of phenotypes? How important are factors that are intrinsic to the neuron, including its genetic endowment, and how important are factors that arise progressively during development of the dendrites through interaction between the neuron and its environment? To what extent is the pattern of branching and the distribution of synapses on the dendritic tree a matter of chance and to what extent are these determined by the genome? During normal development we may regard the invariant features of the dendrites of any given type of neuron as indications of the rigid components of development, and the variable features may be regarded as indications of the plastic elements.

By experimentally increasing the range of the conditions it is hoped to reveal the full extent of the resulting responses in the developing nervous system. Responses that are qualitatively similar to, although quantitatively greater than, the normal responses of the nervous system to physiological challenges are properly termed plastic changes to distinguish them from pathological changes that obviously result in malformations and malfunctions. This is emphasized here because in many experiments the conditions which are imposed on the organism often exceed the range of conditions to which the developing nervous system can respond adaptively, and the responses to such extreme conditions not only are magnified quantitatively, but also may be qualitatively different from normal plasticity. For this reason, the experiments in which plasticity is studied in response to changes in sensory stimulation are preferable to those in which the

plasticity occurs in response to surgery. The latter sort of experiments can be designed to show which functions and structures are rigid under defined experimental conditions and can show the full extent of compensatory and adaptive changes that can be achieved before maladaptive changes occurs.

That dendritic growth has a large measure of rigidity or autonomy is shown by the conservation of many features of normal dendritic morphology in neurons that are deprived of their normal axonal inputs and in neurons that are improperly aligned or are malpositioned. In the mammalian cerebral cortex, 15–20 percent of the pyramidal cells in the rabbit, cat, and macaque monkey are improperly oriented, and in some cases are totally inverted. In these neurons the pattern of dendritic arbors conforms with the axis of the cell body and not with the axis radial to the cortical surface. By contrast, the axon often arises from an unusual position on the cell body or from a dendrite and arches back to run in the usual direction, as is shown in Fig. 5.15 (Van der Loos, 1965; A. Globus and Scheibel, 1967c). This indicates that the orientation of the dendrites is intrinsically determined for each class of neurons, but the direction of axonal growth is more under the control of external factors. Such inverted pyramidal cells in the visual cortex of the mouse have a normal distribution of spines on their apical dendritic shafts, but the absolute number of spines is diminished (Valverde and Ruiz-Marcos, 1969). This shows either that the distribution of dendritic spines on pyramidal cells may depend on factors that are intrinsic to the neuron and may be relatively independent of external factors such as axonal contacts, or that the appropriate axonal connections with the spines are made regardless of their orientation. The latter alternative is more likely in light of the evidence that normal synaptic connections form on disoriented and misplaced cells in the cerebral cortex of the reeler mutant mouse (see Section 10.15).

Dependence of developing dendrites on transsynaptic stimulation is shown by failure of dendrites to develop fully in the absence of axons that normally terminate on them. This is discussed at length in Section 6.14. The regressive changes that occur in dendrites deprived of afferent connections during development may be illustrated by the effects of destruction of the cerebellar granule cells whose axons (the parallel fibers) normally synapse

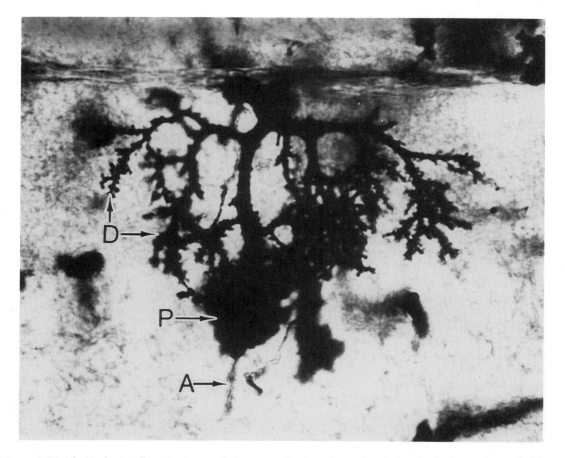

Figure 6.15. The Purkinje cell retains its typical phenotype after loss of granule cells but the dendrites, deprived of their main excitatory afferents, are stunted and deformed. A Purkinje cell is shown in the cerebellar cortex of a rat at P12, after destruction of external granule cells by X-rays at P1. The dendrites have greatly diminished branches and dendritic spines, and are abnormally oriented laterally and away from the surface. A = axon; D = dendrite; P = Purkinje cell. From R. J. Shofer, G. D. Pappas, and D. P. Purpura, in *Response of the Nervous System to Ionizing Radiation*, T. J. Haley and R. S. Snider (eds.), Little, Brown, Boston, 1964.

on the dendritic spines of the Purkinje cells. If the cerebellar granule cells fail to develop because of a genetic abnormality, or are destroyed by a virus infection, irradiation by X-rays, or cytotoxins, the Purkinje cell dendrites fail to develop normally. After removal of the granule cells in neonatal mammals, the immature pattern of Purkinje cell dendritic branching persists in the adult, the dendritic spines survive but are reduced in size, and the Purkinje cell dendrites are not oriented toward the outer surface of the cerebellum but are deflected laterally and downward as if making an attempt to contact fibers in the deeper layers of the cerebellum (Fig. 6.15). It

seems as if the synaptic sites on the Purkinje cell dendrites left vacant by the horizontal fibers may be occupied by synapses from mossy fibers. Such heterologous synapses have been seen with the electron microscope (Altman and Anderson, 1972; Sotelo, 1975). This is supported by the electrophysiological evidence that after virus destruction of granule cells there is abnormal direct excitation of Purkinje cells by mossy fibers (Llinás *et al.*, 1973).

In spite of the failure of the Purkinje cell dendrites to develop fully, they remain surprisingly typical and are unmistakable even when they are incorrectly positioned and disoriented in the weaver mouse, as discussed in Section 10.15. The effects of such insults to the Purkinje cell provide a measure of its plasticity in the sense of its dependence on the external environment and especially its dependence on normal synaptic inputs, while the residual structural and functional integrity of the Purkinje cells gives a measure of its rigidity or autonomy.

6.12. Effects of Stimulation and Deprivation on Development of Dendrites and Synapes

The role of function in morphological development of the nervous system has been demonstrated in many ways: firstly, by showing that the brains of domesticated mammals are significantly smaller than those of comparable species in the wild; secondly, by showing changes in brain morphology of animals reared in conditions of sensorimotor "impoverishment," compared with normal controls or with animals reared in "enriched" environments; thirdly, by showing changes in brain morphology of animals subjected to sensory deprivation or increased stimulation compared with normal controls; fourthly, by determining the effects of pharmacological blockade of nervous activity in intact animals or in nervous tissue *in vitro*.

As Darwin (1868) was the first to point out, the size of the brain tends to be considerably reduced in animals as a result of domestication. The effects of an "enriched" environment on brain weight appear to have relevance to the well-known observation that domesticated animals have smaller brains than the same species in the wild (Kruska, 1987, review). This has been shown by comparing captive and wild birds (Senglaub, 1959), rabbits (Choinowski, 1958), European polecats and ferrets (Schumacher, 1963), cats (Röhrs, 1955), dogs and wolves (Schultz, 1969; Röhrs and Ebinger, 1978), alpacas and llamas (Herre, 1958, 1966; Herre and Thiede, 1965), sheep (Ebinger, 1974), pigs (Herre, 1936; Stephan, 1951; Lunau, 1956; Kruska, 1970a,b, 1972; Kruska and Rohrs, 1974), and donkeys (Herre, 1958, 1966). In all these species the brain weight of the domesticated animals is 15–30 percent less than the brain weight of those in the wild. The maximum effect is on the cerebral isocortex, while the allocortex is less severely affected. The most marked effect is on the visual cortex, which may be reduced by 35 percent in domesticated animals compared with those in the wild. This may be related to the smaller size of the eye and retina in domesticated animals (Wigger, 1939). The cerebellum is reduced by about 15 percent and the medulla by about 10 percent in animals in captivity compared with those in the wild.

Differences in brain weight between different breeds of domestic animals are well documented in pigeons (Haase *et al.*, 1977; Rehkämper *et al.*, 1988), ducks (Senglaub, 1959), rabbits (Moeller, 1975), and dogs (Ebinger, 1980). Homing pigeons have bigger brains than other breeds (Haase *et al.*, 1977), and the tectum, hippocampus, paleostriatum, and especially the neostriatum and olfactory bulb are considerably larger in homing pigeons (Rehkämper *et al.*, 1988). These differences in brain weight are much greater than those reported between animals exposed to "enriched" and "impoverished" environments in the laboratory (Bennett *et al.*, 1969; Rosenzweig *et al.*, 1971, 1972; Walsh *et al.*, 1971, 1973; Cummins and Livesey, 1979).

The difference between brain size in domesticated and wild animals is probably a combination of inherited and environmental effects. An environmental effect is indicated by the fact that the brain weight of the first generation of animals born in captivity is 10–20 percent less than the brain weight of the parents raised in the wild (Herre, 1966, review). The effect seems to be produced by factors acting early in life, since animals born in the wild and domesticated later have the same brain size as animals raised in the wild. However, the conditions required to stimulate brain growth in the wild and the critical period during which the environment might stimulate growth of the brain have not been investigated.

A much slower reduction of only about 5 percent in brain weight after several generations in captivity occurs in polecats (Rempe, 1970) and bank voles (Runzheimer, 1969). Kruska (1987) estimates that it has taken 1000 generations under domestication for the ferret's brain weight to decrease 30 percent compared with wild ancestors, whereas the brain weight of farm minks has diminished by only 5 percent during 100 generations of domestication, which is within the normal range of variability. An inherited effect is shown by the fact that the return of domestic pigs to life in the wild several generations ago has produced no increase in brain size

(Krushka and Röhrs, 1974). For additional discussion of the relation of brain weight to body weight see Section 2.12.

There are many reports of changes in dendritic spines in the cerebral cortex following either sensorimotor deprivation or increased functional activity. The significance of such changes has to be considered in the light of the facts that dendritic spines in the cerebral cortex form excitatory synapses almost exclusively, and that cerebral cortical dendrites and synapses develop postnatally. Rats raised in an enriched environment for 30 days after weaning have increased density of dendritic spines on pyramidal neurons of the visual cortex compared with rats raised under impoverished conditions (Globus et al., 1973). Continuous visual stimulation of rats from birth to 80 days results in higher density of dendritic spines on pyramidal cells in layers IV and V of the visual cortex, starting on P16 on the proximal part of the apical dendrite and extending to the entire dendritic tree by P20 (Parnavelas, 1978). In adult cats, long-term electrical stimulation of the cerebral cortex results in higher density of dendritic spines and increased branching of apical dendrites of pyramidal cells of the suprasylvian gyrus on the opposite side (Rutledge et al., 1974). Increased branching of dendrites of cortical pyramidal cells occurs after young or adult rats are raised in an enriched environment compared to impoverished conditions (Holloway, 1966; Volkmer and Greenough, 1972; Greenough and Volkmar, 1973; Uylings et al., 1978; Juraska, 1984).

A number of studies show that some dendritic spines develop in the absence of visual stimulation while other spines depend on visual input for their development. Thus the dendritic spines and synapses on them start developing before birth in all mammals, and the number of dendritic spines continues to increase after birth before the eyes open in mice, rats, and cats (Cragg, 1975a,c). However, a large increase in the number of dendritic spines occurs at the time of eye opening on postnatal days 10–19, and this increase is almost completely prevented by keeping the mice in the dark, as is shown in Fig. 6.16 (Ruiz-Marcos and Valverde, 1969). In mice reared in the dark, the characteristic spatial distribution of dendritic spines is maintained (exponential increase in numbers of spines with increasing distance from the cell body), but the absolute number of spines is reduced along the whole length

of the dendritic shafts (Valverde and Ruiz-Marcos, 1969). The majority of spines are apparently unaffected by visual deprivation. The effect is reversible: returning the dark-reared mice to normal visual stimulation results in a return to nearly normal numbers of spines within a week (Valverde, 1971). The number of spines on pyramidal cells in layers IV and V of the rat's visual cortex can be increased above control levels by raising the rats in constant dim light (Parnavelas et al., 1973).

Increase in brain weight and thickness and weight of cerebral cortex occurs in rats raised under environmentally enriched conditions (Bennett et al., 1964, 1969; Diamond et al., 1964, 1966, 1967; Rosenzweig et al., 1971, 1972; Walsh et al., 1971, 1973; Cummins and Livesey, 1979; D. G. Jones and Smith, 1980, review; Walsh, 1981, review). The effect occurs in blinded rats (Krech et al., 1963). No changes in thickness of visual cortex were found in mice reared in continuous light from birth to 51 days compared with controls reared under normal lighting conditions (Egert, 1975). The enriched environmental conditions may have complex effects, including nutritional and hormonal changes (Juraska, 1984), and are thus not exactly comparable to sensory stimulation. Moreover, the changes produced in the cerebral cortex by environmental enrichment are complex and include increased glial cell proliferation in the cortical radiations and corpus callosum (Altman and Das, 1964), increased number of cortical astrocytes (Diamond et al., 1966; Szeligo and Leblond, 1977), and an initial reduction in glial cells followed by increases of astrocytes and oligodendrocytes in rats handled for the first 10 days after birth (Sturrock et al., 1983). Evidence of increased numbers of cortical neurons is conflicting: no changes were found in rats raised under enriched conditions (Diamond et al., 1966; Szeligo and Leblond, 1977), whereas rats handled daily for 11 days after birth were found to have increased nerve cell proliferation in the neocortex, hippocampus, and cerebellar cortex (Altman et al., 1968a,b).

The number of neurons per unit volume of visual cortex is reduced in rats raised with enriched experience, indicating that the neurons are more widely separated (Turner and Greenough, 1985). In the visual cortex of the cat raised with enriched experience, the numerical density of symmetrical synapses containing flattened vesicles is nearly twice the density found in the visual cortex of cats with

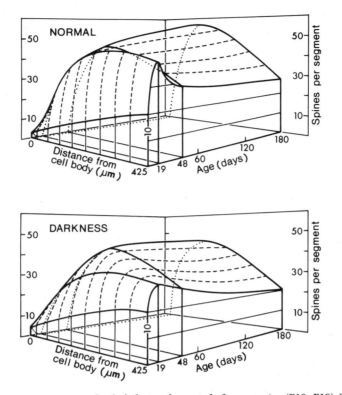

Figure 6.16. An effect of rearing mice in the dark during the period of eye opening (P10–P19). This results in a reduction in the number of spines on apical dendritic shafts of pyramidal cells in the visual cortex, but the characteristic spatial distribution of spines is relatively unaffected when compared with normal. From A. Ruiz-Marcos and F. Valverde, *Exp. Brain Res.* 8:284–294 (1969).

impoverished experience (Beaulieu and Colonnier, 1987). This is especially significant because most of the symmetrical synapses with flattened vesicles in the visual cortex are inhibitory GABAergic (Wolff *et al.*, 1984; Somogyi and Hodgson, 1985), and because many of the receptive field properties of visual cortical neurons are GABA dependent (Sillito *et al.*, 1980). The numerical density of boutons with flattened vesicles is 17 percent lower and the number of contacts per bouton is lower in enriched cortex, but the total number of boutons remains unchanged. The effect of enriched experience is to reduce the number of contacts per bouton, but the contact area remains unchanged (Beaulieu and Colonnier, 1988).

Deprivation of olfactory receptors produced by blocking one of the external nostrils of the rat from postnatal days 1–30 results in a 25 percent reduction in volume of the ipsilateral olfactory bulb (Brunjes and Frazier, 1986). The number of granule

cells is greatly decreased in the deprived olfactory bulb (Benson *et al.*, 1984; Skeen *et al.*, 1985; Frazier and Brunjes, 1988) but it is not clear whether this is the result of diminished proliferation or increased cell death or both. The granule cells are the last neurons to be generated and the effect is delayed until P20 (Frazier and Brunjes, 1988). Changes in mitral and tufted cells in the olfactory bulb have been reported after olfactory deprivation (Meisami, 1976; Meisami and Safari, 1981; Meisami and Noushinfar, 1986; Skeen *et al.*, 1986), but those changes were not found by others (Benson *et al.*, 1984; Frazier and Brunjes, 1988).

The most revealing studies on the effects of sensory input have been on development of the visual system, because the quantity and quality of the visual stimulus can be precisely controlled, because the anatomy of the system is known in sufficient detail to permit accurate localization of any effects, and, above all, because the relationship between structure and function is securely established for many types of identified neurons and synapses in the visual system. The pertinent information about the various types of neurons in the visual pathways of mammals is given in Section 11.17.

Synaptogenesis occurs in the retina of the cat and the rat before birth, although the receptor outer segments become evident only on the 5th day after birth (Cragg, 1975a). This shows that synaptogenesis can occur without visual experience. Other studies have shown that all types of retinal cells and synapses develop in rats reared in total darkness for up to 3 years (Burke and Hayhow, 1968). Rats raised with the eyelids sutured closed for 12–18 months develop normal retinal ganglion cell activity (Sherman and Stone, 1973). The only retinal changes that have been found consistently in rats raised from birth in darkness or with the eyes occluded is an increase in the number of amacrine cell to bipolar cell synapses (Fifková, 1972, 1973; Sosula and Glow, 1970) and an increase in the number of amacrine to ganglion cell synapses in the inner plexiform layer (Sosula and Glow, 1970; Chernenko and West, 1976). It should also be noted that exposure to continuous illumination damages the photoreceptors and causes degenerative changes in the retina of rats (Noell et al., 1966; Noell and Albrecht, 1971; Olstein and Anderson, 1972).

It is necessary to make some distinctions between those components whose development is sensitive and those that are insensitive to visual stimulation and deprivation. This is illustrated by the effects of visual experience on the visual cortex. In the cat's visual system, the majority of synapses develop in the absence of stimulation. Cragg (1975a) reported that binocular lid suture in cats from the time of opening the eyes to 45 days of age results in 30 percent reduction of the number of synapses in the visual cortex. Visual deprivation produces a reduction in the thickness of layers II and IV of the visual cortex (Gyllensten, 1959; Gyllensten et al., 1965), a reduction in the number of synapses in the visual cortex (Cragg, 1967, 1969, 1972c, 1975a,b), or a reduction in the dendritic spines of pyramidal neurons in layer IV of the striate cortex (Valverde, 1967; A. Globus and Scheibel, 1967b; Ruiz-Marcos and Valverde, 1969; Parnavelas et al., 1973). Coleman and Riesen (1968) reported that stellate cells in layer IV of the visual cortex of cats reared in darkness have fewer and shorter dendrites than the same

cells in normal cats. Valverde (1976) found shorter axons of local-circuit neurons in the visual cortex of mice reared in darkness for 19 days.

There is good evidence that neuronal activity plays an important role in maintenance and elimination of synapses (see Sections 6.5, 11.15, 11.16, and 11.21). However, the role of nerve activity in the initial formation of synapses is uncertain. Probably this is a reflection of the complexity of many of the experiments, in which it is difficult to identify all the dependent variables, and probably different types of synapses have different functional requirements for their development. Neuromuscular synapses develop even though patterns of nerve activity are not normal, in tissue culture, after pharmacological blockade of action potentials, or after blockade of synaptic transmission. Neuromuscular junctions develop in tissue culture of nerve and muscle of amphibians (Harrison, 1907b; Corner and Crain, 1964; M. W. Cohen, 1972), chicks (Szepsenwol, 1947; James and Tresman, 1969; Fischbach, 1972), and rats and mice (S. M. Crain, 1966; Bornstein et al., 1968; Robbins and Yonezawa, 1971). Functional neuromuscular junctions develop between separate pieces of spinal cord and muscle of the chick embryo (Veneroni, 1968; Veneroni and Murray, 1969; Nakai, 1969) and mammalian fetus (S. M. Crain, 1964, 1966, 1968; E. R. Peterson and Crain, 1968), cultured in close proximity (S. M. Crain, 1974, 1976, reviews). Neither release of acetylcholine from the nerve ending nor binding to receptors on the muscle is required for the development of neuromuscular junctions. Neuromuscular junctions form in the chick embryo injected with agents that block release or uptake of acetylcholine—curare, botulinum toxin, hemicholinium, alphabungarotoxin, or absence of calcium—although severe muscular atrophy occurs (Giacobini et al., 1973; S. S. Freeman et al., 1976; Henderson et al., 1984). Neuromuscular connections develop in cocultures of skeletal muscle and nervous tissue in the presence of curare in concentrations which greatly reduce the sensitivity of the muscle to acetylcholine (S. M. Crain and Peterson, 1967, 1974; M. W. Cohen, 1972; Steinbach et al., 1973). Neuromuscular connections also develop in rat skeletal muscle that is mechanically immobilized (Juntunen, 1973a). However, immobilized skeletal muscle later undergoes atrophy (Jirmanová and Zelená, 1970; Riley and Allin, 1973; Tomanek and Lund, 1974).

The mere fact that synapses develop between neurons in tissue culture indicates that highly specific patterns of impulse traffic are not required for that level of development, but it does not prove that the same holds for normal development. Similarly, synapses that appear to be morphologically normal develop *in vitro* after blockade of action potentials with xylocaine (Model *et al.*, 1971) or tetrodotoxin (Huizen *et al.*, 1985). Those negative results should be contrasted with the following positive results: blockade of action potentials by means of tetrodotoxin results in failure of development of retinogeniculate synapses (Kalil *et al.*, 1986), and blockage of electrical activity by means of ketamine–xylazine anesthetic results in failure of development of ocular dominance columns in kittens (Rauschecker and Hahn, 1987). There is also evidence of activity-dependent sharpening and stabilization of the goldfish retinotectal projection (Schmidt, 1985; Eisele and Schmidt, 1988; Schmidt *et al.*, 1988) and the mammalian retinogeniculate system (Dubin *et al.*, 1986; Kalil *et al.*, 1986). For additional examples see Sections 11.16. 11.18, and 11.21.

Removal of an eye results in the well-known transneuronal degeneration of lateral geniculate neurons (Minkowski, 1920; M. R. Matthews *et al.*, 1960) and transneuronal changes in the striate cortex, as discussed in Section 6.14. These changes consist of diminution of dendritic spines at the base of the apical dendrites of pyramidal cells in layer IV of the striate cortex (A. Globus and Scheibel, 1966, 1967a–d; Valverde, 1968; Valverde and Esteban, 1968). Changes in the orientation of dendrites of stellate cells in the visual cortex have been seen after removal of the eye of the mouse at birth (Valverde, 1968). The stellate cells have dendrites that normally radiate in all directions through layers III, IV, and V of the striate cortex. After removal of the eye at birth, layer IV is rendered virtually free of stellate cell dendrites, which radiate mainly into layers II and III. The geniculostriate visual afferent axons are also absent from layer IV; hence Valverde concluded that the dendrites of stellate cells that normally connect in layer IV undergo compensatory growth to connect in layers II and III with recurrent collaterals of superficial pyramidal neurons and in layer V with horizontal collaterals of deep pyramidal cells. The adjustment of synaptic associations in the striate cortex deprived of afferent optic fibers seems

to be similar to the occupation by aberrant presynaptic terminals of synaptic sites on dendrites that have been left vacant by the failure of development of the normal contingent of afferent fibers. Many other examples are given later of relocation of nerve endings from their normal synaptic sites to occupy vacant postsynaptic sites. In general, these examples show that degeneration of developing presynaptic terminals may leave synaptic sites vacant and, therefore, "up for grabs." Ingrowing axonal terminals may occupy the vacant postsynaptic sites and form aberrant connections. Preemption of vacant synaptic sites by sprouts from neighboring axons occurs in the peripheral nervous system (Section 9.9) and in the CNS, as discussed in the following section.

6.13. Synaptic Reorganization in the CNS

William James (1890) was bold enough to conjecture *"why collateral innervation would establish itself after loss of brain tissue, and why the incoming stimuli would find their way out again, after an interval, by their former paths"* (W. James, 1890, Vol. II, p. 592). He wrote: *"The normal paths are only paths of least resistance. If they get blocked or cut, paths formerly more resistant become the least resistant paths under the changed conditions. . . . My conclusion then is this: that some of the restitution of function (especially where the cortical lesion is not too great) is probably due to genuinely vicarious function on the part of the centres that remain; whilst some of it is due to the passing off of inhibitions"* (W. James, 1890, Vol. I, pp. 71–72).

Preemption of vacant synaptic sites by axonal sprouts from uninjured neighboring afferents shows that the conditions under which sprouting occurs are similar in many cases. Regeneration of injured nerve fibers must be distinguished from collateral sprouting of uninjured axons. Axonal sprouting in the CNS is almost invariably of the latter type (Raisman, 1966, 1969; Raisman and Field, 1972; Lynch *et al.*, 1972, 1974; Cotman *et al.*, 1973; Gentschev and Sotelo, 1973; Rustioni and Sotelo, 1974; Steward *et al.*, 1974, 1976; Gage *et al.*, 1983a,b). The development of collateral sprouting from uninjured axons in the vicinity of CNS injuries is an indication of release of sprouting factors from the denervated neurons and possibly from associated glial cells, but the exact mechanism of stimulation of axonal sprouting in the CNS is still a matter of conjecture.

In the first modern study of collateral sprouting in the CNS, C. N. Liu and Chambers (1958) partially denervated the spinal cord of adult cats by cutting dorsal roots or by section of the corticospinal tract on one side. About 10 months later, after all debris of degeneration had been removed, an adjacent dorsal root was sectioned bilaterally. The animal was killed 4–5 days later, and the axonal degeneration resulting from the section of the final dorsal root was determined. The authors reported an increase in the quantity and extent of degeneration on the side opposite the severed corticospinal tract and on the same side as the chronically sectioned dorsal roots. This shows that sprouting of axons in the spinal cord occurs from the intact dorsal roots. This has been confirmed autoradiographically (M. Murray and Goldberger, 1974) in cats and monkeys. McCouch *et al.* (1958) found that presynaptic dorsal root potentials are increased below a hemisection of the spinal cord compared with the normal side, and they suggest that this arises from sprouting of dorsal roots in the spinal cord.

Collateral sprouting occurs in the septal nuclei of the adult rat (Raisman, 1969; Raisman and Field, 1973b). The two main inputs to this nuclear complex are from the brainstem via the medial forebrain bundle and from the hippocampus via the fornix. Their synaptic endings are sufficiently different to be easily distinguishable in electron micrographs. Removal of the hippocampal afferents results in their replacement by collateral sprouts from septal afferents from the medial forebrain bundle (Fig. 6.17). Sprouting has been demonstrated with the electron microscope in the ventral cochlear nucleus of the adult rat (Gentschev and Sotelo, 1973) and in the nucleus gracilis of the cat (Rustioni and Sotelo, 1974). In the cochlear nucleus of the adult rat, removal of the primary afferents results in reinnervation by sprouting of uninjured afferents in 5–9 days (Gentschev and Sotelo, 1973). In these cases, the sprouting occurs over a distance of about 250 μm or less. The reinnervation is heterologous (as the ultrastructure of the reinnervating synaptic boutons in each case is different from the original synaptic terminals) and does not lead to functional recovery. There is no evidence, except the presence of normal

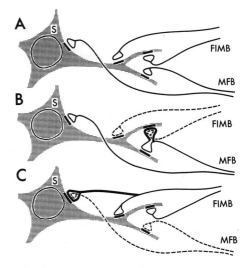

Figure 6.17. Rearrangements of synaptic connections of neurons in the septal nuclei after section of either one of the two afferent systems. (A) The normal situation: afferents from the medial forebrain bundle (MFB) terminate in boutons on the septal neuron soma (S) and dendrites, whereas some fimbrial afferents (FIMB) are restricted in termination on dendrites. (B) Several weeks after section of fimbrial afferents, the MFB axons extend from their own terminal sites to occupy the vacated sites, thus forming double synapses. Degenerated afferents and synapses are shown by dashed lines, presumed plastic changes by heavy lines. (C) Several weeks after a MFB lesion, the fimbrial fibers now give rise to terminals occupying somatic sites which are presumably those vacated as a result of the former lesion. From G. Raisman, *Brain Res.* 14:25–48 (1969).

components of the synapse, that effective transmissions occurs at these new synapses.

Extensive collateral sprouting of intact adrenergic neurons occurs after neighboring adrenergic neurons in the CNS have been cut (Stenevi *et al.,* 1973; R. Y. Moore *et al.,* 1973, review). These adrenergic neurons also regenerate vigorously. Their axons can innervate tissues that normally receive adrenergic innervation, such as the iris, when these tissues are implanted in the region of cut central adrenergic neurons in the medial forebrain bundle and adjacent nigrostriatal tract of adult rats and rabbits. Sprouts from central adrenergic neurons can be detected histochemically 5–7 days postoperative (R. Y. Moore *et al.,* 1971). In all these cases, the recovery is quite rapid, because the distance over which sprouts have to grow is quite small, usually less than 250 μm, and because the degenerating boutons which the sprouts replace are removed rapidly. However, delayed reinnervation has been reported in the nucleus gracilis of the cat: the primary afferents degenerate within a few days but reinnervation, by axons of unknown origin, occurs only after 1–6 months (Rustioni and Sotelo, 1974).

The hippocampal formation lends itself particularly well to studies of specific formation of synapses on granule and pyramidal cells and for studies of the plasticity or rigidity of those axodendritic synapses. There is a topographically organized arrangement of inputs to the granule cells of the dentate gyrus, as shown in Fig. 6.14, and each of the inputs can easily be removed experimentally. The dentate gyrus serves as a relay between the entorhinal cortex and the regio inferior of the hippocampus. In the adult rat, lesions of the entorhinal cortex, from which the perforant or temporoammonic pathway originates, denervate the distal half of the dendrites of granule cells of the fascia dentata. This results in sprouting of the cholinergic endings, which originate in the septum and normally end on the distal segment of the granule cell dendrites. It also results in sprouting of the commissural fibers that normally terminate on the proximal part of the granule cell dendrites. The same phenomenon occurs when other afferents to the granule cell dendrites are removed. In all cases, the deafferented dendrites are reafferented by sprouts from neighboring terminals on the same dendrites (Lynch et al., 1973a–c, 1974). These sprouts are, therefore, no longer than 250 μm. Somewhat more extensive sprouting has been seen from the entorhinal system of the opposite side, which normally sends a very sparse projection to the contralateral dentate gyrus. These sprouts may extend as much as 2 or 3 mm across the hippocampal fissure to reinnervate the deafferented granule cell dendrites (Steward et al., 1974). The cells of origin of these reinnervating sprouts from the contralateral cortex are of the same type as those which normally innervate the dentate granule cells from the ipsilateral cortex (Steward et al., 1976).

These experiments show that the precise regional localization of the different inputs to the granule cell dendrites is unlikely to be due to an exclusive biochemical affinity of each type of afferent for a specific dendritic zone. Rather, the topographical segregation of afferents on the dendrites may develop as the result of a temporal order

of arrival of each type of afferent in relation to outgrowth of the dendritic tree, and possibly due to a competition between the afferents for the available synaptic sites on the dendrites (D. I. Gottlieb and Cowan, 1972).

The anatomical correlate of the formation of new connections is the almost complete reappearance of dendritic spines 20–80 days after entorhinal lesions (Parnavelas et al., 1974). These experiments also show that the number of spines is a function of the dendrites—deafferentation results in a reduction of spines and therefore the axons are required for their maintenance, but regardless of the type of reinnervating axons, the number of dendritic spines returns to a constant numerical density. These observations show that the dendritic spines in the cerebral cortical granule and pyramidal cells are very labile and dependent on synaptic input for their development and survival. For example, removal of the entorhinal afferents, which occupy the distal half of the dendrites of granule cells in the dentate gyrus, results in loss of 30 percent of spines. However, the spines return to normal by 60 days after the lesion (Parnavelas et al., 1974). Valverde (1971) has shown that there is a loss of spines from the apical dendrites of pyramidal cells of mice raised in the dark from birth to 20 days of age. However, when these animals are returned to normal visual experience, there is a partial recovery of the number of apical dendritic spines. Raisman and Field (1973b) have reported that the spines in the septal nuclei are reduced by 50 percent 7 days after removal of their hippocampal afferents, but the spine density returns to normal by 30 days postoperative. Functional connections are formed by sprouts which can first be detected on the dendrites of granule cells in the hippocampal dentate gyrus 10–14 days after a lesion of the entorhinal cortex (Steward et al., 1974).

Another type of synaptic reorganization occurs after removal of the primary visual cortex of the rabbit. This operation results, during the following 2 weeks, in death of almost all the neurons in the dorsal nucleus of the lateral geniculate nucleus (LGN). One year postoperative, Ralston and Chow (1973) observed synaptic reorganization in the LGN so that the optic afferents that form axodendritic synapses on the LGN neurons, when deprived of their normal postsynaptic sites, form axoaxonal synapses, probably with surviving interneurons of the nucleus. Such synaptic reorganization can hardly be regarded as a form of physiological compensation or adaptation, as it is certain that no recovery of visual function occurs.

Anomalous connections in the visual system of the golden hamster develop if lesions are made in the optic tract in the newborn animal but not when similar lesions are made in adults. No reconnections appear to form after lesions of the visual system in adult mammals. By contrast, when the superior colliculus is damaged soon after birth, some optic axons grow into the residual part of the colliculus. Others cross the midline to form functional connections in the opposite, undamaged colliculus. Here the axons from the two eyes segregate in separate regions of the colliculus. These connections result in maladaptive turning of the head away from a visual stimulus. Other optic axons connect anomalously with two regions of the thalamus, the nucleus lateralis posterior and the ventral lateral geniculate nucleus, which normally receive inputs from the superior colliculus but do not normally receive direct retinal projections. In the review of his observations, G. E. Schneider (1973) attributes these anomalous sprouts to the tendency, first noted by Ramón y Cajal (1928), for axons to conserve the total quantity of their terminal arborizations (also see Devor and Schneider, 1975). It should be noted, however, that not all the optic axons have reached the colliculus at the time of the operation, and the anomalous projections might arise not as a result of pruning of their axonal terminals in the colliculus, but as a result of misrouting before arrival at the colliculus. Such misrouting of optic axons to the wrong side of the brain has been found after removal of the eye in newborn rats, an effect that is not observed when the eye is removed after the 10th day after birth (R. D. Lund et al., 1973; R. D. Lund and Lund, 1973). As in the initial report of axonal sprouting in the visual system following eye removal in the 3-month-old rat (D. C. Goodman and Horel, 1966), subsequent reports have confirmed and extended the evidence showing that the anomalous sprouts are more extensive when the eye is removed shortly after birth (Guillery, 1972; Kalil, 1972, 1973; Chow et al., 1973; R. D. Lund et al., 1973; R. D. Lund, 1978; Finlay et al., 1979). The effects are due to a combination of survival of retinal ganglion cells that would normally have died (see Section 8.3), sprouting from the optic tract of the remaining eye in areas that normally receive inputs from both eyes, and

also due to misrouting of retinal axons that have not yet completed their growth to the visual centers (D. C. Goodman et al., 1973; Stanfield and Cowan, 1976).

The functional effectiveness of collateral sprouting varies from nonfunctional to grossly malfunctional, as after lesions to the visual pathways of newborn hamsters. These animals are extremely immature at birth and show the most rapid and extensive collateral sprouting that has been observed in the CNS of mammals. Yet, despite considerable recovery of function, the ultimate effect is maladaptive behavior. For example, after unilateral removal of the superior colliculus in the newborn hamster, G. F. Schneider (1970, 1973, review) found that optic axons destined for the ablated superior colliculus form functional connections with the remaining superior colliculus. This results in misdirected visual pursuit behavior which is not corrected by experience. A functional deficit also follows partial transsection of the lateral olfactory tract in the newborn hamster; mating behavior in adult life is impaired, apparently as a result of collateral sprouts from residual axons that form aberrant connections (Devor, 1975).

Another sort of malfunction resulting from collateral sprouting is the spasticity and hyperreflexia that occur after lesions of the descending spinal fiber tracts: these tracts do not regenerate and thus their target neurons are reinnervated by sprouting of segmental afferents (Chambers et al., 1973; M. Murray and Goldberger, 1974). In the cerebellar cortex, the synaptic reorganization that occurs to a limited extent after loss of parallel fibers does not result in any improvement of the cerebellar ataxia (see Section 10.14). These observations are consistent in principle, if not in all details, with Cajal's pessimistic appraisal of the functional value of the abortive regeneration he observed in the mammalian CNS as expressed in the frequently cited statement that "in adult centers the nerve paths are something fixed, ended, immutable. Everything may die, nothing may be regenerated" (Ramón y Cajal, 1928, p. 750).

The question of whether failure of the CNS to support axon regeneration is due to inability of the central neurons to regenerate or to the nonpermissive conditions of the environment is considered at great length by Cajal in his masterpiece, Degeneration and Regeneration of the Nervous System (1928).

He discusses the experiments of Tello (1911) in which peripheral nerves were grafted in the CNS of the rabbit. After 12 days Tello observed growth of central axons into the graft. Cajal comments: *"They behaved in their growth, branching, orientation, energetic progress, etc., exactly like the sprouts of the central stump of a cut nerve. . . . These newly formed fibres converge from various points of the cortex, as though they were attracted by an irresistible force."* Cajal concludes that this is a transient trophic stimulus because some months later the graft as well as the newly formed fibers disappear (Ramón y Cajal, 1928, pp. 738–744). The use of peripheral nerve grafts to enhance CNS regeneration was reviewed by Ramón y Cajal (1928). The idea was revived by Kao (1974) and Kao et al. (1977), who showed that axonal regeneration in the mammalian spinal cord can be enhanced by implanting peripheral nerve or ganglion. This result has been extended by Aguayo and colleagues (Aguayo et al., 1979, 1982, 1984, 1985; Richardson et al., 1980, 1982; David and Aguayo, 1981; Benfey and Aguayo, 1982; Aguayo, 1985; Sceats et al., 1986; Bray et al., 1987; Vidal-Sanz et al., 1987). They have shown that peripheral nerves grafted into the CNS stimulate regeneration of CNS axons into the graft. This probably occurs as a result of both release of neurotrophic factors from Schwann cells and the presence of permissive conditions in the graft. Therefore, the abortive regeneration of central axons is not due to their intrinsic inability to regenerate, but to nonpermissive conditions in the CNS, especially contact of regenerating axons with oligodendroglial cells (Caroni and Schwab, 1988a,b, 1989; Schwab and Caroni, 1988).

The problem of the long-term survival and function of heterologous synapses remains unsolved. The little evidence that is now available shows that some heterologous synapses may persist structurally and functionally although they result in dysfunction, while other heterologous synapses are eliminated or become functionally ineffective. In terms of the hypothesis of functional validation of synaptic connections (M. Jacobson, 1970a,b, 1974b; Hirsch and Jacobson, 1975), newly formed synapses are labile unless stabilized by function (see also Changeux and Danchin, 1976). Some heterologous synapses may not become stabilized and may therefore degenerate or become functionally ineffective. For example, in the cerebellum of the staggerer mutant

mouse, there is a failure of development of Purkinje cell dendritic spines that normally connect with the parallel fibers of the granule cells. The parallel fibers develop and form transient contacts with the dendritic shafts of Purkinje cells, but eventually, as the animal matures, the parallel fibers degenerate and the granule cells die.

To balance these examples of collateral sprouting and reinnervation in the CNS, there are as many cases where sprouting and reinnervation have not been detected following partial deafferentation of central nuclei. For example, in adult cats and kittens, no sprouting of cervical primary afferents onto the spinal nucleus of the trigeminal nerve could be found a year or more after trigeminal denervation (Kerr, 1972, 1975a,b). In that instance, sprouting of cervical primary afferent axons was expected because it is known that trigeminal denervation results in deafferentation of the dorsal horn of the spinal cord at the level of C1. Absence of sprouting has also been reported in the dorsal column nuclei after chronic deafferentation (Rustioni and Molenaar, 1975). Sprouting of the auditory nerve into the medial superior olive is not seen after removal of the anteroventral cochlear nucleus (C. N. Liu and Liu, 1971; E. L. White and Nolan, 1974). In the adult cat, after removal of the optic input, the lateral geniculate nucleus is not reinnervated by collateral sprouts (Guillery, 1972b), although in kittens a slight amount of translaminar sprouting has been reported (Hickey, 1975). In general, reinnervation of deafferented neurons in the mammalian visual system does not occur in the adult. Finally, there are many cases, reviewed by Stenevi et al. (1973), of failure to detect sprouting of central aminergic neurons into deafferented regions such as the superior colliculus, lumbar spinal cord, hypothalamus, and other regions of the CNS in which there is a low density of adrenergic innervation. These regions are far removed from a region of high density of adrenergic nerves, and no sprouting can be expected over such distances.

There are thus almost as many reports of failure to find sprouting as there are reports of successful sprouting in the mammalian CNS, and there seems to be a reason for this difference. In the cases where sprouting is expected but is not found, the axons which are expected to sprout are in close proximity to the denervated zone but they are segregated from the axonal terminals that are removed, whereas in the successful cases the sprouting axons share part of the same postsynaptic zone. The lack of sprouting may be due to a failure of release, transmission, or reception of the signal that must arise from the denervated zone. Obviously, the transmission of the necessary signals will be facilitated if the responding axonal terminals are already connected to or close to the denervated cell, and that is the situation in most cases of sprouting in the CNS. In all cases, proximity is a vital factor, and the distances are very short (usually less than 250 μm) over which sprouts have to grow for reafferentation to occur. In most but not all cases, the sprouts arise from axons that belong to the same system as the axons that they replace. As a general rule, afferents which are deprived of their normal targets prefer alternative targets in the same functional system, but if those are removed, the afferents may connect with other anomalous targets and may even be misrouted into foreign functional systems and form connections there (see Section 10.9). For example, rearrangements within the hippocampus, septal nuclei, or spinal cord are confined in each case to a single functional system. This is also true of the visual system: optic tract axons sprout to anomalous positions but remain confined to the visual system.

The extent of anomalous projections after injury during development depends on the stage of development and the extent of the normal transient redundant axonal projections at that stage. If the transient projections cross between pathways that are later restricted to a single modality (see Section 10.9), removal of the definitive pathway or target may result in persistence of alternative pathways. Alternatively, if the redundancy is restricted to a single modality, the plasticity will likewise be restricted.

The stimulus for collateral sprouting in the CNS is still a matter of conjecture. There are three alternative theories: first, that sprouting is stimulated by products of degeneration; second, that sprouting is stimulated by trophic factors produced by the postsynaptic cells or their associated glial cells; third, that sprouting is due to an inherent tendency of neurons to conserve their protoplasmic volume. One observation makes it unlikely that sprouting is stimulated by products of degeneration, namely, that the sprouts can grow into a region that is not denervated. For example, in the newborn hamster, after unilateral removal of the

superior colliculus, sprouts of optic nerve fibers grow into the residual uninjured superior colliculus.

The theory that sprouting is due to an inherent tendency of the neuron to conserve its original protoplasmic volume applies only to cases in which part of the axon is cut away and sprouts emerge from the residual part to compensate for the loss of volume. This theory cannot account for the cases in which sprouting occurs from uninjured neurons in the neighborhood of a denervated region. Neither can that "pruning" hypothesis (G. E. Schneider, 1973; Devor and Schneider, 1975; Sabel and Schneider, 1988) account for sprouting of motoneuron endings after treatment with botulinum toxin (M. R. Bennett, 1983, review). On the other hand, the latter observation is consistent with a mechanism in which botulinum toxin prevents activity of the muscle and thus increases production or release of a trophic factor or factors (see Section 9.8).

Suggestive of the theory that the postsynaptic cells (and associated glial cells) release a trophic factor that is utilized or neutralized by nerve endings is the observation that reinnervation of vacated synaptic sites is delayed until the original nerve endings have disappeared. This is also consistent with the theory that presynaptic endings inhibit production or release of one or more trophic factors, possibly by depolarization of the postsynaptic cell. This theory also has the virtue of parsimony in that it applies to sprouting in the CNS as well as to sprouting in the peripheral nervous system (see Section 9.9). The theory of alternative sources of trophic support can also explain why retraction of initially redundant axonal and dendritic branches occurs: the branches persist which receive the strongest trophic support, but if those are removed experimentally, axons and dendrites may persist and grow to the next best source of trophic support.

6.14. Role of Transneuronal Stimulation on Developing Neurons

As connections develop between neurons, the possibility arises of one neuron stimulating the development of another across the synapse. As a result of such transsynaptic or transneuronal stimulation, neurons may exercise an influence on others, either directly across a single synapse or indirectly via interneurons in a chain or circuit.

Transneuronal stimulation is required by many types of neurons to complete their development. If the direction of the effect is from the presynaptic to the postsynaptic neuron, it is referred to as *anterograde transsynaptic or anterograde transneuronal stimulation*, whereas if the stimulation is in the reverse direction, it is termed *retrograde transsynaptic or retrograde transneuronal stimulation*. The evidence shows that cellular proliferation and the initial stages of cellular differentiation in the nervous system can occur in the absence of intracentral, afferent, or efferent connections, but the final maturation and continued vitality of neurons depend on transsynaptic stimulation. The transsynaptic effects continue throughout life and can be demonstrated in adult mammals by showing that some neurons atrophy after removal of their afferent nerves or their postsynaptic targets (see Section 6.11).

There is a wealth of evidence that transsynaptic trophic stimulation is required for survival of neurons, that removal of afferents leads to neuronal atrophy and death, and that the effect of deafferentation is more severe in the young than in the adults of the same species (reviewed by Cowan, 1970; Guillery, 1974; Globus, 1975; Smith, 1977). Deafferentation has been shown to result in neuronal atrophy and death in the avian isthmo-optic nucleus (Sohal, 1976); the avian nucleus magnocellularis, nucleus angularis, and nucleus tangentialis (Levi-Montalcini, 1949; Peusner and Morest, 1977; Rubel, 1978; Lippe *et al.*, 1980; Durham and Rubel, 1983; Born and Rubel, 1985; see Section 6.4); the cochlear nucleus (Kane, 1974; Trune, 1982a,b); the dorsal lateral geniculate nucleus (Tsang, 1937; Kupfer and Palmer, 1964; Guillery, 1973; Heumann and Rabinowicz, 1980; Kalil, 1980); the ventral lateral geniculate nucleus and ectomamillary nucleus (Peduzzi and Crossland, 1983); optic tectum (Larsell, 1931; Filogamo, 1950; Kelly and Cowan, 1972); pontine nuclei (Trumpy, 1971); somatosensory relay nuclei; and cerebral cortex (see Section 11.7). This vast diversity of neurons have at least one feature in common that predisposes them to atrophy after deafferentation: they receive afferent stimulation predominantly or exclusively from a single presynaptic source.

Where the targets of one set of neurons are the presynaptic inputs to another set, the transsynaptic effects may extend across more than one synapse, and the effect is then called primary, secondary, tertiary, etc. Thus, after removal of an eye, the atrophy of cells in the lateral geniculate nucleus which occurs across one synapse is called primary transneuronal anterograde degeneration (Minkowski, 1920; W. H., Cook *et al.*, 1951; M. R. Matthews *et al.*, 1960; Kupfer and Palmer, 1964; Guillery, 1973; Heumann and Rabinowicz, 1980; Kalil, 1980), while the loss of dendritic spines in the visual cortex which occurs across two synapses is an example of secondary transneuronal anterograde degeneration (Tsang, 1937; A. Globus and Scheibel, 1966, 1967b; Valverde, 1967, 1968; Valverde and Esteban, 1968). The effect in the reverse direction is known as transneuronal retrograde degeneration. It is seen, for example, in the retinal ganglion cells after removal of the striate cortex in primates (Van Buren, 1963).

Presynaptic stimulation may have trophic effects. For example, afferents from the optic tectum help to maintain neurons of the isthmo-optic nucleus in the chick embryo (P. G. H. Clarke, 1985). In the ciliary ganglion of the chick embryo, death of postganglionic neurons is increased by blocking synaptic transmission in the ganglion (L. L. Wright, 1982). Retrograde transsynaptic effects occur in a direction opposite to that of nerve impulse traffic and synaptic transmission. Therefore, synaptic transmission cannot itself be the trophic stimulus. However, a retrograde transsynaptic effect may be coupled to anterograde synaptic transmission, as it is at the neuromuscular synapse: anterograde stimulation of muscle by motoneurons regulates synthesis of acetylcholine receptor mRNA in the muscle (Schuetze and Role, 1987, review; Goldman *et al.*, 1988). Neuromuscular junctions are required for retrograde transmission of neurotrophic factor(s) from muscle to motoneurons (see Sections 8.7 and 9.7).

Secondary transneuronal anterograde degeneration occurs in those relay nuclei which form a closed system, that is, in which the relay nuclei are exclusively or nearly totally limited to connecting with one another. The retinogeniculostriate system has already been mentioned. Other systems in which secondary and tertiary transsynaptic degeneration is seen are the secondary auditory relay nuclei, such as the lateral superior olive in newborn mammals (Powell and Erulkar, 1962), and the nucleus laminaris in birds (Rubel *et al.*, 1976; Parks, 1979), which degenerate after destruction of the cochlea. Secondary transneuronal anterograde degeneration may occur in the presence of the presynaptic cells, for example, in the second- and third-order neurons of the olfactory bulb after destruction of the olfactory epithelium (Graziadei and Graziadei, 1978). This suggests that the mere physical presence of the presynaptic endings is not sufficient to stimulate the postsynaptic cell.

An advantage of studying transsynaptic effects during development is that they occur more rapidly and more severely in the developing than in the mature nervous system. Developing neurons are much more sensitive than mature neurons to direct injury as well as to deafferentation and to removal of their targets. Although the time course of transsynaptic degeneration varies in different organisms and in different neuronal systems in the same organism, for any given system the latency is less and the severity of degeneration is greater in younger than in older animals. Thus anterograde transsynaptic atrophy that occurs after deafferentation, for example, of the lateral geniculate nucleus is slow in adult cats: after an initial period of a few weeks during which little atrophy is apparent, the degeneration reaches a peak in the 2nd month and then levels off by about 60–90 days. By contrast, in newborn cats degeneration of deafferented neurons occurs within a few days and results in death of a considerable percentage of the affected neurons within a few weeks (Torvik, 1956; Kupfer and Palmer, 1964).

The reasons for these differences between younger and older animals can only be surmised. First, older neurons may have a larger store of the supposed trophic agent, or younger neurons may have a greater rate of utilization of the putative agent. A reservoir of the trophic agent may be larger in mature than in developing neurons because a longer segment of afferent axon is left in connection with the mature than the immature neurons. This, however, could hardly account for the large differences in the latent period before onset of degeneration in young neurons compared with mature neurons. Older neurons may receive an alternative source of trophic stimulation from glial cells and Schwann cells. Thus, Schwann cells are a source of NGF and of CNTF, both of which have a potent survival effect on neurons after axotomy (Kromer, 1987; Montero and Hefti, 1988; Sendtner et al., 1990). They may also have sustaining axonal col-

laterals which protect them from retrograde transsynaptic degeneration, and multiple sources of afferents may protect older neurons from the effects of removal of a single afferent system. These protections might not have developed in the younger neurons.

Another factor that has to be taken into consideration is the completeness of the deprivation, either of afferents or of target organs. The severity of the degeneration tends to be directly proportional to the number of afferents that are removed. This rule is best exemplified in the various auditory relay nuclei in the chick embryo, which will be discussed later. However, the rule does not appear to apply to some other cases. For example, in young kittens, unilateral lesions in the brainstem result in virtually complete loss of cells in the inferior olive on both sides, indicating that some cells die after deprivation of only half their afferents (Torvik, 1956). Another apparent exception to the rule is the relatively mild effect of complete deafferentation of cells of the superior cervical ganglion. The postganglionic cells do not die even after they are deafferented during development, but they are reduced in size and have reduced levels of tyrosine hydroxylase and a reduced number of axonal terminals in the iris (Black et al., 1976; Black and Mytilineou, 1976a). The postganglionic cells survive because they are maintained by NGF transported retrogradely from the peripheral targets (see Section 8.16). Although NGF and anterograde transsynaptic stimulation appear to have different mechanisms of sustaining the superior cervical ganglion cells, they are able to survive after total deprivation of their afferents because NGF functions as a residual maintenance factor (Thoenen et al., 1972; Black and Mytilineou, 1976b).

The inferior olivary neurons which project to the cerebellum die in the absence of their targets. This is an example of retrograde transsynaptic degeneration. The neurons of the inferior olive are generated normally, migrate to their positions in the olive, and sprout axons in the absence of the cerebellum, which is the central projection field of the olivocerebellar axons. The neurons of the inferior olive normally project in somatotopic order onto cells of the cerebellum. The olivary neurons in the chick originate and migrate from the rhombic lip on E5–E11 (Harkmark, 1954). Destruction of the cerebellum of the chick embryo before E13 has no effect on the production, migration, and early differentiation of neurons of the inferior olive (Harkmark, 1956). However, the olivary neurons degenerate between E16 and E19, after their axons fail to form connections with neurons in the cerebellum.

Mauthner neurons in amphibian embryos provide some advantages for studying transsynaptic effects during development: the Mauthner neuron is produced and starts its differentiation before its afferents develop and before its axons makes synaptic connections in the spinal cord. However, the development of the lateral dendrite of the Mauthner neuron requires transsynaptic stimulation from the vestibular nerve. Thus excision of the vestibular apparatus in salamander larvae results in failure of development of the Mauthner neuron on the affected side (Piatt, 1947). When the vestibular apparatus is grafted to the region of the eye, an additional Mauther neuron frequently develops at the point of entrance of the vestibular nerve into the midbrain (Piatt, 1947, 1969). This remarkable occurence of an ectopic Mauthner neuron can be explained if part of the hindbrain had been included in the graft. It might show, however, that either the vestibular input induces the formation of the Mauthner neuron *de novo* (which would be the only known instance of induction of a neuronal type by axonal endings) or the vestibular afferents prevent the death of a Mauthner neuron precursor that would otherwise have died in the absence of adequate vestibular input. That the vestibular input is not absolutely necessary is demonstrated by the fact that Mauthner neuron may develop and sprout an axon in the isolated medulla grafted to the flank of *Ambystoma* (Piatt, 1944).

Another case of relevance to this discussion is the pair of abdominal sensory appendages called cerci in the cricket. In this insect the cerci are connected to two giant interneurons so that each cercus makes an excitatory connection with the ipsilateral giant interneuron and an inhibitory connection with the contralateral interneuron. Removal of one or both cerci during development results in transsynaptic atrophy of the interneurons (J. S. Edwards and Palka, 1974), while covering one cercus with a cream which reduces sensory stimulation during development also results in transsynaptic changes in the interneurons (S. G. Matsumoto and Murphey, 1977).

Transneuronal trophic effects during development have been well studied in the auditory relay nuclei of the chick embryo (Levi-Montalcini, 1949; Rubel et al., 1976; Rubel, 1978; Parks, 1979; Lippe et al., 1980; Durham and Rubel, 1983; Born and Rubel, 1985). After removal of the otocyst in the chick embryo on E2, Levi-Montalcini (1949) found that neuron production and differentiation are unaffected in the primary auditory relay nuclei, known as the nucleus angularis and the nucleus magnocellularis. However, cell degeneration becomes evident at E11 after deafferentation in both the latter nuclei, all their neurons having been produced and being well differentiated. Neuron production and death have been carefully studied in the nucleus magnocellularis and in the secondary auditory relay nucleus, known as n. laminaris (Rubel et al., 1976). The neurons of n. magnocellularis are all produced between 48 and 72 hours of incubation, with a peak at 60 hours. Nucleus laminaris neurons are produced in the period from 72 to 108 hours, with a peak at 84 hours. By E7 the neurons have migrated from their germinal zone in rhombic lip to their positions in the brainstem. By E9 a total of about 5400 magnocellularis neurons and about 4500 laminaris neurons are present, but during the following 4 days the number of neurons decreases by 18 percent in n. magnocellularis and by 84 percent in n. laminaris (Rubel et al., 1976). After removal of the otic vesicle there is a further cell loss of 30 percent in n. magnocellularis and of 80 percent in n. angularis, compared with the normal side, according to Levi-Montalcini (1949). She also found that removal of various intracentral afferents to the primary auditory relay nuclei has little or no effect on their development and survival, provided that the primary afferents from the organs are intact.

The secondary auditory relay nucleus, n. laminaris, receives its afferents from two sources: the dorsal dendrites receive afferents from the ipsilateral n. magnocellularis, while the ventral dendrites receive input exclusively from the contralateral n. magnocellularis (Rubel and Parks, 1975). The fact that no loss of cells of n. laminaris was observed by Levi-Montalcini (1949) after removal of the primary auditory neurons is probably due to the sustaining effect of the remaining input via the crossed dorsal cochlear tract from the contralateral n. magnocellularis. Cutting the crossed dorsal cochlear tract of chicks results within 96 hours, at P5–P7, in virtually complete atrophy of the ventral dendrites of n. laminaris cells (Benes *et al.*, 1977). The importance of this observation is that it shows that the transsynaptic degeneration is localized to the dendritic branches from which the presynaptic terminals have been removed (Deitch and Rubel, 1984), as shown in Fig. 6.5.

Sensory stimulation is undoubtedly required for the maturation of some neuronal circuits, and in those cases failure of neural maturation may occur after sensory deprivation. Although the neurons originate and form connections according to a developmental timetable that is not contingent on stimulation or experience, the connections may break down or fail to become fully mature in the absence of the appropriate sensory stimulation. This final phase of development of connections has been termed *functional validation* (M. Jacobson, 1969, 1970a; Hirsch and Jacobson, 1975). The effects of early sensory stimulation on the development of neuronal connections and on the development of behavior will be discussed at length in Chapter 11.

The experiments performed by Weiss (1941b) show that limb buds transplanted in reverse orientation in salamanders move in reverse, and the experiments of Sperry and others, which are discussed fully in Chapter 11, show that the neuronal connections that develop after excision and inversion of the eyes of amphibians result in permanent inversion of visual reflexes. These maladaptive reflexes are not changed by experience or learning. In these cases, the genetic and developmental programs have a sovereign role in controlling the basic patterns of reflex behavior, and functional adaptations are subordinate or absent. The evidence that anatomical development of a part of the nervous system can occur in the absence of sensory stimulation does not necessarily mean that normal functional maturation occurs. Where sensory stimulation is deficient or absent during development, motor patterns develop in accordance with genetically determined potentialities and restrictions. These do not guarantee the development of fully integrated behavior. "Nature" and "nurture" will have different relative importance in different species and in the development of different kinds of behavior. As the evidence presented in Chapter 11 shows, genetic and developmental mechanisms are necessary for the formation of organized CNS circuits, but in the absence of sensory input they are not always sufficient to result in maturation of adaptive behavior.

The following generalizations can now be made. There are reciprocal interdependences between the presynaptic and postsynaptic neurons. The strength of these interdependences between neurons is proportional to the exclusivity of their association. Survival of neurons may require transsynaptic stimulation. By contrast, the production, migration, initial differentiation, and outgrowth of axons depend on a developmental timetable that is intrinsic to the developing neurons and is unaffected by sensory input or by retrograde or anterograde transsynaptic stimulation. The basic patterns of reflex activity develop without reference to sensory stimulation, experience, or adequacy of the reflexes for survival of the animal.

6.15. Transneuronal Influence of the Eye on Development of Visual Centers

The eye exerts a twofold influence on the development of the neurons with which it connects in the brain, namely, a transneuronal trophic stimulating effect and an effect that depends on visual activity. The main function of the latter is to organize the functional operations of neurons in the visual centers so that inputs from the two eyes are congruent in animals that have binocular vision. Removal of one eye creates an imbalance in the binocular functional activity arriving in the visual centers. The imbalance results in various defects that are considered in Sections 11.15 and 11.21.

The effect of the optic nerve fibers that will be considered here is their transneuronal stimulation of differentiation and growth of neurons in the visual centers. Withdrawal of this trophic influence results in enhanced cell death and in retarded differentiation of the surviving cells. The effects on cell death in the retina are considered in Section 8.3. The precise effects of removal of some or all of the retinal axons depend on the stage of development of the operation and on the phylogenetic status of the experimental animal. To generalize, it can be said that the operation has its most catastrophic effects earlier in development and in animals higher on the phylogenetic scale. In no case has any effect of optic afferents been found on the production of cells in the visual centers. This is what may be predicted from the fact that production of neurons in the visual centers is virtually complete in birds and mammals before the arrival of optic nerve fibers. This is not the case in submammalian vertebrates, in which neuron production in the retina and visual centers continues in adults.

The debate about the effects of afferent axons on cell proliferation in the brain was already settled at the time of writing the 1st edition of this book (Jacobson, 1970b, pp. 257–260) on the logical grounds given above and also on the evidence that removal of the eye affects mitosis only during the phase of glial cell production. This issue has now been conclusively settled in the frog (Currie and Cowan, 1974b) and the chick (Cowan *et al.*, 1968; Kelly and Cowan, 1972), and there are no reasons to believe that other vertebrates behave differently. Removing an eye has been shown to alter neuron differentiaton and growth and to affect gliogenesis. The effect on glial cell production is secondary to reduced growth of the deafferented neurons and to absence of the axons which would normally be en-sheathed and myelinated by neuroglial cells. The opposite effect results from increasing the afferent supply to the visual centers, either by grafting an additional eye or by deflecting optic afferents from one side to superinnervate the visual centers on the other side.

Removal of an eye during embryonic develop-ment results in changes in the visual centers which have been described in all the vertebrate classes, although most often in the submammals. In the sub-mammalian vertebrates, the majority of optic nerve fibers terminate in the contralateral optic tectum, although some end in the contralateral dien-cephalon and mesencephalic tegmentum, and a small percentage terminate in the ipsilateral thalamus. There is also a projection from the retina to the ipsilateral optic tectum in the frog, but the pathway to the ipsilateral tectum is an indirect one through the contralateral tectum and via the nucleus isthmus. All modalities of visual perception—such as the sense of direction and location in visual space, the perception of patterns, and the detection of movement -are functions of the optic tectum in the submammals. Its homologue in mammals, the supe-rior colliculus, also subserves many of these func-tions. Electrophysiological experiments have shown that there is a point-to-point (or area-to-area) projection of the retina on the optic tectum, thus confirming the older anatomical evidence for a reti-notopic projection onto the tectum (see Sections 11.9–11.11).

There are several reports of reduction in vol-ume of the contralateral optic tectum in fish after removal of an eye during embryonic development (E. L. White, 1948; Leghissa, 1951; Pflugfelder, 1952; Schmatolla, 1972), but the causes of the shrinkage of the affected tectum cannot be deter-mined from those reports.

The effects of removing an eye in frog embryos and larvae have been studied by Dürken (1913, 1930), Larsell (1929, 1931), and Kollros (1953). Af-ter ablation of one eye in the embryo of the frog *Rana fusca*, Dürken (1913, 1930) reported that the contralateral optic tectum fails to develop fully: there is virtual absence of the superficial layer in which the optic nerve fibers run and a slight thin-ning of the deeper layers. Larsell (1929, 1931) re-moved one eye in larvae of the tree frog *Hyla regilla* and observed a reduction in size and thickness of the contralateral optic tectum after metamorphosis. He distinguished nine tectal layers, numbered 1–9 from the periventricular cell layer to the superficial layer, in which the optic nerve fibers run. He reported that the number of cells in layer 9 of the de-afferented tectum hardly increases between the time of eye removal and metamorphosis, whereas the number of cells in layer 9 of the control tectum almost doubles in the same time. The deep layers of cells surrounding the ventricles are virtually un-affected. In addition to the absence of optic nerve fibers from the affected tectum, the growth of den-drites in the superficial tectal layers is greatly re-duced (Larsell, 1931), thus providing yet another example of the failure of dendrites to develop in the absence of the axons that synapse on them.

Kollros (1953) removed one eye from embryos of the frog *Rana pipiens* and found a reduction of 50 percent in the volume and number of cells in the superficial layers 7, 8, and 9 and a reduction of 25 percent in the deep cellular layers of the affected tectum when compared with the control side at the end of metamorphosis. There are fewer mitotic fig-ures in the affected tectum than in the normal tec-tum. The difference in the number of mitotic fig-ures amounts to 10 percent by early larval stages and to 60 percent by the end of metamorphosis. Kollros attributed the hypoplasia of the tectum to a reduc-tion in proliferation and migration of neurons. This is unconvincing, not only because of the large indi-vidual variations in the counts of mitotic figures re-ported by Kollros, but also because no distinction was made between mitosis giving rise to neurons or to glial cells. The main effect was found in the rostral half of the tectum at late larval stages when production of tectal neurons has virtually ceased in that part of the tectum but when gliogenesis is probably at its maximum. Moreover, it is difficult to imagine how the optic axons, which terminate in the superficial layers of the tectum and do not extend as far as the ventricular germinal zone, can influence production of neurons. What Kollros (1953) and later investigators (McMurray, 1954; Terry and Gordon, 1960; Eichler, 1971) seem to have demonstrated is that removal of the optic afferents has a transsynaptic effect on tectal neurons. This almost certainly results in a slowing of their growth, thus removing a potent stimulus for glial cells to divide, namely, their associations with growing neurons (see Section 3.4).

Currie and Cowan (1974b) have shown that removal of an eye during embryonic stages has no effect on the subsequent production and migration of tectal neurons in the frog. However, a reduction in the number of mitoses in the tectum starts at the beginning of metamorphosis. Most of the reduction in mitotic activity, amounting to about 16 percent, is seen in the rostral part of the tectum, whereas proliferation continues at the caudomedial margin of the rectum. Most or all of the cells that are formed in the rostral part of the tectum after the onset of metamorphosis are glial cells.

Increase in volume of the amphibian optic tectum occurs after the tectum has formed connections with an additional eye or with a large eye transplanted in place of a small one. P. Pasquini (1927) transplanted an additional eye to the embryo of the salamander *Pleurodeses waltlii* and found cellular hyperplasia of the tectum roughly proportional to the increase in the additional visual input to the tectum. An increase in tectal size has also been seen after both optic nerves have grown into the tectum on one side in the frog (Hirsch and Jacobson, 1973) and in the goldfish (R. Levine and Jacobson, 1975). An increase in tectal size also occurs in the frog when an additional eye is grafted into the eye socket and superinnervates the contralateral tectum (M. Jacobson and Hunt, 1973). Heteroplastic grafting of eyes between the salamanders *Ambystoma tigrinum*, which has large eyes, and *Ambystoma punctatum*, which has small eyes, shows that the size of the tectum is proportional to the size of the eye that connects with it (Harrison, 1929; Twitty, 1932; L. S. Stone, 1930, 1953). It is not known whether the

increase in these cases consists of an increase in the number or size of cells or is the result of a combination of factors.

There have been several studies of the development of the optic tectum in the chick embryo and of the effects of removing an eye during development. Filogamo (1950) removed the optic vesicle of the chick embryo during the first 3 days of incubation and detected no changes in the differentiation and growth of neurons in the optic tectum until embryonic day 12. Then the dendrites of the deafferented tectal neurons fail to develop, followed by degeneration of a large number of tectal neurons. After removal of the optic vesicle at E3, the acetylcholinesterase (ChE), which is detected histochemically, develops normally in all layers of the tectum until E12 (Filogamo, 1960). However, there is a failure of development of ChE in the layer into which optic nerve fibers normally grow on E12–E14. Subsequently, the ChE diminishes during the period when the synaptic connections develop in the tectum (Marchisio, 1969). Electrical potentials in the optic tectum, evoked by photic stimulation of the eye, are first detectable on E18 in the chick embryo (Sedlacek, 1967; Corner *et al.*, 1967). However, optic nerve fibers first reach the tectum on E6–E12, as shown histologically (Cowan *et al.*, 1968). On E13, optic nerve fibers in the tectum can be demonstrated by autoradiography of materials that have entered the tectum as a result of axonal transport from the eye (Bondy and Madsen, 1971).

Several investigators have observed no changes in cellular proliferation after removal of the optic vesicle in the early chick embryo (Filogamo, 1950; Leghissa, 1951, 1959; Pflugfelder, 1952; Cowan *et al.*, 1968). The first changes in the number of tectal cells are found after E12, whereas mitoses have virtually ceased after E10 (Cowan *et al.*, 1968). S. Fujita (1964) has shown by means of autoradiography after the injection of [³H]thymidine that neurons of the chick embryo tectum originate before E9, the deep cellular layers being formed before the superficial cellular layers. After E9, only glial cells are produced in the tectum.

Cellular proliferation in the optic tectum of the chick embryo is completely independent of the developing eye (Cowan *et al.*, 1968; Currie and Cowan, 1974b). No change in either the total number of mitotic figures in the tectum or their spatial distribution is found after removal of the optic vesicle at the end of E2. The total number of mitotic figures

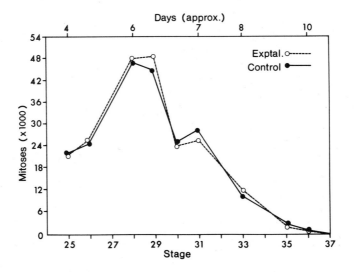

Figure 6.18. Total number of mitotic figures in the optic tectum of chick embryos at different embryonic stages following removal of the optic vesicle on one side at Stages 10–13 of the Hamburger and Hamilton (1951) series, between 34 and 50 hours of incubation. There were no significant differences between the experimental and control sides of the tectum. From W. M. Cowan *et al., J. Exp. Zool.* **169**:71–92 (1968).

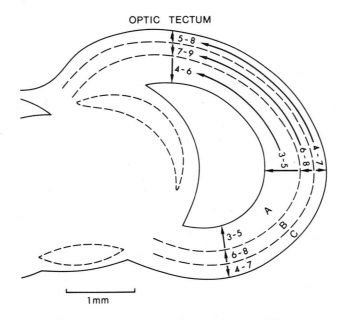

Figure 6.19. Time of origin of cells in the three major developmental strata of the optic tectum (A, B, C) of the chick embryo, determined autoradiographically. The times are given for the rostral part of the tectum: cells originate 1–2 days later in the equivalent parts of the caudal part of the tectum. Arrows indicate the ventrolateral-to-dorsomedial gradient of time of cell origin in each stratum, and the apparent inside-out gradient in stratum C, and the outside-in gradients in strata A and B. Modified from J. H. LaVail and W. M. Cowan, *Brain Res.* **28**:421–441 (1971).

in the optic tectum of the chick embryo increases from about 20,000 on E4 to a maximum of about 45,000 on E5–E6, and then declines to 2000 on E9 and to about 18 on E12 (Fig. 6.18). The number of mitotic figures in the caudal part of the optic tectum exceeds that in the dorsomedial half between E4 and E7. This proliferative gradient is reversed during E8–E12, while neuron production declines and glial cell production increases.

Gradients of time of origin of tectal neurons in the chick embryo were demonstrated by Cowan *et al.* (1968) by labeling with tritiated thymidine. These studies indicate that tectal neurons originate in the rostral and ventrolateral pole of the tectum on E3–E7. At progressively later times from E7 to E12 the cells originate in a gradient extending caudally and dorsomedially (Fig. 6.19). These gradients of cellular proliferation are unaffected by removal of the optic vesicle.

Removal of the eye in mammalian embryos has no discernible effect on the proliferation, migration, or differentiation of neurons in the superior colliculus, which is homologous with the optic tectum. In a strain of mice in which the eyes fail to develop at an early embryonic stage, H. B. Chase (1945) found that the superior colliculi atrophy later.

In an experiment study using tritiated thymidine autoradiography, DeLong and Sidman (1962) described how removal of the eye of the mouse at birth affects the superior colliculus. They showed that cells of the superior colliculus originate in two bursts: the majority of neurons originate prenatally on E11–E13, whereas most of the cells originating postnatally are neuroglia. Therefore, removal of the eye at birth cannot change the production of neurons but might change glial cell production.

The optic nerve fibers first reach the colliculus of the mouse at about day 14 of gestation. Therefore, removal of the eye at birth involves transection of the optic nerve. DeLong and Sidman (1962) found that this results in severe transneuronal atrophy and degeneration of about 40 percent of the cells in the contralateral colliculus between 4 and 7 days after birth. In addition, there is a large reduction in the production of glial cells of the colliculus 4 days after birth. Thereafter, an increase in the production of glial cells results in restoration of the number of cells in the colliculus to 86 percent of normal in the adult.

The experiments with eye–brain connections show that the neurons of the visual centers are dependent on adequate connections from the eye. The dual effects of removal of an eye should be noted: a combination of anatomical deafferentation and functional deprivation. Deafferentation results in transneuronal atrophy and degeneration of neurons in the visual centers followed by glial cell proliferation. Production of neurons in the visual centers is unaffected by eye removal. There is evidence, discussed in Chapter 11, that deprivation of visual activity alone, without disruption of anatomical connections between the eye and the brain during development, results in profound physiological and anatomical changes in the neurons of the visual centers.

7 Dependence of the Developing Nervous System on Nutrition and Hormones

He who admits the principle of sexual selection will be led to the remarkable conclusion that the nervous system not only regulates most of the existing functions of the body, but has indirectly influenced the progressive development of various bodily structures and of certain mental qualities. Courage, pugnacity . . . bright colours and ornamental appendages, have all been indirectly gained by the one sex or the other, through the exertion of choice, the influence of love and jealousy . . . and these powers of the mind manifestly depend on the development of the brain.

Charles Darwin (1809–1882), *The Descent of Man and Selection in Relation to Sex*, 2nd Ed., 1875

7.1. Vulnerability of the Human Brain to Malnutrition

The destiny of nations depends on the manner of their nutrition.
Jean Anthelme Brillat-Savarin (1755–1826), *The Physiology of Taste, or Meditations on Transcendental Gastronomy*, 1825

A large percentage of children in the "Third World," and a significant number in the rich industrial countries, are unable to obtain food necessary for normal development, and many pregnant women suffer from malnutrition. It is therefore a question of the highest importance whether fetal or childhood malnutrition retards or otherwise alters neurological development. If so, the types of changes, their causal mechanisms, and the permanence or degrees of reversibility of the lesions are of very great moral and social con-

cern. Ethical values are an important component of this research program. It should have attracted great scientific interest and generous public support, yet relatively little money and effort have been expended to answer important questions about causes, prevention, and treatment of physical and functional neurological damage resulting from fetal and neonatal malnutrition. This is evident from the small number of publications in this field in the past decade compared with the efflorescence of publications from other research programs of no greater scientific importance and of lesser human significance. The pregnant phrase of Brillat-Savarin at the beginning of this section should be written on the doorposts of every national legislative assembly.

The effects of maternal malnutrition on the human fetus are not well understood but can result in placental insufficiency causing premature birth, which carries a high risk of mental retardation. Children subjected to chronic malnutrition from birth to 18 months of age, severe enough to result in growth retardation, suffer permanent deficits in emotional, cognitive, and intellectual functions. Acute episodes of neonatal malnutrition also may result in permanent brain damage. The lesions caused by malnutrition in children are not well characterized but are most likely reduction in glial cell numbers and functions, retardation of growth of dendrites and synaptogenesis, and defective myelination. These effects may be totally reversed by nutritional therapy and enriched social conditions provided before age 2 but only partially reversed if therapy is delayed to later ages.

Retardation caused by malnutrition has a complex etiology in which malnutrition and socioeconomic deprivation interact to produce the syndrome of physical and mental retardation and dysfunction. All the organ systems may be affected. The effects on the nervous system are both direct, due to insufficient nutrients required for growth, as well as indirect, due to lack of trophic and growth factors and hormones required for normal development.

It is necessary to conduct epidemiological studies of the populations at risk in order to discover the causal factors and to design and implement programs to prevent and treat childhood malnutrition. The biological mechanisms can also be analyzed in animal models chosen because they are believed to be relevant to human conditions. However, animals in the wild rarely, if ever, suffer from malnutrition, which is a condition created by the human species on a global scale.

At least half the world's population has suffered a period of nutritional deprivation during childhood, and at present about 300 million children throughout the world are malnourished (World Health Organization, Scientific Publication No. 251, 1972). The majority of these children suffer from chronic lack of proteins and calories punctuated by episodes of acute malnutrition caused by illness and exacerbated by wars and other adverse political and economic conditions. Assessment of any direct effects of chronic malnutrition on the nervous system is difficult because of the other disadvantages of poor children (Pollitt and Thomson, 1977, review).

There is no doubt that economic poverty and malnutrition interact to stunt physical and mental development. For example, in a study of more than 7000 children in the United States, Edwards and Grossman (1980) found intelligence quotient (IQ) and scholastic achievement test scores significantly correlated with height and weight, and a history of chronic nutritional deprivation was correlated with subnormal test scores. The fact that sociocultural factors play such an important role in intellectual and scholastic development makes it necessary to analyze the variables, including the contribution of malnutrition to the retardation of impoverished children (Cravioto and DeLicardi, 1972; Herzig *et al.*, 1972; Manocha, 1972; Greene and Johnston, 1980; Margen, 1984; Brozek, 1985). The methodological problems of such a research program are thoroughly discussed by Barrett and Frank (1987).

Prenatal nutritional deprivation of the human fetus may occur in multiple pregnancy as a result of competition between the fetuses for nutrients. Birth weight of twins is lower than that of singletons, and birth weight is significantly correlated with later intelligence (Churchill *et al.*, 1966). Birth weights below 2000 g invariably affect behavioral and intellectual development, whereas birth weights between 2500 and 4500 g have variable adverse effects on development of higher nervous functions, depending on other factors such as adequate infant care, disease, nutrition, and sociocultural conditions (Drillien, 1958; Wiener, 1962; Scarr, 1969). Twins average about 7 IQ points below singletons (Stott, 1960; Vandenberg, 1966; Inouye, 1970). The importance of intrauterine competition for nutrients is shown by the fact that identical twins with the same birth weight have the same IQ, but if their birth weights are unequal, the twin with the lower birth weight has the lower IQ in later life (Willerman and Churchill, 1967). The number of variables that enter into human intelligence makes these results difficult to interpret. Thus, in a review of the effect of very low birth weight (1500 g or less) on later intelligence, Francis-Williams and Davies (1974) point out that as many of the harmful factors in the treatment of such infants have been eliminated (excessive use of oxygen, hypothermia, prolonged starvation, infections), there has been progressive improvement of the ultimate IQ attained by children with low birth weight. When babies with low birth weight are cared for under optimal conditions, mental retardation or significant deficits in IQ do not occur (P. A. Davies and Stewart, 1975).

In humans, it is not known whether twins have

a lower brain weight or fewer brain cells than singletons, as would be predicted if animal experimental results, to be described later, can be extrapolated to humans. The deficit is unlikely to be due to failure of nerve cell production because production of nerve cells ceases by 25 weeks of gestation (Dobbing and Sands, 1970), whereas differences in the weight of multiple fetuses compared with a single fetus become apparent only after 26 weeks of gestation (McKeown and Record, 1952). The deficit is more likely to be due to some failure of glial cell production plus retarded neuronal cell growth and differentiation rather than to a reduction in neuronal cell numbers. Nevertheless, there is good evidence that loss of brain cells can occur after severe malnutrition in human infants. Children who die of severe malnutrition in the first 2 years after birth have greatly reduced quantities of DNA in the cerebrum, cerebellum, and brainstem (Fig. 7.1) compared with well-nourished children of the same age (Winick and Rosso, 1969; Winick *et al.*, 1970). It is not known whether the deficit is in the number of neurons or glial cells, but it is more likely to be a glial cell deficit which is known to occur in malnourished rats (Robain and Ponsot, 1978; Bhide and Bedi, 1984).

Assessment of the effects of malnutrition on nervous development in children is complicated by at least three main difficulties. First, the effects of malnutrition cannot be entirely separated from the effects of other harmful conditions, such as maternal neglect, environmental impoverishment, and lack of stimulation and incentive. Second, malnourished children show behavioral abnormalities which are variable and are difficult to measure accurately, such as reduced social responsiveness, increased irritability, and emotional disturbances. Third, the effects of malnutrition on the human brain can rarely be assessed directly by postmortem physical and chemical measurements. Instead, less reliable indices, such as physical status, ratio of weight to height, head circumference, and IQ, are generally used. These indices are themselves complex variables, and their interpretation is usually difficult and frequently ends in controversy. For example, general intelligence is a complex product of many variable factors, one of them being the size of the brain. As a result, authorities disagree about the relationship between brain size and intelligence—the relationship can be shown in animals (see Section 2.13) but in humans it tends to be overridden by other factors that vary in different sociocultural contexts. In those cases where IQ is found to be reduced in malnourished children, it is often difficult, if not impossible, to determine whether the reduced IQ is the result of retarded brain development due to mal-

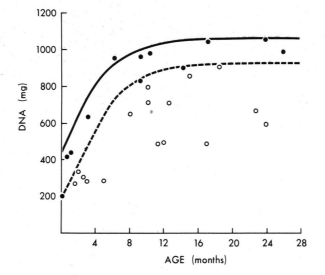

Figure 7.1. Severe childhood malnutrition can result in a reduced DNA content of the brain. The DNA content of the cerebrum of normal children (dark line, black dots) and severely malnourished children (dashed line, circles). From M. Winick, P. Rosso, and J. Waterlow, *Exp. Neurol.* **26**:393-400 (1970), copyright Academic Press, Inc.

nutrition and associated conditions such as disease, or whether the poor performance is largely or entirely due to social and economic disadvantages. Moreover, a single IQ test has little value, particularly if it is done at an early age: IQ at 1 year of age has no correlation with the IQ at age 17 (B. S. Bloom, 1964). Besides, the IQ is subject to change during childhood: changing the educational level of children can result in increase or reduction of their IQ by as much as 28 points (Skeels, 1966). Obviously, the rate of development of general intelligence is a more revealing index than a single measurement.

Occipitofrontal circumference of the head is another index that is often used to assess the effects of malnutrition on brain development. However, the circumference of the head is also related to the thickness of the skull and scalp, so that it has been claimed that there is a poor correlation between head size and brain size (Eichhorn and Bayley, 1962). Intelligence is normal in a small percentage of microcephalic children (H. P. Martin, 1970), and reduced head circumference in infants and young children may not be irremediable (H. P. Martin, 1970; Stoch and Smythe, 1976). Nevertheless, there is a linear relationship between occipitofrontal head circumference over a range of 24–44 cm and brain weight over a range of 100–700 g from 25 weeks of gestation to 8 months postnatal (Lemons *et al.*, 1981). Head circumference is significantly correlated with brain size in cases of intrauterine growth retardation (Battisti *et al.*, 1986) and in cases of nutritional deprivation during the first 2 years of life, when most of the growth of the brain occurs (Johnston and Lampl, 1984).

In view of criticisms of the validity of IQ tests, especially that they are racially and culturally biased, it is significant that deficits in IQ of malnourished children have been reported from countries which differ in race, culture, economic, and social conditions: India (Champakam *et al.*, 1968), Indonesia (Liang *et al*, 1967), Lebanon (Botha-Antoun *et al.*, 1968), Latin America (Pollit and Granoff, 1967; Birch, 1972; Cravioto and DeLicardi, 1975; Klein *et al.*, 1977; Barrett and Frank, 1987), Yugoslavia (Cabak and Najdanvic, 1965; Cabak *et al.*, 1967) and Africa (Stoch and Smythe, 1963; Fisher *et al.*, 1978). In one such study, Stoch and Smythe (1963, 1967) found that severely undernourished South African children from 1 to 8 years of age were 20 points lower in IQ than well-nourished children of

similar parentage. When these children were studied 15 and 20 years later, the same severe intellectual deficits were found, and physical abnormalities of the brain were found by computerized tomography scans in some cases, showing that the changes are permanent (Stoch and Smythe, 1976; Handler *et al.*, 1981; Stoch *et al.*, 1982). Similar conclusions were reached in another study of the effects of severe undernutrition during infancy on subsequent intellectual functions in Yugoslavian children (Cabak and Najdanvic, 1965; Cabak *et al.*, 1967). There were marked deficits in IQ in 36 children who had been hospitalized between the ages of 4 and 24 months because of malnutrition but had not suffered from chronic illness thereafter, and who had no significant reduction in body growth. The mean IQ of the malnourished children was 88, in contrast to 101 and 109 for two groups of comparable normal children. Significantly, none of the malnourished children had an IQ above 110 (Fig. 7.2). No correlation was found between the age of hospitalization and subsequent intellectual impairment. Hospitalization during the 1st year of life is frequently associated with sensory deprivation and separation of the child from the mother, and these contribute to subsequent emotional disturbances and intellectual impairment (Spitz and Wolf, 1946; Coleman, 1957).

Malnourished children have learning and scholastic difficulties. This is a complex syndrome in which apathy, emotional disturbances, and impaired cognitive and intellectual abilities are synergistic in producing dysfunction (Lester, 1979). Children who are severely malnourished in the 1st year of life subsequently show behavior disturbances and difficulties with reading, spelling, and arithmetic (Richardson *et al.*, 1973; Barrett and Frank, 1987). Reduced ability to integrate inputs from various sensory modalities, for example, auditory–visual integration, has been found in children suffering from malnutrition before 3 years of age (Birch, 1964; Kahn and Birch, 1968; Cravioto and DeLicardie, 1975). Lester *et al.* (1975) studied effects of acute malnutrition in 1-year-old children in Guatemala and found much slower habituation to repeated stimulation. Comparable changes in habituation have been reported in malnourished rats (Bronstein *et al.*, 1974; Frankovà and Zemanovà, 1978).

Language development is a significant indication of general intellectual status in children (Cameron *et al.*, 1967). Findings which are from differ-

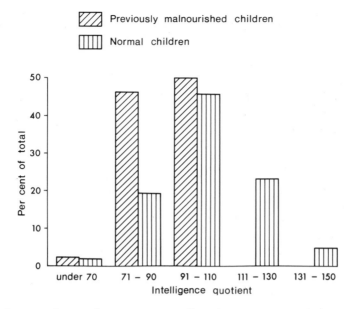

Figure 7.2. Severe malnutrition during infancy may cause intellectual impairment. Distribution of IQs of 36 children aged 7–14 years who had been severely malnourished between the ages of 4 and 24 months, compared with the IQs of normal children of the same ages. Adapted from V. Cabak and R. Najdanvic, *Arch. Dis. Child.* 40:532–534 (1965).

ent countries, and therefore unlikely to be culturally or racially biased, show retarded language development in malnourished children (Barrera-Moncada, 1963; Monckeberg, 1968; Champakam *et al.,* 1968; Chase and Martin, 1970). Retardation of language development has a complex etiology, which includes social deprivation, illness, and maternal deficits as well as malnutrition.

Several studies have provided evidence supporting the concept of a critical period from birth to about 2 years of age during which the nervous system is most vulnerable to malnutrition and most responsive to nutritional therapy. The amount of reversibility of impairment following childhood malnutrition is of great practical importance in planning food supplementation programs and other forms of prevention and treatment. The time and duration of malnutrition, as well as the time at which nutritional therapy and environmental enrichment are started, may be critical.

One study shows that there can be negligible long-term effects of acute starvation—no physical or mental deficits were found in victims of the severe famine in Holland from 1944 to 1945 when they were examined 19 years later (Stein *et al.,* 1975). The famine was very severe but of relatively

short duration and the amount of intrauterine or neonatal growth retardation is not known. However, it seems that any effects were later reversed by nutrition, education, and good sociocultural conditions. This should be compared with the significant intellectual impairment reported in German schoolchildren who were severely undernourished during and after World War I (Blanton, 1919).

Several studies have shown that severely malnourished children can benefit from early nutritional therapy and enhanced sociocultural conditions (Yatkin and McLaren, 1970; McKay *et al.,* 1972; Chavez *et al.,* 1974; Irwin *et al.,* 1979; Monckeberg, 1979; Mora *et al.,* 1979). Winick *et al.* (1975) found that IQ and scholastic performance between age 6 and 12 were normal in malnourished Korean children adopted into American families before the age of 2 but were significantly below normal in children adopted after 2 years of age.

Cravioto and Robles (1965) reported that severely malnourished Mexican children admitted to hospital before 6 months of age showed the slowest rate of recovery and greatest loss of intellectual ability compared with malnourished children who entered hospital between ages 37 and 42 months, who recovered more rapidly and had least intellectual deficit. McKay *et al.* (1978) found that food supplements given to chronically malnourished Colombian children improved their cognitive, language, and social abilities. The greatest gains were made when treatment was started at age 3, and the gains were progressively less when treatment started at ages 4 and 5. In a study of chronically malnourished pregnant women and children in Louisiana (Hicks *et al.,* 1982), a positive relationship was found between the age at which food supplementation was started and subsequent gains of IQ. Mothers received extra food during pregnancy, and their children who continued to receive it from birth to 4 years had higher IQ scores at 6 years of age than their siblings who started receiving extra food after 1 year of age for 3 years.

Other studies have failed to find any evidence of a critical period although they clearly show that malnutrition and poor socioeconomic conditions result in physical and intellectual impairment. Chase and Martin (1970) reported that children in the United States who were admitted to hospital in a severely malnourished condition before 4 months of age were subsequently less impaired than children who entered hospital after 4 months of age, although both groups later showed significant retardation. This could be interpreted to mean that starting therapy early during the critical period is more effective that starting treatment later. Jamaican children who were hospitalized with severe malnutrition at ages 3–24 months were found to have no correlation between the age of admission to hospital and retardation of IQ at 5–11 years of age (Hertzig *et al.,* 1972). Presumably severity of malnutrition and age of onset are only two variables among many, including social and educational deprivation, family instability, and maternal illiteracy, all of which combine to retard child development.

The biological mechanisms of the dysfunction and retardation caused by malnutrition in humans are not well understood, but they are likely to be complex. The nervous system may be affected both directly and indirectly. Nutrients are required for growth as well as to provide materials for synthesis of growth factors, trophic factors, and hormones required for normal development of the nervous system and the other supporting systems. Severe malnutrition directly affects the heart muscle, resulting in cardiac insufficiency and reduced blood supply to the brain. The reduced plasma proteins cause edema in all the tissues including the brain. Anemia, which is often associated with malnutrition, may diminish the oxygen supply to the brain. Neonatal malnutrition results in retarded development of the immune system and consequently in greater risk of infectious disease. Those who survive the insults of malnutrition during infancy and childhood frequently remain with physical and mental disabilities as well as social and economic disadvantages.

7.2. Effects of Malnutrition on Brain Development in Experimental Animals

The effects of maternal undernutrition on fetal brain development have been studied most often in rats, which differ significantly from humans in several important ways: multiple births are the rule in rats, and production of neurons continues throughout gestation. By contrast, production of neurons in humans is virtually completed by about the midpoint of gestation, after which glial cell production continues to the end of gestation and into the 2nd postnatal year. As neurons and glial cells in the fetal nervous system may not be equally susceptible to the effects of maternal undernutrition, and as the malnutrition may have different secondary effects on the placenta and on the endocrine system in different species, extrapolation from the rat to humans should be made with considerable caution.

The vulnerability of the developing nervous system to radiation, poisons, viruses, undernutrition, or hyperthermia is determined by the cellular activities in the developing system that respond to the insult under consideration. Therefore, the effects of the agents or conditions will be different at different times in development, and the vulnerable periods may not be the same for all agents and may differ according to the timetable of developmental events in the nervous system in different species (Dobbing, 1971, 1973, 1976).

It is fairly obvious that nutritional deprivation is most likely to have maximum effects on those developmental processes that are most active at the time of the deprivation; during what has been called the "brain growth spurt" (Dobbing and Sands, 1971, 1979). Thus malnutrition produces severe deficiencies in the number of neurons if it occurs during the period of neuronal production, maximal effects on glial cell number if it coincides with the period of glial cell proliferation, and maximal effects on myelination if it occurs during the period of myelination. However, these processes occur in different species at different times in relation to the time of birth, so that the outcome of neonatal malnutrition will be considerably different in the mouse than in humans. Therefore, when making extrapolations from experimental animals to humans, one should try to relate the effect of malnutrition to the developmental processes occurring during the time of malnutrition rather than to the time of birth.

Animal models of human cognitive, intellectual, and linguistic skills are notoriously inadequate. I do not think that impairment of maze running or aversive responses or other behavior in malnourished laboratory animals is relevant to impairment of reading and numerical calculation in malnourished children. However, there is considerable evidence that severe malnutrition during development results in behavioral disturbances in adult rats and other laboratory animals (Bronfenbrenner, 1968; Frankovà and Barnes, 1968; Frankovà, 1973; Barnes and Moore, 1970; Levitsky and Barnes, 1970; Barnett et al., 1971; Smart et al., 1975; Smart, 1977).

The effects of malnutrition on the cerebral cortex of the rat are correlated with the times of development of different neurons: layer V pyramidal cells are affected most in the early postnatal age; layer III pyramidal cells at early and later postnatal ages; and interneurons during the late postnatal age (Schönheit, 1982). The most striking effects at all ages are reduction of the number of dendritic spines (Schönheit, 1982) and a deficit in the number of synapses per neuron (Thomas et al., 1979; Bedi et al., 1980, 1989; Warren and Bedi, 1982). Malnutrition of rats for 2–3 weeks after birth results in a deficit of about 30 percent in the synapse-to-neuron ratio in layers II–IV of the visual cortex (Warren and Bedi, 1982). Nutritional therapy until 200 days of age results in about 20 percent increase in the number of synapses per neuron compared with normal controls. This increase is converted to a 30 percent reduction in the synapse-to-neuron ratio in rats reared in isolation (Bedi et al., 1989), indicating that social and nutritional deprivation are additive in their detrimental effects on synaptogenesis in the cerebral cortex. Other effects of neonatal malnutrition on the cerebral cortex of the mouse are loss of

neurons and axon terminals (Cragg, 1972). Delay in development of the cortical barrels and reduction of the number of neurons in the cortical barrels in malnourished rats (Vongdokmai, 1980) could be due to a direct effect on the cerebral cortex or to an effect on the sensory relay nuclei or on the vibrissal follicles (see Section 11.7).

The cerebellar cortex, which develops rapidly in the neonatal period in humans and other altricial mammals, is particularly vulnerable to the effect of neonatal malnutrition (Persson and Sima, 1975; Griffin et al., 1977a,b; McConnel and Berry, 1978a,b, 1981; Clos et al., 1979; Hillman and Chen, 1981; Vitiello et al., 1989; Normand et al., 1989). Undernutrition of the newborn rat and mouse results in stunting of growth of Purkinje cell dendrites (Griffin et al., 1977a; McConnell and Berry, 1978a; Pysh et al., 1979; Bedi et al., 1980). As illustrated in Fig. 7.3, underfeeding rats for the first 20 days after birth results in reduction of Purkinje cell dendritic length and branching which persists into adulthood (McConnell and Berry, 1978a,b, 1981). Neonatal underfeeding results in a 20 percent reduction in the density of Purkinje cell dendritic spines (Pysh et al., 1979; Hillman and Chen, 1981b). The effects on

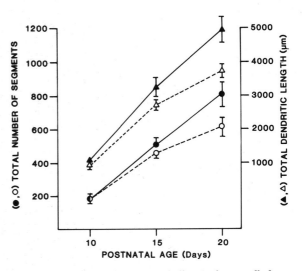

Figure 7.3. Alterations in cerebellar Purkinje cell dendrites of undernourished rats. Rats were undernourished from birth by limiting their access to the mother's milk, killed at 10, 15 or 20 days after birth, and the total length and segment frequency of Purkinje cells were measured in groups of normal control and undernourished rats. From P. McConnell and M. Berry, *J. Comp. Neurol.* **200**:463–479 (1981).

Purkinje cell dendrites probably have a complex etiology, including direct effects on synthesis and assembly of membrane and cytoskeletal components of dendrites and indirect effects of loss of granule cells (Rebière and Legrand, 1972; Barnes and Altman, 1973a,b; Lewis *et al.*, 1975; Gopinath *et al.*, 1976; Hillman and Chen, 1981a,b), and loss of glial cells (Robain and Ponsot, 1978). The effects of malnutrition on hormones also have to be taken into account. Neonatal undernutrition has a more severe effect on myelination, synaptogenesis, and total volume of the cerebellum in females than males (Hillman and Chen, 1981a,b). Refeeding neonatally undernourished rats leads to complete recovery of Purkinje cell dendritic morphology and Purkinje-to-granule cell ratios if therapy is started at P10 or P15, but significant deficits remain if feeding is begun after P20 (McConnell and Berry, 1981). To the limited extent to which extrapolation is justifiable, this is consistent with the concept of a critical period in rats as well as in humans (see Section 7.1).

Myelination is one of the few processes that can be studied best in rats and may be extrapolated to humans. In both human and rat, myelination occurs mainly postnatally and continues for about the same time relative to lifespan (Wiggins, 1982, review). Myelination in the central nervous system as well as

in peripheral nerves of rats is greatly reduced as a result of neonatal malnutrition (Dobbing, 1963; Culley and Mertz, 1965; Benton *et al.*, 1966; H. P. Chase *et al.*, 1967; Clos and Legrand, 1969, 1970; Hedley-Whyte, 1973; Sima, 1974a,b; Krigman and Hogan, 1976; Sima and Sourander, 1978; Lai and Lewis, 1980a,b; Wiggins, 1982, review; see Section 3.17). As illustrated in Fig. 7.4, reduced myelination in the corpus callosum of undernourished rats is strongly correlated with reduced numbers of oligodendrocytes (Lai *et al.*, 1980; Lai and Lewis, 1980; Clos *et al.*, 1982a,b). Malnutrition also results in reduction of myelin protein content (Wiggins *et al.*, 1976) and reduction of myelin gangliosides (Yusuf and Dickerson, 1979). The ultrastructure of Schwann cells is abnormal and the number of myelin lamellae is reduced in the sciatic nerve of 12-day-old rats underfed from birth (Clos and Legrand, 1970). There is evidence that similar deficits occur in severely malnourished human infants. J. H. Fox *et al.* (1972) found that the total quantity of myelin is reduced in malnourished infants, but the chemical composition of the myelin is not altered, and similar findings have been reported in experimentally undernourished rats (Krigman and Hogan, 1976).

Zamenhof *et al.* (1968) showed that restriction of protein in the diet of rats for a month before

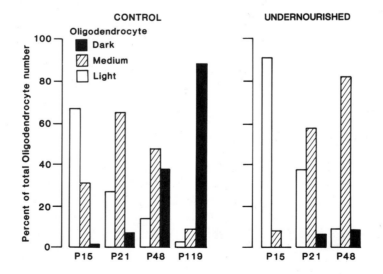

Figure 7.4. Effects of undernutrition on oligodendrocyte maturation in the rat corpus callosum. Halving of the mother's food intake from the 6th day of pregnancy through lactation and halving of the food intake of the young rats after weaning resulted in an increased percentage of immature (light) and decreased percentage of mature (dark) oligodendrocytes in the corpus callosum at P15, P21, and P48. An increased ratio of astrocytes to oligodendrocytes in the corpus callosum of undernourished rats was also observed (not shown). From M. Lai, P. D. Lewis, and A. J. Patel, *J. Comp. Neurol.* 193:965–972 (1980).

mating and during pregnancy results in 30 percent reduction in body weight and 10 percent reduction in brain DNA of the offspring compared with normal newborn rats. Similar results have been obtained by Winick (1969) and by Zeman and Stanbrough (1969). The authors recognize that their results neither show which types of brain cells are reduced nor show their regional distribution. These experiments also do not show whether the reduction in DNA (cell number) results from nutritional deficiency directly or indirectly, for example, due to placental insufficiency or hormonal effects.

To determine the time of maximal susceptibility of the fetus to maternal malnutrition and the extent of recovery after normal nutrition is restored, Zamenhof et al. (1971d) deprived groups of pregnant female rats of protein for 5-day periods at different times during gestation. Abortion occurred in the majority of cases deprived before 10 days of gestation, and in all groups the offspring had significant reductions of body weight, cerebral weight, and cerebral DNA. The effect cannot be due to the protein requirement of the fetuses, which constitutes a very small fraction of the maternal protein requirement. It must be due to other factors such as placental insufficiency and deficiency in maternal gonadotropic hormones, which results in lower levels of estrogen and progesterone. These results also show that even a short, 5-day period of maternal protein deprivation results in irreversible loss of fetal brain cells. That hormonal factors may play a role in this effect is shown by the reversal of the effect of undernutrition by growth hormone injections (Zamenhof et al., 1971c).

There is considerable evidence that placental growth is stunted by maternal malnutrition (Winick, 1967, 1970a; Winick et al., 1967; Dayton et al., 1969; Zamenhof et al., 1971a). The complexity of the effects of maternal malnutrition is shown by the phenomenon of transfer of the effects from one generation to the next. It has long been suspected that poor nutrition of the female infant may affect the neurological development of her offspring born much later (Cowley and Griesel, 1963; R. H. Barnes et al., 1966). In rats, Zamenhof et al. (1971e) obtained evidence that the normally nourished female offspring (F_1) of a mother (F_0) which had been malnourished during pregnancy will produce offspring with significantly reduced brain DNA. The transfer is not genetic, as it occurs only through F_1 females

but not through F_1 males. The most likely explanation is that the F_1 females, although well nourished postnatally, suffer some permanent physical deficiency *in utero* that restricts the development of their (F_2) progeny. The physical defect in the F_1 generation has not been discovered, but the effect might be caused by a deficiency of pituitary hormone-releasing factors in the F_1 females. Even in experimental animals the effects of malnutrition may be difficult to separate from those of hormones, even when well-designed control experiments are performed. The effects of hormones on development of the nervous system are considered in the following sections.

7.3. Thyroid Hormone Actions on Neural Development

The thyroid gland produces two hormones, L-thyroxine (T^4) and L-triiodothyronine (T^3) which are small hydrophobic molecules and therefore require carriers (thyroxine-binding globulin and thyroxine-binding prealbumin) for their transport in the blood and extracellular fluid to their cellular targets. Thyroxine is the main circulating form but it is converted to (T^3) which is the active hormone. This conversion is done by enzymes in the tissues, as demonstrated in cultured astrocytes (Cavalier et al., 1986) and neurons in primary culture (Leonard and Larsen, 1985).

Thyroid hormone release is regulated by thyrotropin (TSH) secreted by the anterior pituitary, which is under the control of hypothalamic TSH-releasing hormone. Pituitary and hypothalamic cells have thyroid hormone receptors which mediate the negative feedback action of thyroid hormones on hypothalamus and pituitary (Menezes-Ferreira et al., 1986). The thyroid hormone–receptor complex regulates transcription of RNAs encoding TSH (Shupnick et al., 1985; Carr et al., 1987).

Steroid and thyroid hormones act by binding to specific intracellular receptors belonging to the same receptor superfamily which also includes the retinoic acid receptor (Evans, 1988, review). The hormone–receptor complexes bind to specific sites with high affinity ($K_d \sim 0.5$ nM) and low capacity (few thousand sites per nucleus) on DNA and act as transcriptional regulators of specific sets of genes. Two thyroid receptors have been identified, and there may be more which are tissue specific. One of these is an abundant neuronal form of the thyroid hormone receptor (C. C. Thompson *et al.*, 1987). T^3 receptors are expressed on neurons in the mammalian brain during the fetal period while neuron production is underway in many brain regions. T^3 receptors continue to be expressed at high levels in neurons and glial cells throughout perinatal and postnatal development. Thyroid hormone stimulates neural development in several ways: increasing cell proliferation, synthesis of microtubule-associated proteins (MAPS) and tubulin, increasing microtubule assembly, axonal and dendritic outgrowth, synaptogenesis, and myelination.

T^3 receptors are present in rat brain on prenatal day 20 (Schwartz and Oppenheimer, 1978). The density of T^3 receptors in the rat brain reaches a maximum at birth in the cerebellum and at P9 in the cerebrum and then falls to adult levels by about 30 days of age (Eberhardt *et al.*, 1978; Schwartz and Oppenheimer, 1978a,b; Naidoo *et al.*, 1979). T^3 receptors are present on glial cell and neuronal cell lines (Ortiz *et al.*, 1986) and the receptors have the same affinity for TB in both neurons and glial cells but the binding capacity is three times greater in neurons (Luo *et al.*, 1986).

In the human brain T^3 receptors are detectable at 10 weeks of gestation and increase sixfold in the following 6 weeks (Bernal and Pekonen, 1984). It should be remembered that neuron production in the human cerebral neocortex continues until 25 weeks of gestation (Dobbing and Sands, 1970).

The high level of expression of the T^3 receptor in specific regions of the adult mammalian nervous system, particularly the hippocampus, amygdala, and cerebral neocortex (Dratman *et al.*, 1982; Ruel *et al.*, 1985), raises the possibility that some derangements of the central nervous system (CNS) could be caused by abnormalities of the receptors as well as by the well-known changes in levels of thyroid hormones (Sapolsky, 1986).

Thyroid hormone stimulates a 10- to 15-fold increase in Na^+, K^+-ATPase activity in neonatal rats (Schmitt and Donough, 1986). This is part of the general increase in metabolic rate which is one of the main actions of thyroid hormones (Guernsey and Edelman, 1983). Another general action of T^4 is to enhance tubulin synthesis and thus to promote neurite outgrowth. Synthesis of tubulin is enhanced

by T^4 in organ cultures of neonatal rat brain (Chaudhury and Sarkar, 1983). It has been proposed that T^4 stimulates neurotubule assembly by an action on MAPs (Francon *et al.*, 1977; Tellons *et al.*, 1979; Nunez, 1985; see Section 5.5). T^3 stimulates synthesis of MAP1B and induces neurite outgrowth in cultured neuroblastoma cells (Hargreaves *et al.*, 1988). These effects of thyroid hormone on microtubules are consistent with several reports of reduced axonal and dendritic growth in hypothyroid rats and of the converse in hyperthyroid rats. For example, cerebellar parallel fibers are reduced in length (Lauder, 1978, 1979) and Purkinje cell dendrites have diminished branching (Nicholson and Altman, 1972a–c) in hypothyroid rats. The density of microtubules is reduced to half normal in the large dendritic trunks of Purkinje cells in thyroid-deficient rats (Faivre *et al.*, 1983). The stimulation of dendritic growth by thyroid may be mediated by its action on microtubules. Thyroid hormone treatment of rats during the neonatal period results in an increase in size of the cell body and dendrites of pyramidal cells in area CA3 of the hippocampal formation (E. Gould *et al.*, 1990).

7.4. Role of Thyroid Hormones in Mammalian Brain Development

In mammals the thyroid starts functioning in the fetus, at 10–12 weeks in the human fetus, for example, and there is no transfer of thyroid hormones from mother to fetus. As a result, maternal hypothyroidism does not affect the fetus. However, children born with abnormalities of the thyroid resulting in congenital hypothyroidism have a high incidence of congenital mental deficiency. This deficiency is correlated with the severity of hypothyroidism and the age at which treatment is started (Klein *et al.*, 1972; Quirido *et al.*, 1978). Treatment of congenital hypothyroidism with thyroid hormones given from birth results in development of IQ within the normal range, whereas treatment of severe hypothyroidism started between 6 and 12 months of age results in normal IQ in only 15 percent of children (Smith *et al.*, 1957; Van Gemund and de Angulo, 1971; Glorieux *et al.*, 1985).

Thyroidectomy or the administration of antithyroid drugs to rats during the postnatal period results in failure of growth and maturation of the cerebral cortex (Eayrs, 1955, 1960; Gomez et al., 1966; Rabié et al., 1979; Rami et al., 1986a,b) and in a delay in the maturation of the cerebellar cortex (Legrand, 1965; Legrand et al., 1961; Hamburgh, 1968; Nicholson and Altman, 1972a–c; Rebière and Dainat, 1976; Lauder, 1977a,b, 1978, 1983; Dussault and Ruel, 1987, review).

Neonatal thyroidectomy of rats results in marked reduction in the growth of the brain after 14 days of age. This is due to a decrease in myelination (Balázs et al., 1969) and a reduction in volume of neurons, but not to a reduction in the number of cells (Geel and Timiras, 1967; J. M. Pasquini et al., 1967; Balázs et al., 1968). The development of dendrites is retarded and the degree of dendritic branching is reduced in the cerebral cortex of hypothyroid mammals (Eayrs, 1955). The number of axodendritic synapses in the cerebral cortex also seems to be reduced in rats after neonatal thyroidectomy (Balázs et al., 1968). These changes are associated with behavioral changes (Eayrs and Lishman, 1953; Eayrs, 1960) and changes in the electroencephalogram (P. B. Bradley et al., 1960a,b).

Reduction in the number of synapses in the molecular layer of the cerebellum of hypothyroid rats, as seen by electron microscopy (Nicholson and Altman, 1972 b,c) or as shown by assay of the synaptosomal fraction of cerebellar homogenates (Rabié and Legrand, 1973), has been considered to indicate a direct effect of thyroid hormones on synaptogenesis. However, evidence to the contrary is that cerebellar axodendritic synapses appear normal in hypothyroid rats (M. C. Brown et al., 1976) and that the primary effect of hypothyroidism seems to be on dendritic growth. This illustrates the difficulty of distinguishing between primary and secondary effects of the hormone on synaptogenesis.

The effect of thyroid hormone on cell proliferation in the cerebellar external granule layer is now fairly clear. Thyroidectomy of newborn rats results in a 25 percent reduction in the cerebellar DNA content by the end of the 2nd week, but the external granule layer persists longer in hypothyroid rats and the normal DNA content of the cerebellum is ultimately reached in the 4th or 5th postnatal week (Legrand, 1967a,b; Balázs et al., 1968; Patel et al., 1976). Nicholson and Altman (1972a) suggested that lack of T[4] results in a reduced rate of cell proliferation, but careful observations have shown no

changes in the length of the cell cycle and duration of phases of the cell cycle (P. D. Lewis et al., 1976).

There are changes in the relative numbers of different classes of cerebellar cells in hypothyroidism (Nicholson and Altman, 1972a; Clos and Legrand, 1973; Lauder, 1977a,b). In hypothyroid rats the rate of migration of granule cells and the outgrowth of their parallel fibers are slowed, resulting in a permanent deficit in their length (Lauder, 1978, 1979). Retarded migration of granule cells may be related to retardation of differentiation of cerebellar astrocytes (Clos et al., 1982a,b), including the Bergmann glial cells, which are required for granule cell migration. Death of granule cells occurs as a result of failure of their axons, the parallel fibers, to make adequate connections with Purkinje cell dendritic spines. The primary effect of hypothyroidism on the neonatal cerebellum is to produce stunting of dendrite development, reduced outgrowth of parallel fibers. The secondary consequences are failure of synaptogenesis, death of some granule cells, basket cells, and stellate cells, followed by reactive hypertrophy of astrocytes, reduced proliferation of oligodendrocytes, and consequent failure of myelination. The amount of isoenzyme II of carbonic anhydrase, a specific marker for oligodendroglial cells, is greatly decreased in the cerebellum of hypothyroid rats and moderately decreased in undernourished rats (Clos et al., 1982a,b). The myelin deficiency could be caused by a reduction in activity of insulin-like growth factor 1, which is a potent inducer of oligodendrocyte proliferation (McMorris et al., 1986).

Synaptogenesis in the molecular layer of the cerebellum is retarded in hypothyroid rats (Rebière and Legrand, 1970; Nicholson and Altman, 1972b,c; Rebière and Dainat, 1976). Administration of T[4] can correct the deficit if given in the first few weeks after birth, but after that age the deficit is refractory to treatment and is permanent (Rabié and Legrand, 1973; Rabié et al., 1979).

The effects of neonatal thyroid deficiency on development of the cerebrum are primarily retardations of differentiation and growth, resulting in a reduction of dendritic growth and synaptogenesis. Thyroid deficiency produces no changes in the length of the cell cycle, the phases of the cycle, or DNA synthesis in the subependymal layer of the lateral ventricle (P. D. Lewis et al., 1976). Cell proliferation in the subependymal layer mainly or exclusively produces glial cells (see Section 2.2), so that lack of thyroid apparently does not impair neuron production in the forebrain. This is also consistent with the observation that postnatal increase in DNA content of the forebrain is not altered by thyroid deficiency (Patel *et al.*, 1976). However, the DNA content of the olfactory bulb is reduced after neonatal hypothyroidism, indicating that some reduction in the number of cells, probably granule cells, occurs there.

There appears to be a critical period during which thyroid hormone is required for development of dendritic spines on apical dendrites of pyramidal cells in the visual and auditory cortex of the rat (Ruiz-Marcos *et al.*, 1979, 1983). Rats were thyroidectomized at P10 and treated with thyroid hormone starting at different times after the operation. Normal dendritic spines developed when treatment started at P12, but an irreversible reduction of spines occurred when treatment started at P15 and was more severe when treatment began at P20. Some of the effects of hypothyroidism may be caused by degenerative changes in pituitary eosinophil cells which synthesize or store growth hormone (Contopoulos *et al.*, 1958; Herlant, 1964; Schooley *et al.*, 1966). However, treatment of neonatally thyroidectomized rats with growth hormone does not reduce the effects of thyroidectomy on the brain (Eayrs, 1961; Hamburgh, 1968; Krawiec *et al.*, 1969; Geel and Timiras, 1970).

Postnatal treatment of rats with T⁴ results in a decrease in brain weight and body weight, accelerates the histogenesis and morphogenesis of the cerebellar cortex (Nicholson and Altman, 1972a–c; Clos *et al.*, 1974), increases the number of dendritic spines in layer IV of the visual cortex (Schapiro *et al.*, 1973), and increases S100 protein, an astrocyte marker, in the cerebellum (Clos *et al.*, 1982). T⁴ stimulates DNA synthesis in the cerebellum of the rat 2–6 days postnatally, but by 12 days of age the cerebellar DNA content is reduced below normal levels (Weichsel, 1974). A similar early increase by 6 days of age, before a later decline in DNA content of the cerebellum, was noted by Gourdon *et al.* (1973) and by Patel *et al.* (1979). The decrease has also been found by Balázs *et al.* (1971), who administered large doses of T³ to newborn rats and recorded a 20–30 percent reduction in the body weight and brain weight at 50 days of age. The reduced brain weight was found to be due to a 30–40 percent

reduction in the number of brain cells formed after birth. The effect is probably caused by acceleration of cell differentiation after 12 days of age (Patel *et al.*, 1979).

The hippocampal formation is very sensitive to changes in levels of thyroid hormones during the neonatal period in rats. Thyroid hormone receptors are present in neurons of the hippocampal formation (Dratman *et al.*, 1982). Hyperthyroidism in newborn rats results in overgrowth of the hippocampal granule cell axons, the mossy fibers, which synapse on the hippocampal pyramidal cell dendrites (Lauder and Mugnaini, 1977, 1980). The mossy fibers appear to be normal in rats made hypothyroid from birth, but there is a reduction of volume of the hippocampus (Rabié *et al.*, 1979), which may be the result of either diminished production or increased death of granule cells. Hypothyroidism during neonatal development in rats causes reduction of production of dentate granule cells and stunting of pyramidal cells in area CA3 (Rami *et al.*, 1986a,b). Hyperthyroidism in rats during the neonatal period results in considerable growth of the cell body and dendrites of CA3 pyramidal cells but little change in CA1 pyramidal cells (E. Gould *et al.*, 1990). Sexual dimorphism of pyramidal cells in area CA3 but not in CA1 is seen after neonatal thyroid treatment: in males the pyramidal cells have more apical dendritic spines whereas in females the basal dendrites are increased in length. These differences might also have functional significance because the apical dendritic spines receive inputs from granule cell mossy fibers (Fig. 6.15) whereas the basal dendrites receive inputs from neighboring pyramidal cells. These changes in morphology of CA3 pyramidal cell dendrites may either be caused by a direct action of thyroid hormone on tubulin synthesis, MAP synthesis, and microtubule assembly (see Section 7.3 for references), or indirectly, by stimulating development of basal forebrain cholinergic neurons which project to the hippocampal formation (E. Gould and Butcher, 1989).

7.5. Changes in the Nervous System during Amphibian Metamorphosis

Thyroid hormones control metamorphosis in the amphibians and thus play a special role in the developmental changes that the nervous system undergoes during metamorphosis. The change from an aquatic to a terrestrial mode of living requires remodeling of many parts of the nervous system correlated with the changes in behavior that are entailed by emergence from water onto land. Studies of these changes can provide opportunities for enlarging our knowledge of the neuroanatomical and neurophysiological foundations of behavior. The change from a sluggish aquatic browser to a voracious terrestrial predator that occurs when the tadpole changes into a frog involves changes in all the sense organs and sensory systems and development of the central nervous mechanisms controlling posture and locomotion on land. These changes require modification or elimination of some of the nervous structures used by the tadpole, for example, the Mauthner neuron (Stefanelli, 1950) and the neurons supplying the tail (M. F. Brown, 1946). New structures arising during metamorphosis include addition of the major part of the retina (Pomeranz, 1972; M. Jacobson, 1976a,b, 1977; D. H. Beach and Jacobson, 1979a–c) and the associated visual central projection neurons in the diencephalon and mesencephalon (Currie and Cowan, 1974a; M. Jacobson, 1977; Hoskins and Grobstein, 1984), development of the cerebellum (Gona, 1972, 1973, 1975, 1976) and the mesencephalic nucleus of the trigeminal nerve (Kollros and McMurray, 1956), changes in the sensory innervation of the skin (M. Jacobson and Baker, 1969), and changes in the spinal cord segments connected to the limbs (Beaudoin, 1956; Race, 1961; Reynolds, 1963; A. F. Hughes, 1966). Thyroid hormones play a part in regulating all these changes. In few other cases can the effects of a hormone on nerve cell production, differentiation, and death be correlated with the changes in behavior so effectively as they can during amphibian metamorphosis.

Administration of T[4] to amphibian larvae results in precocious maturation of the nervous system. T[4] applied locally to various parts of the nervous system of amphibians hastens the development of the neurons that are directly affected by the hormone. A direct effect of T[4] has been shown on the corneal reflex center (Kollros, 1943a), the trigeminal mesencephalic nucleus (Kollros and Pepernik, 1952; Kollros and McMurray, 1956), Mauthner neurons (Weiss and Rossetti, 1951; Pesetsky and Kollros, 1956; Pesetsky, 1960, 1962), and retina (Kaltenbach

and Hobbs, 1972; D. H. Beach and Jacobson, 1979b).

In the retina of *Xenopus* the change from a radially symmetrical pattern of cell proliferation at the retinal margin to a pattern of cell proliferation mainly at the ventral retinal margin occurs during metamorphosis (M. Jacobson, 1976a,b, 1977; D. H. Beach and Jacobson, 1979a) and is stimulated by T[4] (Kaltenbach and Hobbs, 1972; D. H. Beach and Jacobson, 1979b), as shown in Fig. 7.5. Analysis of cell cycle kinetics shows that the increase in mitosis at the ventral retinal margin is not due to a dorso-

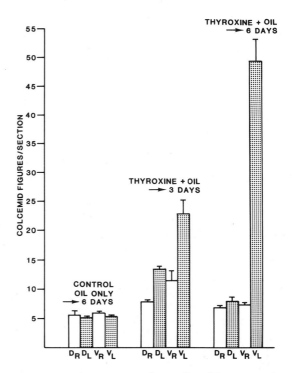

Figure 7.5. Thyroxine stimulates cell proliferation in the retina of the frog tadpole. Average numbers of colcemid figures per histological section are shown in the dorsal and ventral halves of right and left retina (D_R, V_R, D_L, V_L) of three groups of *Xenopus* tadpoles during early metamorphosis (Stage 54). A control group received 38 nl oil injected in the left eye. This produced no significant effect. Two more groups received 38 nl oil + thyroxine (2.5 mg/ml) into the left eye: one group was fixed 3 days later, the other group 6 days later. The number of colcemid figures in the thyroxine-treated eyes increased five-fold after 3 days and 10-fold after 6 days, compared with the untreated eyes of the same animals. All animals were fixed 4 hours after colcemid injection. Bars show standard error of the mean. From D. H. Beach and M. Jacobson, *J. Comp. Neurol.* 183:615–624 (1979).

ventral gradient of difference in the duration of the mitotic cycle (Fig. 2.6), but to a difference in the number of proliferating cells (D. H. Beach and Jacobson, 1979b). T^4 applied to the medulla of the frog tadpole causes precocious development of the corneal reflex on that side compared with the opposite side (Kollros, 1942, 1943a). The corneal reflex consists of retraction of the eye in response to mechanical stimulation of the cornea. It starts during metamorphosis and is not present in younger tadpoles, although all the peripheral mechanisms are present, presumably because the central reflex mechanisms mature only during metamorphosis (Kollros, 1958).

Kollros and McMurray (1956) showed that T^4 implanted in the midbrain of the frog tadpole results in a graded increase in size of the trigeminal mesencephalic neurons. Increase in size of the neuron perikarya varies inversely with the distance from the source of the hormone. Hypophysectomy or administration of thiourea to frog tadpoles results in a reduction in size of the trigeminal mesencephalic neurons, which indicates that the growth of the neurons depends on continuous stimulation by T^4 (Kollros and McMurray, 1956).

Effects of T^4 on mitosis in the CNS of amphibians have been described by Baffoni (1957b, 1959, 1960). After administration of T^4 to frog tadpoles, he observed an initial increase, followed by a decrease, in the number of mitotic figures in various parts of the brain. No increase in the final size of the brain appears to result from treatment with T^4. Although thyroidectomized tadpoles may attain giant size, they have brains smaller than normal controls (B. M. Allen, 1924). It is not known whether the reduction in brain size is due to a reduction in cell number, cell size, or myelin formation. Ferguson (1966) found that after unilateral excision of the medulla of frog tadpoles, T^4 increases the mitotic activity that occurs during regeneration of the medulla. However, the extent of restitution of the excised half is the same in animals treated with T^4 as in untreated frogs.

The effects of T^4 on neurons in the spinal cord and spinal ganglia are complicated by the fact that T^4 directly stimulates growth of the limbs and resorption of the tail, and this in turn results in an increase in the size and number of neurons in the spinal cord and ganglia supplying the limbs and in degeneration of the neurons supplying the tail. During metamorphosis the neurons that supply the tadpole tail degenerate. There is some evidence that the primary action of T^4 is on the tail (R. Weber, 1962), whereas the degeneration of neurons in the tail occurs secondarily as a result of the loss of their peripheral connections (M. E. Brown, 1946). Histolysis of muscles of the tadpole tail is well advanced before degenerative changes appear in the neurons of the spinal cord that supply the tail. Moreover, nerve degeneration starts peripherally, and retrograde degeneration proceeds slowly toward the cell bodies, which suggests that the primary cause of degeneration is the loss of peripheral connections in the tail rather than a direct effect of T^4 on the spinal neurons during metamorphosis (M. E. Brown, 1946).

The difficulty of distinguishing local or primary effects of T^4 on neurons from its general or secondary effects is illustrated by the conflicting reports of the hormone's effects on the Mauthner neurons in the medulla of larval anurans. During normal metamorphosis the Mauthner neurons increase in size and then slowly degenerate after normal metamorphosis (Fig. 7.6) or after precocious metamorphosis induced experimentally with T^4 (Baffoni and Catte, 1950, 1951; Baffoni, 1953; Stefanelli, 1950, 1951; H. Fox and Moulton, 1968; Moulton *et al.*, 1968). Stefanelli (1950) concluded that degeneration of Mauthner neurons is a secondary effect of degeneration of the motor neurons in the tail and lateral lines. However, there is evidence that Mauthner neurons do not depend for their growth and maintenance on the size of their peripheral field. Thus, the size of Mauthner neurons in the frog tadpole is not affected by removal of the tail (Weiss and Rossetti, 1951) or by unilateral ablation of posterior lateralis nerves (Pesetsky, 1960). Mauthner neurons also develop normally in grafts of rhombencephalic portions of embryonic *Rana pipiens* heads in which the Mauthner neurons are isolated from motor centers and are connected with a reduced number of lateral line organs (Pesetsky, 1960).

Since the regression of Mauthner neurons following amphibian metamorphosis cannot be attributed to a reduction of their axonal load, one has to consider whether it may be due to direct action of T^4 on the neurons, or whether death of Mauthner neurons is predetermined by a mechanism like that of the "death clock," which results in cell death in the developing limb (Saunders, 1966; Saunders and Fallon,

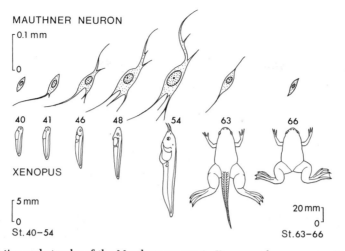

Figure 7.6. Differentiation and atrophy of the Mauthner neuron in *Xenopus*. The upper row shows development of the Mauthner neuron during larval Stages 40–54 of the normal series of Nieuwkoop and Faber (1964), shown in the lower row. Mauthner neuron grows during larval stages, and then atrophies during metamorphic climax and in the adult.

1966; see Section 8.2). That the death of Mauthner neurons is not preordained is indicated by the fact that the neurons survive indefinitely if metamorphosis is delayed with thiourea. Evidence that Mauthner neurons respond directly to T^4 is that implantation of a T^4 pellet on one side of the medulla results in decrease in the size of the Mauthner neuron and increase in the size of the surrounding medullary neurons on the side of the thyroxine implant (Weiss and Rossetti, 1951; Pesetsky and Kollros, 1956). Pesetsky (1962) has suggested that the decrease in size of Mauthner neurons observed after implantation of thyroid pellets is due to withdrawal of the hormone when the implanted pellet becomes depleted of T^4. He found that Mauthner neurons increase in size when tadpoles are immersed in high concentrations of thyroxine (Pesetsky, 1962) and diminish in size in thyroidectomized tadpoles (Pesetsky, 1966). He proposed that the growth of Mauthner neurons is stimulated by T^4 during the late larval stages and that the neurons develop a dependence on the hormone; therefore, he thought, the reduction in the level of T^4 in the blood that occurs at the climax of metamorphosis (Etkin, 1964) may result in involution of Mauthner neurons. The Rohon–Beard neurons in the spinal cord of frog tadpoles also increase in size in response to T^4 (L. B. Stephens, 1965). In both these cases, the initial increase in size of the neuron may be a pathological swelling, not

growth, and may thus be an early change leading to cell death.

Beaudoin (1955) observed that the cells of the lateral motor column of the spinal cord of *R. pipiens* are generated, migrate, and grow steadily until mid-larval stages, but at the time when T^4 causes rapid growth of the hindlimbs, more than two-thirds of the lateral motor neurons degenerate while the surviving neurons increase in size. Beaudoin (1956) showed that T^4 can influence the development of the spinal motor neurons of the frog, directly or indirectly, by stimulating limb growth. Implantation of T^4 into one hindlimb of a frog tadpole causes precocious growth of the limb and an increase in the size of the neurons of the lateral motor column on that side. However, T^4 also has a direct effect on the frog spinal motor neurons, as was shown in two ways by Beaudoin (1956). First, amputation of the limb bud at early larval stages, followed later by immersion of the tadpole in T^4 solutions, results in more rapid loss of motor neurons on the operated side than that occurring without the influence of T^4. Second, T^4 implanted adjacent to the spinal cord results in an increase in the size of the lateral motor neurons on that side.

A. F. Hughes (1966) showed that differentiation of lateral motor neurons in the frog *Eleutherodactylus* is accelerated by T^4 and retarded by treatment with thiourea. However, thyroidectomy or hypophysectomy in *Eleutherodactylus* does not prevent the loss of lateral motor neurons, whereas hypophysectomy prevents the reduction in the number of lateral motor neurons in *R. pipiens* (Race, 1961). Hypophysectomy arrests the differentiation of neurons of the lateral motor column of the spinal cord of *R. pipiens* (Race, 1961). Immersion of *R. pipiens* embryos or early larvae in T^4 solutions results in precocious maturation of the lateral motor column neurons (Reynolds, 1963). T^4 is not necessary for the initial formation, migration, and early differentiation of lateral motor column neurons, as a typical column forms in hypophysectomized tadpoles (Race, 1961). Reynolds (1963) concluded that the capacity of the lateral column neurons to respond to T^4 is not present before late embryonic stages (Stage 25 of Shumway, 1940, 1942).

Xenopus tadpoles treated with the antithyroid drug propylthiouracil grow much larger than normal. When treated with thyroid hormone they metamorphose into giant frogs in which the cells, including neurons, are increased in size but not in number (Sperry and Grobstein, 1985). Those findings are not consistent with the theory that cell death regulates neuron numbers to match the size of the peripheral field. This is discussed further in Chapter 8.

7.6. Effects of Adrenal Glucocorticoids on Brain Development

Corticosteroids cross the placenta and blood–brain barrier by simple diffusion. They bind to specific cytoplasmic receptors in neurons and glial cells. The hormone–receptor complexes are translocated into the nucleus, where they regulate transcription of certain sets of genes (Schmidt and Litvak, 1982, review; Evans, 1988, review). There are two types of glucocorticoid receptors in the mammalian CNS: type 1 and type 2 (Reul and De Kloet, 1985; Funder and Sheppard, 1987, reviews). Type 1 receptors have a high affinity for corticosterone, while aldosterone is a competitive antagonist; they are localized mainly in the dentate gyrus granule cells and CA1 and CA2 pyramidal cells of the hippocampal formation. Type 2 receptors have highest affinity for synthetic glucocorticoids and about 10 times lower affinity than type 1 receptors for corticosterone and are localized on glial cells and neurons throughout the nervous system.

The sites of action of corticosteroids in the brain are mainly localized to the septum and other limbic structures. This was first shown by injection of [³H]corticosterone into adrenalectomized rats followed by measurements of the uptake of labeled hormone in various brain regions (McEwen et al., 1969). By means of autoradiography of tissue sections after injection of [³H]corticosterone the sites of uptake have been localized to essentially the same regions in mice (Coutard and Osborne-Pellegrin, 1979), rats (Stumpf, 1971a; Gerlach and McEwen, 1972; McEwen et al., 1974; Rhees et al., 1975; Stumpf and Sar, 1975; Warembourg, 1975; Sapolsky et al., 1983), and rhesus monkeys (Pfaff et al., 1976). Cells are heavily labeled in the hippocampal formation, especially pyramidal cells of CA1 and CA2 and granule cells of the dentate gyrus. Lighter labeling is seen over structures in the limbic system: the indusium griseum, septal nuclei, pyriform cortex, and parts of the amygdala. Light labeling also occurs outside the limbic system in the cerebral neocortex, cerebellar cortex, motor nuclei of the brainstem, and dorsal horn of the spinal cord. In all these regions only neurons were labeled with [³H]corticosterone or with [³H]aldosterone (Gerlach and McEwen, 1972; Warembourg, 1975; Pfaff et al., 1976; Birmingham et al., 1979, 1984). Therefore, those neurons were mainly expressing type 1 glucocorticoid receptors. Labeling of neuroglial cells or Schwann cells (Warembourg et al., 1981) is not seen in autoradiographs although there is ample evidence, given later, that they have type 2 glucocorticoid receptors and respond to glucocorticoids.

Glucocorticoid receptors can first be detected in rat brain on E17 (Kitraki et al., 1984) and increase gradually to adult levels by P15–P30 (Olpe and McEwen, 1976; Clayton et al., 1977) except in the cerebellar cortex, where the expression of glucocorticoid receptors is correlated with the growth and disappearance of the external granular layer (Pavlik and Buresova, 1984).

The effects of glucocorticoids administered during the neonatal period are inhibition of proliferation of neurons and neuroglial cells; retardation of cell differentiation, especially of outgrowth of dendrites, synaptogenesis, and myelination; induction of the catecholamine synthetic enzymes tyrosine hydroxylase (TH), dopamine beta-hydroxylase (DBH), and phenylethanolamine N-methyltransferase (PNMT) in neurons of neural crest origin; induction of glutamine synthetase

(GS) in astrocytes and glycerol-3-phosphate dehydrogenese (GPDH) in oligodendrocytes (Meyer, 1985, review).

Administration of glucocorticoids to newborn rats results in a reduction of DNA content and of incorporation of thymidine into DNA (Cotterell et al., 1972; Howard and Benjamin, 1975; Burdman et al., 1975; Ardeleanu and Sterescu, 1978). Tritiated thymidine autoradiography shows inhibition of cell proliferation in the rat cerebellar external layer during corticosterone injections in the neonatal period (Bohn and Lauder, 1978, 1980) as well as reduction of granule cell proliferation in the hippocampal dentate gyrus (Bohn, 1980). Recovery occurs after cessation of treatment from P1 to P4 and is greater than recovery after treatment from P7 to P18. Temporary inhibition of glial cell production occurs after neonatal hydrocortisone treatment in the rat optic nerve (Bohn and Friedrich, 1982) and cerebral subependymal zone (Bohn, 1979). Myelination in the pyramidal tract is reduced after a single injection of prednisone given to rats at P6 (Gumbinas et al., 1973). A reduction of cerebral cortical dendritic spines follows neonatal hydrocortisone treatment in the rat (Schapiro et al., 1973; Oda and Huttenlocher, 1974).

Adrenalectomy of neonatal rats on P11 accelerates brain growth, increases total brain DNA (Meyer, 1983, 1985), and increases myelination, probably permanently (Meyer and Fairman, 1985). Adrenalectomy of adult male rats results in selective and complete loss of hippocampal granule cells 3–4 months after surgery, and the loss is completely prevented by corticosteroid treatment (Sloviter et al., 1989).

7.7. Role of Glucocorticoids in Development of Neurons of Neural Crest Origin

The most thoroughly studied parameters of neuronal differentiation modulated by glucocorticoids are inductions of neurotransmitter synthesizing enzymes in cells of neural crest lineage. Expression of these enzymes is also regulated by thyroxine and by nerve growth factor (NGF).

Tyrosine hydroxylase (TH) expression in sympathetic postganglionic neurons is under control of corticosteroids and NGF (Thoenen et al., 1971). In the rat superior cervical ganglion in vitro TH induction by NGF is potentiated by corticosterone (Otten and Thoenen, 1976, 1977).

Dopamine β-hydroxylase (DBH) is increased in rat superior cervical ganglion treated with dexamethasone in culture (Otten and Thoenen, 1976). Corticosterone potentiates NGF induction of DBH in the superior cervical ganglion in vitro (Otten and Thoenen, 1977). Immunocytochemical studies show that the corticosterone-induced DBH in the superior cervical ganglion is mainly in the small intensely fluorescent (SIF) cells (Eränkö et al., 1982). There are about 200 SIF cells and about 20,000 postganglionic neurons in the superior cervical ganglion of the newborn rat (Päivärinta and Eränkö, 1982). The number of ganglionic neurons remains constant whereas the SIF cells increase to about 600 in the adult (Eränkö and Soinila, 1981). In the adult the SIF cells secrete dopamine or norepinephrine. However from E17 to about P14 the SIF cells transiently contain the enzyme phenylethanolamine N-methyltransferase (PNMT), which catalyzes formation of epinephrine from norepinephrine (Bohn et al., 1982). Glucocorticoids administered neonatally to rats increase the number of SIF cells about 10-fold (Eränkö and Eränkö, 1972; Eränkö et al., 1972; Päivärinta and Eränkö, 1982) and greatly increase PNMT activity in the superior cervical ganglion (Ciaranello et al., 1973; Ciaranello and Axelrod, 1975; Moore and Phillipson, 1975; Luizzi et al., 1977; Bohn et al., 1982, 1984; Eränkö et al., 1982). These effects disappear rapidly after cessation of treatment at 2 weeks of age but can be reinduced by a second course of glucocorticoids administered several weeks later (Bohn et al., 1982; Päivärenta et al., 1982). These effects could be caused either by transient induction of PNMT in preexisting SIF cells (Eränkö et al., 1982) or by proliferation of new SIF cells. That the latter probably occurs is shown by the fact that cytosine arabinoside prevents the increase in PNMT cells induced by glucocorticoids (Bohn and Friedrich, 1982).

7.8. Role of Glucocorticoids in Glial Cell Development

The effect on glial cell differentiation is shown by glucocorticoid induction of two glial cell enzymes, glutamine synthetase (GS), which is localized in astrocytes, and glycerol-3-phosphate dehydrogenase (GPDH) which is primarily found in oligodendrocytes.

Glutamine synthetase is specifically localized in astrocytes throughout the nervous system (Norenberg, 1979; Norenberg *et al.*, 1980) where its function is to catalyze synthesis of glutamine from glutamic acid and ammonia. Astrocytes store glutamate for use by glutaminergic neurons. Astrocytes themselves have glutamate-sensitive ion channels and respond to glutamate with an increase in intracellular calcium (Cornell-Bell *et al.*, 1990).

In the chick embryo retina GS activity normally increases rapidly from E16 to E21 but can be induced by hydrocortisone to increase as early as E7 (Moscona and Piddington, 1966, 1967; Piddington and Moscona, 1967; Moscona *et al.*, 1972). The GS is localized in the Müller cells of the retina (Linser and Moscona, 1979; Noremberg *et al.*, 1980). Hydrocortisone binds specifically to Müller cells and enters their cell nuclei by a temperature-dependent process (Chader, 1973; Diamant *et al.*, 1975).

In the rat CNS, GS activity increases gradually throughout embryonic development and the neonatal period (Wu, 1964; Vaccaro *et al.*, 1979; Patel *et al.*, 1983). Corticosteroids increase GS activity in neonatal rat forebrain only until about P15 (Wu, 1964) whereas induction of GS in the cerebellum was found as late as P87 (Patel *et al.*, 1983). Glutamine synthetase is induced by glucocorticoids in mouse astrocytes in primary culture and in rat C6 glioma cells but not in rat neuroblastoma cells (Hallermeyer *et al.*, 1981; Juurlink *et al.*, 1981; Caldani *et al.*, 1982).

GPDH is greatly enriched in oligodendrocytes (Leveille *et al.*, 1980; Cammer *et al.*, 1982a,b; Meyer *et al.*, 1982) although lower levels of GPDH activity have been found in Bergmann glial cells (Fisher *et al.*, 1981). The function of the enzyme in the nervous system is to provide glycerol-3-phosphate for lipid synthesis, especially during myelination (Laatsch, 1962; Leveille *et al.*, 1980). GDPH activity in the rat brain increases in parallel with myelination in various regions, from very low levels at birth to adult levels by about P40 (DeVellis and Schjeide, 1968; DeVellis and Inglish, 1973). A similar correlation between myelination and GPDH is observed in chick brain (Adler and Klucznick, 1982). The normal increase in GDPH is inhibited by hypophysectomy and stimulated prematurely by corticosteroid administration (DeVellis and Inglish, 1968, 1973). Induction of GPDH by glucocorticoids has been demonstrated in primary cultures of rat oligodendrocytes but not in primary astrocyte cultures (McCarthy and DeVellis, 1980). There is evidence that GDPH expression in oligodendrocytes is regulated by interaction with neurons. Thus GDPH activity in rat optic nerve increases during optic nerve degeneration (Meyer *et al.*, 1982), and GPDH induction by glucocorticoids is inhibited in rat C6 glioma cells cocultured with rat neuroblastoma cells (Ciment and DeVellis, 1982).

7.9. Role of Growth Hormone in Neural Ontogeny

Studies of the effects of growth hormone on the developing nervous system have been limited not only by technical difficulties such as contamination of the growth hormone with other trophic hormones of the anterior pituitary, but also by uncertainties regarding the site and mode of action of the hormone on the nervous system. Some of these limitations are apparent in the study of the effects of growth hormone on *R. pipiens* tadpoles (Zamenhof, 1941). A preparation of growth hormone was injected for 12–22 days on alternate days into tadpoles at the stages of limb growth. The treated animals showed a 44–126 percent increase in the number of cells (neurons and glial cells) in the cerebral hemispheres, in comparison with normal controls. It was concluded that the growth hormone stimulates cellular proliferation in the brain. However, the alternative, that the hormone might reduce cell death, was not considered. Moreover, an impure preparation of growth hormone was used, and the increase in cells might have been produced by adrenocorticotropin, thyrotropin, and prolactin that were probably present in the injections. The effects of purified prolactin or growth hormone on the brain of the frog *R. pipiens* during development were studied by R. K. Hunt and Jacobson (1970, 1971). Six injections of prolactin (5 μg) administered to early frog tadpoles produced a 20–25 percent increase in brain weight and 35–43 percent increase in total brain DNA at metamorphosis. In contrast, six injections of growth hormone (25 μg) increased brain weight by 12–20 percent and brain DNA by 10–15 percent. Additional studies with [³H]thymidine suggest that the effects of both hormones are at least partially due to increased cellular proliferation, although the patterns of precursor incorporation are quite different in the two cases. The rate of incorporation of [³H]thymidine into DNA in the brain nearly doubles during the period of growth hormone injections, but returns to the control rate shortly thereafter. Conversely, prolactin only slightly increases the rate of DNA synthesis in the brain during the injection period, but the rate of DNA synthesis is markedly increased during the following 10-day period, when it normally declines.

Growth hormone administered to rats after birth does not increase the size or weight of the nervous system (Rubenstein, 1936; Zamenhof, 1942; M. C. Diamond et al., 1969). Hypophysectomy of rats a few days after birth does not alter brain weight, brain protein content, thickness of the cerebral cortex, or branching of basal dendrites of cortical pyramidal cells (M. C. Diamond et al., 1964, 1969; Gregory and Diamond, 1968a,b). These negative results are in contrast to the reported 70–90 percent reduction of myelination in newborn rats treated with growth hormone (Pelton et al., 1977).

By contrast with the negative results of injecting growth hormone postnatally, administration of growth hormone to pregnant female rats has been shown to affect the nervous system of the offspring. Zamenhof (1942) injected pregnant female rats with an impure preparation of growth hormone daily from days 7 to 20 of gestation and examined the brain of the fetuses at birth (delivered by cesarean section at term) or after reaching maturity. Compared with control rats, the offspring of the treated females had an increase of 18.7 percent in body weight, 36 percent in cerebral hemisphere weight, 21 percent in the thickness of the cerebral cortex, and 86 percent in the number of cells in the entire cortex. The rats that developed to adults had an increase of 15–28 percent in cell density and 38–41 percent in the total number of cells in the cerebral cortex as compared with counts in untreated rats. The accuracy of these cell counts is questionable because no corrections were made for shrinkage of the brains during fixation or for the increase in cell size in the treated animals, which may be sources of serious error (Abercrombie, 1946; Hendry, 1976). Moreover, the preparation of growth hormone used in the experiments was contaminated by detectable amounts of other hormones of the anterior pituitary (footnote in Clendinnen and Eayrs, 1961).

In a later series of experiments, Zamenhof et al.

(1966) reported that purified growth hormone administered to pregnant rats resulted in a 10–20 percent increase in the weight and DNA content of the brain of the offspring and comparable increases in density of cells in the cerebral cortex, in number and length of dendrites of cortical pyramidal cells, and in the ratio of neurons to glial cells. Therefore, they concluded that prenatally administered growth hormone primarily effects the neurons and results in a relatively greater increase in the number rather than the size of neurons. This conclusion is not supported by the results of Clendinnen and Eayrs (1961), who studied the offspring of rats given daily injections of purified growth hormone from day 7 to day 20 of gestation. These offspring are slightly heavier at birth, and their motor activity matures somewhat earlier than normal controls. At 33 and 60 days of age, the cell gray-coefficient (the proportion of cortex occupied by cell bodies) was found to be increased by 20 percent above the normal value in the treated rats. There was a 22 percent increase in the mean length of dendrites and a 23 percent increase in the mean number of dendritic branches of cerebral cortical neurons (Fig. 7.7). These observations indicate that an increase in neuronal size and probably of connectivity occurs, but there is no evidence of an increase in the number of neurons. Because the histology of the cerebral cortex was studied at 33 and 60 days, after the growth of dendrites and the formation of synapses in the cerebral cortex are virtually completed in normal rats, these observations do not show whether the maturation of the cortex occurs earlier in rats treated prenatally with growth hormone or whether maturation occurs at the usual time postnatally, with a time lag after prenatal administration.

Whether the effects represent the primary response to the hormone or a secondary response is often impossible to decide. Secondary effects may be on the general metabolism or nutrition of the animal or on the hypothalamopituitary axis, resulting in changes in other hormones. Interactions between thyroid hormone and growth hormone have been demonstrated in the control of skeletal growth and the control of RNA content in the cerebral cortex in rats (Geel and Timiras, 1970). Growth hormone (400 μg/100 g body weight per day) produces no increase in body or brain growth in hypothyroid rats in the first 25 days after birth. A similar problem regarding the mode of action of the hormone arises

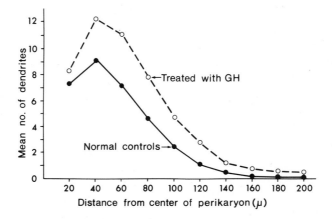

Figure 7.7. Growth hormone stimulates growth of dendrites of cerebral cortical pyramidal cells. The mean number of basal dendrites of pyramidal cells in layer IIIc of the sensorimotor cortex of rats at P30 and P60 treated prenatally with growth hormone, compared with normal controls. From B. G. Clendinnen and J. T. Eayrs, *J. Endocrinol* 22:183–193 (1961).

in connection with reports of stimulation of brain development in the fetus after administration of growth hormone to the mother (Zamenhof *et al.*, 1966, 1971c; Sara and Lazarus, 1974; Sara *et al.*, 1974). The problem with these results is that growth hormone does not cross the placenta from mother to fetus (Gitlin *et al.*, 1965; Laron *et al.*, 1966). The growth hormone may affect the fetus indirectly by mobilizing maternal nutrient supplies, may increase uterine size and blood supply, may increase placental size, or may enhance maternal hormonal mechanisms that stimulate total growth.

Another factor that may confound the assessment of the prenatal action of growth hormone is the fact that the hormone prolongs gestation (Croskerry and Smith, 1975). In many of the reports of increased brain weight at birth, the animals may well have been postmature. No increase in body or brain weight is found in rats after prenatal treatment with growth hormone when the fetuses are delivered by cesarean section near term (Croskerry *et al.*, 1973).

The conflicting results obtained by different investigators are indicative of the uncertainties and sources of error in such experiments, in which there are many uncontrolled variables. Variables such as the length of gestation and the size of the litter may be controllable. More difficult to control are the effects of the hormone on the mother's nutrition, metabolism, hormonal function, and placental function. These may have much greater indirect effects

on the fetus than any direct effect of the hormone on fetal brain development.

7.10. Sex Hormones in Brain Development

Sex determination is primarily genetic. In mammals a gene on the Y chromosome controls differentiation of the indifferent gonad into a testis. The Leydig cells secrete testosterone, which stimulates differentiation of the male reproductive organs and secondary sexual characteristics, and the Sertoli cells secrete Müllerian inhibitory substance, which inhibits development of the female reproductive organs. In the female, in the absence of testosterone, the Müllerian duct develops into Fallopian tubes, uterus, and vagina.

The nervous system in both sexes is initially indifferent and intracellular estradiol receptors develop in neurons of both sexes. In the male, testosterone is converted to estradiol in the brain. The estrogen–receptor complex is translocated to the nucleus where it regulates transcription of genes that organize the brain as male. Masculinization of the brain can occur only during a short critical period (in rats, birth ± 5 days). Female brain organization ensues in the absence of testosterone during the critical period. Sexual dimorphism of CNS occurs as the result of sex hormones increasing the number of neurons formed, reducing the number that normally die, increasing cell growth, dendritic branching, increasing synaptogenesis, and regulating patterns of synaptic function and neuronal electrical activity. Differential cell death is the major mechanism for development of sex differences in the nervous system.

Testosterone is the only androgen formed by the fetal testes, and it is enzymatically converted to dihydrotestosterone. These two androgens have different peripheral and nervous target tissues both prenatally and postnatally. In the fetus, testosterone promotes virilization of the urogenital tract by acting on the Wolffian duct to induce the development of the epididymis, vas deferens, and seminal vesicle. In the nervous system testosterone is aromatized to estrogen, which binds to intracellular receptors and organizes male brain functions during a short critical period of brain development. Dihydrotestosterone has no effect on sexual behavior, although it can stimulate gonadotropin release in adult rats.

The secondary sexual characteristics that are organized by gonadal hormones include not only those of the genitalia and secondary sexual organs but also the appropriate brain functions that subserve sexually dimorphic behavior in birds as well as mammals. The subsequent development of sexual behavior in mammals is determined by or modified by sex hormones that bind to specific receptors in the brain regions which subserve sexual behavior and gonadotropin release from the pituitary, namely, the medial preoptic area, limbic forebrain structures, and ventromedial hypothalamic nuclei.

A single injection of testosterone given to a female or castrated male rat within the first few days after birth results in male sexual behavior at maturity (Segal and Johnson, 1959; G. W. Harris and Levine, 1962, 1965; Grady et al., 1965; S. Levine and Mullins, 1966). There is considerable evidence that prior to a critical period the central nervous structures controlling sexual behavior in mammals of both sexes are indifferent (G. W. Harris, 1964; G. W. Harris and Levine, 1965; Gorski, 1966; Arnold and Gorski, 1984, review). The brain contains estrogen receptors before birth in both sexes. During the critical period, sexual differentiation of the neural tissues mediating masculine sexual behavior occurs under the influence of estrogen derived from neural aromatization of testosterone. Feminine sexual behavior ensues in the absence of testosterone.

It has long been known that a small percentage of normal female mammals of many different species will exhibit male sexual behavior, while the spontaneous display of female sexual behavior by male mammals is much rarer (F. A. Beach, 1975). It now appears that such "atypical behavior" may be due to the fact that, in both sexes, the hormone which alters sexual behavior is estradiol and the effect of estradiol on the developing brain is to produce male sexual behavior.

Naftolin et al. (1971a,b, 1972) originally proposed that testosterone is converted to estradiol in the brain and that the masculinizing effect of testosterone is mediated by estradiol which binds to estradiol receptors in neurons (Feder et al., 1974; Krey et al., 1982). Fetal and neonatal blood contains an estrogen binding protein, identical to alpha-fetoprotein, that prevents the estrogen from entering the developing brain (Raymond et al., 1971; B. Attardi and Ruoslahti, 1976). Testosterone, or synthetic estrogen such as diethylstilbestrol, does not bind to this protein and is free to enter the developing brain (McEwen et al., 1975). In the brain, testosterone is converted to estradiol particularly well in the hypothalamus, amygdala, and preoptic area, but not in the cerebral cortex, which nevertheless contains specific nuclear estrogen receptors (Lieberburg and McEwen, 1975; McEwen et al., 1976). The masculinizing effects of testosterone as well as estrogen in the fetus and neonate are apparently mediated by the brain estrogen receptors. These effects refer to the developing brain only. In the adult, testosterone is preferentially bound by the hypothalamus in the male whereas estradiol is preferentially bound by the female hypothalamus (Plapinger and McEwen, 1973; Plapinger et al., 1973). This selectivity is not present in prenatal and neonatal rats before sexual differentiation of the hypothalamus occurs (Tuohimaa and Niemi, 1972). Experimental androgenization of female rats as well as the normal masculinization of the brain of male rats results in loss of the capacity of the hypothalamus to accumulate estradiol in the adult (Tuohimaa and Johansson, 1971; Vertes et al., 1973).

Estradiol is the primary determinant of brain sexual organization in birds as well as mammals (Arnold and Gorski, 1984, review). However, during a critical period of development, estrogen masculines the mammalian brain, whereas it feminizes the avian brain.

In the quail or the chicken, injection of estradiol into the egg on E10 results in no change of sex behavior of females but results in complete reversal of sex behavior of males. The critical period for feminization of copulatory behavior of males by estradiol is before the 12th day of an 18-day incubation period in the quail (Adkins-Regan, 1987, review).

In canaries and zebra finches only the male sings, and this behavior is androgen dependent and learned during development. Females can learn to sing if given estradiol during the first 2 weeks after hatching and treated with testosterone as young adults. Sex differences in singing behavior are subserved by sexually dimorphic nuclei in the telencephalon and brainstem. Sexual dimorphism in the brain of the zebra finch develops as the result of a greater rate of cell death in the females than in the male robust nucleus of the archistriatum (RA) and the magnocellular nucleus of the neostriatum (MAN), as well as continued production of more neurons in the male hyperstriatum ventralis pars caudalis (HVc) and Area X. Addition of neurons to HVc and Area X in males, but not in females, occurs between P20 and P55. More neurons die in females than males in RA and MAN between 15 and 45 days after hatching (Nordeen and Nordeen, 1988; Kirn and DeVoogd, 1989). Androgen prevents the loss of neurons that normally occurs in female birds (Bottjer *et al.*, 1985; Bottjer, 1987; Nordeen *et al.*, 1987). How these differences give rise to differences in development of song of males and females remains unknown.

In mammals, androgens rescue neurons from death in the bulbocavernosus nucleus in the lumbar spinal cord. This nucleus contains motoneurons innervating the levator ani and bulbocavernosus muscles. These muscles are attached to the penis of the male and are absent in adult female rats. Adult males have three times the number of bulbocavernosus neurons found in females. At birth males and females both have large numbers of bulbocavernosus motoneurons and the perineal muscles they innervate. The sex differences develop in the 1st postnatal week as the result of more death of motoneurons in the female (Nordeen *et al.*, 1985; Sengelaub and Arnold, 1986), as shown in Fig. 7.8. Females treated perinatally with testosterone propionate have a reduced amount of motoneuron death, resulting in a permanent increase in the number of bulbocavernosus motoneurons (Nordeen *et al.*, 1985) and their bulbocavernosus and levator ani

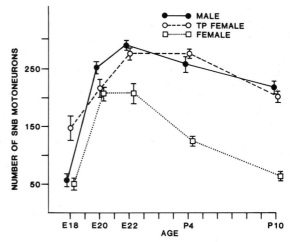

Figure 7.8. Androgens prevent normally occurring neuronal death in the female spinal nucleus of the bulbocavernosus. Counts of motoneurons in the spinal nucleus of bulbocavernosus from E18 through P10 for normal females (n = 24), females treated with testosterone propionate from E16 through E22 (n = 27) and normal males (n = 23). Points show means ± standard errors; n = 3–7 per data point. From E. J. Nordeen, K. W. Nordeen, D. R. Sengelaub, and A. P. Arnold, *Science* 229:671–673 (1985), copyright American Association for the Advancement of Science.

muscles are preserved (Breedlove and Arnold, 1983b). Their bulbocavernosus motoneurons are larger than those of normal females (Breedlove *et al.*, 1982; Breedlove and Arnold, 1981, 1983b; Lee *et al.*, 1989). Treatment of males perinatally with antiandrogens results in increased death of bulbocavernosus motoneurons and atrophy of the perineal muscles they innervate (Breedlove and Arnold, 1983a). The bulbocavernosus motoneurons remain sensitive to androgens throughout life; castration results in atrophy and administration of androgens results in increase in size of bulbocavernosus motoneurons and increase in dendritic length and branching (Breedlove and Arnold, 1981; Kurz *et al.*, 1986, 1990; Goldstein *et al.*, 1990). During normal development of the male rat, circulating testosterone levels change from high levels before birth to low levels during the first 4 postnatal weeks, and then gradually rising to about half adult levels at 7 weeks and reaching adult levels a few weeks later (Resko *et al.*, 1968; Ketelslegers *et al.*, 1978; Corpechot *et al.*, 1981). Growth of dendrites of bulbocavernosus neurons appears to follow the changes in circulating testosterone: dendrites reach maximum length by the 4th postnatal week and then retract to adult length by 7 weeks of age (L. A. Goldstein *et al.*, 1990). Castration or treatment with testosterone results in reversible changes in dendritic length of bulbocavernosus motoneurons (L. A. Goldstein *et al.*, 1990). The peripheral connections of these motoneurons are also androgen dependent: the levator ani muscle normally retains multiple innervation under the influence of testosterone, and elimination of multiple endplates occurs after castration (Jordan *et al.*, 1989a,b). The sexual dimorphism of the bulbocavernosus nucleus is regulated by androgens and is insensitive to estrogens (Breedlove *et al.*, 1982; Breedlove and Arnold, 1980, 1981, 1983). This is consistent with the absence of the bulbocavernosus and levator ani muscles in testicular feminization rats, which are sensitive to estrogens but lack normal androgen receptors (Breedlove and Arnold, 1980, 1981).

Testicular feminization (pseudohermaphroditism) is caused by a mutation which produces defects in cytosolic androgen receptors (Bardin *et al.*, 1973; Naess *et al.*, 1976; Wieland and Fox, 1981). The result is a male genotype with a female phenotype in humans (Morris, 1953), cattle (Nes, 1966), dogs (Schultz, 1962), rats (Stanley *et al.*, 1973), and mice (Lyon and Hawkes, 1970). In testicular feminization the brain is masculinized (or defeminized) by estrogens, as in normal males, although the peripheral targets are feminized (Shapiro *et al.*, 1980).

In mammals the level of testosterone in the blood increases in the male during the perinatal period, declines after birth, and rises again at puberty. The perinatal rise in testosterone levels is required for the *organization* of neural mechanisms subserving male sexual behavior, while the increased testosterone at puberty is required for *activation* of some of the neural mechanisms resulting in masculine behavior. The perinatal testosterone has a priming effect on tissues whose full expression of male function is triggered by the increased testosterone normally secreted at puberty.

Thus it is customary to distinguish between the *organizing action* of the hormone on the brain during development and the *activating action* of the hormone in the adult. Some types of behavior require an action of the hormone only during development, for example, the leg lifting during micturition in male dogs or mounting in male monkeys. These forms of behavior are displayed by females that are masculinized by testosterone given prenatally or neonatally. Other types of behavior require hormonal activation as well as organization, for example, mounting in the rat. Thus females that are masculinized by testosterone at birth exhibit male mating behavior only when it is activated by hormones. Yet other kinds of sexually dimorphic behavior, such as the masculine "yawn" in the monkey, require activation but not organization, and therefore can be produced in normal adult females treated with androgens (F. A. Beach, 1975, review).

One difficulty of studying the effects of neonatal castration arises from species differences in the effects of prenatal androgens, because the duration of exposure of the fetus to androgens varies with the length of gestation. In hamsters, in which gestation lasts only 16 days, castration of males on the day of birth results in abolition of the activating effect of testosterone given to the adult (Noble, 1973). By contrast, castration of male rats (gestation 22 days) on the day of birth does not abolish the mounting that results from testosterone treatment in adults (Grady *et al.*, 1965). Conversely, in the female rat, administration of testosterone prenatally and postnatally results in a marked increase in mounting behavior. Even a single injection of testosterone given to female rats on the 4th day of life can result in increased mounting under certain conditions (Södersten, 1973), whereas dihydrotestosterone given prenatally or postnatally has no such effect on female rats (Whalen and Luttge, 1971a,b). This difference has been attributed to the fact that testosterone is converted to estradiol, whereas dihydrotestosterone is not. The conversion of testosterone to estradiol occurs *in vitro* in brain tissue incubated with some androgens (Reddy *et al.*, 1974), as well as in the intact perfused brain (Flores *et al.*, 1973). Estradiol accumulates in neonatal rat brain cell nuclei after administration of testosterone, indicating that estradiol is a normal metabolite of testosterone (Lieberburg and McEwen, 1975).

The uptake of $[^3H]$testosterone from the bloodstream by the brains of male rats and of $[^3H]$estradiol by the brains of female rats was first shown by scintillation counting of extracts of brain, and these studies indicate that the hormones are concentrated in the anterior hypothalamus and preoptic region (Eisenfeld and Axelrod, 1965; Kato and

Villee, 1967; Resko *et al.*, 1967). Binding of sex steroids also occurs in the septum, amygdala, and hippocampus (McEwen and Pfaff, 1970).

Evidence of more precisely localized nervous uptake of sex hormones has been obtained by autoradiography of sections of brain following intravenous injection of [³H]testosterone or [³H]estradiol (Pfaff, 1968a–c; Pfaff and Keiner, 1973; Morrell *et al.*, 1975, review). There is a remarkable similarity in the anatomical distribution of sex hormone binding sites in males and females and in all vertebrate orders, and the brain sites of sex hormone accumulation are also implicated in species-specific sexual behavior. For example, mating behavior, song, and other vocalizations in the male chaffinch are dependent on testosterone, and testosterone binding to neurons is found in the midbrain and other regions that are implicated in the hormone-dependent behavior (R. E. Zigmond *et al.*, 1973). The pattern of labeling of the male brain with [³H]testosterone (Morrell *et al.*, 1975) is quite similar but not identical to that of the female brain with [³H]estradiol. Most, if not all, of the label seems to be associated with the nuclei of neurons, although some glial cells are also labeled (Pfaff and Keiner, 1973). The preoptic region, tuberal region of the hypothalamus, rostral regions of the limbic system and hypothalamus, and the mesencephalon underneath the tectum are sites of sex steroid binding in all vertebrates, and these are also regions that have been implicated in sexual behavior and in gonadotropin release (Fig. 7.9).

Androgenized females of nonhuman mammalian species exhibit masculine sexual behavior, but in human females who have been androgenized *in utero* the suppression of feminine behavior is minimal, although there is some behavioral masculinization. The remarkable observation on such human females who have been exposed to androgens prenatally, and also female pseudohermaphrodites with the adrenogenital syndrome, is that they have unusually high IQ (Ehrhardt and Money, 1967; V. G. Lewis *et al.*, 1968; Money, 1971; P. A. Walker and Money, 1972; Money and Ehrhardt, 1972, review). In a sample of seven boys and girls with the adrenogenital syndrome, Money and Lewis (1966) reported a slightly increased mean IQ of 109.9, indicating that prenatal androgens have an elevating effect on the ultimate IQ. The effect is greater in girls exposed to androgens prenatally as a

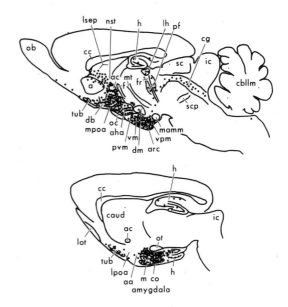

Figure 7.9. Distribution of estrogen-concentrating neurons in the brain of the female rats represented schematically in two sagittal sections. Most labeled neurons could be represented in a medial plane (bottom drawing). Estradiol-concentrating neurons in the amygdala and hippocampus are represented in a more lateral plane (top drawing). Locations of estradiol-concentrating neurons are represented by black dots. a = nucleus accumbens; aa = anterior amygdaloid area; ac = anterior commissure; aha = anterior hypothalamic area; arc = arcuate nucleus; caud = caudate nucleus; cbllm = cerebellum; cc = corpus callosum; cg = central gray; co = cortical nucleus of the amygdala; db = diagonal band of Broca; dm = dorsomedial nucleus of the hypothalamus; f = fornix; fr = fasciculus retroflexus; h = hippocampus; ic = inferior colliculus; lh = lateral habenula; lot = lateral olfactory tract; lpoa = lateral preoptic area; lsep = lateral septum; m = medial nucleus of the amygdala; mamm = mammillary bodies; mpoa = medial preoptic area; mt = mammillothalamic tract; nst = bed nucleus of the stria terminalis; ob = olfactory bulb; oc = optic chiasm; ot = optic tract; pf =nucleus parafascicularis; pvm = paraventricular nucleus (magnocellular); sc = superior colliculus; scp = superior cerebellar peduncle; tub = olfactory tubercle; vm = ventral premammillary nucleus. From D. W. Pfaff and M. Keiner, *J. Comp. Neurol.* 151:121–158 (1973).

result of administration to the mother of steroids with an androgenic action, to prevent abortion. Ehrhardt and Money (1967) reported that in 10 such girls the mean IQ was 125 (S.D. 11.8), and six had an IQ above 130. A similar increase in IQ is found in males exposed to excess androgen *in utero* (Money and Ehrhardt, 1972, p. 102). Such findings raise tantalizing questions about the relationships between human intelligence and the brain structures and functions sensitive to hormone stimulation. Are there specific structures stimulated by hormones that increase IQ, or is the effect a general one, resulting in an increase in the total number of neurons or total number of synaptic connections, or is the effect due to some as yet unknown type of process?

There are numerous anatomical differences between the brains of males and females (reviewed by Arnold and Gorski, 1984; Toran-Allerand, 1984; Swaab and Hofman, 1984). The weight of the human brain at birth is greater in males. The ratios of brain-to-body weight and brain-to-body height are the same in both sexes at birth but males develop increasingly higher ratios (Bayley, 1956; Tanner *et al.*, 1966; Dekaban and Sadowsky, 1978; Voigt and Pakkenberg, 1983).

The splenial part of the corpus callosum in the human female is larger and more bulbous than in males (de Lacoste-Utamsing and Holloway, 1982; de Lacoste *et al.*, 1986; Holloway and de Lacoste, 1986). The difference is reported to be present in the fetus by 28 weeks of gestation (Baack *et al.*,

1982). This may be correlated with the observation that cerebral hemispheric asymmetry is greater in males than females (Wada *et al.*, 1975; McGlone, 1980), and with sex differences in cerebral hemispheric dominance (Witelson, 1976, 1985; Harris, 1978; Kimura, 1980, 1983; Kimura and Harshman, 1984).

The nuclei in the anterior hypothalamus that are involved in the control of endocrine function are several times larger in male than in female mammals. Sexual dimorphism in the hypothalamus is present in the quail (Viglietti-Panzica *et al.*, 1986), in rats (Gorski *et al.*, 1978, 1980; Robinson *et al.*, 1986), guinea pigs (Hines *et al.*, 1985; Byne and Bleier, 1987), ferrets (Tobet *et al.*, 1986), gerbils (Commins and Yahr, 1984), and humans (Swaab and Fliers, 1985; Swaab and Hofman, 1988; Allen *et al.*, 1989; Hofman and Swaab, 1989). The sexual dimorphism of the human preoptic hypothalamic area is caused by a large loss of cells in females (Fig. 7.10) between the ages of 4 and 10 years, followed by a second period of cell loss, greater in females, after 50 years of age (Swaab *et al.*, 1985; Swaab and Hofman, 1989).

Sexual dimorphism has also been found in the

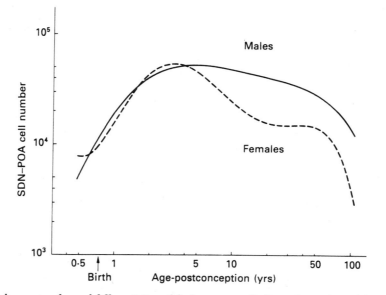

Figure 7.10. Development and sexual differentiation of the human sexually dimorphic nucleus of the preoptic area (SDN–POA). Cell numbers reach a peak value around 2–4 years postnatally, after which a sexual differentiation occurs due to a reduction in cell number in the SDN–POA in females, whereas the cell number in males remains approximately unchanged up to the age of 50 years. The curves are 5th degree polynomial functions fitted to the data compiled from Swaab and Hofman (1988), with F_s (5,49) = 10.05, $p < 0.001$ for males and F_s (5,39) = 7.32, $p < 0.001$ for females. From M. A. Hofman and D. F. Swaab, *J. Anat. (London)* 164:55–72 (1989).

branching patterns of dendrites of the preoptic area in the hamster, rat, and rhesus monkey (Greenough *et al.*, 1977; Meyer and Gordon, 1982; Ayoub *et al.*, 1983). There are sex differences in the synaptic organization in the preoptic nucleus of the rat, with the male and androgenized female having more synapses than the female (Raisman and Field, 1971, 1973a). Similar sex differences in synaptic organization in the rat brain have been found in the hypothalamic arcuate nucleus (Ratner and Adamo, 1971; Matsumoto and Arai, 1981) and in the medial amygdala (Nishizuka and Arai, 1981; Arimatsu and Seto, 1982).

8 Neuronal Death and Neurotrophic Factors

According to tradition, the development of the vertebrate nervous system has hither-
to seemed to proceed straight on in a gradually ascending path, without turnings,
temporary expedients, or regressive changes. As a consequence none were looked for
and none were found.

John Beard (1858–1918), *The History of a Transient Nervous Apparatus in*
Certain Ichthyopsida, 1896

8.1. Prolegomena to a History of Nerve Cell Death during Development

Men make their own history, but they do
not make it just as they please; they do not
make it under circumstances chosen by
themselves, but under circumstances di-
rectly encountered, given and transmitted
from the past. The tradition of all the dead
generations weighs like a nightmare on the
brain of the living.

Karl Marx (1818–1883), *The Eigh-*
teenth Brumaire of Louis Bonaparte, 1852

The tyranny of theory over the evidence is nowhere more glaringly evident than in the history of the delayed discovery of neuronal death during normal development. The tyranny in this case was imposed by the theory that both ontogeny and phylogeny are progressive, from lower and less organized to higher and more organized nervous systems. Evidence of neuronal death during normal development was reported but was ignored because it was in conflict with the idea of progressive development. Reports of neuronal death were buried in the literature, to be unearthed much later as curious historical relics. Such reports come back to haunt us as they haunted previous generations

who could not accept evidence that conflicted with their cherished theories.

Neuron death during normal development was discovered and described in considerable detail by John Beard in 1896 in the Rohon–Beard cells of the skate: *"This normal degeneration of ganglion-cells and of nerves is now for the first time described and figured for vertebrate animals, in which hitherto such an occurrence is without precedent"* (Beard, 1896a). Rohon–Beard cells had been discovered by Balfour (1878), who illustrated them in the spinal cord of elasmobranch embryos, and they were further described by Rohon (1884) in the trout and in other fish embryos by Beard (1889, 1892). Beard traced their origin from *"immediately laterad to the medullary plate,"* in other words, from the neural crest. He described their differentiation, outgrowth of their neurites, discovered their degeneration (Beard, 1896a), and tried to build a general theory on that evidence. Beard (1896b) thought that cell death occurs generally during what he called "critical periods" (the first time that term was used in neuroscience). According to Beard, the critical period represents a period of regression and reorganization of embryonic structures and a transition to the definitive structures of the adult. The quotation from Beard that forms an epigraph to this chapter shows that he recognized the prejudice against the idea of normal regressive developmental stages. He noted that his evidence contradicted the biogenetic law of Ernst Haeckel according to which the embryo simply climbs up the phylogenetic tree, recapitulating the structures of its ancestors as it ascends to its appropriate level.

After Beard's definitive work on death of Rohon–Beard neurons, the few reports of neuron death during normal development were consigned to obscurity not altogether undeserved in view of their inability to relate the facts to a general theory of neuron death. Cell death during normal development of the nervous system was first reported in the amphibian spinal cord by Barbieri in 1905 and in the chick embryo neural tube by Collin (1906a,b).

Ernst (1926) was the first to recognize that overproduction of neurons was followed by death of a significant fraction of neurons in many regions of the nervous system of vertebrates. For example, he reported death of a third of the neurons in the dorsal root ganglia. The originality of his findings may be appreciated from the following brief extracts. After discussing the report by Sánchez y Sánchez (1923) of massive cell death during metamorphosis of insects (now undeservedly forgotten, e.g., in the review by Truman and Schwartz, 1982), Ernst says: *We find ourselves in agreement with Sánchez y Sánchez. He states that he found such extensive cell death in all ganglia of appropriate stages that he at first hesitated to publish descriptions, because he could not believe that such results were not already well known. We too found such massive cell death, above all in the retina, in the trigeminal and facial ganglia, in the upper jaw, and in the anterior horn, that we were at first doubtful whether we were dealing with normal events. . . . We have at the same time the explanation of why ganglia of older embryos always have fewer cells than those of very young stages. . . . The results are in complete agreement in showing that degenerations always occur most strongly in the ganglia from which the nerves grow out to the extremities. . . . There remains only a group of degenerations which are always found, namely in the anterior horns of the spinal cord, the floor of the third and fourth ventricles and at the transition from the thick lateral wall of the brain to the thin roof of the ventricle. . . . Characteristic of all these degenerations is the timepoint of their occurrence: it consists of a striking correspondence be-*tween the vascularization of these regions and the occurrence of degenerations. . . . For all these cases we must for the present be satisfied with confirmation of the facts that in the named regions a large number of cells are available for differentiation into nerve cells but that only a fraction of them are used for that purpose whereas the remainder are destined for disintegration.*

Ernst (1926) deserves credit for proposing a general theory of neuron death during normal development and for obtaining a diversity of evidence to support it. The work of Glücksmann (1940, 1951, 1965) merely confirmed the findings of Ernst and others and provided an incomplete but convenient summary in English of some of the literature in other languages. This led to the deplorable practice (e.g., Saunders, 1966, but soon followed by others, e.g., P. G. H. Clarke, 1985a; Hurle, 1988) of ignoring the work of Ernst and his predecessors and crediting Glücksmann with the concept of three different modes of cell death, when all he did was to give them names.[1]

Ernst (1926) had provided good evidence of his own and reviewed the previous evidence showing that there are three main types of cell death during normal development: the first occurring during regression of vestigial organs; the second occurring during cavitation, folding, or fusion of organ anlage; the third occurring as part of the process of remodeling of tissues. These were later named phylogenetic, morphogenetic, and histogenetic cell death by Glücksmann (1940, 1951, 1965).

The great neurocytologists of the 19th and early 20th century were in a position to see the death of cells in the developing nervous system but failed to discover it. Why scientists fail to see important things that are staring them in the face is notoriously difficult to understand. Cajal was fond of saying that the truth is revealed to the prepared mind, and I should agree that the minds of the great neurocytologists of his time were not prepared for the

---

[1]"In spite of all the flatteries of self-love, the facts associated at first with the name of a particular man end by being anonymous, lost forever in the ocean of universal science. The monograph permeated with individual human quality becomes incorporated, stripped of sentiments, in the abstract doctrine of the general theories." (Ramón y Cajal, 1923)

truth about neuronal death during normal vertebrate development. Another important reason for their failure to see neuronal death was their reliance on Golgi and silver impregnation techniques which do not show cellular debris clearly or obscure it with metallic precipitates. The Nissl stain could have revealed neuronal death to the unprejudiced observer, but the observers were prejudiced by the idea of progressive development. Death of embryonic cells was recognized as a phenomenon of significance only during disintegration of vestigial organs and during metamorphosis. Cajal was, of course, well aware of the massive death of neurons that occurs during insect metamorphosis brilliantly studied by his student Domingo Sánchez y Sánchez. It is remarkable that the concept of regression of axonal and dendritic structures was easily accepted whereas death of large numbers of neurons in the vertebrate nervous system was not an acceptable fact. Cajal relished the analogy between regression of axonal and dendritic branches and pruning of excessive branches from trees and bushes in a formal garden, but he never conceived of uprooting and destroying large numbers of trees in the process of laying out the garden.

The long delay in accepting the evidence of developmental neuronal death has been regarded as an historical enigma. Here is how the puzzle may now be solved. Nineteenth-century biologists saw that development has an overriding *telos*, a direction, and a gradual approach to completion of the embryo, and also saw a terminal regression and final dissolution of the adult; but a fallacy arose when the progression and regression, which coexist from early development, were separated in their minds. Development was conceived in terms of progressive construction, of an epigenetic program—from simple to more complex. For every event in development they attempted to find prior conditions such that, given them, nothing else could happen. The connections and interdependencies of events assure that the outcome is always the same. Such deterministic theories of development made it difficult to conceive of demolition of structures as part of normal development, and it was inconceivable that construction and destruction can occur simultaneously. It became necessary to regard regressive developmental processes as entirely purposeful and determined. For example, elimination of organs that play a role during development but are not required in the adult or

regression of vestigeal structures such as the tail in humans were viewed as part of the ontogenetic recapitulation of phylogeny. Regression in those cases is determined and is merely one of several fates: cellular determination may be either progressive or regressive. The idea of progress in all spheres, perhaps most of all in the evolution and development of the vertebrate nervous system, has appealed to many thinkers since the 18th century. Such ideas change more slowly than the means of scientific production; thus new facts are made to serve old ideas. That is why the history of ideas, even if it does not exactly repeat itself, does such a good job of imitation.

In the realm of ideas held by neuroscientists, the idea of progressive construction, of hierarchically ordered programs of development, has always been dominant over the idea of a plenitude of possibilities, from which orderly structure develops from disorderly initial conditions by a process of selective attrition (M. Jacobson, 1970b, 1974b; Changeux *et al.*, 1973; Changeux and Danchin, 1976; Edelman, 1985). Progressive development implies increasing orderliness gained by the organism, *"sucking orderliness from its environment,"* and by *"feeding on negative entropy"* (Schrödinger, 1944, p. 74). Schrödinger did not recognize that the organism can lose entropy (that is, gain orderliness) by ridding itself of internal disorder as effectively as by *"attracting, as it were, a stream of negative entropy upon itself"* (Schrödinger, 1944, p. 74). Cell death may be a quick way for the embryo to reduce its entropy level.

The idea of development of organization by means of selective cellular attrition has gained popularity since the 1970s. Before that time, the dominating idea was that matching between nerve centers and peripheral structures or between different nerve centers is achieved by programs of cell proliferation, migration, and differentiation in which orderly progress always prevails. But this early period of construction is now known to be followed by a period of deconstruction.

Another dominant idea from the beginning of the century until now (e.g., Cowan *et al.*, 1984) was that the number of neurons is matched to the size of their targets as a result of reciprocal trophic interactions between nerves and their peripheral innervation fields: neuronal proliferation, migration, and survival were conceived to result from trophic influences coming from the target tissues, and a reciprocal trophic influence of nerves on the target tissues ensured the vitality of muscles and sense organs (reviewed historically by Oppenheim, 1981). For the past 200 years the nutritional functions of nerves have generally been regarded as distinct from their roles in sensation and movement. For example, Procháska (1784) states: *"Sylvius, Willis, Glisson and others considered that there were two fluids in the nerves, one thick and albuminous, subservient to nutrition, the other very thin and spiritous, intimately connected with the former, and subservient to sensation and movement . . ."*

A century ago the word "trophic" was on everyone's lips to signify the mysterious life-giving effects of nerves on one another and on the tissues which they supply. In Foster's *Text-Book of Physiology* (3rd ed., 1879), trophic action is defined as *"the possibility of the nervous system having the power of directly affecting the metabolic actions of the body, apart from any irritable, contractile or secretory manifestations."* The first experimental evidence of a trophic action of sensory nerves was the demonstration that taste buds degenerate after denervation and regenerate only if sensory nerves are present (von Vintschgau and Hönigschmied, 1876; von Vintschgau, 1880; Hermann, 1884; see Section 9.14). Wilhelm Roux (1881) discusses *"the trophic action of functional stimuli"* under which he has a section *"on trophic nerves"* (p. 125). There he reviews the trophic effects of nerves on the muscles and other tissues, and he makes the distinction between a direct trophic action of the nerves on these tissues and the indirect effects of lack of stimulation, disease, changes in blood flow, etc. He concludes that nerves have a trophic effect which is not entirely due to excitation. He maintains that not only are the peripheral organs provided with a trophic stimulus independently of the nervous activity, but also *"the central nervous substance likewise is influenced in its nourishment by the peripheral organs with which it has formed an excitation-unity"* and that *"the central nervous tissue should be regarded, so to speak (practically) not as a one-sided provider but at the same time as the nutritive provider by the peripheral tissues."* In 1899 L. F. Barker could write, *"The more thought one gives to the subject the more he will find in the trophic relations of neurones to make him hesitate before he denies the possibility of conduction of impulses or influences in either direction throughout the neurone."* Gold-

scheider (1898) first conjectured that materials are transported from the nerve cell body to the axon terminals. During the following decades evidence built up to support the theories that trophic factors flow from the nerve cell body to the axonal endings (Olmsted, 1920a,b, 1925; May, 1925) and that nerves release specific trophic factors into the tissues they innervate (Parker, 1932; see M. Jacobson, *Conceptual Foundations of Neuroscience*, in preparation, for a discussion of the significance of those premature theories. Perhaps here I should say that those premature conjectures fell on deaf ears and unprepared minds. To arrive on the scene with a message prematurely might be like someone in the position of shouting "fire" in an empty theater).

Experimental analysis of the changes in the developing nervous system resulting from altering peripheral sensory and motor fields was pioneered by Braus (1905) and Shorey (1909) and followed by many others (see Sections 8.6 and 8.10). Removal of limbs or grafting additional limbs was shown to result in hypoplasia or hyperplasia, respectively, and those results were interpreted consistently in terms of regulation of cellular proliferation. Regulation of cell death was never considered, as the reader can easily verify from the general textbooks dealing with the subject, such as Samuel Detwiler's *Neuroembryology* (1936) and *Principles of Development* by Paul Weiss (1939). The appearance of Glucksmann's 1951 review of cell death during normal development prompted a reconsideration of the effects of limb amputation. Prior to the publication of Glücksmann's review, Hamburger and Levi-Montalcini (1949) concluded that *"two basically different mechanisms operate in the control of spinal ganglion development by peripheral factors: (a) the periphery controls the **proliferation** and **initial differentiation** of undifferentiated cells which have no connections of their own with the periphery; (b) the periphery provides the conditions for **continued growth** and **maintenance** of neurons following the first outgrowth of neurites"* (Hamburger and Levi-Montalcini, 1949). After the discovery that a mouse sarcoma implanted in the chick embryo results in neuronal hyperplasia and hypertrophy (Bueker, 1948) the effect was consistently misinterpreted as a primary action of the factor on neuronal proliferation (Levi-Montalcini and Hamburger, 1951, 1953).

Victor Hamburger (1958) was able to show that the number of motoneurons in the chick embryo decreases after limb amputation as a result of increased cell death, not because of failure of mitosis or of motoneuron differentiation. However, he did not yet recognize the significance of death during normal development. Arthur Hughes (1961) was the first in recent times to show that a large overproduction of motoneurons occurs during normal development and that motoneuron death is a major factor regulating their final numbers, and Martin Prestige (1965) was the first to demonstrate the same in spinal ganglia. Yet the belief persisted that the periphery controls cell proliferation, even after the discovery of nerve growth factor (NGF), which was at first said to have mitogenic effects (Levi-Montalcini, 1965, 1966; Levi-Montalcini and Angeletti, 1968; see Section 8.12). The confusion was resolved only after [^{3}H]thymidine autoradiography showed that changes in mitotic activity in the nervous system, following limb grafting or amputation, is confined entirely to glial cells (Carr, 1975, 1976; see Section 8.12). The path to discovery of the biological effects of NGF and other neurotrophic factors detoured around the difficulties and confusions created by surgical manipulation of limbs (see Section 8.12). Those were prologues to the biochemical identification of NGF—the rest is history, that ultimate act of imaginative reconstruction.

8.2. Cell Death during Development of the Nervous System

Ernst (1926) showed that cell death during normal development of vertebrates has three main forms with special functions: the first occurs during disintegration of tissues that develop transiently in the embryo; the second during morphogenesis at regions of separation, fusion, folding, bending, or cavitation; and the third during remodeling of tissues and adjustment of the final numbers of cells of different kinds after an initial period of excessive cell production. These three types of cell death were called *phylogenetic*, *morphogenetic*, and *histogenetic* by Glücksmann (1951, 1965). These terms serve, at present, to make distinctions that appear to be significant in the present state of our ignorance about the mechanisms of cell death during development. We should be prepared to abandon such terms without compunction when the basic mechanisms and functions

of nerve cell death during development are more completely known.

Phylogenetic cell death in the vertebrates occurs during the regression of vestigial organs such as the pronephros (Fox, 1970) and mesonephros (Salzegeber and Weber, 1966; Haffen and Salzegeber, 1977), the tail in the human embryo (Fallon and Simandl, 1978), and many structures of amphibians during metamorphosis (Lockshin, 1981), for example, the Rohon–Beard neurons (Hughes, 1957; Lamborghini, 1987) and the Mauthner neurons (Stefanelli, 1950, 1951). Programmed degeneration of Rohon–Beard cells is an example of phylogenetic cell death. Rohon–Beard neurons are derived from the neural crest and form a transient primary sensory system linking the ectoderm and neural tube in fish and amphibian embryos. The Rohon–Beard neurons degenerate as their place is taken by spinal dorsal root ganglia (Beard, 1892, 1896a; Hughes, 1957; Lamborghini, 1987). The cause of their degeneration is unknown. It is unlikely to be due to thyroxine (Stephens, 1965). The number of Rohon–Beard neurons is diminished only slightly by removal of the ectoderm with which they connect (Stephens, 1965; Bacher, 1973), which shows that they are not maintained exclusively by contact with their peripheral targets or that they may receive trophic support from within the central nervous system.

There are many structures present in the nervous system of all vertebrate embryos that persist in the submammalian species but degenerate in the mammalian embryo, for example, the paraphysis (Ernst, 1926), nervus terminalis (J. B. Johnston, 1914; J. W. Brown, 1980), and the vomeronasal nerve and organ, which degenerates during human development (Humphrey, 1940). The death of nerve cells which occurs in the caudal end of the spinal cord of vertebrate embryos, leaving only glial cells in the filum terminale, is another such case (Streeter, 1919).

During insect metamorphosis, phylogenetic cell death occurs of neurons such as those which operate larval musculature and function only during embryonic development (Truman, 1983, 1984, review). For example, there are two pioneer neurons whose axons are the first to extend from the limb bud to the CNS of the grasshopper (Bate, 1976). These pioneer neurons die after they have performed their function of guiding other axons to form one of the main nerve trunks of the leg (Kutsch and Bentley, 1987).

Morphogenetic cell death occurs in many developing organs, for example, the limbs (Saunders and Gasseling, 1962; Saunders, 1966; Hurle and Hinchliffe, 1978), and in many parts of the developing nervous system during cavitation, fusion, folding, and bending of organ anlage such as the neural plate and neural tube and during formation of the optic and otic vesicles.

A considerable number of cells die during reduction in thickness of the dorsal part of the neural tube which accompanies the formation of the dorsal raphe in the mesencephalon and the choroid plexuses of the 3rd and 4th ventricles (Ernst, 1926; Källén, 1955; Maruyama and D'Agostino, 1967; Mattanza, 1973). Morphogenetic cell death also occurs during formation of the optic vesicle and choroid fissure (von Szily, 1912; Ernst, 1926; Glücksmann, 1951). Zones of cell death, termed the suboptic death center (Källén, 1955, 1965) or suboptic necrotic centers (Navascués *et al.*, 1988), are seen ventral to the emergence of the optic stalk from the diencephalon. In the chick embryo they appear during Stages 14–24. They appear to have some mechanical function during morphogenesis of the optic stalk and may play a role in guidance of optic nerve fibers at the chiasma (Navascués *et al.*, 1988). Cell death also occurs in the ventral midline of the embryonic retina during formation of the choroidal fissure, which provides a passage for intraocular blood vessels and retinal axons (Ernst, 1926; J. Silver and Hughes, 1973; Garcia-Porrero and Ojedo, 1979; Shook, 1980; Garcia-Porrero *et al.*, 1984; Horsburgh and Sefton, 1986; Cuadros and Rios, 1988).

Cell death in the retina and optic stalk starts before and continues during the initial outgrowth of optic nerve fibers in the rat and mouse (J. Silver and Hughes, 1973; Silver and Robb, 1979; J. Silver and Sapiro, 1981; Horsburgh and Sefton, 1986) and in the chick embryo retina (Navascués *et al.*, 1985; Cuadros and Rios, 1988). The exact relationship between cell death and axon outgrowth is not known. Von Szily (1912) suggested that the products of cell degeneration may attract optic nerve fibers. Macrophages that invade the area of retinal cell death may release neurotrophic factors that stimulate axon outgrowth. Retinal cell death may result in formation of axon guidance channels (J. Silver and Robb, 1979, J. Silver and Sidman, 1980), but Suburo *et al.*

(1979) failed to see any channels until much later, after differentiation of retinal Muller cells. Scott and Bunt (1986) found that in *Xenopus* neural tube the extracellular spaces are not aligned to form channels (see Sections 5.12 and 5.14). Death of retinal ganglion cells occurs at a later stage, after their axons have contacted the visual centers. This is discussed in Section 8.3 as an example of histogenetic cell death.

Cell death during morphogenesis of the chick wing is a well-studied case of morphogenetic cell death (Saunders, 1966, review; Hurle and Hinchliffe, 1978). Fallon and Saunders (1968) have shown that when cells of the posterior necrotic zone (PNZ, a region of mesodermal cell death at the posterior junction of the wing bud and body wall) from chick embryos at Stages 17–23 are grafted to another embryo or are explanted to a culture medium, cell death occurs on schedule, when the PNZ cells reach Stage 24. Death of PNZ cells appears to be preprogrammed. However, the PNZ cells can be saved from death by grafting them before Stage 22 to the dorsal side of the wing bud or by placing them *in vitro* in association with dorsal wing bud mesoderm. Although the causes of survival of PNZ cells in those cases are not known, it can be concluded that death of cells in the PNZ need not be inevitable. Programmed death of cells occurs in the placenta, in which the trophoblastic giant cells die in tissue culture at an age that corresponds with their lifespan *in vivo* in the rat (Dorgan and Schultz, 1971).

Morphogenetic cell death is a widespread phenomenon found, for example, during changes in shape in the formation of the otocyst pit (Ernst, 1926; Glücksmann, 1951). It also occurs during degeneration of the interdigital tissue in reptiles (Fallon and Cameron, 1977) and birds (Saunders, 1966, review; Saunders and Fallon, 1966, 1967, review; Whitten, 1969; Hurle, 1988, review). In amphibian embryos formation of the digits does not involve cell death but occurs by means of differential growth (Cameron and Fallon, 1977). This shows that the same result can be achieved by different morphogenetic processes, including cell differentiation, migration, changes of cell shape, and changes in the intercellular matrix.

Histogenetic cell death occurs during histogenesis and remodeling of tissues such as cartilage, bone, various cell groups in the CNS and ganglia of the peripheral nervous system (PNS).

This is the common type of cell death during development of the nervous system. It is strongly contingent on conditions outside the cells that die, that is, on interactions with other cells, and on nutritional, hormonal, and trophic influences. There are several mechanisms known to cause histogenetic neuronal death, in particular excitatory amino acids which cause cytotoxic increases of intracellular calcium ions. The effects of trophic factors may be to counteract such destructive mechanisms.

Cell death during normal development of the vertebrate nervous system has been reported in the following locations: ciliary ganglion (Landmesser and Pilar, 1974, 1978; Narayanan and Narayanan, 1978; Pilar et al., 1980; L. L. Wright, 1981); sympathetic ganglia (Levi-Montalcini and Booker, 1960; L. L. Wright and Smolen, 1983, 1987; Maderdrut et al., 1984, 1988); dorsal root ganglia (Hamburger and Levi-Montalcini, 1949; Hughes, 1961; Prestige, 1965; Carr and Simpson, 1970; Hamburger et al., 1981); cranial and spinal visceromotor neurons (Levi-Montalcini, 1950; Dubey et al., 1968; L. L. Wright, 1981; Oppenheim et al., 1982; Arens and Straznicky, 1986); cranial motoneurons (Cowan and Wenger, 1967; Sohal, 1977; Sohal and Weidman, 1978; Sohal et al., 1978); spinal somatic motoneurons (Hamburger and Levi-Montalcini, 1949; Levi-Montalcini, 1950; Hughes and Tschumi, 1958; Hughes, 1961, 1974; Prestige, 1967a,b; Hamburger, 1975; Chu-Wang and Oppenheim, 1978a,b; Oppenheim, 1981, 1985, 1989, reviews; Tanaka and Landmesser, 1986; Oppenheim et al., 1989a,b); trigeminal mesencephalic neurons (L. A. Rogers and Cowan, 1973; Alley, 1974; Kollros, 1984; Kollros and Thiesse, 1985; Hiscock and Straznicky, 1986); habenular nuclei (Wree et al., 1981); optic vesicle (von Szily, 1912; Ernst, 1926; Glücksmann, 1930, 1951; J. Silver and Hughes, 1973; Garcia-Porrero and Ojedo, 1979; Shook, 1980; Garcia-Porrero et al., 1984; Cuadros and Rios, 1988); retinal neurons (Rager, 1978, 1980; Rager and Rager, 1978; W. F. Hughes and McLoon, 1979; Cunningham et al., 1981; Cunningham, 1982; Jeffery and Perry, 1982; Lam et al., 1982; Potts et al., 1982; Sengelaub and Finlay, 1982; Dreher et al., 1983; Spira et al., 1984; R. W. Young, 1984; Horsburgh and Sefton, 1986; Stone and Rapaport, 1986; Dunlop and Beazley, 1987; Dunlop et al., 1987; Provis, 1987; Wong and Hughes, 1987b,c; S. R. Robinson, 1988; Harman et

al., 1989); optic tectum and superior colliculus (Cantino and Daneo, 1972; Arees and Aström, 1977; Giordano et al., 1980; Cunningham et al., 1981; Finlay et al., 1982); isthmo-optic nucleus (Cowan and Wenger, 1967; Sohal and Narayanan, 1974; P. G. H. Clarke and Cowan, 1976; P. G. H. Clarke et al., 1976); basal ganglia (Janowsky and Finlay, 1983); acousticovestibular nuclei (Levi-Montalcini, 1949; Rubel et al., 1976); Pontine nuclei and inferior olive (Armstrong and Clarke, 1979); cerebellum (Janowska and Finlay, 1983); and cerebral cortex (Finlay and Slattery, 1983; Heumann and Leuba, 1983; Price and Blakemore, 1985).

No doubt many other sites of cell death remain to be discovered in the vertebrate nervous system during normal development. It is not known whether the mechanism of cell death is the same or different in all those locations and at various times during development. To illustrate the universality and yet the diversity of neuronal death in the vertebrate nervous system, seven sites of neuronal death will be discussed in detail, including examples of sensory and motor neurons in the CNS and PNS: retina, isthmo-optic nucleus, trochlear nucleus, spinal motoneurons, ciliary ganglion, mesencephalic trigeminal nucleus, and dorsal root ganglia. In all those sites neurons are produced in excess and a large percentage die when their axons are close to or in contact with their postsynaptic targets. Those neurons are themselves targets for other neurons which are also subject to death. In general, nerve cell survival depends on both afferent transneuronal trophic support and retrograde trophic support. In addition, neurons can receive trophic support from glial cells and from circulating hormones. The strengths of these sources of trophic stimulation are different in the various sites that will be considered, and different experimental operations can alter one or other sources of trophic support.

The role of hormones in cell death is very important (see Chapter 7). In many regions of the nervous system there are relatively large differences between males and females in the number of neurons, and there is increasing evidence that these differences develop under the influence of sex hormones, in some cases as a result of control of cell death (see Section 7.10). The superior cervical ganglion of the rat, in which there are more neurons in the male, has been well studied. All the superior cervical ganglion neurons originate prenatally and the difference between the sexes is not present at birth. It develops as a result of loss of about 40 percent of the neurons during P3–P7, with more cell death occurring in the female rat (Dibner and Black, 1976; Hendry and Campbell, 1976; L. L. Wright and Smolen, 1983a,b, 1985, 1987). Castration of males at birth results in increased cell death (Wright and Smolen, 1985). Treatment of male or female rats with testosterone or estradiol during the 1st week after birth reduces cell death in the superior cervical ganglion (Dibner and Black, 1976; Wright and Smolen, 1983, 1987). Cell death in the superior cervical ganglion can also be reduced by treatment with NGF (Levi-Montalcini and Booker, 1960; Hendry and Campbell, 1976; see Section 8.18). This example is given here to emphasize that neuron death during normal development is under the control of several factors, and sex differences have to be taken into account.

It is not yet clear whether the mechanisms of nerve cell death during development are the same as the mechanisms of cell death during development of other systems (Schweichel and Merker, 1973; Lockshin and Beaulaton, 1974a,b; R. D. Pollack and Fallon, 1974, 1976; Wyllie et al., 1980; Beaulaton and Lockshin, 1982; Umansky, 1982; Hurle, 1988). What is not known about nerve cell death during development can be stated in the form of a few questions which are briefer but no less significant than the mass of facts that will be given on the following pages. When and where do neurons die under genetic control and when and where are they killed by external conditions? Are there naturally occurring toxins which cause neuronal death? What are the roles of oxidizing agents and of increased intracellular free calcium ions? What are the intracellular sites of damage leading to neuronal death? What roles are played by excitatory amino acids and their cell membrane receptors? How do trophic factors protect neurons from death? How long does it take for different types of neurons to die and what is the significance of such differences? These are some of the questions that remain to be answered.

Cell death has been found in many parts of the vertebrate CNS and PNS at various stages of development. Cell death has been demonstrated by counting the total number of cells at different stages and by counts of dying cells. A useful way of labeling dying cells is by intravascular injection of horseradish peroxidase (HRP) into embryos: the HRP is taken up by brain macrophages and some dying neurons, but not by healthy neurons (P. G. H. Clarke, 1984). The HRP is localized in membrane-bound vacuoles, which shows that dying cells endocytose extracellular proteins and transport them to lysosomes for destruction. Dying neurons show other evidence of self-destruction, so-called autophagy (Ericcson, 1969) or apoptosis (Kerr et al., 1972; Wyllie et al., 1980), including condensation and dissolution of chromatin and transfer of chromatin into cytoplasmic autophagic vacuoles (P. G. H. Clarke and Hornung, 1989). Cells undergoing self-destruction during normal development are mingled among normal cells and the cells condense before death. By contrast, cellular necrosis as the result of external toxins affects all cells in a population and the cells swell prior to death (Wyllie et al., 1980).

It is necessary to know how long it takes for pyknotic cells and debris to be cleared away in order to measure the rate of neuron death from counts of pyknotic cells, which usually constitute only 1–5 percent and rarely approach 10 percent of the total neurons in the population undergoing histogenetic death. Arthur Hughes (1961) made a guess of 3 hours for clearance of dead spinal motoneurons in *Xenopus*. Digestion of cell debris by microglial cells may occur in about 3 hours, but not all dead cells are associated with microglial cells. Flanagan (1969) estimated that degeneration of spinal motoneurons in the mouse required 1.4 hours, but this is certainly an underestimate. Such underestimates of the time for death and removal of pyknotic cells lead to large overestimates of the total number of cells lost. Horsburgh and Sefton (1987) made an estimate of 24–48 hours for clearance of dead retinal ganglion cells after a kainate injection into the superior colliculus of the rat. Wyllie et al. (1980) estimated that all debris is cleared in 12–18 hours in the rat adrenal cortex. Wong and Hughes (1987c) estimated that removal of all degenerating cells from the retinal ganglion cell layer of the cat takes 10–20 hours.

According to the competition theory of neuron death, neurons have unequal success in competing for limited supplies of trophic factors provided retrogradely from their target tissues, or anterogradely from their afferents, or from both sources. Accordingly, neuronal death may be caused by failure of some neurons to obtain critical amounts of neurotrophic factors in competition with other neurons. This theory is inadequate in the simplistic form in which neurons merely compete for a limited supply of a trophic factor which they require to support differentiation (Oppenheim, 1981; Purves, 1988, reviews). It is now evident that the young neuron is subject to a battery of potentially lethal conditions but can withstand those if, and only if, it can obtain certain exogenous factors. Whether a particular neuron lives or dies will depend on the balance between the strength of the potentially lethal mechanisms and the access to neurotrophic factors from several sources. In such a sophisticated view of nerve cell death, competition for trophic factors is only one link in a complex causal network.

Evidence consistent with the competition theory is that cell death in the chick isthmo-optic nuclei is increased when two isthmo-optic nuclei are made to innervate a single retina (P. G. H. Clarke and Cowan, 1976; P. G. H. Clarke et al., 1976; O'Leary and Cowan, 1984). This increased death occurs in spite of the fact that both isthmo-optic nuclei also receive trophic support from afferents arising in the optic tectum. Other evidence consistent with the competition hypothesis is that cutting one of the three nerves which connect the ciliary ganglion with the ciliary muscle results in rescue of about 40 percent of the ciliary neurons that would have died during normal development (Pilar et al., 1980).

The experimental evidence may be difficult to interpret if the neurons are sustained by afferent transneuronal trophic stimulation as well as by retrograde trophic stimulation from the target tissues (Cunningham, 1982; Linden and Serfaty, 1985). For example, in *Xenopus* tadpoles, when the motoneurons that supply both hindlimbs are made to supply a single limb, the number of surviving motoneurons is normal (Lamb, 1981). This evidence may refute the competition theory, at least for *Xenopus* motoneurons, or it may imply that the motoneurons received additional support from the CNS and from afferents which overide the effects of competition for trophic support from the muscles. Other significant evidence that is not consistent with the competition theory is that in both the frog and chick embryo some neurons are being born while others are dying in the dorsal root ganglia and the lateral motor column of the spinal cord, for example, so that only a fraction of the neurons in the same population could compete at one time. The evi-

dence for and against the theory of competitive interaction between motoneuron axons is discussed further at the end of Section 8.7.

The frequently used experimental strategy of removing peripheral tissues in order to see the effects on the neurons innervating them has limitations. One limitation is that surgical excision of an organ such as the limb or eye interrupts both afferent and efferent nerves. The resulting changes in the nervous system are complex and may include loss of neurotrophic factors originating in the ablated organ, loss of afferent neurotrophic stimulation, and imbalance between excitatory and inhibitory synaptic activity. Removal of an eye produces changes in the visual centers that receive afferent nerve fibers from the eye, and in addition, neurons are affected that send their axons to the eye (see Section 8.4). Neuron survival may depend on a proper balance between anterograde and retrograde trophic support and not only on competition for trophic factors in the peripheral tissues (Cunningham, 1982). Thus, amputation of a limb disconnects somatic and autonomic motoneurons from their targets in the limb and also removes afferents originating from various sense organs in the limb.

Many examples show that neurons originate, migrate, and differentiate in the absence of their normal targets, but die after axons fail to connect with their targets. After removal of the cerebellum of the chick embryo, the neurons of the inferior olivary nucleus originate, migrate, and differentiate normally, but degenerate when their outgrowing axons fail to find connections in the absent cerebellum (Harkmark, 1956). Similarly, in the staggerer mutant mouse, the cerebellar granule cells die after their axons, the parallel fibers, fail to find their normal synaptic targets, the dendritic spines of the Purkinje cells, because the spines are defective in the mutant (see Section 10.15). These examples of the most exaggerated forms of death of neurons deprived of their synaptic targets suggest that the so-called histogenetic death of nerve cells during normal development may also occur because the cells fail to find synaptic targets. It seems that this may not be the only factor, as is shown by the finding that all the isthmo-optic axons (P. G. H. Clarke et al., 1976) and probably all the spinal motoneuron axons (A. F. Hughes and Egar, 1972; Prestige and Wilson, 1974) reach the proximity of their targets, and the axons that arrive at the target zone last do not appear to have a lower probability of survival than those that arrive there first (P. G. H. Clarke et al., 1976).

The evidence that death of embryonic neurons can be reduced by providing them with additional postsynaptic targets or after treatment with neuromuscular blocking agents (see Section 8.7) or by inhibition of RNA or protein synthesis *in vitro* (Martin *et al.*, 1988) shows that the cells that die are neither intrinsically defective nor preprogrammed to die.

The first evidence showing that neurons can be rescued from death was obtained by Shieh (1951), who transplanted cervical spinal cord in chick embryos in place of thoracic spinal cord at a stage before the onset of death of the ventrolateral motoneurons and found that some motoneurons survive that normally would have died. Hollyday and Hamburger (1976) showed that an additional leg grafted near the normal hindlimb in chick embryos results in an increased number of motoneurons innervating the extra limb, and that those neurons, derived from thoracic and rostral lumbar spinal cord levels, are a

different population from those that innervate the normal hindlimb (Fig. 8.1). Rescue of motoneurons that would normally have died also occurs in frogs with supernumerary limbs (Maheras and Pollack, 1985). Grafting additional periphery also saves neurons that would normally have died in the trochlear nucleus and isthmo-optic nucleus of the chick embryo (Narayanan and Narayanan, 1978; Boydston and Sohal, 1979).

It has been suggested that histogenetic cell death is ubiquitous in all parts of the developing CNS (e.g., Hollyday and Hamburger, 1976). However, cell death has not been seen in most parts of the nervous system. In some regions, this may reflect the rapidity of degeneration and the efficiency of removal of cellular debris. **There are good reasons for suspecting that cell death is not ubiquitous but is found in those neurons that have a limited source of trophic support, for example, which form connections only with a single postsynaptic target and are unable to make connections elsewhere if that target is unavailable. The type of neuron that does not die during normal development is one that can obtain trophic**

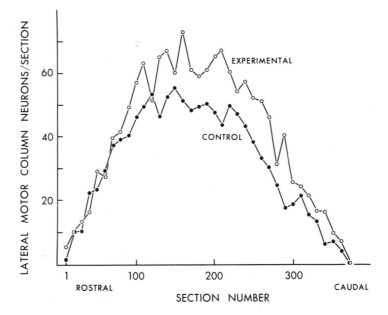

Figure 8.1. Motoneurons can be rescued from death by grafting an extra limb for them to innervate. Counts of lateral motor column neurons on the right (experimental) and left (control) sides of the spinal cord of a chick embryo at E12 after grafting an extra leg on the right side at E3.5. The extra leg was innervated by spinal cord segments 22, 23, 24, and 25 (see Fig. 8.8C). There was a 25.5 percent increase in the number of lateral motoneurons on the right side, mainly in spinal segments not normally supplying the limbs. From M. Hollyday and V. Hamburger, *J. Comp. Neurol.* **170**:311–320 (1976).

support from more than one source, for example, the neuron which sends axonal branches to connect with several targets of the same type or whose axon connects with more than one type of postsynaptic cell. Such neurons die only when deprived of more than one source of trophic support. Adjustments of connections by such neurons can be made by retraction or elimination of the axon or of the collaterals without death of the neuron.

Axonal projections which are diffuse initially may be refined to a point-to-point projection either by cell death, as in the retinotectal and retinogeniculate projections (Bunt and Lund, 1981; Jeffery and Perry, 1982; Bunt et al., 1983; Martin et al., 1983; O'Leary et al., 1983; Insausti et al., 1984; Jacobs et al., 1984; Jeffery, 1984), or by retraction of axonal branches without neuron death, as in the cerebral cortex (Innocenti, 1981; O'Leary et al., 1981; Ivy and Killacky, 1981, 1982; Stanfield et al., 1982; Koppel and Innocenti, 1983; Bates and Killacky, 1984; Innocenti and Clarke, 1984; Dehay et al., 1985; Olavarria and Van Sluyters, 1985; Innocenti et al., 1986; O'Leary and Stanfield, 1986; Killacky and Chalupa, 1986; Chalupa and Killacky, 1989). This is considered in more detail in Section 10.9.

There are many cases showing that retraction of nerve fibers during development occurs without death of neurons. In some cases it can be inferred that axonal retraction results from competition between fibers, but it is not certain whether the competition is for neurotrophic factors available in limited quantities or for other limiting conditions. For example, in the cerebellum of newborn rats many climbing fibers innervate each Purkinje cell but these fibers are retracted during the early postnatal period, leaving a single climbing fiber in possession of each Purkinje cell in the adult (Crepel et al., 1976). This retraction appears to result in part from competition between climbing fibers and granule cells (Crepel, 1982), as discussed in Section 10.12. Evidence for such competition is that multiple climbing fibers on individual Purkinje cells persist in mutant mice deficient in granule cells or after destruction of granule cells with X-rays (see Section 10.14). There are other cases in which elimination of axonal branches occurs without death of neurons, possibly as a result of competition between axon terminals: the thalamocortical and callosal innervation of the visual cortex (Rhoades and Dellacroce,

1980; Lund et al., 1984; Olavarria and Van Sluyters, 1985; Innocenti et al., 1986), and the ipsilateral corticocortical projections (Dehay et al., 1985); and callosal projections to the somatosensory cortex (Caminiti and Innocenti, 1981; Ivy and Killacky, 1981, 1982; O'Leary et al., 1981), and corticospinal projections (Bates and Killacky, 1984; O'Leary and Stanfield, 1986). These are discussed in Sections 10.9 and 11.7.

8.3. Developmental Death of Retinal Ganglion Cells

The retinal ganglion cells form a crucial relay between intrinsic retinal circuits and the visual centers. Therefore, the death of retinal ganglion cells is involved in a number of essential adjustments of the visual projections. The first of these is the convergence of bipolar and amacrine cells on retinal ganglion cell dendrites. Secondly, retinal ganglion cell death is involved in development of the gradient of numerical density of retinal ganglion cells from the area centralis to the peripheral retina. Elimination of misrouted optic axons and of the initially diffuse projections to visual centers also involves death of retinal ganglion cells. Establishment of the nasotemporal division in the projection of the retina to the left and right sides of the brain requires elimination of anomalous retinal ganglion cells. Development of segregated projections from the two eyes to the visual centers is related to the period of retinal ganglion cell death in mammals. Retinal ganglion cell death is the result of many factors, including competition between their dendrites for afferent stimulation from bipolar and amacrine cells, competition for trophic factors supplied by their central targets, and correspondence between the impulse traffic in adjacent neurons.

Death of retinal ganglion cells during normal development has been reported in the chick (Rager and Rager, 1976, 1978; W. F. Hughes and McLoon, 1979; Straznicky and Chehade, 1987), wallaby (Dunlop and Beazley, 1987; Coleman and Beazley, 1989; Harman et al., 1989), kangaroo (Dunlop et al., 1987), rat (Cunningham et al., 1982; Jeffery and Perry, 1982; Potts et al., 1982; Fawcett et al., 1984), mouse (R. W. Young, 1984), hamster (Sengelaub et al., 1982, 1986; Sengelaub, 1983, 1986; Insausti et al., 1984), cat (Stone *et al.*, 1984; Stone and Rapaport, 1986; Wong and Hughes, 1987b,c; Leventhal *et al.*, 1988a), and human (Provis *et al.*, 1985a,b; Provis, 1987). Cell death in other retinal layers has been reported in the wallaby (Harman *et al.*, 1989), mouse (Young, 1984), rat (Spira *et al.*, 1984; Beazley *et al.*, 1987), and cat (S. R. Robinson, 1988). Loss of retinal ganglion cells coincides with loss of optic axons during development in the rat (Lam *et al.*, 1982; Dreher *et al.*, 1983; Perry *et al.*, 1983; Fawcett *et al.*, 1984), cat (Ng and Stone, 1982; Williams *et al.*, 1983; Stone and Rapaport, 1985; Lia *et al.*, 1986; Wong and Hughes, 1987b,c), wallaby (Braekevelt *et al.*, 1986), rhesus monkey (Rakic and Riley, 1983), and human (Provis *et al.*, 1985b).

Death of retinal ganglion cells has several different functions. First, it is involved in establishing intraretinal connections (Linden and Perry, 1982; Young, 1984). Second, cell death starts and ends earliest in the area centralis. Retinal ganglion cell death changes the initial uniform distribution of ganglion cells into the center-to-peripheral gradient of ganglion cell numerical densities, with the highest numerical cell density in the area centralis (Sengelaub and Finlay, 1982; Stone *et al.*, 1982; Beazley and Dunlop, 1983, 1985a; Provis *et al.*, 1984; Dunlop and Beazley, 1985a, 1987; Dunlop, 1987; Wong and Hughes, 1987c), as shown in Fig. 8.2. Third, death of retinal ganglion cells results in refinement of the retinotopic projection and elimination of incorrectly projecting axons from the retina to the ipsilateral optic tectum or superior colliculus (Bunt and Lund, 1981; Jeffery and Perry, 1982; Bunt *et al.*, 1983; Martin *et al.*, 1983; O'Leary *et al.*, 1983; Insausti *et al.*, 1984; Jacobs *et al.*, 1984; Jeffery, 1984). Fourth, retinal ganglion cell death is involved in changing the retinogeniculate inputs from the two eyes from an initially diffuse projection to separate projection of each eye to different layers of the lateral geniculate nucleus (Rakic, 1981, 1986, review; Rakic and Riley, 1983).

Cell death in the retina occurs earliest in the ganglion cell layer (which contains displaced amacrine cells as well as ganglion cells), followed by death of amacrine and bipolar cells and finally by death of receptors. This inside-out gradient has been observed in the frog (Glücksmann, 1940), quail (Yew, 1979), and mouse (Young, 1984). Cell death in the retinal ganglion cell layer consists predominantly of ganglion cells, but evidence for death

of displaced amacrine cells has been found in the rat (Horsburgh and Sefton, 1985), hamster (Sengelaub *et al.*, 1986), and possibly in the cat (Wong and Hughes, 1987c).

At the time of onset of cell death the retina possesses a ventricular germinal layer in which pyknotic nuclei can be seen in the mouse (Young, 1984) and cat (Wong and Hughes, 1987c), as shown in Fig. 8.2. The period of retinal cell death coincides with vascularization of the retina and with invasion of microglial cells, which are macrophages that remove the cellular debris (Hume *et al.*, 1983; Wong and Hughes, 1987c). Cell death in the ganglion cell layer of the mouse retina occurs during the first 11 days after birth, peaking on days 2–5; amacrine cell death peaks between days 3 and 8; bipolar and Müller cell and inner rod degeneration peaks at 8–11 days; and death of outer rods continues to about 3 weeks after birth (Young, 1984). There is also a central-to-peripheral gradient of retinal cell death, corresponding with the gradient of cell generation and differentiation in the chick (Rager and Rager, 1978), mouse (Young, 1984), cat (Wong and Hughes, 1987c), and human (Provis, 1987).

Natural death in the retinal ganglion cell layer lasts from E8 to E17 in the chick (Rager and Rager, 1976; W. F. Hughes and McLoon, 1979) and results in loss of up to 40 percent of ganglion cells. This is the same time during which retinal axons grow into the tectum (Crossland *et al.*, 1975; Rager and Von Oeynhausen, 1979; Thanos and Bonhoefer, 1987), and remodeling of their terminals occurs in the tectum (Nakamura and O'Leary, 1989). Retinal ganglion cell death eliminates axons that project aberrantly to the ipsilateral side of the brain in chick embryos (McLoon and Land, 1982; O'Leary *et al.*, 1983; Thanos and Bonhoefer, 1984).

Loss of about 50 percent of retinal ganglion cells occurs in the rat during the 2 weeks after birth (Potts *et al.*, 1982; Lam *et al.*, 1982; Perry *et al.*, 1983). This is comparable with 49 percent loss of ganglion cells in the newborn hamster (Sengelaub and Finlay, 1982). Pyknotic nuclei in the cat retinal ganglion cell layer, constituting 3–5 percent of the ganglion cells, can be seen at E40, reach a peak close to birth at E57, and decline rapidly after birth (Wong and Hughes, 1987c).

In humans, retinal ganglion cell death during normal development occurs between 14 and 30 weeks of gestation, with more ganglion cells dying in

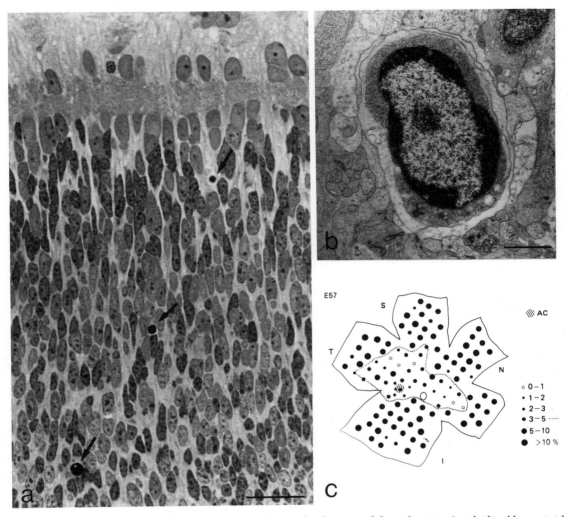

Figure 8.2. Cell death is a naturally occurring process during development of the cat's retina. In toluidine blue–stained semithin sections of embryonic retina, darkly staining profiles are often observed in the ventricular or germinal layer (arrows, a). Such profiles are also present in the ganglion cell layer and are confirmed by electron microscopy to be pyknotic nuclei (b). The proportion of cells that are pyknotic in the presumed ganglion cell population reaches a maximum 1 week before birth (E57). The topographic distribution map (c) of the percentage of presumed ganglion cells that are pyknotic at E57 demonstrates a region of relatively low percentage death in the area centralis (AC) and along the visual streak (broken contour). It suggests that cell death plays a significant topogenic role in sculpting the adult peripheral ganglion cell distribution from its precursors. Magnification bars: a = 25 μm; b = 2 μm. From R. O. L. Wong and A. Hughes, *J. Comp. Neurol.* **262**:496–511 (1987).

the central retina between 14 and 16 weeks and more in the peripheral retina between 16 and 30 weeks of gestation (Provis, 1987). Loss of retinal ganglion cells coincides with loss of optic nerve fibers, showing that the dying ganglion cells had projected their axons into the optic nerve and probably to the visual centers (Provis *et al.*, 1985b). The period of retinal ganglion cell and optic axon loss in

humans corresponds with the period in monkeys, the 3rd quarter of gestation, during which inputs from the two eyes are segregated in different layers of the lateral geniculate nucleus (Rakic, 1976, 1977). This loss of neurons occurs prenatally and therefore cannot be related to visual experience (see Section 11.20 and Fig. 11.29).

Removal of one eye during the period of retinal

ganglion cell death results in an increased survival of ganglion cells and optic nerve fibers of the remaining eye in hamsters (Sengelaub and Finlay, 1981, 1982; Insausti *et al.*, 1984) and cat (Williams *et al.*, 1983; Chalupa *et al.*, 1984). There is some controversy over the amount of saving of retinal ganglion cells that occurs after unilateral eye removal in the rat: some workers report slight savings (Lund *et al.*, 1973; Cunningham, 1976; Jeffery and Perry, 1982; Fawcett *et al.*, 1984), while others report no savings (Sefton and Lam, 1984; Crespo *et al.*, 1985). This is probably related to the small binocular visual field in rats. However, the rule that the amount of retinal cell death is proportional to the size of the binocular visual field, and thus to the amount of interaction between the afferents from two eyes in the visual centers, is not obeyed by the wallaby. That marsupial has an extensive binocular visual field, but removal of one eye does not result in a reduction of retinal cell death in the other eye (Coleman and Beazely, 1989). The saving in the remaining eye is no more than 35 percent in the monkey, which has the most extensive binocular visual field (Rakic and Riley, 1989). Therefore, the segregation of retinal axons from left and right eyes cannot be the only function of retinal ganglion cell death. This is discussed further in Section 11.20. The increased optic nerve fiber count does not result from increased branching of optic axons (Cunningham, 1976; Lia *et al.*, 1986) but results from increased survival of retinal ganglion cells and their axons (Jeffery and Perry, 1982; Chalupa *et al.*, 1984).

The evidence is consistent with the theory that retinal ganglion cells compete for trophic factors released from their targets in the lateral geniculate nucleus and superior colliculus. One of these is likely to be brain-derived neurotrophic factor (BDNF) (see Section 8.17). In addition, retinal ganglion cell dendrites compete for inputs from bipolar and amacrine cells in the retina (Linden and Perry, 1982; Linden and Serfaty, 1985). In the cat, optic axon loss starts while the lateral geniculate nucleus and superior colliculus are only sparsely innervated by optic axons (Williams and Chalupa, 1982; Shatz, 1983), which may indicate that the axons do not compete for synaptic space but rather for trophic factors. Evidence that competition involves electrical activity was obtained by Fawcett *et al.* (1984). Blockade of electrical activity of one eye by means of tetrodotoxin in neonatal rats results in persistence

of a projection from the opposite eye to the entire superior colliculus and in survival of a substantial number of the ipsilaterally projecting ganglion cells that would normally have died. Rescue of retinal ganglion cells by preventing them from firing suggests that cell death normally occurs because retinal axon terminals are unsuccessful in their competition for a trophic factor that is down-regulated by nerve activity (see Section 8.6 for a possibly analogous effect of neuromuscular blockade in preventing death of spinal motoneurons). The identity of the trophic factor(s) remains unknown. NGF has been reported to enhance regeneration of optic axons in the goldfish and newt (Turner and Glaze, 1977; Turner and Delaney, 1979; Turner *et al.*, 1980; Yip and Grafstein, 1982), but Humphrey (1988) found no such enhancement in the frog. Enhanced survival of retinal ganglion cells after section of the optic nerve has been reported in response to repeated intraocular injection of NGF in adult rats (Carmignolo *et al.*, 1989). These effects of NGF are far less than expected if NGF is a survival factor for retinal ganglion cells. BDNF is one of the trophic factors necessary for survival of chick embryo retinal ganglion cells (Johnson *et al.*, 1986; Rodriguez-Tébar *et al.*, 1989; Thanos *et al.*, 1989; see Section 8.17).

There is considerable evidence of reciprocal interdependence between retinal ganglion cells and their targets. Retinal ganglion cell death coincides with death of neurons in the superior colliculus of the rat (Giordano *et al.*, 1980; Cunningham *et al.*, 1982) and hamster (Finlay *et al.*, 1982). Increased death of cells in the optic tectum occurs after removal of retinal input (De Long and Sidman, 1962; Kelly and Cowan, 1972; Ostrach and Mathers, 1979).

Cutting the optic nerve in birds and mammals results in death of virtually all the retinal ganglion cells (Eayers, 1952; Munchnick and Hibbard, 1980; Perry, 1981; Grafstein and Ingoglia, 1982; McConnel and Berry, 1983). Retinal ganglion cells die in the chick after surgical removal of their target, the optic tectum (Hughes and McLoon, 1979), or after transplantation of the eye to the chorioallantoic membrane (McLoon and Hughes, 1978). In fish, it appears that ganglion cells do not die after optic nerve section (Murray, 1982). In frogs, optic nerve section results in death of almost half of the retinal ganglion cells (Beazley, 1981; Humphrey and

Beazley, 1985; Scalia *et al.,* 1985; Beazley *et al.,* 1986; Jenkins and Straznicky, 1986; Stelzner and Strauss, 1986; Humphrey, 1988; Humphrey *et al.,* 1989), but the surviving ganglion cell axons regenerate and reestablish an orderly retinotectal projection map (see Section 11.13). Retinal ganglion cell death in the frog is not prevented by blocking retinal ganglion cell activity by means of tetrodotoxin (Sheard and Beazley, 1988). For discussion of the possible role of impulse traffic of retinal ganglion cells in formation of retinotectal projection maps see Section 11.15.

8.4. Neuronal Death in the Isthmo-Optic Nucleus

The neurons of the avian isthmo-optic nucleus (ION) project their axons to the amacrine layer of the contralateral retina where they synapse mainly on amacrine cells (Dowling and Cowan, 1966; An-

gaut and Raffin, 1981). The isthmo-optic neurons receive afferents from the optic tectum (Crossland and Hughes, 1978). All the neurons of the ION originate as postmitotic cells over a period of less than 48 hours, from E5 to E7 in the chick embryo (Cowan and Wenger, 1968a; P. G. H. Clarke *et al.,* 1976; Cowan and Clarke, 1976). The cells assemble to form the nucleus in temporospatial order, from ventrolateral to dorsomedial. Migration is completed by about E9.5, and all the isthmo-optic axons have grown into the retina by E12. At E12.5 the ION contains about 22,000 neurons, but 60 percent of the cells die during the period from about E12.5 to E16.5. Cell death occurs uniformly throughout the nucleus, showing that death of a cell is not determined by the time of its origin. At hatching about 9500 cells remain in the isthmo-optic nucleus (Fig. 8.3) and a further 1500 "ectopic" isthmo-optic neurons in the isthmus and midbrain tegmentum also project their axons to the contralateral retina. In addition, about 40 neurons project from the ION to

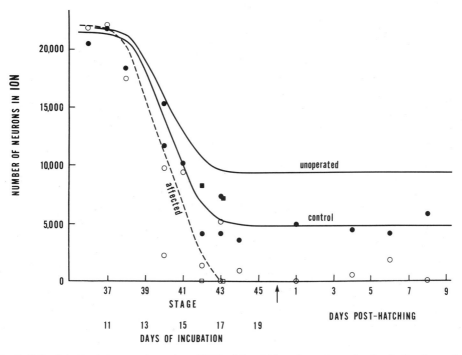

Figure 8.3. Cell death in the isthmo-optic nucleus (ION) of the chick embryo shown by the decline in numbers of ION cells in normal embryos ("unoperated" curve). After removal of one eye at 2–3 days of incubation, the number of cells declines to virtually zero in the ION contralateral ("affected" curve) and declines to about half normal numbers in the ION ipsilateral to the enucleated eye ("control" curve). Circles and squares denote removal of the eye and removal of the retina, respectively. The arrow shows the time of hatching. From P. G. H. Clarke, L. A. Rogers, and W. M. Cowan, *J. Comp. Neurol.* **167**:125–142 (1976).

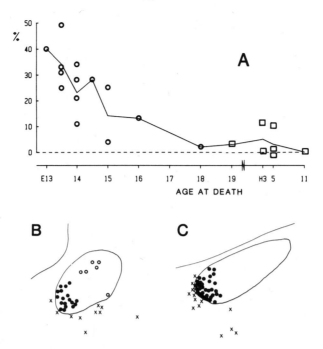

Figure 8.4. Many isthmo-optic neurons project to topographically incorrect positions in the contralateral retina, and they all die. (A) Percentage of aberrantly projecting isthmo-optic neurons at different ages, retrogradely labeled after placing of the tracer DiI at a localized position in the peripheral part of the contralateral retina of the chick embryo at E10. Circles indicate times during the period of death of isthmo-optic neurons, while squares are at ages after cell death in the ION. (B and C) Computer plots in coronal sections through the ION after DiI placement in VL retina at E10 followed by fixation at E13.5 (B) or at E18 followed by fixation at P5 (C). Filled circles denote labeled neurons in the correct region, open circles are aberrantly projecting neurons, and X's are labeled neurons outside the isthmo-optic nucleus. Kindly provided by Peter G. H. Clarke.

the ipsilateral retina (O'Leary and Cowan, 1982, 1984). Many isthmo-optic neurons initially project their axons to the incorrect positions in the retina, and all of those die (Fig. 8.4). In the duck ION there is a similar sequence of events: the number of neurons reaches a maximum of about 6000 cells on E15, but cell death on the following 3 days reduces the number of cells to almost 3500 by 21 days of incubation (Sohal and Narayanan, 1974).

The percentage of ipsilaterally projecting neurons is greatly increased at E13 after removal of one eye on E3 (P. G. H. Clarke and Cowan, 1975; O'Leary and Cowan, 1984). However, the total number of surviving ION neurons from both sides projecting to the residual eye does not exceed the number normally projecting from the contralateral ION (O'Leary and Cowan, 1984). This is evidence in favor of the competition hypothesis discussed near the end of Section 8.2.

There are three lines of evidence showing that the factors causing death of ION neurons are in the retina and not in the nucleus. However, as will be shown below, the afferent supply from the tectum is also a critical factor. Firstly, after removal of the retina or optic cup on E3 in the chick embryo, the ION forms normally until E13 and then the loss of cells in the contralateral ION is greatly increased so that no neurons remain in the nucleus at E18 (Cowan and Wenger, 1967; P. G. H. Clarke *et al.*, 1976; O'Leary and Cowan, 1984). The proliferation, migration, and differentiation of ION neurons are not affected by removal of their targets, the amacrine and displaced ganglion cells in the retina. The neurons die only after they fail to connect with those targets. Secondly, the isthmo-optic neurons die after intraocular injection of kainate, which kills the retinal amacrine cells, or after intraocular injection of colchine, which blocks axonal transport, if these drugs are injected before the time of normal cell death in the isthmo-optic nucleus (P. G. H. Clarke, 1982a, 1985b; Catsicas and Clarke, 1987a,b). Zero cell death occurs after kainate injection on E19, 2 days after the time of normal cell death in the ION (Catsicas and Clarke, 1987b). Therefore, either the isthmo-optic neurons lose their dependence on trophic factors from the retina or obtain trophic support from elsewhere. Ectopic isthmo-optic neurons, which may project to displaced retinal ganglion cells, are unaffected by kainate injections into the retina (Catsicas and Clarke, 1987b). Additional evidence that the factors supporting ION neurons are in the retina is that ION neurons can be saved from death by providing them with an additional eye grafted on E3 (Boydston and Sohal, 1979).

These results support the theory that the isthmo-optic neurons are maintained by a trophic factor transported from their endings in the eye and die if they are deprived of the ocular trophic factor (Cowan and Wenger, 1968; P. G. H. Clarke *et al.*, 1976; O'Leary and Cowan, 1984; Catsicas and Clarke, 1987b). The isthmo-optic neurons also receive anterograde transneuronal trophic support from their main source of afferents coming from the optic tectum.

The role of tectal afferents to the ION was not sufficiently recognized in earlier work in which the effects of unilateral eye removal were thought to result almost entirely from deprivation of trophic factors originating in the eye (P. G. H. Clarke and Cowan, 1976). Natural cell death in the ION is increased after lesioning of the optic tectum (P. G. H. Clarke, 1985b; P. G. H. Clarke and Egloff, 1988). The additional neuronal death occurs only during the latter half of the period of natural cell death, which suggests that tectal afferents have a trophic effect at that time. After unilateral eye removal there are not only aberrant ipsilateral projections from ION to retina, but also from retina to tectum. This appears to be the cause of survival of some ION neurons on the deprived side observed by P. G. H. Clarke and Cowan (1976). Hence, the almost total loss of neurons in the ION deprived of its ocular targets is partly caused by deafferentation of the tectum, which is the main source of afferents to the ION. The ION neurons do not survive in the absence of tectal afferents (P. G. H. Clarke, 1985b).

8.5. Dependence of Motoneurons on Muscles: Neuronal Death in the Trochlear Nucleus

The trochlear nucleus is composed of a homogeneous population of neurons clearly separate from surrounding structures and with a single peripheral target, the superior oblique muscle on the opposite side. This appears to be a relatively simple case of matching of the size of the motoneuron population with the size of the muscle. There is an initial overproduction followed by death of about 50 percent of trochlear neurons. They can be rescued from death by grafting additional target muscle, or by treatment with neuromuscular blocking agents.

The trochlear nucleus of the chick is a small nucleus composed of about 1000 neurons, according to Dunnebacke (1953), and about 1400, according to Cowan and Wenger (1967). At 72 hours of incubation the trochlear nucleus can first be recognized lying immediately dorsolateral to the medial longitudinal bundle in the floor of the aqueduct of Sylvius. The trochlear nerve fibers start sprouting on E4, decussate, and emerge from the brain to innervate the superior oblique muscle on the opposite side. The fibers reach the muscle by E10 and sprout profusely on E11 and E12 (Sohal *et al.*, 1978). There is no evidence of addition of neurons to the trochlear nucleus after E4 or E5, and the nucleus attains its maximal complement of neurons at E5 (Dunnebacke, 1953). Dendrites appear on the trochlear neurons on E5, and the neurons continue growing until hatching.

There is a progressive decrease in the number of trochlear neurons, resulting in the survival of only 50 percent of the original number of neurons (Cowan and Wenger, 1967; Sohal, 1976). The largest loss of neurons occurs between E9 and E17 (Fig. 8.5). No significant reduction occurs after hatching. Grafting an extra optic vesicle rescues about 40 percent of the trochlear motoneurons that would have died (Narayanan and Narayanan, 1978; Boydston and Sohal, 1979).

Creazzo and Sohal (1979) found that trochlear neurons are rescued from death by injection of alpha-bungarotoxin into the yolk sac of duck embryos during the period of trochlear neuron death (E11–E17) and until E24, but the rescued neurons

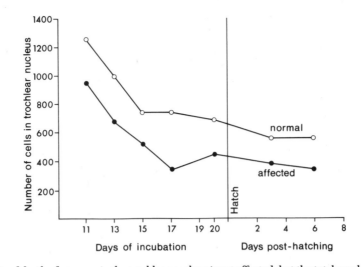

Figure 8.5. The rate of death of neurons in the trochlear nucleus is not affected, but the total number of surviving neurons is reduced, after removal of their targets. Number of neurons in the trochlear nucleus of the chick after removal of the optic vesicle on one side on embryonic Stages 11–13 (34–50 hours of incubation). From W. M. Cowan and E. Wenger, *J. Exp. Zool.* 164:275–280 (1967).

die if the toxin is discontinued after E17. After toxin treatment, all the trochlear neurons project to the superior oblique muscle, as shown by retrograde transport of HRP from the muscle to the trochlear nucleus. This indicates that if a retrograde trophic factor controls trochlear neuron death, its action requires muscle activity. Pittman and Oppenheim (1979) found that curare, alpha-bungarotoxin, alpha-cobratoxin, and botulinum toxin are all equally effective in preventing death of spinal motoneurons in the chick embryo if the treatment is given on E6–E9, during the period of cell death, but not effective if it is started after E12 (see Section 8.7).

Extirpation of the optic vesicle and surrounding mesoderm at E1.5, including the anlage of the superior oblique muscle, results in development of only 10–26 percent of the superior oblique muscle and causes death of up to 83 percent of the trochlear neurons supplying the reduced muscle (Dunnebacke, 1953). Although the superior oblique muscle has been removed at E1.5, there is no effect on proliferation, migration, and differentiation of trochlear neurons until after E5, when they normally begin innervating the muscle. A less radical extirpation of the optic vesicle and superior oblique anlage results in loss of about 80 percent of trochlear neurons (Cowan and Wenger, 1967). The number of neurons is reduced from an estimated

1300 at E9, to 1000 at E11, and finally to 300 at 6 days after hatching (Fig. 8.5). Degenerating cells are only rarely seen, even when the loss of cells is at a maximum (Dunnebacke, 1953; Cowan and Wenger, 1967), and signs of glial proliferation or invasion by macrophages have not been reported. Obvious signs of neuron death are absent in this situation because the loss of neurons is slow in the trochlear nucleus. By contrast, cell debris accumulates and macrophage activity is evident in the spinal cord and spinal ganglia after amputation of a limb. The severity of neuronal death after limb amputation is increased by the combination of retrograde and anterograde transneuronal effects resulting from stimultaneously depriving both the motor and sensory neurons of their peripheral fields. This is considered in the next section.

8.6. Regulation of the Number of Spinal Motoneurons

During vertebrate embryonic development an excess number of spinal motoneurons is generated, followed by the death, depending on species, of half to three-quarters of spinal motoneurons after their axons have entered the limb and during the period of development of limb reflex movements. The normal maturation and subsequent vitality of the motoneurons depend on their connections with muscle. Proliferation, migration, and initial differentiation of motoneurons, including outgrowth of their axons to contact muscles, occur autonomously and are not affected by removal of the muscles. Removal of the limb during a critical period results in death of nearly all the neurons deprived of peripheral targets. Motoneurons can be rescued from cell death by grafting additional target tissue, or by treatment with neuromuscular blocking agents.

Overproduction followed by death of spinal motoneurons has been found in frogs (Hughes, 1961, 1965, 1974; Prestige, 1967a,b, 1970; Lamb, 1981), birds (Hamburger, 1975; Chu-Wang and Oppenheim, 1978a,b; Oppenheim et al., 1978, 1989a,b; Landmesser, 1980), and mammals (Romanes, 1946; Harris-Flannagan, 1969; Rootman et al., 1981). A gradual loss of about 30 percent of the motoneurons in the ventral horn of the spinal cord occurs in normal mice between days 2 and 12 after birth (Romanes, 1946).

The number of motoneurons that survive can be reduced by amputating a limb, which removes the peripheral targets (muscles) and also eliminates afferents from the limb to the motoneurons. Amputation of the developing limb can result in additional loss of most or all motoneurons in amphibians (May, 1930; Stultz, 1942; Beaudoin, 1955; Perri, 1951; Hughes and Tschumi, 1958; Hughes, 1961; Prestige, 1967a,b; Decker, 1978; Lamb, 1981; Kett and Pollack, 1985; Stebbins and Pollack, 1986; Farel, 1989), birds (Shorey, 1909; Hamburger, 1934, 1958, 1975; Barron, 1948; Oppenheim et al., 1978; Oppenheim, 1981, 1984), and mammals (Barron, 1945; Romanes, 1946). Grafting an additional limb results in survival of many of the motoneurons that normally would have died in frogs (R. M. May, 1933; Hollyday and Mendell, 1976; Lamb, 1979b) and in the chick (Hollyday and Hamburger, 1976). Polydactyly in the chick (Baumann and Landauer, 1943) and the mouse (Tsang, 1939) is also associated with an increased number of motoneurons in the spinal cord segments supplying the extra digits.

These changes in the final number of neurons might eventuate from changes in cellular proliferation, migration, differentiation, and death. After a period of initial uncertainty about the relative effects of these four processes and mistaken identification of mitoses in glial cells for neuronal proliferation, it has now been shown that proliferation and early differentiation of motoneurons are not influenced by the limb and that glial cell proliferation occurs as a response to the growth of motoneurons. Outgrowth of motor axons occurs in the absence of the limb, and the axons grow out to the vicinity of the peripheral targets, but more than half the total number of neurons subsequently die. These results suggest that at least one of the causes of motoneuron death is failure of their axons to make peripheral synaptic connections and consequently failure to obtain trophic support from the muscle.

The motoneurons in frogs form a column in the ventrolateral part of the spinal cord (M. L. Silver, 1942; D. W. Kennard, 1959; Cruce, 1974). The normal development of this lateral motor column in frogs has been described in *Rana* (Beaudoin, 1955; Race and Terry, 1965; Hughes, 1968a–c; Pollack, 1969), *Xenopus* (Hughes, 1961; Prestige, 1967b), and *Eleutherodactylus* (Hughes, 1966, 1968a). Newly formed motoneurons migrate from the ventricular germinal zone laterally into the mantle layer of the spinal cord. This migration occurs during the early development of the limb bud, and the motoneurons grow slowly until midlarval stages. Lateral motoneurons at lumbosacral levels develop earlier than those in the brachial cord (Pollack, 1969). There is no evidence of death of young motoneurons until midlarval stages, but thereafter, through metamorphosis, 60–80 percent of the lateral motor column neurons degenerate.

Hughes (1961) counted the motoneurons in the lumbar ventral horn of the spinal cord in the clawed frog *Xenopus* at different stages during development and found that for every neuron that finally survives to metamorphosis about eight degenerate. Before metamorphosis at Stage 53 of the normal series of Nieuwkoop and Faber (1965) there are about 4000 neurons in the lumbar region of the spinal cord, whereas after metamorphosis there are only 1200 (Fig. 8.6). Microglial cells appear at Stage 53 and phagocytose degenerating neurons. The peak of degeneration at larval Stages 54–56 coincides with the onset of movements in the hindlimbs, and this can be correlated with the formation of neuromuscular junctions as determined by cholinesterase staining (Hughes, 1961). The surviving neurons are presumably those that have formed peripheral connections. Their nuclear size almost

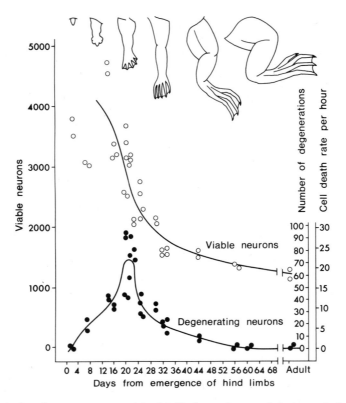

Figure 8.6. Death of spinal cord motoneurons supplying hindlimbs reaches a peak during early development of the limbs and declines during metamorphosis in *Xenopus*. The number of degenerating neurons is based on a degeneration time of 3.2 hours. Modified from A. F. Hughes, *J. Embryol. Exp. Morphol.* 9:269–284 (1961).

doubles from midlarval stages to the completion of metamorphosis (Beaudoin, 1955; Race and Terry, 1965). Pollack (1969) observed a further increase in nuclear size after metamorphosis in the brachial lateral motoneurons of *Rana*.

The development of the motoneurons in amphibians is partly under the control of the thyroid gland (Hughes, 1974, review). Although the production and initial differentiation of the motoneurons can occur in the absence of thyroxine in hypophysectomized frogs (Race, 1961), their full growth depends on the presence of thyroxine. High doses of thyroxine given to metamorphosing frogs (*Rana pipiens*) result in precocious cytodifferentiation and death of spinal motoneurons (Reynolds, 1963). The corollary to this experiment is that an antithyroid drug, thiourea, prevents the cell death that normally occurs in the spinal cord and spinal ganglia of *Xenopus* from larval Stage 53 to metamorphosis (Prestige, 1965).

Beaudoin (1955) found that removal of the hindlimb bud of the frog *R. pipiens* at an early larval stage (I or III of the normal stages of A. C. Taylor and Kollros, 1946) does not affect normal development of the motoneurons until after midlarval stages (IX), when rapid disappearance of motoneurons occurs on the operated side of the spinal cord and results in an 82 percent loss of motoneurons by Stage XVI. Production, migration, and the initial stages of differentiation of motoneurons in the frog spinal cord do not appear to be affected by amputation of the hindlimb.

Prestige (1967b, 1970) removed a hindlimb from *Xenopus* embryos before Stage 53, when the limb is in the palette stage. Limb bud amputation at that stage has no effect on the production and early maturation of spinal motoneurons (Hughes and Tschumi, 1958; Prestige, 1967b). Axons can be seen in the limb bud as early as Stage 49 (Hughes and Tschumi, 1958), and these have been shown to be motoneuron axons which transport HRP from the limb bud to the motoneurons in the ventral horn of the spinal cord (Lamb, 1974). At these stages, the ventral horn neurons have not established neuromuscular connections in the limb. Peripheral neuromuscular connections are made soon after Stage 53 and movements of the hindlimb start at Stage 54. At the same time, histogenetic degeneration of neurons is first seen in the ventral horn of the spinal cord as well as in the spinal sensory ganglia supplying the hindlimbs. Amputation of a hindlimb at Stage 54, when the leg has reflex movements and therefore has sensory and motor connections, results within 3–4 days in massive degeneration of neurons in the ventral horn of the spinal cord. Death of spinal motoneurons during normal development in *Xenopus* reaches a peak at larval Stages 54–56 and then declines gradually to metamorphosis (Hughes, 1961).

It has been known for decades that the effects of amputation of the developing limb differ according to the stage of maturation of the neurons and more recent evidence shows that young and old neurons have different requirements for trophic support. In *Xenopus*, before larval Stage 53, the ventral horn consists entirely of recently formed neurons. Outgrowth of axons from some of these neurons has commenced and some axons have entered the limb bud by Stage 50 (Hughes and Tschumi, 1958; Lamb, 1974), but neuromuscular connections are not made until Stage 54. Prestige (1967b) found that the earlier the limb is removed, the shorter the latent period before the motoneurons start to degenerate. If the limb is amputated at larval Stage 54, when the majority of ventral horn cells are in the process of forming neuromuscular junctions, the resulting degeneration occurs within 3–4 days of amputation. Limb amputation at still later stages, after Stage 56, when the motoneurons are in the final stages of maturation, results in a gradual onset of chromatolysis and cell death. The latent period between limb amputation and death of spinal motoneurons depends on the maturity of the neurons at the time of amputation. When this is performed at Stages 55–56, final loss takes place after about 3 weeks; after amputation at Stage 57, during the 4th week; after amputation at Stage 61, during the 3rd and 4th months; and after amputation as juveniles, not until the 4th–7th months. "*Young neurons therefore die after amputa-*

tion very quickly, while older ones take longer. Thus the times at which cells die after amputation plot out a maturity spectrum for the cells in the ventral horn at the time of the operation" (Prestige, 1967b). The very low threshold of young motoneurons to limb amputation shortly after the nerves have formed neuromuscular connections and the high threshold of mature motoneurons may be due to the absence of a survival factor at earlier stages or to lower sensitivity of the motoneurons to such a factor. Ciliary neurotrophic factor (see Section 8.18) applied to the cut central stump of the facial nerve has been shown to protect the facial neurons from chromatolysis and death in the neonatal rat (Sendtner *et al.*, 1990). Ciliary neurotrophic factor (CNTF) or a similar factor released by muscle or cells of injured mature peripheral nerves may protect neurons from death.

Limb bud amputation before the time at which their axons grow into the limb has a paradoxical effect on the young neurons, resulting in a transient increase in their numbers until the stage when their axons normally form connections with the limb muscles (Beaudoin, 1955; Hughes, 1961; Prestige, 1967b; Decker, 1978). In the absence of these muscles the motoneurons eventually die at Stages 54–56 in *Xenopus*. This shows that injury to the axon as a result of amputation of the limb bud is not the primary cause of cell death, because when the limb is amputated after the motoneurons have grown into it but before they have made neuromuscular connections, their death is delayed until the stage when they normally would have formed connections (Prestige, 1967b). Hindlimb amputation or section of ventral roots supplying the hindlimbs does not affect motoneuron number when the operations are done after metamorphosis (Farel, 1989). In *Xenopus*, amputation of both hindlimbs results in death of all the motoneurons supplying the limbs (Lamb, 1981).

In frogs, amputation of one hindlimb early in development results in a small increase in number of lateral motoneurons during the period of limb regeneration (Beaudoin, 1955; Kett and Pollack, 1985; Stebbins and Pollack, 1986). This may mean that regenerating limb tissue produces a neurotrophic factor. Increased survival of motoneurons also occurs after section of the ventral spinal nerve roots to the hindlimb of the bullfrog during the period of histogenetic motoneuron death (Farel, 1989), as shown in Fig. 8.7. In the bullfrog,

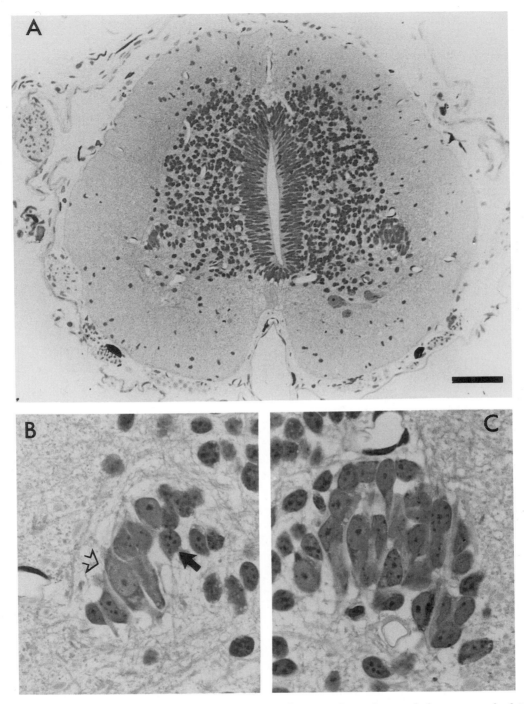

Figure 8.7. Motoneurons can be rescued from death by cutting their axons during the period of motoneuron death in the frog. (A) Cross-section through the lumbar spinal cord of the tadpole of the bullfrog, *Rana catesteiana*, whose lumbar ventral roots on the right side were cut 6 weeks earlier. (B and C) Lumbar motoneurons on the unoperated and operated sides: the increased number of motoneurons is mainly of what appear to be a more differentiated type (white arrow in B), not the immature type (black arrow). Rescue of lumbar motoneurons from death occurs only if the tadpoles do not enter metamorphic climax during a 6–7 week postoperative period. These results are consistent with a theory that motoneuron death normally results unless prevented by a change of metabolic state which can be produced by a number of conditions, one of which is axotomy. From P. B. Farel, *J. Neurosci.* 9:2103–2113 (1989), copyright Society for Neuroscience.

catastrophic death of motoneurons occurs only if the ventral roots are cut during metamorphic climax, even if the nerves regenerate and reconnect with muscles (Farel and Bemelmans, 1985, 1986), and amputation of the hindlimb has no effect on motoneuron number if the tadpoles do not enter metamorphic climax (Farel, 1989).

The cellular mechanisms of rescue of motoneurons that would normally have died are not revealed by the aforementioned observations. Contact of the motoneurons with peripheral tissue targets during a critical stage of development sets in motion the events leading to motoneuron death. The trophic factors required by motoneurons undoubtedly change during development in ways that have not yet been defined. One of the likely mechanisms may involve calcium-mediated cytotoxicity gated by the N-methyl-D-aspartate (NMDA) subclass of glutamate receptors (reviewed by Cotman and Iversen, 1987; Rothman and Olney, 1987; Choi, 1988; Choi and Rothman, 1990). Neurons are rendered more sensitive to lethal Ca^{2+} entry by hypoxia and injury, such as axotomy (Choi, 1988; Novelli et al., 1988). Frog motoneurons possess NMDA receptors (McClellan and Farel, 1985; King et al., 1987). Cell death can result from a lethal influx of extracellular Ca^{2+} through cell membrane channels gated by NMDA receptors. This hypothesis could be tested by seeing whether neuronal death is reduced by NMDA antagonists.

8.7. Developmental Regulation of Motoneuron Numbers in Chick Embryos

Motoneurons are generated during a short period (E2–E5) in the chick embryo followed by a period of motoneuron death (E6–E9), resulting in the survival of about half the original number of motoneurons. Glial cell proliferation coincides with the period of neuronal death and continues afterward. At any given level of the spinal cord, there is asynchrony in the time of generation and the rate of development of different types of motoneurons. Some motoneurons are already in an advanced stage of differentiation while production of motoneurons by division of ventricular germinal cells is still in progress. Death of some motoneurons begins while others are still projecting their axons toward the periphery and synapses are forming on the motoneurons.

Motoneurons originate in the chick embryo between E2 and E5 in the lateral motor column of the spinal cord (Hollyday and Hamburger, 1977), dorsal motor nucleus of the vagus (L. L. Wright, 1981), trigeminal motor nucleus (Heaton and Moody, 1980; Arens and Straznicky, 1986), and in the duck oculomotor, trochlear, and abducens nuclei (Sohal and Holt, 1977). Generation of glial cells continues after neuron production has ceased. Death of motoneurons during normal development starts as birth of motoneurons ceases. In the chick lumbar lateral motor column approximately half the motoneurons die during E6–E9 (Hamburger, 1975; Oppenheim et al., 1978; Lamb, 1981a; Lance-Jones, 1982). From E8 to E21, glial cells increase steadily in the white matter of the spinal cord of the chick embryo (Bensted et al., 1957; H. Fujita and Fujita, 1964), and only the glial cells are labeled by tritiated thymidine injected into the chick embryo during this period of development (S. Fujita, 1963, 1965b).

The initial differentiation of motoneurons begins while they are still in the course of migration out of the ventricular germinal zone. At 40 hours of incubation, the first silver-impregnated neurofibrils can be seen in young motoneurons in the hindbrain near the otic invagination and in the cranial nerve nuclei (Cowdry, 1914). By 59 hours, silver impregnation can be seen in commissural fibers in the cord and in spinal ventral roots (Tello, 1922a; Hughes, 1955). Axons of the motoneurons continue to grow into the ventral roots during E3, E4, and E5. The first motor axons make contact with anterior trunk muscles at E3.5. The first motor axons arrive at the proximal muscles of the limb on E5. Many of the axons which grow out on E6 are commissural, but some exit via dorsal and ventral roots (Windle and Orr, 1934). Barron (1943, 1946, 1948) observed that the development of dendrites of spinal motoneurons occurs shortly after their axons connect with the muscles and conjectured that the sprouting of dendrites is triggered by the contact of the axon with muscle fibers. However, afferent connections to the motoneurons also form at about the same time as their axons contact muscles, and both may be related to the onset of motoneuron death.

Synaptogenesis on lumbar spinal motoneurons in the chick embryo begins at E4 at about the same time as the motoneurons form connections with muscles. Synaptogenesis continues during the period of cell death from E6 to E12 (Oppenheim *et al.*, 1974). Deafferentation of those motoneurons increases the number that die (Okada and Oppenheim, 1985). Normal axosomatic synapses can be seen on dying motoneurons, and this is an indication that motoneuron death is not caused by presynaptic degeneration (Okada *et al.*, 1989). Reflexes can first be elicited by stimulating the skin of the chick embryo on E6, and this can be correlated with the growth of the central processes of dorsal root ganglion cells into the spinal cord on E5 and E6 and the first appearance of synapses in the spinal cord on E5. The reflex arcs from the skin, which pass via the dorsal root ganglia and spinal interneurons to motoneurons ending in muscles, are completed on E5–E7 at different spinal levels. The onset of stretch reflexes is delayed until E10 and E11, when the monosynaptic reflex circuit from the muscle spindles to motoneurons is completed (see Section 9.11).

In the chick spinal cord the motoneurons are arranged as follows: The lateral somatic motor column, which supplies the limbs, is present only in the brachial (segments 12–16) and the lumbar (segments 22–30) enlargements of the cord. The medial somatic motor column, which innervates the axial musculature, extends throughout the length of the cord (Fig. 8.8). The visceral preganglionic neurons lie in the ventrolateral column (of Terni) and send axons to the prevertebral autonomic ganglia. There are also segmental groups of neurons situated laterally in the spinal cord just beneath the pia mater, which have been called *marginal nuclei* or *Hofmann's nuclei*. They are probably preganglionic visceromotor neurons. All the young neurons in the ventrolateral motor column appear to be identical when stained with hematoxylin or silver at E2–E3

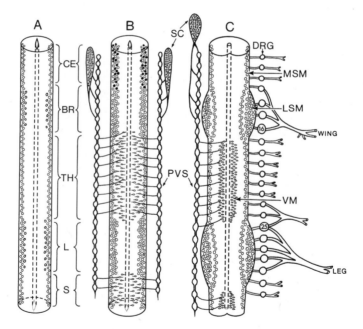

Figure 8.8. Motoneuron origin and migration in the spinal cord of the chick embryo (A at E3; B at E4.5; C at E8). Motoneurons originate and migrate from the ventricular germinal zone at all levels, with more accumulation in the lateral motor columns at limb levels. Visceromotor neurons (spindle-shaped) migrate toward the central canal to form the visceromotor column at thoracic levels. Degenerating motoneurons at cervical levels are shown in black. The somatic motoneurons form into a medial column that supplies axial muscles and proximal limb muscles, and into a lateral motor column that supplies distal limb muscles. In C, the spinal nerves and DRG have been omitted on the left side and the sympathetic ganglia on the right. BR = brachial; CE = cervical; DRG = dorsal root ganglia; L = lumbar; LSM = lateral somatic motor column; MSM = medial somatic motor column; PVS = sympathetic ganglia; S = sacral; SC = superior cervical ganglion; TH = thoracic; VM = visceromotor. Adapted from R. Levi-Montalcini, *J. Morphol.* 86:253–283 (1950).

However, Levi-Montalcini (1950) has shown that they are functionally heterogeneous: some young neurons differentiate further into somatic motoneurons whose axons grow into the ventral roots to the muscles, whereas others differentiate into visceral preganglionic neurons whose axons run in the rami communicantes to the prevertebral autonomic ganglia. The growth of the rami communicantes occurs at E3–E4 at all levels of the spinal cord except the brachial and lumbosacral, where they are absent. In the cervical region of the spinal cord, all the preganglionic visceral neurons degenerate and disappear in a short period of about 12 hours between E4.5 and E5 (Fig. 8.8). This occurs at the same time as the headward migration of the prevertebral cervical sympathetic ganglia to form the orthosympathetic cervical ganglia.

The visceromotor neurons are generated, differentiate, and die on the same time schedule as the somatic motoneurons at the same levels. Arens and Straznicky (1986) showed that about 3500 visceromotor neurons in the trigeminal motor nucleus of the chick are generated from E2 to E5 with about 50 percent of the neurons born on E3, and they start degenerating on E5. Death of trigeminal motor neurons peaks on E7 and then gradually declines to cease by E13. About 50 percent of the visceromotor neurons die, leaving a final count of about 1800 neurons. Treatment with curare from E5 results in survival of most of the neurons that would have died, showing that they were not programmed to die. The significance of this finding is discussed later in this section. An even more catastrophic death of virtually all visceromotor cells in the cervical spinal cord occurs between E4 and E5 in the chick embryo during normal development (Levi-Montalcini, 1949). Less dramatic loss of neurons, amounting to about 70 percent of the original number of visceromotor neurons, occurs during normal development of Hofmann's nuclei of the chick spinal cord in the last 10 days of incubation (Dubey et al., 1968). Formation of separate somatomotor and visceromotor neuron columns in the spinal cord of the chick embryo starts at E4.5 as follows: At E4, all the young motoneurons of the chick spinal cord form a compact ventrolateral column of cells. The most medial neurons at thoracolumbar levels start migrating medially from the ventrolateral column at E4.5 (Fig. 8.8). They form a column of preganglionic visceral neurons which become visibly differentiated after E5, and they can be distinguished from the somatic motoneurons by the much larger size of the latter. From E5, the young somatic motoneurons grow much more rapidly than the young visceral neurons, so that at hatching, the visceral motoneurons are about one-tenth the size of the somatic motoneurons.

The ventrolateral motor column is formed by migration of neurons from the ventricular germinal zone of the basal plate starting on E2. Migration starts at the cervical level and rapidly extends caudally so that mitotic figures are uniformly distributed in the basal plate throughout the cord (Levi-Montalcini, 1950). Neuron production reaches a maximum on E3 as determined by mitotic counts (Hamburger, 1948; Corliss and Robertson, 1963), and neuron production is virtually completed by E4 as shown by [³H]thymidine labeling (Hollyday and Hamburger, 1977). Neurons appear to develop uniformly throughout the spinal cord, apparently as a result of a uniform rate of mitosis in the germinal zone of the basal plate (Hamburger, 1948; Corliss and Robertson, 1963). More reliable recent counts of motoneurons have revealed greater numbers of motoneurons at brachial and lumbosacral levels in chick embryos at E4 before the beginning of cell death (Oppenheim et al., 1989). This indicates that segmental specializations develop very early in the spinal cord, presumably as a result of early inductive interactions, and those segmental differences are not due to influences of the limbs. The initial segmental differences also originate independently of cell migration and cell death (Fig. 8.9).

The initial growth of capillaries into the neural tube of the chick embryo at E4.5 occurs at the same time as the onset of cell death (Ernst, 1926; Ramón y Cajal, 1929b; Hughes, 1934; J. F. Feeney and Watterson, 1946). Capillarization of the spinal cord of Xenopus (Sims, 1961) and of the cat retina (Wong and Hughes, 1987c) also occurs during the period of maximal cell death (Sims, 1961). The correlation of ingrowth of capillaries and the appearance of macrophages that remove the debris of dead cells is consistent with the concept of the hematogenous origin of macrophages in the CNS (Cammermeyer, 1970; Ling et al., 1980; Hume et al., 1983; Perry et al., 1985; see Section 3.2).

The brachial and lumbosacral enlargements of the ventrolateral motor column of the spinal cord are greatly increased as a result of growth of the somatic motoneurons, starting at E5. At the same

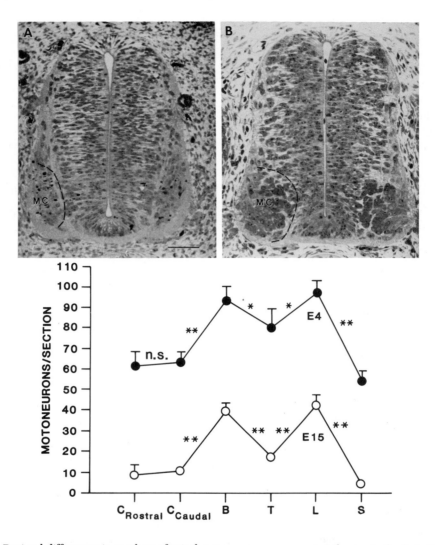

Figure 8.9. Regional differences in numbers of spinal motoneurons are present at the onset of cell death. Photomicrographs of transverse sections of cervical (A) and lumbar (B) spinal cord from E4 (Stage 24) chick embryos illustrating the difference in size of the motor column (MC). Scale bar = 50 μm. Dense profiles in the MC in A are dying neurons that occur in this region between E4 and E4.5. (Below) Numbers of presumptive motoneurons (mean ± S.D.) in the motor column at different segmental levels of the spinal cord: C = cervical; B = brachial; T = thoracic; L = lumbar; S = sacral, on E4 (black symbols) and E15 (white symbols). $C_{Rostral}$ and C_{Caudal} refer to the rostral and caudal halves of the cervical spinal cord. Sample size = 6–7 for each data point. ° $p < 0.01$; °° $p < 0.001$ (t-test). Modified from R. W. Oppenheim, T. Cole, and D. Prevette, *Dev. Biol.* **133**:468–474 (1989), copyright Academic Press, Inc.

time, the somatic motoneurons segregate into a small medial and a large lateral column. The medial column runs through all levels of the spinal cord. The lateral column is absent at the thoracolumbar and cervical regions, having degenerated in the cervical region and having migrated medially to form the visceromotor column in the thoracolumbar re-

gion of the cord, as is illustrated in Fig. 8.8 (Levi-Montalcini, 1950, 1964a,b).

The development of Hofmann's nucleus major of the chick spinal cord has been described by Dubey *et al.* (1968). The cells that form these nuclei arise by separation of the most lateral neurons of the marginal layer of the spinal cord at about 6 days of incubation.

At E7–E10, there are 25–27 pairs of nuclei, arranged segmentally, one on each side of the spinal cord just beneath the pia mater. The eight pairs of nuclei in the lumbosacral region enlarge during E8–E14 and form bilateral prominent bulges on the ventrolateral aspect of the spinal cord. Between E10 and E14, the number of cells in Hofmann's nuclei is greatly reduced, but the surviving cells increase in size. Dubey *et al.* (1968) found that only 31 percent of the cells present in Hofmann's nuclei of the embryo survive in the adult. They also determined that the number of cells is not affected by amputation of the limb buds or by grafting of an additional limb, and they concluded that neurons of Hofmann's nuclei do not supply the limbs, but are probably visceral preganglionic neurons.

There is considerable evidence that proliferation of neurepithelial germinal cells and the initial stages of neuron differentiation are independent of the periphery. Thus amputation of a limb bud in anuran amphibians has no effect on the proliferation and early differentiation of cells in the spinal cord and spinal ganglia (Beaudoin, 1955; Perri, 1956; Hughes, 1961; Prestige, 1967a,b, 1974). In amphibians, amputation of a limb results in death of neurons at the stage of development when they would normally have formed peripheral connections. In the chick embryo the evidence, given later, leads to the same conclusion.

Removal of muscles in the chick embryo does not affect the proliferation and initial differentiation of the motoneurons. For example, after excision of the superior oblique muscle anlage in the chick embryo at E1.5, the proliferation, migration, and differentiation of trochlear motoneurons proceed normally until the full complement of trochlear neurons is formed at E5. No difference is found at E5 between the trochlear nucleus on the side that is in possession of its peripheral field and the nucleus on the side that lacks its peripheral field (Dunnebacke, 1953, Cowan and Wenger, 1967).

The effects of amputation of a limb bud in the chick are similar to those in frogs and are considered in Section 8.6. Shorey (1909) first showed that removal of a limb in chick embryos results in cellular hypoplasia of the spinal motoneurons and the spinal sensory ganglia. Hamburger (1934) also found that removal of the wing bud of the chick embryo at E2.5–E3 results, after 5 or 6 days, in reduction of between 28 and 61 percent in the number of motoneurons in the ventrolateral column of the spinal cord. The loss of motoneurons is roughly proportional to the amount of muscle that is removed. However, even the most radical excision of the limb results in survival of about 10–20 percent of the somatic motoneurons. This probably results from subtotal amputation and projection of some motoneurons to the opposite limb. Limb amputations done at E2.5–E3 do not injure axons because the motor axons grow into the hindlimbs after the time of the operation (Heaton, 1977). After amputation of a hindlimb bud of a chick embryo at E2.5, Hamburger (1958) found that the development of the lateral motor column continues normally up to E5, but the majority of lumbosacral lateral motoneurons die at E5–E8, during the period that they would normally have made connections in the leg.

The evidence does not support the theory that the periphery can influence the centers from a distance, before the outgrowing axons make peripheral contacts. On the contrary, the evidence shows that proliferation of neurepithelial germinal cells and the initial differentiation of neurons occur normally in the absence of the peripheral organs. The degeneration of neurons occurs only after their axons have reached close to their targets in the peripheral organs or have actually formed connections with them. Contacts between terminals of the axons and the peripheral organs is essential for the maturation of the neuron and for the maintenance of the neurons. The evidence supports the theory of trophic factors originating in the tissues and transported retrogradely in the axon.

The first direct observations of flow of materials in axons from axonal endings toward the cell bodies were reported by Hughes (1953) in isolated spinal dorsal root ganglia in culture and by Nakai (1956) in isolated neurons from dorsal root ganglia. More recent studies of retrograde axonal flow are discussed in Section 5.10. Prestige (1967a,b) suggested that a factor is transported by retrograde axonal flow from the periphery to the developing cell body. The delay in degeneration after removal of the limb bud may indicate that the "maintenance factor" is stored in the neuron and that it dies when its stores are exhausted. This idea had earlier been proposed to account for the delayed onset of atrophy of muscle and cutaneous sense organs after cutting of a peripheral nerve: the longer the peripheral stump of the nerve, the larger the reservoir of trophic factor and the longer the delay before the onset of atrophy in the muscle and sensory cells (J. M. D. Olmsted, 1920b; Parker, 1932; Parker and Paine, 1934; J. V. Luco and Eyzaguirre, 1955).

A role for retrograde transneuronal trophic stimulation of motoneurons by muscles is shown by evidence of several kinds in chick and mouse embryos (see Section 9.8). Muscle contraction regulates the extent of sprouting and branching of motoneuron terminals and the formation of neuromuscular junctions (Jansen *et al.*, 1973, 1975; Srihari and Vrobová, 1978). Muscle contraction regulates the levels of acetylcholine receptor (AChR) mRNA and the distribution of AChRs on muscle fibers throughout life (Klarsfeld and Changeux, 1985; Schuetze and Role, 1987, review; Goldman *et al.*, 1988).

Survival of embryonic chick spinal motoneurons is enhanced *in vivo* and *in vitro* by soluble survival-promoting factors from myotubes or cells associated with myotubes. These factors have been extracted from embryonic muscle (Dohrmann *et al.*, 1986, 1987; Tanaka, 1987; Oppenheim *et al.*, 1988) and from the CNS (Dohrmann *et al.*, 1987). At least one of these neurotrophic factors comes from astrocytes rather than from neurons (Eagleson and Bennett, 1986). Double trophic support from both the peripheral targets and the central connections and the possibility that they act at different times complicate interpretations of the available evidence.

Pharmacological blockade of transmission at the neuromuscular junction results in increased number of muscle AChRs and increased number of motoneuron branches (see Section 9.7). If the blockade occurs during the period of natural motoneuron death, it results in increased survival of motoneurons, as shown in Fig. 8.10 (Laing and Prestige, 1978; Creazzo and Sohal, 1979; Pittman and Oppenheim, 1979; Oppenheim and Maderdrut, 1981; Ding *et al.*, 1983; Arens and Straznicky, 1986; Dahm and Landmesser, 1988; Okada *et al.*, 1989; Oppenheim *et al.*, 1989b). There is no effect on motoneuron number if curare treatment is started after the end of motoneuron death (which lasts from E4 to E15 in chick embryos). However, the effect is reversible if the dose of curare does not exceed 1 mg/day, and if treatment is stopped on E6 motor activity begins and motoneuron numbers decline to

normal values. The role of muscle contraction in mammalian development is also shown by the evidence of increased number of motoneurons, increased branching of motoneuron axons, and increased AChRs on muscle fibers of mice with a muscular dysgenesis mutation in which muscles do not contract in the embryo (Rieger and Pincon-Raymond, 1981; Powell *et al.*, 1984; Oppenheim *et al.*, 1986).

Treatment of the chick embryo with curare not only blocks transmission at the neuromuscular junction, but also blocks cholinergic transmission in the CNS, including transmission at synapses on motoneurons (Landmesser and Zente, 1986). Chick embryos treated with curare from E6 to E9 have about 35 percent more motoneurons than controls, but the numerical density of axosomatic and axodendritic synapses on motoneurons is the same in curare-treated embryos and controls at E10 (Okada *et al.*, 1989). This shows that a compensatory increase of synapses occurs on surviving motoneurons at E10. This is transient because at E16 the numerical density of synapses on motoneurons treated with curare is reduced to half the control values. The curare-treated motoneurons do not differ from controls in either size or dendritic branching. Therefore, it can be inferred that the absolute number of synapses decreases on curare-treated motoneurons. This does not appear to be the result of death of interneurons (S. McKay and Oppenheim, 1988). Rather, it may be due to a limited number of synapses that can form on each motoneuron.

The available evidence may support alternative theories of the actions of motoneuron-survival factors derived from the peripheral tissues and from the CNS. The CNS and peripheral neurotrophic factors may be available in limited quantities, able to prevent death of only a fraction of the number of motoneurons that are normally generated. Alternatively, the access of neurons to the factors may be limiting. In addition, the competition for neurotrophic factors may depend on motoneuron activity, which may be spontaneous or may be driven by afferent stimulation. Furthermore, glial cells may have trophic actions on neurons. There is some evidence that an astrocyte-derived neurotrophic factor can maintain motoneurons (Eagleson and Bennett, 1986), and the possibility should also be entertained that neurotrophic factors are released by macrophages (microglial cells).

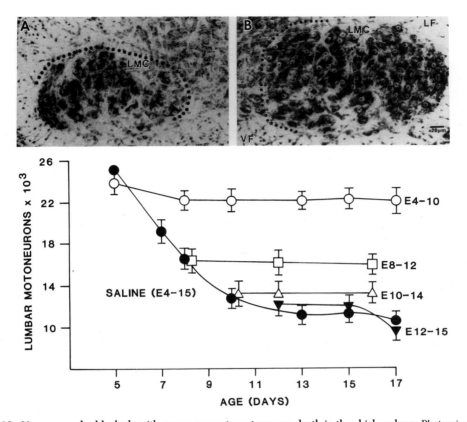

Figure 8.10. Neuromuscular blockade with curare prevents motoneuron death in the chick embryo. Photomicrographs of motoneurons in comparable regions of the lumbar lateral motor column (LMC) on E10 following daily treatment of chick embryos with saline (A) or curare (B, 2.0 mg/day) from E4 to E10. LF, VF refer to lateral and ventral funiculi. (Below) Numbers of motoneurons (mean ± S.D.) on one side of the lumbar spinal cord at different ages following treatment with saline or curare (2.0 mg/day) for varying durations and at different periods of development. Treatment from E4 to E10 rescues virtually all motoneurons. Treatments from E8 to E12 or E10 to E14 rescues that portion of motoneurons that have not yet died. Treatment from E12 to E15, when normal cell death has ceased, has no effect on motoneuron numbers. Although not shown, curare treatment from E3 to E5, which is before the onset of cell death, has no effect on motoneuron numbers at E6. Sample size for each data point ranges from 6 to 12. Except for the E12–E15 group, curare treatment significantly increased motoneuron numbers at each time point examined ($p < 0.001$, t-test). Modified from R. W. Oppenheim, T. Cole, and D. Prevette, *Dev. Biol.* **133**:468–474 (1989), copyright Academic Press, Inc.

The amount of muscle-derived neurotrophic factors may either be regulated directly by muscle contraction, in a manner similar to regulation of AChR mRNA, or the limiting condition may be in the ability of motoneurons to gain access to the factor. Evidence obtained for the latter alternative is that the level of motoneuron-survival factor in muscle is not increased by chronic curare treatment (Tanaka, 1987). This indicates that the muscle-derived motoneuron-survival factor is not regulated by muscle contraction and, therefore, that motoneuron survival is limited by access to the factor.

The limiting condition may be the number of neuromuscular junctions formed by each motoneuron (Oppenheim *et al.*, 1989b). This limiting condition would have to be related to the number of muscle fibers innervated by each motoneuron (the motor unit), which varies greatly between different muscles and motoneurons.

Specific matching of motoneurons with muscles may be another condition that determines whether motoneurons survive or die. Evidence for such matching is discussed in Section 9.4. Hughes (1965) conjectured that motoneurons die because they fail to form connections with specific muscles. Evidence consistent with this mismatch theory is that partial amputation of a limb before contact with motoneuron axons results in selective death of motoneurons that normally project to that part of the limb (Hughes, 1968; Laing, 1979; Lamb, 1981). After removal of part of the motoneuron population, leaving the limb intact, the remaining motoneurons connect preferentially with appropriate limb regions in *Xenopus* (Lamb, 1979) and the chick (Lance-Jones and Landmesser, 1980). In those experiments the motoneurons have a choice, and some motoneurons may have a competitive advantage over others, as Lamb (1981b) has pointed out, whereas there is no choice in other experiments, when a complete mismatch between motoneurons and muscles is produced. For example, when segments of spinal cord are rotated or additional limb buds are grafted in chick embryos long before motoneurons are born, the motoneurons connect with inappropriate muscles and survive (Hollyday *et al.*, 1977; Morris, 1978; Stirling and Summerbell, 1979, 1981; Lance-Jones and Landmesser, 1981).

Other evidence is inconsistent with the mismatch theory. Motoneurons normally project with considerable fidelity to their matching muscles in the frog but die nevertheless (Farel and Bemelmans, 1985, 1986). There are no errors of connections which have been detected during normal innervation of the hindlimb in the chick (Landmesser and Morris, 1975; Landmesser, 1978; Lance-Jones and Landmesser, 1981a; Hollyday, 1983). Spinal motoneurons which are rescued by curare treatment innervate appropriate limb muscles (Oppenheim, 1981; Laing, 1982), showing that the neurons do not normally die because they form grossly incorrect connections. After limb transplantation or rotation, motoneurons that form connections with the wrong muscles do not necessarily die (Morris, 1978; Hollyday, 1981; Lance-Jones and Landmesser, 1981b; Summerbell and Stirling, 1981; Straznicky, 1983; Landmesser and O'Donovan, 1984).

In summary: About half to three-quarters of the spinal motoneurons that are generated in the lateral lumbar motor column die during normal development. Their death occurs during a relatively short period during which their axons make contact with myotubes in the developing limbs. The number of surviving motoneurons depends on the number of available myotubes.

Amputation of a limb before the motoneurons form connections with muscles results in death, at the normal time, of all motoneurons that normally project to the amputated muscles. Deafferentation alone results in increased motoneuron death. Grafting an additional limb increases the number of surviving motoneurons roughly in proportion to the additional muscle.

Pharmacological blockade of neuromuscular transmission in the intact embryo (and thus also blockade of cholinergic transmission in the CNS) results in rescue of all the motoneurons that would have died in the chick embryo. Ventral rhizotomy rescues motoneurons that would have died in the frog tadpole. Therefore, the motoneurons do not inexorably die because they are defective. Other evidence shows that motoneurons do not make errors of connection with muscle during normal development or after they are rescued from death. Motoneurons can survive even after having had no choice but to connect with incorrect muscles.

These findings must be considered in relation to evidence given in Chapter 9 which shows that while motoneurons project initially to correct muscle groups (or compartments), they compete for limited synaptic space on myotubes, and that terminal branching of motor axons is controlled by a trophic factor whose release from muscle is down-regulated by muscle contraction. The greater the number of terminal branches on a motoneuron axon, the greater its advantage in competing for a synaptic site on muscle and also for obtaining more trophic support.

Therefore, there appear to be at least two mechanisms operating at the periphery which determine the probability of survival of a motoneuron: firstly, the availability of a sprouting factor released by muscle which acts directly on the motoneuron axon; secondly, the number of terminal branches of each axon determines the probability of making functional neuromuscular junctions and thus of obtaining a sufficient quantity of muscle-derived neurotrophic factor. In theory this factor is released only from actively contracting muscle, is transported retrogradely, and enhances the survival of the motoneuron. At this time, it is not clear whether there are several peripherally derived neurotrophic factors or only a single muscle-derived neurotrophic factor which has two different sites of action, namely, stimulating axonal sprouting and enhancing neuronal survival. In addition to peripheral trophic mechanisms, during a certain period the motoneuron may require central trophic stimulation from one or more trophic factors derived from glial cells or afferent neurons or both. Lack of the necessary factors during the critical stage while motoneurons form peripheral connections leads to motoneuron death. One of the likely mechanisms may be a lethal influx of Ca^{2+} through motoneuron membrane channels gated by the NMDA class of glutamate receptors.

8.8. Neuronal Death in the Ciliary Ganglion

The ciliary ganglion has certain advantages for investigations of neuron death: its development, period of cell death, afferent and efferent connections, and functions are well characterized. The ciliary ganglion has two distinct types of neurons of approximately equal numbers: small choroid neurons that innervate vascular smooth muscle in the choroid layer of the eye, and the larger ciliary neurons that innervate striated muscle in the ciliary body and iris (Landmesser and Pilar, 1974, 1978). Both types of neurons originate from the cranial neural crest (Hammond and Yntema, 1958; Narayanan and Narayanan, 1978).

The ciliary ganglion neurons reach their definitive position in the chick embryo at E6–E7, to form a ganglion totaling about 6000 neurons. Afferent axons from the accessory oculomotor nucleus enter the ciliary ganglion by E3–E4, and efferent axons from the ganglion enter the iris and choroid by E5–E6. Cell death occurs equally in the two populations of ciliary ganglion neurons from E7 to E15, reducing the number by about 50 percent to a final population of about 3000 neurons (Landmesser and Pilar, 1974). The fact that preganglionic axons make functional synapses in the ciliary ganglion before death of ciliary ganglion cells (Landmesser and Pilar, 1974, 1976) shows that death is not merely due to failure of anterograde transneuronal trophic stimulation.

Removal of the eye vesicle of the chick embryo on E2 results in greatly increased loss of ciliary ganglion neurons (Amprino, 1943; Levi-Montalcini and Amprino, 1947; Cowan and Wenger, 1968; Land-

messer and Pilar, 1974). Transplantation of an additional eye vesicle at E2 results in considerably enhanced survival of ciliary neurons (Narayanan and Narayanan, 1978).

Survival of ciliary neurons in culture is greatly enhanced by ciliary neurotrophic factor, a protein extracted from the ciliary target tissues (Barbin *et al.,* 1984), as discussed further in Section 8.17. Basic fibroblast growth factor (bFGF) enhances survival of both types of ciliary ganglion cells *in vitro* (Unsicker *et al.,* 1987) and *in vivo* (Dreyer *et al.,* 1989). bFGF is present in striated muscle and may therefore be a genuine neurotrophic factor required by ciliary neurons (see Section 8.18).

8.9. Control of Neuron Numbers in the Trigeminal Mesencephalic Nucleus

The trigeminal mesencephalic (TM) nucleus provides the sensory nerves to the muscle spindles in the jaw muscles and extraocular muscles. The advantages of studying this nucleus are that the neurons are large and easy to count and are clearly distinguishable from glial cells. It is a relatively small and well-circumscribed nucleus, and it has well-defined peripheral target tissues. In all species that have been studied there is a similar program of gradual production and assembly of neurons of the TM nucleus. This is followed by rapid loss of about 50 percent of the cells during metamorphic climax in the frog, *R. pipiens* (Kollros, 1984; Kollros and Thiesse, 1985) and about 75 percent of the TM neurons in the hamster (Alley, 1974) and the chick embryo as described below.

The neurons of the TM nucleus originate from the cephalic neural crest (Piatt, 1945; Narayanan and Narayanan, 1978), as described in Section 4.5. Excision of the mandible from salamander larvae results in marked reduction of the number of cells in the TM nucleus (Piatt, 1946). Conversely, heteroplastic grafting of the large mandible of the tiger salamander in place of the smaller mandible of the spotted salamander during embryonic stages results in considerable increase in the number of neurons in the TM nucleus. The mechanism of the hyperplasia has not been studied in this case. In light of what is known, it is most likely to have resulted from survival of neurons that would have died in the absence of a large enough peripheral field to provide neurotrophic support for all the trigeminal mesencephalic neurons that are produced. As the TM neurons are unresponsive to NGF or anti-NGF antibodies (Straznicky and Rush, 1985), they must depend on some other neurotrophic factor(s).

This has been definitely demonstrated for the trigeminal mesencephalic nucleus of the chick embryo (L. A. Rogers and Cowan, 1973; Arens and Straznicky, 1985; Straznicky and Rush, 1985; Hiscock and Straznicky, 1986). The neurons are produced in the neural folds or neural crest on E3 and E4, and by E6 the total number, about 4500 neurons, has assembled in the TM nucleus. Cell death in the nucleus becomes appreciable during the next 4 days and reaches a maximum on E11–E12. From E13, the number of cells remains stable at about 1000. Thus, of the neurons that are produced and migrate to form the TM nucleus, about 75 percent die.

Retrograde labeling of trigeminal mesencephalic neurons following injection of HRP into jaw and extraocular muscles of chick embryos at E6–E15 shows that axons first reach the periphery at E10. By E14 most of the mesencephalic trigeminal neurons have projected axons to the muscles. A lower percentage of neurons is labeled with HRP during the period of maximum cell death than in older embryos, suggesting that many neurons die before their axons contact the peripheral targets (Hiscock and Straznicky, 1986). These findings indicate that failure to contact their peripheral targets and to obtain trophic support from them is not the only cause of death of mesencephalic trigeminal neurons. Similar observations have been made in dorsal root ganglia (Lance-Jones, 1982; Carr and Simpson, 1982). This is discussed in the following section.

8.10. Neuronal Death in Spinal Dorsal Root Ganglia

The dorsal root ganglia (DRG) are formed by migration of neural crest cells (see Section 4.5). This occurs during the first 2.5 days of incubation in the chick embryo (Weston, 1963; Weston and Butler, 1966; Johnston, 1966). At E2.5, the first signs of neuronal differentiation and growth are visible in the ventrolateral (VL) part of the spinal ganglia, and these VL neurons are then distinguishable from the smaller cells in the mediodorsal (MD) part of the ganglion, which do not start their growth spurt until E9. At the end of E3, the central processes of the VL neurons reach, but do not yet enter, the spinal cord in the brachial region (Tello, 1922a; Levi-Montalcini and Levi, 1943). They enter the spinal cord and form the dorsal roots on E5 just before the spinal motor reflexes can be elicited by cutaneous stimulation on E6, thus indicating that the peripheral processes of the VL neurons in the spinal glanglia form connections in the skin (Visintini and Levi-Montalcini, 1939). The large VL neurons grow in size and gradually assume their characteristic pseudounipolar form on E8–E10. They do not develop an affinity for silver until E9–E10, and neurofibrils can be seen in them from that time (Hamburger and Levi-Montalcini, 1949).

The small MD neurons differentiate and grow in size from E9. Neurofibrils are first seen in silver-impregnated MD neurons at E10 (Visintini and Levi-Montalcini, 1939), coincident with the arrival of the sensory nerves at the muscle spindles (Tello, 1922b). This also coincides with the time when stretch reflexes can first be elicited on flexing the hindlimbs. Therefore, Hamburger and Levi-Montalcini (1949) suggested that at least some of the MD neurons are connected with sensory terminals in muscle spindles (see Section 9.11). Both MD and VL neuron populations contain proprioceptive and exteroceptive neurons (Honig, 1977). Retrograde labeling with HRP injected into the limb show that axons of VL neurons are labeled from E5 and MD neurons a day or 2 later (Oppenheim and Heaton, 1975; Honig, 1977; Scott, 1981). From E9 the MD neurons grow faster than the VL neurons, so that from E15 it is no longer possible to distinguish the two cell types histologically. By E20 cells of all sizes are distributed throughout the ganglion except at its VL margin, where a rim of VL neurons persists.

Differentiation of spinal dorsal root ganglion cells of the chick embryo has been studied with the light and electron microscope (Pannese, 1968, 1969, 1976; Pannese et al., 1971). A most interesting finding is that the VL neurons are bipolar neurons from E4.5 to E7 and that they die at that early stage of their differentiation (Pannese, 1976). Until E5, the young neurons have scant cytoplasm, little rough endoplasmic reticulum, and few polyribosomes. After E5, they show all the signs of mature neurons that are exporting materials into the axon: well-developed rough endoplasmic reticulum, a large number of free ribosomes, mitochondria, and an extensive system of Golgi cisternae. The neurons, which are in close apposition until E5, become separated by ensheathing glial cells. Acetylcholinesterase (ChE), assayed histochemically with the electron microscope, is detectable in the chick embryo spinal dorsal ganglion cells at E3 (Pannese *et al.*, 1971). ChE is present in the spinal ganglia of the rabbit embryo at 10 days of gestation (Tennyson *et al.*, 1967). In these cases, ChE appears before the neurons form either peripheral or central connections.

Mitotic activity in the chick DRG reaches a peak on E5 and E6 and is completed at E9 (Levi-Montalcini and Levi, 1943; Hamburger and Levi-Montalcini, 1949). Proliferation of glial cells is said to start after E9 and to continue through hatching (Bensted *et al.*, 1957), but electron microscopic observations indicate that glial cells are present as early as E5 and that they totally ensheath the neurons by E10 (Pannese, 1969). The earlier studies of histogenesis in the spinal ganglia were made by relatively unreliable methods of counting cells and mitotic figures. Using the more reliable technique of tritiated thymidine autoradiography, Carr (1975, 1976) has shown that production of neurons ceases by E6.5 in the VL region and by E9.5 in the MD region and that after those times only glial cells continue to be produced in the DRG.

Neuron production, differentiation, and death all occur at the same time in the DRG. As a result only a small fraction of the neurons could compete for peripheral target tissues at any time. Unlike motoneurons, which die only after they have contacted their targets, a significant percentage of DRG neurons die before their axons reach their targets. This is also inconsistent with the theory of competition for trophic factors produced by the peripheral target tissues.

Carr and Simpson (1982) showed that after an injection of [³H]thymidine at E5.5 in the chick embryo, which is at the peak of death of VL cells, up to 16 percent of dying cells were labeled 2 hours later. In that short time those labeled neurons could not have projected their axons to the periphery. In the mouse, death of DRG cells occurs in two waves, the first of which peaks at E13, before sensory axons reach the periphery. A 2nd wave peaks at E19–E20 after the axons have reached their targets (Scaravilli

and Duchen, 1980). Those findings suggest that other factors in the DRG itself or factors derived from the CNS are involved before neurotrophic factors from the periphery come into play.

Cell death in DRG of the chick embryo has been studied quantitatively by Carr and Simpson (1978) and by Hamburger *et al.* (1981). The two studies are in agreement, but the former ended at E9.5 while the latter continued to E12. Hamburger *et al.* (1981) found that cell death in thoracic ganglion 18 is considerably greater than in brachial ganglion 15 but occurs over essentially the same time period at both levels. Both the VL and DM neurons die, but considerably fewer degenerating DM neurons than VL neurons can be counted at each stage. Death of DM neurons occurs later than VL neuron death, which correlates with the difference in the times of their origin. In thoracic ganglion 18, death of VL neurons begins very early at E4.5, reaches a peak at E5–E6, and then declines to end at E8. Death of DM neurons begins on E7.5, peaks at E8, and ends at E11 in the thoracic ganglion. In brachial ganglion 15 the VL neurons begin to die on E5.5. Their death peaks at E7 and ends on E9. Death of DM neurons starts at E7.5, reaches a peak at E8.5, and gradually declines to a minimum at E12. A few dying neurons, 1–2 percent of the total neuron population of the ganglion, were found at all stages examined by Hamburger *et al.* (1981), who consider these to represent "sporadic death" due to local factors and not to factors in the periphery. Injection of NGF into the yolk sac daily from E3.5 to E12 results in rescue of all the DM and the majority of VL cells that would have died (Hamburger *et al.*, 1981). This indicates that NGF is a trophic factor that maintains these neurons but does not show the site at which the injected NGF acted on the DRG neurons— directly on the neurons, on their central neurites, or on their peripheral neurites.

Increase or reduction in the size of the peripheral innervation zone has different effects on VL and MD neurons of the chick spinal ganglia. According to Hamburger and Levi-Montalcini (1949), amputation of a limb of the chick embryo at E2.5–E3 results in death of the majority of differentiated VL neurons at E5–E6, while the MD neurons slowly atrophy. This shows that the neurons die in the absence of the limb in which they normally form connections.

Grafting an extra limb on the chick embryo at

E2.5–E3 results in an increase by as much as 80 percent in the number of neurons that differentiate to form VL neurons in the spinal ganglia innervating the extra limb. The MD neurons appear to be unaffected. Hamburger and Levi-Montalcini (1949) also observed an increase of about 20 percent in the number of mitoses in the spinal ganglia at the level of the grafted limb. From these observations they concluded that the periphery stimulates proliferation of young neurons and maintains differentiated neurons (see Section 8.1). Clarification came only after it was realized that growth of neurons stimulates proliferation of neuroglial cells, so that one of the effects of amputation of a limb bud is to reduce glial cell proliferation. This has been shown by tritiated thymidine autoradiography of the brachial DRG after amputation of the wing bud of the chick embryo at E2.5 (Carr, 1976). Neuron production is unaffected by wing bud amputation until E6.5, after which a considerable reduction of proliferation is observed in the VL region only. Carr (1975, 1976) demonstrated that proliferation in the VL region after E6.5 is exclusively neuroglial. Amputation of the wing bud results in diminished production of glial cells but not of neurons. Carr (1976) found that grafting an additional wing bud does not increase proliferation, as shown by no increase in labeling with [³H]thymidine in the ganglia that innervate the graft as compared with the normal ganglia on the other side.

During normal development in *Xenopus* embryos, cell death is first seen in the spinal ganglia S8, S9, and S10, which supply the hindlimbs at larval Stages 53–54 (23–26 days of development), just before movement of the limb begins (Prestige, 1965). Histogenetic degeneration in the ventral horn of the spinal cord starts at about the same time (Hughes, 1961; Prestige, 1967b).

Prestige (1965) counted the total number of cells and the number of degenerating cells during development in the spinal ganglia S8, S9, and S10 of *Xenopus* tadpoles and found that two neurons degenerate for every one that survives to maturity. Degeneration starts at Stage 54 (26 days of development), when the toes of the hindlimb are being formed. The hindlimbs have spontaneous movements at that stage, but they are insensitive until Stage 55 (32 days), when reflex movements can be elicited by stimulating the skin of the legs (Hughes and Prestige, 1967). Degeneration of neurons in spinal ganglia supplying the hindlimb reaches a peak at Stages 55–56 (32–38 days). In *Xenopus* spinal ganglia S8, S9, and S10 on one side, 1500 neurons at Stage 50 (15 days) increase to about 10,000 at Stage 55 (32 days), which are later reduced to about 8000 at Stage 65 (54 days).

In the trunk ganglia S5, S6, and S7, which do not supply the limbs, the number of neurons increases from about 1500 at Stage 50 (15 days) to over 3000 at Stages 55–57 (32–40 days) and decreases to 2500 at Stage 65 (54 days). An estimated 4000 neurons degenerate in these ganglia; that is, two die for every one that matures. This estimate should be regarded with caution because it is based on the unsupported assumption, initially made by Hughes (1961), that the degeneration time is about 3 hours, when, in fact, young neurons probably die more rapidly than older neurons (Prestige, 1967b). However, it is clear that at any time point only a fraction of the neurons could compete with one another because some neurons are being born while others are dying.

Amputation of a developing limb in amphibian larvae results in degeneration of almost all neurons in the DRG supplying the limb in urodeles and anurans (Dürken, 1911; Detwiler, 1924; Wieman and Nussman, 1929; R. M. May, 1930, 1933; Hughes and Tschumi, 1958; Prestige, 1967a, 1974, Hughes and Carr, 1978, review; Bibb, 1988). Although the neurons in the spinal ganglia of the amphibians all have the same histological appearance, there must be at least two functional types that have not been identified histologically. One type must supply the muscle spindles and tendon stretch receptors, and the other type must provide sensory nerves to the skin. Amputation of the limb bud would remove the peripheral field of both types. In addition, limb amputation deafferents neurons in the spinal cord, including spinal motoneurons and motoneurons supplying the intrafusal muscle fibers of muscle spindles.

Increase in the number of neurons in the DRG occurs following surgical operations that produce an increase in the size of the peripheral field. Rescue of neurons shows that the neurons which normally die are not programmed to do so and are not defective. For example, increase in the number of neurons in spinal sensory ganglia occurs after grafting of additional limbs in amphibians (Detwiler, 1920b, 1933a, review; R. M. May, 1933). In a frog with three functional right legs, Bueker (1945b) found hyperplasia of more than 70 percent in spinal ganglia S8 and S9 connected with the extra limbs. Heteroplastic transplantation of a limb from the larvae of a large species of salamander (*Amblystoma tigrinum*) in place of the limb of a smaller species (*Amblystoma punctatum*) results in enhancement of the number of neurons in the spinal ganglia supplying the limb (Detwiler, 1930b; Schwind, 1931). This shows that the effect is not species specific. Heteroplastic transplantation of a limb from *A. tigrinum* to the head of *A. punctatum* results in increased neuronal numbers in cranial ganglia (Detwiler, 1930a). This shows that there is not absolute specificity of connections between sensory ganglion cells and their peripheral fields in urodeles.

It should be noted that there are several authoritative reports of the absence of either sensory or motor hyperplasia in amphibians with additional limbs (Harrison, 1924b; Nicholas, 1924; Weiss, 1937b). The conditions of these experiments must have differed in some unknown way from those that resulted in hyperplasia in other experiments.

In summary: DRG neurons are produced in excess and about half die during normal development. Amputation of a limb results in death of all DRG neurons. Many, but not all, can be rescued by providing additional peripheral target tissue, and 100 percent of DRG neurons in the chick can be rescued by injection of NGF into the yolk sac. These results show that the DRG neurons that normally die are not defective. A significant number of DRG neurons die before their axons reach the periphery, which indicates that they lack a trophic stimulus originating in the ganglion, neighboring tissue, or CNS. Death of DRG neurons occurs in most cases only after their axons reach peripheral targets. Evidence given in Section 8.16 shows that their axons transport NGF retrogradely from the target tissues and that NGF is a neurotrophic factor required for survival and maintenance of all DRG neurons. In addition to NGF, DRG neurons receive trophic support from BDNF and neurotrophin-3 (NT-3), which all belong to the same family of neurotrophic molecules (see Section 8.17).

8.11. Effects of NGF on Development of the Nervous System: Summary

NGF is a neurotrophic factor that is required for survival and neurite growth of cholinergic neurons of the basal forebrain, sympathetic postganglionic neurons, and sensory ganglion cells derived from the neural crest. NGF is a dimer consisting of two identical 13.2-kDa polypeptide chains. NGF is produced by cells in peripheral targets of sympathetic and sensory axons as well as by Schwann cells and macrophages in developing and regenerating peripheral nerves. The highest levels of NGF in the mammalian brain occur in regions of the hippocampal formation and cerebral cortex which are targets for cholinergic magnocellular neurons of the basal forebrain. In the chicken brain the highest levels of NGF are in the optic tectum and cerebellum. Ameboid microglial cells can produce NGF in the brain.

The most direct evidence that certain neurons require NGF *in vivo* for survival is that antibodies to NGF cause death of those neurons during the period when they form connections with their peripheral targets, and exogenous NGF rescues neurons that would otherwise die. Other evidence leading to the same conclusion is that the target cells contain NGF and its mRNA; neurons possess specific NGF receptors; and they convey the NGF–receptor complex to the cell body by means of fast axonal transport.

The effects of NGF are to promote neuronal survival, induce synthesis of specific proteins, especially neuropeptide synaptic transmitters and enzymes that synthesize neurotransmitters, and stimulate axonal and dendritic growth.

The biological functions of NGF are mediated by binding of NGF to specific cell membrane receptors followed by internalization and retrograde transport of the NGF–receptor complex to the cell body. Neurons sensitive to NGF have both low-affinity and high-affinity types of receptors. Only low-affinity receptors are possessed by Schwann cells and many types of CNS neurons which do not require NGF for survival and growth.

Neurons may obtain trophic support from different combinations of trophic molecules at different stages of development. Neurons may also be supported from more than one source via axonal branches which project to different targets. For example, neurons in the DRG and cranial sensory ganglia may receive trophic stimulation both from their peripheral targets and from their connections in the CNS. The peripheral tissues provide NGF whereas the CNS provides BDNF and NT-3 in addition to NGF.

8.12. Discovery of NGF

The history of the discovery of a factor in mouse sarcoma and salivary glands that dramatically increases metabolism, growth, and survival of neurons in sensory and sympathetic ganglia has frequently been reviewed (Levi-Montalcini, 1964d, 1965, 1966, 1975, 1980, 1987; Levi-Montalcini and Angeletti, 1968; Barde and Thoenen, 1979; Greene and Shooter, 1980; Thoenen and Edgar, 1985; Thoenen *et al.*, 1987; Whittemore and Seiger, 1987; Barde, 1989).

In 1948, Bueker reported that mouse sarcoma 180 grafted into the body wall of 3-day chick embryos resulted in a 20–40 percent increase in the size of spinal DRG that innervated the tumor. Bueker's experiment was repeated by Levi-Montalcini and Hamburger (1951), who found that implantation of a mouse sarcoma into 3-day chick embryos results in a two- to threefold increase in the size of the DRG and a five- to sixfold increase in the sympathetic ganglia supplying the sarcoma, as well as in those not supplying the sarcoma. Increased size of the ganglia was first seen on day 6 of incubation, shortly after the nerves had grown into the sarcoma. All the cells appeared to increase in size in sympathetic ganglia, but in the DRG only the small MD cells and not the large VL cells were reported to respond to stimulation by the tumor. This difference was later found to be an experimental artifact resulting from the differences in the trophic support received by the two types of DRG neurons from their targets in the CNS (Lindsay *et al.*, 1985; Johnson *et al.*, 1986). The MD cells are largely or entirely connected to muscle spindles and make monosynaptic connections with spinal motoneurons, whereas the VL cells are connected to cutaneous sense organs and make polysynaptic connections in the spinal cord. The response of DRG of the chick embryo to stimulation by the sarcoma is maximal between days 7 and 9 of embryonic development, declines thereafter, and is no longer apparent after E15. A similar period of responsiveness of explanted chick DRG *in vitro* to purified nerve growth factor has been reported by Winick and Greenberg (1965a,b). It is important to note that production of neurons ceases between days 7 and 9 of incubation in the chick embryo spinal cord, DRG, and sympathetic ganglia, whereas proliferation of glial cells starts only after production of neurons has ceased and continues until hatching (Brizzee, 1949; Bensted *et al.*, 1957; Carr, 1975, 1976). The period of responsiveness to NGF corresponds with the period of glial proliferation, outgrowth of neurites from the neurons, and formation of connections with their target tissues.

Levi-Montalcini (1952) discovered that a diffusible agent released from the sarcoma resulted in overgrowth of sensory and sympathetic ganglia. Using 4- to 6-day chick embryos, she found that the sarcoma produces its effects on the ganglia even when it is grafted on the chorioallantoic membrane so that the sarcoma and the embryo are in communication only through the bloodstream. When sarcoma and ganglion are cultured in the same hanging drop of plasma clot, the sarcoma produces a halo of nerve fibers growing out of the ganglion, but no fiber outgrowth occurs from a ganglion cultured in the absence of a source of NGF, as Fig. 8.11 shows (Levi-Montalcini *et al.*, 1954). The NGF appears to be an absolute requirement for the outgrowth of nerve fibers from explanted sensory and sympathetic ganglia in tissue culture.

The size and density of the halo of fibers growing out of ganglia at 37°C *in vitro* 18–24 hours after the addition of serial dilutions of NGF became a standard biological test of the presence and potency of NGF in tissue extracts (Levi-Montalcini, 1964d, 1966). The biological unit of NGF is defined by this assay as the concentration of NGF (units per milliliter) required to produce maximum outgrowth of fibers from the explanted ganglion. One biological unit corresponds to about 10 ng of NGF.

The NGF was found in a nucleoprotein fraction of the mouse sarcoma (S. Cohen *et al.*, 1954). Phosphodiesterase in the form of snake venom was added to the sarcoma extract in order to break down the nucleic acid, with the unexpected result that growth of nerve fibers was increased. The snake venom yielded preparations of NGF about a thousand times more potent than the crude extract from mouse sarcoma (S. Cohen and Levi-Montalcini, 1956; Levi-Montalcini and Cohen, 1956; S. Cohen, 1958, 1959). Because the snake venom gland is homologous with a salivary gland in mammals, a search was made for NGF in salivary glands. A protein NGF 10,000 times more potent than the sarcoma extract can be prepared from mouse submaxillary glands (S. Cohen, 1960), in which the concentration of NGF is about 400 ng/mg of tissue in adult male mice.

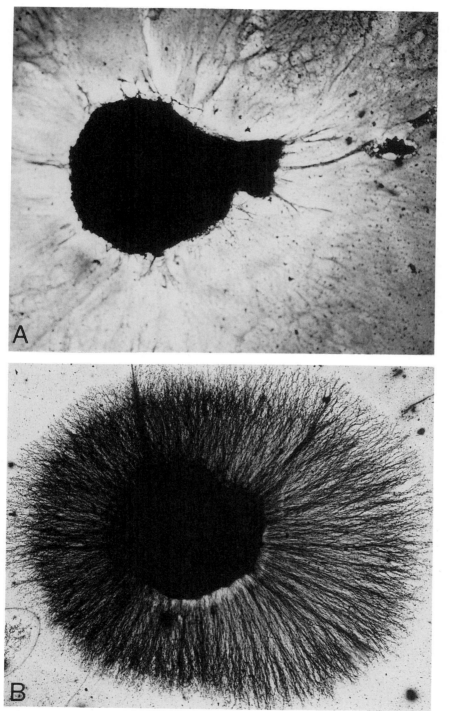

Figure 8.11. Effects of nerve growth factor on DRG in tissue culture. (A) DRG from an E7 chick embryo cultured for 24 hours in control medium; (B) a DRG in the same medium supplemented with NGF (0.01 µg/ml) for 24 hours. Silver stain. From R. Levi-Montalcini, *Science* 143:105–110 (1964), copyright American Association for the Advancement of Science.

8.13. Effects of NGF Antiserum

One of the strongest lines of evidence that NGF is essential for growth and survival of sympathetic adrenergic neurons is that NGF antibodies totally inhibit outgrowth of nerve fibers from chick embryo ganglia cultured in optimal concentrations of NGF and that injection of NGF antiserum into newborn mammals results in selective destruction of sympathetic adrenergic neurons (S. Cohen, 1960; Levi-Montalcini and Booker, 1960b; Levi-Montalcini and Angeletti, 1966; Zaimis, 1964; Zaimis et al., 1965; Zanini et al., 1968). Injections of NGF antiserum into pregnant mice on days 15–17 of gestation result in almost total destruction of the sympathetic nervous system of the newborn offspring (Klingman and Klingman, 1967). Daily injections of NGF antiserum into newborn mammals produce almost complete destruction of the prevertebral and paravertebral ganglia of the sympathetic nervous system (Fig. 8.12), an effect that is termed *immunosympathectomy.*

The first effects of NGF antiserum are observed within a few hours after injection. Synaptic transmission in sympathetic ganglia fails (Larrabee, 1969; Halstead and Larrabee, 1972), and the first cytological abnormalities can be detected (Levi-Montalcini and Booker, 1960b; Sabatini et al., 1965; Levi-Montalcini et al., 1969) within a few hours after injection of antiserum. Degenerative changes in sympathetic nerve cells are seen with the electron microscope 2 hours after antiserum injection, and 12 hours later there are obvious signs of degeneration, such as condensation of chromatin, folding of the nuclear membrane, loss of neurofilaments and neurotubules, reduction of endoplasmic reticulum, and reduction in size of the adrenergic nerve cells. After 2 days many dead cells can be seen. By the end of the 1st week most of the neurons have disappeared, but the glial cells appear to be normal. After a month almost all the glial cells have disappeared, leaving only a few neurons, including the small intensely fluorescent (SIF) cells, which are not affected by NGF, and nonneuronal cells (Levi-Montalcini, 1972).

Functional changes that follow injection of NGF antiserum include loss of synaptic transmission in sympathetic ganglia (Larrabee, 1969; Halstead and

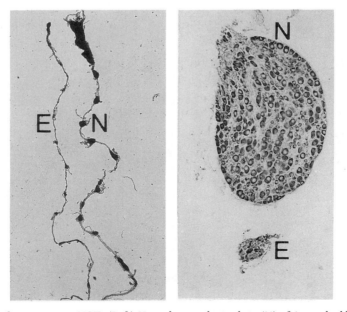

Figure 8.12. Effects of antiserum to NGF. (Left) Normal sympathetic chain (N) of 1-month-old mouse compared with sympathetic chain (E) of 1-month-old mouse treated for 5 days after birth with antiserum to NGF. From R. Levi-Montalcini and S. Cohen, *Ann. N.Y. Acad. Sci.* 85:324–341 (1960). (Right) Transverse section through the superior cervical ganglion of a normal 9-day-old mouse (N) and the superior cervical ganglion (E) of a 9-day-old mouse treated for 3 days after birth with antiserum to NGF. From R. Levi-Montalcini, *Science* 143:105–110 (1964), copyright American Association for the Advancement of Science.

Larrabee, 1972), impaired uptake of [^{3}H]nor-epinephrine into the ganglia (Angeletti *et al.*, 1971a), and rapid depletion of catecholamines from the adrenergic nerve terminals in the organs inner-vated by sympathetic ganglia as well as in central catecholaminergic neurons. There is a parallel de-cline in the catecholamine-synthesizing enzymes tyrosine hydroxylase and dopamine beta-hydroxyl-ase, whose activity is reduced by 40 percent after a single injection of NGF antiserum (Angeletti *et al.*, 1971a; Hendry and Iversen, 1971). In newborn mammals an adequate dose of NGF antiserum pro-duces permanent immunosympathectomy, whereas administration of antiserum to adults does not result in death of adrenergic neurons, and the depletion of catecholamines and other metabolic effects of the antiserum are reversible in adults (Angeletti *et al.*, 1971a). Treatment of adult rats with anti-NGF anti-bodies results in severe reduction of neuropeptides such as substance P in sensory neurons (Otten *et al.*, 1980).

Chronic deprivation of NGF can also be pro-duced in autoimmunized animals: immunization of guinea pigs or other species with mouse NGF results in production by the immunized animal of anti-bodies against its own NGF (Gorin and Johnson, 1979). The developing mammalian fetus can be de-prived of NGF by rendering the pregnant mother autoimmune to NGF (Johnson *et al.*, 1980, 1983).

Death of cultured rat sympathetic neurons caused by deprivation of NGF can be prevented by inhibitors of RNA and protein synthesis (Martin *et al.*, 1988). This shows that neuron death following deprivation of NGF is not a passive, but an active process requiring RNA and protein synthesis. The effects of anti-NGF antibodies on the fetus are to reduce the number of DRG neurons and trigeminal ganglion neurons by up to 80 percent (Johnson *et al.*, 1980, 1986; Pearson *et al.*, 1983). Neurons derived from the ectodermal placodes and those of the nodose ganglion are not affected by anti-NGF in the mammalian fetus (Pearson *et al.*, 1983) and in the chick embryo (Rohrer *et al.*, 1988b).

8.14. Characteristics and Distribution of NGF

There is considerable evidence that NGF is a naturally occurring trophic molecule for sympa-thetic and sensory neurons derived from the neu-ral crest and for some neurons of the basal fore-brain: administration of NGF reduces naturally occurring cell death and promotes axonal sprout-ing of those neurons; NGF and its mRNA are pre-sent in limited quantities in peripheral tissues and their concentrations are proportional to the densi-ty of innervation; those neurons degenerate after anti-NGF treatment or after blocking retrograde axonal transport of NGF.

NGF is encoded by a single gene of 45 kb from which at least four different mRNA transcripts can be made by differential splicing. Two primary trans-lation products (27 and 34 kDa) are glycosylated to produce a 35-kDa precursor without biological ac-tivity (Edwards *et al.*, 1988a). This is processed by proteolytic enzymes to produce the biologically ac-tive form, which can be released immediately or stored in vesicles to be released later by a calcium-dependent mechanism (Edwards *et al.*, 1988b).

The NGF extracted from mouse submaxillary glands occurs in a high-molecular-weight complex known as 7S NGF. This contains the NGF itself, known as βNGF, and two other subunits, alpha and gamma, which do not stimulate nerve growth (Varon *et al.*, 1968). The βNGF alone has all the nerve growth activity of the material first prepared by S. Cohen (1960) and used in the original experiments by Levi-Montalcini's group. The purified βNGF is a dimer consisting of two identical polypeptides which are not covalently linked. Each polypeptide consists of 118 amino acids and has a molecular weight of 13.2 kDa (Angeletti and Bradshaw, 1971; L. A. Greene *et al.*, 1971; Bothwell and Shooter, 1977). The amino acid sequence of NGF (Whittemore *et al.*, 1988) resembles that of proinsulin, which is the protein precursor of insulin, but NGF and insulin have different membrane receptors and different actions (Angeletti and Bradshaw, 1971; Frazier *et al.*, 1972). NGF belongs to a family of basic polypeptide neurotrophic factors, including BDNF and NT-3, which all have about 50 percent amino acid sim-ilarity (see Section 8.19).

Molecular cloning of the gene for βNGF from birds and mammals (Ebendal *et al.*, 1986; Meier *et al.*, 1986; Wion *et al.*, 1986) has made it possible to detect the presence of NGF mRNA by means of Northern blot analysis and *in situ* hybridization. The presence of NGF transcripts can thus be correlated with the appearance of the protein, which can be detected by means of sensitive enzyme immunoassay techniques (Korsching et al., 1985; Whittemore et al., 1986; Lärkfors et al., 1987; Auburger et al., 1987).

NGF is found in all vertebrates except the elasmobranchs (Winick and Greenberg, 1965b), which suggests that it first appeared in evolution in the teleosts. The biological action of mouse, bovine, human, and chicken NGF are identical, showing that the receptor binding site has been conserved. By contrast, there is a very poor immunological cross reactivity between NGF from different species. This shows that the antigenic domains have diverged during evolution in spite of the fact that there is a sequence similarity of about 85 percent between NGF from different species (Meier et al., 1986; Ebendal et al., 1986).

NGF is found in many different peripheral tissues which are targets of sympathetic and sensory nerve fibers (Davies et al., 1987). It is present in the blood serum of all mammals (Levi-Montalcini and Angeletti, 1968), in extracts of normal sensory and sympathetic ganglia of embryos and adults (Bueker et al., 1960; Levi-Montalcini and Angeletti, 1968), and in the urine and saliva of mice (Levi-Montalcini and Booker, 1960a). NGF is an exocrine secretion of the submandibular glands of adult male mice, where its presence is irrelevant to its neurotrophic functions. NGF has not been detected in the salivary glands of the rat, and it is produced in the salivary glands of mice only in the adult male. The concentration of NGF in submaxillary glands of adult male mice (about 400 ng/mg of tissue) is 10 times greater than the concentration in adult female submaxillary glands and about 1000 times greater than in other tissues. Excision of the submaxillary salivary glands of adult mice does not result in any adverse effects (Levi-Montalcini and Cohen, 1960). After removal of the submaxillary glands from adult mice, there is a temporary decline in concentraton of NGF in the blood plasma to about 15 percent of the normal value, but the concentration increases to normal levels after about 4 months, although no regeneration of the submaxillary gland occurs (Hendry and Iverson, 1973).

NGF is found in very low concentrations (1–4 ng/g tissue) in the peripheral target tissues, indicating that its concentration limits the density of innervation of NGF-sensitive neurons. There is a direct proportionality between the density of sympathetic innervation of a tissue and its NGF content (Korsching and Thoenen, 1977; Ebendal et al., 1983) as well as its NGF mRNA content (Shelton and Reichardt, 1984; Heumann et al., 1984). It is predictable that NGF receptor mRNA is present in neurons which respond to NGF whereas NGF mRNA is high in cells which produce NGF. Thus the peripheral target tissues of sympathetic and sensory axons contain both NGF and its mRNA (Korsching and Thoenen, 1983a; Shelton and Reichardt, 1984). By contrast, the level of NGF receptor mRNA is high in the neurons of the basal forebrain which respond to NGF (Lu et al., 1989). In the CNS the levels of NGF and its mRNA are highest in the hippocampal formation and neocortex, which are regions that receive strong projections from cholinergic magnocellular neurons of the basal forebrain (Korsching et al., 1985; Shelton and Reichardt, 1986; Whittemore et al., 1986). In the striatum, cholinergic neurons form local connections exclusively, and thus the levels of mRNA for NGF and for its receptor are coregulated developmentally in that region (Lu et al., 1989).

Levi-Montalcini (1966) noted that NGF may be produced by fast-growing mesodermal tissues, and this is consistent with the large body of evidence that mesenchyme exerts a strong attraction on growing axons (Ramón y Cajal, 1910, 1928, p. 358). Malignant cells of mesenchymal origin secrete NGF (Levi-Montalcini, 1952; Oger et al., 1974), as do fibroblasts in vitro (M. Young et al., 1975), neuroblastoma cells (R. A. Murphy et al., 1975), and glioma cells (Longo and Penhoet, 1974). Synthesis of NGF by Schwann cells is stimulated by interleukin-1 released from macrophages in the degenerating peripheral nerve (Lindholm et al., 1987). The fact that glial cells can be substituted for NGF to maintain neuronal growth in vitro also indicates that glial cells are a source of NGF or a similar substance (Burnham et al., 1972; Varon et al., 1974a). Neuronal growth can be supported by glial cells without the addition of NGF to the tissue culture medium, but NGF alone is unable to sustain the growth of neurons cultured in the absence of glial cells (Varon et al., 1974a; Monard et al., 1975). That NGF antiserum inhibits the effect of glial cells on neuronal outgrowth indicates that the effect is mediated by NGF (Varon et al., 1974b). Ameboid microglial cells (brain macrophages) from embryonic rat brain release large amounts of NGF when stimulated *in vitro* (Mallat *et al.*, 1989). Other trophic molecules synthesized by ameboid microglial cells are interleukin-1 (Giulian *et al.*, 1988; Hetier *et al.*, 1988), which stimulates astrocyte proliferation, and tumor necrosis factor (Leibovich *et al.*, 1987), which promotes angiogenesis.

8.15. Growth Effects of NGF

The biological effects of NGF are maintenance of neuron survival, stimulation of neurite outgrowth, cell growth, induction of enzymes that synthesize neurotransmitters, and trophic influence from target organs on the innervating nerve fibers (Thoenen and Barde, 1980; Yankner and Shooter, 1982; Reichardt, 1986). These biological effects are specific to neurons which possess high-affinity NGF receptors, namely, sympathetic and sensory neurons derived from the neural crest, and some cholinergic neurons in the basal forebrain, namely, the medial septal nucleus, nucleus basalis, and nucleus of the diagonal band of Broca.

Injection of NGF into chick or mouse embryos results in hypertrophy of sympathetic ganglia, which can increase their weight 5–12 times above control values (Levi-Montalcini and Booker, 1960a). Profuse overgrowth occurs of cutaneous sensory nerve fibers, and overgrowth of sympathetic nerve fibers is seen in meso- and metanephros, ovaries, testes, thyroid, spleen, liver, pancreas, and feather bulbs. No increase of nerve fibers occurs in the skeletal muscles, heart, gut, or respiratory tract (Levi-Montalcini, 1952; Levi-Montalcini and Hamburger, 1953). It is not known whether the nerves that supply the latter organs do not respond to NGF at all stages of development or whether they had merely lost their responsiveness at the stages when the experiments were performed.

Sympathetic neurons are unresponsive to NGF early in development and outgrowth of their axons occurs in the absence of NGF (Coughlin and Collins, 1985). NGF is not necessary for survival of sympathetic neurons in adults. However, NGF maintains normal levels of tyrosine hydroxylase in sympathetic neurons throughout development and later life and those levels are markedly decreased after anti-NGF treatment (see Section 8.13). Preganglionic sympathetic neurons are also affected by NGF, probably indirectly as a result of increased survival and

growth of the postganglionic neurons (Johnson *et al.*, 1977; Schäfer *et al.*, 1983). This is an example of a retrograde transneuronal trophic effect.

Administration of NGF to adult rats results in hypertrophy of sympathetic adrenergic neurons (Angeletti *et al.*, 1971b) and increased density of adrenergic nerve terminal plexuses in the iris, salivary glands, heart, intestine, spleen, and pancreas, as well as increased levels of norepinephrine in those organs (Bjerre *et al.*, 1975a). However, those increases require continued administration of NGF, and they subside to normal levels by about 2 months after NGF treatment ceases.

The evidence that NGF is retrogradely transported in the DRG axons in adult mammals and that changes in levels of substance P occur in response to treatment with NGF or with antiserum to NGF shows that the neurotrophic effects of NGF continue into adulthood. All the neurons of the DRG originate from neural crest, and all require trophic support from NGF as well as BDNF as discussed in Sections 4.5 and 8.19. However, cranial sensory neurons derived from placodes are unresponsive to NGF but are responsive to BDNF (neurons of the VL part of the trigeminal ganglion and all the neurons of the vestibuloacoustic, geniculate, petrosal, and nodose ganglia). By contrast, cranial sensory ganglion neurons derived from neural crest are responsive to both NGF and BDNF (Lindsay *et al.*, 1985; Barde, 1989, reviews). Some sensory neurons of neural crest origin do not appear to possess NGF receptors and are not affected by NGF or anti-NGF antibodies: trigeminal mesencephalic neurons (Straznicky and Rush, 1985); the largest neurons in the DRG (Raivich *et al.*, 1985; Richardson *et al.*, 1986); neurons with large-diameter myelinated axons supplying the muscle spindles (Goedert *et al.*, 1984; Miyata *et al.*, 1986).

It is not known when the effect of NGF on axon outgrowth from chick embryo DRG begins, but it first becomes detectable at 6 days of incubation, reaches a maximum at 7–9 days, and is no longer detectable after 16 days of incubation (Levi-Montalcini and Hamburger, 1951; Winick and Greenber, 1965a). In sympathetic ganglia 23–30 of the chick embryo, NGF first produces a detectable effect at 9 days; its effect is maximal at 13–15 days and then gradually declines until it is no longer detectable at 4–17 days after hatching. In the mouse superior cervical ganglion, the effect of NGF on axon outgrowth is maximal during the first 4 postnatal days and then declines until it is no longer apparent after postnatal day 16 (Halstead and Larrabee, 1972). These time periods refer to the outgrowth of axons in response to NGF. NGF support of neurite outgrowth from early stages of development of DRG neurons requires laminin in the substratum (Edgar, 1985). The hypertrophic effect on adrenergic nerve cell bodies and the stimulation of sprouting at adrenergic axon terminals continue in the adult.

After NGF treatment no changes in neuron numbers are found when appropriate corrections are made for increase in volume of the nucleus and cell body (Hendry and Campbell, 1976). The neuron count in the 5-day-old rat superior cervical ganglion is 19,186 ± 539, and after NGF treatment there is an increase to 24,720 ± 885 (Hendry, 1976). Thus the count of 32,000 neurons in the superior cervical ganglion of normal 7-day-old rats and the reported increase to double that number after NGF treatment are considerable overestimates (Levi-Montalcini and Booker, 1960a). Counts of mitotic figures are also liable to the errors mentioned in Section 2.3, and after NGF treatment, counts of mitotic figures in ganglia have to be corrected for increases in cell size as well as for changes in the length of the M phase and of the duration of the cell cycle. For example, the number of mitotic figures in mouse sympathetic ganglia treated *in vitro* with NGF was reported to increase to a maximum of twice that in untreated ganglia (Levi-Montalcini and Booker, 1960a). No corrections for changes in cell cycle time or for increase in cell size appear to have been made, nor was it shown whether the mitotic figures are in neuron or glial precursors. The incorrect conclusion that NGF stimulates neuronal proliferation (Levi-Montalcini and Hamburger, 1951; Levi-Montalcini, 1965, 1966; Levi-Montalcini and Booker, 1960a; Levi-Montalcini and Angeletti, 1968; Thoenen et al., 1971) was based on counting errors and failure to take glial cell proliferation into account.

An increase in the number of neurons (resulting from diminished cell death rather than increased proliferation) and hypertrophy of the surviving neurons would be expected to result in a glioblastic response. Increased proliferation of the glial cells could account for the increase in mitotic activity in ganglia treated with NGF. Another indication that the mitotic activity observed in ganglia treated with

NGF may be glial is that NGF exerts its maximal action after the time when neuron production normally ceases and during the period of increasing production of glial cells.

The young neurons are able to develop normally while their axons are growing toward their targets (Lumsden and Davies, 1983). The trigeminal axons of the rat lack NGF receptors during their initial outgrowth (Davies et al., 1987). In rats NGF and its mRNA only appear in the targets of trigeminal neurons after the trigeminal axons have arrived (Davies et al., 1987). These findings rule out any role of NGF in guiding trigeminal sensory axons to their targets. Nor do the nerves appear to be required for production of NGF by the targets: the level of NGF mRNA in the skin of the chick embryo remains unaffected by early denervation (Rohrer et al., 1988a).

8.16. Mechanism of Action of NGF

Trophic action of NGF-responsive neurons involves synthesis and secretion of NGF by the tissues innervated by those neurons, followed by receptor-mediated uptake of NGF by axonal terminals and retrograde transport of NGF to the cell body (Thoenen and Barde, 1980; Yankner and Shooter, 1982, reviews). NGF receptors have been identified and cloned. There are high-affinity (type 1) and low-affinity (type 2) receptors on all classes of cells which respond to NGF. The high-affinity receptors are internalized and are responsible for mediating the biological effects of NGF. Some types of cells that are not responsive to NGF possess low-affinity NGF receptors, often transiently during development. NGF can act directly in the growth cone, stimulating axon elongation. NGF also acts after retrograde transport to the cell body, increasing RNA and protein synthesis and enhancing growth and maintenance of neurons. Specific actions of NGF are to induce synthesis of tyrosine hydroxylase and dopamine β-hydroxylase in sympathetic adrenergic neurons, of peptide neurotransmitters in DRG cells, and of choline acetyltransferase in cholinergic neurons of the basal forebrain. NGF deprivation can result in death of NGF-responsive cells, but this can be prevented by inhibitors of protein or RNA synthesis. This suggests that neuronal death caused by lack of NGF is an active process requiring new RNA and protein synthesis. The evidence supports the theory that NGF is required for axonal outgrowth, for differentiation and survival of neurons of neural crest origin and certain CNS cholinergic neurons during development, and for their maintenance in the adult.

The peripheral target organs have been shown to contain NGF mRNA and NGF protein (Korsching and Thoenen, 1983a; Shelton and Reichardt, 1984). NGF and its mRNA are also found in a number of regions of CNS, including hippocampal formation, neocortex, midbrain and cerebellum (Korsching et al.,1985; Large et al., 1986; Rennert and Heinrich, 1986; Shelton and Reichardt, 1986; Whittemore et al., 1986; Buck et al., 1988; Lu et al., 1989). The levels of NGF protein and its mRNA correlate with the density of cholinergic innervation in the CNS of the rat (Korsching et al., 1985).

The functions of NGF are mediated by binding to cell surface receptors followed by receptor-mediated endocytosis and retrograde transport of the NGF–receptor complex at a rate of about 2.5 mm/hour (Stoekel and Thoenen, 1975; Ebbott and Hendry, 1978; Palmatier et al., 1984; Johnson et al., 1987). Retrograde transport of labeled NGF has been demonstrated in sympathetic and sensory neurons (Hendry et al., 1974a,b; Stoeckel et al., 1975, 1976; Johnson et al., 1978; Korsching and Thoenen, 1983), in spinal motoneurons (Jan et al., 1988; Wayne and Heaton, 1988), and in basal forebrain cholinergic neurons (Seiler and Schwab, 1984). NGF receptor labeled with a specific antibody is transported retrogradely in NGF-sensitive neurons (Taniuchi and Johnson, 1985; Taniuchi et al., 1986). Intracellularly injected NGF has no biological effect, showing that complexing of NGF with its receptor is a necessary step in mediating its effects (Yankner and Shooter, 1979; Heumann et al., 1981).

The NGF receptor has been detected on many types of neurons in the CNS which do not depend for their survival on NGF (Richardson et al., 1986; Buck et al., 1987), as well as on glial cells (Rohrer, 1985; Bernd et al., 1988) and Schwann cells (Taniuchi et al., 1986a, Di Stefano and Johnson, 1988). All those types of neurons and glial cells appear to express the low-affinity type of NGF receptor and may lack necessary steps in the trophic mechanism, such as receptor-mediated endocytosis of NGF.

Receptors for NGF were originally detected by their binding to ^{125}I-NGF (Banerjee et al., 1973; Herrup and Shooter, 1973; Richardson et al., 1986; Raivich and Kreuzberg, 1987; Riopelle et al., 1987). Specific monoclonal antibodies against NGF receptors (Chandler et al., 1984) have been used to characterize NGF receptors by means of immunoprecipitation (Taniuchi and Johnson, 1985; Marano et al., 1987) or by immunocytochemical staining of tissue section in the rat (Springer et al., 1987), nonhuman primates (Schatteman et al., 1988; Kordower et al., 1988), and human CNS (Hefti et al., 1986). The NGF receptor mRNA has been characterized by Northern blot analysis (Buck et al., 1987) and its tissue distribution mapped by in situ hybridization (Ayer-LeLievre et al., 1988).

Receptors for NGF have been demonstrated in cultured neural crest cells (Bernd, 1985), sympathetic and sensory ganglion neurons (Herrup and Shooter, 1973, 1975; Server and Shooter, 1977; Riopelle et al., 1987), Schwann cells in vitro (Zimmerman and Sutter, 1983) and in vivo (Taniuchi et al., 1986b, 1988), and in the CNS on the magnocellular neurons of the basal forebrain and their axons (Raivich et al., 1985, 1987; Taniuchi et al., 1986a; Yan and Johnson, 1987).

Molecular cloning and sequencing of the NGF receptor (Radeke et al., 1984) shows that it is a 427-amino-acid transmembrane protein that is encoded by a single 3.8-kb mRNA. Its amino acid sequence is dissimilar to all other known membrane receptor proteins. The receptor has intracellular, transmembrane, and extracellular domains, and the presence of the latter is regulated during development (Di Stefano and Johnson, 1988). The NGF receptor is a glycoprotein that exists as a monomer of 70–80 kDa or a dimer of 140–200 kDa (Johnson et al., 1986). Two types have been characterized: type I have high-affinity ($K_d \sim 10^{-11}$ M), slow dissociation rate at 4°C (half-time $\sim$ 30 min), and molecular weight of about 80 kDa; type II have a lower binding affinity ($K_d \sim 10^{-9}$ M), fast dissociation rate (half-time $\sim$ 10 sec), and molecular weight of about 140 kDa (Sutter et al., 1979; Schechter and Bothwell, 1981; Bernd and Greene, 1984; Bukser et al., 1985; Stach and Perez-Polo, 1987). Both types of NGF receptor are the products of a single gene (Hempstead et al., 1989).

Receptors of both types have been found on all classes of cells which are responsive to NGF. Evidently the high-affinity receptors are solely responsible for mediating the trophic effects of NGF (Sonnenfeld and Ishii, 1982; Stach and Wagner, 1982). Interconversion of the two types occurs: receptors on the surface appear to be type II whereas receptors in the process of endocytosis represent type I (Eveleth and Bradshaw, 1988). Differential expression of NGF receptors occurs during development (Buck et al., 1987; Schatteman et al., 1988).

NGF receptors are synthesized in the cell body and transported anterogradely to the nerve endings. After binding to NGF, the NGF–receptor complex is internalized by a mechanism similar to the receptor-mediated endocytosis induced by other polypeptide hormones (Wileman et al., 1985, review). The NGF–receptor complex is transported retrogradely to the cell body, where it associates with rough endoplasmic reticulum and with the nuclear membrane, but does not appear to enter the nucleus (Schwab and Thoenen, 1977; Schwab, 1977).

Evidence that a ras oncogene protein may mediate the effects of NGF is that introduction of ras protein into PC12 cells (Bar-Sagi and Feramisco, 1985) or into embryonic neurons (Borasio et al., 1989) mimics the effects of NGF, including outgrowth of fibers. Moreover, injection of antibody to ras protein into PC12 cells inhibits the effects of NGF (Hagag et al., 1986).

Motoneurons of newborn rats express NGF receptors transiently (Yan and Johnson, 1988), and NGF is transported retrogradely in motoneurons of newborn rats (Yan et al., 1988) but not in adult rats (Stoeckel et al., 1975). Specific binding of ^{125}I-NGF to spinal motoneurons of E4–E10 chick embryos indicates the presence of NGF receptors (Raivich et al., 1985, 1987). NGF is retrogradely transported in spinal motoneurons of E5–E7 chick embryos (Wayne and Heaton, 1988) but not in E10 chick embryos (Brunso-Bechtold and Hamburger, 1979). The NGF receptors are of the low affinity type, and this may be why NGF administered to newborn rats does not result in morphological or biochemical changes in motoneurons, such as increase of choline acetyltransferase, indicative of trophic effects (Yan et al., 1988). Many types of neurons transiently express low-affinity NGF receptors during development (sensory neurons derived from placodes, cerebellar Purkinje cells, external granular, cells and many others, as shown by Richardson et al., 1986; Yan and Johnson, 1988). NGF most probably does not have trophic effects on those types of neurons.

Schwann cells express NGF receptors during development (Zimmerman and Sutter, 1983; Rohrer, 1985; Heumann et al., 1987). There is negligible production of NGF by Schwann cells in adult nerves. However, after cutting of the sciatic nerve in adult rats, all the Schwann cells distal to the lesion express NGF, and this is down-regulated as the axons regenerate (Taniuchi et al., 1986; Heumann et al., 1987).

That NGF acts directly on the nerve endings, stimulating their elongation, was shown by Campenot (1978, 1982a,b): in a tissue culture system designed to expose different parts of the neuron selectively to NGF, application of NGF to the cell bodies maintains the neurons without increasing axonal elongation, whereas NGF applied to the axon increases the rate of elongation. Stimulation of axonal growth toward a source of NGF has been demonstrated in tissue culture (Chamley et al., 1973; Ebendal and C. O. Jacobson, 1976). This suggests that NGF may lure axons toward their targets during normal development. Chick DRG neurites in vitro grow toward a high concentration of NGF released from a micropipette (Gundersen and Barrett, 1980). Stimulation of neurite outgrowth by NGF involves induction of microtubule assembly (Drubin et al., 1985, 1988; Black et al., 1986; Aletta et al., 1988).

The effect of NGF on RNA and protein synthesis has been the subject of considerable research, but the results and conclusions have often been conflicting and difficult to evaluate. Experiments in vivo are difficult to compare with experiments in vitro, and experiments on excised ganglia or primary cell lines which have previously been exposed to NGF in the animal are not strictly comparable with the effects on PC12 cell cultures exposed to NGF for the first time. Greene and Shooter (1980) review the evidence and conclude that NGF stimulation of neurite outgrowth, maintenance, and survival are independent of transcription, but induction of tyrosine hydroxylase by NGF requires transcription.

NGF probably stimulates overall protein synthesis and thus increases neuronal size. It is certain that protein synthesis is required for axon outgrowth and for tyrosine hydroxylase induction. One of the effects of NGF is to induce the synthesis of tyrosine hydroxylase and dopamine β-hydroxylase in sympathetic adrenergic neurons (Hendry and Iversen, 1971; Thoenen et al., 1971; Stoeckel et al., 1974; Kessler and Black, 1980). These enzymes are found specifically in adrenergic neurons and in the chromaffin cells of the adrenal medulla, where they catalyze the synthesis of epinephrine and nor-epinephrine. By contrast, dopa decarboxylase, the 3rd enzyme in the biosynthetic pathway to nor-epinephrine, has a wider cellular distribution and is unaffected by NGF.

Corticosteroids can potentiate the effects of NGF. In superior cervical ganglion cells *in vitro*, induction of tyrosine hydroxylase by NGF is potentiated by corticosterone or dexamethasone but not by estradiol, testosterone, or progesterone (Otten and Thoenen, 1976, 1977). NGF alone is not able to induce tyrosine hydroxylase activity in PC12 cells (Edgar and Thoenen, 1978), but induction of tyrosine hydroxylase by NGF occurs after treatment of PC12 cells by dexamethasone, a synthetic glucocorticoid (Otten and Towbin, 1980).

Sensory ganglion neurons respond to NGF by increased synthesis of the neuropeptide neurotransmitters substance P and somatostatin. Substance P levels are increased in DRG cells in rats treated with NGF and are decreased after treatment with NGF antiserum (Kessler and Black, 1980, 1981; Otten and Lorez, 1983; Hayashi et al., 1985). Cholinergic neurons in the basal forebrain and striatum respond to NGF by induction of choline acetyltransferase, the enzyme responsible for synthesis of acetylcholine (Gnahn et al., 1983; Hefti et al., 1985; Mobley et al., 1985; Auburger et al., 1987). Central catacholaminergic neurons in the locus coeruleus and substantia nigra neither respond to NGF nor possess NGF receptors (Konkel et al., 1978; Schwab et al., 1979).

Magnocellular cholinergic neurons in the basal forebrain and striatum of mammals require NGF for development and maintenance (Honegger and Lenoir, 1982; Gnahn et al., 1983; Mobley et al., 1985; Hefti, 1986; Hefti and Weinger, 1986; Korsching, 1986, review). Striatal neurons are sensitive to NGF (Mobley et al., 1985) but do not contain high levels of NGF or its mRNA, whereas magnocellular neurons of the basal forebrain actively synthesize NGF (Korsching et al., 1985). Retrograde transport of NGF and NGF receptors occurs in those neurons (Seiler and Schwab, 1984; Johnson et al., 1987). Administration of NGF by intraventricular infusion results in elevation of choline acetyltransferase levels in those CNS cholinergic neurons in newborn rats but not in adults (Gnahn et al., 1983; Mobley et al.,

1985). Chromatolysis and death of those neurons occur after they are separated from their targets in the hippocampal formation (Daitz and Powell, 1954; Gage et al., 1986) and cerebral cortex (Pearson et al., 1983; Sofroniew et al., 1983). Those chromatolytic changes can be reduced by intraventricular infusion of NGF (Hefti, 1986; Williams et al., 1986; Kromer, 1987; Montero and Hefti, 1988) or by intracerebral grafting of cells that produce NGF (Springer et al., 1988a,b).

The adult hippocampal formation, especially the dentate gyrus and CA3, contains high levels of NGF (Crutcher and Collins, 1982; Shelton and Reichardt, 1984; Korsching et al., 1984). The NGF is transported from the hippocampal formation to the cholinergic neurons of the medial septal nucleus via the septohippocampal pathway (Schwab et al., 1979). After cutting of that pathway, the level of NGF in the hippocampal formation increases about 50 percent above controls 10 days after the lesion and then declines to control levels after about 1 month (Crutcher and Collins, 1985; Gasser et al., 1986; Korsching et al., 1986; Larkfors et al., 1987). After septohippocampal lesions there is an increase of NGF but not of its mRNA in the hippocampus (Korsching et al., 1986), which indicates that the synthesis of NGF is unaffected and that the NGF accumulates in the hippocampus because it is not taken up and transported by the septohippocampal nerve fibers. Destruction of target neurons in the hippocampal formation by injecting NMDA into the hippocampus in young adult rats does not result in death of basal forebrain cholinergic neurons (Sofroniew et al., 1990). This shows that those neurons either are not dependent on trophic substances derived from the hippocampal neurons, or that they obtain trophic support from other sources, most probably from glial cells which are unaffected by NMDA.

Increased levels of NGF in the hippocampal formation stimulate sprouting of uninjured vascular sympathetic nerve fibers into the hippocampus (Stenevi and Björklund, 1978; Crutcher et al., 1979, 1981). This sprouting is inhibited by intracerebral infusion of antiserum to NGF (Springer and Loy, 1985). Sprouting of uninjured sympathetic nerve fibers from blood vessels into the CNS also occurs after intracerebral injection of NGF in neonatal rats but not in adults (Menesini-Chen et al., 1978).

The present evidence shows that NGF plays an

essential role in stimulating the growth of developing axons from neurons of the spinal sensory ganglia and sympathetic ganglia. NGF may be secreted by the tissues along the route of growth of these axons as well as by the target tissues normally supplied by these neurons.

The fact that neural crest cells require an interaction with somitic mesenchyme in order to differentiate into sympathetic ganglia suggests that NGF, secreted by somitic mesenchyme, stimulates the expression of sympathetic neuron phenotypes in neural crest cells (A. M. Cohen, 1972). NGF stimulates regeneration of peripheral adrenergic nerve fibers and may be required for the regeneration and maintenance of those fibers throughout life (Bjerre et al., 1973, 1974). The presence of NGF in the tissues of adult mammals, the persistence of NGF receptors in adult sympathetic adrenergic neurons, and the high levels of NGF and its mRNA as well as NGF receptors in the adult mammalian CNS imply that NGF has a continued functional role in the adult.

The effect of the NGF–receptor complex in responsive neurons is not directly on the genome but is produced via ras p21 protein. NGF injected directly into the cytoplasm produces no effects (Seeley et al., 1983). NGF-blocking antibodies injected into NGF-responsive cells do not block the neurite-promoting effects of NGF treatment. However, neurite outgrowth from PC12 cells is stimulated by intracellular injection of Ha-ras p21 protein (Bar-Sagi and Feramisco, 1985) or by transfection with the N-ras gene (Guerrero et al., 1986). Introduction of T24-ras protein into freshly dissociated chick embryo neurons by shaking the cells in a high concentration of the protein results in neurite outgrowth from DRG neurons, ciliary ganglion neurons, and nodose ganglion neurons (Borasio et al., 1989). Since these three types of neurons are responsive to three different neurotrophic factors—NGF, CNTF, and BDNF, respectively—these results suggest that the action of all three growth factors are mediated by ras proteins. The ras proteins are located on the inner side of the plasma membrane, where they play a role in signal transduction involving their GTP binding activity (Santos and Nebreda, 1989, review). They are encoded by a family of three genes Ha-ras, Ki-ras, and N-ras, which are expressed very widely in developing and adult tissues, including pancreas, thyroid, and kidney, but the highest levels of ras proteins are found in developing and adult CNS and PNS (Furth et al., 1987; Sudol, 1988).

8.17. Ciliary Neurotrophic Factor (CNTF)

CNTF is an acidic protein of about 24 kDa which is present in peripheral nervous tissues and which promotes the survival of sympathetic, parasympathetic, motor, and sensory neurons during development and in the adult (Barbin et al., 1984; Manthorp et al., 1986; Watters and Hendry, 1987; Blottner et al., 1989; Sendtner et al., 1990). CNTF has been purified and cloned (L-F. H. Lin et al., 1989, 1990). It is entirely different in sequence from any other known neurotrophic factor. The inferred amino acid sequence indicates that CNTF lacks a conventional signal sequence for secretion. This may mean that it is released only after cell damage or that, like fibroblast growth factor (FGF), which also lacks a conventional secretion signal sequence, it is released by an unconventional mechanism.

One role for CNTF may be to control sympathetic ganglion cell proliferation and differentiation. CNTF inhibits proliferation of sympathetic ganglion cells explanted in vitro on E7 and induces the expression of vasoactive intestinal peptide (Ernsberger et al., 1989; Saadat et al., 1989). Another potential role for CNTF may be to control type 2 astrocyte differentiation (Hughes et al., 1988; Lillien et al., 1988). CNTF has a potent survival effect on neurons after injury of their peripheral axons, and it accumulates at the site of axotomy. Although a CNTF receptor has not at this time been identified, its activity at very low concentrations indicates that it enters neurons by receptor-mediated uptake, and that it is probably transported retrogradely. CNTF mRNA is present in peripheral nerves, and as the axons do not contain mRNA, it can be inferrred that CNTF is made by Schwann cells.

8.18. Fibroblast Growth Factors (FGF)

Basic and acidic FGF (bFGF and aFGF), which are proteins of molecular weight 16 kDa that bind strongly to heparin, are found in embryonic brain (Risau et al., 1988) and adult brain (Gospodarowicz, 1987) in relatively large amounts (about 500 μg/kg). FGF is thus about 100 times more abundant in brain than NGF or BDNF. Basic FGF is produced by neurons in normal CNS (Pettmann *et al.*, 1986; Finkelstein *et al.*, 1988) and by astrocytes in culture (Ferrara *et al.*, 1988; Hatten *et al.*, 1988). FGF molecules lack a conventional signal sequence for secretion and yet they pass out of the cell into the extracellular matrix (Blam *et al.*, 1988). Both bFGF and aFGF support *in vitro* survival of embryonic neurons from a variety of regions of the CNS of the rat (Morrison *et al.*, 1986; Walicke *et al.*, 1986, 1988; Knusel *et al.*, 1990), cerebellar external granular neurons of mouse (Hatten *et al.*, 1988), and spinal cord and ciliary ganglion of chick embryos (Unsicker *et al.*, 1987).

Both forms of FGF stimulate outgrowth of neurites from postnatal rat retina (Lipton *et al.*, 1988) and PC12 cells (Togari *et al.*, 1983; Rydal and Greene, 1987; Neufeld *et al.*, 1987). Fiber outgrowth from cultured mouse cerebellar granule cells is inhibited by antibodies to bFGF (Hatten *et al.*, 1988). FGF reduces the effects of injury and enhances regeneration in the mammalian PNS and CNS. Schwann cell proliferation *in vitro* is stimulated by bFGF (Krikorian *et al.*, 1982). Peripheral nerve regeneration in the rat is enhanced by implanted tubes which slowly release bFGF (Aebischer *et al.*, 1989). After cutting of the septohippocampal pathway in the adult rat, the death of cholinergic neurons in the basal forebrain is prevented by administration of FGF (Anderson *et al.*, 1988). The neurotoxic effect of glutamate, resulting from an influx of Ca^{2+} into hippocampal neurons *in vitro*, is prevented by FGF (Mattson *et al.*, 1989). After section of the optic nerve of the adult rat, the death of retinal ganglion cells is delayed after application of FGF to the cut nerve (Sievers *et al.*, 1987). Implantation of bFGF in the eye of Stage 22–24 chick embryos after removal of the neural retina results in regeneration of the neural retina by transdifferentiation of retinal pigment epithelium (C. M. Park and Hollenberg, 1989).

8.19. Brain-Derived Neurotrophic Factor (BDNF) and Neurotrophin-3 (NT-3)

BDNF is a 12.3-kDa basic protein which is found in very low abundance in the CNS. It has been sequenced and shown to belong to the same family of proteins as NGF (Leibrock *et al.*, 1989), which

also includes NT-3 (Maisonpierre *et al.*, 1990). NGF, BDNF, and NT-3 are all basic proteins of about 120 amino acids that have about 50 percent amino acid sequence similarity.

The present lack of antibodies to BDNF has prevented its localization to specific cells, but from its effects on neurite outgrowth, it is likely that BDNF is produced by target cells. The sites of expression of mRNAs coding for BDNF and NT-3 have been identified by means of Northern blot analysis: BDNF mRNA levels are highest in brain of adult rat, with significant levels in heart, lung, and muscle, whereas NT-3 is expressed in all tissues, especially in the brain of the newborn mouse (Maisonpierre *et al.*, 1990). BDNF stimulates outgrowth of neurites from DRG neurons *in vitro* (Davies *et al.*, 1986b). The maximal effect of BDNF occurs during the time when those embryonic neurons contact their targets in the CNS. Dependency of chick embryo retinal ganglion cells on BDNF becomes progressively greater from E5, when the ganglion cell axons have reached the chiasm, to E11, when their axons reach the tectum (Rodriguez-Tébar *et al.*, 1989). Retinal ganglion cells of 17-day rat embryos can be maintained *in vitro* in the presence of BDNF but die in its absence (Johnson *et al.*, 1986). BDNF supports neurite outgrowth from adult rat retinal explants (Thanos *et al.*, 1989). An implication of these findings is that the targets of retinal ganglion cells produce BDNF. Unlike NGF, BDNF does not have any effect on sympathetic or parasympathetic neurons (Lindsay *et al.*, 1985; Davies *et al.*, 1986a; Hofer and Barde, 1988). BDNF supports the survival of the proprioceptive neurons in the DRG that are not responsive to NGF (Davies *et al.*, 1986a). Also unlike NGF, BDNF stimulates neurite outgrowth and supports the survival of sensory neurons derived from ectodermal placodes, namely, nodose ganglion neurons (Hofer and Barde, 1988). NT-3 promotes neurite outgrowth from both nodose ganglion and DRG neurons *in vitro* (Maisonpierre *et al.*, 1990). Neither NGF, BDNF, nor NT-3 promotes neurite outgrowth from explanted ciliary ganglion neurons which respond to CNTF (see Section 8.17). Neurons that are responsive to BDNF possess both high-affinity and low-affinity receptors specific for BDNF (Rodriguez-Tébar and Barde, 1988).

In summary: although the sites of synthesis and mode of transport and transduction of BDNF and NT-3 are incompletely known, the evidence is consistent with the hypothesis that, like NGF, BDNF and NT-3 are produced by target cells, bind to specific receptors, are internalized by receptor-mediated endocytosis, and are transported to the cell body where their effects are to stimulate neurite outgrowth and to support neuro-

nal survival. NT-3, BDNF, and NGF belong to a larger family of neurotrophic molecules. Neurons which project neurites to different targets receive support from different neurotrophic factors produced by each target, and these factors are developmentally regulated (Lindsay *et al.*, 1985; Johnson *et al.*, 1986; Maisonpierre *et al.*, 1990).

9   Development of Nerve Connections with Muscles and Peripheral Sense Organs

> *The quest of a single neuromuscular unit has in fact had many of the dramatic features associated with the quest for a single atom, and the success achieved by the physiologist is in most respects quite as remarkable as that of the physicist.*
>
> John F. Fulton (1899–1960), *Physiology of the Nervous System*,
> 1st ed., p. 40, 1938

9.1. Notes on the History of Ideas about the Connections Made by Peripheral Nerves

> *If any one offers conjectures about the truth of things from the mere possibility of hypothesis, then I do not see how any certainty can be determined in any science; for it is always possible to contrive hypotheses, one after another, which are found to lead to new difficulties.*
>
> Isaac Newton, "Letter to Pardies, 10 June 1672" (In *The Correspondence of Isaac Newton*, H. W. Turnbull, ed., Cambridge University Press, Cambridge, 1959)

We have considered the growth of knowledge about outgrowth of nerve fibers (Section 5.1) and note here only the historical origins and early evolution of ideas about peripheral nerve endings. The history of ideas about the modes of termination of peripheral nerve fibers parallels that of ideas about endings of nerve fibers in the central nervous system (CNS). Until the 1860s it was generally believed that the peripheral nerves end by anastomosing with one another to form plexuses in the skin and muscles. It

was also thought that sensory nerve fibers branch and anastomose in the skin and mucous membranes and then recombine to form fibers that return to the CNS (Beale, 1860, 1862). The concept of anastomosis between the processes of nerve cells in the CNS was supported by the evidence available at that time (see Sections 5.1 and 6.1). Both central and peripheral nervous systems were believed to be organized on the principle of nerve networks. Microscopes could not resolve individual fine unmyelinated nerve fibers in the peripheral nerves. They revealed fascicles which were mistaken for single nerve fibers. Interlacing of such fascicles was misconstrued as true anastomoses between fibers. As we shall see later, this misconception persisted until Ranson (1911) showed that peripheral nerves contain large numbers of unmyelinated fibers and proved that they are sensory (Ranson, 1913, 1914, 1915).

Wilhelm His (1856) was the first to discover free nerve endings in the epithelial layer of the cornea stained with silver nitrate, and this was confirmed in 1867 by Julius Cohnheim, using the recently invented method of staining nerve fibers with gold chloride. The use of gold chloride made it possible to see fine peripheral nerve endings in skin, mucous membranes, and smooth muscle. Free termination of nerve fibers in smooth muscle was demonstrated by Löwit in 1875 using gold chloride followed by formic acid, which is the basis of the modern technique of gold staining. When Friedrich Merkel (1875, 1880) described the cutaneous nerve endings that now bear his name, he thought that the *Tastzellen* (touch cells) were ganglion cells from which the nerve fibers originate. That they are modified epithelial cells in contact with disklike expansions of the nerve endings was shown by methylene blue staining of nerve endings at different stages of development in the skin of the pig's snout (Szymonowicz, 1895). The modern epoch of research on Merkel cells is reviewed in Section 9.12.

The gold chloride method also led to uncertainty about whether nerve terminals penetrate into the peripheral cells, and even into the cutaneous hairs (Bonnet, 1878). The beautiful Golgi preparations of Retzius (1892, 1894) and van Gehuchten (1892) left no doubt that all the different types of nerve endings end freely in the hair follicles and adjacent skin. Very rapid progress in describing peripheral nerve endings was made after introduction of methylene blue staining (Ehrlich, 1885) and after Golgi published his rapid method in 1886. As an indication of the the sudden burst of activity in this field, Kallius (1896) cites 185 papers in his review of the histology of sensory nerve endings. Lenhossék (1892–1893) and Retzius (1892) showed that nerve endings end freely among the cells of the taste bud. Prior to their reports it was believed that the taste cells give off nerve fibers which run to the CNS (see Section 9.13). The periodic varicosities of autonomic nerve endings in the mucous membranes of the bladder and esophagus were clearly demonstrated by Retzius (1892).

The concept of anastomosis between peripheral nerve fibers was not laid to rest by the evidence that they end blindly and that there are one-to-one relationships between some sensory nerve endings and some peripheral sensory cells and organelles. It seems to have passed unnoticed by historians of neuroscience that the concept of anastomosis between peripheral nerve fibers persisted long after the neuron theory was well established. The reason for this is that until the introduction of the pyridine silver method by Walter Ranson (1911), it was not possible to stain unmeylinated nerve fibers reliably and to count them in peripheral nerves. Before Ranson's work the unmyelinated axons were seen only after dissociation of the nerve fibers by soaking pieces of peripheral nerve in weak acid solutions after fixation in alcohol (Ranvier, 1878). Ranson (1911, 1912a,b, 1913, 1914) discovered that the majority of small unmyelinated peripheral nerve fibers are sensory, showed that they have their cell bodies in the dorsal root ganglia, and traced their fine central processes into Lissauer's tract of the spinal cord. He also correctly conjectured that they subserve pain (Ranson, 1915). Ranson's evidence that the majority of unmyelinated peripheral axons are afferent was not accepted immediately and continued to be denied for another 20 years, for example, by Bishop *et al.* (1933), and indisputable evidence that they are afferents was finally published only in 1935 (Ranson *et al.*, 1935).

The nerves growing into the skin appear to be confronted with a large number of potential targets from which each nerve has to select one target. The situation is complicated by the fact that the density of cutaneous innervation and the number of sensory corpuscles are quite constant in each region of the skin. These aspects of the problem were first fully grasped by Ramón y Cajal, who, in a remarkable paper published in 1919, established the theoretical framework into which all subsequent contributions to the problem have ineluctably had to be fitted. He believed that both selective growth (that is, chemotropism) and selective terminal connection (that is, chemoaffinity) probably play a part in regulating the pattern of cutaneous innervation. He pointed out that the density of innervation of each region of the skin is precisely determined and that *"each fiber is destined for an epithelial territory devoid of nerves, and there are no vast aneuritic spaces in some regions nor excessive collections of fibrils in others"* (Ramón y Cajal, 1919). He suggested that the nerve fibers are attracted by chemicals in the epidermis, which are either used up or neutralized by the nerves as they grow into the skin, so that *"after invasion of the epithelium a state of chemical equilibrium is created, by virtue of which the innervated territories are incapable of attracting new sprouts."*

In addition to the general attractive effect of the epithelium, Cajal proposed a more specific neurotropic effect to account for the specific innervation of different types of sensory organelles and muscles. He pointed out that this specificity is unlikely to be the result of mechanical guidance, because then *"it becomes difficult to understand how, of the large nervous contingent arriving at the mammalian snout, some fibers travel without error to the cutaneous muscle fibers, others toward the hair folli-cles, others to the epidermis and finally some to the tactile apparatus of the dermis. A similar multiple specificity is found in the tongue, where hypoglossal fibers invade the muscle, trigeminal fibers innervate the ordinary papillae, and facial (geniculate gangli-on) and glossopharyngeal fibers go to the gustatory papillae"* (Ramón y Cajal, 1919). The research pro-grams constructed on these concepts are considered in Section 9.12.

Motor nerves were described as ending freely in both skeletal muscle and smooth muscle, in the form of loops or plexuses on the surface of the mus-cle fibers. For example, Koelliker (1852) remarks that *"with respect to the ultimate termination of the nerves, it may be stated that in all muscles there exist anastomoses of the smaller branches forming the so-termed plexuses."* At that time the striated muscle fibers were known to be cells called primitive tubes, containing fibrils, and surrounded by a sarcolemma. Schwann (1847) showed that several mononucleate myoblasts fuse to form a multinucleate myotube. Remak (1845) and Lebert (1850) showed that striated muscle fibers differentiate by elongation of myotubes and that self-multiplication of their nuclei occurs. It should perhaps be noted, because it is not well known, that both Remak (1845) and Lebert (1845) were among the first to apply the cell theory rigorously to development and pathology, and in that respect Lebert's *Physiologie pathologique,* pub-lished in 1845, was a forerunner to Virchow's more renowned *Cellularpathologie* published in 1849.

The motor end-plate was discovered and named by Willy Kühne in 1862. He was at first unable to see whether the nerve and muscle are continuous or only contiguous. In 1869 Kühne asked the question: *"In what way do nerves terminate in muscle?"* He came to the wrong conclusion: *"We now believe that we are able to perceive the direct continuity of the contractile with the nervous sub-stance."* He then expressed some doubts: *"Yet it may still happen that, in consequence of further im-provements in our means of observation, that which we regard as certain may be shown to be illusory."* Sixteen years later, in his Croonian Lecture, Kühne was able to say that *"nerves end blindly in the mus-cles. . . . Contact of the muscle substance with the non-medulated nerve suffices to allow transfer of the excitation from the latter to the former"* (Kühne, 1888). Thus, the concept of transmission of nervous excitation by contact rather than by continuity be-

tween nerve and muscle was formed before the con-cept of contact between neurons in the CNS. Once the concept of nervous transmission by contact be-tween nerve and muscle was accepted, it became easier to generalize it to transmission by contact be-tween nerve and nerve in the CNS. The theory was at that time ahead of the evidence, which was ob-tained remarkably quickly during the decade at the close of the 19th century (see Sections 5.1 and 6.1).

The anatomical concept of what is now known as the motor unit originated in the late 19th century. However, the modern term was first used in 1925 by Liddell and Sherrington and later defined by Eccles and Sherrington (1930) as *"an individual motor nerve fibre together with the bunch of muscle fibres it innervates."* Counts of the nerves and muscle fi-bers were made by Tergast (1873), who showed that the ratio of nerve to muscle fibers ranges from 1:80 to 1:120 in limb muscles but is only 1:3 in the extra-ocular muscles of the sheep, but he did not know that nearly half the nerves to muscle are sensory, which was discovered much later (Ranson, 1911). Nevertheless, Tergast (1873) established the princi-ple that muscles which perform fine movements have smaller motor units than those which perform gross movements. This was eventually confirmed by counting muscle and nerve fibers and correlating the counts with the tension developed by each mo-tor unit (Clark, 1931).

The muscle spindle was first identified and named by Willy Kühne (1863). The definitive work on muscle spindles and their sensory and motor nerve endings was accomplished by Ruffini (1892, 1898). After Ruffini there was little that others could add with the methods then available, and Ruffini's account of muscle spindles was not superseded until much later (Denny-Brown, 1929; Boyd, 1960). Sherrington (1894, 1897) proved that muscle spin-dles are proprioceptors of muscle, and the classical experimental analysis of muscle proprioceptive function was done by Mott and Sherrington (1895), who analyzed the effects of cutting various combina-tions of dorsal roots supplying the limb in monkeys.

9.2. Development of Neuromuscular Connections: Summary

The mature neuromuscular synapse consists of the motor axon terminal expanded to form an end-plate, separated from the specialized junctional region of muscle membrane by a cleft 50–100 nm wide. The nerve ending contains round clear vesicles (30–60 nm diameter) which are clustered adjacent to presynaptic membrane specializations called active zones. The postsynaptic membrane is pleated with the thickened tops of the folds juxtaposed with the presynaptic active zones. The tops of the postsynaptic folds are sites of acetylcholine receptor (AChR) molecules which are closely packed at a density of about 10,000 molecules/μm^2. Their density declines steeply to less than 10 molecules/μm^2 a few micrometers from the neuromuscular junction. At the junction each AChR molecule is bound to a molecule of a 43-kDa protein on the cytoplasmic side of the postsynaptic membrane. A basement membrane covers the extracellular surface of the postsynaptic membrane. Molecules of the heavy, tailed forms of acetylcholinesterase (AChE) are anchored to the basement membrane. Several muscle cell nuclei are clustered in the end-plate region of the muscle fiber and other nuclei are located at intervals in the extrajunctional part of the fiber.

Development of neuromuscular connections starts with outgrowth of motoneuron axons in a regular order from pools of motoneurons arranged segmentally in the brainstem and spinal cord. This is coordinated with proliferation of myoblasts and their fusion to form myotubes. Before contacting the myotubes, the motoneurons are active spontaneously and release acetylcholine (ACh) and trophic molecules which regulate myotube differentiation.

AChR molecules start developing in the myoblast and myotubes before contact with nerves. These AChR molecules are mobile in the plane of the membrane and reach a uniform density of about 500 molecules/μm^2 in the myotube membrane. AChR molecules cluster and become immobilized at the site of nerve contact, rapidly increasing in density to about 2000 molecules/μm^2 at the end-plate region. AChE molecules are synthesized by the muscle and are secreted and immobilized in the basement membrane in the cleft of the neuromuscular synapse.

Muscle activity starts prenatally and is necessary for maturation of the neuromuscular junction as well as for differentiation of the functional properties of muscle fibers. Electrical activity of the muscle results in further changes of density of AChR molecules and of their functional charac-

teristics. These changes include increase in the metabolic half-life of junctional AChR molecules (to about 1 week) and reduction of the half-life of extrajunctional AChR (to less than 1 day). These developments involve changes in rates of transcription of the genes coding for the four subunits of the AChR. They also involve changes in control of translation and RNA stability, and posttranslational events such as glycosylation of the AChR molecules, and their assembly to form pentameric functional receptors in the membrane. In the junctional region, AChR gene transcription is enhanced by calcitonin gene-related peptide (CGRP), and probably also by other trophic molecules, coreleased with ACh from the motor nerve ending, taken up by the muscle, and mediated by cyclic AMP. In the extrajunctional region, the electrical activity of muscle results in repression of AChR gene transcription, probably mediated by calcium ions.

Differentiation of the molecular mechanisms determining the speed of contraction of muscle fibers is controlled by the type of motoneurons. Cross-union of nerves to slow and fast muscles results in conversion of their speed of contraction and biochemical functions to match their nerves.

Denervation of muscle or pharmacological blockade of neuromuscular transmission results in reversal of the developmental changes in distribution and functional properties of AChR molecules and other functional characteristics of muscle fibers. These changes can be prevented by electrical stimulation of the muscle. The changes that occur after denervation are reversed after nerve regeneration and reformation of neuromuscular synapses, which usually occurs at the sites of old end-plates.

In adult mammalian skeletal muscle each fiber is supplied by a single motor end-plate, but during early development as many as six motor nerve fibers may occupy the same end-plate region. Elimination of excess motor nerve terminals occurs postnatally and requires muscle activity.

The evidence strongly supports the theory that motor nerve terminals compete for diffusible neurotrophic molecules, produced and secreted by muscle fibers, which promote sprouting of motor nerve endings. The supply of neurotrophic molecules is down-regulated by muscle activity so that motor nerve endings that most effectively ex-cite muscle activity have a competitive advantage over nerve endings that have not formed effective neuromuscular junctions. Less competitive nerve endings retract, and motoneurons die after retraction of a critical number of their axon terminals, as a result of failure to obtain adequate quantities of neurotrophic molecules. Retrograde neurotrophic stimulation may also account for growth and maintenance of motoneurons and for development of their central reflex connections.

9.3. Specificity of Formation of Neuromuscular Connections

The nerve supply of skeletal muscles is very constant, except for rare anomalies, each muscle is innervated by a specific group of motoneurons. Muscles that originate from segmentally arranged myotomes are innervated by motoneurons located in corresponding segmental levels of the brainstem and spinal cord (Fetcho, 1987, review; Lance-Jones, 1988a) These regular relationships between muscles and motoneuron pools have been demonstrated by cutting various peripheral nerves and then observing that chromatolysis is confined to a localized group of motoneurons whose axons have been cut (Romanes, 1946, 1951, 1964; Szentágothai, 1948, 1949). More recently, accurate mapping of relations between muscles and motoneurons has been done by tracing the retrograde flow of horseradish peroxidase injected into the vicinity of motor nerve terminals in the muscles (Kristensson and Olsson, 1971, 1973; Kristensson, 1975, review). Axial muscles as well as limb muscles are innervated in a topographically orderly way by motoneuron groups (Swett et al., 1970; M. C. Brown and Booth, 1983; M. R. Bennett and Lavidis, 1984). Not only do the axons of motoneurons supply specific muscles, but also their dendrites form specific connections within the spinal cord with the neurons that are involved in postural and locomotor reflexes.

Each nerve entering the primary muscle mass in the limb bud innervates a specific group of myotubes. This has been termed a neuromuscular compartment, defined as the subvolume of a muscle innervated by primary nerve branches of the motor nerve as it enters the muscle (English and Letbetter, 1982a,b). Primary motoneurons innervate neuromuscular compartments in the somites of Xenopus

embryos (Moody and Jacobson, 1983). Neuromuscular compartments in the limbs are innervated in a mutually exclusive way by different primary motor nerves in the cat, rat, and frog (English and Weeks, 1984; Noakes et al., 1986; Balice-Gordon and Thompson, 1988; D. R. Brown et al., 1989). Neuromuscular compartments are found before birth in the rat and do not develop from a more diffuse pattern of innervation by postnatal synapse elimination (Donahue and English, 1987, 1989), as shown in Fig. 9.1.

How does matching between motoneurons and muscles develop? The possibility that there is a high degree of affinity between a particular motor nerve and a particular muscle has been ruled out by the many experiments in which limbs grafted to abnormal positions have become functionally innervated by foreign nerves. Many experiments show that motor axons regenerate to reinnervate muscles nonselectively in adult mammals (Bernstein and Guth, 1961; Miledi and Stefani, 1969; Gerding et al., 1977; Riley, 1978; Brushart and Mesulam, 1980; Mizuno et al., 1980; Gillespie et al., 1986; Horvat et al., 1987; Cullheim et al., 1989). Such experiments do not rule out weak affinities between nerve and muscle which may be overridden by other experimental variables. Some degree of selective reinnervation has been found after reinnervation of juvenile, but not adult, mammalian skeletal muscles (Aldskogius and Thomander, 1986; Hardman and Brown, 1987; Laskowski and Sanes, 1988). In frogs the reinnervation of limb muscles after axotomy and nerve regeneration is selective in juveniles but not in adults (Farel and Bemelmans, 1986; Lee and Farel, 1988; D. R. Brown and Everett, 1990). There are also species differences in the selective reinnervation of muscles, with submammalian species showing more selective reinnervation. Selective reinnervation of transplanted muscles can occur in the axolotl, showing that nerves have specific affinities for muscles (Wigston and Kennedy, 1987). After denervation of muscle in the newt and axolotl the motor nerves grow back to their appropriate limb muscles (Holder et al., 1982, 1984; Stephens and Holder, 1987; S. Wilson et al., 1989).

Many experiments show that heterotopic grafts of parts of the nervous system innervate muscles nonselectively (Braus, 1905; Detwiler, 1923, 1925, 1930a; Nicholas, 1930a, 1933; Piatt, 1940). Piatt (1940) showed that when segments of spinal cord of

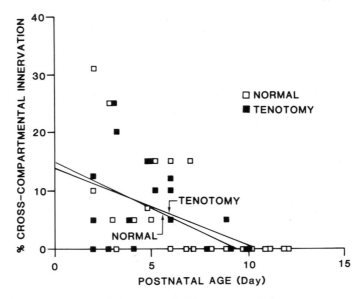

Figure 9.1. Rat lateral gastrocnemius muscle is composed of four neuromuscular compartments, present at birth. About 15 percent of cross-compartmental innervation is eliminated postnatally at the same rate in normal muscle and tenotomized muscle in which synapse elimination is delayed. Therefore, selective elimination of cross-compartmental innervation is not dependent on synapse elimination. From S. P. Donahue and A. W. English, *J. Neurosci.* 9:1621–1627 (1989).

the salamander are grafted to new positions, they can supply any muscle indiscriminately. He concluded that the developing motoneurons of the salamander possess no functional specificity or inherent affinity for the muscles that they normally supply. *"The fact that in normal ontogeny these neurons form constant and regular patterns of distribution must be the result of factors extrinsic to the nerve fibers themselves, but not referably to specific attraction exerted by different muscle groups"* (Piatt, 1940). This is in agreement with the evidence that limb buds devoid of nerves ("aneurogenic limbs") which have been transplanted to the trunk of the frog tadpole become functionally innervated by the spinal nerves at the level of the grafts (Braus, 1905; Harrison, 1907a; Fekete and Brockes, 1987). In the salamander, limb buds transplanted to the head become functionally innervated by cranial nerves (Braus, 1905; Nicholas, 1933; Hibbard, 1965b). The muscles of a limb bud transplanted to the orbit of the newt become innervated by the nerves that normally supply the extraocular muscles (Nicholas, 1930, 1933). Tail muscle transplanted to the position of the limb becomes innervated by limb segments of the spinal cord in the frog tadpole (Letinsky, 1974). Other evidence showing nonselectivity of neu-

romuscular associations is that sartorius muscle transplanted to the thorax of the adult frog may become innervated by the vagus nerve, and these preganglionic autonomic nerve fibers prevent the muscle fibers from atrophying but do not alter the functional characteristics of the muscle. Neither are the properties of the vagus nerve fibers altered by synapsing with skeletal muscle: the vagus nerve fibers retain their small diameters and high threshold for electrical stimulation (Landmesser, 1971, 1972).

In the chick embryo, limb muscles cannot be stably innervated by non-limb bearing segments of spinal cord: if thoracic spinal cord is grafted in place of either brachial or lumbosacral spinal cord before outgrowth of motor nerves, the nerves grow into the limbs but fail to form stable neuromuscular synapses (Strazicky, 1967). When an additional hindlimb is grafted anterior to the normal hindlimb in the chick embryo, the neuromuscular synapses formed in the limb by thoracic nerves are not stable (Hollyday, 1981). However, limb-bearing segments of spinal cord can innervate limb muscles nonselectively, for example, after removal of some of the nerves supplying the limb (M. R. Bennett *et al.*, 1979) or after removal of some spinal cord segments supplying the limb (Lance-Jones and Landmesser, 1980).

The fact that muscle can be experimentally innervated by foreign motor nerves makes it unlikely, but does not rule out the possibility, that the nerve grows to the appropriate muscle as the result of either an attraction or an affinity between individual axons and myotubes in birds and mammals. There is considerable evidence that the initial specificity of connections between nerves and muscles in birds and mammals is mainly the result of guidance of axons to premuscle masses (Landmesser, 1984; Tosney and Landmesser, 1985a,b) and then to individual muscles (Landmesser, 1978; Lance-Jones and Landmesser, 1981; Tanaka and Landmesser, 1986). The stereotyped pattern of peripheral innervation is mainly due to the fact that the nerves are not free to grow at random, but tend to be guided mechanically and by the distribution of extracellular matrix molecules that favor nerve outgrowth (Swanson and Lewis, 1982; Tosney and Landmesser, 1984; Stirling and Summerbell, 1985).

Cell death in the pathways occurs in advance of the outgrowing axons in the chick limb (Tosney and Landmesser, 1985a). The spatial pattern of cell death in the hindlimb coincides with the paths followed by axons growing into the limb and it appears that axons may be attracted preferentially into pathways containing dead and dying cells (Tosney *et al.*, 1988).

Another important factor in determining the pattern of muscle innervation is the order in which the motoneurons sprout their axons. Romanes (1941, 1946) has shown that the motoneurons in the ventral horn of the spinal cord of the rabbit fetus mature and sprout their axons in a spatiotemporal order that is correlated with the order of innervation of muscles in proximodistal sequence in the limbs. The first axons to reach an uninnervated muscle will neurotize it, and at the same time may exclude other nerves and constrain them to terminate elsewhere. The muscles are thus innervated in an orderly segmental sequence in the limb (A. C. Taylor, 1943, 1944; Roncali, 1970; Pettigrew *et al.*, 1979; Bennett, 1983, review). A stereotyped, segmental pattern of innervation can be explained on the basis of a timed outgrowth of motor axons, mechanical guidance, especially by blood vessels, guidance by components of the extracellular matrix, and the exclusion of motor nerves that arrive after the muscles have already been innervated (Braus,

1905; Harrison, 1907a; A. C. Taylor, 1943, 1944; Piatt, 1940, 1957a,b, 1958; Pettigrew *et al.*, 1979). The pattern of nerves in the limb is determined by local conditions in the limb and not by the origins of the nerves: normal nerve patterns develop in chick wing innervated by thoracic spinal cord transplanted in place of brachial spinal cord (Straznicky, 1967) and in wing bud transplanted in place of the leg (Laing and Lamb, 1983a). In chick wing with duplicated segments, the nerve patterns are also duplicated (Lewis, 1978). An additional hindlimb bud grafted anterior to the normal hindlimb bud is innervated in the normal pattern by lumbosacral and thoracic nerves in the chick embryo, but the neuromuscular synapses formed by thoracic nerves eventually degenerate (Morris, 1978; Hollyday, 1981).

Considerable evidence shows that regenerating nerves can recognize specific synaptic sites which determine the pattern of nerve endings on the muscle fibers. Nerves regenerate to innervate their former synaptic sites on the muscle (Gutmann and Young, 1944; Saito and Zacks, 1969; Lullman-Rauch, 1971; M. R. Bennett *et al.*, 1973a,c; D. P. Kuffler, 1986). The basement membrane contains cues which enable axons to regenerate to their original synaptic sites on the muscle (Letinsky *et al.*, 1976; Sanes *et al.*, 1978; Burden *et al.*, 1979; Angant-Petit *et al.*, 1983; Anglister and McMahan, 1985; D. P. Kuffler, 1986). Cross-innervation of muscles with different patterns of nerve endings (e.g., focal, *en plaque* and multiple, *en grappe*) results in formation of the pattern of endings appropriate to the muscle, regardless of the type of nerve, and the regenerated connections are only formed at the old synaptic sites (M. R. Bennett *et al.*, 1973c; M. R. Bennett and Pettigrew, 1974). This dominance of the postsynaptic element has also been reported when retinal axons are forced to connect with somatosensory neurons of the thalamus in hamsters (Campbell and Frost, 1987). In the chick auditory relay nuclei the form of anomalous synapses is determined by both elements (Parks *et al.*, 1989). This is discussed in Section 6.4. However, the relative strength of the motoneuron and muscle in determining the form of the neuromuscular junctions depends on the experimental conditions. If the motor axons have a choice, they have a strong tendency to form the correct type of neuromuscular synapses, but mismatched connections occur if enough muscle fibers are not available or if motor nerves are forced to grow into a foreign muscle.

Recognition by the nerve of the original synaptic sites is neither dependent on the paths taken by the nerve to reach the synaptic sites (M. R. Bennett et al., 1973a) nor on the presence of functional ACh receptors (van Essen and Jansen, 1974). The presence of the muscle fiber and its plasma membrane is also not required for recognition of the synaptic site by the motor nerve ending. After degeneration of nerve and muscle the basement membrane persists, and if muscle regeneration is prevented by X-irradiation, the nerves regenerate to the synaptic sites that they occupied originally on the basement membrane (Sanes et al., 1978). If the nerve is prevented from regenerating but the muscle is permitted to regenerate, normal postsynaptic specializations develop at the original sites on the muscle fibers (Burdon et al., 1979). These results show that the basement membrane contains molecules necessary for the nerve to recognize the synaptic site, and also for localization of the postsynaptic specializations at specific sites on the muscle fiber. Antibodies have been produced that bind specifically to the basement membrane at the sites of neuromuscular synapses (Sanes and Hall, 1979; Sanes and Chiu, 1983; Anderson and Fambrough, 1983; Fallon et al., 1985). This shows that certain molecules are found only at those synapses. One of them is s-laminin, a glycoprotein for which nerve endings have a high affinity. The gene for this molecule has been cloned (Hunter et al., 1989).

Specificity of reinnervation in the invertebrate nervous system has been studied in the cockroach, in which selective reconnection of muscle with regenerated motoneurons occurs (Bodenstein, 1957; Guthrie, 1962, 1967; Jacklet and Cohen, 1967a,b; D. Young, 1972; K. G. Pearson and Bradley, 1972; Denburg et al., 1976). In the leech, nerves can re-form connections either by regeneration or by reconnection. After a lesion to the connectives between sequential ganglia, the axons re-form the appropriate connections (Baylor and Nicholls, 1971; Jansen and Nicholls, 1972). Peripheral nerve lesions are also followed by recovery of the appropriate connections with muscles and skin in the proper positions in the body wall. Sensory nerves regain their former stimulus modality (touch, pressure, or noxious stimuli) and motor neurons reinnervate either circular or longitudinal muscles selectively (Van Essen and Jan-

sen, 1977). We do not know whether formation of such highly specific connections in the leech is the result of chemotaxis, guidance of regenerating axons along their route to their targets, specific recognition between motor nerve terminals and muscles, or a combination of several of these mechanisms.

Sensory nerve fibers cannot innervate vertebrate skeletal muscle. Although the axons of sensory nerves grow in close apposition to the sarcolemma, no neuromuscular junctions are formed (Langley and Anderson, 1904b; Gutmann, 1945; Weiss and Edds, 1945; Zalewski, 1970b). The different specificities of sensory and motoneurons to form neuromuscular junctions are already determined in the neural plate. When pieces of neural plate, jacketed in ectoderm and mesoderm, are cultured in vitro, only the presumptive motor regions and not the presumptive sensory regions are able to form functional neuromuscular junctions in the explant (Corner, 1964).

The ability of a neuron to innervate a skeletal muscle is also limited by its transmitter: as Dale (1935) first suggested, only cholinergic nerves can reinnervate denervated skeletal muscle. Thus, autonomic preganglionic neurons can innervate denervated skeletal muscle (Langley and Anderson, 1940a,b; Landmesser, 1971; M. R. Bennett et al., 1973b), but postganglionic sympathetic nerves cannot (Hinsey, 1934; Bowman and Nott, 1969; L. Olson and Malmfors, 1970; C. F. Luco and Luco, 1971; M. W. Cohen, 1980).

Muscle with its nerves intact will not accept any new innervation (for example, when foreign motor nerves are implanted in the muscle), but will accept such implants after denervation (Aitken, 1950; H. Hoffman, 1951b; J. Koenig, 1971). No neuromuscular junctions are formed by the peroneal nerve implanted into the gastrocnemius muscle when its normal innervation (the tibial nerve) is intact, although the implanted nerve fibers grow freely into the muscle. Preimplantation of the peroneal nerve into the gastrocnemius muscle 30 days before cutting of the tibial nerve is followed by the formation of neuromuscular junctions by the peroneal nerve within 2 days after the tibial nerve has been cut (Fex and Thesleff, 1967). After innervation or after cross-innervation, the neuromuscular junctions are formed at original sites on many muscle fibers, which shows that the position of the original junction has special properties (M. R. Bennett et al.,

1973a,b). Hyperinnervation of muscle has been produced by partially denervating it and allowing regeneration of the cut motor axons. As a result, many end-plates become doubly innervated by the collateral sprouts of residual motor axons as well as by regenerated axons (H. Hoffman, 1950, 1951a; Guth, 1962).

9.4. Development of Skeletal Muscle Innervation

Muscles develop from somitic mesoderm and are segmentally organized, whereas the connective tissues associated with muscle (tendons, collagen, and bone) originate from somatopleure. The fates of these cells, to form either muscle or connective tissue, are already determined before migration into the limb bud (Chevallier, 1978, 1979; Chevallier *et al.*, 1977; M. Jacobson, 1990b, review).

The limb muscles develop from myoblasts which migrate into the fore- and hindlimb buds from the brachial and lumbosacral somites, respectively (Jacob *et al.*, 1978). The myoblasts form a dorsal premuscle mass, which becomes the extensor muscles, and a ventral premuscle mass, which forms the flexor muscles. Individual muscles split off from the premuscle masses. The extensor muscles are innervated by motoneurons in the lateral part of the lateral motor column, the flexor muscles by more medial motoneurons (M. R. Bennett *et al.*, 1980, 1983). Each muscle is innervated by a specific pool of motoneurons in a segmentally organized somatotopic arrangement in the frog (Lamb, 1976, 1977; Kullberg *et al.*, 1977), the chick (Roncali, 1970; Landmesser, 1978; Morris, 1978; Lance-Jones, 1979; Pettigrew *et al.*, 1979); reptiles (Sewertzoff, 1904; Romer, 1942), and mammals (Browne, 1950; Romanes, 1951; Burke *et al.*, 1977).

The first motor axons grow out a few hours before or at the same time as the first myoblasts migrate from the myotome to form the premuscle mass in the frog embryo (A. C. Taylor, 1943; Kullberg *et al.*, 1977), chick embryo (Grim, 1970; Roncali, 1970; Landmesser and Morris, 1975; M. R. Bennett *et al.*, 1980; M. R. Bennett, 1983, review), and rat embryo (M. R. Bennett and Pettigrew, 1974; Dennis *et al.*, 1980). New nerve fibers and myoblasts continue to be added over several days, so that

innervation occurs asynchronously, for example from E13 to E18 in the diaphragm and intercostal muscles of the rat embryo (M. R. Bennett and Pettigrew, 1974).

It is significant that from the beginning of their differentiation the myoblasts are in close proximity to motor nerve endings. It is very probable that trophic molecules released together with ACh play a role in differentiation of myotubes at this stage.

As early as E14 in the rat, fibers of the intercostal nerves release ACh spontaneously, resulting in generation of miniature end-plate potentials by intercostal myotubes as shown in Fig. 9.2 (Diamond and Miledi, 1962; M. R. Bennett and Pettigrew, 1974). At the same stage, before formation of endplates, end-plate potentials can be generated on electrical stimulation of the nerve (Dennis *et al.*, 1980). Neuromuscular junctions do not form until the muscle has differentiated to the myotube stage (Tello, 1917; Filogamo and Gabella, 1976). Neuromuscular contacts have been seen, using silver-impregnation techniques, in the neck muscles of the chick at E2.5, just before the onset of spontaneous motility in the neck muscles on E3 (Visintini and Levi-Montalcini, 1939; De Anda *et al.*, 1963; Filogamo and Gabella, 1967). The first, morphologically undifferentiated, neuromuscular junctions can be seen in chick embryos at E4–E6 (Atsumi, 1971; Sisto-Daneo and Filogamo, 1974, 1975) and in *Xenopus* embryos at Stage 21 (Kullberg *et al.*, 1977). In the rat fetus, the first muscular contractions are seen in the neck at 16 days of gestation and in the muscles of the trunk and limbs at 19 days (Angulo y Gonzalez, 1932; Straus and Weddell, 1940). This is correlated with the stages at which electrical stimulation of motor nerves results in muscle contractions (Windle *et al.*, 1935; Straus, 1939). In the forelimb of the rat fetus, muscular contractions can first be elicited by electrical stimulation at E16, which corresponds with the time at which neuromuscular contacts are first visible histologically (Straus and Weddell, 1940; Kelly and Zack, 1969b). The neuromuscular junctions form later in the hindlimbs than in the forelimbs and are first seen in the muscles of the hindlimbs of the chick embryo only at E7–E13 and continue to form for several days later (H. Hirano, 1967a,b; Landmesser and Morris, 1975).

At the early stage of development of the neu-

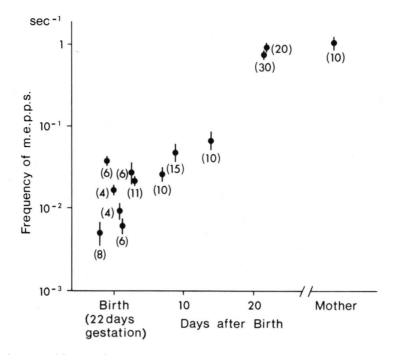

Figure 9.2. Development of functional neuromuscular synapses. Frequency of miniature end-plate potentials (m.e.p.p.) in muscle fibers of the diaphragm of the rat at different ages. The number of fibers examined is given in parentheses. From J. Diamond and R. Miledi, *J. Physiol.* 162:393–408 (1962).

romuscular junction the synaptic cleft is irregular and lacks basal lamina. Few synaptic vesicles are present in the presynaptic ending, and postsynaptic membrane specializations are either absent or starting to develop. Two days later, at E18 in the rat diaphragm the synaptic cleft is about 50–90 nm wide, is partially filled with basement membrane, clusters of synaptic vesicles are present and some mitochondria may be seen in the presynaptic terminal, and the postjunctional muscle membrane is thickened and electron-dense and is starting to become folded. Full morphological maturation of the neuromuscular junction takes several weeks after the first neuromuscular contacts are made (Fig. 9.3).

Development of cholinesterase (ChE) in the cleft of the neuromuscular junction occurs in association with development of the basement membrane in the synaptic cleft. The high-molecular weight, tailed forms of ChE molecules are found specifically at the neuromuscular junction (Hall, 1973; Vigny *et al.*, 1978). ChE synthesis is controlled in the muscle fiber and the nerve is not required for development of ChE. This is shown

by reinnervation of muscle with a foreign nerve which forms new functional neuromuscular junctions at ectopic sites, but the ChE is restored at the sites of original junctions in the absence of the original nerve endings (Weinberg and Hall, 1979; Lømo and Slater, 1980a,b). ChE also develops at sites of contact between cultured muscle fibers and latex beads coated with polylysine or polyornithine (Peng *et al.*, 1988).

ChE can be detected histochemically in the synaptic cleft on E17 in the rat embryo (Bennett and Pettigrew, 1974; Bevan and Steinbach, 1977), in the chick embryo at E6–E7 (Atsumi, 1971), and in the bullfrog after Stages 14–16 (Letinsky and Morrison-Graham, 1980). Appearance of ChE can be correlated with shortening of the duration of the end-plate potential (Rubin *et al.*, 1979; Kullberg *et al.*, 1980; Dennis *et al.*, 1980).

After completion of development, neuromuscular junctions are stable for as long as they have been observed in living preparations, for months at least (Lichtman *et al.*, 1987), and perhaps for a lifetime. After cutting of the motor nerve the

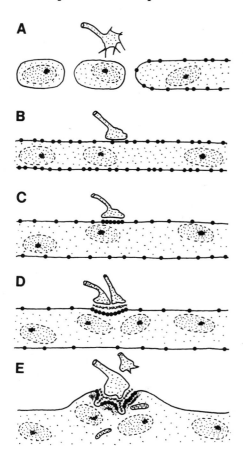

Figure 9.3. Expression of acetylcholine receptor (AChR, black dots) during formation of the neuromuscular junction. (A) Fusion of myoblasts to form myotubes and enhanced synthesis of AChR. Growth cone of motor axon approaches; (B) contact with myotube results in cessation of motor axon elongation. (C) AChR molecules cluster at region of contact of motor axon with myotube; myotube contractions increase and extrajunctional AChR density diminishes; (D) several motor axon terminals occupy the same junctional region of the myotube; (E) a single motor axon ending becomes stabilized and others retract. Subneural folds and postjunctional specializations develop. From R. Laufer, B. Fontaine, A. Klarsfeld, J. Cartaud, and J.-P. Changeux, *News Physiol. Sci.* 4:5–9 (1989), copyright Int. Union Physiol. Sci./Am. Physiol. Soc.

end-plates persist for up to a year (Gutmann and Young, 1944). Six months after denervation the postsynaptic membrane still has maximal sensitivity to ACh (Miledi, 1960) and the number of AChRs has only been reduced by 30–40 percent (Frank *et al.,* 1976). After denervation, cholinesterase persists for at least 7 weeks at about 50 percent of its normal

level (Guth *et al.,* 1964; Vigny *et al.,* 1976; Sanes and Hall, 1979).

Remodeling of motor nerve endings in adult skeletal muscle has been observed in living preparations stained with fluorescent dyes. Considerable morphological changes were seen in the majority of neuromuscular junctions in frog muscle (Herera and Banner, 1987) and in about 40 percent of neuromuscular junctions in adult mouse soleus muscle. By contrast, no change in the shape of neuromuscular junctions was seen in adult mouse sternomastoid muscle observed continuously for several months, although overall growth of neuromuscular junctions occurred (Lichtman *et al.,* 1987). Growth of both the motor nerve terminal and the postsynaptic region appears to be determined by expansion of the muscle fiber membrane as the muscle fiber grows (Balice-Gordon and Lichtman, 1990). Apparently the amount of remodeling varies between different synapses in the same muscle and between different muscles, but the cause of variation is not known at present. The evidence obtained in living muscle is consistent with evidence obtained from fixed tissue showing plasticity at normal neuromuscular junctions (Barker and Ip, 1966; Tuffery, 1971; Kempley and Stolkin, 1980).

In adult mammals, each fast (phasic, type I) skeletal muscle fiber is normally innervated by a single myelinated axon terminating in a single endplate, usually located near the middle of the muscle fiber, the so called *en plaque* nerve ending. By contrast, slow (tonic, type II) muscle fibers tend to have more than one end-plate on each muscle fiber in adult mammals (Lichtman *et al.,* 1985). In birds, the twitch muscle fibers have a single end-plate while the slow-graded muscle fibers are innervated by several *en grappe* nerve endings spaced about 1000 μm apart (Tiegs, 1953; M. R. Bennett and Pettigrew, 1976). In anuran amphibians the twitch muscles may be innervated by a single motor end-plate or by several *en plaque* endings spaced about several millimeters apart, whereas *en grappe* nerve endings are found on slow-graded muscle fibers. In urodele amphibians each muscle fiber is supplied by several end-plates spaced about 800 μm apart on the middle two-thirds of the muscle fiber (McGrath and Bennett, 1979). The comparative morphology of the neuromuscular junction of vertebrates has been reviewed by Couteaux (1963) and Coërs (1967).

During development, each muscle fiber is innervated by more than one motor axon, originating from different motoneurons (Redfern, 1970; M. C. Brown et al., 1976). Elimination of some neuromuscular synapses occurs as a normal event during development of innervation of skeletal muscle in mammals, birds, and amphibians (M. C. Brown et al., 1976; M. R. Bennett, 1983; Betz, 1987, reviews). We should remember that during the postnatal period of elimination of neuromuscular synapses the motoneurons are undergoing protean regressive changes and remodeling: loss of a large percentage of synapses on the cell body (Conradi and Ronnevi, 1975), loss of all synapses on the initial axon segment (Conradi and Ronnevi, 1977), loss of terminal branches of recurrent axon collaterals (Cullheim and Ulfhake, 1982, 1985), and formation and retraction of dendritic branches resulting in transformation of the form of the motoneuron dendritic tree (Ulfhake and Cullheim, 1988a,b).

Although each fast skeletal muscle in adult mammals is innervated by a single motor nerve ending, the initial innervation is polyneuronal, with an average of three to five synapses ending on each muscle fiber in newborn rats (Redfern, 1970; M. R. Bennett and Pettigrew, 1974; M. C. Brown et al., 1976; Korneliussen and Jansen, 1976) and newborn cats (Bagust et al., 1973). Muscle fibers normally grow in length at their ends. New synapses are added at the ends of muscle fibers but most of these synapses are destined to be eliminated (M. R. Bennett and Pettigrew, 1974, 1975; McGrath and Bennett, 1979; Weakley, 1980; Van Essen, 1982, review).

Synapse elimination occurs during the first 3 postnatal weeks in rat skeletal muscle, as shown in Fig. 9.4 (Redfern, 1970; Brown et al., 1976; M. R. Bennett and Pettigrew, 1975; Korneliussen and Jansen, 1976; Betz et al., 1979). Rat soleus muscle fibers are initially innervated by axons from L4 and L5 but those from L4 are selectively eliminated (Miyata and Yoshioka, 1980). This is correlated with the larger size of the synaptic potentials produced by terminals of L5 than of L4 (O'Brien, 1981). In the soleus muscle of the rat, M. C. Brown et al. (1976) found that the percentage of muscle fibers

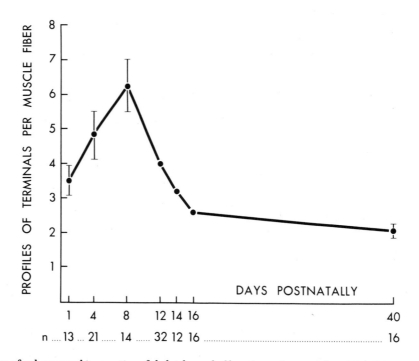

Figure 9.4. Reduction of polyneuronal innervation of skeletal muscle fibers in newborn rats from P1 to P4. n = Number of end-plates examined at each age; error bars = ±1 SEM. From H. Korneliussen and J. K. S. Jansen, *J. Neurocytol.* 5:591–604 (1976).

that are innervated by more than one nerve ending decreases from 91 percent at 10 days after birth to 2.5 percent at 15 days of age. In the levator ani muscle of the rat, which is sensitive to testosterone, as discussed in Section 7.10 (Venable, 1966; Soucar et al., 1982), 18 percent of the muscle fibers are multiply innervated in the adult and synapse elimination is delayed until after 2 weeks of age (Jordan et al., 1988), whereas in the extensor digitorum longus muscle synapse elimination is completed before 2 weeks of age. Elimination of neuromuscular synapses requires muscle contraction and is delayed in the rat soleus after tenotomy (Miyata and Yoshioka, 1980). Synapse elimination does not occur or is diminished if synaptic transmission is blocked in the chick (Gordon et al., 1974; Srihari and Vrbova, 1978).

The mechanism of activity-dependent synapse elimination is not known. It does not require death of motoneurons, because the eliminated nerve terminals are retracted but do not normally degenerate (D. P. Kuffler et al., 1980). Moreover, synapse elimination occurs postnatally, whereas motoneuron death is completed before birth in mammals (Lance-Jones, 1982; Hardman and Brown, 1985; Oppenheim, 1986). Another conjecture is that nerve activity releases proteolytic enzymes or toxic substances that remove newly formed synapses (O'Brien et al., 1981, 1984; Connold et al., 1986). Alternatively, inactive muscle may produce growth factors that maintain motor nerve endings and stimulate their sprouting (Bennett, 1983, review).

Evidence consistent with the hypothesis that a diffusible sprouting factor is released by inactive muscle is that partial denervation of muscle in rats results in sprouting of neighboring, innervated synapses (McBrown and Holland, 1979; M. C. Brown et al., 1980). Terminal sprouting that occurs after botulinum poisoning of mouse soleus is prevented by direct electrical stimulation of the muscle (M. C. Brown et al., 1977). In the frog, terminal sprouting occurs in the intact cutaneous pectoris muscle after denervation of the homologous muscle on the opposite side (Rotshenker, 1979; Reichert and Rotshenker, 1979; Rotshenker and Reichert, 1980). This may conceivably involve a signal transmitted retrogradely from the site of axotomy and transneuronally from injured to normal motoneurons on the opposite side.

Loss of motor axons that have reached the limb

bud and death of their motoneurons is reviewed in detail in Sections 8.6 and 8.7.

9.5. Neural Control of the Differentiation of Skeletal Muscle

Three stages are described in the development of vertebrate skeletal muscle: myoblast, myotube, and myofiber (Boyd, 1960; Bennett, 1983, reviews). The elongated myoblasts differentiate from mesodermal cells that originate from somitic mesoderm. There is considerable evidence showing that different types of adult muscle fibers originate from different populations of myoblasts (reviewed by Stockdale and Miller, 1987). Proliferation of myoblasts is followed by fusion of mononucleate myoblasts to form multinucleate primary myotubes. There are at least two different populations of myoblasts that fuse to form myotubes: primary myotubes are formed early in embryonic development, and secondary myotubes form about 2 days later in rats (Bonner, 1978, 1980). Only the secondary myotubes are dependent on nerve supply in order to differentiate (Duxson et al., 1989). The primary myotubes extend the full length of the muscle and attach to both tendons, whereas the small, secondary myotubes and satellite cells form on the surface of the primary myotubes, all enclosed within the same basement membrane (Kelly and Zacks, 1969; Kelly, 1983; Duxson and Usson, 1989).

Myofibrils appear at the periphery of the myotubes. The primary myotubes differentiate to form myocytes: the membranes of the T system develop; the cell becomes filled with myofibrils, and the nuclei are displaced to the periphery of the mature muscle fiber. The primary myotubes differentiate first and contain slow myosins and they have other characteristics of slowly contracting muscle fibers (acid-stable myosin ATPase, low levels of myofibrillar ATPase, low glycolytic enzyme levels). Secondary myotubes differentiate postnatally and contain fast myosin and possess other characteristics of fast muscle fibers (alkaline-stable myosin ATPase, high levels of myofibrillar ATPase, high glycolytic enzyme levels) (Kelly and Rubinstein, 1980; Whalen et al., 1981; A. J. Harris et al., 1989a,b). Muscle cells are coupled by means of gap junctions from the myotube stage and coupling persists between some skeletal muscle fibers in postnatal rats (Schmalbach, 1982). In developing muscles of higher vertebrates, some myocytes differentiate into the intrafusal muscle fibers of the muscle spindles. This requires the presence of sensory nerves. The development of muscle spindles in relation to their innervation is considered in some detail in Section 9.11. Muscle development in arthropods and annelids is different from development of vertebrate skeletal muscle (Jellies, 1990, review). Individual cells act as muscle organizers which persist after assembly of muscle cells around them. The assembly involves a series of cell–cell interactions resulting in progressively more complex structures. Development of vertebrate and invertebrate muscle is, of course, similar in the respect of epigenetic programs resulting in progressive differentiation.

In all vertebrate species studied, the muscle differentiates to the primary myotube stage before it becomes innervated during normal development (Terävväinen, 1968; A. M. Kelly and Zacks, 1969). **In amphibians the muscles can develop normally to maturity in the absence of nerves** (Harrison, 1904; Hooker, 1911; Hamburger, 1928). **Development of muscle occurs normally during limb regeneration in axolotl larvae continuously immobilized under general anesthesia** (Carlson, 1973). **However, in birds and mammals, only the initial phases of development (to the myotube stage) can occur in denervated muscle and in regenerating muscle** (Allbrook and Aitken, 1951; Jirmanová and Thesleff, 1972), **and full maturation of the muscle is dependent on a motor nerve supply** (Anders, 1921; E. A. Hunt, 1932; Hamburger and Waugh, 1940; Eastlick, 1943; Eastlick and Wortham, 1947). **Apparently there is a phylogenetic increase in the dependence of muscle on nerve supply.**

Regeneration of muscle in many respects recapitulates its ontogeny (Carlson, 1973, review). Satellite cells, which lie between the sarcolemma and basement membrane of the muscle fibers, persist in adult muscle and after muscle injuries are the stem cells which proliferate to provide myoblasts (Mauro, 1961; Church, 1969, 1970; Shafiq, 1970; Moss and Leblond, 1971). Not only large injuries can be repaired, as was known in the last century (Waldeyer, 1865; Volkmann, 1893), but also an entire muscle such as the gastrocnemius can regenerate from minced fragments to regain about one-third of its former mass (Carlson, 1973). Regeneration can proceed to the myotube stage in the absence of nerves,

but the muscle then degenerates if nerves are lacking. The muscle spindles also contain satellite cells which can give rise to intrafusal muscle fibers (Elliott and Harriman, 1974). The failure of muscle spindles to develop in regenerated muscles (Zelená and Sobotková, 1971) is apparently due to absence of type Ia sensory nerves, which are an absolute requirement for the differentiation of muscle spindles (see Section 9.11).

In adult mammals, the skeletal muscles contain fibers of two major types, slow-twitch (tonic, type I) and fast-twitch (phasic, type II) fibers, which have different structures, contract at different speeds, and contain different types of myosin, myosin ATPase, and different amounts of myoglobin and glycolytic enzymes. Some skeletal muscles (for example, soleus) are composed mainly of slow fibers. Other muscles, such as flexor hallucis longus, flexor digitorum longus, and gastrocnemius, are composed mainly of fast fibers, whereas others contain different proportions of slow and fast fibers.

In newborn mammals all the limb muscles are slow. Differentiation into fast (phasic) and slow (tonic) muscles occurs only postnatally. This occurs during postnatal weeks 3–6 in the kitten (Denny-Brown, 1929; Koshtoyantz and Ryabinovskaya, 1935; Buller et al., 1960a; Buller and Lewis, 1964; Buller, 1966) and during the first 5 postnatal weeks in the rat (Close, 1964; Yellin, 1967a,b). After birth all muscles show an increase in the speed of their contractions, but after a few weeks the speed of contraction does not increase in those destined to become tonic muscles while the phasic muscles continue to increase their speed of contraction. Shortening of the contraction time of the muscles is not related to changes in conduction velocity of action potentials in their motor nerves. The conduction velocity of all the motor nerves increases 10-fold from birth to maturity, owing to increase in fiber diameter and to the distance between nodes of the myelin sheath, but the ratio of conduction velocities of motor nerves that supply fast and slow muscles remains constant (Ridge, 1967).

Denervation of slow or fast muscles results in alterations in the speed of contraction, myoglobin content, and enzyme content to levels intermediate between those of normally slow and fast muscle fibers (Romanul and Hogan, 1965; Hogan et al., 1965; McPherson and Tokunaga, 1967; Yellin, 1967a,b). **Reinnervation by the same nerve results in**

a return of the characteristics of the muscles to their normal levels (Buller *et al.*, 1960b; Close, 1965). Like denervation, treatment with botulinum toxin results in a change of the histochemical profile of muscle to a level intermediate between that of fast and slow muscle (Drachman and Romanul, 1970).

The conversion of many major components of slow into fast muscle, and *vice versa*, after cross-union of their motor nerves shows that many functional characteristics of the muscle are determined by the nerve that supplies it. The biochemical differences between slow and fast skeletal muscle are specified by the nerve, and the interconversion from one type of muscle to another can occur at any age. The mechanism by which the motoneuron regulates the function of its muscle is unknown, but several possibilities have to considered: (1) the amount of contractile activity, regardless of how it is produced; (2) the number, frequency, or pattern of nerve impulses in the motor nerves; and (3) the influence of trophic substances produced by the motor nerves.

Cross-innervation of slow muscle by a nerve that normally supplies fast muscle, and *vice versa*, results in reversal of the characteristics of the muscle: speed of contraction (Close, 1965), myoglobin content (McPherson and Tokunaga, 1967), total soluble proteins (Guth and Watson, 1967), and levels of oxidative and anaerobic enzymes (Romanul and van der Meulen, 1967; Yellin, 1967b; Karpati and Engel, 1967). Cross-innervated muscle has mechanical properties intermediate between those of fast and slow muscles. However, the conversion of the mechanical properties of fast to slow muscle is much more complete than conversion of the mechanical properties of slow to fast muscle after cross-innervation (Buller *et al.*, 1960b; Buller and Lewis, 1965). Muscles that are partially reinnervated by their own nerve and partially cross-innervated contain areas of fast and areas of slow fibers. They contract rapidly or slowly depending on the nerve that is stimulated (Romanul and van der Meulen, 1967). The effects of cross-innervation apparently occur only where both slow and fast types of muscle fibers have a single motor end-plate (Tiegs, 1953; Bone, 1964), and they have been observed in mammals and frogs (Miledi and Orkand, 1966).

In birds, the fast and slow muscles differ in their innervation pattern as well as in their ultrastructure, enzymes, myoglobin, and speed of con-traction. Fast-twitch muscles (for example, posterior latissimus dorsi) have focal *en plaque* innervation, while slow-graded muscles (for example, anterior latissimus dorsi) have multiple *en grappe* innervation with motor end-plates occurring every 600–1000 µm along the entire muscle fiber. Cross-innervation of anterior and posterior latissimus dorsi in the chick does not alter the speed of contraction or the ultrastructure of these muscles (Hník *et al.*, 1967). When the muscle and nerve are mismatched, the pattern of innervation is dependent on the muscle rather than on the nerve that supplies it: thus anterior latissimus dorsi muscle of the chicken retains its multiple *en grappe* pattern of innervation when cross-innervated with the nerve to posterior latissimus dorsi (M. R. Bennett *et al.*, 1973c).

An elegant test of whether the form of the neuromuscular junctions is determined by nerve or muscle has been carried out by Grim *et al.* (1989). They grafted quail limb buds in place of chick limb buds and *vice versa*, making use of the different patterns of innervation of the plantaris muscle fibers—multiple innervation in the chick but focal innervation in the quail. The location of motoneurons innervating the grafted limb was later traced by means of horseradish peroxidase (HRP) injected into the limb. They found that the innervation pattern is determined by the motoneurons when the latter are correctly matched with the muscle, regardless of species. However, the species of the muscle determines the pattern of innervation (focal or multiple) when the innervation is incorrect, namely, from motoneuron pools that do not normally innervate the plantaris muscle (Fig. 9.5).

9.6. Matching of Motoneurons with Muscle Fibers

The functional characteristics of the muscle fibers are closely matched with the size and type of the alpha-motoneurons that innervate them. Mammalian fast muscles are innervated by large motoneurons (phasic alpha-motoneurons) and slow muscles are innervated by small motoneurons (tonic alpha-motoneurons) (Granit *et al.*, 1956; Eccles *et al.*, 1958a; Wuerker *et al.*, 1965; Henneman *et al.*, 1965; Henneman and Olson, 1965). The phasic alpha-motoneurons have rapidly conducting axons and respond reflexly with a brief high-frequency

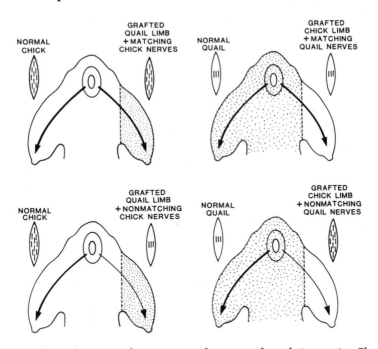

Figure 9.5. A hierarchy of factors determines the species-specific pattern of muscle innervation. Plantaris muscle fibers of the chick are multiply innervated whereas those of the quail are focally innervated. To study the factors determining that species-specific pattern of innervation, chick–quail chimeras were made by grafting a leg bud of one species in place of the leg or wing bud of the other species. The results depended on the matching between species as well as on the matching between nerves and muscles, as shown in this diagram. Modified from M. Grim, K. Nensa, B. Christ, H. J. Jacob, and K. W. Tosney, *Anat. Embryol.* **180**:179–189 (1989), copyright Springer-Verlag.

burst of action potentials. The tonic alpha-moto-neurons have axons with lower conduction velocities, and they have a prolonged low-frequency discharge in response to sustained reflex stimulation. The frequency of repetitive discharge from alpha-motoneurons is thus matched by the speed of contraction of their muscles so that maximum efficiency is achieved. This is the teleological explanation of why the motor nerve induces matching functional characteristics in its muscle (Eccles *et al.*, 1958a,b). One of the consequences of the different functional properties of motoneurons that innervate the two types of muscle is that fast muscles are excited infrequently and for short durations while slow muscles are excited for much longer periods. This difference in the total time of usage has important implications because there is considerable evidence that the properties of the muscle are determined by the total amount and probably also the pattern of contractile activity (Lømo, 1976, review).

The total amount of contraction and probably the temporal pattern of contraction are important in determining the functional properties of muscle. Guth and Yellin (1971) conclude that *"muscle cells undergo continual alterations throughout life in adaptation to changing functional demands and that the histochemically demonstrable 'fiber types' merely reflect each muscle fiber's constitution at a given moment in time."* In normal development and during normal life, the activity is determined by the type of motoneurons. Attention has already been directed to the relationship between the functional characteristics of the muscle and those of the motoneuron that innervates it. The pattern and frequency of nerve impulses may determine the nature of the muscle (Eccles *et al.*, 1958a,b; Vrbová, 1963a,b; Henneman and Olson, 1965; Wuerker *et al.*, 1965; C. B. Olson and Swett, 1966, 1969; Salmons and Vrbová, 1969; Hennig and Lømo, 1985). Muscles that are innervated by large motoneurons contract rapidly and develop large amounts of tension, but are used phasically at irregular intervals. Muscles that are innervated by small motoneurons contract slowly and develop small amounts of tension, but they are used frequently or tonically.

Frequent use of a muscle, regardless of its type of motoneuron, results in slowing of the muscle contraction time (Gutmann et al., 1969; Guth, 1971). By contrast, a slow muscle such as the soleus muscle increases its speed of contraction when it is rested, as occurs after cutting of the achilles tendon (Vrbová, 1963a,b). This increase in the speed of contraction of tenotomized soleus muscle can be prevented by long-term electrical stimulation of the muscle at frequencies of 5 or 10 per second, but not by stimulation at frequencies of 20 or 40 per second (Salmons and Vrbová, 1969). Tenotomy in 4-day-old rats prolongs the period of polyneuronal innervation in the soleus muscle (Benoit and Changeux, 1975). Reduction in the amount of contractile activity of muscles has also been attempted by splinting, casting, or pinning a limb. These procedures result in an increase in the extrajunctional ACh sensitivity (Solandt et al., 1943; Fischbach and Robbins, 1969) and a decrease in the contraction time of slow muscles (Fischbach and Robbins, 1969; Mann and Salafsky, 1970). Another method of reducing the impulse traffic in motor nerves is by isolating the spinal cord connected to the hindlimb of the dog, dividing the cord above and below the lumbosacral segments, and cutting the dorsal roots supplying the hindlimb (Tower, 1937a,b). This results in slow atrophy of the muscle and in an increase in extrajunctional ACh sensitivity which is not as great as that after denervation (Johns and Thesleff, 1961). Other methods of reducing or totally preventing muscle contraction have been to block nerve conduction by injection of tetrodotoxin into the sciatic nerve of rats (Pestronk et al., 1976b) and to maintain cats under deep Nembutal anesthesia (Davis, 1970; Montgomery, 1972). These procedures result in denervation-like changes, including increase of speed of contraction after barbiturate anesthesia and increase in extrajunctional ACh receptors after nerve conduction block.

Finally, the evidence that electrical stimulation of denervated muscle is sufficient to prevent most of the atrophic effects of denervation (Lømo et al., 1974; Eken and Gundersen, 1988; Gorza et al., 1988; Gundersen et al., 1988) is not consistent with the hypothesis that a trophic agent, transmitted from nerve to muscle, is responsible for maintaining the muscle. The appearance of extrajunctional ACh sensitivity can be completely prevented by repetitive stimulation of denervated muscle (Drachman and Witzke, 1972; Lømo and Rosenthal, 1972; R. C. Kauffman et al., 1974; Frank et al., 1975). Reinnervation of denervated rat soleus muscle by foreign nerves is diminished by electrical stimulation of the muscle (Jansen et al., 1973).

If frog skeletal muscle is divided into an innervated and an uninnervated portion, the latter will accept new innervation and the former will not (Miledi, 1962). The presence of an intact neuromuscular junction prevents the muscle fiber from forming new motor end-plates. The formation of new motor end-plates is not due to injury, since a foreign nerve simply laid on a denervated muscle and not implanted into an incision can neurotize the muscle (Gwyn and Aitken, 1964). Nor is the acceptance of new innervation merely the result of muscular inactivity, because implanted nerves cannot form end-plates in tenotomized muscle that has atrophied from disuse but has a normal nerve supply (Aitken, 1950).

Muscle poisoned with botulinum toxin forms functional neuromuscular junctions with an implanted nerve, even when its own innervation is intact (Fex et al., 1966). Botulinum toxin prevents release of ACh from the nerve terminals and thus prevents muscle contraction. However, it is conceivable that the release of some other unidentified molecules from the nerve terminal may also be prevented by botulinum toxin. After botulinum poisoning, the ingrowing foreign nerve fibers form new end-plates quite separate from the old ones, which remain intact (Fex et al., 1966).

Some evidence indicates that there may be some aspects of muscle differentiation that are controlled by a trophic factor released from motor nerve endings. It should be noted, however, that valid interpretations of these experimental results can also be made without invoking a trophic agent. For example, the demonstration that radioactively labeled amino acids are transferred from the motor nerve to the muscle (Kerkut et al., 1967; I. M. Korr et al., 1967; I. M. Korr and Appeltauer, 1974) falls short of showing that the transferred material has any trophic effect. Another type of experimental result suggests, but does not directly demonstrate, that the motor axon has a store of trophic agent which, after cutting of the motor nerve, is gradually depleted in the peripheral nerve stump (Ranish *et al.*, 1980). Thus there is a latent period between cutting of the nerve and the onset of fibrillation in the denervated muscle which is proportional to the length of the peripheral stump (Gutmann *et al.*, 1955). This might mean that the proximodistal flow of the trophic agent is about 2–5 mm/hour (J. V. Luco and Eyzaguirre, 1955; J. B. Harris and Thesleff, 1972). This is within the range of rapid axonal transport (see Section 5.8) and might only indicate that the length of the peripheral stump is related to a reservoir of materials transported distally in the axon for maintenance of the nerve terminal and for release of ACh rather than release of a trophic agent. In fact, Miledi and Slater (1970) have shown that the latent period before onset of fibrillation is the period during which spontaneous release of ACh persists after nerve section. Another type of evidence showing that a trophic agent is transported in the axon to the nerve terminal is that inhibition of axonal transport produces some of the effects of denervation in the muscle but does not prevent traffic of nerve impulses or release of ACh at the neuromuscular junction (Albuquerque *et al.*, 1972; W. W. Hoffman and Peacock, 1973; Juntunen, 1973b; Max and Albuquerque, 1975). The same method, involving application of a cuff containing a local anesthetic, colchicine, or vinblastine, has been used to block flow of a presumed trophic agent in sensory nerve fibers (Aguilar *et al.*, 1973; J. Diamond *et al.*, 1976). The difficulty of interpretation of this type of experiment stems from the direct effects of the colchicine or other agents on the muscle.

In summary, the evidence that muscle contraction is an important, if not the sole, factor that determines the functional properties of muscle is of three kinds. First, there is the evidence that muscles that are used frequently during normal activity tend to have slow speeds of contraction. Second, there is evidence that resting a muscle, which can be achieved by several methods mentioned later, results in denervation-like changes in the functional characteristics of skeletal muscle. Third, there is evidence that direct electrical stimulation of denervated muscle is able to retard or prevent the effects of denervation. This evidence does not rule out the existence of a trophic factor released from motor nerve endings that regulates functional characteristics of muscles, but it shows that muscle contraction alone results in virtually all the effects that might be attributed to such a trophic factor. However, evidence that trophic factor(s) may regulate the number of AChRs is given in the following section.

9.7. Neural Control of Muscle AChRs

During development of the neuromuscular synapse there are large changes in the number, distribution, and density of AChRs in the surface membrane of the muscle cells. Before contact between the motoneuron axon and muscle cells there is a uniformly low density of AChRs along the entire length of the muscle cell. After neuromuscular contact, AChRs rapidly become concentrated in the postsynaptic membrane, whereas the density of extrajunctional AChRs decreases. The total number of extrajunctional AChRs continues to increase as the muscle grows but their density remains low. Intracellular AChRs are uniformly distributed along the length of developing muscle cells, but in mature muscle AChRs and the mRNAs for their subunits are restricted to the subsynaptic region.

The number of AChR molecules on the muscle membrane can be measured by the binding of alpha-bungarotoxin or alpha-cobra toxin labeled with a fluorophore, radioactive iodine, or an electron-dense marker. These toxins bind specifically and irreversibly to the alpha-subunit of the nicotinic AChR. In addition, antibodies to the alpha-subunit of the AChR may be used to label the receptors. Measurements show that at the tops of the junctional folds the AChR molecules are closely packed at a density of about 10,000 receptors/μm^2 (Peper and McMahan, 1972; Mattews-Bellinger and Salpeter, 1978, 1983). There is steep gradient of AChR density, with the packing density declining to about 10 receptors/μm^2 a few micrometers away from the neuromuscular junction (Fertuck and Salpeter, 1976). AChRs form uniformly over the surface of the myotube to reach a density of about 500 receptors/μm^2 before the time of initial contact between the myotube and the nerve terminal. A few hours after contact the AChR molecules rapidly increase in number to about 2000 receptors/μm^2 at the site of contact with the nerve ending, and their ion channels develop mature functions. These changes have been observed in tissue culture (Anderson and Cohen, 1977; Frank and Fischbach,

1979; Olek *et al.*, 1983) and *in vivo* (Bevan and Steinbach, 1977; Burden, 1977; A. J. Harris, 1981; Steinbach, 1981; Weinberg *et al.*, 1981; I. Chow and Cohen, 1983; J. Goldfarb *et al.*, 1990).

The density of extrajunctional receptors decreases rapidly after onset of electrical activity of the muscle (Diamond and Miledi, 1962; Bevan and Steinbach, 1977). The change in AChR density involves lateral diffusion of previously formed receptors in the membrane (Kidokoro and Brass, 1985), as well as insertion of new receptors preferentially at the junctional region. This may be the result of any or all of the following: increased transcription, increased translation, stabilization of transcripts, and posttranslational modification resulting in increased half-life of AChR molecules.

The AChR molecules of the electric organ of *Torpedo* have been well characterized. The AChR is formed of five subunits: two alpha, one beta, one gamma, and one delta, with a total molecular weight of about 275 kDa (M. P. McCarthy *et al.*, 1986, review). The receptor has two ACh binding sites, one on each of the two alpha-subunits. A protein of 43-kDa molecular weight is closely associated with the AChR on the cytoplasmic side of the membrane. In the mouse the genes for the four types of AChR molecules are on different chromosomes and each is translated from a different mRNA. The proteins are glycosylated and undergo further postranslational modifications before their assembly and insertion in the muscle membrane (Salpeter and Loring, 1986, review). The junctional AChRs have a metabolic half-life of about 1 week whereas extrajunctional receptors have a half-life of about 1 day. The AChRs are internalized and degraded by lysosomal enzymes (Fambrough, 1979, 1983, reviews).

Intracellular AChRs are uniformly distributed along the entire length of the muscle fibers during early stages of development in the chick embryo (Atsumi, 1981) and the frog, *Xenopus* (J. Goldfarb *et al.*, 1990). In mature rat muscle fibers the intracellular AChRs are restricted to the synaptic region (Pestronk, 1985). The mRNAs for AChR subunits are also restricted to the synaptic region (Merlie and Sanes, 1985; Fontaine *et al.*, 1988).

Evidence that the initial increase of AChR molecules in the myotubes is the result of new synthesis and is independent of muscle activity has been obtained from molecular genetic studies of primary cultures of muscle cells or of myogenic cell lines

(Merlie and Smith, 1986). The increase in the AChR molecules is preceded by increases in the amounts of mRNA indicating an eightfold increase in rates of transcription of genes coding for the alpha- and delta-subunits (Buonanno and Merlie, 1986). In primary cultures of myotubes that have spontaneous electrical activity, blocking the electrical activity by means of tetrodotoxin results in doubling of the number of AChR molecules in the membrane and in a 13-fold increase in alpha-subunit mRNA. The effect of tetrodotoxin is prevented by actinomycin D, which inhibits transcription (Klarsfeld and Changeux, 1985). Increase in the level of alpha-subunit primary gene transcript, measured during increase of AChR molecules that follows denervation of chick muscle, shows that the effect is caused by increased gene transcription (Shieh *et al.*, 1987). Accumulation of alpha-subunit mRNA around muscle cell nuclei situated beneath end-plates, but not around extrajunctional nuclei in 15-day-old chicks, has been demonstrated by means of *in situ* hybridization (Fontaine *et al.*, 1988). The same technique has shown a marked increase in alpha-subunit mRNA around extrajunctional muscle cell nuclei following denervation. These results could be due to increased transcription or stabilization of transcripts or both.

Evidence shows that a rise in calcium ion levels, which results from electrical activity of the myotubes, represses AChR gene transcription (Salpeter and Loring, 1985, review). This is very likely to be the mechanism of reduction of extrajunctional receptors during normal development and of increase of extrajunctional receptors after denervation of muscle or after pharmacological blockade of transmission at the neuromuscular synapse.

A neuropeptide, calcitonin gene-related peptide (CGRP), has been found to have effects which make it likely to function as a trophic factor regulating AChR gene expression. CGRP is a peptide of 37 amino acids which is found in motoneuron cell bodies and their axon terminals. CGRP applied to chick myotubes in primary culture results in enhancement of alpha-subunit mRNA by 300 percent (Fontaine *et al.*, 1987) and 50 percent increase of surface AChR molecules (Fontaine *et al.*, 1986; New and Mudge, 1986). The effects of CGRP are independent of electrical activity but appear to be mediated by cAMP (Laufer and Changeux, 1987).

A number of soluble factors extracted from

brain have been identified which increase AChR molecules in cultured myotubes (Salpeter and Loring, 1985; Schuetz and Role, 1987, reviews). These are likely to be purified and characterized in the near future.

Some of the effects of motor nerve terminals can be mimicked by latex beads coated with polylysine or polyornithine, applied to *Xenopus* muscle in culture (Peng *et al.*, 1988). AChRs accumulate and cholinesterase activity develops at the region of contact within a few hours of application of the beads (Peng *et al.*, 1981; Peng and Cheng, 1982; Peng, 1986, 1987). Postsynaptic specializations characteristic of neuromuscular junctions differentiate at the sites of contact of muscle with beads (Peng and Cheng, 1982). These results are difficult to interpret but may signify that basic polypeptides have the effects of trophic molecules released from motor nerve endings or that those trophic factors are basic polypeptides.

9.8. Plasticity of Motor Nerve Endings

The growing axon sprouts vigorously when it reaches the field which it is destined to innervate. This observation led Ramón y Cajal (1919, 1928) to postulate that axonal sprouting is stimulated by neurotrophic factors produced by the cells in the terminal field. His concept was that the axons that enter a peripheral field compete for the available neurotrophic factors, using them or neutralizing them in the process of lateral sprouting. According to this theory, the sprouting is self-limiting and results in each terminal field having a characteristic and fairly uniform density of axon branches, with little overlap between the terminal domains of neighboring axons.

The main advance since Cajal's time has been the discovery that inactive, but not active, muscle produces neurotrophic molecules. This evidence supports the theory that neurotrophic molecules released by postsynaptic cells enhance growth of presynaptic nerve terminals, which, after forming functional synapses, inhibit the release or production of neurotrophic molecules. This neurotrophic theory has great heuristic value; it suggests many experiments that might elucidate how the differences in density of innervation of different tissues and in different regions of the CNS develop, and

how sprouting of normal axons occurs after partial denervation in the CNS and PNS.

The neurotrophic theory provides an explanation of the sprouting of neighboring afferents into a surgically deafferented region. This tendency to sprout collaterals from uninjured axons at the margins of a zone of surgically deafferented skin (Wedell *et al.*, 1941; Livingston, 1947; Edds, 1953; Aguilar *et al.*, 1973; J. Diamond *et al.*, 1976) is discussed in Section 9.12 in connection with the development of cutaneous innervation. Motor nerve sprouting occurs after partial denervation of muscle (Wehrmacher and Hines, 1945; Hines *et al.*, 1945; Weiss and Edds, 1946; M. C. Brown *et al.*, 1981, review), or after abolition of muscle activity by blocking impulse conduction in the motor nerve with tetrodotoxin (M. C. Brown and Ironton, 1977a), or after presynaptic blockade with botulinum toxin (Duchen and Strich, 1968), or after postsynaptic blockade with alpha-bungarotoxin (Holland and Brown, 1980). Direct electrical stimulation of muscle prevents or reverses motor nerve sprouting (M. C. Brown and Ironton, 1977b).

Uninjured, neighboring axons sprout collaterals after surgical deafferentation of neurons in the CNS (see Section 6.12). Here it should be emphasized that those examples of sprouting in the CNS can be more easily understood in relation to the theory that has been outlined, but their mechanisms remain to be discovered. Collateral sprouting of neighboring axons into a denervated zone is due either to disinhibition of their tendency to sprout or to stimulation of sprouting in response to sprouting factors released by the cells that they normally innervate.

This neurotrophic theory also provides an explanation for the apparent competition between axons for terminal space. This was elaborated by Ramón y Cajal. He first suggested that the stimulus for collateral sprouting is frequently excessive during the initial phase of innervation, and that the number of nerve endings thus tends to exceed the number of synaptic sites that can be occupied by them. This results in a competition between the nerve endings for synaptic sites on their target cells, followed by elimination of the endings that fail to find a site at which to form a synapse.

Collateral sprouting has been most thoroughly studied in the skin, as described in Section 9.12. The development of collateral sprouts from motoneuron terminals as they grow close to muscles is also well documented. During the initial innervation of mammalian skeletal muscle, there is an excess formation of neuromuscular connections, most of which are destined to disappear during early postnatal life, eventually leaving each muscle fiber connected to a single nerve terminal (Redfern, 1970; M. R. Bennett and Pettigrew, 1974; M. C. Brown *et al.*, 1976; Lichtman, 1977; Purves and Lichtman, 1980; Betz, 1987, review). This is described in Section 9.4 in relation to development of neuromuscular connections. In that situation, the ratio of nerve terminals to muscle fibers changes as new muscle fibers are formed after birth (Chiakulas and Pauly, 1965). It is conceivable that a similar process may occur in the CNS: afferents are present in advance of the stream of migrating neurons and they may make temporary connections with the first neurons to arrive in their field, only to change their connections as more neurons arrive. This occurs in the formation of thalamocortical connections in the subplate of the mammalian cerebral cortex (see Section 10.7). A similar process of transfer of connections in the cerebellar cortex occurs: the climbing fibers form temporary connections with the somatic spines of Purkinje cells before making their permanent synaptic connections on the Purkinje cell dendrites (see Section 10.12).

9.9. Axonal Sprouting in the Peripheral Nervous System

In all mammals so far studied, experimental partial denervation of a skeletal muscle is followed, after a few days, by the sprouting of collateral nerve branches from the surviving, uninjured intramuscular axons. These sprouts arise from the subterminal nodes of Ranvier or from the preterminal, unmyelinated part of the axon or from the end-plate, as shown in Fig. 9.6 (Edds, 1949, 1953, review; H. Hoffman, 1950; Coers and Woolf, 1959; Barker and Ip, 1966; M. C. Brown *et al.*, 1981, review). Exner (1884) first observed that partially denervated muscle, unlike fully denervated muscle, does not degenerate, and he put forward the theory that recovery of function occurs by growth of the residual intact nerves—another example of a premature theory (see footnote 1 in Chapter 1) which was much later put forward as a mature theory by Hines *et al.* (1945). The collateral sprouts

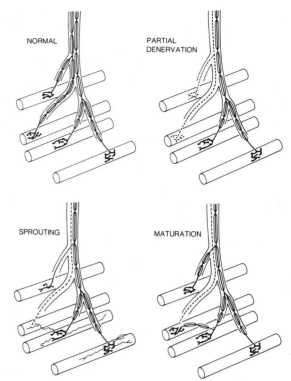

Figure 9.6. Terminal and nodal axonal sprouting of intramuscular nerves. Normal: diagrammatic representation (not to scale) of a branch of an intramuscular nerve with two myelinated axons innervating four muscle fibers. The perineural sheath envelops the axons down to the terminals, which are drawn as they appear after staining with zinc iodide–osmium tetroxide. For simplicity the endoneurium (basement membrane of Schwann cells and collagen within the perineurium) and the perineural sheath and Schwann cells overlying the terminals are not shown. Partial denervation: the severed axons and their terminals degenerate. Sprouting: by 5 days terminal and nodal sprouts have usually appeared and begin to contact previously denervated end-plates. Maturation: 1–2 months after partial denervation, sprouts innervating end-plates are myelinated and all other sprouts have usually disappeared. It is not known whether the original shape of each terminal is restored. From M. C. Brown, R. L. Holland and W. G. Hopkins, *Ann. Rev. Neurosci.* 4:17–42 (1981), copyright Annual Reviews Inc.

enter the neurilemmal sheaths of the severed axons and grow directly to the denervated end-plates, where they form functional neuromuscular junctions. The branches have only to grow a few hundred micrometers to reach the end-plates, and reinnervation is rapid and efficient. The collateral branching starts within a few days of partial denervation in mammals, but is most abundant during the 3rd week, and continues for several weeks. As a result of reinnervation, the tension developed by the muscle on stimulating its residual motor nerve almost completely regains the tension developed by stimulating the normal innervation of the muscle on the other side (Van Harreveld, 1945; Weiss and Edds, 1946). The individual muscle fibers that have been reinnervated become 50–60 percent larger in cross-sectional area than the fibers of the opposite normal muscle (Van Harreveld, 1945). Initially, the collateral axonal branches are of fine caliber, but they rapidly increase in diameter and in the 2nd postoperative month reach diameters within the range of normal nerve fibers (Edds, 1950a; H. Hoffman, 1950). The axons that have become overloaded as a result of forming an excess of terminal branches then increase in diameter after several months (Edds, 1950b; Cavanaugh, 1951). The size of the motor unit, that is, the number of muscle fibers supplied by one motoneuron, is increased four- or fivefold after partial denervation (Thompson and Jansen, 1977). This is independent of the original size or type of the motor unit, and thus probably represents the limits of neuron growth (Brown and Ironton, 1978b).

When the cut nerves regenerate into a partially denervated muscle, they may either be excluded by the collateral sprouts that have formed end-plates, or double innervation of end-plates by collateral sprouts or regenerated fibers may occur (H. Hoffman, 1951a; Guth, 1962), or the regenerated fibers may displace the sprouts in amphibians (Cass *et al.*, 1973; Fangboner and Vanable, 1974; M. R. Bennett and Raftos, 1977; Dennis and Yip, 1978) and in mammals (M. C. Brown and Ironton, 1976, 1978). Displacement and withdrawal of the sprouts occurs only when the nerves regenerate early, but not after delayed regeneration (Slack, 1978; Thompson, 1978). Proposed mechanisms for displacement of sprouts by regenerated axons include competition for a limited supply of trophic agent produced by the muscle (Jansen *et al.*, 1978), competition for a limited area of muscle fiber (Brown and Ironton, 1978), and destruction of one ending by proteolytic enzymes released by the other ending (O'Brien *et al.*, 1978).

The collateral sprouting of residual axons which occurs after partial denervation of the sartorius muscle is increased by total denervation of the neighboring quadriceps muscle (Van Harreveld, 1947). This indicates that collateral sprouting in the sartorius may be stimulated by a diffusible substance liberated from the denervated quadriceps. However, initial attempts to extract such a substance from denervated muscle and inject it into a partially denervated muscle did not produce clear evidence of increased or accelerated reinnervation (Van Harreveld, 1947). Evidence of such an effect was obtained by H. Hoffman (1950) following intramuscular injection of ether extracts of egg yolks, muscle, peripheral nerve, or white matter of the brain. Any of these substances injected into the anterior tibial muscle of the rat results in new outgrowth of collaterals from motor axons and from 30–50 percent of the motor endplates within 3 or 4 days after the injection. Ether extracts of the gray matter of the brain are as inactive as extracts of heart or liver. H. Hoffman (1950) postulated that a lipid is released from degenerating nerve fibers and stimulates sprouting of collaterals from surviving axons and end-plates; he called this hypothetical substance *neurocletin*. The active molecule has not been identified, but it appears to be a monounsaturated fatty acid (Hoffman and Springell, 1951). It is possible that the substance stimulates muscle to release more neurotrophic factor rather than acting as a neurotrophic factor itself.

Schwann cells may have a role in stimulating collateral sprouting and regeneration of motor nerve axons. After axotomy the Schwann cells proliferate and produce nerve growth factor (NGF), which stimulates growth cone activity and axon elongation (see Sections 3.9 and 8.14). Schwann cells precede the motor axons growing into the embryonic chick limb bud (Landmesser, 1987; Noakes and Bennett, 1987) and Schwann cells migrate into the premuscle masses before ingrowth of axons (Noakes and Bennett, 1987). If Schwann cells are eliminated by removal of the neural crest before they migrate out, the spinal nerves grow into the base of the limb but fail to form normal connections with muscles in the chick embryo (Carpenter and Hollyday, 1986). The Schwann cells can stimulate axon outgrowth by releasing NGF and they can act as an adhesive substrate by expressing cell adhesion molecules (especially NgCAM) on their surfaces (Landmesser, 1987).

Collateral and ultraterminal sprouts are seen in normal, uninjured axons supplying the skeletal muscle fibers as well as those supplying the intrafusal muscle fibers in healthy muscles of cats and rabbits where the motor supply is intact (Barker and Ip, 1966; Tuffery, 1971; Brown and Ironton, 1978; Cardasis and Padykula, 1979) (Fig. 9.7). Such sprouts, which end blindly, have previously been regarded as embryonic vestiges that persist after failing to make functional connections (Ramón y Cajal, 1925; Tello, 1922b). However, Barker and Ip (1966) suggest that the motor nerve endings in normal muscle may have a limited lifespan and may be replaced by collateral ultraterminal sprouting. The population of nerve terminals may be in a state of dynamic equilibrium (Weddell and Zander, 1951). It seems to be a property of vertebrate sensory nerve terminals to undergo cycles of degeneration and regeneration, particularly in sites where the sense organelles and nerve terminals are subject to wear and tear, as in the epithelium of the tongue (see Section 9.13).

In the peripheral nervous system, when nerves are cut and allowed to regenerate into their distal stumps, there is considerable reconnection of axons with their proper targets. For example, selective reinnervation of fast and slow muscle fibers occurs after nerve regeneration in the toad *Bufo marinus* (Hoh, 1971). Reinnervation of the superior

cervical ganglion after cutting of the preganglionic fibers results in selective reinnervation of ganglion cells by preganglionic fibers from particular levels of the spinal cord (J. N. Langley, 1895, 1897), and, in the ciliary ganglion, the reinnervating fibers form the correct synaptic connections from the beginning (Landmesser and Pilar, 1970). Even if there is collateral sprouting from neighboring fibers onto denervated ganglion cells, the inappropriate connections are displaced when the appropriate presynaptic fibers regenerate (Guth and Bernstein, 1961). However, several foreign nerves, including peripheral motor nerves and the vagus nerve, can regenerate to form functional heterologous synapses with superior cervical ganglion cells whose own presynaptic fibers have been removed (J. N. Langley, 1898; J. N. Langley and Anderson, 1904a,b; Guth, 1956a,b; Ceccarelli *et al.*, 1971; McLachlan, 1974; Ostberg *et al.*, 1976; Purves, 1976). The specificity of connections in these cases is relative: a variety of foreign cholinergic nerve fibers can take the place of the native presynaptic fibers. When both foreign vagal and native sympathetic fibers innervate the superior cervical ganglion of the guinea pig simultaneously, about half the ganglion cells receive synapses from both sources after about 1 month, and the proportion of doubly innervated cells remains constant for at least 14 months, showing that the foreign synapses are as stable as the native ones on the same neuron (Purves, 1976). There is now considerable evidence that in some situations in the peripheral nervous system the foreign innervation persists and remains functionally effective after the normal nerves are allowed to reinnervate their postsynaptic cells. This result has been reported in mammalian skeletal muscle (Tonge, 1974a–c; Frank *et al.*, 1974, 1975), frog fast muscle (Miledi, 1963), and perch gill muscle (Frank and Jansen, 1976).

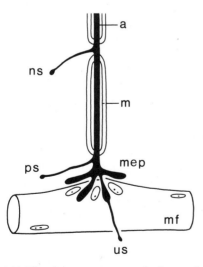

Figure 9.7. The three positions at which axonal sprouts may arise at preterminal and terminal parts of the motor axon. a = axon; m = myelin sheath; mep = motor end-plate; mf = muscle fiber; ns = nodal collateral sprout; ps = preterminal sprout; us = ultraterminal sprout. From D. Barker and M. C. Ip, *Proc. Roy. Soc. (London) Ser. B* 163:538–554 (1966).

9.10. Formation of Connections between Sensory Nerves and Sensory Receptors

Sensory nerves always arrive before sensory receptor cells start differentiating in the skin, taste buds, lateral line organs, muscle spindles, tendon organs, and other chemoreceptors, thermoreceptors, and mechanoreceptors in the viscera and blood vessels. This leads one to suspect that the presence of sensory nerve may be required for the differentiation of sensory receptor cells. The evidence that sensory nerves "induce" the development of sensory receptors is discussed in the following pages.

It is well known that each type of sense organ can respond only to a specific stimulus modality and to a limited range of intensities. An attempt will be made to answer the question of whether the sensory nerve determines the modality specificity of the sense organ, or *vice versa*, or whether a reciprocal interaction between nerve terminal and sense organ determines their functional specificity. At present, no direct evidence has been obtained by recording from developing sense organs, and we have to rely mainly on the evidence from studies of denervation and reinnervation of sense organs.

All types of sensory cells degenerate after denervation and may regenerate or differentiate anew after reinnervation. If the denervated sense organelles survive, the effects of denervation may be completely reversed after reinnervation. A problem that has not been fully resolved is whether regenerating sensory nerves reconnect with the sense organs with which they were originally connected or whether reinnervation is totally nonselective. Some evidence of selective reinnervation is given below.

Some observations show that regenerating sensory nerves may be attracted or guided to the positions occupied by degenerating sensory cells. R. M. May (1925) reported that regenerated nerve terminals return to the positions previously occupied by taste buds in catfish. After cutting the dorsal lateral line nerve and cutaneous nerves in frog tadpoles, Speidel (1964) observed a marked preference for reinnervation of lateral line organs by lateral line nerves rather than by cutaneous nerve fibers. A similar preferential reinnervation is seen after regeneration of cutaneous nerves to the hairy skin of the cat: the nerves show a distinct tendency to regenerate to their original terminal positions in relationship to Merkel cells (Burgess *et al.*, 1974; Horch, 1979). Quite specific targeting of sensory nerve fibers has been observed during development and nerve regeneration in amphibians (S. A. Scott *et al.*, 1981; Mearow and Diamond, 1988). The concept of "target" cells in the skin of vertebrates is similar to the concept of "guidepost" cells which serve as targets for nerve fibers growing along peripheral nerve pathways of insects (Bate, 1976; Ho and Goodman,

1982; Goodman *et al.*, 1982; Bentley and Kishishian, 1982; Taghert *et al.*, 1982).

Two problems are raised by such observations. First, how do the regenerating axons find their way to their original locations? Are they guided there by growth factors produced by the Schwann cells that mark their original paths, or are they attracted by alluring substances emanating from the degenerating receptors? Second, what is the source of the cells that differentiate as new receptors? It is known that the original cells can participate in the formation of receptors after nerve regeneration, but that is impossible in cases where the original receptors have completely degenerated before the nerves return. In that case, the nerves induce differentiation in the epithelial cells, and we wish to know whether all epithelial cells have this capability or whether there are special precursor cells that remain undifferentiated until they are contacted by a sensory nerve fiber. Partial solutions to these problems will be given in the following sections.

9.11. Development of Innervation of Golgi Tendon Organs and Muscle Spindles

Golgi tendon organs are slowly adapting stretch receptors. They are located in series with muscle fibers along tendons and aponeuroses. Each organ is spindle shaped and is composed mainly of bundles of collagen fibers surrounded by a capsule, about 600 μm long and 50 μm at the greatest diameter (Golgi, 1880; reviewed by Matthews, 1972; Barker, 1974; Hunt, 1974). Each Golgi tendon organ is supplied with a single type 1b sensory nerve fiber which branches among the collagen fibers inside the organ.

Development of Golgi tendon organs has been studied with light microscopy in the chick embryo (Tello, 1917, 1922) and with electron microscopy in the rat fetus (Zelená, 1976; Zelená and Soukup, 1977). In the chick embryo the sensory nerve fibers contact myotubes near the ends of muscles at about E9. The nerve fibers branch and the tendon organs differentiate in relationship to the nerves until they resemble mature Golgi tendon organs at the time of hatching. In the leg muscles of the rat, axons contact the aponeuroses at the ends of muscles on E18. Golgi tendon organs can be recognized in relationship to the nerve terminals on E20–E21, as shown

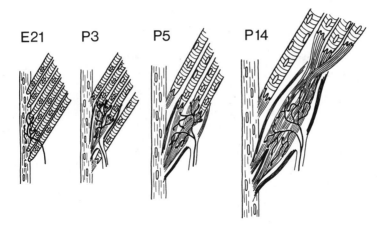

Figure 9.8. Development of the Golgi tendon organ of the soleus muscle of the rat. On E21 the Ib nerve fiber branches on the aponeurosis and around the attaching myotubes. Three days after birth (P3) the Golgi tendon organ is encapsulated, and myotubes no longer extend to the aponeurosis but still occupy the developing Golgi tendon organ. The Ib nerve fiber branches to end on myotubes and among Schwann cells and collagen bundles interposed between the myotubes and the aponeurosis. At P5, axon terminals are only seen among Schwann cells and collagen bundles. Muscle fibers recede from the Golgi tendon organ, their myotendinous region still being enclosed by the capsule. At P14 the Golgi tendon organ is structurally mature. From J. Zelená and T. Soukup, *J. Neurocytol.* 6:171–194 (1977). Copyright Chapman and Hall.

in Fig. 9.8. Most of the differentiation of Golgi tendon organs in the leg muscles of the rat occurs postnatally and they become structurally mature 2–3 weeks after birth (Zelená and Soukup, 1977). This process of development apparently is induced by the sensory nerve ending and its associated Schwann cells. Dense core vesicles are prominent in the nerve endings in contact with myotubes and their role in the induction of the Golgi tendon organ has been suggested by Zelená (1976). Schwann cells and fibroblasts proliferate around the nerve endings. Extracellular matrix and collagen are produced, apparently by Schwann cells as well as fibroblasts. Collagen fibers and some elastin fibers form between the aponeurosis and the myotubes, and the latter gradually retract as the Golgi tendon organ differentiates.

Golgi tendon organs develop normally after neonatal tenotomy which prevents their normal functioning (Zelená, 1963). However, their development is dependent on the sensory nerve and they fail to develop after neonatal denervation (Zelená, 1964, 1975).

Muscle spindles are stretch receptors found in vertebrate skeletal muscle (reviews by Barker, 1974; C. C. Hunt, 1974; Binder *et al.*, 1982; Boyd and Gladden, 1985). They consist of specialized intrafusal muscle fibers innervated by the gamma-motoneurons and by sensory nerve terminals of the type 1a axons from the spinal dorsal root ganglia. These sensory neurons develop predominantly from the small MD neurons of the spinal ganglia (see Section 8.10). There are three types of intrafusal muscle fibers in mammalian muscle spindles: two types of large nuclear bag fibers (bag_1 and bag_2 fibers) and the smaller nuclear chain fibers, so called because of the arrangement of their nuclei. The three types of fibers also have differences in myosin ATP and myosin. The bag_1 fiber contains slow-tonic myosin, whereas the bag_2 and chain fibers contain slow-twitch and fast-twitch myosins, respectively (Rowlerson *et al.*, 1985). Immunocytochemical studies show that all three types of intrafusal fibers express an embryonic form of myosin in adult mammals (Maier *et al.*, 1988). The adult pattern of myosin develops by P3 in the rat and depends on sensory but not motor innervation, as discussed below (Kucera and Walro, 1989). The neuromuscular junctions are confined to the poles of the intrafusal muscle fibers, whereas the sensory axons are confined to the equatorial zone of the spindle where they form the annulospiral and flower-spray nerve endings (Kucera *et al.*, 1988a). The normal development of muscle spindles is illustrated in Fig. 9.9.

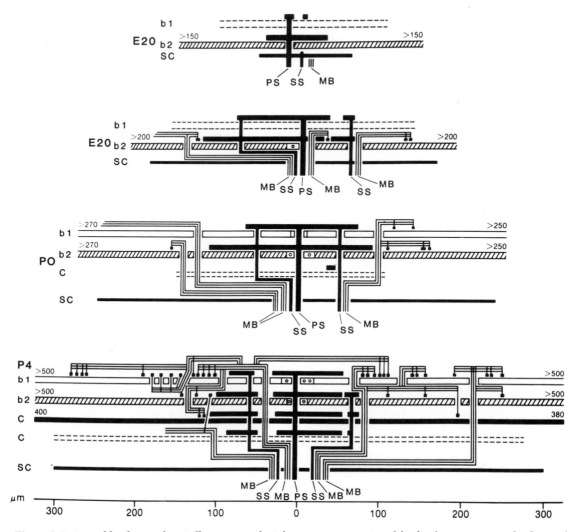

Figure 9.9. Assembly of a muscle spindle nerve supply. Schematic representation of the developing nerve supply of a muscle spindle of the rat soleus muscle from E20 to P4. Intrafusal myotubes are represented by horizontal dashed lines and myofibers by solid lines. Nuclear bag$_1$ (b$_1$), nuclear bag$_2$ (b$_2$), and nuclear chain (C) myofibers are shown as white, hatched, and black, respectively. The equatorial region of the nuclear bag fibers is shown by small circles. Note that the primary (PS) and secondary (SS) afferents innervate all intrafusal fibers, whereas bundles of motor axons (MB) innervate the intrafusal myofibers but not the myotubes. Motor nerve endings are denoted by small black squares. Note that the individual motor endings are polyaxonally innervated. SC = spindle capsule. Scale shows the length of the spindle relative to the equator (zero). Polar lengths of intrafusal fibers are given at the end of the myofiber. From J. Kucera, J. M. Walro, and J. Reichler, *Am. J. Anat.* 183:344–358 (1988).

This complex program of assembly of the muscle spindle has been described in many papers which should be consulted for details of the structural changes that occur during development (Sutton, 1915; Tello, 1922b; Cuajunco, 1927a,b; Kalugina, 1956; Barker and Milburn, 1972, 1984; Landon, 1972a,b; Milburn, 1973a,b, 1984; Kucera *et al.*, 1988a,b).

In the hindlimb of the chick embryo, the muscle spindles can first be seen on E9, and no additional spindles develop after E13 (Tello, 1922b). Because stretch reflexes can be elicited from E10 to E11, sensory nerves must have connected with the spindles before then (Visintini and Levi-Montalcini, 1939; Hamburger and Levi-Montalcini, 1949). The innervation of muscle spindles in the jaw muscles of the chick embryo probably occurs between E10 and E14, as indicated by the retrograde labeling after injection of HRP into the jaw muscles (Hiscock and Straznicky, 1986). Death of neurons in the trigeminal mesencephalic nucleus occurs during the period of innervation of muscle spindles in the jaw muscles, as discussed in Section 8.9.

The muscle spindles develop under the influence of their nerves, but here the problem is complicated by their dual innervation. The initial development of the intrafusal muscle fibers, to the myotube stage, occurs in the absence of innervation. However, the differentiation of mature intrafusal muscle fibers requires both sensory and motor innervation. In the rat, the muscle spindles begin to appear in the limbs on day 18 of gestation and their development is synchronous and is completed during the following 10 days (Fig. 9.9). Rat muscle spindles contain one nuclear bag_1, one nuclear bag_2, and two nuclear chain fibers. These fibers develop in three generations: on E18 some primary myotubes begin to differentiate into the bag_2 fiber; on E20 the 1st generation of secondary myotubes begin to differentiate into the bag_1 fiber; and on E22 the 2nd generation of seecondary myotubes gives rise to the two chain fibers (Zelena, 1957; Landon, 1972; Milburn, 1973a,b). These three types of intrafusal muscle fibers acquire sensory and motor innervation in the same order as they develop (Kucera *et al.*, 1988b). Initially, the intrafusal muscle fibers are innervated only by sensory nerve terminals. These are present on myoblasts, myotubes, and myofibers. No additional sensory endings develop and none are retracted after they form (Kucera *et al.*, 1988b).

In the hindlimb of the rat, sensory innervation of the muscle spindles develops on E18, while the neuromuscular junctions develop at the polar regions of intrafusal muscle fibers only on E20 and on the subsequent days (Fig. 9.9). An excess of motor nerve endings contact the intrafusal fibers initially, followed by retraction of redundant motor nerve terminals (Kucera *et al.*, 1988b). The large alpha-motoneuron axons to the extrafusal muscle fibers arrive at the muscle about 2 days before the small gamma-motoneuron axons arrive at the intrafusal muscle fibers. It is not known whether alpha-motoneurons transiently contact intrafusal muscle fibers, or if not, why they avoid them. Perhaps the alpha-motoneurons are excluded from the muscle spindles by the sensory nerves.

At birth, the muscle spindles are immature, containing two myotubes with nuclear bags and one satellite myotube. Postnatally, intrafusal myotubes fuse to form another satellite myotube. The two myotubes that are formed last develop nuclear chains, and this completes the full complement of intrafusal fibers in the rat by 4 days after birth. However, the polar zones of the spindles do not become fully differentiated until 12 days after birth (Milburn, 1973a,b).

The differentiation of the intrafusal muscle fibers is under control of the sensory nerves and remains so throughout life. Elimination of the sensory nerve supply by cutting the dorsal roots in adult cats and dogs, leaving the motor supply intact, results in degeneration of the muscle spindles (Tower, 1932; Kucera and Walro, 1987). The nuclei of intrafusal muscle fibers are clustered in the equatorial zone beneath the sensory nerve endings. Their location is regulated by the sensory nerve, as shown by the fact that clustering of myonuclei does not occur after deafferentation of muscle in the newborn rat (Kucera and Walro, 1987). The myonuclei disintegrate in adult muscle spindles deprived of sensory innervation (Kucera, 1980). Denervation of rat muscle spindles on day 19 or 20 of gestation (60–72 hours before birth) results in rapid degeneration (Zelená, 1957). Since the only innervation present at the time of the operation on E19 are the sensory nerves, they must be required for differentiation of the muscle spindles. On the other hand, if the sensory nerves remain intact, spindle development is little affected following selective motor denervation (Zelená, 1964, 1965; Zelená and Soukup, 1973, 1974a,b). Therefore, the sensory nerve itself must exert the trophic effect. The observation that there are specialized junctions, resembling synapses, between the sensory nerve and the intrafusal muscle suggests that the sensory nerves may release a trophic agent that stimulates the muscle, and the presence of light- and dense-cored vesicles in the sensory nerve ending and of coated pits in both the muscle and axonal membrane is consistent with this hypothesis (Zelená and Soukup, 1973). The synapse-like structure may also mediate transmission from the muscle to the sensory nerve.

There is a critical period, lasting up to 2 weeks after birth, during which muscle spindles depend on their sensory nerves for development and survival. With increasing age, muscle spindles in the rat hindlimb have a progressively decreasing dependence on their nerve supply (Zelená, 1957,

1964). In newborn rats, sensory denervation results in atrophy and degeneration of the muscle spindles within 10 days. Denervation in rats 20 days after birth, when the muscle spindles are fully differentiated, merely results in slight atrophy of the intrafusal muscle fibers 10 days later. There is a critical period during which muscle spindles will degenerate if deprived of their innervation, but the spindles will survive if they are denervated after that period. In the gastrocnemius muscle of the rat, the spindles require innervation until 6–8 days postnatally, after which they survive if denervated (J. K. Werner, 1973). Similar critical periods have been defined for dependence of taste buds on their nerves (Hosley *et al.*, 1987b) and for dependence of Pacinian corpuscles on sensory nerves (Zelenà *et al.*, 1978; Zelenà, 1980).

9.12. Development of Cutaneous Sensory Innervation

There are three main problems, each with several auxiliary problems, that have to be considered in the development of cutaneous innervation: outgrowth of sensory nerves along stereotypical pathways, localization of cutaneous nerves to domains or dermatomes in body space, and formation of nervous connections with specific peripheral sense organelles. The first is part of the general problem of axonal growth considered in Chapter 5. The second is also considered in Sections 11.6 and 11.7 with respect to development of somatosensory projection maps. The third problem is considered here.

The skin and mucous membranes contain many different types of sense organelles, each innervated in a characteristic pattern, as well as numerous free nerve endings. How do the different sense organelles become associated with the appropriate nerve endings, and how is the numerical density of sense organelles and nerve endings controlled?

The following experimental strategies have been used to answer those questions. Firstly, studies of normal development have been done to see whether sense organelles develop before, during, or after arrival of nerves. Secondly, there have been studies of the effects of denervation and reinnervation on sense organs. Thirdly, the effects of cross-

innervation of sense organs have been observed. Fourthly, the changes in sense organs after the grafting of skin or mucous membrane to unusual locations have been investigated. Fifthly, sprouting of intact nerves into a neighboring denervated region has been studied.

Peripheral sensory nerve patterns, the most complex of which are in the limbs, are determined by the epigenetic landscape composed of the tissues through which the nerves grow (G. J. Swanson and Lewis, 1982; J. Lewis *et al.*, 1983; Tosney and Landmesser, 1985a). The stereotyped patterns of peripheral nerve pathways and the domains occupied by their nerve endings in body space are the result of complex epigenetic programs. The dorsal root ganglia (DRG) are arranged segmentally with respect to the primary mesodermal segmentation (see Section 1.2). The neural crest from which the DRGs orginate is not primarily segmented. That is one of the reasons why surgical reversal of segments of neural crest in the early embryo results in normal development of DRGs and has no effect on peripheral sensory nerve patterns. The latter form with reference to the tissues through which the nerves grow. The motor nerves, which start growing out before sensory nerves, also act as guides for the latter. When motoneurons are removed early in development in the chick embryo, the sensory nerves to muscle fail to develop (A. C. Taylor, 1944) but cutaneous sensory nerves form normally (Landmesser and Honig, 1986; G. J. Swanson and Lewis, 1986; S. A. Scott, 1988). Thus, sensory nerves can grow selectively along normal pathways in the absence of motor nerves. However, when limb-bearing segments of spinal cord plus neural crest are excised and reimplanted with rostrocaudal inversion, both sensory and motor nerve patterns are reversed (Honig *et al.*, 1986).

The regular segmental arrangement of dermatomes develops as a result of several factors: the origin of sensory nerves from the segmentally arranged DRGs; the short initial distance, less than 1 mm, which the nerves have to traverse to reach the periphery (although the trajectory of segmental nerves through the brachial and lumbosacral plexuses is complex, the distances are small); and competition between the nerves for peripheral territory, resulting in regular domains finally occupied by them. The density of innervation which can be supported by any region of skin appears to be the limiting factor, not the number of available DRG neurons. Thus, DRG neurons are rescued from death by giving them a larger peripheral domain into which to grow after elimination of the DRGs which normally occupy that domain (Carr, 1984).

The density of cutaneous innervation and the number of sensory corpuscles in each region are remarkably invariant. These appear to be regional characteristics of the epithelium and are probably determined during early development, before entry of the nerves, by interactions between the epithelium and underlying mesenchyme (McLoughlin, 1968; Sengel, 1976, 1983). The distribution of hairs and feathers is also determined by interactions between epithelium and mesenchyme, probably involving extracellular matrix molecules (Wessells, 1965; Wessells and Roessner, 1965; Hay, 1981; Bernfield, 1981; Saxén *et al.*, 1982; Sengel, 1983). Virtually nothing is known about the early stages of development of the epithelium when its local properties are determined which control the density of innervation and of sensory corpuscles.

Ramón y Cajal (1919) established two of the basic theories on which the modern research program on development of cutaneous innervation has been built: first, that different cutaneous nerves subserving different sensory modalities are specifically attracted to the appropriate sensory receptor organs; second, that the final number of sensory nerve fibers is limited by availability of substances required for their growth in the periphery (see Section 9.1). A number of observations indicate that there may be some kind of biochemical control of the density of cutaneous innervation, for example, denervation of a region of skin results in collateral sprouting of adjacent nerve fibers, which grow into the denervated region (Weddell *et al.*, 1941; Livingston, 1947). This kind of growth adjustment of nerve endings was studied in the tail fin of the frog tadpole by Speidel (1941), who concluded that *"in some manner the denervated zone constitutes a local stimulus with sufficient influence to evoke new sprouts from nearby fibers which otherwise would not have given rise to them."* Collateral nerve sprouting is the normal method of innervation during development and growth of the skin. Regulation of the density of cutaneous innervation continues throughout life. Nerve endings and sense organelles in the skin and mucous membranes are continually destroyed as a result of normal wear and tear. The

innervation of these tissues remains in a steady state because replacement of epidermal cells, nerve endings, and sense organelles exactly compensates for their loss (Tello, 1932; Cowdry, 1932, Vol. 1, p. 24; Fitzgerald, 1962; Beidler, 1963; Beidler and Smallman, 1965). The observation by Fitzgerald (1961, 1962) that during development of the pig snout the number of axonal branches increases in proportion to the number of epidermal ridges is consistent with Cajal's concepts of the control of cutaneous innervation density.

Direct observation of the process of growth adjustment of peripheral nerves can be made in the tail fin of the living tadpole. Speidel (1933, 1935a,b, 1941, 1942) observed the growth of nerves in the dermis of the tail fin of the living tadpole almost continuously over a period of several weeks (Figs. 5.9 and 5.10). Collateral branches occur at any position in unmyelinated axons and at the nodes of Ranvier in myelinated axons. The branches may extend, retract, or degenerate, and as a result the pattern of innervation is constantly changing. Speidel (1942, p. 63) concluded: *"It seems very probable to me that the endings of terminal arborizations within the central nervous system undergo adjustments quite like those of terminal arborizations of the skin."* This has proved to be true, and evidence is given in Section 6.13 of sprouting of presynaptic terminals which occupy synaptic sites on partially denervated neurons in the CNS.

The alternative hypotheses of mechanisms of innervation of the skin and formation of cutaneous sensory corpuscles are the following: First, there may be a coincidence between the time of arrival of nerves and the time at which their targets originate or are mature enough to accept innervation. The evidence does not show any regular pattern of temporal coincidence of the sort that would be consistent with such a hypothesis. Second, guidance or attraction to the appropriate endings or attraction by them may account for the specificity of innervation, and there is evidence of such targeting of nerve fibers on Merkel cells in the skin of amphibians and mammals. In salamanders the Merkel cells can be seen with the electron microscope before they become innervated (E. Cooper and Diamond, 1977; E. Cooper *et al.*, 1977). The Merkel cells of salamanders and *Xenopus* and of the glabrous skin of the rat's footpad differentiate independently of nerves. In that respect they differ from some Merkel cells in cutaneous touch domes of the rat and from other sensory organelles such as taste buds and Herbst corpuscles, discussed below, which differentiate under the influence of nerves.

There are marked differences between various types of sensory organelles with respect to their dependence on nerves. We can make the distinction between organelles which differentiate under inductive influence of nerves, those which also require continuous trophic support by nerves, and those which can differentiate and survive without nerves.

Merkel cells are specialized cells of vertebrate skin found abundantly in regions which are very sensitive to touch, such as the digits, lips, nose, and hairs (Merkel, 1875, 1880; Munger, 1965; Iggo and Muir, 1969; Breathnach and Robins, 1970; Hashimoto, 1972; Breathnach, 1977, 1980; English *et al.*, 1980; Tachibana and Nawa, 1980; Halata, 1981; Tachibana *et al.*, 1983; Pác, 1984; Nafstad, 1986) and tentacles of *Xenopus* embryos (Eglmeier, 1987). Merkel cells in birds are located in the dermis and have been shown by means of quail–chick grafts to originate from neural crest in the chick (Saxod, 1978). In mammals, both dermal and epidermal Merkel cells are found (Breathnach and Robins, 1970; Hashimoto, 1972; Winkelman and Breathnach, 1973; Halata, 1979, 1981), whereas in amphibians, the Merkel cells originate exclusively in the epidermis (Nafstad and Baker, 1973; Tweedle, 1978; Eglmeier, 1987).

The origin of Merkel cells is controversial: many authors consider them to originate from neural crest (Breathnach and Robins, 1970; Hashimoto, 1972; Breathnach, 1977, 1980; Saxod, 1978; Moll *et al.*, 1984; Hartschuh *et al.*, 1986); others favor an epidermal origin of Merkel cells (Munger, 1965; Tweedle, 1978; Tachibana *et al.*, 1983; Pác, 1984; Klauer, 1986; Nafstad, 1986; Eglmeier, 1987). It seems likely that Merkel cells have a dual origin: those located in the dermis originating from neural crest while those in the epidermis originate locally. With the exception of birds (Saxod, 1978) and amphibians (Tweedle, 1978), their origins have not been traced by means of definitive experimental methods.

Each Merkel cell is associated with a single sensory nerve ending and its associated Schwann cell to form a Merkel disc. This is a mechanorecep-

tor complex with low threshold and rapid adaptation to stimulation. The Merkel cell contains dense core vesicles, the nerve endings contain clear vesicles, and there are synapse-like junctions between them. Merkel cells have been considered to have neuroendocrine functions on the evidence of immunocytochemical staining for Met-enkephalin and vasoactive intestinal polypeptide (Hartschuh *et al.*, 1979, 1980, 1983) and on the basis of their presence in carcinomas (Gould *et al.*, 1985). However, the Met-enkephalin does not have a neurotransmitter function in Merkel cells (Gottschaldt and Vahle-Hinz, 1982). Initiation of the sensory nerve impulse on stimulating the Merkel cell–nerve complex does not involve a conventional chemical synaptic transmission step in salamander skin (Diamond *et al.*, 1986). Merkel cells can be destroyed by enzymatic treatment of the epidermis or by irradiation following uptake of quinacrine by the Merkel cells. After elimination of Merkel cells, Mearow and Diamond (1988) found that essentially normal mechanosensory responses can be initiated in the cutaneous nerve endings. This shows that Merkel cells are not required for mechanosensory transduction.

Merkel cells serve as highly specific targets for low-threshold mechanoreceptor cutaneous nerve endings during development and during nerve regeneration in the salamander and frog (Scott *et al.*, 1981; Mearow and Diamond, 1988) and rat (Mills *et al.*, 1989). In the cat, regenerating sensory nerve fibers grow directly to their original Merkel cells (Horch, 1979). After nerve regeneration in the rat, Merkel cells in cutaneous touch domes are reinnervated exclusively by the appropriate low-threshold mechanosensory nerve fibers, and the high-threshold mechanosensory fibers do not contact Merkel cells although they are in the immediate vicinity of the touch domes (Doucette and Diamond, 1987). After reinnervation of cutaneous sensory nerves in the cat (Burgess and Horch, 1973; Burgess *et al.*, 1974; Horch, 1979), and the rat (J. Diamond, 1982), reinnervation of Merkel cells occurs with virtually complete recovery of structure and function. Touch domes of the rat contain two Merkel cells, each innervated by its own nerve ending. Elimination of one nerve ending does not result in collateral sprouting from the other, but when the other axon is crushed and allowed to regenerate it sprouts to innervate both Merkel cells in the dome (Yasargil *et*

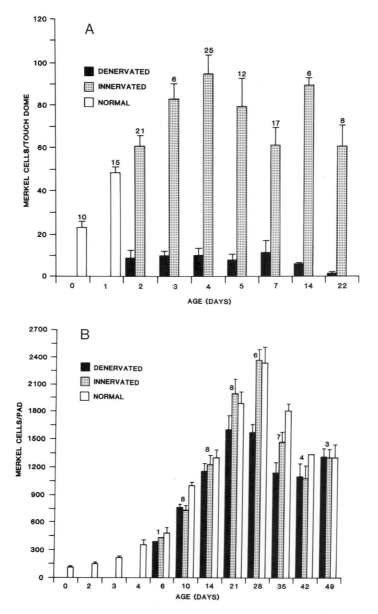

Figure 9.10. Merkel cells in touch domes of rat skin are very dependent on innervation for development and survival (A), whereas Merkel cells in the skin of the footpad are relatively independent of innervation (B). The mean numbers of Merkel cells in rats at different ages are shown in normal, innervated, and denervated touch domes (A) and in the skin of the footpad (B). Error bars show the standard error of the mean for each group. The differences between innervated and denervated domes were significant at all ages in (A). In (B) there were significant differences between denervated and innervated footpads in the groups at 21, 28, and 35 days of age, but the overall pattern of Merkel cell development was unchanged by denervation of the footpads. Equal numbers of innervated and denervated domes were examined (A), and the numbers of denervated footpads examined (B) are given above the histograms. Modified from L. R. Mills, C. A. Nurse, and J. Diamond, *Dev. Biol.* 136:61–74 (1989), copyright Academic Press, Inc.

al., 1988). Therefore, the Merkel cells function as targets for regenerating axons but cannot provide a sprouting stimulus for intact axons.

Merkel cells can develop and survive independently of nerves in the skin of salamanders and *Xenopus* (Scott *et al.*, 1981; Mearow and Diamond, 1988) and in the glabrous skin of the footpad of the rat (Mills *et al.*, 1984, 1989). By contrast, Merkel cells of rat touch domes are dependent on nerves for their differentiation and survival in the early postnatal period, as shown in Fig. 9.10 (Mills *et al.*, 1984, 1989). In adult rats about 40 percent of the Merkel cells survive denervation (Nurse *et al.*, 1984a) and reinnervation restores the Merkel cells that were reduced by denervation (Nurse *et al.*, 1984b).

There may be a critical period for dependence of cutaneous sensory organelles on their nerves. Thus, Pacinian corpuscles in the rat degenerate after denervation performed before 5 days of age (Zelená, 1978, 1980) but persist intact after denervation in adult rats (Zelená, 1982), although most Pacinian corpuscles become multiply reinnervated in adults (Zelená, 1984). In the rat the nerves induce the formation of Pacinian corpuscles and are required for maintenance only up to 5 days after birth but do not maintain Pacinian corpuscles in the adult. There is also a critical period, from birth to 10 days of age in the rat, when taste buds require nerves for their normal differentiation (Hosley *et al.*, 1987b). A critical period has also been defined in newborn rats in which muscle spindles are dependent for survival on their nerve supply (Zelená, 1957, 1964).

Denervation of a region of skin results in collateral sprouting from neighboring undamaged nerves. The collateral branches grow into the denervated region of skin, which then regains its sensitivity (Speidel, 1941; Weddell *et al.*, 1941; Livingston, 1947). This type of collateral sprouting is clearly adaptive, and one is struck by the correlation between the degree of degeneration and the number of extra axonal branches that restore the original density of cutaneous innervation. Restoration occurs only during early development and is limited in adult mammals: in the adult rat collateral sprouting is very sparse and extends for only a short distance into the neighboring denervated skin (Kinnman and Aldskogius, 1986). During development, there seem to be homeostatic mechanisms which regulate the density of innervation of skin or muscles so that after

the peripheral organs become saturated with nerves, no more axon collaterals are produced and the excess collaterals degenerate.

Ramón y Cajal's concept that the epithelium regulates axonal sprouting by producing a neurotropic factor that is neutralized by the nerve has been corroborated by evidence that an antisprouting factor may be transported in the axon to the nerve terminal. Aguilar *et al.* (1973) and J. Diamond *et al.* (1976) blocked axonal transport by means of colchicine applied to one of the three cutaneous nerves to the leg of the salamander and observed collateral sprouting of neighboring undamaged nerves into the peripheral field of the colchicine-treated nerve. Collateral sprouting can be prevented by treatment with antiserum to nerve growth factor. The axons sprout normally after cessation of the anti-NGF treatment (J. Diamond *et al.*, 1987).

The studies of Saxod (1978, review) on the development of innervation of Herbst and Grandry corpuscles in the duck beak show that those cutaneous receptors, which normally form at the endings of the ophthalmic branch of the trigeminal nerve, can be made to form *de novo* in relation to spinal sensory nerves. This makes it unlikely that there is an all-or-none affinity between the nerve ending and its target cells in the skin. Of course, all such cross-innervation experiments, in which only one kind of nerve fiber innervates the target cells, cannot rule out the possibility that nerve terminals of one kind have a greater affinity than those of another kind for the target cells, but if both kinds innervate the targets, those with the greater affinity will displace those with less affinity.

Another experiment to determine whether there is any specificity in the formation of connections between sense organelles and sensory nerves was performed by Kadanoff (1925). He exchanged hairy skin of the snout and hairless skin of the soles of the feet in mice and guinea pigs. Reinnervation of both types of grafts occurs. In some cases, the innervation pattern of the graft resembles what was normal for the grafted skin and not for the skin that the nerves originally supplied. This is most clearly seen in the case of hair follicles that are innervated normally in snout skin transplanted to the soles of the feet.

In birds, sensory nerves arrive in the skin long before the development of the feather follicles and the sensory corpuscles which they innervate. The first sensory nerves arrive in the skin of the back as early as day 4 of incubation in the chick embryo (Saxod, 1978). From E4 to E10 the nerves form a dense plexus which surrounds and innervates the developing feather follicles. The cutaneous sensory corpuscles begin to appear synchronously in different regions at E17 in the chick and at E20 in the duck embryo.

Herbst and Grandry corpuscles are specialized, encapsulated sensory corpuscles in the dermis which function as rapidly adapting mechanoreceptors. There are several thousand corpuscles situated on the beak and tongue of the duck, where they are supplied by the ophthalmic branch of the trigeminal nerve. Similar corpuscles are found on the skin of other parts of the body in many birds. Studies of their morphogenesis with the light microscope (Heringa, 1918; Tello, 1932) have been greatly extended by Saxod (1967, 1970a,b) using the electron microscope. Their development has been thoroughly reviewed by Saxod (1978).

Saxod (1973a) used autoradiography to study the histogenesis of Herbst and Grandry corpuscles in the duck beak. Injection of [³H]thymidine as a pulse any time before E16 results in equal probability of labeling any of the types of cells in the corpuscles as well as other cells of the dermal mesenchyme. From E18 to E20 the sensory cells associated with the nerve endings undergo their final mitosis (inner bulb cells of Herbst corpuscles and Grandry cells of Grandry corpuscles). The inner space cells and capsular cells of the Herbst corpuscle and the satellite cells of the Grandry corpuscle are generated as postmitotic cells on E20–E24.

Herbst and Grandry corpuscles thus start developing at E20 on the duck beak, and they are fully developed by the final 3 days of embryonic development (E26–E28). The constituent cells are assembled progressively from the center to the periphery around the nerve fiber, and they also differentiate in an inside-out order (Fig. 9.11). This seems to be the rule for other encapsulated sensory corpuscles, for example, Pacinian and Meissner corpuscles.

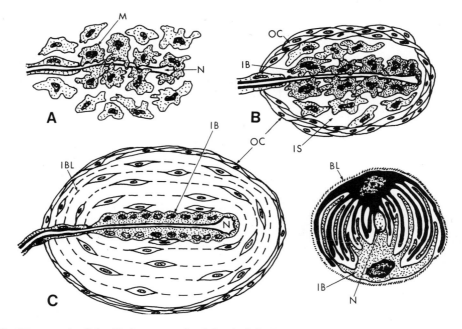

Figure 9.11. Histogenesis of the Herbst corpuscle of the duck beak occurs in an inside-out sequence. (A, day 20 of incubation) Large multipolar cells are grouped around the sensory nerve terminal. (B, 23–26 days of incubation) These cells form two rows of lamellar cells of the inner bulb. Flat cells form an outer bulb. The inner space is narrow. (C, at hatching, day 28) The inner bulb consists of about 20 lamellar cells, shown in transverse section on the lower right. The inner space contains concentric perforated lamellae. BL = basal lamina; IB = inner bulb; IBL = perforated lamellae of inner bulb; M = multipolar cells; N = nerve ending; OC = outer capsule. By courtesy of R. Saxod.

The origins of the various types of cells that compose the sensory corpuscles, such as the Herbst corpuscle and the Pacinian corpuscle, remained the subject of surmise and speculation until the chick-quail chimera techniques made it possible to analyze this question. There are three cell types in Herbst corpuscles, which are arranged concentrically. The nerve ending, in the center of the corpuscle, is surrounded by inner bulb cells, the latter are surrounded by inner space cells, and those are surrounded by capsular cells (Saxod, 1970b, 1971, 1978). Grandry corpuscles are composed of a nerve ending, flattened in the shape of a disc, on either side of which is a large Grandry cell. These are surrounded by satellite cells which are enclosed by a capsule. The various hypotheses of the origins of these cells are reviewed by Saxod (1978), and it is necessary only to point out that until the cells could be identified by radioactive or cellular markers their origins remained a matter of surmise. Thus Shantha and Bourne (1968) suggested that the corpuscles are modifications of the sheaths of the peripheral nerves; Pease and Quilliam (1957) thought that the inner bulb and inner space cells are modified fibrocytes of mesodermal origin; while others, correctly as it now seems, believed the inner bulb cells to be modified Schwann cells and thus derived from the neural crest (Rhodin, 1963; Polacek, 1966; Chouchkov, 1971). The capsular cells were generally thought by these authors to be modified fibrocytes. The origins of these cells in the Herbst corpuscle have been finally determined by Saxod (1973a,b). He combined the frontal bud (which gives rise to the beak) from the quail with Gasserian ganglion from the duck, or frontal bud from the quail with sensory ganglion from the chick. Chimeric Herbst corpuscles are formed in which the quail cells can be identified by a large chromatin granule made visible by Feulgen staining. Saxod (1973a,b) showed that all, or almost all, the inner bulb cells and some inner space cells accompany the nerve during its outgrowth from the Gasserian ganglion and are thus of neural crest origin, while all the other cells are derived from dermal mesenchyme. The origins of the cells of the two other types of corpuscles in birds, the Grandry and Merkel corpuscles, have not yet been resolved.

The influence of the nerve on development of Herbst and Grandry corpuscles has been studied in a number of ways: by determining whether the corpuscles will develop in the absence of nerves; by observing the effects of denervation on the developing and mature corpuscles; by determining whether the corpuscles can be innervated by foreign nerves. The results of all these experiments show that the sensory corpuscles require nerves for initial development and continued maintenance. Saxod and Sengel (1968) transplanted skin before the development of innervation from the duck beak to the chorioallantoic membrane, where the skin grows but no corpuscles develop in the absence of nerves. Moreover, removal of the innervation of the corpuscles during their development results in their degeneration. Likewise, in the adult chick, crushing the ophthalmic branch of the trigeminal nerve results in atrophy of the sensory corpuscles to about one-third their normal size in 14 days. The corpuscles become reinnervated at about 14 days after the nerve crushing, and the sensory corpuscles double in size during the following 14 days and attain parity with normal corpuscles at the end of a month (Quilliam, 1962).

The reinnervation of corpuscles by foreign nerves was first clearly demonstrated by Dijkstra (1933), who transferred skin containing Herbst and Grandry corpuscles from the duck's beak to its foot, which normally lacks these corpuscles. Many of the corpuscles degenerate after transplantation but reform when the graft is reinnervated by sensory nerves of the foot. This suggests that the foot sensory nerves can exert the same trophic effect as the trigeminal nerve in maintaining the corpuscles. Because these experiments were done on adult ducks, they do not show whether cutaneous nerves of the foot can induce the formation of Herbst and Grandry corpuscles *de novo*. This question was answered by Saxod and Sengel (1968) by showing that Herbst and Grandry corpuscles develop *ab initio* in beak skin grafted to other parts of the body and innervated by spinal nerves. The question of which nerve fibers (sensory, motor, sympathetic) innervate the corpuscles was dealt with by Saxod (1972a) by associating frontal buds with various sources of innervation in grafts grown in the extraembryonic coelom (Fig. 9.12). Coelomic grafts of frontal bud alone or frontal bud and sympathetic ganglia develop no corpuscles. Similarly, no corpuscles develop when frontal bud is innervated by motoneurons growing from the ventral half of the neural tube. By contrast, corpuscles develop in all frontal buds that are innervated by Gasserian or spinal ganglia (Saxod, 1972a).

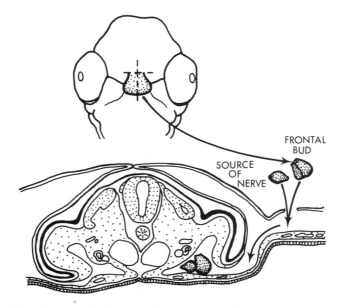

Figure 9.12. Herbst and Grandry corpuscles develop only when supplied by sensory nerves, not by motor or sympathetic nerves. Grafts of frontal bud (donated from a 2-day duck embryo, shown above) combined with nervous tissue (e.g., spinal ganglion) develop in the extraembryonic coelom (shown in transverse section of a 35-somite host embryo at the level of the 20th somite). By courtesy of R. Saxod.

The same results are obtained when xenoplastic combinations of frontal buds and sensory ganglia are made between chicken, duck, and quail but not between duck and mouse or lizard embryos.

Pacinian corpuscles develop in the cat mesoderm innervated by the saphenous nerve (Ilyinsky *et al.*, 1973) or by the hypogastric nerve (Schiff and Loewenstein, 1972) or by dorsal spinal root axons (Zelená and Jirmanová, 1988). The maintenance of taste buds after cross-innervation, discussed later, is also consistent with the other evidence showing the nonspecific inductive or trophic influence of sensory nerves on sensory end-organs.

Saxod (1972b) made heterochronic associations of pieces of duck beak at various embryonic ages with nerves at a fixed age (E4.5). In other experiments, the frontal bud was allowed to develop in the coelom in the absence of innervation for 7 to 20 days before grafting the frontal bud to the wing of a 4.5-day embryo, where it becomes innervated. The results of those experiments show that the stage at which corpuscles begin to develop depends on the absolute age of the skin and not on the time of innervation. The nerves must be more than 14 days of embryonic age in order to respond to the action

of the cutaneous mesenchyme that controls the proliferation and differentiation of the inner bulb cells, which are modified Schwann cells. The corpuscles can develop under the influence of the nerve ending only after the skin reaches the age of E19–E20. These morphogenetic interactions, leading to differentiation of Herbst corpuscles, thus seem to occur some days before the time of origin of the inner bulb cells on E18–E20 and of the inner space cells on E20–E24, according to Saxod (1973a). Knowing the time of the cellular interactions should make it easier to discover the mechanisms by which the nerve induces development of the corpuscle. The regional specificity of the dermal mesenchyme, which determines the types and numbers of corpuscles, is acquired at a much earlier age—it is present in the frontal bud at E4.5—and the origin of that specificity remains completely unknown.

These experiments show that the presence of sensory nerves is an absolute requirement for the initial formation, maturation, and subsequent maintenance of sensory organelles. Although the grafts are innervated by foreign sensory nerves, the types of sensory organelles, their number, and their spatial distribution are determined by the origin of the skin graft. Other experiments also indicate that the sensory organelles have an inherent capacity to differentiate in a special way and that the nerves provide only the stimulus and do not determine the mode of differentiation of the sensory organelles that they innervate.

9.13. Development of Nervous Connections of Taste Buds

The sensory nerve supply to the epithelium always develops before the taste buds appear. The gustatory nerve supply to the fungiform taste buds on the anterior two-thirds of the tongue epithelium is the chorda tympani branch of the seventh cranial nerve, while the glossopharyngeal nerve supplies the taste buds in the vallate and foliate papillae on the posterior third of the tongue and on the nasopharynx. Taste buds on the soft palate are supplied by the greater superficial petrosal branch of VII. There is also a nongustatory sensory nerve supply by the lingual nerve to the anterior two-thirds of the tongue, by the vagus nerve to the posterior third, and by sympathetic fibers which enter the papillae (Gabella, 1969). The majority of vallate taste buds are bilaterally innervated in the rat (Hosley *et al.*, 1987a).

The time of development of the taste papillae which bear the taste buds, their number, and their distribution are remarkably invariant in all individuals of the same species. Their morphological development in the embryo has been studied most thoroughly in the rat (Farbman, 1965, 1971; Mistretta, 1972) and hamster (Belecky and Smith, 1990), and essentially the same developmental sequence, on a longer time scale, is seen in the human taste papillae and taste buds (Bradley and Stern, 1967; Bradley, 1972). Fungiform taste buds on the anterior part of the tongue develop before the taste buds in the vallate and foliate papillae on the posterior part of the tongue and nasopharynx. The latter develop postnatally in rodents. In the rat, the fungiform papillae all appear on the same day at 14–15 days of gestation. Initially, they are small eminences on the surface of the front of the tongue, formed by a cluster of epithelial cells in which taste buds have not yet differentiated. There is a single circumvallate papilla in the rat, on the posterior surface of the tongue, which also appears on day 15 of gestation. Papillae can be seen in the 6- to 7-week human fetus

as thickenings of the epithelium, which acquire a connective tissue core and become raised in the next few weeks. The distribution and number of taste papillae in the embryo are the same as those of the adult, are quite invariant, and are probably determined by interaction between epithelium and mesenchyme during early development. At that stage, the epithelium is not innervated.

The gustatory nerves grow into the papillae and innervate the epithelium at the same time as taste buds appear. This first occurs on day 20 of gestation in the rat (Farbman, 1965, 1971), and taste buds can be seen on the fungiform papillae of the human fetus at 7 weeks and have been seen on circumvallate papillae at 11 weeks *in utero* (Bradley and Mistretta, 1975; review). All the taste buds do not appear simultaneously. Their numbers increase in relation to branching of the gustatory nerves into the epithelium. Prenatal maturation of taste buds occurs in the sheep (Bradley and Mistretta, 1973; Mistretta and Bradley, 1978). Maturation of the taste buds and development of a taste pore, by which each bud communicates with the oral cavity, occur during the 3rd month of gestation in the human fetus (Bradley and Stern, 1967; Bradley, 1972). By contrast, in the rat the percentage of taste buds with pores on fungiform papillae is about 1 percent at 1 day after birth and gradually increases to 92 percent at 12 days of age (Mistretta, 1972). The number of taste buds increases during postnatal development in the rat: about 91 foliate taste buds develop by 45 days of age, and about 610 vallate taste buds are formed by postnatal day 90 (Hosley and Oakley, 1987; Hosley *et al.*, 1987a,b). Electrical responses in the chorda tympani nerve in response to various chemical stimuli applied to the tongue are present from 2 days of age in the rat, when only 1–7 percent of taste buds on fungiform papillae have pores (Hill and Almli, 1980). Maturation of the taste buds in the rat correlates with their ability to discriminate between differently flavored solutions. Newborn rats show no preference between water and solutions of saccharin or quinine until 9 days of age, when they begin to prefer the sweet solution, but they reject the bitter solution only after 14 days of age (H. L. Jacobs and Sharma, 1969).

It is not known whether the gustatory nerves have an effect on cellular proliferation in the taste buds. Guth (1963) proposed that epithelial cell proliferation is independent of nerves and that nerves stimulate only differentiation of taste cells. N. Robbins (1967a) found that DNA synthesis in the taste buds of the frog is almost totally abolished by cutting the lingual nerve. However, as the rate of mitosis is very slow in the frog's taste buds, the difference between the normal rate and that after denervation is barely significant. In any case, the taste buds of frogs are sufficiently different from those of other vertebrates for Roper (1989) to decide to exclude them from comparison with those of other vertebrates.

Treatment of castrated male rats with testosterone for 30–60 days results in the development of taste buds in abnormal locations—on the upper surface of the vallate papillae of the tongue (Allara, 1952; Zalewski, 1969b). This phenomenon was investigated by Zalewski (1969b,c), in order to determine whether testosterone might be a trophic agent for taste buds. He found no obvious change in the number of taste buds after castration. Testosterone

does not maintain old taste buds or stimulate the formation of new ones in the absence of gustatory nerves. The action of testosterone on taste buds depends, in some unknown way, on the presence of normal innervation.

There are three types of gustatory papillae that bear taste buds in mammals, namely, fungiform, foliate, and circumvallate papillae on the tongue, and there are numerous fungiform-like papillae on the soft palate and epiglottis. The fungiform papilla has two or three taste buds on its oral surface. The circumvallate papilla has a circular moat, the walls of which can contain up to 279 taste buds in humans and 375 taste buds in the rat. The taste bud consists of flask-shaped cells of epithelial origin grouped like staves of a barrel composed of four types of cells (Fig. 9.13). Types I (dark cells), II (light cells), and Type III cells are long and narrow and extend from the base of the taste bud to the apical pore which communicates with the exterior. Basal cells are flat-

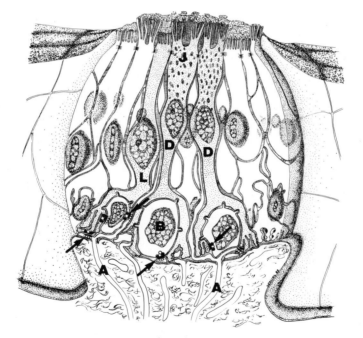

Figure 9.13. Diagram of receptor cells and synaptic connections in a taste bud from the urodele, *Necturus maculosus*. This drawing illustrates the taste cells and the synapses that they form. A taste bud from this species is shown as a summary figure, since, with only a few differences in cytological details, examples of these connections have been shown to occur in many species. Type I, or dark cells (D), and type II, or light cells (L), synapse with gustatory axons (A). Synaptic sites (arrows) often appear to be bidirectional, based on ultrastructural observations. Apical junctional complexes (J) may be the sites of electrical connections between adjacent dark cells. Basal cells (B) form synapses with other taste cells and with gustatory axons, suggesting that they may be a form of interneuron in the taste bud. From S. D. Roper, *Ann. Rev. Neurosci.* 12:329–353 (1989), copyright Annual Reviews Inc.

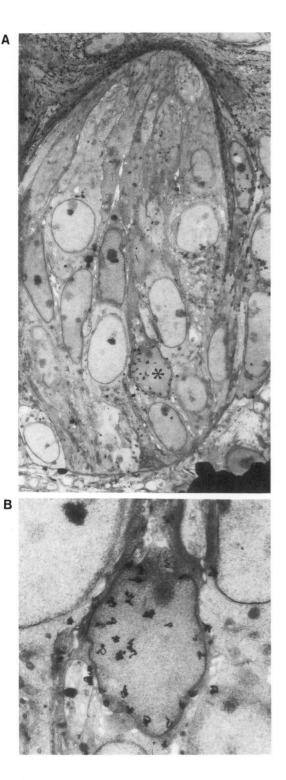

tened, lie at the base of the taste bud, and do not extend to the taste pore (Murray, 1973, 1986; Delay *et al.*, 1986; Delay and Roper, 1988; Roper, 1989, review). Type I cells comprise 55–75 percent of the population, and the other types each constitute 5–15 percent. Type III cells are marked by the presence of numerous dense-cored vesicles which may contain monoamines. All these types of cells have chemical synapse-like junctions with nerve endings and also are electrically coupled to each other. The ultrastructure of the chemical synapses is atypical and their polarity is often ambiguous (de Lorenzo, 1963; Uga and Hama, 1967; Graziadei, 1970). Roper (1989) suggests that these are features of immature synapses which are unable to develop fully before the taste cells complete their short lifespan, averaging 10–12 days in the rat (Beidler and Smallman, 1965; Conger and Wells, 1969; Delay *et al.*, 1986).

The problem of the origins of the different types of taste cells and the lineage relationships between them has been debated for almost a century (Parker, 1922, review). There are two theories to account for the origins of the different types of cells in the taste bud. The first is that the different types represent different stages of maturation of a single lineage (Kolmer, 1910; Parker, 1922). The alternative theory is that each type represents a different path of differentiation from an indifferent progenitor cell (Farbman, 1980). The evidence obtained by means of electron microscopic [3H]thymidine autoradiography (Delay *et al.*, 1986) is consistent with the 1st but not with the 2nd theory. The basal cells are the first to incorporate [3H]thymidine after a single injection and are thus the progenitor cells. This is followed by labeling of type I cells followed by an intermediate cell type and type II cells on the succeeding days (Fig. 9.14). This evidence supports the theory that the different types are stages of maturation of a single

Figure 9.14. Evidence supporting the hypothesis that there is a single cell lineage in mouse vallate taste buds. High voltage electron microscopic autoradiograph of a taste bud (A), in longitudinal section with a radioactively labeled type I (dark) cell (asterisk), from a mouse fixed 3 days after injection of [3H]thymidine. Magnification 1840×. (B) The labeled dark cell at magnification 5800×. From R. J. Delay, J. C. Kinnamon, and S. D. Roper, *J. Comp. Neurol.* 253:242–252 (1986).

lineage and not separate lineages (reviewed by Roper, 1989, but see Murray, 1986, for an alternative opinion that the terminally differentiated cell is type III).

There is a continual turnover of all the epithelial cells of the tongue, including those of the taste buds. The average lifespan of a taste bud in the tongue of the rat and mouse is about 10 days (B. E. Walker, 1960; Beidler, 1963; Beidler and Smallman, 1965; Conger and Wells, 1969). The cells in the taste bud are displaced from the periphery of the bud, where mitosis occurs, to the center of the bud, where they degenerate. This has been observed in the taste buds of the catfish (R. M. May, 1925), frog (N. Robbins, 1967a), and rat (Beidler, 1963; Beidler and Smallman, 1965). Presumably the nervous connections do not change as the cell moves, but it is not known how the nerve endings make connections with new taste cells and disconnect from those that die.

The olfactory receptor cells pose a similar problem (Graziadei, 1973, 1974; Graziadei and Monti Graziadei, 1978, review): they undergo continual replacement in all vertebrates (Fig. 9.15). The receptor cells in the olfactory mucosa are neurons whose axons form the olfactory nerve. Newly formed olfactory cells have to send their axons in the olfactory nerve to the olfactory bulb to make synaptic connections with the 2nd-order neurons. It is not known whether olfactory receptors with different response properties reconnect selectively with matching 2nd-order neurons, but that seems to be necessary if this continual disconnection and reconnection of synapses in the glomeruli of the olfactory bulb occur without any change in the overall functions of the olfactory system.

9.14. Trophic Action of Nerves on Taste Buds

Dependence of taste buds on their sensory nerves was first demonstrated more than a century ago by showing that the taste buds degenerate after denervation (Von Vintschgau and Hönigschmied, 1876; Von Vintschgau, 1880). This was the first experimental evidence of a trophic action of sensory nerves on sense organs. However, the concept of the trophic actions of nerves on a variety of tissues has a venerable history, summarized in Section 8.1. Her-

mann (1884) first proposed the theory that nerves are required for development of taste buds. Since then, there have been numerous reports of the degeneration of denervated taste buds and their regeneration and restoration of their structure and function after reinnervation (J. M. D. Olmsted, 1920a; R. M. May, 1925; Torrey, 1934; Zelená, 1964; Zalewski, 1968, 1969a–c, 1970a; Guth, 1958, 1971, review; Cheal and Oakley, 1977; Hosley et al., 1987a,b). Degeneration occurs only if the gustatory nerve itself degenerates (Torrey, 1936); if the nerve is cut proximal to the ganglion, degeneration does not occur (Kamrin and Singer, 1953; Donegani and Gabella, 1967).

The rate of degeneration of taste buds after denervation depends on the species and on the length of the distal nerve stump (see below). In the rat and rabbit, reduction in size of taste buds on the tongue is evident 8 hours after denervation, and the taste buds disappear completely in 4–7 days (Beidler, 1963). The taste buds on the barbels of the catfish show atrophic changes within a few days of denervation and disappear in 11–19 days, with the proximal taste buds degenerating before the distal buds (J. M. D. Olmsted, 1920a,b; R. M. May, 1925; Torrey, 1934; Geraudie and Singer, 1977). Complete degeneration of the frog taste buds is delayed for up to a year after denervation (N. Robbins, 1967a).

The evidence given above does not show whether the trophic effect is specific or nonspecific, that is, whether a particular type of gustatory nerve can exert a trophic effect on only one or on all types of taste buds and whether the effect can also be produced by nongustatory nerves. This has been investigated in mammals by reinnervation of taste buds by other gustatory nerves or by nongustatory nerves (Guth, 1958; Zalewski, 1969a,c, 1981; Oakley, 1974a,b; Dinger et al., 1985), and in submammals by heterotopic grafting of the tongue to regions where it is reinnervated by foreign nerves.

In the rat, the taste buds normally supplied by the glossopharyngeal nerve degenerate after denervation and regenerate after innervation by another gustatory nerve, namely, the chorda tympani or the vagus (which contains gustatory fibers to the pharynx and larynx) (Guth, 1958; Zalewski, 1969c). However, the taste buds do not regenerate after reinnervation by the hypoglossal, which is a pure motor nerve (Guth, 1958; Zalewski, 1969c). Another nongustatory sensory nerve, the auriculotemporal, is not

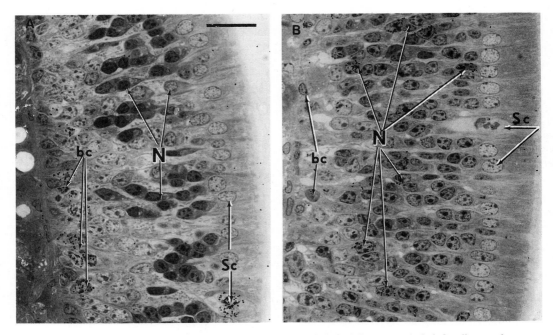

Figure 9.15. Turnover of neurons in the olfactory epithelium of the adult mouse. Labeled cells are shown auto-radiographically after injections of [³H]thymidine, in (A) at 12, 18, and 24 hours before death, and in (B) after injections twice daily for 5 days and survival for 14 days after the final injection. In (A), many basal cells (bc) and one supporting cell (Sc) are labeled but neurons (N) are unlabeled. In (B), many neurons are labeled but no basal cells remain labeled because they have either differentiated into neurons or diluted their label by repeated mitoses. Labeled neurons disappear from the olfactory epithelium 30–35 days after incorporation of the label. Bar equals 10 μm. Courtesy of P. P. C. Graziadei and A. Monti Graziadei.

able to maintain old taste buds or induce the development of new ones in the rat tongue (Zalewski, 1969c; Oakley, 1974a,b). Therefore, the trophic action required for the induction and maintenance of taste buds seems to be restricted to gustatory nerves and to be absent in motor nerves or nerves of general sensation. However, some nongustatory nerves can maintain taste buds in mammals after CNS innervation (Zalewski, 1981; Dinger *et al.*, 1985) and taste buds reappear in tongues transplanted to the anterior chamber of the eye when combined with lumbar dorsal root ganglia or after innervation by trigeminal nerve fibers from the iris (Zalewski, 1973, 1976, 1980; Gómez-Ramos *et al.*, 1979). The specificity of trophic action of gustatory nerves on taste buds is also absent in urodele amphibians. In newts and salamanders, taste buds, innervated by foreign nerves, develop in tongue transplanted to the side of the body (L. S. Stone, 1933, 1940) or the orbit (Mintz and Stone, 1934; Poritsky and Singer, 1963). Taste buds also develop in tongue transplanted to

the liver of the newt, apparently in the absence of innervation (Wright, 1964).

There are several types of taste receptor cells, and the nerve fibers from each type (sweet, salt, bitter, etc.) are largely segregated in their central projections via the chorda tympani and glossopharyngeal nerves (H. Burton and Benjamin, 1971). The way in which the appropriate connections are formed between receptor cells and nerves is not known. In theory, there are three ways in which the receptors of different types may form connections with matching taste nerve fibers: the nerve may determine the specificity of the receptors or vice versa, or both nerve and receptor may be specified independently. The first alternative is that specific types of nerve fibers impose their functional specificity on the taste cells with which they connect. This is not entirely ruled out by the evidence given below that cross-innervated taste buds in adult rats retain their original specificity, because the initial specification that occurs during embryonic development may be imposed by the nerves but may not be modifiable thereafter. The second alternative is that the receptors have inherent functional specificities which they impose on the unspecified nerves. If the receptor cell has an inherent transducer action and imposes this action upon its nerves, how is the information dealt with centrally? This is the question asked by 19th-century psychologists: If the optic and auditory nerves were crossed, would the thunder be seen and the lightning be heard? Or would there be a compensatory change in the CNS? That question is considered further in Chapter 11 in relation to afferent influences on the organization of sensory projections in the CNS. The afferent influences from the facial vibrissae, for example, determine the organization of their projections to thalamus and somatosensory cortex (see Section 11.7). When afferents from a specific sensory modality are experimentally rerouted to occupy the thalamocortical pathways normally occupied by fibers subserving different sensory modalities, the centers become substantially reorganized to conform to the modality of the afferents (see Section 11.7).

There may be no need for central reassociation of gustatory nerves during normal development because from the onset of their growth into the tongue the chorda tympani and glossopharyngeal nerves segregate to suppy different regions of the epithelium, with little overlap. This peripheral segregation of nerves occurs independently of the taste buds, which develop only after the nerves reach the epithelium. This eliminates the need for large adjustments of central connections but does not account for the formation of nervous connections with different functional types of receptors within the area supplied by one nerve. The third alternative is that both receptors and nerve fibers are specified independently, in parallel, and that nerve fibers of each type recognize the appropriate type of receptor cells and selectively connect with them. Oakley's (1967, 1970) observations on the responses of cross-innervated taste buds in the rat tongue do not greatly help to distinguish between these alternatives: the fact that the responses of the receptors are not altered after cross-union of the glossopharyngeal and chorda tympani nerves might be interpreted as evidence that the receptors can accept any gustatory nerve indiscriminately, or it could mean that, because fibers with the same functional specificity are present in both nerves, connections are formed only

between matching nerve fibers and receptors. The same problem of interpretation arises in connection with the cross-innervation experiments on the frog, performed by N. Robbins (1967b). He showed that taste buds on the tongue can be prevented from degenerating after denervation when they are reinnervated by a cutaneous branch of the trigeminal nerve. This may signify either that the trophic action of sensory nerves on taste buds is nonspecific in frogs or that the trigeminal nerve, which innervates chemoreceptors on the skin of the frog head, contains gustatory nerve fibers.

In theory, the most attractive feature of the hypothesis of independent parallel specification of nerves and receptors is that it can account for the way in which nerves form connections with a continually changing population of receptor cells. Provided that all types of receptors are continually produced, each nerve ending has only to select a receptor of a type that matches its own.

The question that remains to be answered is how the nerve exerts its trophic effect on the taste receptor cells. In the absence of direct evidence, only very tentative conclusions based on indirect evidence are possible. The hypothesis that the trophic effect is mediated by an agent transmitted from the nerve to the taste cells originated with J. M. D. Olmsted (1920a,b, 1925), who proposed that some substance *"of the nature of a hormone"* is released by the gustatory nerve endings. This hypothesis was elaborated by R. M. May (1925), who postulated the *"flow of a hormone-like substance from the cell body of the neuron to its terminations,"* and by Parker (1932).

These were the first suggestions in modern times of a flow of materials in nerve fibers. The theory of axonal transport of trophic factors was premature: for 30 or more years the theory was not widely accepted because of its resemblance to the ancient belief in the flow of vital spirits in the nerves and because of a preoccupation at that time with the mechanisms of transmission of action potentials that drew attention away from other functions of the neuron. The trophic factor theory only began to have a strong heuristic value, stimulating new research, after the serendipitous discovery of NGF (see Section 8.12).

Parker (1932) and Torrey (1934) discovered that the latent period between cutting of nerve and the onset of atrophic changes in denervated sense organs is proportional to the length of the distal stump of nerve, and they conjectured that a trophic factor is stored in the nerve and transported distally to supply the sense organs. Their observations were repeated and confirmed during the next 50 years. In the rabbit there is a correlation between the length of the distal stump of the transected glossopharyngeal nerve and the time of onset of degeneration of the taste buds (State and Dessouky, 1977). In the gerbil, after section of the glossopharyngeal nerve there is a linear relationship between the length of the peripheral nerve stump and the decline of taste response in the tongue to 50 percent of control level (Oakley *et al.*, 1980). The results are consistent with the theory that a trophic substance is depleted from the distal nerve stumps at a rate of about 4 cm/day. Other evidence supporting that theory are that after the lateral line nerve of the catfish has been cut, degeneration of the lateral line organs spreads proximodistally from the cut at a rate of about 2 cm/day (Parker, 1932; Parker and Paine, 1934). A similar correlation has been found between the length of the peripheral stump of a severed motor nerve and the time of onset of atrophic changes in muscle (J. V. Luco and Eyzaguirre, 1955; Emmelin and Malmfors, 1965). J. V. Luco and Eyzaguirre (1955), after cutting the motor nerve to the tenuissimus muscle of the cat, showed an apparent proximodistal flow of trophic factor at the rate of 2 mm/hour for the first 73 hours, and from 1.4 mm/hour to 0.5 mm/hour thereafter. These results suggest that the latent period might be due to the gradual depletion of a reservoir of trophic factor in the peripheral stump of the nerve, which is released at the nerve terminals. It seems that a trophic factor may flow proximodistally in sensory and motor nerves at about the same rate, that is, on the order of 2–4 cm/day. Additional evidence supporting that theory is that block-

ade of axonal transport by means of colchicine applied to the glossopharyngeal nerve of the gerbil results in a marked reduction of taste responses 2–3 hours after application of the colchicine (Oakley *et al.*, 1981). Chronic blockade of axonal tranport completely eliminates taste response and results in degeneration of taste buds (Sloan *et al.*, 1983).

In summary: Development of peripheral sensory organelles and formation of connections between them and sensory nerve endings are complex processes involving at least five developmental programs. Firstly, inductive cellular interactions between epithelia and underlying mesenchyme specifies the types of structures that may differentiate in epithelia, for example, the different types of Merkel cells, Pacinian corpuscles, taste buds, and other specialized cell types. Secondly, sensory nerves are stimulated to grow into epithelia by extracellular matrix molecules and probably by diffusible trophic factors synthesized by cells in the epithelia. Thirdly, there is evidence that ingrowing sensory nerve endings are attracted to certain cells which serve as targets, and specific connections form between those targets and certain types of sensory nerves. Fourthly, sensory nerves stimulate differentiation of specific types of sensory organelles with which they connect. The sensory organelles fail to differentiate or degenerate in the absence of nerves during a critical early period of their development. The role of Schwann cells in these processes may be significant but has not been adequately studied. Fifthly, nerves are required for maintaining the differentiated state and vitality of the sensory organelles, temporarily during development or permanently throughout life depending on the type of sensory organelle.

10 Histogenesis and Morphogenesis of Cortical Structures

That the cortex of the cerebrum, the undoubted material substratum of our intellectual activity, is not a single organ which enters into action as a whole with every psychical function, but consists rather of a multitude of organs, each of which subserves definite intellectual processes, is a view which presents itself to us almost with the force of an axiom. . . . If . . . definite portions of the cerebral cortex subserve definite intellectual processes, there is a possibility that we may some day attain a complete organology of the brain-surface, a science of the localization of the cerebral functions.

Alexander Ecker (1816–1887), *Die Hirnwindung des Menschen*, 1869

10.1. Historical Orientation[1]

In my opinion there are only quantitative differences, not qualitative differences, between the brain of a man and that of a mouse. Accordingly, all cortical regions which are vested with a specific structure and a specific function and are differentiated in humans are also represented—with the corresponding simplification and reduction—in the mammals and probably even in the lower vertebrates.

Ramón y Cajal (1852–1934), Estudios sobre la corteza cerebral humana. III. Cortez motriz. *Revista trimestral micrográfica* 5:1–11 (1890)

Three important theories of nervous organization, valid for our time, emerged from the cell theory. Firstly, the demonstration that the nerve cell and fiber are parts of the same structure (first claimed by Remak, 1838) was the first step in the formulation of the neuron theory, which is discussed in Sections 5.1 and 6.1. Secondly, recognition that there are different types of nerve cells, even in the same region, was the beginning of the theory of neuronal typology. Thirdly, realization that there are regionally specific patterns of nerve cells and fibers, especially in the cerebral cortex, was the beginning of a theory of cytoarchitectonics (reviewed by Brodmann, 1909; Lorente de Nó, 1943; Kemper and Galaburde, 1984).

Those extensions of the cell theory were linked to the theory of evolution of the nervous system and, especially as seen from the viewpoint of this chapter, to the theory of evolution of the

[1]A wealth of information about the history of the cerebral and cerebellar cortex can be obtained from the primary authors as well as from easily available and reliable secondary sources (E. Clarke and O'Malley, 1968; R. M. Young, 1970; A. Meyer, 1971; E. Clarke and Jacyna, 1987). The purpose of this historical orientation is to identify the leading ideas and to relate them to a conceptual framework (see M. Jacobson, in preparation).

401

forebrain. Evolution of the telencephalon was understood as a process which exploited the neural structures—cell groups and their connecting fiber tracts—laid down during earlier stages of evolution. Telencephalization involves selective expansion and elaboration of the front end of the neural tube. This starts phylogenetically with the evolution of the floor plate which becomes the huge basal cell masses of fishes. The later phylogenetic advances may be seen as successive additions of new pallial formations: first the primordial pallium of fishes, next the primary hippocampo-pyriform pallial formation of Amphibia, thereafter the secondary hippocampal and pyriform cortices of reptiles, and finally the neopallium of mammals. Efforts were made to trace the phylogenetic order of emergence of different fields in the neopallium and to relate phylogeny to ontogeny. This research program was constructed, around the end of the 19th and beginning of the 20th centuries, by many workers, notably L. Edinger, C. J. Herrick, Elliot Smith, and Ariëns Kappers.

The two quotations standing at the head of this chapter emphasize the early historical origin of two major concepts of organization of the cerebral cortex: firstly, the concept of parcellation of the cerebral cortex into different areas which subserve specialized functions; secondly, the concept of a common organizational scheme for the entire cortex. Questions arising out of the first concept relate to how the different regional specializations develop. For example, to what extent are the specialized areas preformed from the time of their origin and to what extent do they differentiate epigenetically from a simple primordial pattern to a more complex final organization? Karl Ernst von Baer recognized that *"each step in development is made possible only by the immediately preceding state of the embryo. . . . From the most general in form-relationships the less general develops, and so on, until finally the most special emerges"* (Entwickelungsgeschichte der Thiere, Part 1, pp. 147, 224, 1828). Subsequent studies of brain development were made within the framework of the theory of epigenesis—from simple to more complex stages of ontogeny—and also within the framework of a theory of ontogeny recapitulating phylogeny.

The concept that the mature organization of the cortex develops from a more uniform early state and the final state emerges by addition as well as elimination of components was already well established by the beginning of this century. Korbinian Brodmann (1909, p. 226) summarized that concept of progressive versus regressive differentiation as follows: *"Considered genetically it is partially new production of anatomical cortical fields, partially their regression or reversion which are combined here. . . . Undoubtedly both processes, that is progressive and regressive differentiation, occur concurrently during development of cortical fields."* This was a premature theory which could not be substantiated until more than 70 years later.

Several questions emerged regarding the conservation of certain features of cortical organization in different regions in all mammals. For example, how have the six layers and their characteristic cell types, inputs, and outputs been conserved? Are the similarities based on homology, meaning that they share the same evolutionary ancestry, or are they based on analogy, meaning that they evolved under similar functional and adaptive pressures regardless of ancestry?

Franz Joseph Gall (1825) first theorized that different mental faculties are represented in separate regions of the surface of the human brain. Although he claimed to be able to relate the cortical representations to bumps on the cranium, he did not claim to be able to delimit separate cortical areas subserving different faculties. Before the 1860s it was generally believed that the cerebral cortex is the seat of psychic and mental functions while motor functions were believed to be controlled by the brainstem. Those beliefs were established by Jean-Pierre-Marie Flourens (1794–1867) on the basis of his surgical ablation experiments. One of his principal achievements was to demonstrate that the cerebellum functions to coordinate voluntary movements. That was then the strongest refutation of Gall's phrenological theory which localized sexual functions in the cerebellum (Gall, 1835, Vol. 3, pp. 141–239; for a brief history of concepts of cerebellar function see Dow and Moruzzi, 1958, pp. 3–6). Flourens concluded that the cerebrum is the seat of sensation but is not directly involved in control of voluntary movements. Flourens understood that different functions are localized in different parts of the brain, but he concluded that the cerebral cortex functions as a whole, as the organ of sensory perception, intellect, the will, and the soul. (For detailed consideration of Flourens' views, which changed in the two editions of his *Recherches*, see R. M. Young, 1970.)

There were two opposing schools of thought about cerebral localization—we can call those "lumpers" who saw unity in diversity, and we can call those "splitters" who saw diversity in unity. The prevailing views at different moments of history have tended to oscillate between the extreme lumper and splitter positions. Flourens belonged to the school of lumpers who believed that the cerebral hemispheres function as a whole.

Those beliefs were put in doubt by the observations of Hughlings Jackson (1863) that tumors and other disease processes involving the cerebral cortex sometimes cause seizure movements that progress from distal to proximal limb muscles, often involve the facial muscles, and resemble fragments of purposeful movements. Jackson proposed that the cerebral cortex directly controls body movements, especially of the face and distal limbs. He theorized that cerebral cortical control of movements is organized in terms of coordinated movements and not of individual muscles, for any muscle could be brought into play in a variety of different movements.

Experimental support for part of Jackson's theory was provided by Fritsch and Hitzig (1870), who evoked coordinated movements of body parts in the dog in response to galvanic stimulation around the cruciate sulcus of the cerebral cortex on the opposite side. Much better evidence of a somatotopic motor representation was obtained by Faradic stimulation of the cerebral cortex of the monkey (Ferrier, 1875, 1876, 1890) and higher apes (Grünbaum and Sherrington, 1902, 1903; Leyton and Sherrington, 1917). The latter also showed that the postrolandic area is inexcitable, contrary to the general belief at that time that the rolandic area is both sensory and motor (Mott, 1894; Bechterew, 1899; see Fulton, 1943, and A. Meyer, 1978, for the history of the concept of sensorimotor cortex and of the efforts to delimit sensory regions of cortex). Cushing (1909) provided the first evidence that stimulation of the postcentral gyrus in humans can result in somatic sensation without movement. It was only after it became possible to record electrical cortical re-

sponses evoked by peripheral stimulation that the somatotopic sensory projections to the cortex could be mapped physiologically in cat, dog, and monkey (Adrian, 1941; C. N. Woolsey, 1943).

The area of cerebral cortex from which body movements could be evoked with shortest latency and lowest threshold was defined physiologically as the primary motor cortex. However, it was known that movements can be elicited from widespread cortical areas by using suprathreshold electrical stimuli (Fulton, 1935; Hines, 1947a,b). Mapping those cortical areas led to the discovery of the supplementary motor cortical area, which was found first on the mesial surface of the frontal lobe of the human brain (Penfield and Welch, 1949, 1951; T. C. Erickson and Woolsey, 1951) and later confirmed in experimental animals (C. N. Woolsey, 1952, 1953, 1958; G. Goldberg, 1985, review). The areas defined physiologically were correlated with the anatomical localization of giant pyramidal cells and with the origins of the pyramidal and extrapyramidal pathways (Bechterew, 1899; Brodmann, 1905). The structure–function correlations were strengthened by observations of functional deficits and the extent of nerve fiber degeneration following cortical lesions (Fulton and Kennard, 1934; Fulton, 1935; Hines, 1947b).

From those studies the motor cortex appeared to be organized as a mosaic in which each body part is represented in somatotopic order. Whether fundamental units of cortical organization are movements or individual muscles (e.g., H.-T. Chang *et al.*, 1947) is an important question that has been reviewed by Kaas (1983) and D. R. Humphrey (1986), but is beyond our scope.

Let us now briefly summarize the evolution of modern concepts regarding the cellular organization of the cerebral cortex (see M. Jacobson, in preparation). The principal concepts regarding cellular organization evolved in parallel with construction of the neuron theory as summarized in Sections 5.1 and 6.1. **There were five crucial conceptual advances made surprisingly rapidly in the final 60 years of the 19th century: recognition that the nervous system is composed of many types of nerve cells and fibers grouped in characteristic morphological patterns; understanding that nerve fibers are outgrowths of nerve cells; making the distinction between axons and dendrites in terms of** differences in structure and in the direction of transmission of nervous activity; understanding that nerve cells are linked by contact at synaptic junctions; and conceiving of function in terms of integration of excitatory and inhibitory actions mediated by different synapses. Making allowances for the inevitable overlap between them, it may be useful to consider these concepts evolving in the order given above, and as parts of a research program, advancing to progressively higher levels of understanding.

Koelliker, in the 1st edition of his *Handbuch der Gewebelehre*, 1852, was already able to classify nerve cells according to shape (pyriform, fusiform, etc.) and according to the number of processes emerging from the cell body (apolar, unipolar, or bipolar). Koelliker's cellular typology was originally based on the appearance of unstained neurons dissociated from fixed brain. The first evidence confirming that similar differences between cell types occurs in a regular histological pattern in sections of the cerebral cortex stained with carmine was reported by Berlin (1858). The concept of structural types was linked to that of functional differentiation, termed by A. Milne-Edwards (1857, Vol. 1) the *"physiological division of labour,"* one of the dominant concepts of biology in the latter half of the 19th century (see Herbert Spencer, 1876, p. 166; Oscar Hertwig, 1893-1898, Vol. 2, p. 79). In adopting that concept, Cajal (1900) also emphasized that the *"principle of division of labor, which holds sway more in the brain than in any other organ, requires that the organs which register sensations are different from those which register memories."*

In addition to the **principle of functional differentiation**, 19th-century studies of the cerebral cortex were guided by two other principles, namely, the **principle of functional and structural homology** of cortical areas in different mammals, and the **principle of divergent differentiation** of homologous parts in relation to their use and disuse in different mammals. These three principles are discussed at length by Brodmann (1909, Chapter 7), and they continue to influence our current ideas about development and evolution of the cerebral cortex. For example, evidence that cells with similar functional properties are clustered together anatomically in the cerebral cortex is consistent with the principles of functional differentiation and of functional and structural homology. Examples in the visual cortex are the ocular dominance and orientation columns in the primary visual cortex (Hubel and Wiesel, 1962, 1968) and color clusters in the primary visual area (Livingstone and Hubel, 1984; Tootell *et al.*, 1988c) and 2nd visual area (Hubel and Livingstone, 1987). Horizontal and corticocortical connections also link clusters or groups of neurons with similar functional specificities (Gilbert and Wiesel, 1989).

The first schemata of cortical architectonics were guided by the principle of regional structural–functional differentiation and were based on differences in sizes and shapes of cell bodies and by their horizontal layering. Those features dominate the histological picture in sections of cerebral cortex stained with carmine, which was the best method of staining then available (Berlin, 1858; Meynert, 1872; Lewis, 1878; Lewis and Clarke, 1878). Despite the limitations of the histological techniques (see Section 6.2), the architectonics of the cerebral cortex was first worked out in remarkable detail by Theodor Meynert (1867–1868, 1872). Cajal (1911, p. 601) says that Meynert's *"study was so exact that, notwithstanding the imperfection of his methods, it is still the best we possess."* Meynert (*Bau der Grosshirnrinde*, 1868, p. 58) subdivided the cortex into two main types: one with a white surface layer and the other with a gray surface layer. The latter he subdivided into five-layered cortex ("general type" and "claustrum formation") and eight-layered cortex (e.g., calcarine cortex). The white-surface cortex he also called "defective cortex" (including Ammon's horn, uncus, septum pellucidum, and olfactory cortex).

Another guiding principle was that certain cortical regions have been conserved during evolution in all mammals and can be recognized by their functions and structures, especially with respect to layering of certain types of neurons and their afferent and efferent connections. This principle of structural and functional homology generated a terminology in which the homologies are implied. Terminology often reflects the theoretical prejudice of the users. Edinger (1908a,b) coined the term paleencephalon to mean the phylogenetically most ancient part of the central nervous system (CNS), and the only part in most fishes, as contrasted with what he termed the neencephalon, of which the neocortex is the most recent culmination. The concept that the CNS of modern amniotes contains a core of ancient structures that are overlaid by layers of structures that evolved at later times was originated by L. Edinger (1908a,b) and Ariëns Kappers (1909). This concept has been extended by McLean in his theory of the triune brain. According to McLean (1970, 1972), the brain of higher primates is formed of three systems that originated in reptiles, early mammals, and late mammals. A related concept is that the cerebral cortex enlarges during evolution simply by addition of new areas (Smart and McSherry, 1986a). But evolution does not simply add new levels of organization on top or by the side of the old levels, so to say, like strata in an archeological site. No, the old adapts to the new and they all continue to evolve. Progression of the old and new occur together. The progression is not A→AB→ABC but A→A′B→A″B′C and so on. Terms such as paleocortex, neocortex, and archicortex imply a phylogenetic progression which is not well based on evidence, and I use those terms only with certain qualifications. Those terms were coined by Ariëns Kappers (1909) on the basis of comparative studies of lower vertebrates, and their transferral to the mammals, and especially to primates, is a questionable practice. The terms rhinencephalon and pallium were adopted by Koelliker (1896) in his monumental attempt to attach ontogenetic and phylogenetic significance to the different regions of the cerebral cortex.[2] The term "rhinencephalon," for example, was associated with the concept of macrosmatic, microsmatic, and anosmatic brains, that is, with the importance of the sense of smell in the evolution of the species (Broca, 1878; Turner, 1891; Retzius, 1898). The rhinencephalon was seen as

either hypertrophied or atrophied in different species, depending on their use of the sense of smell. For example, the olfactory tubercle, prepyriform area, retrosplenial area, and amygdaloid nucleus were regarded as atrophied in the primates, in which the sense of smell is relatively weak.

Finally, the principle of divergent differentiation embraces the concepts of differentiation of several cortical areas from a protocortex, of progressive adaptation of cortical differentiation as a result of natural selection during evolution and as a result of use and experience of the individual, and also includes the concept of plasticity of the cortex after injury. As Brodmann (1909, p. 243) clearly understood, all these can occur as a result of progressive or regressive transformations.

We should also remember that a theory prevalent at the end of the 19th century held that nerve cells are all multipotential or even equivalent at early stages of development, and that nerve cell differentiation is controlled by afferent stimulation. Koelliker (1896, Vol. 2, p. 810) summed up the evidence in no uncertain terms: "*So I am finally forced to the conclusion that all nerve cells at first possess the same function, and that their differentiation depends solely and entirely on the various external influences or excitations which affect them, and originates from the various possibilities that are available for them to respond to those contingencies.*" This concept has attained current validity with the evidence that cerebral cortical functions can be specified by afferent nerve fibers (see Sections 10.9 and 11.7). The concept that localization of functions in the cerebral cortex is determined by the input from the periphery and is not autonomously determined within the CNS has endured for more than a century and continues to receive support (e.g., D. D. M. O'Leary, 1989, review). This theory was held by Golgi and Nissl among anatomists, Flourens and Goltz among physiologists, and S. Exner, Wundt, W. James, and Lashley among psychologists (reviewed by Neuberger, 1897; Soury, 1899; Lashley, 1929; Holt and Riese, 1950, 1951; Walker, 1957; Tizard, 1959). For example, Wundt (1904, p. 150) says, "*We know, of course, that the cell territories stand, by virtue of the cell processes, in the most manifold relations. We shall accordingly expect to find that the conduction paths are nowhere strictly isolated from one another. We must suppose, in particular, that under*

[2]The successive editions of *Handbuch der Gewebelehre* by Koelliker (six editions from 1852 to 1896) are invaluable for tracing progress during the 2nd half of the 19th century. A very useful single source of information, in English translation, about the mid-19th-century levels of understanding of development and structure of the nervous system is the *Manual of Histology* edited by S. Stricker (English ed., 3 Vol., 1870–1873). It contains chapters on research techniques, the cell theory, and embryonic development by S. Stricker, spinal cord by J. Gerlach, the retina by M. Schultze, and on brains of mammals by T. Meynert. In his autobiography, Cajal refers to Stricker's treatise as "*a model . . . invaluable for the devotee of the laboratory*" and notes that he acquired a copy in 1883, before he started his investigations of the histology of the nervous system, and considerably earlier than his initial use of the Golgi technique in 1887–1888.

altered functional conditions they may change their relative positions within very wide limits." As Brodmann (1909) says, *"All these theories are in fundamental agreement in their concept that the ganglion cells are equivalent forms, unencumbered by their origins, their positions, or their external forms."*

The concept of an organology of the cerebral cortex, as expressed by Ecker in the epigraph to this chapter, for example, attained maturity with the cytoarchitectonic and myeloarchitectonic maps, which aimed at showing the structural and presumed functional parcellation of the cortex. This concept can be traced back to the phrenological theory of Gall and Spurzheim, whose *Anatomie et Physiologie due Système Nerveux* (1810–1819), especially in Volumes 1 (1810) and 2 (1812), tried to establish a relationship between the intellectual functions and the shape of the cranium and the underlying convolutions. The phrenological theory, while incorrect in the localization of so-called intellectual and moral functions, was based on much correct anatomical observation, especially that of Gall. Its main significance was to have given an impetus to studies of the relationship between structure and function of the cerebral cortex (see E. Clarke and O'Malley, 1968; R. M. Young, 1970). Out of such studies has come the principle that the magnification of cortical representation is proportional to the functional importance of the peripheral sensory or motor fields and that the primary gyri correspond fairly well, although not precisely, with cytoarchitectonic fields and with functional representation in the cortex (Connolly, 1950, pp. 264–269; Kaas, 1983).

The cortical cytoarchitectonic map of Campbell (1905) is the prototype based on the differences in layering of the cell bodies revealed in Nissl-stained sections. Campbell's structure–function correlations had the virtues of simplicity and reasonableness and were initially communicated to the Royal Society of London by Sherrington in 1903 before publication in book form in 1905. The introduction of the Weigert stain in 1882 resulted in an efflorescence of studies of the fiber tracts of the CNS (Bechterew, 1894; Edinger, 1896) and of the cerebral cortex (Vogt, 1904; Poliak, 1932). Difference in the time of development of myelin in the cerebral cortex was another criterion that was pressed into service to demarcate different regions of the cortex (Flechsig, 1898, 1901, 1903, 1927; Zunino, 1909). This direction of research led to the publication of cerebral cortical maps of increasing complexity, in which the relevance to function and development tends to be inversely proportional to the number of cortical regions demarcated (Campbell, 1905, shows 20; Brodmann, 1909, shows 52; Von Economo and Koskinas, 1925, delimit more than 100). We may ask whether the trend shows an increasing departure from reality or a progressive approach to the truth. Neither fits snugly into any theory of history of neuroscience, unless it is a theory of evolution of hypertrophic species which results in the ultimate extinction of the monstrosities. The last in the line of progressively more complicated cortical maps by Von Economo and Koskinas (1925) and the myeloarchitectonic studies of the Vogts (1902, 1904, 1919, review) are probably destined to remain forever enshrined in their gigantic volumes, to be opened by the curious bibliophile, but ignored by the working scientist looking for useful information.

Distrust of the validity of cortical maps was based on what the mappers left out as much as on their excessive zeal to split fields. The reaction to these errors of omission or errors of commission took an extreme, almost nihilistic form in the statement by Lashley and Clark (1946) that in some cases, *"architectonic charts of the cortex represent little more than the whim of the individual student."* Their skepticism was aroused by the evidence available at that time showing lack of correspondence between electrophysiologically defined cortical areas and anatomically defined architectonic areas. The correspondence has more recently been shown to be quite precise (Kaas, 1983, review). Moreover, quantitative computerized morphometric analysis of cortical cytoarchitectonics has eliminated subjective evaluation and has largely confirmed the validity of classical cytoarchitectonic and myeloarchitectonic maps (Fleischhauer *et al.*, 1980; Zilles *et al.*, 1980, 1982; Wree *et al.*, 1983). The more criteria used to distinguish between different cortical areas, the more subdivisions tend to be revealed: in addition to classical cytoarchitectonics, modern cortical maps take into consideration cortical inputs and outputs, intracortical connections, histochemical and immunocytochemical markers, electrical activity and functional properties of the constituent neurons, overall functions, and the effects of lesions (Braak, 1980; Wise and Goschalk, 1987).

Cajal (1922) was alert to the problem of errors of omission resulting from the use of highly selective stains: *"There is little value, therefore, in dealing with the differentiation of cortical areas based exclusively on the revelations of the Nissl and Weigert methods, because they show an insignificant portion of the constituent features of the gray matter."* In Cajal's hands, the Golgi technique, complemented by staining with methylene blue and reduced silver nitrate, led to the discovery of the dendritic spines and many new types of neurons. The breadth of his observations on the anatomical relationships between different types of neurons in the cerebral cortex and his views on the functional subdivisions of the cortex (for example, he argued that precentral and postcentral gyri are both sensory and motor) can now be appreciated more easily in the English translation by De Felipe and Jones (1988) of a large selection of Cajal's writings on the cerebral cortex.

Koelliker was the pivotal figure connecting the epochs before and after the general use of the Golgi technique. I agree with the assessment by Lorente de Nó (1938) that *"Kölliker's account of the structure of the human cortex (1896) is one of the masterpieces of neuroanatomy and it marks the end of an historical period of research on the cerebral cortex."* Golgi occupies a unique position in the earlier epoch as a solitary worker who discovered his marvelous technique prematurely in 1873 and worked with it in virtual isolation unaided by critique, until the significance of his work was first recognized by Koelliker in 1887 (see Section 6.2). Cajal occupies a different position as the person uniquely capable of using the Golgi technique to build on the foundations laid by those in the earlier epoch.

The wealth of information about the cellular organization and functions of the nervous system that had been amassed by the end of the 19th century was codified in the large textbooks published at that time (Koelliker, 1896; Bechterew, 1899; Soury, 1899; Ramón y Cajal, 1899–1904; Sherrington, 1906; Van Gehuchten, 1906). It was finally possible to consider the organization of the CNS in terms of functional assemblies of different types of neurons linked together by synaptic junctions and to analyze their input and output relationships anatomically and physiologically. This synthesis is set forth in Sherrington's lectures on *"The Integrative Action of the Nervous System"* (1906), in which he gives the evidence showing the importance of reflex inhibition and the concept of the final common path. For a history of the concept of nervous inhibition see Fearing (1930, pp. 187–217) and Fulton (1938, p. 77). We may ask how it was possible for Fearing (1930),

in his masterly history of reflex action, to make only two passing references to the work of Cajal.

It is curious that Cajal appears to have failed to grasp the significance of inhibition: he does not refer to it, and he did not accept the challenge of trying to identify the structural substrates of inhibitory functions in the CNS. The question of whether entire neurons or only parts of them had inhibitory functions seems to have eluded him. This may have been because his grasp of anatomical organization was descriptive, albeit at a very high level of insight. His concept of functional organization was dominated by the notion of polarized flow of excitation, which could be altered by changes at the synapses, but he failed to see the significance of inhibition and the final common path as they were worked out by Sherrington (1897, 1904, 1906). By contrast, Sherrington was one of the first to fully understand the significance of Cajal's discoveries.

It has often been said that achievements in neuroscience in recent years are unprecedented. Never before has so much been discovered by so many at such great expense, but I am unable to affirm that we are witnessing a golden age such as that which took place a century ago.[3] The flow of discoveries in neuroscience has never been stronger than in the 1890s, and it must have been exhilarating to live in a time when the tide came rushing in day after day bearing new gifts. In at least one other respect it resembles our own molecular biological era: priority for discovery is determined by speed of publication as much as by the moment of discovery.[4] The smart investigator joins the rush to publish every new find, but few can match Cajal, who pub-

---

[3]It should be remembered that almost all of Ramón y Cajal's important work was done in the 4 years from the beginning of 1888 to the end of 1891. Cajal said that he reached the height of his powers in 1888, and that he *"celebrated his Palm Sunday,"* acclaimed by the multitude, in 1890 and 1891. Other giants of that era, Koelliker, Lenhossék, van Gehuchten, and Retzius, were also phenomenally productive in the first decade after 1887, following their use of the Golgi technique.

[4]Bruce Alberts (1989) believes that *"today's biologist faces an easy harvest of riches. For the next twenty years or so, one need not be especially clever or wise to make major contributions to biology. With luck, even the random cloning of a new gene—which requires little skill and no insight—can turn out to be exciting."* The opportunistic use of powerful techniques generates much exciting data but leaves little time for reflection on their relation to theories and values.

lished 19 of his 28 papers in 1890 and 1891, at the rate of one almost every month, in the *Gaceta Médica Catalana* and other local journals, to establish priority. Later he expanded and republished many of them in journals with international distribution. Not all his contemporaries had the advantage of rapid publication (see Section 6.1).

By the closing decades of the 19th century less than 100 workers had laid the secure foundations on which neuroscience continues to be upheld. This can be confirmed by perusal of the great textbooks that appeared at the end of that golden age. To go back in search of the golden age is not to deny, but rather to affirm, the values of the present. That more than half my references are to works published since 1980 shows that I have chosen to put my money on the future. A final comment—we cannot simply compare the past with the present. Each has to be dealt with on its own terms. We have new problems, and even when we take up their old problems we arrive at new solutions, different from theirs.

10.2. Comments on Assembly of Complex Neuronal Systems

Attempting to reduce the massive and intricate body of knowledge about neuromorphogenesis to a single chapter, the author is reminded of Samuel Johnson's sentence in the Preface to his *Dictionary of the English Language* (1755): *"Wherever I turned my view, there was perplexity to be disentangled and confusion to be regulated: choice was to be made out of boundless variety."* We are faced with an almost impenetrable thicket of data. We might show some humility in the face of this mass by considering one fact at a time, but slow progress is one of the penalties exacted by humility. Instead, we have to push on as fast as possible and stand ready to answer for mistakes. When Samuel Johnson was asked why he had made a mistake in his dictionary, he replied, *"Ignorance, madam, pure ignorance."* The following comments are made in that undogmatic spirit.

My first comments have to do with how fates of neurons are specified. Neuronal fates in vertebrates are indeterminate and probabilistic (M. Jacobson, 1980, 1985, review; see Section 2.11). Even neurons that are generated in small numbers such as Rohon–Beard neurons and the Mauthner neuron in fishes and amphibians, have an indeterminate lineage (Jacobson, 1981a,b; Jacobson and Moody, 1984; Kimmel and Warga, 1986). Neurons in the cerebral and cerebellar cortex have indeterminate lineages (Walsh and Cepko, 1988; Luskin *et al.*, 1988; Price and Thurlow, 1988). Their fates are decided by epigenesis, which involves a sequence of determinative events which are contingent on their positions at the time of generation, their pathways of migration, interaction with afferent fibers, interactions between their axons and targets, and transsynaptic effects of afferents. We conceive of neuronal specification as a sequential and progressive process and have provided evidence to that effect (M. Jacobson and Moody, 1984; also see Sections 10.3 and 11.7 for evidence of progressive specification of cerebral cortical neurons).

Morphogenesis of the cerebral cortex and cerebellar cortex illustrates the main phases of neuromorphogenesis: first, consecutive production of different types of neurons and glial cells and their migration to characteristic positions; second, a period of growth which includes production of redundant dendritic and axonal branches and the formation of transient connections; and, finally, pruning of the excessive growth and death of redundant neurons. The establishment of the final definitive pattern of cellular relationships is thus the resultant of several processes that are patterned in space and time, namely, histogenesis, cell migration, cell interactions, cell differentiation, elimination of neuronal processes and synapses, and cell death.

The temporal sequence of neuron production and differentiation in neuronal sets is correlated with the temporal sequence of formation of connections between those sets. Considerable evidence supporting that concept has come from studies of the temporospatial gradients of time of neuron origin, using [^{3}H]thymidine labeling as discussed in Section 3.10. This is a fundamental concept concerning assembly of complex neuronal systems. It raises questions regarding the coordination of programs of histogenesis and cell differentiation in different neuronal sets that are initially separate but finally connect together, reciprocally in some cases as between the corpus striatum and substantia nigra (Bayer and Altman, 1987, review), as shown in Fig. 10.1. I conceive of the entire nervous system sharing the same reference coordinates which are established in the early embryo (see Section 2.2), as illustrated in Fig. 11.6.

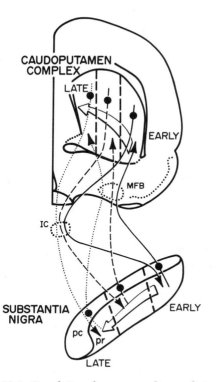

CAUDOPUTAMEN
COMPLEX

LATE

EARLY

MFB

IC

SUBSTANTIA
NIGRA

EARLY

pc

pr

LATE

Figure 10.1. Correlations between gradients of time of neuron origin, time of nerve fiber outgrowth, and formation of connections in the nigrostriatal system. Axons of the early-originating nigral neurons (continuous lines) project via the medial forebrain bundle (MFB) to form connections with neurons originating earliest in the ventrolateral caudoputamen complex. Reciprocal connections develop from superficial neurons in the lateral part of the complex projecting via the internal capsule (IC) to synapse with neurons in the dorsolateral substantia nigra. Thus, early-originating neurons in both structures are interconnected. The same temporospatial relationships hold for neurons that are intermediate in age (dashed lines) and those which originate late (dotted lines). From S. A. Bayer and J. Altman, *Prog. Neurobiol.* 29:57–106 (1987).

One may conceive of these programs of assembly of complex neuronal systems having evolved gradually to attain some degree of optimization. The tendency to optimization is reflected in certain features of histogenesis and morphogenesis that are common to many parts of the CNS of vertebrates: spatial and temporal gradients of cell production, migration, and differentiation; separate origins of neighboring regions that are different cytoarchitectonically; a predisposition for phylogenetically older parts of the brain to originate earlier in ontogenesis. Optimization of development of complex neu-

ronal systems always requires constraints. In the first place the system is limited by physical constants. For example, diffusion coefficients set limits to the scale of patterns that can be set up in the embryo by diffusible morphogens; the upper and lower limits of cell size are set by various physical constants, and so on. The total number of variables is enormous. What may be optimal for one process is certain to be suboptimal for many others, so that the entire structure and its global functions, not separate components, are the units on which natural selection works. Combinations, not each process separately, tend to be optimized. Indeed, the word "optimized" conveys a false meaning unless it is understood in relative rather than absolute terms. Evolution is a process of making do, of finding provisional working solutions, and very rarely attaining optimal solutions. One way to conceive of evolution of the nervous system is in terms of a series of incomplete solutions. Each new partial solution can only exploit what is already given by previous incomplete solutions. I think this is similar to what Jacob (1982) means when he states that evolution causes changes in development by "tinkering."

Neuronal groups are elementary units composed of a small number, usually about five, of different types of neurons. Complexity arises from iteration of neuronal groups and from elaboration of the patterns of connections between neuronal groups, rather than from the variety of neuronal types. Iteration of a neuronal group to form a regular array is seen most clearly in the retina, cerebellar cortex, and cerebral cortex. Complexity of this kind is achieved with great economy of structural and regulatory genes. Lorente de Nó (1938) introduced the concept that *"the cortex is composed of an enormous number of elementary units, not simply juxtaposed but also overlapping."* How such reiterated patterns may develop is considered in Section 11.5. The elementary unit may provide the primordial, pluripotential organization from which a potential diversity of final patterns of organization can develop epigenetically. Complexity may be achieved by constructive processes or by deconstructive processes, by addition or elimination of neuronal groups or of individual cells, fibers, and synaptic connections. Generation of redundancy and later elimination of many components also reduces the genetic load that would be required for constructing invariant patterns of organization.

Morphogenesis literally means the generation of form, and all the processes and mechanisms that are involved in forming the nervous system can be subsumed under that term. Constructive processes include generation of cells, cell migration, changes in cell shape, cell growth, cell interactions, cell differentiation, assembly of cells, and formation of synaptic connections. Regressive or deconstructive processes include elimination of many temporary structures and down-regulation of molecules that subserve transient functions. Morphogenesis is essentially epigenetic: each state is both the cause of future states and the result of prior states of the system. While identification of individual types of neurons is necessary, and recognition of their taxonomic relationships is useful, the latter is artificial because the nervous system is not an assembly of single cells but of cell groups, or populations. Cells do not normally develop in isolation, but as groups. Therefore, development should be considered in terms of cell groups, and mechanisms identified by which cell groups are established and by which cells develop collectively, rather than individually.

Cell interactions are required to form nerve cell collectives and to coordinate and integrate their development. Interactions between the cells are of many kinds and involve many different molecular mechanisms. There are short-, medium-, and long-range interactions. Short-range interactions occur between cells in direct contact and between cells and components of the intercellular matrix. They include cell interactions mediated by cell surface adhesion molecules and cell surface recognition molecules. There is an attractive parsimony in the concept of morphogenesis being accomplished by a few different cell adhesion molecules that are regulated with respect to the molecular species, quantities, and time and place of expression during development (see Section 1.7). However, this oversimplified concept needs to be enlarged to accommodate the medium- and long-range morphogenetic molecules and the regulation of their expression during development. One has to add that short-range interactions between cells, by means of cell surface recognition and adhesion molecules, could not alone suffice to produce a complex organism in which all parts develop and function in correlation. To achieve such coordination it is necessary to have medium- and long-range interactions by means of diffusible molecules, such as growth factors and

trophic agents. Medium-range interactions over a distance of about 100 μm are mediated by diffusible morphogens released from specific cells and taken up by other cells bearing specific receptors. Long-range interactions involve molecules that are released, diffuse, or are transported over long distances in relation to the size of the embryo (several hundred microns to several millimeters) and affect cells bearing specific receptors. Long-range cellular interactions are mediated by growth factors and hormones. The functional specificity of these mechanisms may result from differences between the molecules that are involved, their quantities, spatial distributions, and the time and duration of their expression.

Concerning the order of genesis of various types of neurons, the cerebellar cortex illustrates the differences between two main classes of neurons. In most regions of the CNS there is one type of neuron, termed the *principal neuron* or type I neuron or macroneuron, which is surrounded by a constellation of *local circuit neurons*, also called type II neurons or microneurons. The cells with long axons, first called *projection cells* by Schäfer, have long been recognized as having significantly different functions from the local-circuit neurons. The latter have also been named switching or connecting cells (*Schaltzellen*) by von Monakow, *intermediate cells* by Schäfer, association cells (*Vereinigungszellen*) by Bechterew, and cells with short axons (*células de cilindro-eje corto*) by Ramón y Cajal (1897). The principal neuron is usually the largest neuron in its neuronal group, is the first neuron to originate and differentiate in that set, and is usually the only neuron to project its axon outside its neuronal group. All these criteria of a principal neuron are met by the cerebellar Purkinje cell. All inputs converge, either directly or indirectly, on the Purkinje cell, and it is the sole pathway for outflow of information from the cerebellar cortex. The local circuit neurons, namely, Golgi type II, stellate, basket, and granule cells, all originate later than the Purkinje cell, and all make their axonal connections entirely within the cerebellar cortex.

The Purkinje cells have already lined up in an orderly layer before the local circuit neurons originate or migrate to their final positions. We do not know how these cells assemble in their correct spatial relationships, but it is a plausible hypothesis that, in each system, the principal neuron, being the first in the field, serves as the main organizing influence on the assembly of the local-circuit neurons. The principal neuron has greater autonomy than the local-circuit neurons, and this is shown by the fact that the program of development of principal neurons is relatively insensitive to changes in external conditions (see Section 10.14) or to mutations that primarily affect local-circuit neurons (see Section 10.15).

The complexity of the mammalian brain prompted a search by several of the founders of modern neuroscience, especially Gustaf Retzius, for "simple" nervous systems in which the analysis of neuromorphogenesis might be accomplished more easily. While such simple systems as are found in the nematodes, some molluscs, and some arthropods may provide the advantages of large neurons and relatively small total numbers of cells, the complexity in such nervous systems is no less than it is in the basic set of five neurons in the mammalian cerebellum. Indeed, there are no more than a few thousand different types of neurons in the entire mammalian brain, and each part of brain can be reduced to a neuronal set that contains about five types of neurons, as in the neuronal set that is the basic circuit module of the cerebellar cortex.

It is not the variety of cell types that makes the cerebellar cortex and cerebral cortex more complex than the kidney, for example. Both are built on the principle of modular construction, that is, by iteration of a basic morphological module or cellular group. Rather, complexity arises from the variety of interconnections between the different cell types belonging to a neuronal group (intramodular complexity), from the combinations of connections between similar neuronal groups within the cortex (intermodular complexity), and from the connections of neuronal modules with different modules in other parts of the CNS. Regional differences in complexity can also occur as the result of regionally different amounts of cell death. Complexity arises from iteration of neuronal groups and, therefore, in expansion of neuronal fields, in the cerebral cortex, for example. The thickness of the cortex remains fairly constant throughout the mammalian series but the cortical area increases progressively. This is one indication that complexity evolved by addition of neuronal groups rather than by increase in complexity of the individual elementary neuronal group.

10.3. Development of the Cerebral Cortex: Overview

The complexity of this topic makes a *tour d'horizon* desirable to identify some of the more significant observations and concepts.

The structure of the cerebral cortex is similar in all mammals. Brodmann (1909, p. 198) shows that the similarity between all mammals in the organization of cerebral cortical fields is evident in three ways: (1) in the similarity of the overall pattern; (2) in the constancy of structure of individual regions; (3) in the persistence of individual fields in the entire mammalian series.

Cautious extrapolation of data from one mammalian species to another is quite defensible. However, extrapolation to submammalian species is more difficult to justify. Reptiles and birds have a relatively simple telencephalic cortex, whose structure varies in different species, and which has been said to be homologous to the mammalian hippocampus, but may indeed have evolved quite separately from the mammalian cerebral cortex (Ariëns Kappers *et al.*, 1936; Pearson, 1972; Northcutt, 1981; Tsai *et al.*, 1981; Goffinet, 1983; Molla *et al.*, 1986). An indication of separate evolution of submammalian and mammalian cerebral cortex is that the sequence of origin of cortical layers in birds is outside-in (Tsai *et al.*, 1981) but it is the reverse in mammals.

There are enormous species differences in area of the cerebral cortex in different mammals, but the cortical thickness varies relatively little (average ranges from 1.5 mm to 3.5 mm) in species as different as mouse and humans in which brain weight averages 1 g and 1350 g, respectively. In a phylogenetic series of mammals there is marked increase in the area of cerebral cortex, and in the complexity of cortical organization as shown by increases in the glia-to-neuron ratio and in the proportion of local-circuit neurons. This is discussed more fully in Section 2.12.

There are two general types of mammalian cerebral cortex, named homogenetic and heterogenetic by Brodmann (1909) and subsequently referred to as isocortex and allocortex by Oskar Vogt (1911). According to Brodmann (1909, p. 243) all homogenetic cortex is initially based on the six-layered basic pattern but can be subdivided into homotypic and heterotypic regions, depending on whether the initial plan is preserved or lost. Homotypic regions preserve the six-layered pattern throughout ontogeny, but heterotypic regions pass through a six-layered stage during development and either gain additional layers by splitting of the original embryonic layers (e.g., striate cortex) or lose layers as a result of atrophy or fusion of embryonic layers (e.g., precentral area). By contrast, heterogenetic cortical formations lack a six-layered pattern during ontogeny and phylogeny (e.g., olfactory bulb, hippocampal formation, subiculum, induseum griseum, septum pellucidum, entorhinal area, presubicular and prepyriform area).

The isocortex has significant regional variations in the numbers of different types of cells, but all isocortex, which constitutes most of the cerebral cortex in humans, has six layers when viewed in Nissl-stained sections and has a uniformity of structure in all regions (Brodmann, 1909; Vogt, 1911; Rockel *et al.*, 1980). The allocortex has less distinct and variable lamination and has a well-developed superficial tangential fiber layer. The allocortex receives its afferents, especially olfactory, through the tangential layer, whereas the isocortex receives its afferents from the thalamus or elsewhere through the underlying white matter. As a general rule, the proportion of allocortex is larger in animals in which olfaction is dominant over vision, and the reverse applies to the isocortex.

Attempts to classify cortical regions according to their ontogenesis have been made by Flechsig (1876, 1927) on the basis of myelination, and by Brodmann (1909) and M. Rose (1926) on the basis of cytoarchitectonics, but their results, especially the latter, are limited by incomplete and often erroneous data about histogenesis that was available to them. Cytoarchitectonic maps of the cerebral cortex aim to reflect functional and ontogenetic differences between cortical areas. Campbell (1905) shows about 20 different cortical areas; Brodmann (1909) shows 52; Von Economo and Koskinas (1925) delimit more than 100. All three are in essential agreement on the main areas of the isocortex, but they differ mainly on the number of subdivisions of allocortex (for critical reviews of cortical cytoarchitectonics see Lorente de Nó, 1943; Bailey and Bonin, 1951; for an extreme reaction against the validity of cytoarchitectonic mapping see Lashley and Clark, 1946). The transitions between regions of the cerebral cortex are not in question, but we still do not understand their mechanisms of development.

Historically, the question of how different areas of the cerebral cortex develop their unique characteristics has led to two opposing theories: either the specializations emerge from an initially equipotential state or they originate from predetermined rudiments (see Section 10.1). According to one recent version of the latter theory, the ventricular germinal zone consists of a mosaic of proliferative units that are the basis for development of cortical microcolumns and are organized as a protomap of prospective cytoarchitectonic areas (Reznikov *et al.*, 1984; Rakic, 1988). These theories, which may be called epigeneticist and preformationist theories of cortical ontogeny, both allow plasticity, but by different means—under varied conditions the preformed rudiments may develop at different rates and to different degrees, whereas specialized functions can emerge by progressive specification of neurons within the equipotential cortex. In both cases the relative positions of the final boundaries between functionally specialized areas may shift under different normal or experimental contingencies. One question is whether the boundary shifts are caused by differential growth of the parts or by the assumption by one part of the characteristics of another. In the first case an expansion of one area (e.g., by sprouting of axons, dendritic expansion, increased cell proliferation) occurs to compensate for a contraction of another area. In the second case reorganization of existing components occurs. The two cases are not mutually exclusive.

There are at least four ways in which differences between cortical areas may develop: neuronal fates, intracortical connections, cortical inputs, and cortical outputs may be determined differently. Each of these can occur by different mechanisms. For example, neuronal fates may be determined by lineages from specified progenitors, by epigenetic interactions, by progressive and regressive differentiation. Intracortical circuits may change as a result of expansion or contraction of dendritic trees, formation and elimination of synaptic connections, and changes in synaptic functions. Fiber projections may be organized differently in the final state as the result of regionally selective outgrowth or selective elimination of an initially diffuse projection. The latter may take the form of death of neurons, elimination of entire axons, or only retraction of collaterals.

The patterns of histogenesis will undoubtedly prove of value in defining different cytoarchitectonic regions and the relationships between structure and function of the cerebral cortex. The cerebral hemispheres develop from the region of the rostral dorsal part of the neural tube named the telencephalic pallium. The wall of the pallium is at first formed of clonogenic neuroepithelial germinal cells (see Section 2.2) whose continued proliferation is the main cause of outward bulging of the pallial walls to form the cerebral vesicles. The radial alignment of these neuroepithelial germinal cells imposes a primary radial pattern on histogenesis of the pallium. This primary radial organization is progressively distorted by generation, differentiation, and growth of neurons and glial cells, and by formation of afferent and efferent nerve fibers, all of which impose a horizontal lamination on the primary radial pattern. The distortion of the simple radial pattern makes it necessary for neurons to be guided by radial glial cell processes that maintain uninterrupted paths from the zone of neuronal generation to the zones in which the neurons finally settle.

Postmitotic neurons migrate from the ventricular zone towards the surface of the cerebral vesicles. These young neurons meet ingrowing corticopetal axons, mainly monoaminergic fibers from the midbrain and pons, that form a primordial superficial plexiform layer and form the first horizontal layering. Neurons enter the superficial plexiform layer to form the cortical preplate. The cortical plate develops within the preplate as neurons continue to migrate out of the ventricular germinal zone. The cortical plate splits the cortical preplate tangentially to form layer I of the cerebral cortex and a subplate formed from the deeper fibers and some neurons of the preplate. The first neurons to enter the plexiform layer differentiate as the Cajal–Retzius cells and some other types of neurons, which, together with the superficial fibers, form layer I of the cortex. Neurons continue to migrate from the ventricular and subventricular zones into the cortical plate, where they assemble in an "inside-out" order (layers VI–II in sequence), as described in Section 10.6.

During the early stage of development of the cerebral cortex, young neurons are guided from the ventricular zone into the cortical plate by the radially aligned neuroepithelial cells. As the pathway of migration increases in length after formation of the cortical plate, and as the cortical neurons have to migrate past those that originated

earlier, they are guided toward the surface by radial glial cells. Thalamocortical axons arrive at the cortical plate before many of their target neurons in layer IV are generated. These axons may synapse temporarily on neurons located in the subplate before transferring their synaptic connections to cortical plate neurons. Neurons arrive in the deep layers of the cortex and start forming circuits while those of layers II and III are still migrating. In addition to the inside-out gradient, there are also anterior–posterior and lateral–medial gradients of cell production and differentiation.

During development of the cortex there is a period of reorganization of transient structures during which neurons die and many corticopetal nerve fibers and their synaptic connections are eliminated. After formation of all the definitive layers of the cerebral cortex the ventricular zone disappears. No neurons are produced postnatally in the cerebral isocortex but production of granule cells in certain parts of allocortex continues for some time after birth. Generation of macroglial cells continues in the subventricular zone throughout life (see Sections 2.10 and 3.3).

10.4. Formation of the Cortical Preplate

During the development of the cerebral cortex four transient tangential zones can be recognized in the wall of the cerebral vesicle, named, from the ventricle outward, the ventricular, subventricular, intermediate, and marginal zones (Boulder Committee, 1970).[5] In terms of that concept, cell proliferation occurs in the ventricular zone during early

---

[5]Revision of nomenclature is a necessary and ongoing process to keep the terminology consistent with new knowledge. The Boulder Committee terminology now requires further revision to include the role of the preplate in cortical ontogeny. Revision of nomenclature has always been controversial (His, 1895; Herrick and Herrick, 1897; Wilder, 1897; Warwick, 1978), but we no longer always deserve the judgment that *"the anatomic nomenclature coming from America in recent years I hold to be completely wrong. . . . One should hope that a scholar who has enjoyed an adequate schooling, should not lightly accept the many barbarisms of this nomenclature such as . . . cephalad, caudad, dorsad, cephalo-dorsad . . . hemicerebrum etc . . . but would first go out and learn what these terms mean"* (Koelliker, 1896, p. 814).

stages and in the subventricular zone at later stages of development; the intermediate zone becomes the white matter; the marginal zone consists of tangential fibers and the first neurons to be generated, and becomes layer I of the cortex. According to that concept the cortical plate (the future layers II–VI) develops as neurons migrate to lie *between* the marginal and intermediate zones. However, that scheme has had to be modified by the evidence originally obtained by Marin-Padilla (1971, 1978, 1983, 1988) that the cortical plate develops *within* a preplate. The preplate is formed of a superficial plexus of corticopetal nerve fibers and the earliest generated neurons. The later-generated neurons migrate to form a layer within the preplate, thus splitting it into a superficial superplate (layer 1) and a deep subplate (interstitial layer VII). Both superplate and subplate contain neurons that were generated earliest. Those in layer I differentiate as Cajal–Retzius cells and other types of neurons that have not yet been characterized (see Section 10.5). Some authors propose that many of the cells in the interstitial layer die (Luskin and Shatz, 1985a; Valverde and Facal-Valverde, 1987; Shatz *et al.*, 1988, review), but others suggest that their decrease in numerical density results from growth of the brain (Marin-Padilla, 1972; Rickmann *et al.*, 1977). Many neurons of the embryonic interstitial layer differentiate as interstitial neurons in the white matter of the adult (Kostovic and Rakic, 1980; Valverde and Facal-Valverde, 1988).

10.5. The Cajal–Retzius Cells and Layer I

Cajal–Retzius cells are the first neurons to mature in all regions of the cerebral cortex of mammals, and cells of similar appearance and position also occur in the cerebral cortex of submammals. The presence of the external plexiform layer and Cajal–Retzius cells before development of the cortical plate has been reported in the mouse (Goffinet and Lyon, 1979), rat (König *et al.*, 1975, 1977, 1981; König and Marty, 1981; Raedler and Sievers, 1976; Raedler and Raedler, 1978; Raedler *et al.*, 1980; Rickman *et al.*, 1977; Rickman and Wolf, 1981), cat (Marin-Padilla, 1971, 1978), and in human embryos (Larroche, 1981; Larroche and Houcine, 1982; Marin-Padilla and Marin-Padilla, 1982; Marin-Padilla, 1983, 1990).

The Cajal–Retzius cell has a large stellate cell body in the upper part of layer 1 of the cerebral cortex. It has a single axon descending vertically, extending many collaterals in all directions horizontally to run for a long distance in the middle level of layer 1, and finally terminating as a horizontal myelinated fiber in the lower half of layer 1, making synaptic contacts with apical dendrites of pyramidal neurons. Usually it has several horizontal dendrites, 500 μm–1 mm long radiating in all directions parallel to the surface of the cortex, which apparently make contacts with axons in the external plexiform layer. These afferent fibers of unknown origin, possibly mesencephalic, are already present before the arrival of the Cajal–Retzius cells. The Cajal–Retzius cells have the morphology of horizontal multipolar neurons, as seen in Golgi preparations (Marin-Padilla, 1970a, 1990) and in electron micrographs (Raedler and Sievers, 1976; Edmunds and Parnavelas, 1982; Parnavelas and Edmunds, 1983), and they express neuronal but not glial cell markers (König and Schachner, 1981). Their functions remain an enigma.

Cajal–Retzius cells were discovered in the rabbit by Ramón y Cajal (1891) and in the same year in the human fetus by Retzius, who at first thought they were glial cells. Retzius (1893, 1894) recognized that they are neurons and called them "Cajal's cells." Cajal later jokingly referred to them as "Cajal's cells of Retzius" (see F. Clarke and O'Malley, 1968, p. 443). The relationship of those cells to the primordial tangential nerve fibers of the cerebral cortex was shown by Koelliker (1896; see Fig. 10.2). They are the first neurons to be generated, starting on E12 in the rat temporal cortex (König *et al.*, 1977), and have already arrived in the marginal zone of the rat occipital cortex on E13 before any other neurons of the isocortex have been born, and differentiate rapidly to reach maturity before the rat's birth.

There is some controversy regarding the fate of Cajal–Retzius cells and whether they atrophy and disappear or merely become greatly reduced in numerical density as the cortex increases in volume. They may also become altered in position and morphology after birth. According to Marin-Padilla (1970a, 1990), the Cajal–Retzius cells form the first neuronal circuits to be found in the motor cortex, and these persist through life. They appear during the intrauterine period in humans and have been

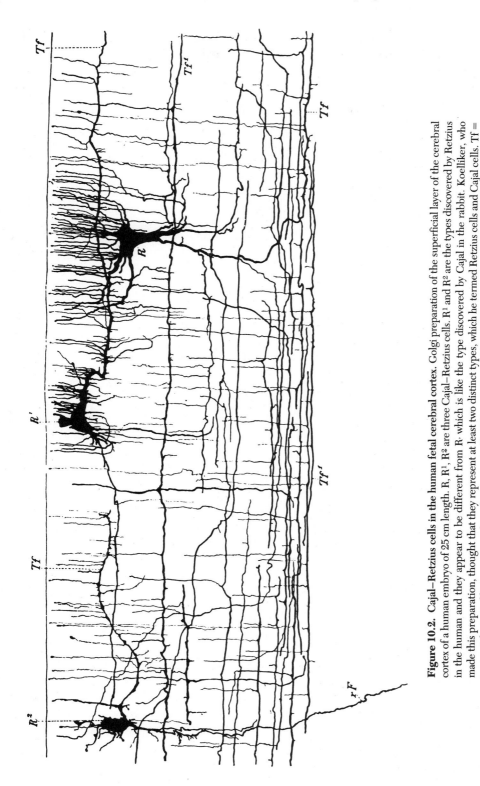

Figure 10.2. Cajal–Retzius cells in the human fetal cerebral cortex. Golgi preparation of the superficial layer of the cerebral cortex of a human embryo of 25 cm length. R, R¹, R² are three Cajal–Retzius cells. R¹ and R² are the types discovered by Retzius in the human and they appear to be different from R: which is like the type discovered by Cajal in the rabbit. Koelliker, who made this preparation, thought that they represent at least two distinct types, which he termed Retzius cells and Cajal cells. Tf = tangential nerve fibers connected to the Retzius cells; Tf¹ = tangential nerve fibers without visible connections, therefore regarded by Koelliker as afferents; rF = radial fiber of the cell R². From A. Koelliker, *Handbuch der Gewebelehre des Menschen*, Vol. 2, p. 661 (1896).

said to atrophy and disappear shortly after birth (Noback and Purpura, 1961; Duckett and Pearse, 1968). In the human fetus during the last months of gestation and early postnatal period, the Cajal–Retzius cells have been reported to lose their dendritic attachments to the pia and move more deeply into the molecular layer, and to disappear shortly after birth (Conel, 1939-1963: Vol. I, p. 103; Vol. II, p. 9; Vol. III, p. 9; Vol. IV, p. 7). However, in the adult, there are horizontal cells in layer I which are called the "horizontal cells of Cajal." Ramón y Cajal (1909–1911) distinguished between the fetal and adult forms of horizontal cells in layer I and suggested that the fetal type matures and persists as the adult type of horizontal cell. Molliver and Van der Loos (1970) reported that Cajal–Retzius cells can be found only until 12 days after birth in the dog, but similar cells have been reported in the adult dog brain (M. W. Fox *et al.*, 1966). Thus, while it is possible that some of these cells may atrophy and disappear, it is certain that many survive in a modified form as a class of horizontal cells in the superficial layer of the cerebral cortex, where their dendrites receive inputs from axons in the superficial plexiform layer and their axons make synaptic contacts with the apical dendritic branches of pyramidal neurons (Marin-Padilla and Marin-Padilla, 1982; Marin-Padilla, 1990).

10.6. Histogenesis of the Cortical Plate

The time of origin ("birthdates") of neurons in the mammalian cerebral cortex has been determined by injecting the gravid female with tritiated thymidine, killing the fetuses at intervals after the injection, and determining the pattern of labeled neurons in autoradiographs of histological sections of their brains (see Section 2.10).

Labeling with [³H]thymidine reveals a very orderly pattern of generation, migration, and assembly of neurons in tangential strata. Neurons of the cerebral preplate originate first and later differentiate as Cajal–Retzius cells and other neurons of layer I and as interstitial neurons of the subplate. Neurons of the cortical plate are generated continuously by mitosis of germinal cells, first in the ventricular zone and later in both the ventricular zone and subventricular zone. The first neurons to be generated migrate outward to con-

tact layer I. Neurons that arrive near the surface of the cortical plate are displaced to deeper levels by those that arrive later. Thus, the cortical layers are assembled in an inside-out sequence. Different classes of cells in the cerebral cortex are generated over different time periods and from different germinal cell populations. How this developmental timetable is coordinated and controlled by genetic and epigenetic mechanisms remains one of the most compelling problems yet to be unraveled.

The finding that neurons of the cerebral isocortex are assembled in a sequence in which the oldest neurons occupy the deepest cortical layers (Sidman *et al.*, 1959; Uzman, 1960; Angevine and Sidman, 1961) falsified the hypothesis that the layers of the cerebral isocortex develop sequentially from superficial to deeper layers, which had been continually repeated after it was first proposed by His (e.g., Tilney, 1933).

Since 1959, the mapping of neuron birthdates has given rise to volumes of data. With rare exceptions most of these catalogues of neuron birthdates, bereft of even the most timid conceptual analysis, read like the minutes of a committee meeting. They can be summarized in general terms in a few sentences. Neurons of the cerebral isocortex in most mammals originate over a restricted prenatal period occupying about one-third of the gestation time. They are generated, migrate, and differentiate relatively slowly, so that there are significant disparities between the first and last neurons to be generated. The neurons of the cortical plate assemble in an inside-out sequence and also show regional differences (spatial gradients) of time of origin. The temporal order of generation of neurons is quite well correlated with the order of outgrowth of their axons and the formation of synaptic connections between neurons within a set and between different sets (Bayer and Altman, 1987, review). The birthdates given below should be regarded as averages—the actual time of origin of neurons depends on their position in the spatial gradients, and in the case of the commonly used experimental animals, on the genetic strain.

In the mouse, all the neurons of the cerebral isocortex originate over a period of about 7 days of a 19-day gestation period, from E11 to E17 (Angevine and Sidman, 1961). In the rat, with a gestation time of 21 days, the neurons of the preplate originate on E12 (König *et al.*, 1977), and neurons of the cortical plate are generated on E16–E21 in an inside-out order (Berry and Rogers, 1965; Berry *et al.*, 1964a,b; Hicks and D'Amato, 1968; Derer, 1974). Histogenesis of the cerebral cortex has been described in detail in the rat. This is considered later. In the visual cortex of the ferret, which has a 41-day gestation, neurons are generated from E20 to P14 (C. A. Jackson *et al.*, 1989) In the cat, the gestation time is 65 days, and the majority of neurons of the cerebral cortex originate between E30 and E57 (Luskin and Shatz, 1985a,b) as shown in Fig. 10.3. In humans with a gestation time of 265 days, all the neurons of the cerebral isocortex originate over a period of about 100 days during midgestation starting at about E40 and continuing to about E125 (Poliakov, 1965; Rakic, 1978); in rhesus monkey, they are generated over a corresponding 60-day period in a gestation time of 165 days (Rakic, 1974). For example, all neurons in the visual cortex (areas 17 and 18) originate between E40 and E100 in the rhesus monkey (Rakic, 1974, 1977).

There are also anterior–posterior and lateral–medial gradients of cell proliferation in the cerebral isocortex such as are found in other regions of the CNS. The spatial origin of the gradients in the somatosensory cortex seems to correspond with the eventual location of the oropharyngeal region of the sensorimotor somatotopic representation (Smart, 1983). Anterior-to-posterior and lateral-to-medial gradients of neuron origin have also been found in the visual cortex of the monkey (Rakic, 1976), cat (Luskin and Shatz, 1985b), and ferret (McSherry, 1984; McSherry and Smart, 1986). There appears to be no relationship between those gradients and the retinotopic projection to the cortex in the cat (Luskin and Shatz, 1985b) or ferret (C. A. Jackson *et al.*, 1989).

The regularity of genesis of neurons and glial cells in the cerebral cortex of the rat has provided data with which to arrive at some general principles of cortical histogenesis (Bayer and Altman, 1987, review). During the earliest period of cortical histogenesis in the rat, from E13 to E14, mitosis occurs exclusively close to the ventricle. Neurons produced during that time arrive in the primordial plexiform layer on E16–E17. The subventricular germinal zone forms on about E16 (see Section 10.8). After E16 the ventricular and subventricular zones produce young neurons and probably also glial cells which migrate into the cortical plate over a period of

several days from E17 to E21. There they eventually occupy the deep cortical layers.

A transition in the program of cortical cell generation occurs at about E19. After E19 mitosis is greatly reduced in the ventricular germinal zone, which ceases to produce neurons. Neurons and glial cells continue to be generated in the subventricular zone from which cells migrate into the superficial layers of the cortical plate where they settle between E21 and P3. After about E21, only glial cells are generated in the subventricular zone of the isocortex. Cell production, migration, and assembly in the cerebral isocortex is extended over many days (in contradistinction to the short time, usually 1 or 2 days, required for the same processes to take place in nuclear neuronal structures).

Prenatal ontogenesis of the human cerebral cortex (Fig. 10.4) follows the same program as homologous regions of the cerebral cortex in other mammals, taking into consideration the prolonged period of human gestation, the altricial state of the human newborn, the delayed development of manual dexterity and of language, and the vastly increased numbers of neurons in the human cerebral cortex (Poliakov, 1953, 1956, 1959, 1961, 1965; Sarkisov and Preobrazhenskaya, 1959; Marin-Padilla, 1970a, 1983, 1984, 1988; Marin-Padilla and Marin-Padilla, 1982; Larroche, 1981; Larroche and Houcine, 1982). Generation of neurons starts at about E40 and lasts for about 2 months: it stops at about E100 in the primary visual cortex (Brodmann's area 17), and at E70 in the limbic cortex (area 24) (Rakic, 1978).

In the motor cortex (precentral gyrus, area 4) of human embryos the arrival of afferent fibers follows a regular sequence, occurring in each layer before and during the time of arrival of neurons in that layer (Marin-Padilla, 1970a). The first fibers arrive in layer I and are followed by the Cajal–Retzius cells, which are the first neurons to originate and to differentiate in the human motor cortex. Thereafter, the pyramidal cells of layer VI and layer V can be seen at 5 months of gestation. These are followed by the interneurons of layer IV (cortical basket cells) about the 7th prenatal month. Then follow the pyramidal cells of layer III, and finally those of layer II can be readily recognized at 7.5 months of gestation. Various types of local-circuit neurons and small neurons of diverse forms appear in all cortical layers during the late prenatal period.

Temporospatial gradients of genesis of neu-

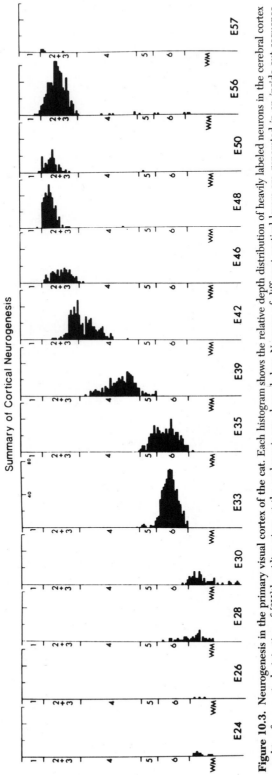
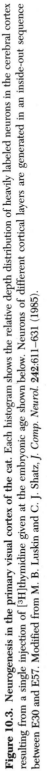

Figure 10.3. Neurogenesis in the primary visual cortex of the cat. Each histogram shows the relative depth distribution of heavily labeled neurons in the cerebral cortex resulting from a single injection of [³H]thymidine given at the embryonic age shown below. Neurons of different cortical layers are generated in an inside-out sequence between E30 and E57. Modified from M. B. Luskin and C. J. Shatz, *J. Comp. Neurol.* **242**:611–631 (1985).

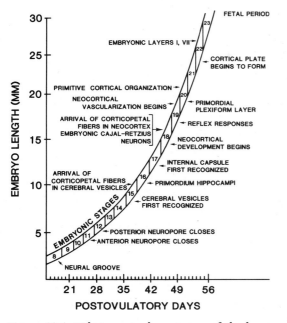

Figure 10.4. Milestones in the ontogeny of the human neocortex. Adapted from M. Marin-Padilla, *Anat. Embryol.* 168:21–40 (1983).

rons in the allocortex of the hippocampal formation have been elucidated in considerable detail. There is a very close correspondence between developmental patterns and cytoarchitectonic divisions of the hippocampal formation (Fig. 2.8). The pattern of histogenesis may thus be of considerable value in helping to delimit cytoarchitectonic regions of the cerebral cortex. There are three gradients of neurogenesis in the hippocampal region: deep to superficial, sandwich, and rhinal to dentate.

Deep neurons are generated before superficial neurons throughout the hippocampal region (consisting of Ammon's horn, dentate gyrus, entorhinal cortex, subiculum, parasubiculum, and presubiculum). The first neurons of the hippocampus are generated from the ventricular germinal zone on E10 in the mouse fetus (Angevine, 1965; Stanfield and Cowan, 1979a) and E15 in the rat (Schlessinger *et al.*, 1975; Bayer, 1980a). The hippocampus displays the "inside-out" sequence of time of neuron origin similar to that described in other regions of the cortex. The younger neurons migrate through previously formed layers to form more superficial layers. In many structures the neurons formed later are sandwiched between those formed earlier (Bayer

and Altman, 1987, review). In the hippocampal region the granule cells of the dentate gyrus are sandwiched between the early-forming large neurons in the hilus and medium-sized neurons in the molecular layer; the pyramidal cells in Ammon's horn are sandwiched between early-formed neurons, for example. Finally, there is a lateral-to-medial gradient, with cells originating first closer to the rhinal fissure and later closer to the dentate gyrus (Angevine, 1965; Schlessinger *et al.*, 1978; Bayer, 1980a). The precise significance of these gradients is still not clear—presumably they are adaptations to facilitate assembly of complex neuronal systems, as discussed in Section 10.2.

Neuron formation in the hippocampal region is completed before birth in the fetal mouse and rat (Bayer, 1980a). However, neurons in the dentate gyrus continue to be formed until postnatal day 20. In the hippocampal formation of the rhesus monkey the first neurons originate almost simultaneously in all regions on E38 but formation of neurons destined for each region ceases at different times: production of pyramidal cells ends between E70 and E80 in area CA1, between E56 and E65 in area CA2, between E65 and E70 in area CA3, and between E75 and E80 in area CA4. Generation of granule cells of the dentate gyrus continues throughout the second half of gestation and gradually declines until it ends about the 3rd postnatal month in the rhesus monkey (Rakic and Nowakowski, 1981a).

In the stratum granulosum of the dentate gyrus there is an "outside-in" order of formation. The primary germinal zone for these cells is in the wall of the lateral ventricle, whence cells migrate along the fibers of the hippocampal fimbria to the dentate gyrus. These displaced germinal cells continue to divide in the dentate gyrus to produce glial cells and granule cells. The granule cells that originate first migrate to the outer edge of the stratum granulosum, and the stratum granulosum grows simply by addition of new neurons to its inner edge.

The granular neurons of the dentate gyrus that are formed postnatally originate locally and are derived from germinal cells within the cortex (Angevine, 1965; Altman and Das, 1967). In the newborn guinea pig labeled granule cells appear in the inner layer of the stratum granulosum of the dentate gyrus 6 hours after injection (Altman and Das, 1967). Clearly, these labeled granule cells must have originated locally, for they could not have migrated from the wall of the lateral ventricle in the short period of 6 hours. In the mouse and rat, progenitors of the granular neurons of the dentate gyrus originate from the ventricular zone for a relatively short period of embryonic development (before E14), and they then migrate to the dentate gyrus, where their proliferation continues for a long time, at least until P20 (Schlessinger *et al.*, 1975; Stanfield and Cowan, 1979a; Bayer, 1980a). This is the only example known at present of a germinal zone within the cortex itself giving rise to neurons of the cerebral cortex, and it should be noted that only granular neurons originate in that way. The external granular layer of the cerebellum is rather similar in that it consists of germinal cells that have migrated from the rhombic lip (ventricular germinal zone in the alar plate of the medulla) over the surface of the cerebellum, where they give rise to the local circuit neurons of the cerebellum. This cerebellar external granular layer is continuous with the germinal zone in the lateral wall of the fourth ventricle and with the pontobulbar body caudally. This extensive germinal zone gives origin to the granular neurons of the cerebellum, cochlear nuclei, and pontobulbar nuclei (Essick, 1907, 1909, 1912; Harkmark, 1954; Taber Pierce, 1966, 1967a,b).

In the mouse, granule cells originate from this extensive germinal zone until at least 20 days after birth (Stanfield and Cowan, 1979). Different inbred strains of mice have markedly different numbers of dentate granule cells, and there are also differences between males and females (R. E. Wimer *et al.*, 1978; C. C. Wimer and Wimer, 1989). Genetic analysis using reciprocal crosses between strains with high and low granule cell numbers and either with or without sexual dimorphism with respect to granule cell numbers shows that 80 percent of the variability in granule cell numbers is attributable to autosomal differences in genotype. The sex differences appear to involve a cytoplasmic factor operating only in females. The factor appears to operate by increasing granule cell death in females, which occurs in both sexes between P20 and P27 (R. E. Wimer *et al.*, 1988).

10.7. Migration of Neurons into the Cortical Plate

There are two different modes of migration of cerebral cortical neurons from the ventricular zone to cortical preplate and cortical plate. During early stages neurons migrate either freely or along neurepithial cells. Late-migrating neurons such as hippocampal granule cells are guided by radial glial cells. This is an adaptation allowing the late-migrating neurons to navigate through a complex tissue via increasingly tortuous pathways.

F. C. Sauer (1935a,b, 1936) has shown that neuroepithelial cells lose their external (pial) attachment and round up toward the ventricle before mitosis. This may also occur in the telencephalon during the early stages of its development before a thick mantle layer has developed. Neurons formed at that stage might lose attachments to internal and external surfaces of the telencephalon and therefore migrate into the mantle layer free of attachments, as Angevine and Sidman (1961) and Stensaas (1967b) suggest. The germinal cells of the telencephalon have numerous branching cytoplasmic processes that are attached to the pial surface, and it is improbable that these external connections break down during every mitotic cycle as the nucleus moves toward the ventricle during metaphase. In the Golgi and silver preparations of the developing cerebral cortex of the rat, Berry and Rogers (1965) found that the germinal cells retain their attachment to the pial and ventricular surfaces, and cells that detach from the pia and round up toward the ventricle during mitosis were not seen. They proposed that the cytoplasm of the germinal cell may not divide immediately after mitosis, but that the daughter nucleus may migrate within the cytoplasm of the maternal cell toward the pial surface where cytoplasmic division may occur. This proposal was founded on light microscopic evidence that neuroepithelial cells occasionally appear to have two nuclei.

Golgi studies of neurogenesis in the forebrain of the opossum (Morest, 1969a, 1970a) do not reveal any evidence of free, ameboid migration of young neurons. According to Morest, the young neuron remains attached by a cytoplasmic process to the germinal zone and extends a cytoplasmic process to the external surface of the forebrain. The nucleus and perikaryon then move into the cytoplasmic process toward the external surface. Next, the primitive processes disappear and the axon and dendrites differentiate. In many cases, the axon and dendrites begin to form before the primitive process entirely disappears. It thus seems likely that at least some neurons remain attached to the pial surface, and their migration from the ventricular germinal zone to the cortex may be the result of shortening of the external cytoplasmic process that is anchored at the pial surface. According to that concept, some neurons would undergo a translocation similar to that undergone during transformation of radial glial cells into astrocytes (Fig. 3.1).

The rate of migration of young neurons from the ventricular zone to the cortical plate is initially fairly uniform, but later becomes spread over a longer time. The relatively slow rate of migration and long migration pathway has significant implications: it means that the cortex is assembled slowly in all mammals. For example, in the rat at birth the neurons in layers IV–VI have arrived at their final positions while those of layers II and III (which are mainly Golgi type II neurons) are still migrating and only reach their final positions 4–6 days after birth (Fig. 10.5).

In the rat, Hicks and D'Amato (1968) reported that young neurons labeled at E14–E18 migrate to the cortical plate in about 2 days, almost synchronously, whereas cells labeled at E19–E21 take from 3 to 10 days to arrive at the superficial layer of the cortex. In the ferret visual cortex the neurons generated early complete their migration in less than 1 week but those generated late require 2

weeks (C. A. Jackson *et al.*, 1989). This lag in the migration of neurons formed late in development also occurs in the rhesus monkey visual cortex (Rakic, 1974). Young neurons labeled at early stages (E46–E53) move about 200 μm from the ventricular zone to the cortical plate in about 3 days (5.5 μm/hour) and almost all arrive at their destinations in less than 7 days. But with advancing age, as the cortical plate thickens, the spatial dispersion is found to be much greater. In a fetus injected at E92 and killed 5 days later, only a few labeled neurons have migrated the full distance, about 1.2 mm, to the superficial layers of the cortex, and the majority of cells are still *en route*, either in the deep cortical layers or in the subventricular and intermediate zones.

It seems likely that the rapid and almost synchronous migration of neurons born together at early stages occurs because all the cells span the full thickness of the cortical plate in a simple radial alignment. At late stages of histogenesis of the cortex, the cells have to migrate a longer distance and to traverse a more complex terrain. At those stages, Rakic (1971a) has demonstrated that the migrating neurons use radial glial cells as guides (Fig. 10.6). However, it is not known whether those neurons originate from the ventricular zone or from

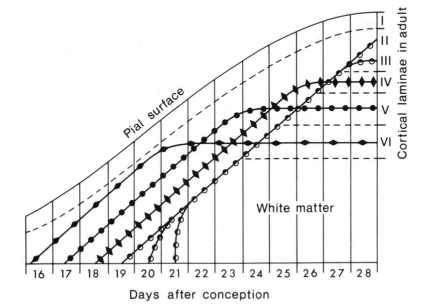

Figure 10.5. Inside-out sequence of origin of neurons in layers of the cerebral isocortex of the rat fetus. The time of origin and pattern of migration of young neurons as shown by labeling of cells with [³H]thymidine injected on E16, E17, E18, and E19–21. From M. Berry, A. W. Rogers, and J. T. Eayrs, *Nature* 203:591–593 (1964).

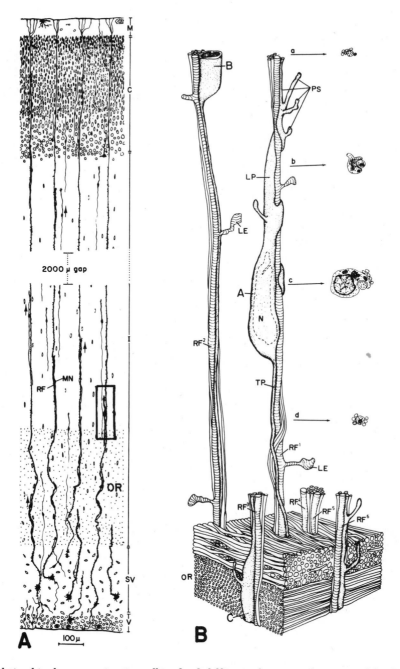

Figure 10.6. Relationships between migrating cells and radial fibers in the intermediate zone of the developing cerebral neocortex of the fetal monkey. The subventricular zone (SV) lies some distance below the area selected for reconstruction in (2) shown in the rectangle in (1), whereas the cortex (C) is more than 1000 μm above it. The lower portion of (2) contains uniform, parallel fibers of the optic radiation (OR) and the remainder is occupied by more variable and irregularly disposed fiber systems; the border between the two systems is easily recognized. Except at the lower portion of the figure, most of these fibers are not shown in order to expose the radial fibers (striped vertical shafts RF[1]–[6]) and their relationships to the migrating cells (A, B, and C) and to other vertical processes. The soma of migrating cell A, with its nucleus (N) and voluminous leading process (LP), is within the reconstructed space, except for the terminal part of the attenuated trailing process and the tip of the vertical ascending pseudopodium. Cross-sections of cell A in relation to the several vertical fibers in the fascicle are drawn at levels "a" to "d" at the right side of (B). The perikaryon of cell B is cut off at the top of the reconstructed space, whereas the leading process of cell C is shown just penetrating between fibers of the optic radiation (OR) on its way across the intermediate zone. From P. Rakic, *J. Comp. Neurol.* **145**:61–84 (1972).

the subventricular zone. The ventricular germinal cells probably maintain their full span from pial to ventricular surfaces, but the cells of the subventricular zone do not appear to be attached to the inner and outer surfaces of the brain. It is possible that neurons originating in the ventricular zone migrate independently, because they span the full thickness of the telencephalon whereas neurons originating in the subventricular zone or in other extraventricular sites such as the cerebellar granular layer can only migrate with the assistance of radial neuroglial cells.

The radial glial cells can be identified with the Golgi technique as well as by staining with GFAP antibody. They stop dividing during the period that they are involved in guidance of migrating neurons (Schmechel and Rakic, 1979a), and after that period they are transformed into protoplasmic or fibrillary astrocytes (Koelliker, 1893; Lenhossék, 1894; Ramón y Cajal, 1894, 1911; Bignami and Dahl, 1974a,b; Rakic, 1975a; Choi and Lapham, 1978; Schmechel and Rakic, 1979b; Misson *et al.*, 1988a,b; Voigt, 1989), as shown in Fig. 3.1. Oligodendrocytes may also originate from radial glial cells in the spinal cord (Choi, 1981; Choi *et al.*, 1983; Choi and Kim, 1984; M. Hirano and Goldman, 1988). Lineages of macroglial cells are considered in detail in Section 3.3.

The behavior of cultured granule cells from cerebellar cortex or hippocampal formation migrating along astrocytic processes is quite like their behavior *in vivo* (Edmondson and Hatten, 1987; Hatten, 1990). The migrating neuron elongates in close contact with and partially enfolding the glial cell process. Its advancing cytoplasmic process, covered with short filopodia and lamellipodia, extends and retracts rapidly as the entire neuron moves at an average speed of 20–60 μm/hour. This is considerably faster than estimates of the speed of neuronal migration *in vivo*, which range around 4 μm/hour (Altman, 1966; S. Fujita *et al.*, 1966; La Vail and Cowan, 1971b; Rakic, 1974; P. G. H. Clarke *et al.*, 1976). Under the conditions *in vitro*, neurons are able to migrate in either direction along a given glial fiber. Electron microscopic examination of migrating granule cells shows an extensive area of close contact and some specialized membrane junctions between the neuron and glial cell (Gregory *et al.*, 1988). Heterotypic combinations between cerebellar and hippocampal neurons and glial cells exhibit normal migratory behavior (Hatten, 1990), showing that the neuron–glial association is not region-specific. However, neuron–glial associations are disrupted by antibodies to astrotactin, a cell surface molecule that mediates neuron–glial interactions (Edmondson and Hatten, 1987).

Migrating cells secrete proteases that break down components of the extracellular matrix in their migratory pathways. For example, plasminogen activators are secreted by migrating cerebellar granule cells (Krystosek and Seeds, 1981a), and by growth cones (Krystosek and Seeds, 1981b; Pittman, 1985; Monard, 1988; Pittman and Buettner, 1989). Plasminogen activators start a cascade of proteolytic cleavages which result in activation of many different proteolytic enzymes that break down components of the extracellular matrix such as fibronectin and collagen. In migrating cells membrane recycling occurs by endocytosis at the base of elongating pseudopodia and addition of new membrane to the leading edge of the cell (Singer and Kupfer, 1986).

The organization of the developing cerebral cortex is primarily radial: the axis of the glial cells is initially radial; cells migrate along radially aligned paths in the cortical plate. The organization of radial glial cells forms a point-to-point projection system between the ventricular germinal zone and the overlying cortical mantle (Rakic, 1971a, 1972a, 1974). The fact that neuronal migration is constrained by the radial glial cells has led to the conjecture that the germinal zone is a mosaic subdivided into "proliferative units" which are related one-to-one to cortical units (Reznikov *et al.*, 1984; Rakic, 1988, review). This radial arrangement presages the columnar functional organization of the mature isocortex in which neurons in the same radial column synapse directly with each other but not directly with neurons of adjacent columns (Lorente de Nó, 1938; Mountcastle, 1957, 1979; Hubel and Wiesel, 1962, 1968, 1972).

The main axis of the cell bodies of the pyramidal cells is radial and their axons and apical dendritic shafts are oriented radially and develop before the lateral dendritic branches. The *maturation* of cortical neurons also occurs in a radial inside-out sequence starting in layer V and subsequently progressing through layers IV, III, and II, as first noted by Vignal (1888) and confirmed later by others (Koelliker, 1896; Stefanowska, 1898; Ramón y Cajal, 1906; Lorenté de Nó, 1933b, 1938). The general validity of the principle of inside-out maturation has been criticized by Molliver and Van der Loos (1970) in that it applies only to the differentiation of basal dendrites of pyramidal cells, which starts earlier in the deeper than in the more superficial pyramidal cells, whereas it is well known that the apical dendritic bouquets of superficial pyramidal neurons mature earlier than those of deep pyramids and that the apical dendritic bouquet is the first and the basal dendrites are the last to appear in ontogeny as well as phylogeny (Ramón y Cajal, 1906, Fig. 17). However, as Marin-Padilla (1978) has emphasized, the apical dendritic bouquets of pyramidal cells develop precociously in relation to the primordial superficial plexiform layer. The tangential organization of dendrites develops only during the postnatal period–for example, during the first 3 postnatal weeks in the mouse (Kobayashi *et al.*, 1964; Meller *et al.*, 1968b) and kitten (Noback and Purpura, 1961), during the first months in the dog (M. W. Fox *et al.*, 1966), and during the first 24 months after birth in humans (Conel, 1939–1963; Schadé *et al.*, 1962). An important part of the tangential connectivity of the cerebral cortex is provided by the Golgi type II neurons, whose dendrites develop much later than those of the pyramidal neurons (Morest, 1969a,b).

The normal pattern of lamination of the cerebral cortex is not essential for the development of normal connectivity, as is shown by the studies on the reeler mouse in which migration of cortical neurons is prematurely arrested. In the reeler mutant mouse, the cortical neurons are conspicuously malpositioned but their connections develop almost normally (Caviness and Sidman, 1972, 1973; Devor *et al.*, 1975; Stanfield *et al.*, 1979; Stanfield and Cowan, 1979a,b; Dräger, 1981; Simmons *et al.*, 1982). The neurons are also malpositioned in the cerebellar cortex, optic tectum, facial nucleus, and several other parts of the brain of the reeler mouse (see Section 10.15). The defect in this mutant appears to be in the mechanism of migration of the young neurons from the ventricular zone to a subpial position. The various types of neurons are produced at the normal times and apparently in normal numbers, but the cells fail to migrate outward past those that were formed earlier. Thus the polymorphic neurons, which originate earliest in the retrohippocampal cortex, normally lie in the deepest stratum, but in the reeler mutant they lie in a subpial position. A class of large neurons is generated next. These fail to migrate past the polymorphic neurons as they normally do, but take up positions deep to the polymorphic neurons. The granular neurons originate last and also fail to complete their migration to a subpial position, but instead come to lie deepest in the cortex. The inside-out order is thus reversed in the reeler. One result of this malpositioning of cortical neurons is that the neurons in the isocortex receiving input from vibrissae do not assemble into the usual barrel formations in reeler mice (Cragg, 1975b), as discussed in Section 11.7.

Despite the malposition of all neuron somata of the cortex in the reeler mouse, their local connections, intracortical, interhemispheric, and thalamocortical projections, develop normally (Devor *et al.*, 1975; Caviness, 1976; Caviness and Yorke, 1976; Simmons *et al.*, 1982). These anatomical observations of normal connectivity despite disordered positioning and orientation of cell bodies are in agreement with the electrophysiological evidence showing normal connectivity in the hippocampus of the reeler mouse despite gross cell malpositioning (Bliss and Chung, 1974). To this conservation of the connectivity should be added the preservation of the characteristic morphology of the pyramidal neurons despite their malpositioning and disorientation in the reeler mouse cerebral cortex (Devor *et al.*, 1975). The characteristic phenotype of cerebral cortical pyramidal neurons is also conserved in the few percent of pyramidal neurons that have improper orientations, including totally inverted neurons, in the otherwise normal cerebral cortex (Fig. 5.15; Van der Loos, 1965). The malpositioned pyramidal neurons project their axons via the corpus callosum to form connections at the proper positions in the opposite hemisphere (Caviness, 1976; Caviness and Yorke, 1976). This shows that the cellular recognition mechanisms can easily overcome large extracellular perturbations in order to link neurons according to their intrinsic specificities (also see R. Levine and Jacobson, 1974). These observations show that the principal neurons of the cerebral cortex, namely, the pyramidal neurons, have considerable autonomy in expressing their phenotypes. It is well to emphasize this aspect of the neuron's differentiation while also pointing out that there are some structures, such as the dentritic spines, that tend to be fewer and smaller in the absence of their afferent axons, and complete maturation of the dendrites may require adequate functional stimulation. This topic is discussed more fully in Section 6.11.

These findings on reeler mice are of the utmost significance. They greatly help to resolve

several difficult and controversial questions. First-ly, they throw light on the problem of the condi-tions necessary for determination of neuron cell types. Normal differentiation of cell types at ab-normal positions in reeler mice shows that cell types are not necessarily determined by interac-tions along their migration routes or by interac-tions at their final positions, or by some kind of "positional information" in the cortex itself. Ap-parently the necessary interactions occur in the ventricular germinal zone and early migration pathways. Determination of cell types must start in the ventricular zone before the cells start migra-tion. This is not consistent with the limited data from cell lineage studies which have been inter-preted to mean that neurons are only determined at their final positions (see Section 2.11). Sec-ondly, the reeler mice shed further light on the problem of the factors that guide axons to their targets. They show that prespecified "substrate pathways" are not required for axons to track along. Rather, axons of malpositioned neurons find their targets regardless of the pathways they have to traverse. Moreover, there is no evidence that axons in reeler mice branch more profusely or extensively than in normal mice. This indicates that the targets emit diffusible signals that are rec-

ognized with high specificity at a distance by out-growing nerve fibers.

10.8. Development of the Cerebral Subventricular Germinal Zone

The *subventricular zone* develops in the later stages of embryonic development of the CNS of mammals as a second zone of proliferating cells between the ventricular germinal zone and the mantle or intermediate zone. This proliferative zone has been called the *subependymal zone* (Kershmann, 1938; Smart, 1961), the *subependy-mal cell plate* (J. H. Globus and Kuhlenbeck, 1944), or the *subventricular zone* (Boulder Com-mittee, 1970). This zone has been described only in the mammalian forebrain, but may be present in other parts of the CNS at some stage of devel-opment. The subventricular zone progressively di-minishes during development. It persists in a ves-tigial manner in the lateral ventricles of the forebrain into adult life (Fig. 10.7) in mice (B. Messier *et al.*, 1958; Smart, 1961), rats (Bryans, 1959; Altman, 1963; P. D. Lewis, 1968a; Privat and Leblond, 1972), cats (Altman, 1963), dogs (K. Fischer, 1967; W. F. Blakemore and Jolly, 1972), and

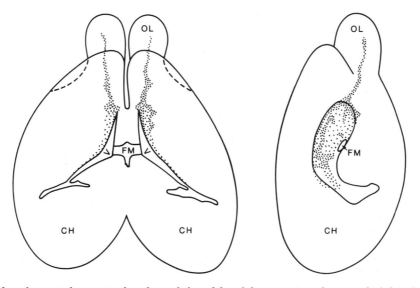

Figure 10.7. The subventricular zone in the telencephalon of the adult mouse. Dorsal view on the left; right lateral view on the right. The extent of the subventricular zone is shown by stippling, and denser stippling shows where it is thickest. CH = cerebral hemisphere; FM = foramen of Monro; V = lateral ventricle; OL = olfactory lobe. From I. Smart, *J. Comp. Neurol.* **116**:325–347 (1961).

primates (Opalski, 1933; J. H. Globus and Kuhlen-beck, 1944; Noetzel and Rox, 1964; P. D. Lewis, 1968a; Rakic, 1974).

The subventricular cells are a potential source of gliomas (Globus and Kuhlenbeck, 1944; K. Fischer, 1967; P. D. Lewis, 1968a). The subventricular zone is one of the commonest sites of brain tumors induced by chemical carcinogens, and it is significant in relation to the origin of glial cells that the induced neoplasms are almost all gliomas. This is in marked contrast to the great rarity of neoplastic transformations of neurons, either spontaneous or induced by carcinogens (Kleihues *et al.*, 1976, review).

According to Rakic (1974), the subventricular zone can be recognized in the rhesus monkey's telencephalon as early as 45 days of gestation (E45) and its thickness increases markedly during the next 10 days. The ventricular zone coexists with the subventricular zone for the next 5 weeks, both zones giving rise to cells that migrate into the overlying cortical plate. It is usually assumed that the subventricular zone gives rise to neurons as well as glial cells during this period, while glial cells only are produced in the subventricular zone after birth. During the period from E50 in the rhesus monkey, the ventricular zone gradually diminishes and has disappeared by E90, while at the same time the subventricular zone increases in width and continues to provide glial cells to the cortex until the end of gestation (about 165 days after conception) and probably for a short time postnatally.

The presence of mitotic figures shows that the subventricular zone retains its capacity to generate new cells in the adult. The germinal cells of the subventricular zone divide *in situ* and do not exhibit interkinetic nuclear migration. The generation time of subventricular cells in the adult rat is 18 hours (P. D. Lewis, 1968a), which is considerably longer than the generation times of 9.5–12 hours found in the ventricular zone of the mouse and rat (Table 2.1). Some of the cells that arise in the subventricular zone are destined never again to divide, as is shown by their persistent heavy labeling after exposure to tritiated thymidine during their final round of DNA synthesis. These cells may differentiate into small neurons. Other cells continue to divide and to dilute their label after migrating from the subventricular zone into the overlying mantle zone. Some of these cells may give rise to neurons, but most or all give

rise to macroglial cells. Cell lineage tracing (see Section 2.11) shows that an indifferent cell is formed that could give rise by division to both glial cells and neurons, as Schaper (1897a) and J. H. Globus and Kuhlenbeck (1944) proposed.

The neurons and glial cells originating in the subventricular zone migrate out through the white matter to the overlying gray matter. Smart (1961) and Altman (1963) have emphasized the role that fiber tracts such as the corpus callosum play in guiding the migrating cells to their destinations. The role of radial glial cells in guiding these cells to their destinations in the telencephalon has been stressed by Rakic (1971a,b, 1972a).

Two types of cells are seen in the subventricular zone at all stages (Smart, 1961; K. Fischer, 1967; W. F. Blakemore and Jolly, 1972). One has a small, deeply stained nucleus (dark-nucleated type) and the other has a lighter, larger nucleus (light-nucleated type). Smart (1961) found a series of transitional forms from the light-nucleated cells leading to immature neurons and considered the dark-nucleated type to be precursors of glial cells. Mitotic figures are present in both types. The subventricular germinal cells have the ultrastructural characteristics of immature cells: they have a high nuclear–cytoplasmic ratio, many free ribosomes and polysomes, and little endoplasmic reticulum (W. F. Blakemore, 1969). In adult mice the two types are uniformly dispersed and present in equal numbers, but at earlier stages the dark-nucleated cells predominate (Smart, 1961). Cumulative labeling with tritiated thymidine in adult mice results in labeling of only 1.5–1.6 percent of the light nuclei, and a maximum of 41 percent of the dark nuclei are labeled (Smart, 1961). Smart concluded that the subventricular zone produces granular neurons ("microneurons") and macroglial cells for a postnatal period that varies in different species; thereafter, a gradual reduction in the production of neurons occurs, but macroglial cells continue to be produced into adult life. Privat and Leblond (1972) found that in young rats the subventricular layer is composed of a few microglial cells and a single cell type, which they term the "subependymal cell," which gives rise to astrocytes and oligodendrocytes. Macrophages in large numbers (so-called ameboid microglia) invade the subventricular zone from the blood and are probably concerned with removal of the debris of degenerating cells (see Section 3.2). Many degenerating cells with pyknotic nuclei are found in the subventricular zone of the adult brain. Because the number of pyknotic nuclei seen in the adult subventricular zone is approximately equal to the number of metaphase figures, Smart (1961) concluded that the majority of cells formed in the subventricular zone of the mouse are destined to degenerate and that the subventricular zone does not add significantly to the cell population of the adult brain. However, P. D. Lewis and Lai (1974) found that there are twice as many mitoses as degenerating nuclei in the subventricular zone of postnatal rats up to 21 days of age and estimated that only 18 percent of the newly formed cells degenerate.

The function of the subventricular zone in adult mammals is not known. While its role in gliagenesis during the early postnatal period is well established, its only role in adult life may be to replace glial cells. This role is consistent with the fact that the incidence of glial tumors in different species is directly related to the size of the residual subventricular zone in the adult brain of that species. There is no evidence showing that neurons are formed in the subventricular zone in adult mammals, although granular neurons continue to be formed in various other germinal zones for a relatively short period after birth.

10.9. Development of Cortical Nerve Fibers

Cerebral and cerebellar cortical inputs are remarkably conserved between species and between different areas. For example, inputs from thalamic nuclei terminate mainly in layer IV and to a lesser extent in layers I and VI of the cerebral neocortex. The outputs also are similar, regardless of functional specializations of different areas: neurons in layer VI project to the thalamus and claustrum, layer V neurons project to all other subcortical targets, and neurons in layers II and III project to other areas in the ipsilateral neocortex and via the corpus callosum to the contralateral cortex. These highly specific projections develop from initially widespread projections as a result of selective retraction of axon collaterals.

Extensive pruning of initially diffuse axonal projections to produce a highly specific somatotopic projection occurs in the corpus callosum. The change from an embryonic projection in which each cortical neuron sends many branches via the corpus callosum to several regions of the opposite cerebral cortex, to result in the adult condition in which each cortical neuron sends a single axon to a specific contralateral region, occurs in the late fetal and early postnatal period in rats (Ivy and Killacky, 1982) and cats (Innocenti et al., 1977, 1986) and in the late fetal period in monkeys (Killacky and Chalupa, 1986; Berland et al., 1987). Nerve fibers in the corpus callosum connecting the two cerebral hemispheres project very specifically in adult mammals. There are very few cortical cells that project to more than one cortical area in the adult monkey (R. A. Anderson et al., 1985). However, in the monkey fetus the callosal projection is relatively diffuse and uniform. The change to a discontinuous projection occurs in the monkey from about E119 to achieve the state resembling that of the adult by about E133, 1 month before birth (Killackey and Chalupa, 1986; Chalupa and Killacky, 1989). This change occurs as a result of retraction of axon collaterals and does not involve significant death of cortical neurons. This is considered again near the end of Section 8.2. Transient connections also occur between regions within a cerebral hemisphere, and these too are removed by axon elimination and not by cell death (Dehay et al., 1984; Innocenti and Clarke, 1984; S. Clarke and Innocenti, 1986; Dehay et al., 1988). In the newborn cat injections of retrograde tracer into area 17 will backfill axons belonging to neurons in the auditory, somatosensory, and motor cortex, but these diffuse projections disappear by 5 weeks of age as the result of axon retraction, not cell death (Fig. 10.8). The function of these transient axonal projections is not yet clear, nor is it certain that they make synaptic connections in the cortex. Although transient synapses in the cortex have been reported (Kostovic and Rakic, 1980; Chun et al., 1987), synaptic transmission may not be necessary: transient axons could function by releasing transmitters and trophic factors from their growth cones (Hume et al., 1983; Young and Poo, 1983; Takahashi et al., 1987).

In the occipital cortex of the rat, cells in layer V initially project axon collaterals into the pyramidal, corticopontine, and corticotectal tracts, but the pyramidal tract collaterals are all lost (Stanfield et al., 1982), while either the corticopontine or corticotectal collaterals or both are retained (D. D. M. O'Leary and Stanfield, 1985). By contrast, neurons

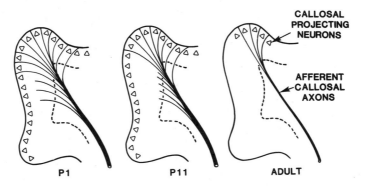

Figure 10.8. Schematic representation of the maturation of callosal connections in the visual cortex of the cat. On the day of birth afferent callosal fibers penetrate the cortical gray matter to the very most superficial layers over a wide area centered on the apex of the gyral axis. Elsewhere transient axons do not ascend higher than layer 4. Cell bodies projecting to the callosum are widely distributed throughout area 17. By P11 a considerable reorganization of callosal connections has occurred. Although at this age callosal projecting cells continue to be distributed throughout area 17, afferent callosal fibers only penetrate gray matter at the axis of the gyrus. Elsewhere transient axons stop abruptly at the white matter/gray matter boundary. As the callosal pathway matures, callosal projecting axons become progressively more restricted, and cells on the medial bank of the lateral gyrus lose these callosal projecting axons. The adult situation is achieved between 1 and 3 months of age. These results show that transient callosal axons, like ipsilateral transient axons, do penetrate the cortical gray matter. Adapted from H. Kennedy, C. Dehay, and C. Bourdet (1988).

in layer V of the rostral part of the neocortex retain their pyramidal tract collaterals. The specificity of cortical inputs and outputs can be assayed by heterotopic transplantation of pieces of cortex. When cortex of E15 rats is transplanted heterotopically into the cortex of newborn rats, rostral (somatosensory) cortex to occipital (visual) cortex, and vice versa, the transplanted neurons behave like the neurons of the host region with respect to retention or loss of pyramidal tract collaterals but they retain their original behavior with respect to projection via the corpus callosum (D. D. M. O'Leary and Stanfield, 1989).

Those findings support the theory that the position of the neuron determines which of its axon collaterals will be eliminated and which will survive, but the mechanisms are not yet known. It would seem likely that such selective elimination or survival of axon collaterals must be effected by mechanisms operating at the axon terminals and/or the postsynaptic target rather than at the cortical neuron giving rise to collaterals. Respecification of cortical neurons can, in principle, occur with respect to its outputs, to the cortical afferents, and to neighboring cells in the cortex. Some cortical characteristics are more sensitive than others to deprivation of afferents. Thus, removal of an eye in the rhesus monkey results in the well-known transneuronal

atrophy of area 17, of the visual cortex. Nevertheless the layering in area 17, the sharp boundary between area 17 and area 18 the absence of callosal projections from area 17 and their presence from area 18, remain essentially normal at birth after eye removal on E77 or E122 (DeHay *et al.*, 1989). The observation that the above-mentioned characteristics are relatively unaffected by absence of the main afferents shows that those characteristics are probably determined in the cortex itself. By contrast, the number of neurons projecting from area 18 via the corpus callosum is considerably increased after eye removal, showing that their development is under control of afferent input from the retina. Evidence that somatosensory maps in the cerebral cortex can alter in response to peripheral injury, even in adult mammals, is given in Section 11.7.

In the adult monkey there are very few cortical cells that project via the corpus callosum to more than one cortical area (M. L. Schwartz and Goldman-Rakic, 1982; R. A. Anderson *et al.*, 1985). This condition develops by selective elimination of an initially widespread collosal projection starting at about E119 and leading to the mature state by E133 in the rhesus monkey (Killacky and Chalupa, 1986). In the rhesus monkey the regionally selective callosal projections develop as a result of retraction of axon collaterals to the contralateral cortex while at the same time preserving collaterals projecting to the ipsilateral cortex (Chalupa and Killacky, 1989). Selective elimination of some axonal collateral has also been demonstrated during refinement of the projections that cross via the corpus callosum in the cat (Innocenti *et al.*, 1986) and rat (Ivy and Killacky, 1982).

Projection of monoaminergic neurons to specific regions and laminae of the cerebral cortex occurs very early in development, and there is some evidence that these afferents have trophic effects and that they may be involved in functional specification of cortical neurons. In the rat, there are three sources of monoaminergic afferents to the cerebral cortex: noradrenaline-containing axons originating from the locus coeruleus project to the entire cortex but most densely to the somatosensory cortex; dopamine-containing axons originating from the rostral mesencephalon project widely but most densely to the prefrontal and temporal cortex; axons containing serotonin (5-hydroxytryptamine), originating in the mesencephalic raphe nuclei, are widely and more uniformly distributed (Parnavelas and Papadoupoulos, 1989, review). In addition to this regionally specific distribution the serotonin-containing axons are among the first to invade the cortical plate when they are organized in patches resembling barrels (see Section 11.7) in the somatosensory cortex of the rat (Rhoades *et al.*, 1990). Noradrenaline-containing nerve fibers invade the primordial plexiform layer and the intermediate zone of the developing cerebral cortex on E17 in the rat (Seiger and Olson, 1973; Lidov *et al.*, 1978; Levitt and Moore, 1979; Schlumpf *et al.*, 1980). From E18 the noradrenaline-containing nerve fibers invade the cortical plate (Coyle and Molliver, 1977; Kristt, 1979). This occurs much earlier than the invasion of thalamocortical afferents, which start entering the cortical plate on P1–P4 in the rat (Wise *et al.*, 1979).

Contrary to earlier concepts of nonspecific, diffuse nonsynaptic termination of varicosities of mono-aminergic axons in the cortex (Descarries *et al.*, 1975, 1977; Iversen, 1984, review), recent electron microscopic immunocytochemical studies show that nearly all labeled varicosities and axon terminals form conventional synapses with cortical neurons in specific laminar patterns of organization (Papadopoulos *et al.*, 1989a,b). The noradrenergic axons project initially to layers I and VI and in the

adult mainly to layers V and VI, which project out of the cortex, whereas the serotonergic axons are directed at layers IVa and IVc, which also receive thalamocortical afferents (Morrison *et al.*, 1982; Morrison and Foote, 1986).

One way of studying the role of noradrenaline-containing fibers during cortical development is to destroy those fibers selectively. This can be accomplished prenatally or shortly after birth by injections of 6-hydroxydopamine which enters the brain of prenatal or newborn rats before development of the blood–brain barrier. Virtually complete elimination of noradrenaline-containing fibers has given conflicting results. No significant effects were observed after administration of 6-hydroxydopamine on E17 (Lidov and Molliver, 1982) or on P1–P3 (Blue and Parnavelas, 1982), whereas large changes have been reported in morphology of pyramidal cells (Felten *et al.*, 1982) and in the numerical density of cortical neurons (Onteniente *et al.*, 1980; Imamoto *et al.*, 1982). Nonspecific toxic effects of 6-hydroxydopamine may account for the latter results. Lack of effect of noradrenaline depletion has been attributed to compensatory changes such as increased sensitivity to circulating noradrenalin and to increased dopamine-containing nerve fibers in the cerebral cortex.

Dopamine-containing nerve fibers are first detectable in the rat neocortex at E17 in the cortical subplate. Like the thalamocortical afferents, the dopaminergic fibers wait for several days in the cortical subplate before entering the cortical plate on postnatal days 1–3 (Lindvall *et al.*, 1974; B. Berger *et al.*, 1976; Verney *et al.*, 1982). The thalamocortical afferents form temporary synapses on interstitial neurons in the cortical subplate (Molliver *et al.*, 1973; König *et al.*, 1975; Wolff, 1978; Friauf *et al.*, 1990) before transferring their synapse directly to neurons in the cortical plate (Luskin and Shatz, 1985a,b; Shatz and Luskin, 1986). There is evidence that the transient connections between thalamic afferents and subplate neurons are required for later formation of thalamocortical connections because they fail to develop after early destruction of the subplate neurons (Ghosh *et al.*, 1990).

A dense transient serotonergic innervation of primary sensory (visual, auditory, and somatosensory) cortex develops during the first postnatal month in the rat (D'Amato *et al.*, 1987). This coincides with the period of maximal dendritic growth and synaptogenesis in the cortex, which may mean that serotonin acts as a trophic agent. More direct evidence of such an effect is the observation that low concentrations of serotonin (20 μM) stimulate neuronal differentiation and synaptogenesis in culture (Chubakov *et al.*, 1986). The noradrenergic afferents to the visual cortex modulate plasticity in cats (see Section 11.21; Kasamatsu, 1983, review). The primordial corticopetal fibers probably have a trophic influence on development of cortical neurons (M. F. Bear *et al.*, 1985; Zagon and McLaughlin, 1986; K. F. Hauser *et al.*, 1987). This has led to the concept that neurotransmitters are released by neurons which have a transient existence, and which function as organizers of the definitive cortical circuitry.

The role of cerebral cortical afferents in determining regional functional specificity has been studied experimentally by misrouting afferents destined for one region into the pathways normally taken by afferents destined for another region of the cerebral cortex. Thus, removal of the superior colliculus and occipital cortex on the day of birth in the hamster or ferret and at the same time deafferenting the medial geniculate nucleus of the ventrobasal nucleus of the thalamus results in retinal axons invading the deafferented thalamic nucleus. Visual-evoked responses can then be recorded in the auditory cortex or somatosensory cortex (Frost, 1982; Sur *et al.*, 1988). Because the rerouted axons extend only to the thalamic relay nuclei, the thalamocortical projection is not anatomically replaced, but relays visual input to nonvisual cerebral cortex. The rerouted retinotopic projection would conform to some extent with the topographical order of the original thalamocortical projection and some evidence is consistent with that prediction (Sur *et al.*, 1990).

10.10. Development of the Cerebellum

This section deals mainly with the development of the cerebellar cortex, which has a similar pattern of organization in all vertebrates (Nieuwenhuys, 1964; Eccles *et al.*, 1967; Larsell, 1967; Palay and Chan-Palay, 1974; Ito, 1984). The adult cerebellum has three cortical layers—named in order from the outer surface: the molecular layer, the Purkinje neuron layer, and the granular neuron layer. The relationships of the cells in these layers in the mammalian cerebellar cortex are shown diagrammatically

in Fig. 10.9. The connectivity of the cerebellum and the functions of the five types of neurons of which it is constructed are known in considerable detail.

The Purkinje cell is the principal neuron and the sole pathway out of the cerebellar cortex. Impulses are conducted into the cerebellar cortex by the climbing fibers, which originate in the inferior olive, and by the mossy fibers, which are mostly the terminals of spinocerebellar and pontocerebellar fibers. There are also axons containing monoamines that originate in the locus coeruleus, raphe nuclei, and substantia nigra that enter the cortex and target on Purkinje cells. The afferent mossy and climbing fibers synapse with unerring precision on their postsynaptic targets: the climbing fibers terminate on spines on the large dendritic branches of Purkinje cells and the mossy fibers terminate in structures called glomeruli in which they form synapses with dendrites of granule cells and the axons of Golgi type II cells.

The local-circuit neurons of the cerebellar cortex, so-called because all their connections are within the cortex itself, are the Golgi, basket, stellate, and granule cells. The granule cell receives input from the mossy fiber. The granule cell axon, called the parallel fiber because it has a trajectory parallel with the axis of the folium, forms synaptic connections on dendritic spines of a row of Purkinje cells. The parallel fibers also synapse on the dendrites of stellate, basket, and Golgi neurons. The parallel fibers are approximately the same length, about 6 mm in chicken, rabbit, cat, and rhesus monkey, which is another indication of the very conservative phylogeny of cerebellar circuitry (Mugnaini, 1983).

The stellate neuron forms synapses on Purkinje cell dendritic shafts, while the basket cell makes synapses with the soma of the Purkinje cell. The Golgi neuron forms a local circuit that does not directly include Purkinje cells: the Golgi cell dendrites receive inputs from parallel fibers, while the Golgi cell axon synapses with granule cell dendrites within the glomerulus. In addition to these types of neurons, the cerebellum has specialized astroglial cells, called Golgi epithelial cells, which have a soma in the Purkinje cell layer, and five or more processes known as the Bergmann glial fibers, extending radially, like a palisade towards the pial surface.

The development of the cerebellar cortex proceeds in a similar order but at quite different rates in different vertebrates (Fig. 10.10). Thus development

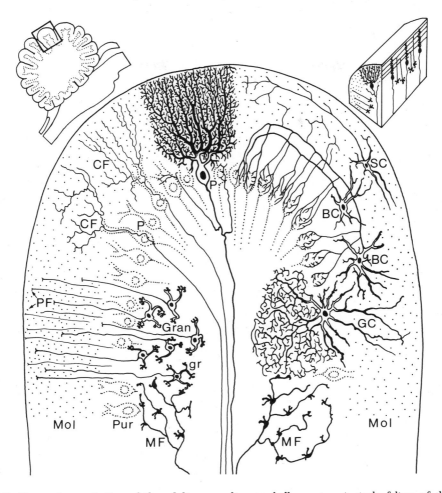

Figure 10.9. Neuronal organization of the adult mammalian cerebellar cortex. A single folium of the mammalian cerebellum (a magnified section of the region shown in the rectangle). BC = basket cell; CF = climbing fiber; Gran = granule cell layer; GC = Golgi II cell; gr = granule cells; MF = mossy fiber; Mol = molecular layer; P = Purkinje cell layer; Pur = Purkinje cell; PF = parallel fibers; SC = stellate cell.

of the Purkinje cell dendritic tree at birth is more advanced in precocial mammals than in altricial mammals: Purkinje cells are more fully developed at birth in sheep (Reese and Harding, 1988), less well developed in the rhesus monkey (Rakic, 1971) and humans (Zecevic and Rakic, 1976), and much less well developed in the mouse (G. Weiss and Pysh, 1978), the rat (Altman, 1972; Berry and Bradley, 1976), the hamster (Oster-Granite and Hendon, 1976), the opossum (Laxon and King, 1983), and the cat (Calvet *et al.*, 1985). An extreme example is the bullfrog *Rana catesbeiana*. During the premetamorphic stages lasting about 2 years, the cerebellum

remains in the form of a cerebellar plate containing undifferentiated Purkinje cells but no external granular layer. Only with the onset of metamorphosis does the external granular layer form and do the Purkinje cell dendrites grow and branch. These events occur rapidly at the same time as growth of the limbs (Gona, 1972, 1973, 1975, 1976). Other structural changes related to changes of function also occur after metamorphosis in the frog; the lateral line input to the auricular lobe (homologous with flocculus in mammals) disappears, and spinal and vestibular inputs develop as the frog emerges onto land (Larsell, 1923, 1925).

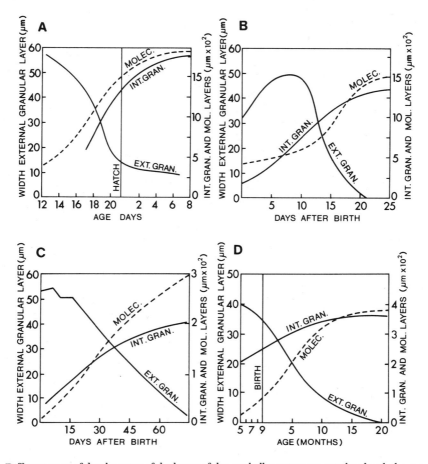

Figure 10.10. Different rates of development of the layers of the cerebellar cortex are correlated with the state of maturity at birth in the chick (A), the rat (B), the dog (C), and the human (D). Plotted from data in Addison (1911), Raaf and Kernohan (1944), Saetersdal (1956), Phemister and Young (1968).

In general, the stage of development of the cerebellum at birth can be correlated with the development of an animal's powers of locomotion and motor coordination. In precocial animals that are able to walk soon after birth (such as the chick, guinea pig, and ungulates), the cerebellum is well developed at birth, whereas in altricial animals (such as the mouse, rat, and human) that are helpless at birth, the cerebellum is in a corresponding state of immaturity, and its histogenesis and morphogenesis mainly occur after birth. That birth itself does not trigger the postnatal events of cerebellar neurogenesis and morphogenesis is shown by the fact that those events occur at the normal time after birth in mammals born prematurely or before birth in rat fetuses in which

gestation is prolonged for 3 days beyond its normal duration (Zagon, 1975).

10.11. Histogenesis of the Cerebellar Cortex

The times and sites of origin of the Purkinje cell and of the four types of cerebellar local-circuit neurons, as well as their migration routes to specific positions in the cortex, their distinctive patterns of differentiation and growth, and their synaptogenesis, have been described in several species. These observations show that assembly of such a complex system follows an invariant timetable.

Well-defined germinal zones can be demarcated, giving origin to different types of neurons in a regular timetable. Histogenesis of large principal neurons occurs first, followed by genesis of local-circuit neurons (Fig. 10.11). The pattern of histogenesis of the cerebellar cortical neurons is complicated by the fact that cells originate from two separate germinal zones. A zone in the roof of the fourth ventricle (the rhombic lip) gives origin to deep cerebellar neurons in addition to the Purkinje and Golgi II cells and the Golgi epithelial cells. The neurons of the deep cerebellar nuclei migrate medially whereas the Golgi epithelial cells and young Purkinje cells migrate outward toward the pia mater to form the mantle layer of the cerebellar plate. Somewhat later, another germinal zone, called the external granule layer, is formed immediately beneath the pia covering the cerebellar plate, and this gives origin to granule cells, stellate and basket cells, and some glial cells, all of which migrate deeper into the cerebral cortex. The fact that cerebellar cells arise from two quite separate germinal layers, each of which generates different classes of neurons, is a special case of the general principle that different types of neurons have separate origins.

Migration of cells out of the ventricular germinal zone to form the cerebellar plate mantle layer occurs before E6 in the chick embryo (Saetersdal, 1956, 1959; Forströnen, 1963; Hanaway, 1967), from E11 to E13 in the mouse fetus (Miale and Sidman, 1961), before E17 with a peak on E15 in the fetus of the albino rat (Addison, 1911; Altman

and Bayer, 1978, 1985c), and from E60 to E80 in the human fetus (Ellis, 1920; Raaf and Kernohan, 1944; Woodard, 1960; Rakic and Sidman, 1969, 1970). In the mouse and rat fetus, by E17, the cerebellar plate is composed of an inner, ventricular germinal layer, a middle mantle or intermediate layer, and an outer marginal layer. The mantle layer of the cerebellar plate is composed of two strata. The deeper stratum of larger immature neurons differentiates to form the large neurons of the roof nuclei. The young neurons of the more superficial stratum of the mantle develop into Purkinje cells.

The Purkinje cells in the chick embryo are generated between E3 and E6, and DNA synthesis ceases in the ventricular germinal zone of the chick on E12 (Hanaway, 1967; Yurkewicz et al., 1981). Their origin from the ventricular germinal zone of the cerebellar plate has been confirmed in chick–quail chimeras (Hallonet et al., 1990). Neurons of the deep cerebellar nuclei originate during the same period (Stages 17–27) as the Purkinje cells in the chick embryo (Kanemitsu and Kobayashi, 1988). Using [³H]thymidine autoradiography, Miale and Sidman (1961) showed that the Purkinje cells of the mouse cerebellum originate—as postmitotic cells no longer able to incorporate tritiated thymidine—on E11, E12, and E13 and migrate out into the superficial part of the mantle from E17. In pyridine-silver preparations of the 14-day embryonic mouse brain, fibers may be seen to have grown into the cerebellum in the path of migrating Purkinje cells (Sidman, 1968). These are probably climbing fibers from the inferior olive and possibly also mono-

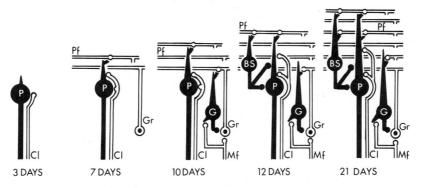

3 DAYS   7 DAYS   10 DAYS   12 DAYS   21 DAYS

Figure 10.11. Diagram showing assembly of functional cerebellar cortical circuits during development in the rat at P3–P21. Inhibitory cells are shown in black, excitatory cells in white. BS = basket and stellate cells; Cl = climbing fiber; G = Golgi cell; Gr = granule cell; Mf = mossy fiber; P = Purkinje cell; Pf = parallel fiber. From T. Shimono, S. Nosaka, and K. Sasaki, *Brain Res.* **108**:279–294 (1976).

aminergic fibers from the locus coeruleus, raphe nuclei, and substantia nigra (Seiger and Olson, 1973; Lauder and Bloom, 1974, 1975).

The other cerebellar cells that are derived from the ventricular germinal zone are the Golgi II neurons, the small neurons of the roof nuclei, and probably some glial cells. The precursors of the Golgi II neurons complete their final DNA synthesis and mitosis on E12–E15 in the albino mouse and migrate directly from the ventricular germinal zone to the molecular layer of the cerebellar cortex (Miale and Sidman, 1961). In the mouse, cells originating in the ventricular germinal zone after E13 differentiate into small neurons of the roof nuclei (Miale and Sidman, 1961; Taber Pierce, 1967b). Mitotic activity in the ventricular germinal zone decreases between E13 and E15 and ceases by E17 in the mouse fetus (Miale and Sidman, 1961). Development of cells derived from the external granular layer (the granule cells, basket and stellate cells, and probably some glial cells) will be discussed following the next section on the development of Purkinje cells.

10.12. Purkinje Cell Ontogenesis

Development of Purkinje cells has five main phases in all vertebrates; the first is embryonic, all the others are postnatal.

1. During the embryonic phase Purkinje cells originate from a ventricular germinal zone in the rhombic lip and migrate to form the first neurons in the cerebellar plate, which, at that phase, also contains radial glial cells.
2. Purkinje cells initially form an irregular layer up to 12 cells deep, but over a period of several days to weeks they become aligned to form a single, regularly spaced layer.
3. Axonal outgrowth from Purkinje cells occurs during the period of alignment and the axon forms synaptic connections with neurons in the deep cerebellar nuclei.
4. A single apical dendrite grows from the Purkinje cell body toward the pial surface, followed by dendritic branching (secondary, tertiary and spiny) during the next phase.
5. Development of synaptic connections with climbing fibers and granule cell axons continues over an extended time, during which elimination of synapses also occurs.

Purkinje cells originate from the germinal zone of the rhombic lip on E10–E13 in the mouse (Uzman, 1960; Miale and Sidman, 1961; Inouye and Murakami, 1980), and from E12 to E15 in the rat (Das and Nornes, 1972; Altman and Bayer, 1978). In all cases the production of Purkinje cells commences and ceases before that of any other type of cell in the cerebellar cortex. They grow very slowly until the proliferation of external granule cells occurs. The Purkinje cells begin to differentiate rapidly after the granule cells migrate past them from the external granule layer to the internal granule layer. These events occur 4–20 days after birth in the albino mouse and albino rat, and from fetal month 4 to well into the 2nd postnatal year in humans. The Purkinje cells form a single row at E18 in the chick (Kanemitsu and Kobayashi, 1988), about P4 in the rat (Addison, 1911; Altman and Winfree, 1977), and P10 in the mouse (Miale and Sidman,, 1961; Hendelman and Aggerwal, 1980). Their nuclei continue to increase in size until P10 in the mouse and P14 in the rat.

Several markers of Purkinje cells have been found, such as cGMP-dependent protein kinase (DeCamilli et al., 1984), cerebellin (Slemmon et al., 1984, 1985), PEP-19 (Mugnaini et al., 1987; Sangameswaran et al., 1989), UCHT-1 and Leu-4 (Garson et al., 1982), vitamin D–dependent calcium-binding protein (Jande et al., 1981; Roth et al., 1981; Baimbridge and Miller, 1982), motilin (Nilaver et al., 1982), mabQ113 (Hawkes et al., 1985), Purkinje cell-specific glycoprotein (Reeber et al., 1981; Langley et al., 1982), and zebrin I and II (Brochu et al., 1990; Wassef et al., 1990). Although all Purkinje cells have similar morphology and connectivity, they have diverse patterns of expression of histochemical markers (Scott, 1964; Maraini and Voogd, 1973, 1977) and antigens (Chan-Palay et al., 1981, 1982; Nilaver et al., 1982; Hawkes et al., 1985; Hawkes and Leclerc, 1987). Purkinje cells positive or negative for different markers form alternating longitudinal, parasaggital bands in the cerebellum in adult and fetal rats (Wassef and Sotelo, 1984; Wassef et al., 1985, 1990; Brochu et al. 1990). One of these markers, zebrin I, a 120-kDa polypeptide, is expressed autonomously in Purkinje cells grown in the anterior chamber of the eye or transplanted into the cerebral cortex (Wassef et al., 1990).

In spite of earlier reports (Sandritter et al., 1967; Lapham, 1968; Nováková et al., 1968; Herman and Lapham, 1968; Lentz and Lapham, 1969,

1970), the Purkinje cells do not become polyploid (Mann and Yates, 1973a; S. Fujita, 1974; J. Cohen *et al.*, 1973; Manuelides and Manuelides, 1974). Polyploid glial cells discovered in the Purkinje cell layer by Lapham and Johnstone (1963) have been confirmed in the human cerebellum by Mann and Yates (1973b). They found that polyploidy is not age dependent and reported a strict numerical ratio between these glial cells and Purkinje cells: for each Purkinje cell they found one octaploid, 50 tetraploid, and 250 diploid glial cells.

The axon of the Purkinje cell can be seen at the time of birth in the rat, and the axonal collaterals that spread transversely from one Purkinje cell to the cell bodies of neighboring Purkinje cells develop shortly after birth (Chan-Palay, 1971).

Dendritic growth of the Purkinje cells is shown by the increase in width of the molecular layer of the cerebellar cortex. This occurs from P4 to P14 in the mouse and in the first 21 postnatal days in the rat. Growth of the Purkinje cell dendrites and increase in their branching have been described in detail in the frog (Uray and Gona, 1982), opossum (Laxson and King, 1983), mouse (Hendelman and Aggerwal, 1980), rat (Addison, 1911; Altman, 1972b; Berry and Bradley, 1976; Mjaatvedt and Wong-Riley, 1988), and human (Zecevic and Rakic, 1976). Growth of the Purkinje cell dendrites is delayed until after birth and occurs over a prolonged period during which the external granular layer gives origin to granule cells. Levels of cytochrome oxidase activity and numbers of mitochondria in rat Purkinje cell dendrites reflect the levels of oxidative energy metabolism. The levels are high during formation of excitatory synapses and reduced during development of inhibitory synapses, as discussed near the end of Section 6.4 and illustrated in Fig. 6.9 (Mjaadvedt and Wong-Riley, 1988).

In the newborn rat the Purkinje cells have an apical dendritic process, which may or may not have a few branches. The first outgrowths from the apical pole of the Purkinje cells become resorbed. The tips of the Purkinje cell dendrites reach only as far as the inner layer of external granule cells, and as the external granular layer becomes depleted, so do the Purkinje cell dendrites extend to reach the pia at 20–25 days after birth, at the time of disappearance of the external granular layer. According to Addison (1911), the number of terminal branches of Purkinje cell dendrites continues to increase up to 110 days after birth in the rat.

Growth of the Purkinje cell dendrites in the cat has been described by Purpura *et al.* (1964). At birth, the Purkinje cells of the cat have a short, unbranched dendrite. Branching of the dendrites occurs especially between 8 and 12 days after birth, and this happens simultaneously with the inward migration of the granule cells. By postnatal day 40 in the cat, the Purkinje cell dendrites have developed dendritic spines, and the dendrites are fully developed by 60 days after birth.

The differentiation of Purkinje cells in humans follows the same sequence as in other mammals, but the human Purkinje cells differentiate and grow more slowly (Zecevic and Rakic, 1976). During the 4th fetal month (12–16 weeks), the Purkinje cells are distributed in several rows and have smooth somas and dendrites which are short and unbranched. During the period from 16 to 28 weeks of gestation, the Purkinje cells become aligned as a single layer, spines develop on somata, and further branching of dendrites occurs. The first synapses develop on the somatic spines and on the dendritic shafts at about 16 weeks and continue to form thereafter. The somatic spines disappear, the dendrites branch, and spines start appearing on the secondary and tertiary branches between the 24th and 28th fetal weeks and continue to form until the dendrites have completed their growth and assumed the adult form at the end of the 1st postnatal year.

The relationship between the migration of granule cells, the growth of Purkinje cell dendrites and the synapses between the axons of the granule cells (the parallel fibers), and the dendritic spines of Purkinje cells has been discussed by Ramón y Cajal (1929a, Chapter 12). He proposed the hypothesis that the growth of the Purkinje cell dendrites is stimulated by the appearance of the parallel fibers and the migration of the granule cells. This is rather similar to Sidman's (1968) notion that an interaction may occur between the Purkinje cells and the granule cells that migrate past them, resulting in the formation of specific connections between them. Although these proposals are still in the realm of speculation, there is evidence that the development of Purkinje cell dendrites is stimulated in some unknown way by the migration of granule cells and the development of parallel fibers. That the matter is not quite so simple as the hypothesis would suggest is shown by the fact that in the human fetus the growth of Purkinje cell dendrites commences before the first migration of granule cells, thus demonstrating an aspect of the Purkinje cell's autonomy (Rakic and Sidman, 1970). The Purkinje cell dendrites do not develop normally but remain stunted in pieces of cerebellum isolated from birth *in vitro* (Aggerwal and Hendelman, 1980) and after the external granule cells are destroyed by X-rays (Purpura *et al.*, 1964) or by a virus (Kilham and Margolis, 1964, 1965, 1966a,b).

Development of climbing fibers has been described by Athias (1897a), Ramón y Cajal (1909–1911), and J. L. O'Leary *et al.* (1971). They grow into the cerebellum from the contralateral inferior olive, are one of the two afferent systems of the cerebellar cortex, and exert a strong excitatory effect on Purkinje cells. The climbing fibers, with their characteristic varicosities, can be seen in reduced silver or Golgi preparations during the early postnatal period from the time of onset of growth of Purkinje cell dendrites. At first, the climbing fibers have numerous redundant branches, which later disappear. Initially, the climbing fibers form a plexus in the granular layer, contributing to the *lamina dissecans*, a layer that appears transiently between the Purkinje and granular layers in the human cerebellum. This is described at the end of this section. The terminal branches of the developing climbing fibers contact Purkinje cell bodies, apparently making transient synaptic connections there (Mugnaini, 1969, 1970; Larramendi, 1969; Altman, 1972b). As the growth of Purkinje cell dendrites occurs, the climbing fibers extend over the surface of all the dendritic branches. At that stage the climbing fibers largely leave the cell body, clearing the way for the later growth of basket cell processes onto the Purkinje cell body. This development extends from the age of P5 to P30 in the rat.

The mechanism of selective association between climbing fibers and Purkinje cells is unknown. Ramón y Cajal cited this as a prime example in support of his theory of chemotaxis or neurotropism, suggesting that the climbing fibers, *"upon arriving from distant centers, smell out, so to speak, the bodies of the Purkinje elements, which they embrace, by means of varicose nests, the rudiments of the future arborization. Once in contact with it, the branches of the nerve nests positively* **climb** *along the principle stem of the dendrites until they finally generate the complicated plexus characteristic of the adult conductors"* (Ramón y Cajal, 1917). In the normal adult there is a one-to-one relationship between climbing fibers and Purkinje cells, but during development a transient period of innervation of each Purkinje cell by several climbing fibers occurs. In the rat this redundant innervation of 3 or 4 climbing fibers to each Purkinje cell is maximal at P5 then regresses rapidly and disappears by P15 (Mariani and Changeux, 1981a,b).

Regression of redundant climbing fibers requires functional synaptic connections between Purkinje cell dendrites and axons of granule cells. Multiple innervation of Purkinje cells by climbing fibers persists for longer than normal in a number of conditions in which the Purkinje cells are deprived of granule cell inputs. This occurs in hypothyroidism, in which development of granule cells is delayed (Crepel *et al.*, 1981). Multiple innervation persists into adulthood after destruction of granule cells by X-rays (Woodward *et al.*, 1971; Puro and Woodward, 1978; Crepel *et al.*, 1981) or in weaver and reeler mutant mice (Crepel and Mariani, 1976; Siggins *et al.*, 1976; Mariani *et al.*, 1977; Puro and Woodward, 1977; Mariani, 1982). There is also persistence of redundant climbing fibers in staggerer mice, where the Purkinje cells fail to form synaptic contacts with parallel fibers (Mariani and Changeux, 1980; Crepel *et al.*, 1980; Mariani, 1982), as discussed in Section 10.15. These observations suggest that the regression of climbing fibers in some way results from competition with the granule cell axons, which are the other main input to Purkinje cells.

A layer of cytoplasmic processes lying between the Purkinje cell bodies and the internal granular layer develops transiently in the human cerebellum. This layer, called the *lamina dissecans* by Hayashi (1924), has been studied more recently by Verbitskaya (1969) and by Rakic and Sidman (1970). It has also been shown in the developing cerebellum of the blue whale (Korneliussen, 1967) and is probably found in all primates and other mammals with a long period of gestation. In the human cerebellum the lamina dissecans first appears at 20–21 weeks of gestation as an acellular layer 15–20 μm thick. In humans it persists for about 10 weeks and then disappears. Its presence can thus be used as an indication of fetal age. The lamina dissecans contains axonal terminals of mossy and climbing fibers and transient cytoplasmic outgrowths from developing granule and Purkinje cells (Rakic and Sidman, 1970).

10.13. Ontogenesis of Cerebellar Local-Circuit Neurons

The granule cells, stellate cells, basket cells, and probably some of the cerebellar glial cells are derived from germinal cells that originate from the rhombic lip and migrate over the surface of the cerebellar plate to form a germinal zone, the external granular layer. The granule cells are generated in the external granular layer and migrate through the molecular layer and Purkinje cell layer to form the internal granular layer (Obersteiner, 1883, Ramón y Cajal, 1890a,b; Schaper, 1894a,b; 1895).

The external granular cells migrate over the surface of the cerebellum from the rostral part of the rhombic lip, a germinal zone in the alar plate forming the wall of the 4th ventricle (Schaper, 1894a,b, 1895; Ramón y Cajal, 1909–1911; Addison, 1911; Raaf and Kernohan, 1944). The germinal zone giving rise to the external granular layer is the most rostral part of the rhombic lip, the more caudal parts of which give rise to cells that migrate to form the inferior olivary nuclei, cochlear nuclei, and pontine nuclei (Harkmark, 1954; Taber Pierce, 1966, 1967a,b, 1973). The cells migrating from the rhombic lip form a continuous sheet extending rostrally over the cerebellar plate and medially into the brainstem, where the mass of migrating cells is termed the *pontobulbar body* in the human fetus (Essick, 1907, 1912).

The mechanism of migration of external granule cells is not well understood. A role of extracellular matrix molecules is quite likely but remains unproven. Fibronectin is not abundant in their migration pathway (Hynes *et al.*, 1986). Migrating external granule cells maintain contact with the basal lamina which may stimulate their motility and mitosis (Hausmann and Sievers, 1985). They are also in contact with axons (of unidentified origin) that may act as guides (Hynes *et al.*, 1986). It is not known what stops their migration after they arrive at their destination.

DNA synthesis and mitosis in the ventricular germinal zone decrease during the 13- to 15-day fetal period in the mouse, while at the same time the number of cells increases in the external granular layer (Miale and Sidman, 1961). In the chick embryo, mitotic activity declines in the ventricular germinal zone after E8 and ceases on E12, while the external granular layer appears only on E6 and increases in thickness between E8 and E15 (Saetersdal, 1956, 1959). Moreover, the DNA content, and hence the number of cells, of the chick cerebellum increases 400 percent between E11 and E21 (Margolis, 1969), as is shown in Fig. 2.19. This increase must be due entirely to proliferation of external granule cells because proliferation in the ventricular germinal zone ceases on E12 (Hanaway, 1967; Kanemitsu and Kobayashi, 1988).

The histogenesis of granule cells in the external granular layer has been described in the chick (Ramón y Cajal, 1890a; Saetersdal, 1956, 1959; Forströnen, 1963; Hanaway, 1967; Mugnaini and Forströnen, 1967; Kanemitsu and Kobayashi, 1988), the mouse (L. L. Uzman, 1960; Miale and Sidman, 1961; S. Fujita *et al.*, 1966; S. Fujita, 1967; Mares *et al.*, 1970), the rat (Addison, 1911; Altman and Das, 1966; Altman, 1966b, 1972c), the dog (Ramón y Cajal, 1929a; Phemister and Young, 1968), the cat (Purpura *et al.*, 1964), the monkey (Kornguth *et al.*, 1967, 1968), and the human (Ellis, 1920; Raaf and Kernohan, 1944; J. S. Woodard, 1960; Rakic and Sidman, 1970).

The external granular layer appears first over the posterolateral part of the cerebellum and spreads anteromedially to cover the entire cerebellar plate. In all vertebrates the external granular layer increases in thickness from a single layer of cells to a layer six to eight cells deep as a result of proliferation of external granule cells. Mitotic figures are scattered throughout the external granular layer during the period of its increase in thickness. In this respect the external granular layer does not resemble the ventricular germinal zone in which cells retract toward the ventricle during mitosis. Therefore, it appears unlikely that interkinetic nuclear migration occurs in the external granular cells. The external granular layer persists for a period that varies according to the species, but eventually it becomes reduced in thickness to a single layer of cells and ultimately disappears.

The external granular layer disappears at about the time of birth or soon after birth in precocial animals such as the chick or guinea pig, but it persists for some time after birth in altricial animals. For example, the external granular layer disappears only 20–25 days after birth in the albino mouse and rat, at about 60 days after birth in the cat, at about 75 days after birth in the dog, and at about 600 days after birth in humans (Fig. 10.10). During the initial period of increase in thickness of the external granular layer, cumulative labeling with [³H]thymidine results in labeling of 100 percent of the external granular cells (S. Fujita *et al.*, 1966). This shows that all the cells are engaged in DNA synthesis and mitosis. However, in the second half of the period of development of the external granular layer, a zone of cells without mitotic figures has been described, lying between the actively proliferating external granular cells and the molecular layer (Ramón y Cajal, 1909–1911; Addison, 1911). The cells in this zone do not incorporate [³H]thymidine, thus showing that they have ceased mitosis (S. Fujita *et al.*, 1966).

Migration of the granule cells was known to pose a difficult problem; because they arise late in development, they have to migrate along paths apparently blocked by obstacles in the form of cells that have developed earlier, and yet, as Cajal showed (Fig. 10.12), they follow a straight radial path. That problem was solved with the discovery that the Bergmann glial fibers act as guides for migrating granule cells (Mugnaini and Forströnen, 1967;

Rakic, 1971b) as shown in Fig. 10.13. In Golgi preparations, Cajal recognized the changes in shape and position of the granule cells as they migrate from the external granular layer. The cells in the superficial half of the external granular layer, which are in various phases of the generation cycle, were named the *"phase embryonale ou indifferent"* by Cajal. In the deeper part of the external granule layer the cells are bipolar, with two processes oriented parallel to the surface in the direction of the folia similar to the parallel fibers of the mature cortex (*"phase de la bipolarité horizontale"*). Cajal recognized that these were postmitotic granule cells at the beginning of their inward migration. By the use of tritiated thymidine autoradiography, it has been shown that these granule cells have ceased DNA synthesis, since they remain unlabeled after a period of exposure to the [³H]thymidine that results in labeling of all the cells in the superficial zone of the external granule layer (S. Fujita *et al.*, 1966; S. Fujita, 1967). A 3rd cytoplasmic process grows from the granule cells vertically down into the molecular layer, and the nucleus migrates into this process. The cells assume a T shape (*"phase de la bipolarité verticale"*),

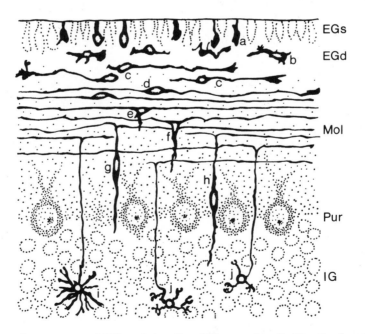

Figure 10.12. Phases in the migration and differentiation of cerebellar granule cells. Migration from the superficial zone of the external granule layer (EGs) to the deep zone of the external granule layer (EGd), through the molecular layer (Mol) and Purkinje cell layer (Pur), to the internal granule layer (IG) of the mammalian cerebellum. Modified from S. Ramón y Cajal (1909–1911).

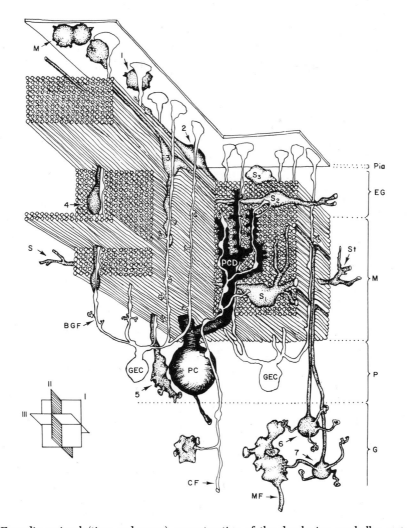

Figure 10.13. Four-dimensional (time and space) reconstruction of the developing cerebellar cortex in the rhesus monkey. The geometric figure in the lower left corner indicates the orientation of the planes: I, transverse to the folium (sagittal); II, longitudinal to the folium; III, parallel to the pial surface. On the main figure, the thicknesses of the layers are drawn in their approximately true proportions for the 138-day-old monkey fetus, but the diameters of the cellular elements, particularly the parallel fibers, are exaggerated to make the reconstruction more explicit. A description of the temporal and spatial transformations of the postmitotic granule cells (designated by numerals 1–7) and stellate cells (S), as well as other details, is given in Rakic (1971, 1987). BGF = Bergmann glial fiber; CF = climbing fiber; D = dividing external granule cell; EG = external granule layer; GEC = Golgi epithelial cell; M = molecular layer; MF = mossy fibers; P = Purkinje layer; PC = Purkinje cell; PCD = Purkinje cell dendrite; S_{1-3} = stellate cells; S = stellate cell dendrite.

as the nucleus migrates within the vertical cytoplasmic process and through the molecular layer and Purkinje cell layer. When the granular cell reaches its position in the internal granular layer, its migration ends, and some short, clawlike telodendria sprout from the cell body. This was termed the *"phase du grain profond ou jeune"* by Cajal. The

telodendria of the granule cells and of the Golgi cells, together with terminals of the mossy fibers, form the cerebellar glomeruli, which are first seen in the inner nuclear layer at 12–14 days after birth in the rat (Addison, 1911). As the granule cells continue to be formed into the 3rd week, and as additional time is taken by their migration and the growth of their dendrites, the formation of glomeruli continues for more than 30 days postnatally (Altman, 1972c).

It seems, from the arrangement of the internal granule cells, as if the deepest granule cells are generated first and the internal granule layer is formed in "inside-out" order. The axons of granule cells in the outer layer of the internal granular layer ascend to the surface of the molecular layer, while the granule cells lying progressively deeper send their axons to correspondingly deeper levels of the molecular layer (C. A. Fox et al., 1967; Altman, 1972b).

Mugnaini and Forströnen (1967) studied the ultrastructural changes that occur in the cerebellar cortex of the chick embryo at E17–E20 and found a continuous series of transitional forms of granule cells between the external and internal granular layers. Electron microscopy has thus confirmed the description of migrating granule cells illustrated by Ramón y Cajal (1890a,b, 1909–1911) and has shown that the radially oriented Bergmann glial fibers are used as guides by the granule cells (Fig. 10.13) as they migrate from the external to the internal granular layer (reviewed by Sidman and Rakic, 1973).

Proliferation and migration of cerebellar granule cells have been studied in the newborn mouse by means of [3H]thymidine autoradiography (Miale and Sidman, 1961; Altman, 1966b; S. Fujita et al., 1966). S. Fujita et al. (1966) determined the percentage of labeled cells in the internal and external granular layers of the cerebellum of the newborn mouse at different times after a single injection of [3H]thymidine (pulse labeling) and after the cells had been exposed to the labeled nucleotide for longer periods (cumulative labeling). The percentage of cells in the external granular layer which are labeled 2 hours after a single injection of [3H]thymidine increases from 30 percent at birth to 44 percent at P7 and then diminishes to zero at P20 (S. Fujita et al., 1966). Proliferation in the cerebellar ventricular germinal zone ceases after P10 in the mouse cerebellum, and labeling after P10 is confined almost entirely to the external granule cells, which makes it relatively easy to follow their migration.

The transit time of migrating external granule cells can be determined from the time of a pulse of [3H]thymidine to the time of first appearance of labeled granule cells in the internal granular layer. Altman (1966b) estimated that the maximum transit time of external granule cells over a distance of 200

μm is 3 days; the minimum speed of migration is 1.7–2.5 μm/hour. According to S. Fujita et al. (1966), the transit time is 42 hours, and the speed of migration of cerebellar granule cells is approximately 100 μm/day in the mouse (4.2 μm/hour). These rates of migration should be compared with the rate of 5.5 μm/hour of neurons migrating from the ventricular germinal zone to the cortical plate of the rhesus monkey (Rakic, 1974) and the migration rate of 4 μm/hour of neurons in the chick optic tectum (LaVail and Cowan, 1971b) and chick isthmo-optic nucleus (P. G. H. Clarke et al., 1976). The similar rates found independently in several different systems and species indicate that the underlying mechanisms of neuronal migration are probably similar in all these cases. By contrast, in vitro the rate of migration of granule cells on astrocytic processes is 20–60 μm/hour (Edmondson and Hatten, 1987; Hatten, 1990).

Concerning the origins of cerebellar glial cells, Ramón y Cajal concluded that only neurons are derived from the external granular layer, whereas all cerebellar glial cells are derived from the periventricular germinal layer. Schaper (1894a,b, 1895) proposed that the external granular layer consists of "indifferent cells" that may give rise to glial cells as well as neurons. From the results of [3H]thymidine audioradiography, S. Fujita et al. (1966) conclude that glioblasts originating from the ventricular germinal zone have already dispersed throughout the cerebellum of the mouse at birth before any cells have migrated from the external granular layer. The pulse-labeling experiments make it clear that a great deal of cell proliferation occurs in the internal granular layer of the mouse cerebellum from birth to P5. Between birth and P5, labeling of 5–10 percent of cells in the internal granular layer occurs within 2 hours after a single injection of [3H]thymidine. In that short period, labeled cells could not have migrated into the internal granular layer, and they must therefore be glioblasts, proliferating in the internal granular layer. Because cell migration from the external granular layer does not commence until P3 in the mouse, S. Fujita et al. (1966) concluded that the glioblasts of the internal granular layer originate from the ventricular germinal zone. They suggested that only after the cells of the external granular layer cease producing neurons do they change into glioblasts, which form the oligodendrocytes and astrocytes of the molecular layer. This is supposed to occur several days before the disappearance of the external granular layer, which occurs about P20 in the mouse.

Some of the cells produced in the external granular layer migrate only as far as the molecular layer and there differentiate into basket cells and small stellate cells. According to Altman (1972a), the basket and stellate cells are impeded from penetrating deeper than the underlying bed of parallel fibers because their processes are oriented at a right angle to the parallel fibers. In the rat the basket cells originate mainly on P6 and P7 while the stellate cells originate mainly on P8–P11 (Altman, 1972a). Some indication of the proliferative activity of the external granular layer may be gained from the observations that the DNA content of the mouse cerebellum increases 580 percent in the first 2 weeks after birth (Howard, 1968) and the DNA content of the chick cerebellum increases 400 percent in the last 10 days of incubation (Margolis, 1969). These increases can be attributed largely to the formation of granule cells and, to a far lesser extent, to glial proliferation. With a generation time of 16–20 hours, the external granule cells of the mouse can produce at least 14 generations in the first 14 days after birth, while in fact the total number of cells (DNA content of the cerebellum) increases 6 times. This indicates that many external granule cells cease DNA synthesis and mitosis before P14.

10.14. Selective Effects of Harmful Agents on Developing Cerebellar Cortical Neurons

An aspect of the specificity of neuronal types is their selective sensitivity or resistance to infections, cytotoxic agents, and ionizing radiation. Differences in the effect of such agents may thus help to reveal singularities in structure and function or in the developmental programs of the cerebellar neurons. Cells undergoing rapid mitosis and migrating cells are particularly susceptible to damage or destruction by radiation, cytotoxins, or virus infections. The external granule layer of the cerebellum is one of the sites of the most intense proliferative and migratory activity in newborn mammals. Agents acting in the perinatal and early postnatal period are thus likely to interfere with the development of cerebellar granule cells, and the other cerebellar cells may change as a result of loss of granule cells. Such changes have

been reported in the mammalian cerebellum as a result of postnatal X-irradiation (Hicks, 1958; Hicks et al., 1961; Hicks and D'Amato, 1966; Altman et al., 1968, 1969; Altman and Anderson, 1972), viruses (Kilham and Margolis, 1964, 1965, 1966a,b; Herndon et al., 1971a,b), cytotoxic chemicals such as nitrogen mustard, triethylene melamine, methylazoxymethanol, and other toxins (Hicks, 1954; Herndon, 1968; Nathanson et al., 1969; Shimada and Langman, 1970; Chanda et al., 1973; Lovell et al., 1980; Chen and Hillman, 1989), the thymidine analogue 5-bromodeoxyuridine (Zamenhof et al., 1971b; Webster et al., 1973; Yu, 1977), and fluorodeoxyuridine, which inhibits DNA synthesis (Maruyama et al., 1968; Shimada and Langman, 1970; Webster et al., 1973). External granular cells that survive the effects of X-rays or fluorodeoxyuridine can proliferate and reconstitute the external granule layer (Altman et al., 1969; Shimada and Langman, 1970; Altman and Anderson, 1972). This is a good example of plasticity in the developing brain of mammals.

Cytotoxic depletion of Purkinje cells results in a proportional reduction in granule cells but the reverse does not occur, showing that while granule cell survival is dependent on Purkinje cells, the latter originate and survive independently of granule cell influences. After destruction of the cerebellar granule cells, a variety of changes have been seen in the other cells of the cerebellum. Some of the changes, for example, the stunting of Purkinje cell dendrites, may be ascribed to removal of the normal afferents to the dendrites of Purkinje cells. The number of Purkinje cells is not reduced and the dendritic spines persist after removal of their afferents. The deafferented spines remain permanently disconnected as a rule, but in rare cases they have been found making anomalous synapses with mossy fibers (Altman and Anderson, 1972; Llinás et al., 1973). In the cerebellar cortex of ferrets after infection with panleukopenia virus, which destroys the granule cells, Llinás et al. (1973) found some evidence indicating that the mossy fibers, deprived of the granule cells which are their normal postsynaptic targets, may form anomalous synapses on stellate, basket, and Golgi cells. This is of interest in relation to mechanisms of development of neuronal connections, but the pathological changes that occur after virus infection should not be extrapolated too freely to normal development, and the term "neuronal plasticity" should not be used in such cases. To apply the term to all reactions of the nervous system in response to injury, regardless of the mechanism of the neuronal reaction, would only corrupt the meaning of the term. The term "neuronal plasticity" is better reserved for adaptive modifications of neurons within the normal physiological range and is thus a form of homeostasis. In the pathological case, the "specificity" of the mossy fibers themselves or of the cerebellar neurons may have been altered by the virus so that mossy fibers fail to recognize their correct postsynaptic targets.

Anomalous connections may be interpreted to support the theory that specificity of connections is not absolute but merely relative; connections may normally be made on the basis of the best fit between pre- and postsynaptic elements, but if the normal best fit cannot be achieved, a 2nd best fit may be a viable alternative. This and other hypotheses of the mechanisms of selective formation of synapses and of neuronal plasticity are discussed in Sections 6.10 and 6.13.

10.15. Mutations Affecting the Development of the Cerebellum

The times and sites of origin, migration, differentiation, and synaptogenesis of all the types of neurons in the cerebellar cortex, as well as those projecting to and receiving projections from the cerebellar cortex, have been described. However, the genetic, molecular, and cellular mechanisms remain largely obscure. One of the most promising ways of uncovering those mechanisms is to analyze mutations that alter development of specific components of the cerebellum. The genetic loci of these mutations have been mapped and molecular mechanisms can now be analyzed by molecular genetic technology.

Mutations affecting the cerebellum are autosomal recessive with the exception of lurcher, which is a dominant mutation. It is noteworthy that they all have their influence on terminal stages of differentiation, not on histogenesis. The various cerebellar neurons originate at the normal times and apparently in normal numbers, but the mutations produce changes in cell migration and differentiation. It is likely that mutations that affect histogenesis will have such widespread repercussions as to preclude fetal survival, even in the

heterozygous condition. This is entirely in accord with the concept that almost all mutations affecting development do so at late stages because mutations affecting early stages of development are usually lethal (Huxley and De Beer, 1934; M. Jacobson, 1974b, 1975a).

Over 20 mutations that affect the cerebellum have been described in the mouse (review, Sidman, 1983). Many of these mutations have been mapped on the mouse chromosomes (Roderick and Davisson, 1984). They are not clustered on any chromosome. Of the seven best studied mutations known to affect cerebellar development only reeler has widespread effects on many parts of the brain, but others also have pleiotropic effects. For example, Purkinje cell degeneration and nervous both result in slow retinal degeneration. Another example is the loss of dopaminergic neurons in the substantia nigra in the weaver mutant. A 3rd example is the degeneration of the principal neurons of the dorsal cochlear nucleus as well as Purkinje cells in lurcher, staggerer, nervous, and Purkinje cell degeneration. Purkinje cells are targets for monoamine-containing fibers. In all the cerebellar mutants there is a reduction in volume of the cerebellar cortex, and this results in an increased density of monoaminergic (NA and 5-HT) fibers. In Purkinje cell degeneration, the monoaminergic fibers persist after loss of their targets, the Purkinje cells (Landis et al., 1975; Kostrozewa and Harston, 1986; Triarhou and Ghetti, 1986).

The salient features of the mutant mice with cerebellar abnormalities are summarized as follows. The effects are described in the homozygous condition unless otherwise noted.

Swaying (gene symbol sw, Sidman, 1968). Mice with the swaying mutation show hypotonia of the limbs and ataxia from birth. Parts of the anterior cerebellar vermis are missing, and the remainder of the vermis is malformed and fused with the colliculi. The cerebellar cortex is broken into islands of cells by aberrant fascicles of nerve fibers. Despite the disruption of the normal morphology, the individual cell types preserve their proper anatomical relationships. This is in marked contrast to the abnormal intercellular relationships found in all the other cerebellar mutants.

Weaver (gene symbol wv, Sidman et al., 1965; Sidman, 1968). In the homozygous weaver mutant the cerebellum is small due to loss of almost all the granule cells during the 1st and 2nd weeks after birth. There is massive death of catecholaminergic neurons in the substantia nigra and loss of dopamine in the caudoputamen. The mice are small, hypotonic, ataxic, and have a severe tremor, but some survive to adult age. In the cerebellum, in addition to the loss of granule cells, the Bergmann glial cells are reduced in size and irregular in shape. Other abnormalities of the cerebellum include reduction of the numbers of Golgi II cells and Purkinje cells, failure of alignment of Purkinje cells, and stunting of the dendrites of Purkinje cells, which form a layer that is several cells deep. Despite the absence of the parallel fibers that normally synapse on the Purkinje dendritic spines, the latter appear unaffected (A. Hirano and Dembitzer, 1973; A. Hirano *et al.*, 1977). Innervation of individual Purkinje cells by several climbing fibers persists in weaver mice (Mariani, 1982). Climbing fibers retain their connections with somatic spines of Purkinje cells (Landis, 1973). There are abnormal connections between mossy fibers and Golgi II cells. The granule cells originate at the normal time and apparently in normal numbers, but they die at the inner margin of the external granular layer. The fact that granule cell death starts on the day of birth and that the majority of them die before starting their migration suggests that their defect may be expressed at that early stage (Smeyne and Goldowitz, 1989).

The primary defect in weaver was first recognized to be in the granule cells by Sidman (1968), and this hypothesis received additional support from the evidence that the small percentage of granule cells that migrate as far as the internal granular layer die nevertheless (Sotelo and Changeux, 1974). More direct evidence that the granule cells are defective is that dissociated *wv/wv* granule cells die in tissue culture whereas +/+ granule cells survive under the same conditions (Willinger *et al.*, 1981; Willinger and Margolis, 1985a,b). Also, in cocultures of +/+ and *wv/wv* neurons and glial cells, the +/+ granule cells migrate on *wv/wv* glial cells, but not vice versa (Hatten *et al.*, 1984, 1986). Analysis of *wv/+* ↔ +/+ chimeras shows that 100 percent of the malpositioned granule cells have the weaver genotype, indicating that they are primarily affected but that granule cells that survive and migrate successfully to the internal granular layer of chimeras are all wild-type. Malpositioned Purkinje cells and Bergmann glial cells can be of either genotype,

showing that they are not primarily affected by the mutation (Goldowitz and Mullen, 1982; Goldowitz, 1989).

The role of Bergmann glial fibers as guides for migrating granule cells first proposed by Mugnaini and Forströnen (1967), and later much amplified by Rakic (1971b), indicated that the primary effect of the mutation might be on the Bergmann glial fibers, which are reduced in number and morphologically abnormal (Rakic and Sidman, 1973a–c). The Bergmann fiber abnormalities are first seen after the 3rd postnatal day in homozygotes as well as in heterozygotes. The Bergmann glial fibers are enlarged 2–4 times in diameter and have a variety of cytoplasmic abnormalities (Rakic and Sidman, 1973b,c; Bignami and Dahl, 1974b; Sotelo and Changeux, 1974b). The available evidence indicates that the defect in Bergmann glial fibers is probably secondary. Differentiation of Bergmann glial cells depends on interactions with Purkinje cells (M. Fisher, 1984; M. Fisher and Mullen, 1988). Rezai and Yoon (1972) found a severe loss of Purkinje and Golgi II cells, which are reduced by about 40 percent, in a gradient with 100 percent loss in the medial half of the cerebellar cortex (Herrup and Trenkner, 1987).

Selective loss of dopamine in the nigrostriatal fibers occurs in weaver mutant mice. Although severe depletion of dopamine in the dorsal striatum occurs, dopamine in the ventral striatum is relatively unaffected (M. J. Schmidt *et al.*, 1982; Roffler-Tarlov and Graybiel, 1984, 1986, 1987; Graybiel *et al.*, 1990; Roffler-Tarlov *et al.*, 1990). Loss of dopamine-containing neurons occurs in the substantia nigra and in the limbic midbrain (Pullara *et al.*, 1986; Kaseda *et al.*, 1987; Roffler-Tarlov and Graybiel, 1987; Ohta *et al.*, 1989). Therefore, the widespread effects make it difficult to assign the defect primarily to any single type of cell. In spite of the excellent morphological studies, we still have no indication of the primary gene products that are altered in weaver or any of the cerebellar mutants.

Staggerer (gene symbol *sg*, Sidman, 1968). The staggerer mutant is clinically similar to weaver, including the ataxia, slight tremor, hypotonia, and a small cerebellum deficient in granule cells, but the pathogenesis is entirely different in the two mutants. In staggerer the defect is first seen in the Purkinje cells, which are small and have stunted dendrites almost devoid of spines (Sidman, 1968, 1972; Landis and Sidman, 1978). Analysis of *sg/sg* ↔ +/+

chimeric mice shows that only the mutant Purkinje cells are abnormal, indicating that the defect is localized to the *sg/sg* Purkinje cells (Herrup and Mullen, 1979, 1981). Multiple innervation of Purkinje cells by climbing fibers persists (Mariani and Changeux, 1980; Crepel *et al.*, 1980). The disease is associated with defective sialic acid metabolism and with defective sialylation of the neural cell adhesion molecule (NCAM), possibly perturbing cell adhesion (Wille *et al.*, 1981; Edelman and Chuong, 1982).

The granule cells originate on schedule and migrate normally but then die in the 2nd–5th weeks after birth. The external granular layer persists for several days longer than normal (Sonmez and Herrup, 1984) as if attempting to compensate for the loss of granule cells. This may indicate that the granule cells normally exert a negative control of external granule cell proliferation. Sidman (1974) and Sotelo and Changeux (1974a) have suggested that the granule cells die because they are dependent on the formation of connections with their usual postsynaptic elements, the spines of Purkinje cell dendrites, which are absent in staggerer (Landis and Sidman, 1978). However, this dependence is not reciprocal, for Purkinje cell dendritic spines are not dependent on the granule cell inputs. This is demonstrated by the survival of the dendritic spines in the absence of granule cells in weaver as well as after depletion of granule cells by irradiation, virus infection, or cytotoxins (Altman *et al.*, 1969; A. Hirano *et al.*, 1972; Llinas *et al.*, 1973).

Reeler (gene symbol *rl;* Falconer, 1951; Hamburgh, 1960, 1963; Meier and Hoag, 1962; Sidman *et al.*, 1965). Reeler mutant mice have ataxia, hypotonia, and a fine tremor. The mutation results in malpositioning of neurons in many parts of the brain, including cerebral cortex, cerebellar cortex, deep cerebellar nuclei, and dorsal cochlear nucleus. The dorsal cochlear nucleus and cerebellar cortex have analogous circuit logic and it is therefore probably significant that they are both affected in several mutations in mice, namely, nervous, lurcher, staggerer, and Purkinje cell degeneration. Certain molecular markers are also common to cerebellar cortex and dorsal cochlear nucleus. Cerebellin is a neuropeptide hexadecapeptide which is a specific marker for Purkinje cells and is found in only one other location, the dorsal cochlear nucleus (Mugnaini and Morgan, 1987). PEP-19 is a polypeptide marker found in Purkinje cells and in cartwheel neurons in the dorsal cochlear nucleus (Mugnaini *et al.*, 1987).

In reeler mice the cerebellum is small and the fissures are greatly reduced. The Purkinje cells are misplaced, misaligned, and reduced to about 82,000, less than half the number found in normal mice. About 5 percent of Purkinje cells are in the normal position, 10 percent are located in the granular layer, and the remainder form deep cerebellar masses (Heckroth *et al.*, 1989). Purkinje cells have stunted dendrites with few small branchlets and gross disorientation of the dendritic tree (Fig. 10.14). The granule cells are reduced in number, and most lie external to the Purkinje cells. The Golgi epithelial cells are malpositioned in the molecular layer and their Bergmann glial fibers are conspicuously disoriented (Rakic, 1975; Mikoshiba *et al.*, 1980; Terashima *et al.*, 1985b), as shown in Fig. 10.15. The primary defect seems to be in the interactions between the Golgi epithelial cells and Purkinje cells (and possibly other types of neurons) which are necessary for migration and alignment of the neurons. There are abnormalities of positions and shapes of neurons in the deep cerebellar nuclei (Mariani *et al.*, 1977; Goffinet *et al.*, 1984). Synaptogenesis appears to occur normally, despite the cellular disarray (Rakic and Sidman, 1972; Bliss and Chung, 1974).

Chimeric *rl/rl* ↔ +/+ mice have no brain abnormalities although the cerebellar cortex is formed of cells of both genotypes (Terashima *et al.*, 1986). This shows that the *rl/rl* phenotype is not expressed autonomously but can be modified by interaction with cells of the wild type (Figs. 10.14 and 10.15).

Developmental malfunctions similar to those in the cerebellum occur in the cerebral cortex (Caviness and Rakic, 1978; Rakic, 1978, review; see Section 10.7). Just as the granule cells fail to migrate past the cerebellar Purkinje cells, the granule cells of the fascia dentata fail to migrate to their proper positions (Meier and Hoag, 1962; Stanfield and Cowan, 1979), the young neurons of the cerebral isocortex fail to migrate outward past the neurons that preceded them, and the thalamocortical projections take aberrant courses, but nevertheless make connections with their correct targets to establish topographically normal afferent and efferent projections (Hamburgh, 1960, 1963; Caviness and Sidman, 1972, 1973; Devor *et al.*, 1975; Caviness,

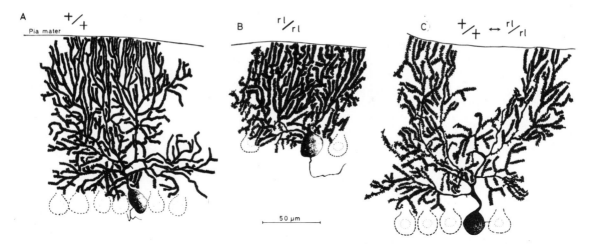

Figure 10.14. Purkinje cell dendrites are stunted in reeler mice but can be restored to normal size by interaction with normal cells in chimeric cerebellum. (A) Normal Purkinje cell; (B) Purkinje cell of a homozygous reeler; (C) Purkinje cell of a chimeric rl/rl ↔ +/+ mouse. Golgi–Stensaas stain. From T. Terashima, K. Inoue, Y. Inoue, M. Yokoyama, and K. Mikoshiba, *J. Comp. Neurol.* **252**:264–278 (1986), copyright Alan R. Liss, Inc.

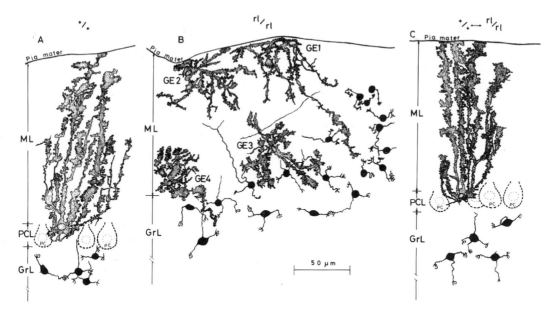

Figure 10.15. Displacement of Golgi epithelial cells and misalignment of their Bergmann fibers in the cerebellar cortex of reeler mice are corrected by interactions with normal cells in chimeric mice. (A) Golgi epithelial cell in the cerebellar cortex of a normal mouse with its cell body in the normal relationship to the Purkinje cell layer (PCL) and its Bergmann fibers extending radially out in the molecular layer (ML) to the pia mater. (B) Golgi epithelial cells in a homozygous reeler mouse with their cell bodies displaced to various positions in the molecular layer (ML) and with disoriented Bergmann fibers. Note the displaced granule cells in the molecular layer. (C) In a chimeric *rl/rl* ↔ +/+ chimera the normal arrangement is restored. Golgi–Stensaas stain. From T. Terashima, K. Inoue, Y. Inoue, M. Yokoyama, and K. Mikoshiba, *J. Comp. Neurol.* **252**:264–278 (1986), copyright Alan R. Liss, Inc.

1976, 1977; Dräger, 1981; Simmons *et al.*, 1982). The patterns of monoaminergic projections to the cerebral cortex are normal in reeler mice (Caviness and Korde, 1981).

Abnormalities also occur in several laminated structures in the forebrain to which the olfactory bulbs project, namely, anterior olfactory nucleus, olfactory tubercle, and cortical nucleus of the amygdaloid complex (Caviness and Sidman, 1972), as well as in the dorsal cochlear nucleus (Martin, 1981), the inferior olivary complex (Goffinet, 1981, 1983), the optic tectum (Frost *et al.*, 1982), and the facial nucleus (Goffinet, 1984). Histogenesis is normal in all these structures, but the mutation changes the positions of the principal neurons in relation to local-circuit neurons and to afferent fibers.

Despite cellular malpositioning, there are only minor abnormalities in the principal connections in the hippocampus, in so far as they can be detected by electrophysiological or anatomical methods (Bliss and Chung, 1974; Stanfield *et al.*, 1979; Dräger, 1981). Conservation of essentially normal synaptic associations between malpositioned and disoriented neurons in the reeler cerebral and cerebellar cortex is a good example of the selective growth of axons to their postsynaptic targets in a situation where failure of such selective synaptogenesis might be predicted (Rakic, 1976; Caviness and Rakic, 1978, reviews). A mutant Japanese quail has been found that is similar to reeler mutant mouse in clinical features and histopathology (Ueda *et al.*, 1979).

Lurcher (gene symbol *Lc*; Phillips, 1960; Wilson, 1975, 1976). This is an autosomal dominant mutation, which in the homozygous condition results in death shortly after birth. Heterozygous (*Lc/+*) mice are smaller than normal, but have a normal lifespan. They have a lurching gait and tend to walk backward. The cerebellum is reduced in size, and has an abnormal pattern of foliation. Heterozygous lurcher mice lose almost all Purkinje cells during the 2nd and 5th weeks after birth (Caddy and Biscoe, 1975, 1979). Analysis of *Lc/+* ↔ +/+ chimeric mice shows that the *Lc* gene acts only in the *Lc/+* Purkinje cells, all of which degenerate (Wetts and Herrup, 1982a,b). Loss of about 90 percent of the granule cells and neurons of the inferior olive occurs secondary to death of Purkinje cells (Wetts and Herrup, 1982a,b, 1983).

Nervous (gene symbol *nr*; Landis, 1973) and

Purkinje cell degeneration (gene symbol *pcd*; Mullen et al., 1976). These two mutants are similar in that death of Purkinje cells is the major abnormality and slow retinal degeneration occurs in both mutations, yet they differ in a number of significant ways (Sidman and Green, 1970; Landis, 1973; Sidman, 1974; Wassef *et al.*, 1986, 1987). In both mutants the majority of Purkinje cells degenerate in the first 2 months after birth, but the mice show only moderate ataxia. The rate of Purkinje cell loss also differs in the two mutations: in *pcd* the loss is very rapid and almost total, whereas in *nr* the loss is slower and incomplete. In Purkinje cell degeneration (Mullen *et al.*, 1976; Landis and Mullen, 1978), cerebellar histogenesis and morphogenesis are normal until cell degeneration begins at about P18, reaches a peak at P22–P28, and results in virtually complete loss of Purkinje cells by P30. Death of Purkinje cells occurs only after formation of synaptic contacts between Purkinje cell dendritic spines and parallel fibers, between P7 and P15. The possible significance of this is discussed later.

There is remarkably little functional loss considering that the Purkinje cells are the only cells projecting out of the cerebellar cortex. There is no evidence of compensatory changes in the deep cerebellar nuclei (Roffler-Tarlov *et al.*, 1979). Almost all retinal photoreceptors degenerate, starting at E13, and Müller glial cells are also abnormal (Blanks *et al.*, 1982). Degeneration of mitral cells of the olfactory bulbs occurs. Secondary to loss of Purkinje cells there is a gradual degeneration of granule cells, resulting in loss of about 90 percent of granule cells by the end of the 1st year. Adult males have abnormal sperm and are thus infertile.

Nervous mutants show mitochondrial abnormalities in all Purkinje cells at about P15, and this is followed by loss of 85–90 percent of the Purkinje cells in the cerebellar hemispheres and more than 50 percent in the vermis, mainly from P23 to P50 (Landis, 1973). Months after loss of most of the Purkinje cells, the parallel fibers survive essentially normally but with a loss of about half of their presynaptic varicosities. Nevertheless, the relatively long survival of parallel fibers in Purkinje cell degeneration and nervous is in sharp contrast with their rapid degeneration in staggerer mice, in which death of Purkinje cells occurs before they form synaptic contacts with parallel fibers. In Purkinje cell degeneration and nervous, the short period of synaptic contact with Purkinje cells apparently stabilizes the parallel fibers (Sotelo, 1980).

Analysis of *pcd/pcd* ↔ +/+ chimeras shows that all the *pcd/pcd* Purkinje cells die, leaving the +/+ cells unaffected (Mullen, 1977). Further evidence that the mutation is intrinsic to Purkinje cells is that when normal E12 cerebellum is grafted into the cerebellum of 2- to 4-month-old *pcd/pcd* hosts, the grafted Purkinje cells survive and form synaptic connections with host neurons (Sotelo and Alvarado-Mallart, 1987; Gardette *et al.*, 1990a,b). Mitochondrial abnormalities are seen in some Purkinje cells in *nr/nr* ↔ +/+ chimeras but it has not yet been shown whether the mutation is cell autonomous (Mullen, 1982).

What has been learned from these cerebellar mutants? Perhaps it is easiest to say what has not been learned: it has not yet been possible to identify the primary gene product that is absent or defective in any of the mutants. Molecular cloning of the genes for these mutations will enable their translation products to be identified. It will then be known whether they are regulatory or structural products. The pleiomorphism of many cerebellar mutations indicates that they are likely to affect "housekeeping" gene products in many types of cells. The phenotypic expression is liable to be misleading, as the history of weaver has shown, and we should not be surprised to find that the primary defect is remote from the phenotypic expression of the mutant allele.

There is not a good correlation between the severity of the anatomical defect and the functional derangement in these mutant mice. Loss of neurons, even on a massive scale, can result in essentially normal organization. For example, massive loss of Purkinje cells occurs in lurcher (Caddy and Biscoe, 1979), Purkinje cell degeneration (Ghetti *et al.*, 1987), reeler (Goffinet *et al.*, 1984; Heckroth *et al.*, 1989), and staggerer (Shojaeian, 1985a,b; Blatt and Eisenman, 1985). This results in loss of inferior olivary neurons. In spite of this loss, topographic organization of the olivocerebellar projection is essentially normal in the mutant mice. Perhaps the fact that total loss of Purkinje cells in *pcd/pcd* mice is associated with mild ataxia whereas persistence of about 15 percent of Purkinje cells in *st/st* mice is associated with severe dysfunction may illustrate the general principle that total and rapid loss of a structure without formation of aberrant connections may be less crippling than the effects resulting from malconnections between surviving cells.

In defense of the use of mutants that affect the nervous system, it can be said that the only means of mapping the genetic loci that influence development of the nervous system is by finding mutant alleles. In addition, the study of the defective morphogenesis of the brain has led to further understanding of the mechanisms of normal morphogenesis. Thus, while the role of Bergmann glial cells in guiding granule cells was suggested by Mugnaini and Forströnen (1967) from studies of normal material, the concept of guidance of migrating neurons by radial glial cells has obtained greater credence from the studies on the weaver mutant. Cloning the *wv* gene and identification of the biochemical lesion(s) in the weaver cerebellum will give additional insight into the molecular basis of neuronal recognition.

The mutants illustrate the considerable autonomy of the Purkinje cells: their phenotype remains recognizable in spite of their gross malpositioning in reeler, and they retain their dendritic spines in spite of the depletion of granule cells in weaver and reeler. In the absence of their normal input these naked dendritic spines rarely accept alternative presynaptic inputs. This and other observations have a bearing on the problem of specificity of synaptic connections. Synapses are formed with surprising normality in mutants in which cells are grossly malpositioned, provided that the cells are present (Rakic, 1975b). In weaver mice the mossy fibers target accurately on heterotopic granule cells (Rakic and Sidman, 1973b), and the malpositioned Purkinje cells in reeler cerebellum receive all the usual synaptic inputs (Rakic and Sidman, 1972). However, aberrant synaptic connections may be formed by presynaptic cells whose postsynaptic targets are absent. For example, in weaver cerebellum, if the depletion of granule cells is slight, the mossy fibers form synapses correctly on granule cells, although the latter are malpositioned. But the mossy fibers synapse aberrantly on Golgi II cells if the granule cells are very severely depleted or virtually absent, as they may be after irradiation or in some regions of the homozygous weaver cerebellum.

The mutants show the limits of malconnections, for when the Purkinje cell dendritic spines are devoid of parallel fiber inputs they do not accept anomalous inputs from neighboring axons such as mossy fiber terminals. Nor do the basket and stellate cells, which synapse on the smooth parts of the Purkinje cell dendrites, occupy the synaptic sites on the spines left vacant by the parallel fibers. It is also very significant that, despite malpositioning of the neurons in the reeler cerebral cortex, the appropriate classes of neurons are connected within the cortex, and the interhemispheric connections through the corpus callosum are normal (Caviness, 1976; Caviness and Yorke, 1976). These observations are consistent with the concept that presynaptic terminals will target with great precision and efficiency on matching postsynaptic targets even if the latter are malpositioned (M. Jacobson and Levine, 1975b), but if the targets that fit normally are inaccessible the next best fit may sometimes be a viable alternative. One has to proceed cautiously with this line of reasoning in cases where poisons or radiation might well have disturbed the postsynaptic membrane markers that enable the axon terminals to recognize their appropriate targets.

In summary, the mutants may be said to have given considerable evidence of the stability of the mechanism that results in selective synaptic association and to have given some evidence of the formation of functional connections between neurons that do not normally form such connections. The possible roles of such malconnections in the evolution of the nervous system is discussed in Section 2.13.

10.16. Development of Cortical Folds in the Cerebrum and Cerebellum

Although the convolutions of the cerebral and cerebellar hemispheres have excited interest since antiquity, scientific studies of the development of the convolutions may be said to have started with Friedrich Tiedemann (1781–1861), who, in 1816, correctly described the order of development of the main *primary, secondary,* and *tertiary* fissures in the human fetus during the final trimester of gestation. The terms primary, secondary, and tertiary were introduced later by Alexander Ecker in 1869,

and an accurate and almost complete description of their development in the human fetus was given by Wilhelm His (1890a, 1904).

Primary sulci are quite invariant in all members of the species (Connolly, 1950; Bailey and von Bonin, 1951), secondary sulci show more individual variation even in identical twins, and tertiary sulci show great variability. Bailey and von Bonin (1951) list the following primary cerebral sulci in the primate brain: hippocampal, Sylvian, calcarine, parieto-occipital, callosomarginal, central, interparietal, superior temporal, olfactory, and rhinal. Secondary sulci include precentral, postcentral, lunate, superior frontal, and orbital.

There is a large literature devoted to the individual and racial variability in the pattern of cerebral convolutions in humans, but in summarizing the literature Bailey and von Bonin (1951) conclude that there is no evidence of racial differences and that the basis of the individual variations, whether genetic or developmental, is not known.

The developing primate cerebral cortex is smooth during the period of neuron genesis and migration, and only shallow primary fissures are present at the time when virtually all cortical neurons have been formed (Schaffer, 1923; Bok, 1929; Smart and McSherry, 1986b). The primary sulci start developing earlier than the secondary sulci, and finally the tertiary sulci. Primary sulci appear after the 20th week of gestation in the human fetus, starting with the calcarine and parieto-occipital sulci on the medial surface of the occipital lobe in all primates. Gyri become well defined between 26 and 28 weeks in the human fetus and are fairly constant in their positions. The tertiary sulci, which start developing in the 8th and 9th months of gestation and become fully developed only in the 1st year after birth, are quite variable. Folding does not occur while the neurons are being produced, but only afterward during the phase of glial cell production, growth of nerve cell processes, and myelination.

By the end of the 4th month of gestation the human brain has developed the characteristic shape and fissuration of the cerebral hemispheres that make it possible to distinguish the human brain from the anthropoid brain by virtue of macroscopic features (Retzius, 1896, 1906b). The density of fissuration is greater at birth than in the adult and the sulci become separated as the cortex expands during the neonatal period. As the brain grows, its surface area would increase as the two-thirds power of brain weight or volume if the surface remained smooth. In fact, as a result of folding of the surface, the surface area increases as the 1st power of brain weight. As a result of cortical folding the cortical surface area of the human brain, relative to a mouse brain, is 12 times larger than would be predicted if the cortex was not folded (Prothero and Sunsten, 1984). Surface area of the cortex can increase relative to brain weight by increasing the number and height of the gyri.

There are two theories of development of cerebral cortical gyri. The 1st is that folding occurs because of the greater growth of the flexible cortex relative to the rigid internal structures such as the corpus callosum, thalamus, and basal ganglia (Le Gros Clark, 1945). According to the other theory, cortical folding is due to relative differences in growth within the cortex itself: differences between layers and between regions (Bielschowsky, 1923; D. H. Barron, 1950; Welker and Campos, 1963; Richman et al., 1975; Smart and McSherry, 1986a,b). Development of convolutions is clearly correlated with the maximal rate of increase in the volume of the cortex, but it seems unlikely that the relatively invariant pattern of gyri can be explained simply by differences in rates of growth between the cortex and the underlying tissues.

An experimental analysis of the problem, by D. H. Barron (1950), shows that the cerebral convolutions develop normally in the sheep fetus after removal of the basal ganglia and corpus callosum or after undercutting of the cortex has separated it from the relatively rigid structures beneath. Barron concluded that the deep brain structures are not involved in cortical folding but that the mechanism of folding is within the cortex. The same conclusion has been reached from a different direction: Richman et al. (1975), from a consideration of congenital defects of cortical folding in human fetuses, concluded that gyri develop because of unequal growth of the superficial and deep layers of the cortex. In microgyria the cortex is thrown into an increased number of small folds, whereas the cortex is smooth in lissencephaly. In both malformations the cortex is thinned and the number of layers is reduced (Richman et al., 1973; R. M. Stewart et al., 1975). In the normal cortex the three outer cortical layers grow at a slightly faster rate than the three inner layers. In the lissencephalic cortex the growth of all cortical

layers is greatly reduced, and there is no significant difference in growth rate between inner and outer layers, whereas in microgyria the inner cortical layers grow more slowly than normal.

Although the difference in rates of growth of cortical layers can explain why the cortex buckles, it does not indicate why the primary and secondary fissures occur at relatively constant positions. That constancy is likely to result from differences in growth rates between different parts of the cortex. Folding of the cortex occurs during the growth of dendrites of cortical neurons, and it is likely that the geometry of dendritic growth and of the fiber trajectories within the cortex will be found to have a constant relationship to the geometry of the gyri. The shape of each gyrus may give an indication of the functional organization of the underlying cortex in the sense that some cellular elements have a constant geometrical relationship to the axes of the gyrus.

Welker and Campos (1963) have cogently reasoned that the invariance of the primary and secondary fissures is due to the differences in the density of the thalamocortical projection to functionally distinct regions of the cortex. Gyri receive strong projections from the thalamus, while sulci receive weak thalamic projections. The major gyri tend to receive projections from distinct peripheral body regions, so that the invariant pattern of primary and secondary fissures can be correlated with functional mapping onto the cortex (Fig. 10.16).

Folding of the cerebellar cortex must occur as the result of proliferation in the external granular layer which leads to tremendous expansion of the cortex over the relatively slowly growing white matter. A role of meninges is suggested by the observation the cerebellar cortical folding is grossly abnormal in rats after destruction of meningeal cells by injection of 6-hydroxydopamine (Sievers et al., 1986). The main pattern of cerebellar gyri and sulci is established early in postnatal development. The cerebellar fissures are all identifiable at P2 in the mouse (Mares and Lodin, 1970), and in the human fetus all the lobules of the cerebellar vermis can be identified as the major fissures develop at about 15 weeks of gestation. Thereafter, the number of folia increases until about 2 months postnatally, as shown in Fig. 10.17 (Loeser et al., 1972).

As the cerebellar cortex grows, the fissures deepen and the gyri become more pronounced. The

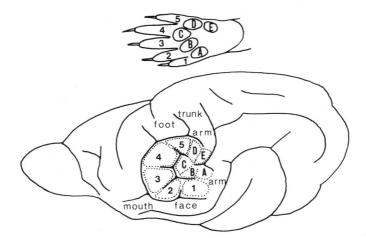

Figure 10.16. Correspondence of gyri in the left cerebral hemisphere with sensory representation of the right side of the body in the raccoon. The area of cortex representing a unit area of skin varies with the receptor density, afferent nerves, and thalamocortical projection. The plantar skin of the footpads of the front paw has a greatly magnified cortical representation. This is correlated with the raccoon's use of its front paws as sensory organs. From W. I. Welker and S. Seidenstein, *J. Comp. Neurol.* 111:469–501 (1959).

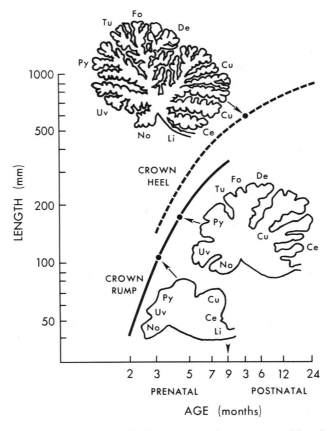

Figure 10.17. Development of folia in human cerebellar vermis in relation to age and length of the fetus and newborn infant. The total number of folia in the cerebellar vermis is about 10 at 15 weeks of gestation, increases to about 50 at 20 weeks, 250 at 40 weeks, and attains the adult number of 300 at about 30 weeks after birth. From J. D. Loeser, R. J. Lemire, and E. C. Alvord, Jr., *Anat. Rec.* 173:109–114 (1972).

mechanisms of gyrification are not known. Many models have been proposed (Harman, 1947; Stephan, 1960; Elias *et al.*, 1969; Haug, 1970; Elias and Schwartz, 1971; Schlenska, 1974; Todd, 1982; Prothero and Sundsten, 1984). It is easy to conceive qualitatively of the mechanics of folding of a sheet of tissue as the result of differences in rates of growth within the cerebellar cortex or between the cortex and underlying brain. More rapid growth of the cortex than the underlying brain is considered to be the principal cause of cerebellar folding (Saetersdal, 1956; Haddara and Nooreddin, 1966).

The pattern of fissuration may be due to differences in rates of cell proliferation or to growth and cell death at different depths in the cortex and in different cortical regions. The causes of such regularities of cell proliferation, growth, and death are entirely unknown. In the cerebellar cortex of the mouse the proliferation rate in the external granular layer is slightly greater in the sulci than on the gyri (Mares and Lodin (1970), which may be the cause of the cortical thickening in the depth of the sulcus and cortical thinning at the convexity of the gyrus.

The pattern of folding of the cerebellar cortex is definitely related to the cellular architectonics: the folia develop in the axis of the parallel fibers, while the Purkinje cell dendrites are in the plane orthogonal to the long axis of the folium. In mutant mice with cerebellar defects that result in reduced growth of the cerebellar cortex, the fissures are also reduced. The secondary cerebellar fissures are almost absent in the reeler mutant mice, in which malpositioning and disorientation of cerebellar cells result in serious disruption of the normal pattern of cortical lamination.

11   Neuronal Specificity and Development of Neuronal Projection Maps

Theorists almost always become too fond of their own ideas. It is difficult to believe that one's cherished theory, which really works rather nicely in some respects, may be completely false. . . . It is amateurs who have one big bright beautiful idea that they can never abandon. Professionals know that they have to produce theory after theory before they are likely to hit the jackpot.

Francis Crick (1916–), *What Mad Pursuit*, 1988[1]

11.1. Theories of Neuronal Specificity and Plasticity in Historical Perspective

Man has been trained in the same way as animals. He has become an author, as they became beasts of burden. A geometrician has learned to perform the most difficult demonstrations and calculations, as a monkey has learned to take his little hat off and on, and to mount his tame dog. All has been accomplished through signs. . . . But who was the first to speak? Who was the first teacher of the human race? Who invented the means of utilizing the plasticity of our organism?

Julien Offroy de la Mettrie
(1709–1751), *Man a Machine*, 1748

During the 17th century science was at first concerned only with formulating mechanical and mathematical models to explain natural phenomena. Philosophy retained its traditional role of explaining how it is possible for a person to perceive objects in the physical world. During the seventeenth and eighteenth centuries a mechanistic picture of the physical universe was gradually extended to include the sense organs and nervous system of the perceiving subject. At first this extension was limited to the direct actions of physical stimuli on the sense organs. These were regarded as the boundary between the physical world and vital processes which were believed to be properties uniquely belonging to living beings. The interactions could be conceived as a penetration of atoms into the sense organs resulting in movements of vital spirits in the nerves of sensation. Descartes conceived of these nervous spirits as material atoms or particles whose movements in

---

[1]Indeed, the probability of a gambler hitting the jackpot is about the same as that of the so-called professional hitting on the "correct" theory. Willingness to abandon refuted theories is a sign of professionalism, but the critera for refutation must be sophisticated, otherwise the true theories are as likely to be abandoned as the false. Theories need to be held with some tenacity to enable them to gather sufficient corroborative evidence to protect them from premature refutation.

the nerves were governed by their physical properties and by purely mechanical processes. The boundary between the external world, conceived as mechanism, and the psyche, conceived as a vital agent, was moved progressively more deeply into the nervous system, until, according to Descartes, the interaction between physical and psychical occurs in the pineal gland.

This neural internalization of the mechanistic universe was the crucial conceptual advance toward mechanization of the brain picture and was the essential point of departure leading to modern neuroscience. Prior to that conceptual advance, neuroanatomical and neurophysiological observations were heavily encumbered with vitalistic preconceptions. After the step had been taken, the boundary between the physical universe and the psyche could be looked for deep in the nervous system, and the nerves linking the psyche to the external world could be regarded safely and simply as mechanisms.

In the 19th century, starting with Helmholtz and du Bois-Reymond, the idea of such a mechanical–vital neural boundary could finally be abandoned. It was at that historical juncture that the concept of nerve cells as components of a neuronal machine became well established. This concept, which required that different components of the neuronal machine must have structural and functional specificity, originated immediately before the histological and physiological evidence was obtained to support the theory.

The theory of neuronal specificity holds that there are different classes of nerve cells which can be distinguished from one another by certain structural and functional properties which may belong collectively to cell groups (e.g., as expressed by the specific pattern of connections between cells in a group and between different groups) and may even be restricted to individual cells.

Throughout the history of the concept of biological specificity we can recognize two distinct and opposing views: emphasis on the importance of structural and functional specificity is associated with the mechanistic view of the organism, whereas the opposite is associated with the vitalistic view.[2]

---

[2]Vitalism is a term of convenience for a number of different concepts that share the notion that life cannot be

Historical progress of the concept of neuronal specificity is closely linked to construction of a mechanistic view of the brain. This program is associated with repudiation of vitalism, denial of teleology, and with understanding specificity in terms of mechanistic causal relationships between structure and function of nerve cells.

There is a relationship between completion of mechanization of the picture of the physical universe and the comparable advance in neuroscience which I have called the mechanization of the brain picture. By this is meant the concept that the brain can be entirely understood in mechanistic terms and the historical development of that concept and growth of knowledge supporting it. Mechanization of the brain picture has closely followed the mechanization of the world picture (M. Jacobson, in preparation). Mechanization of the world picture (Dijksterhuis, 1950) was started in 1543 with Copernicus' work *De Revolutionibus Orbium Coelestium*. The same year Andreas Vesalius published *De Humani Corporis Fabrica*, which marks the first stage

---

explained only by known physical mechanisms. For example, Bichat (1800) proclaimed that vital processes could never be reduced completely to physics and chemistry. Vitalist theories have been reviewed by L. R. Wheeler (1939) and T. S. Hall (1969). One vitalist theory is that nonmaterial causal agents operate only in living matter, e.g., the "entelechy" of Driesch (1908). Proponents of this theory are caught in a paradox: the vital force is believed to be free of the laws of matter but its freedom is impossible without matter. Another vitalist idea is that physical forces operate in a unique way in living matter, and the related idea that unique vital properties emerge as a result of complexity. Varieties of these ideas have been held by numerous scientists, including Johannes Müller, Virchow, Justus Liebig, and Hans Spemann. This kind of belief has been called "vital-materialism" by Temkin (1946) to distinguish it from the mechanical materialism of Helmholtz and du Bois-Reymond, who believed that the mode of organization, not the complexity itself, distinguishes living from dead matter. Some modern inheritors of the idea of emergent properties maintain that consciousness cannot be explained completely by physiology, biochemistry, or molecular biology but only in terms of quantum mechanics (Lockwood, 1989) or by understanding the operation of the brain as a "quantum computer" (Penrose, 1989). But it remains to be seen whether such efforts will go beyond the Cartesian or La Mettrian mechanization of the brain picture to a postmechanistic quantumization of the brain picture.

in mechanization of the picture of the human body and brain. According to Dijksterhuis (1950), the mechanization of the world picture was completed in 1687 with Isaac Newton's *Philosophiae Naturalis Principia Mathematica.*

René Descartes brought the mechanization of the brain picture almost to its logical completion in his late work *Passions of the Soul (Les Passions de l'âme,* 1649) and his *Treatise of Man,* first published posthumously in 1664. Within the limits of his knowledge of the actual workings of the brain, Descartes could conceive of it as a pure mechanism in lower beasts, but he recoiled from saying that the human brain is a self-sufficient machine. He perceived of the human performing some involuntary actions, later to be called reflexes, without the intervention of the soul. In performing such actions the human acts like a machine, but consciousness, thought, reasoning, and free will require the action of the soul. He conceived of the central nervous system (CNS) as an orderly and invariant arrangement of nerve fibers which conduct animal spirits in the form of *"very small bodies that move very fast"* into the brain from the sense organs and out to the muscles. These microscopic entities, tiny bodies travelling in hollow nerve fibers, were purely conjectural—the nerve fiber was first identified by means of the microscope by Fontana in 1781 and particles moving in nerve fibers were observed for the first time almost two centuries later. Here is an example of the conjecture coming first, the experimental evidence following much later (see epigraph to Section 1.1).

Descartes thought that movements of the tiny bodies in the nerves, and life itself, occur without intervention of the soul. The function of the soul is to change the direction of flow. Variable linkages between input and output are made by the command of the soul moving the pineal gland (Fig. 11.1). The soul as conceived by Descartes can be characterized in the words used by Newton to describe gravitation—it is either an occult force or a perpetual miracle. By introducing a nonmaterial agent, Descartes left the mechanistic view of the brain in a compromised position—the mechanism is necessary for life but not sufficient for consciousness, ratiocination, and free will. For Descartes, material objects in the external world produce changes in the material structure of the nervous system which evoke the appropriate mental states as a result of the action of the soul. He affirms the existence of the external world but denies that we can perceive it directly. The Cartesian concept of self is of a soul locked inside the brain receiving information about the external world via remote sensors.

Descartes' legacy enriched and encumbered his intellectual heirs. It encumbered us with a dualistic brain picture (cf. Popper and Eccles, 1977; Eccles, 1989); it enriched us with at least five valuable ideas. These ideas are that the brain is a machine; that variability of brain action is accomplished by switching transmission between the ends of different nerves; that reflex movements, purposeful and adaptive, occur without conscious control; that reflex activity requires a nervous circuit—an afferent nerve linking the sense organ with the brain, transmission in the brain between input and output, and efferent nerves linking the brain to the muscles. Finally, and most important, Descartes saw science and philosophy as essentially interrelated and he formulated two fundamental principles of modern science: the invariability of laws of nature and the power of human reason to understand them. From these premises Descartes argued that progress in science is possible if nature is investigated by the right methods.

It was not until almost a century after publication of Descartes' *Treatise of Man* that a totally uncompromising mechanistic picture of the brain was sketched in outline by Julien Offroy de la Mettrie. In his *Natural History of the Soul (Histoire naturelle de l'âme,* 1745) and in his polemical essay *Man a Machine (L'Homme machine,* 1748) La Mettrie argues that the human is a self-regulating machine, entirely self-sufficient and without a soul or any nonmaterial spirit. Mental faculties, such as volition, imagination, emotion, memory, and consciousness, can be reduced to mechanisms ultimately based on irritability, which is the fundamental attribute of living organisms. Irritability can itself be reduced to motion of the particles and fibers of which the organism is made. La Mettrie obtained his ideas about irritability from Francis Glisson (1597–1677), Giovanni Borelli (1608–1679), Albrecht von Haller (1708–1777), and Hermann Boerhaave (1668–1738) under whom he studied briefly and whose works he translated into French. But La Mettrie went far beyond the timid materialism of his predecessors, who were careful to restrict the application of their theory to purely physical functions such

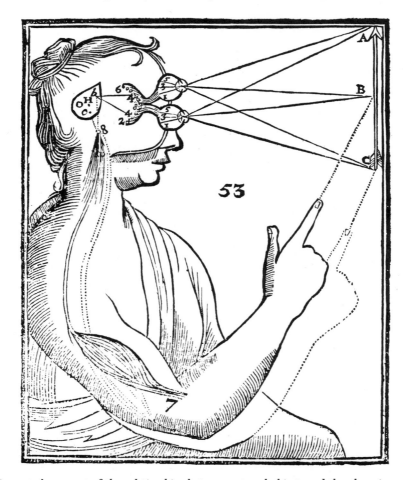

Figure 11.1. Descartes's concept of the relationships between external objects and the observing and acting subject. Several ideas are illustrated in this figure from Descartes's *Treatise of Man* (1st ed., 1664): the image of the external object is inverted on the retina; corresponding points on the retina (e.g., 3 and 3̃) project via intermediate relays 4 and 4 to the same place (b) in the brain, in the pineal gland, in which Descartes thought that the incoming messages from the sense organs were routed along outgoing nerve fibers (8) to either a flexor muscle (7) or extensor (dotted nerve and muscle), thus moving the arm to point the finger precisely to the external object. These events may be entirely automatic, or the soul, located in the pineal (H), can control the action voluntarily. The soul is locked inside the brain, receiving messages from remote sensors and relaying them to remote effectors via fixed pathways.

as movements of the muscles. La Mettrie could say *"Matter is self-moved"* (*Histoire naturelle de l'âme*, V, 1745), and *"The brain has muscles for thinking, as the legs have muscles for walking"* (*L'Homme machine*, 1748). He would have been immensely pleased with the recent discovery of contractile proteins in neurons and with the evidence that dendritic spines change shape in response to stimulation (see Section 6.3). But La Mettrie's writings are mere firecrackers compared with the big guns of Newton and Descartes. His flashes of brilliance only highlight the logical weakness of his arguments. Then, too, there were social, cultural, religious, and politi-

cal conditions which made a mechanistic view of the brain without a soul seem disreputable.[3]

I find it remarkable that the research program to establish ever more precise relationships between structures and functions in the cerebral cortex

[3]This is not the place to consider La Mettrie's successors such as Baron P. H. D. von Holbach (1723–1789), whose *Système de la nature*, first published in 1770 under a pseudonym, further advanced the philosophical position of mechanistic materialism and determinism. For the history of materialism see F. A. Lange (1877–1881), J. T. Merz (1904–1912)., A. Wolfe (1952), J. Roger (1962).

should have moved along two different, and seemingly irreconcilable, tracks: one aimed at total mechanization, the other at finding a refuge for the soul. By the end of the 19th century the Cartesian soul, seated in the pineal gland, could be dismissed either as an error of localization or as a more fundamental error of the dualist philosophical position. For dualists, then, the question was where to locate the soul, and the cerebral cortex was to be its final refuge. The scientific program to define the functions of the cerebral cortex in purely mechanistic terms became an assault on the citadel of the soul. By the end of the 19th century, as the functions of more and more parts of the cortex became defined, it seemed to some as if the soul had finally been driven from its refuge. However, for others the soul continued to inhabit those parts of the cortex to which functions could not yet be assigned. For example, Eccles (1989) conjectures that the place where the human soul interacts with the brain is in the dominant cerebral hemisphere. This is a strong conjecture but it is easily refuted. It is based on the mistaken belief that cerebral hemispheric asymmetry is uniquely human, and on the debatable belief that the immaterial soul needs a localized point of interaction with the material brain. But if one believes in the existence of a soul, there is no good reason also to believe with the Cartesians that the soul enters into functional relationship with the brain only at one anatomical location. Flourens (1824, 1842) believed that the soul is functionally related to the brain as a whole, and that is as credible as the belief that it has a local abode in the cerebral cortex or any other part of the brain.

There was a strong reaction by vitalists to the rise of materialism in the 18th and 19th centuries. The reaction centered on two points: the development of complexity and the purposefulness of development. Both were said to be explicable only in terms of formative vital forces. We have space only for a few examples showing that the same phenomena were interpreted quite differently by vitalists and mechanists: regeneration and pattern regulation in hydra, Wolffian lens regeneration, the specificity of serological reactions, and recovery of function after nerve regeneration.

Abraham Trembley published his book on regeneration and pattern regulation in hydra in 1744 and made the observation that two small, but complete, hydra are reconstituted after bisecting the animal. This was variously interpreted in terms of

different theories: Bonnet saw it as an example of preformation; La Mettrie regarded it as a case of epigenesis (see Nordenskiöld, 1928; Cole, 1930; Needham, 1934; Meyer, 1939). Johann Friedrich Blumenbach (1752–1840) considered the performance of the hydra to be due to a formative effort (*Bildungstrieb*, or *nisus formativus*), and in his *Institutions of Physiology* (1816) he says: *"The word nisus I have adopted chiefly to express an energy truly vital and therefore to distinguish it from powers merely mechanical by which some physiologists formerly endeavoured to explain generation. [The nisus is a union of] two distinct principles in the evolution of the nature of organized bodies— of the PHYSICOMECHANICAL, with the purely TELEOLOGICAL."* This concept of the dual nature of the organism is essentially similar to Descartes' concept of the duality of the brain. It is not mere coincidence that from the 17th to the 20th century vitalists have tried to find similarities between embryonic development and psychic processes, and some illustrative examples of this are given in the following pages.

The experiments by Hans Driesch in the 1890s showing that a whole embryo can develop from a single blastomere and that normal embryos can develop after rearrangements of blastomeres (reviewed by Oppenheimer, 1970b) seemed to him to show the operation of a nonmaterial force operating purposefully to restore that original pattern. Driesch recognized this type of regulative behavior to be typical of what he named the *"harmonious equipotential system."* He states: *The harmonious system then, is not a 'machine'; it is, in fact . . . something that is governed by Invidualizing Causality. Entelechy, as a non-mechanical agent of nature, is at work in the harmonious–equipotential system"* (Driesch, 1914, p. 210). By "individualizing causality" Driesch meant causality with a purpose, namely, teleology (see Churchill, 1969, for a discussion of Driesch's theory of causality). The brain was considered to be a harmonious–equipotential system and to show properties of such a system during recovery from injury. If Driesch had known about the expansion and compression of retinotectal maps (see Section 11.13) or plasticity of somatotopic maps following peripheral nerve injury (see Section 11.7), he would have regarded them as harmonious–equipotential systems.

Wolffian lens regeneration is another example showing how the phenomenon could be given different meanings in the context of different theories. After removal of the lens from the eye of a newt, a new lens grows from the outer edge of the iris in a way which does not correspond with its normal development from surface ectoderm of the embryo. When Gustav Wolff published this result in 1894 he claimed that it demonstrated teleology and vitalism (also see Wolff, *Mechanismus und Vitalismus*, Leipzig, 1902).[4] E. S. Russell (1946) considered Wolffiann lens regeneration to be irrefutable evidence of *"the directiveness"* of regenerative processes in which *"the same end result is achieved as in ontogeny, but from a totally different starting point."* Driesch also considered this to be incapable of explanation in mechanistic terms because he thought that the competence of the tissue to produce entirely different structures from those that they formed during normal development could not have evolved by natural selection. We shall see shortly how this problem can be resolved in terms of teleonomy.

Embryonic regulation was generally conceived by Hans Spemann to be akin to psychic processes. Formation of a lens after ablation of the primary lens-forming cells in the embryo drew from him this interpretation: *" . . . we have from various sides the explanation of the ability of the upper iris margin to produce a lens, which points to the fact that these cells have the same ectodermal origin as the cells of the epidermis. Now, they are even more closely related to the cells of the brain, and from those or their products we may suppose . . . that the processes in them run parallel with psychical process, thus certainly teleological, which means that they can be judged to be analagous to the psychic"* (Spemann, 1905, p. 432). He continued to believe in a similarity between psychic and embryonic regulatory processes until the end of his career. In the final summary of his work, *Embryonic Development and Induction* (Spemann, 1938), he makes this declaration (pp. 371–372): *"Again and again terms have been*

[4]It is significant that Gustav Wolff later turned from embryology to neurology and especially to the problem of aphasia resulting from brain injury. He expressed his anti-mechanistic prejudice in a theory of brain plasticity based on his clinical experience with aphasic patients (Wolff, *Beiträge zur Lehre von den Sprachstörungen*, Leipzig, 1902). Spemann tells us in his autobiography that as a student he was acquainted with Wolff, with whom he shared vitalistic beliefs.

used which point not to physical but to psychical analogies. This was meant to be more than a poetical metaphor. It was meant to express my conviction that the suitable reaction of germ fragments, endowed with the most diverse potencies, in an embryonic 'field,' its behavior in a definite 'situation,' is not a common chemical reaction, but that these processes of development, like all vital processes, are comparable, in the way they are connected, to nothing we know in such a degree as to those vital processes of which we have the most intimate knowledge, viz., the psychical ones."

Discovery of the specificity of serological reactions by Landsteiner (1899) initiated the research program that finally established the mechanistic basis of biological specificity. Incredible as it now seems, specificity of immune reactions was understood by Driesch as evidence in support of vitalism. He states that *"the organism is not of the type of a machine. . . . It is precisely in the field of immunity that such a machine-like preparation of the adaptive effects seems almost impossible to be imagined. How indeed could there be a machine, the chemical constituents of which were such as to correspond adaptively to almost every requirement"* (Driesch, 1908, p. 209). Once again we encounter the notion that mechanistic explanations are inadequate to account for adaptation to novel conditions never before experienced in the evolution of the species. This notion has had many supporters (Driesch, 1908; Bergson, 1911, especially Chapter 1 on mechanism and teleology; H. F. Osborn, 1929; E. S. Russell, 1946; Teilhard de Chardin, 1965). Elsasser (1989) suggests that in biology causality is replaced by creativity. All these writers are hung up in one way or another on the idea of teleology. They conceive of adaptation and fitness of the organism and its parts in terms of design and thus of purpose. This is an important general problem and is of particular interest because of the prevalence of teleological thinking in our field of neuroscience, especially in relation to the design and purpose of nervous organization and the recovery of that organization after injury.

Philosophers of science do not agree on the use of teleological explanations in biology. There are those who consider teleology to be permissible and to be entirely consistent with mechanistic causality (Nagel, 1961; Beckner, 1969; Wimsatt, 1970, 1972; Ayala, 1970; Hull, 1974). Others reject teleological explanations because of the se-

mantic difficulties created by the use of the term "teleology," which has various meanings (Woodger, 1952), and because they claim that use of teleological explanations obfuscates an understanding of how goal-directed processes have evolved by natural selection (Pittendrigh, 1958; Mayr, 1965, 1974, 1981). It seems best to me to regard embryonic regulations and neuronal plasticity as *teleonomic processes,* which are defined as physiological processes that owe their goal directedness to programs that have been adjusted during evolution by the selective value of the goal or end-point (Pittendrigh, 1958; Mayr, 1981). Now it is possible to understand that adaptive responses of the embryo or of the nervous system in response to injury can only make use of the goal-directed programs which have evolved for normal ontogeny, which are teleonomic processes.

The importance of this problem of evolution of nervous plasticity that could have been of no advantage to the species under conditions of natural selection is shown by many examples of plasticity after nervous system injury. Expansion or compression of the retinotectal map in response to size disparities between retina and tectum is one example in amphibians and fishes (see Section 11.13). Even if plasticity results in functional recovery in the laboratory, the time required would nullify any practical advantage under natural conditions. These kinds of plasticity cannot be understood in terms of teleology. But they are understandable as examples of teleonomy: the cellular mechanisms of neuronal plasticity have evolved because they are advantageous in accomplishing normal development. They are fortuitously brought into play after injury and not because they evolved for that purpose.

Reflexes are another example of goal-directed functions that have been interpreted teleologically but are better regarded as teleonomic processes. Reflex action poses the same dilemma as other goal-directed processes—whether to repudiate teleology or to use it as a convenient explanatory principle. Sherrington (1906, p. 236) summed this up as follows: *"Older writings on reflex action concerned themselves boldly with the purpose of the reflexes they described. The language in which they are couched shows that for them the interest of the phenomena centered in their being regarded as manifestations of an informing spirit resident in the organism, lowly or mutilated though that might be.*

Progress of knowledge has tended more and more to unseat that anthropomorphic image of the observer himself which he projected into the object of his observations. The teleological speculations accompanying such observations have become proportionately discredited." But Sherrington could offer nothing to replace teleology, and he reluctantly used it as an explanatory principle. He argues in favor of coming to terms with teleology: *"The purpose of a reflex seems as legitimate and urgent an object for natural inquiry as the purpose of the colouring of an insect or blossom. And the importance to physiology is that the reflex cannot be really intelligible to the physiologist until he knows its aim."* But then he admits that *"the assigment of a particular purpose to a particular reflex is often difficult and hazardous because it is a fractional reaction that may belong to any of many general reactions of varied aim"* (Sherrington, 1906, pp. 235-239). The point can also be made that different reflexes which are not normally coordinated during natural behavior can be integrated by training to produce behavior that could neither have served any functional goal nor have been of any adaptive value in evolution: parrots can be trained to talk and sing and circus animals to perform their tricks, as La Mettrie says (see epigraph to Section 11.1). The trainer can reprogram the existing repertoire of behaviors that have evolved by natural selection. The parrot's repertoire of vocalizations can be reprogrammed to sound like words, but the parrot can never understand the meaning of its utterances.

From Descartes to the neurophysiologists Marshall Hall, Sherrington, and Pavlov, analysis of reflex action has been at the center of all attempts at building models of the nervous system (Fearing, 1930; Liddell, 1960). The words "reflexion," meaning reflex action, afferent (*aufleitend*), and efferent (*ableitend*) were used by Unzer (1771), who follows Descartes in referring to nervous systems as animal machines (*thierische Maschinen*). In Descartes' theoretical construct the sensory and motor nerves are shown entering and leaving the nervous system quite separately, and his model required independent nervous channels in the brain for different functions. However, one well-recognized difficulty with the concept of separate sensory and motor nerves was the observation that stimulating or cutting a peripheral nerve results in a mixture of sensory and motor effects. Resolution of this problem is conventionally said to begin with Charles Bell

(1811), who first proposed the idea that although sensory and motor nerves are mingled in peripheral nerves they are separated in the CNS (Gordon-Taylor and Walls, 1958). Bell had an aversion to experiments on live animals and thus could only show the motor functions of nerves in freshly killed animals. Experimental analysis of the problem by François Magendie (1822), using living animals, proved that the ventral spinal nerve roots are motor and the dorsal roots are sensory (Olmsted, 1944; Cranefield, 1974).[5]

The relationship between structure and function of the spinal nerve roots became known as the *Bell–Magendie law*. It is arguably equivalent in the history of neuroscience to Harvey's discovery of the circulation of the blood in the history of physiology (Foster, 1899; Olmsted, 1944; Cranefield, 1974). Parallels between the two discoveries exist but should not be drawn too closely. They were both generalizations in which direction of flow to or from the center is the essential principle of operation of the whole system. However, the blood was seen to circulate in a closed loop whereas the nerves were at first dimly conceived in terms of an open loop, and the concept of reflex circuits gradually grew out of the Bell–Magendie Law. The Bell–Magendie law started an era of theorizing about the organization of the nervous system in terms of input and output functions of different nerves, each of which subserves a logical function in the whole system. A century later Sherrington (1933, p. 21) could still affirm that *"we have seen the brain as an input–output signalling system."*

During the 19th century the sensory and motor pathways in the CNS were traced experimentally by observing functional impairment caused by CNS lesions. The method of experimental ablation of parts of the CNS was perfected by Flourens, although it had been used by others before, notably by Rolando (1809; see E. Clarke and O'Malley, 1968). The results of ablation experiments provided further con-

[5]In 1811 and 1821 Bell concluded that the anterior spinal roots and columns are both sensory and motor in function and the posterior spinal roots and columns have autonomic ("vital") functions. Magendie (1822) was the first to identify correctly the sensory and motor functions of the anterior and posterior roots. The priority dispute arose in 1824 when Bell published new versions of his 1811 and 1821 reports altered to conform with the results of Magendie's 1822 paper.

firmation of the specificity of separate sensory and motor pathways in the brainstem and spinal cord. Longet (1842) showed that lesions of the dorsal columns of the spinal cord result in loss of sensation but not of movements. By 1851 Brown-Séquard had convincingly demonstrated that hemisection of the spinal cord in guinea pigs results in anesthesia on the opposite side of the body below the lesion and motor paralysis on the same side, thus proving that the nerve fibers conveying sensation cross to the opposite side of the spinal cord while the motor nerve fibers run on the same side.

The concept of functional specificity in the nervous system, that is, that specific functions are subserved by specific types and groupings of neurons, can be said to have originated between 1835 and 1845 with Johannes Müller and his students. After the establishment of the Bell–Magendie law, the question arose as to whether different sensory modalities are subserved by the specificity of the stimulus in addition to the central connections made by the nerves. Johannes Müller (1826) found that the retina will give rise to the sensation of light no matter what kind of stimulus is applied, and this was later generalized to all sensory modalities as the *"law of specific nerve energies."* Theodor Schwann worked in Müller's laboratory for the 4 critical years (1834–1838) which led to his final synthesis of the cell theory in 1839 (for a critical appraisal of Schwann's contribution see Sections 3.6 and 5.1 and footnote 3 in Chapter 8). At that time, Hermann Helmholtz and Emil du Bois-Reymond were also students of Müller and carried out the program of defining the functional specificity of the nervous system by biophysical and psychophysical methods. Within Müller's school there was a progressive movement toward materialism and away from vitalism, to which Müller himself adhered until near the end of his life. In 1844 Helmholtz and du Bois-Reymond formed a group of physiologists, the "organic physicists," who undertook to eliminate all traces of vitalism from their neurophysiological research which would be founded purely on physics and chemistry. Under their influence Müller finally repudiated vitalism. The historical development of the organic physics of 1844 to the biophysics of today is traced by Cranefield (1951).

Nerve regeneration is another large domain of research in which the two antithetical concepts of rigidity (specificity) and plasticity were opposed from the earliest work (Arnemann, 1787) to the modern era (Langley, 1918; Ramón y Cajal, 1928; Weiss, 1937; Young, 1942; Sperry, 1945). Reports of recovery of function in the presence of random regeneration of peripheral nerves were taken to indicate that orderly function can occur in the presence of disordered structure or that reorganization occurs in the periphery or centers or both (reviewed by Sperry, 1947). Many believed that the precise pattern of nerve connections is unimportant: correct function will follow as long as some connections develop in the embryo or regenerate after injury. This was the conclusion of Bethe (1905), Bethe and Fischer (1931a), Anokhin (1935a,b, 1940), and Goldstein (1939). During the 1930s the prevailing opinion was that the central and peripheral nervous systems of mammals, including humans, can recover from injury by adaptive and regulative processes. The restorative processes were conceived of as a form of resonance between the periphery and the nerve centers (Anokhin, 1935a,b), or as a kind of *plasticity* (the word used by Bethe and Fischer, 1931a,b).

During the 19th century plasticity meant modification of the organism by the environment. This was the sense in which Charles Darwin understood the meaning of plasticity, which he rejected in favor of selection of variations as the cause of evolution. Plasticity and selection were considered to be the two causes of adaptation. Lamarck made plasticity, as a result of use and disuse, a central thesis of his theory of evolution by inheritance of acquired characters. In his *Histoire Naturelle* (1815–1822) Lamarck states the *"Law of Use and Disuse"* in the following terms: *"The development of organs and their force or power of action are always in direct relation to the employment of those organs."*

This principle of functional adaptation forms the central thesis of the biological system of Herbert Spencer (1820-1903). In *"The Development Hypothesis"* (1852) Spencer states that *"any existing species—animal or vegetable—when placed under conditions different from its previous ones, immediately begins to undergo certain changes fitting it for the new conditions."* This idea was generalized in Spencer's *Principles of Biology* as the *principle of functional adaptation*. It implies a principle of design and purpose, thus of teleology. Spencer's philosophical works exerted tremendous influence on 19th-century biologists. One of these was Wilhelm Roux, who followed the mechanistic and Darwinian

theories of his teachers Haeckel and Weismann. In his book *Der Kampf der Theile im Organismus* (1881) Roux makes the distinction between functional adaptation, resulting from direct action of the environment on the organ or tissue, namely plasticity, and competitive adaptation, resulting from selection of favorable cellular variations in a Darwinian struggle for survival of the fittest.

During the 19th century an important difference in the understanding of biological plasticity emerged between those who, like Driesch, understood plasticity in terms of the operation of a single continuously variable parameter—a plastic force distributed in some way through the system—and those who conceived of rearrangements of discontinuous entities such as molecules and cells. One might even characterize these as wave theories and particle theories. What decides whether the organization is a continuous gradient or a series of discontinuous patches or blobs? Scale of the pattern is one determining factor: waves and gradients operate only over small dimensions. Thus the gradients in the embryo have to be translated into the stripes or patches on the adult. Wave and particle theories have to some extent been unified in biology with the discovery that a diffusible morphogen can specify cell fates in a concentration-dependent way (Eichele and Thaller, 1987). A continuous gradient is thus translated into discrete molecular labels, and cells specified by possession of those labels may then be free to act autonomously and to express their specificity even after moving to different positions.

Systems that exhibit wavelike or gradient-like behavior also tend to show cooperative interactions between the components whereas in other systems plasticity may be the outcome of competition between the components. Wilhelm Roux (1881) pointed out the difference between these two types of plasticity and drew attention to the functional adaptation resulting from cellular competition and cellular selection on the basis of functional optimization. Historically, Roux's concept was derived from the dichotomy between the Lamarckian and Darwinian theories of evolution. Roux translated those theories into a theory of cellular plasticity: one type of plasticity occurs as the result of use and disuse, the other from a struggle for survival between cells competing for limited supplies of nutrients. In neither case, Roux insists, is it necessary to involve nonmaterial vital forces or to invoke the operation of teleology.

The concept of biochemical specificity of the cell developed historically with the rise of cell biology and physiological chemistry in the second half of the 19th century. Such important cases as the specificity of cellular and bacterial chemotaxis, the specificity of fertilization of the egg by the sperm, serological reactions, and tissue graft rejection were recognized as examples of cellular specificity based on cell type-specific molecules. By the first decade of the 20th century the components necessary to build biochemical molecular models of neuronal specificity were available. For example, Jacques Loeb (1916) wrote: *"What is the nature of the substances which are responsible for and transmit this specificity? . . . There can be no doubt that on the basis of our present knowledge proteins are in most or practically all cases the bearers of this specificity"* (Loeb, 1916, p. 60). Loeb considered *"specificity due to specific proteins"* to be one of the *"two characteristics of living matter,"* the other being the ability to synthesize macromolecules.[6]

The concepts were available which indicated that a biochemical and biophysical analysis of neuronal specificity was desirable. Thus, Weiss (1946) provided a molecular model in which nerve cell specificity was conceived as *"selective adhesion and non-adhesion among cells in terms of molecular configurations along the contact surfaces"* (Fig. 11.2). This model was developed further by Sperry (1963) as the *"chemoaffinity theory."* However, direct tests of that theory could not be done because the tools to do the necessary molecular biological experiments were only invented more recently.

The concept of cellular specificity has a venerable history, supported by classical observations such as those on the specificity of chemotaxis of

[6]Loeb wrote this after he had started his work on protein chemistry at the Rockefeller Institute and after his celebrated address of 1911 on *"The Mechanistic Conception of Life."* Before 1911 his work had been guided by the vitalistic philosophy of his teachers, the botanist Julius Sachs and the neurologist Friedrich Goltz (cf. Pauly, 1987). Loeb did experiments with Goltz on functional representation in the cerebral cortex and came to the conclusion that the cortex functions as a whole. This aspect of Loeb's work is well reviewed by Lashley in *Brain Mechanisms and Intelligence* (1929), in which he reaches the conclusion that the cerebral cortex functions as a whole, as an harmonious–equipotential system, in the sense of that term as used by Driesch.

sperm, first reported by Pfeffer in 1884, and the specificity of serological reactions (Landsteiner, 1899, 1936). Such observations and the general idea of cellular specificity were in the minds of those who tried to explain the selectivity with which neurons connect with one another and with muscles and sense organs (*cf.* Ramón y Cajal, 1909, p. 658, 1928, p. 392).

Cell specificity can be recognized by the preference shown by any type of cell for associating with other cell types. The evidence that cell recognition plays an important role in morphogenesis comes largely from studies of reaggregation of sponge cells (H. V. Wilson, 1907; Humphreys, 1967; Burger, 1974; Burger *et al.*, 1975) and reaggregation *in vitro* of cells from amphibian, avian, and mammalian embryos (Holtfreter, 1939, 1944; Townes and Holtfreter, 1955; Moscona, 1962, 1968; Steinberg, 1962a,b, 1963, 1970). Johannes Holtfreter was the first to show how differential cellular affinities and migrations could account for many aspects of morphogenesis of vertebrate embryos (Holtfreter, 1939, 1944; Townes and Holtfreter, 1955). He found that different types of cells sort themselves out when dissociated cells are mixed and allowed to reaggregate. In experiments in which fragments from different tissues are fused or in which isolated cells of different types are mixed under conditions that allow them to reassemble, the cells of different tissues tend to regain the relative positions in the aggregate that they normally occupy in the embryo. By using mixtures of cells with different appearances, Holtfreter was able to demonstrate that sorting out is due to cell migration. Selective cellular reaggregation is also shown by chick cells segregating from mouse cells (Moscona, 1962) and by sorting out of chick embryo cells labeled with tritiated thymidine from unlabeled chick cells of a different type when the two dissociated cells types are mixed and then allowed to reaggregate (Trinkaus and Gross, 1960).

Holtfreter regarded the sorting out of cells as a manifestation of *"tissue affinities"* or of *"cell specific differences in surface tension"* (Holtfreter, 1939, 1944), while Weiss (1941a) referred to *"selective adhesiveness"* as an important factor in morphogenesis. Townes and Holtfreter (1955) concluded that sorting out of embryonic cells is due to selective cell adhesion and to chemotactic migration of cells along a radial concentration gradient. Steinberg (1962a,b)

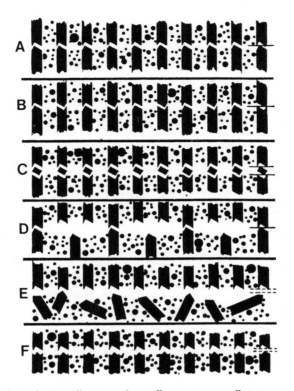

Figure 11.2. Diagram to explain selective adhesion and nonadhesion among cells in terms of molecular configurations on the contact surfaces. The key molecules, which numerically constitute only a small and variable fraction of the surface population, are symbolized as bars with characteristically shaped adhesion sites. In (A) and (B) the adhesion molecules are complementary. In (C) a linker molecule is interposed. (A), (B), and (C) are assumed to result in strong adhesion. (D) shows weak adhesion. (E) and (F) show nonadhesion. From P. Weiss, *Yale J. Biol. Med.* 19:235–278 (1947).

ruled out the latter and showed that sorting out can be due entirely to differential cell adhesion. He found that when two types of cells are sorting out they do not move directly, by radial pathways, to their correct positions but rather form small clusters which gradually fuse to form a single aggregate of one cell type which becomes enveloped by cells of the other type. Steinberg (1963) tested all 15 pairs that can be formed among six different types of chick embryo cells in sorting-out experiments and demonstrated a hierarchical order of affinity in which cells of higher rank in the hierarchy always envelop those of lower order.

The observation that reaggregating cells tend to sort out to regain their former intercellular relations in the tissue made it obvious that nerve cells may exercise a similar selectivity in choosing a pathway along which to migrate or to extend axonal or dendritic processes and in selecting other neurons with

which to form synaptic connections. It was a small step from Holtfreter's demonstration of *"Gewebe-affinität"* ("tissue affinity") to the notion that the self-assembly of nerve circuits results from intercellular recognition, which is, in turn, based on distinctive cytochemical properties of nerve cells (Weiss, 1941, 1947). Those concepts form the basis for the chemoaffinity theory of neuronal specificity (Sperry, 1950a, 1963).

Paul Weiss (1941, 1947) was the first to formulate a molecular theory of the ontogeny of neuronal specificity. He refers to the *"specification"* of neurons by their terminal organs, and he made a molecular model to represent the mechanism of specificity and specification. This model (Fig. 11.2) is obviously a forerunner of the cell adhesion theory of Edelman (1983, 1984). *The chemoaffinity theory of neuronal specificity* as proposed by Roger Sperry (1950a, 1951a,b, 1963, 1965) is essentially derived from the theory of his teacher Paul Weiss, who conjectured that neuronal circuits are assembled as a result of selective biochemical affinities and disaffinities between nerve cells. Its origins from concepts of cell biology have been outlined, but historically the significance of the chemoaffinity theory is that it was a reaction to the extreme empiricist view, widely held in the 1930s, that use and experience organize neuronal circuits out of initially equipotential networks. In emphasizing the predominant role of nature in the nature–nurture controversy, Sperry (1963) suggested that *"the patterning of synaptic connections in the nerve centers, including those refined details of network organization heretofore ascribed mainly to functional molding in various forms, must be handled instead by the growth mechanism directly, independently of function, and with very strict selectivity governing synaptic formation from the beginning. The establishment and maintenance of synaptic association were conceived to be regulated by highly specific cytochemical affinities that arise systematically among the different types of neurons involved via self-differentiation, induction through terminal contact, and embryonic gradient effects."*

Sperry's theory has had considerable heuristic value, although it is now apparent that nerve activity has a larger role in development of the nervous system than Sperry's formulation allowed, especially in the refinement of topographical maps by means of elimination of aberrant and redundant synapses, axons, and entire neurons, as discussed in Sections 11.15 and 11.21.

The principal criterion of neuronal specificity, according to the chemoaffinity hypothesis, is the selective formation of synaptic connections. This specificity is shown with respect to the *types* of neurons that form connections, with respect to their *positions* in the cell population, and, on a finer level of resolution, with respect to the *positioning of the postsynaptic sites* on the neuron. The selective association between different types of neurons is an expression of *neuronal phenotypic specificity*. In addition, a neuron may have an affinity or disaffinity for other neurons depending on its position in the multicellular context, and thus express its *locus specificity*. Finally, the formation of synapses at specific places on the cell is an expression of *synaptic site specificity*.

That some readers may find these terms rather high-sounding ways of asserting the obvious shows how thoroughly the concept of neuronal specificity has permeated our thinking about the nervous system. The reader can easily think of many examples to illustrate the different levels of neuronal specificity. Phenotypic specificity is manifested, for example, by the invariant association between the different types of neurons in the cerebellar cortex (see Section 10.10).

Locus specificity is expressed in the formation of topographical maps in the brain in which the topographical order of the presynaptic set of neurons is reflected by the spatial order of their connections with the postsynaptic set of neurons, for example, the somatotopic projection to the mammalian cerebral cortex (C. N. Woolsey, 1958; Kaas, 1983, reviews; see Section 11.7), and the retinal ganglion cell projection to the visual centers (see Section 11.10). It seems as if each element (generally a group of neurons) has a local address, defined with reference to certain coordinates or boundaries. It should be clear that because an individual neuron has a specific property it does not necessarily mean that the property is held exclusively by one neuron or that it is independent of the presence of other neurons. The specificity is then said to be dependent on context, just as the meaning of a word is a contextual function.

Synaptic site specificity can be illustrated by the localized distribution of inputs to different parts of the Mauthner neuron (Mauthner, 1863, 1895; Beccari, 1907; Bartelmez, 1915; Bartelmez and Hoerr, 1933; Bodian, 1937, 1952; Stefanelli, 1951; Whiting, 1957; Otsuka, 1962, 1964; Rovainen, 1967; Diamond, 1971; Billings, 1972; Kimmel and Schabtach, 1974; Celio *et al.*, 1979; Hackett *et al.*, 1979; Zottoli and Faber, 1979; Cochran *et al.*, 1980; Zottoli, 1981; Kimmel *et al.*, 1981; Jacoby and Kimmel, 1982; Lin *et al.*, 1983). This is one example showing the efflorescence of evidence for specificity of synaptic connections. Many other examples can be given, such as the distribution of synapses on Purkinje cells and other cerebellar neurons, hippocampal pyramidal cells, and spinal motoneurons, each with a multiplicity of authorities to support it (Shepherd, 1990, review).

While specificity implies a certain element of selectivity in the association between neurons, it does not mean that in all cases the association is one-to-one. Unique one-to-one associations are

rarely found. For example, because the Mauthner neuron is a unique cell, it is obliged to have some one-to-one associations. One-to-many and many-to-many associations between neurons are the rule, and many different combinatorial effects are thus made possible. To the extent that the association between any presynaptic and any postsynaptic element may be influenced by other elements, the association is context sensitive and the specificity is contextual (R. K. Hunt and Jacobson, 1974c). Within any given context, the association between presynaptic and postsynaptic elements is invariant. Variability within such systems may be attributed to random perturbations in the genetic and developmental processes, that is, to noise in the system. The amount of such variability will depend on the level of resolution at which the system is observed. Thus the Mauthner neuron, which is a neuronal class consisting of one cell, at the cellular level of resolution exhibits microprecision and invariance of connectivity. However, the differences in size and shape of the two Mauthner neurons in the same brain are visible even at the level revealed by light microscopy, and one does not require computerized morphometric analysis to determine the Mauthner neurons on the two sides are not identical in all subcellular details or in their response to injury (Zottoli et al., 1984) or to regeneration in the same individual (Katz, 1984).

Microvariability is seen when comparing homonymous neurons in genetically identical organisms. For example, in the small crustacean *Daphnia* (Macagno et al., 1973), there are great similarities between individuals and between corresponding cells on the two sides in the same animal when the position of the cell bodies and the branching and synaptic pattern of nerve fibers are recorded to a resolution of a few micrometers. However, when the resolution is increased 5- to 10-fold, variations are recorded which are as large between the two sides of the same animal as between different animals of the same genotype. Such microheterogeneity may be regarded as an indication of the noise level of the genetic control of structure (Waddington, 1957). Microheterogeneity may be seen in every system, and apparently is functionally neutral. In some systems, such as the motoneuron supply to muscles in urodeles (Czéh and Székely, 1971) and in frogs (Lichtman et al., 1984), there may be less requirement for functional precision, and therefore

less constraint is put on precise connectivity (Piatt, 1939, 1942; Székely and Czéh, 1967; M. Jacobson, 1969, 1970a) so that what may be termed *"macroheterogeneity"* can be tolerated without resulting malfunction.

11.2. Assays of Neuronal Specificity

No single method for assaying neuronal specificity has yet been devised that can deal with all its different levels. This is especially true under experimental conditions that alter the context in which the specificities originate and are expressed during normal development. The problems of behavioral or microelectrode mapping assays arise because of their indirectness. They cannot provide direct assays of the molecular and cellular properties or functions in which the specificity resides, but merely give some indication of the effective expression of neuronal specificity in the organized multicellular system.

Direct assays of the cytochemical basis of neuronal specificity have been devised. The specificity of attachment of retinal to tectal cells can be assayed fairly directly by measuring the adherence of cells from dorsal or ventral retinal halves to halves of the tectum of chick embryos (Barbera *et al.*, 1973; Marchase *et al.*, 1975; Barbera, 1975). Cells from the ventral half-retina adhere selectively to dorsal half-tectum, and cells from the dorsal half-retina adhere preferentially to the ventral half-tectum. No selectivity is shown in adhesion of nonretinal nerve cells to tectum. Thus the adhesive selectivity of retinal cells to tectum in these experiments mimics the selectivity of retinal axons for tectal neurons. If the mechanisms of selectivity in this experiment are similar to those in real life, the results show that the molecules responsible for neuronal adhesive selectivity are present on the cell bodies as well as on the tips of axons. Because cells of the retinal pigment epithelium derived from dorsal or ventral retinal halves also show adhesive selectivity for dorsal or ventral tectal halves (Barbera *et al.*, 1973), the specificity appears to depend on retinal position, not on cell type. The biochemical basis of the selective adhesion between cells of the neural retina and tectum of the chick embryo has been investigated by Marchase (1976). The cell adhesion is reduced by low temperature and by inhibition of general metabolism. Treatment of retinal cells with proteases reduces the adhesion of ventral retina to dorsal tectum, but does not affect adhesion of dorsal retina to ventral tectum. However, the latter is affected by treating the tectum with proteases, which suggests that adhesion of dorsal retina to ventral tectum depends on protein located on the ventral half of the tectum.

Another assay of retinotectal selective adhesion has been invented by D. L. Gottlieb *et al.* (1976). They assayed the adhesion of individual ventral or dorsal retinal cells to monolayers of ventral or dorsal retinal cells and report that dorsal retinal cells adhere selectively to ventral retinal cells and ventral retinal cells adhere to dorsal retinal cells. McClay *et al.* (1977) have demonstrated similar specificity of adhesion of dissociated tectal cells.

Many experiments show that retinal axons respond to a gradient in the anterioposterior axis of the retinotectal system. Retinal axons associate preferentially with and grow preferentially on other retinal axons from the same retinal locus, and retinal axons express preferences for associating with homotopic tectal cells or membranes of tectal cells (Halfter *et al.*, 1981; Bonhoeffer and Huf, 1982, 1985; Bonhoeffer and Gierer, 1984; Thanos and Dütting, 1987; J. Walter *et al.*, 1987a,b). Those observations have a bearing on the retinotopic order of optic nerve fibers in the chick optic nerve (Thanos and Bonhoefer, 1983): optic nerve fibers that originate close together in the retina may associate preferentially with one another during their outgrowth from retina to tectum in the chick embryo. However, in frogs and mammals the optic nerve fibers do not maintain retinotopic order in the optic nerve, although they regain it in the optic tract and in the tectum (see below). Another tissue culture experiment of Bonhoefer and Huf (1982) has a bearing on the selective association of retinal axons and tectal cells in chick embryos. They found that axons from the temporal retina grow preferentially on the appropriate, rostral tectal cells and not on inappropriate, caudal tectal cells. This preference is not species specific as it is shown by growing combinations of mouse retinal axons and chick tectal membranes and vice versa (Godement and Bonhoeffer, 1989).

Both the polarity and the position-dependent properties in neuronal sets have been demonstrated in several different experiments which indicate a variable parameter extending gradientwise across the retinal and tectal cell populations. Trisler *et al.*

(1981) have raised monoclonal antibodies that recognize a retinal antigen called TOP (toponymic) which extends as a gradient with a maximum at the temporodorsal and minimum at the nasoventral margin of the retina in the chick embryo. This retinal gradient is complementary to a tectal gradient which extends from a maximum in the ventral tectum to a minimum in the dorsal tectum (Trisler and Collins, 1987), as illustrated in Fig. 11.3. Thus there are matching levels of TOP in the retinal and tectal cells at the same positions in the retinotectal map. TOP satisfies an essential requirement of a positional marker, namely, that the number of molecules/cell varies as a function of the cell's position (Trisler and Collins, 1987). This requirement is not satisfied by another antigen that is present in higher concentration in dorsal than in ventral retina of the perinatal rat and seems to be a function of the number of cells rather than molecules of antigen per cell (Constantine-Paton *et al.*, 1986). Nor does that requirement appear to be met by the regional differences in binding of peanut agglutinin to the plexiform layers of the chick embryo retina (Liu *et al.*, 1983). Any gradients of physiological parameters in a population of nerve cells such as the retina or tectum have to be shown to be related to formation of connections between the two populations, and this has not been accomplished in the aforementioned cases. It has also to be shown that the polarity or gradient is the cause of such connectivity between neuronal populations and not its effect.

One of the attractive features of the differential affinity hypothesis is that it demands little genetic information to control the expression of a few cell adhesion molecules and cell recognition molecules, and thus the genetic control of morphogenesis may be substantially simplified. Specificity may result from a few cell adhesion and cell recognition molecules which are developmentally regulated with respect to their biochemical characteristics, quantities, and spatial distribution. It is much simpler for the zygote to contain instructions for a program of development than to contain all the information to specify the structure of the fully developed organism.

The amount of information required to specify the structure of the fully developed brain in every minute detail cannot be contained in the genome (Bremmermann, 1963; M. Jacobson, 1966, 1969). A more parsimonious use of genetic information to

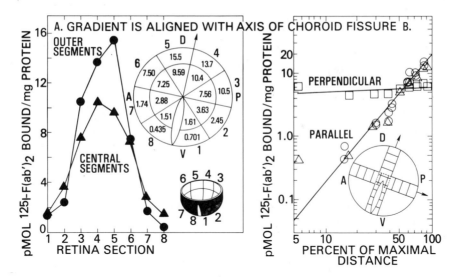

Figure 11.3. Dorsoventral gradient of TOP antigen in the retina of E14 chick embryo. (A) Each retina was divided into eight 45° sectors (7.25 mm in length from center to periphery of retina), and each was subdivided into central (4.9 mm) and peripheral (2.35 mm) portions. Specifically bound $^{125}I\text{-}F(ab')_2$ was measured in each portion. (B) Demonstration that TOP concentration varies with the square of the distance from the ventroanterior margin of the retina (the position of the choroid fissure). Strips of retina in the plane parallel with and perpendicular to the choroid fissure were cut into sections which were assayed for TOP antigen (triangles and squares). Circles show data in (A). From D. Trisler, M. D. Schneider, and M. Nirenberg, *Proc. Natl. Acad. Sci. USA* 78:2145–2149 (1981).

specify a program of histogenesis, cell migration, and cellular interactions, including a sequence of changes in affinities and disaffinities between cells, could result in self-assembly of neural circuits without requiring genetic control of the cell movements and interactions or genetic specification of all the details of the fully developed structure.

A substantial fraction of the genome is devoted to specifying the structure of the nervous system. By extracting the mRNA from the CNS and measuring the fraction of genome DNA to which it hybridizes the fraction has been estimated to be from about 10 percent to more than 30 percent (Sutcliffe, 1988, review). The fact that RNA from mouse brain hybridizes with about 10 percent of nonrepeated mouse DNA, while the comparable figure for mouse liver or kidney is 3 percent, indicates that a greater proportion of the genome is expressed in the brain than in the other organs (Hahn and Laird, 1971; Grouse *et al.*, 1972, 1978; Brown and Church, 1972; Soga and Takahashi, 1975, 1976; Bantle and Hahn, 1976; Chakaraishi, 1979; Van Ness *et al.*, 1979; Coleman *et al.*, 1980; Beckmann *et al.*, 1981; Chaudhari and Hahn, 1983). About one-third of the mammalian genome is ex-

pressed exclusively in the nervous system (Bantle and Hahn, 1976; Chikaraishi *et al.*, 1978). However, the sequence complexity of brain mRNA does not vary greatly among different mammals (Kaplan and Finch, 1982). Most of the mRNAs in the brain are not abundant, and most appear only after birth (Sutcliffe, 1988).

It would be trite to say that "heredity" plays a role in all biological processes and structures: the problem is to trace the causal chain from genes to final structures and functions. This is difficult because there is no single correspondence (isomorphism) between genetic information and the neuronal structures that it generates. This is because the neuronal structures are not specified in detail in the genome. The latter contains only instructions for a developmental program leading to the formation of the nervous system. **The relationship between the genes and the nervous system is not isomorphic but homeomorphic; one-to-one correspondences are found between genes and proteins but genes and higher levels of cellular organization are connected by many-to-many relationships.** The path of migration of the neuron, the direction of growth of its axon and dendrites, the orientation of the dendritic branches, and the precise location of synapses have not been traced back to the genes. Mutations have been found that affect a large variety of structures and functions in the developing nervous system, but in no case has the causal nexus from mutant gene to mutant phenotype yet been unraveled completely (see Section 10.15).

11.3. Development of Neuronal Specificity in Spinal Cord Segments Controlling Limb Movements

Integrated movements, such as those during walking, depend on the development of central generators of patterned motor output (reviewed by Grillner, 1981; Stein, 1984). Such a motor pattern generator consists of a set of neurons that can produce sequences of activity without sensory feedback. Sensory input, while it is essential for adaptive motor behavior in an animal's natural environment, is not necessary for coordinated motor behavior (Weiss, 1937c; Székely *et al.*, 1969; Harcombe Smith and Wyman, 1970; Grillner and Zangger, 1974). In principle, there are two ways in which the central programming of coordinated motor activity could be organized during development. Either the central circuits develop their organization independently of the muscles and sense organs, or the central programs are organized as a result of connections with the peripheral tissues.

The first way we may call central specification of motor activity. The first alternative presupposes that the central circuits controlling coordinated limb movements develop in parallel with the peripheral targets, but there is no presumption regarding the selection of those targets by motoneurons or sensory neurons. We have to discover whether the peripheral connections are formed at random or whether the central neurons form connections selectively with muscles and sense organs. The 2nd alternative does imply that the peripheral tissues are specified and that their specificity is somehow responsible for organizing the activities of the central neurons.

The evidence to be adduced in this section shows that species-specific patterns of motor coordination develop according to an intrinsic program within the CNS. Patterns of movement that develop in transplanted limbs or in transplanted muscles or after cross-union of nerves to antagonistic muscles are in accordance with the inherent specificity of the motoneurons regardless of their peripheral connections and regardless of the functional utility of the movements.

Studies of the motility of grafted limbs have played an important part in research on the development of locomotion in tetrapods. Braus (1905) and Harrison (1907a) observed movements in limbs transplanted in amphibian embryos and showed that nerves that are not normally destined for the limb can innervate limb muscles. Coordinated movements in transplanted limbs were first studied and carefully analyzed by Detwiler (1920a, 1925) and later by Weiss (1922, 1924, 1937a–d). They found that when a limb bud from donor urodele amphibian embryo is grafted caudal to the normal limb bud of another embryo of the same species, it often develops movements that are coordinated with those of of the limbs of the host.

This phenomenon was later called "*homologous response*" or "*myotypic response*" by Weiss (1937 a–d). The movements of the grafted limb are coordinated with those of the host regardless of the orientation of the limb or its functional efficiency. For example, limbs transplanted with their axes reversed develop a coordinated sequence of movements that tend to propel the animal backwards (Weiss, 1937d). These maladaptive movements are unaffected by experience and are not corrected by learning. Sensory input does not play an essential part in the development of the coordinated movements of grafted limbs, as they are unaffected by deafferenting the limb (Weiss, 1937c). The coordinated movements occur even when the grafted limb is supplied by a single nerve that branches to supply all the muscles at random (Weiss, 1928b), provided that the nerve is one that normally supplies the limb (Detwiler, 1920a).

Detwiler (1920a) observed a gradual loss of function of the grafted limb as it is transplanted farther away from its normal position. Normally, the forelimbs of salamanders or newts are supplied by the 3rd, 4th, and 5th nerves arising from the brachial segments of the spinal cord. Detwiler (1920a) showed that some coordinated movements of the grafted limb develop even when it receives a single limb nerve. In cases where the limb grafted to the trunk is supplied by the trunk nerves as well as the 5th spinal nerve, section of the latter abolishes the coordinated movements of the grafted limb (Detwiler and Carpenter, 1929). Limbs grafted to the trunk and innervated exclusively by trunk nerves display feeble and incoordinated movements (Detwiler, 1930b). Limbs grafted to the head and innervated by cranial nerves do not develop movements that are coordinated with those of the normal limbs, but display mass contractions associated with movements of the eyes, jaw, or gills, depending on the source of innervation of the limb (Nicholas, 1933; Detwiler, 1930a,b; Székely, 1959b; Hibbard, 1965b).

The foregoing experiments show that although limb muscles can be innervated functionally by motoneurons at any level of the spinal cord, the mechanisms for coordinated limb movements are restricted to the brachial and lumbosacral regions of the spinal cord; thoracic segments of the spinal cord or cranial motor nuclei are unable to participate in the control of limb movements. Additional evidence showing that the limitation is in the spinal cord and not in the limb is given below. For example, W. M. Rogers (1934) found that limbs may be innervated by a supernumerary segment of the spinal cord grafted between the normal cord and the limb bud in salamander embryos. Normally integrated limb movements occur when the graft consists of the 3rd, 4th, and 5th segments of the cord, which normally innervate the forelimbs, but feeble and uncoordinated movements occur when the limb is innervated by a graft of the 7th, 8th, and 9th spinal cord segments.

Other experiments, showing that the character of limb movements is determined by the region of spinal cord from which it is innervated, were performed by Székely (1963) on newts and by Straznicky (1963) on the chick embryo. Székely showed that an extra limb grafted on the trunk of a newt embryo develops coordinated movements if innervated by a segment of brachial cord transplanted in place of thoracic spinal cord. An extra hindlimb grafted on the trunk and innervated by lumbosacral segments of the spinal cord transplanted in place of thoracic cord moves synchronously with the normal hindlimbs. Straznicky (1963) showed that after brachial segments of the spinal cord have been transplanted in place of lumbosacral

segments in the chick embryo, the leg moves synchronously with the wing on the same side. If a leg is grafted in place of a wing, the leg, innervated by brachial spinal nerves, makes winglike movements.

In all the experiments that have been described, the difference between limbs with integrated locomotor movements and those with uncoordinated movements is not in the adequacy of neuromuscular connections, because the limb muscles appear to receive an adequate supply of nerves. The differences have been shown to reside in the functional organization of the spinal cord supplying the limb. Other experiments have established that early in development the spinal cord segments at limb levels develop functional specificity either for forelimbs or for hindlimbs.

There is evidence that the motor functions of the spinal neuron are specified in the late neurula and that specification increases progressively during development. This evidence has been obtained by transposing segments of the spinal cord in a series of amphibian and chick embryos at different stages of development. Székely (1963) showed that interchanging the brachial and lumbosacral regions of the spinal cord of newt embryos shortly after the time of closure of the neural tube results in reduced and uncoordinated movements of the limbs. Normal limb movements develop if the interchange of presumptive fore- and hindlimb regions of the spinal cord is made at earlier stages of development. Specification of spinal cord segments controlling limb movements also occurs in the early neural tube of the chick embryo. Straznicky (1967) has shown that interchanging brachial and lumbosacral segments of the spinal cord in chick embryos on day 3 of incubation results in development of limb movements corresponding to the origin of the spinal segments innervating the limb.

In the chick embryo it is not certain whether the control of limb movements by spinal cord segments is already irreversibly specified before the motoneurons have made contact with muscles (see Sections 9.3 and 9.4). The axons of motoneurons can be seen in the ventral roots at 50 hours of incubation, and they reach proximal muscles at E2.5 and distal muscles on E3 and E4 (Levi-Montalcini, 1950; Grim, 1970; Roncali, 1970; Swett *et al.*, 1970; Landmesser and Morris, 1975; M. R. Bennett *et al.*, 1980; M. R. Bennett, 1983; M. R. Bennett and

Booth, 1983; M. R. Bennett and Lavides, 1984; Tanaka and Landmesser, 1986). The first, morphologically undifferentiated neuromuscular junctions appear at E4–E6 (Atsumi, 1971; Sisto-Daneo and Filogamo, 1974, 1975). Spontaneous, uncoordinated movements of the trunk start on E3.5, before spinal reflex circuits have been established. The movements of the limbs commence on E6. They are spontaneous, are not coordinated, and are due to random discharges in the spinal motoneurons. Reflex movements of the hindlimbs can be elicited only after E7–E7.5, when the reflex circuits are completed in the brachial and lumbar segments of the spinal cord. The motility of chick embryos is considered fully in the masterful review by Hamburger (1973).

Landmesser and Morris (1975) have shown, by electrophysiological recording from individual muscles and motor nerves in the chick embryo, that the nerves always connect with the appropriate muscles from the beginning, that the innervation is quite invariant for each muscle, and that there is no proximodistal sequence of innervation. The specific pattern of innervation is seen from the time movement can first be elicited on E6 (Stages 27–28). These observations tend to rule out random innervation of limb muscles followed by death of motoneurons that make connections with inappropriate muscles (see Section 9.3).

In the newt, too, the specification of limb-moving segments of the spinal cord occurs either shortly before or during the period of innervation of limb muscles. From the evidence now available, it is not possible to decide whether contact of the motor axon with the muscle precedes specification of the motoneuron and thereby causes motoneuron specification, as Weiss (1928b, 1941b, 1947) has proposed. In newts and salamanders there is a relatively long period during which the spinal cord is not specified as regards limb movements, and transposition of segments of the cord does not affect the subsequent development of limb movements. Detwiler (1923) showed that thoracic segments of the spinal cord are able to regulate when transplanted in place of brachial cord at tailbud stages of the salamander embryo so that normally integrated limb movements result. Straznicky and Székely (1967) have shown that this capacity of thoracic segments of the cord to sustain coordinated limb movements is gradually lost at later stages of development. They showed

that grafting thoracic segments in place of brachial segments of spinal cord in newt embryos at Stage 22 results in the development of normal forelimb movements. Progressively poorer limb movements develop when the limbs are innervated by thoracic segments of spinal cord grafted at Stages 23–27. Incoordinated movements develop when the spinal cord grafts are made after Stage 27. No forelimb movements develop when thoracic cord from an embryo at Stage 28 is grafted in place of brachial spinal cord of a Stage 22 embryo (Straznicky and Székely, 1967). These experiments establish that spinal cord segments at limb levels are at first unspecified as regards limb movement, but later develop functional specificity for fore- or hindlimb movements.

Homologous response develops in the transplanted limb only if it is grafted before a critical stage, which in the frog *Xenopus* is at Stage 54 (Hollyday and Mendell, 1976). This is when the death of motoneurons in the lateral motor column has reached a peak (see Section 8.7), so that one of the limitations may be an inadequate motoneuron pool in the regions of spinal cord not normally connected to limbs. Stage 54 is also when neuromuscular connections develop, hindlimb movements commence, and limb reflexes can first be elicited. Hollyday and Mendell (1975) have suggested that it becomes impossible to form new spinal reflex connections once normal reflex connections are established in the spinal cord. The problem of whether these specificites develop before the spinal nerves form connections in the limbs has not been resolved. Therefore, we still have to consider the hypothesis that the primary specificities are in the muscles, which impart their specificities to the motor nerves that innervate them (Weiss, 1924, 1928a,b, 1931, 1941b, 1947, 1952).

11.4. Theories of Motoneuron Specification

To explain the phenomenon of myotypic response, that is, the movement of muscles in a normal limb in apparent synchrony with homologous muscles in a nearby grafted limb, Weiss at first suggested that *"the nervous system does not form connections with muscles by means of special pathways, but by specific forms of excitation"* (Weiss, 1928a). This theory of selective signaling he called the *"resonance theory"* (Weiss, 1928b, 1931). The nerves were believed to connect indiscriminately with muscles, but the muscles were supposed to be "tuned" to receive only a specific pattern of impulses. This theory had to be abandoned when Wiersma (1931) showed that impulse traffic is present only in motor nerves to muscles involved in reflex contraction, whereas nerves to inactive muscles are quiescent. Weiss then shifted the selective role from the muscle or neuromuscular junction to the motoneuron as a whole. He proposed that *"each muscle gradually transforms ('modulates') its motor neurons into what from then on will be selective receivers admitting only the one type of impulse proper for that particular muscle. Such a modification affecting the neuron in a centripetal direction might gradually extend beyond the motor neurons and spread to other central neurons"* (Weiss, 1935).

The idea of the motoneuron as a selective filter of nerve impulses eventually gave way to the concept of myotypic modulation or specification (the terms are synonymous) of the synaptic connections between motoneurons and premotor neurons in the CNS. The return of normal limb movements after nerve regeneration, even when the pattern of peripheral innervation appears grossly abnormal, was taken by Weiss as evidence that rearrangement of synaptic association must occur. As no such rearrangement was evident at the neuromuscular junctions, Weiss assumed that synaptic plasticity must occur centrally in response to modulation by the muscle. This concept was elaborated by Sperry, who agreed that contact of the nerve with the muscle might result in the formation of central synaptic associations that are appropriate to the actions of the muscle (Sperry, 1950a,b, 1951a,b). He introduced the idea that matching specificities develop independently in the muscles and premotor neurons; the muscles then confer their specificities on the motoneurons, causing them to synapse with the premotor neurons that have matching or homologous specificities.

Temporal and spatial restrictions to the process of myotypic specification have been considered in Section 11.3. There also appear to be important phylogenetic restrictions. In salamanders and newts, myotypic specification seems to occur after grafting of limbs at any stage of development, even in the adult, provided that the grafted limb is supplied by some nerves from lumbosacral or brachial segments of the spinal cord. In anurans and the higher verte-

brates, myotypic specification appears to be restricted to early stages of development and to become irreversibly lost during maturation—earlier in the higher vertebrates than in the lower. If this is indeed correct, switching peripheral connections later in life would not be expected to result in any compensatory adjustments of central synapses. For example, cross-innervated muscles would be expected to contract in accordance with the original connectivity of the motoneuron, with resulting incoordination of movement.

Cross-innervation of muscle fibers inevitably occurs after nerve regeneration in mammals. Even if the cut ends of the nerve are carefully sutured together, the nerve fibers are disarranged during regeneration and they innervate muscle fibers at random. After nerve regeneration in mammals, at any age after birth, recovery of voluntary or reflex movements is always incomplete; muscle power is diminished, and the timing and sequence of muscle contractions are permanently disordered. The incoordination is most marked in muscles involved in fine and complex movements. Reeducation may lead to compensatory use of muscles that are not affected by the injury, but careful studies have shown that, in humans, incoordinated movements of the affected muscles are not improved by practice, even after many years. For detailed documentation of this conclusion, the reader should refer to the masterly review by Sperry (1945a).

Sperry's experiments on the effects of cross-uniting nerves to antagonistic muscles have shown the lack of plasticity in the neuronal circuits mediating coordinated movements of skeletal muscles in mammals. After crossing nerves to antagonistic muscles in the limbs of rats and monkeys, Sperry (1941, 1942, 1947) observed that reversal of movements and malfunction of the limb persist permanently. Reorganization of reflex movements is never observed even when the operations are performed on young animals. However, it remains to be seen whether any functional adaptation may occur in the mammalian fetus after rearrangement of connections between motor nerves and muscles.

The greater functional recovery that occurs in lower vertebrates after rearrangements of muscle innervation indicates that there may be important differences in the recovery process between lower and higher vertebrates. So much of the evidence of myotypic specification has been obtained from salamanders and newts that it is important to emphasize that *"urodeles so differ from other tetrapod vertebrates respecting nerve–muscle relationships that they form a group unto themselves"* (Straus, 1946). In all vertebrates except urodeles the motoneurons of the ventral horn of the spinal cord are arranged in a ventromedial longitudinal column supplying trunk muscles and muscles in the proximal part of the limb, and in a lateral longitudinal column supplying distal limb muscles. There is no distinct columnar arrangement or even a distinct ventral horn in urodeles. This should be compared with the motor system of the frog, in which the columnar arrangement of spinal motoneurons is similar to that in tetrapod reptiles, birds, and mammals (M. L. Silver, 1942; Stussi, 1960; Cruce, 1974). In addition to these differences, the motoneurons are not so well arranged in somatotopic order (according to the relative positions of their muscles) in urodeles as they are in mammals. The significance of this in the analysis of homologous limb movements will be discussed later.

Székely and Czéh (1967) have provided evidence that questions the validity of the phenomenon of homologous response and that calls for a reappraisal of the theory of myotypic specification. They determined the arrangement of the brachial spinal motoneurons innervating the forelimb of the axolotl, *Ambystoma mexicanum*, by observing muscle contractions elicited by microelectrode stimulation in the spinal cord. The motoneurons in rostrocaudal sequence in the cord project to muscles in anteroposterior sequence in the shoulder girdle and proximodistal sequence in the forelimb. However, within this sequence there is considerable overlap of the central representation of different muscles, which blurs the precision of the somatotopic arrangement of motoneurons (Fig. 11.4). The overlap is such as to bring together the motoneurons of functionally related muscles. Székely and Czéh concluded: *"In the light of our results it seems that an extra limb, being innervated by the 4th or 5th spinal nerve, has a good chance to receive the complete set of nerves which are necessary for the control of walking movements without assuming any kind of specification. Some probable shift in the phase of muscle action will be too small to be detected, and the movement of the grafted limb will appear to be synchronized with that of the normal limb."*

Their final point is important because it raises grave doubts about the adequacy of naked-eye observations of the movements of grafted limbs. Czéh and Székely (1971), recording muscle activity from freely moving normal and supernumerary limbs, report that the electromyograms show asynchrony of contraction of homologous muscles when the move-

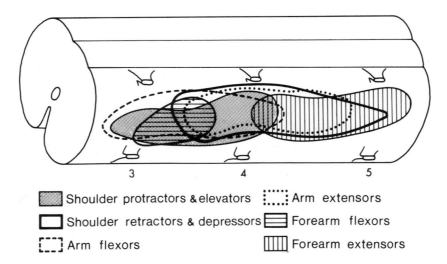

Figure 11.4. Extensive overlap of the spinal cord representation of forelimb muscles in a urodele. Projection to the lateral surface of the spinal cord of the positions of motoneurons supplying muscles moving the forelimb via spinal roots 3, 4, and 5. The positions of motoneurons were mapped by observation of movements of individual muscles in response to electrical stimulation with a microelectrode in the spinal cord. From data in G. Székely and G. Czéh (1967) and G. Székely (1968).

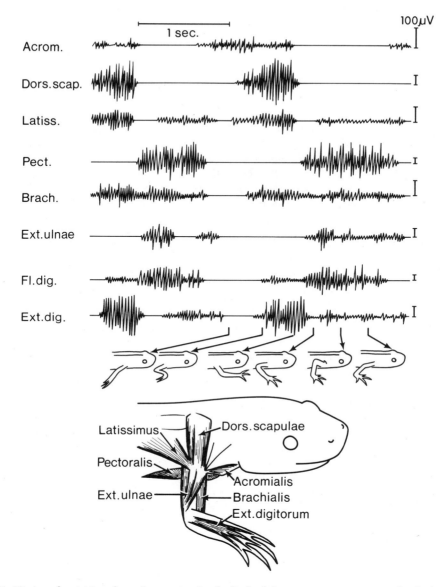

Figure 11.5. Timing of activities of muscles moving the forelimb of the newt. Activity patterns of eight forelimb muscles were recorded electromyographically in the freely moving newt. Electrical recordings from the muscles shown were recorded at different phases of the step. From G. Székely, G. Czéh, and G. Vörös, *Exp. Brain Res.* 9:53–62 (1969).

ments look synchronous. Electromyography reveals incoordination of contraction of extensor muscles innervated by flexor nerves in the cat hindlimb, even though no abnormality is apparent to the naked eye (McIntyre and Robinson, 1958). Electromyography also shows the complexity of timing of contraction, including cocontraction, of agonists and antagonists in the limb during locomotion (Paillard, 1960; Eng-

berg and Lundberg, 1962; Székely *et al.,* 1969), as is shown in Fig. 11.5. These studies show that slight differences in the timing of contractions of individual muscles in the normal and grafted limb, which can be revealed by electromyography, might escape detection by naked-eye observation or even by the slow-motion cinematography used by Weiss (1941b).

At variance with the conclusions drawn from electromyographic recordings from freely moving salamanders are observations of Hollyday and Mendell (1976) of homologous reflex movements evoked by mechanical stimulation of the skin. These authors report synchronous electrical activity in nerves to homologous muscles as well as in the muscles themselves. A full range of reflex movements occur despite a limited sequential innervation of the grafted limb. This, and the finding that homologous reflex movements occur only if the limbs are grafted before Stage 54, is evidence in favor of myotypic specifications of motoneurons connected to the transplanted limb. However, the possibility has not been excluded that the grafted limb receives a nerve supply from collateral branches from spinal nerves normally supplying the limb. The capacity of nerve fibers to find their proper muscle targets, even after deflection of the nerve, has to be considered in all such cases (Grimm, 1971).

Finally, there are considerable variations in the pattern of innervation of specific muscles of the limbs in urodeles (Piatt, 1939, 1942), as well as multiple innervation of muscle fibers by *en grappe* motor nerve terminals (Bone, 1964; Mark *et al.*, 1966). Mark *et al.* (1966) have suggested that selective connections between motor nerves and muscle fibers might be possible in muscles with multiple *en grappe* innervation, but are not possible in muscles with local *en plaque* innervation (see Section 9.5). Each mature mammalian muscle fiber has a single motor end-plate, and as a rule will accept no more. Therefore, the first motor nerve terminal to arrive at the muscle fiber will innervate it, regardless of whether or not it is functionally suitable (see Section 9.6). In fish and urodeles, on the contrary, multiple innervation of muscle fibers occurs normally in the adult as well as after nerve regeneration. In these animals, each muscle fiber is supplied by several nerve terminals, either branches of one axon or branches of different axons belonging to the same motor nerve. The hypothesis is that if motor nerve fibers of different central origin grow into the urodele or fish muscle, the nerve terminals with the greatest selective affinity for the muscle will compete with fibers having less affinity and will displace the latter from the muscle. A similar competitive growth process has been postulated to explain the selective reestablishment of synapses in the superior

cervical ganglion of the cat and guinea pig after regeneration of the preganglionic nerve fibers (Guth and Bernstein, 1961; Lichtman *et al.*, 1979).

The nerve–muscle specificity in fish and urodeles is not "all or none," but appears to be graded. This is indicated by the observation that motor nerves will connect with any muscle if forced to do so by surgical cross-union of nerves or by implantation of motor nerves into foreign muscles, but selective connections tend to be made if the nerve fibers regenerate at random and are permitted to compete for the correct muscle fibers. For example, selective reconnection with extraocular muscles occurs after regeneration of the oculomotor nerve in a fish (Sperry and Arora, 1965). Regeneration of the nerves supplying the fin muscles of a fish results in recovery of coordinated fin movements, but incoordinated movements occur after cross-union of the nerves to the pectoral and pelvic fins (Sperry and Deupree, 1956). Mark (1965) confirmed that simply cutting the nerves of the brachial plexus in a teleost fish results in regeneraton of the motor nerves and recovery of normal movements. However, reversed fin movements result when the nerve to the retractor muscle is implanted into the protractor muscle, and vice versa. The reversed fin movements persist for at least 18 months, but normal movements are restored by cutting the brachial plexus and allowing the nerves to regenerate at random into the fin muscles. These experiments indicate that recovery of coordinated movements of fin muscles in teleosts is due to selective reconnection between motor nerves and muscles rather than to myotypic specification of the central connections of the motoneurons.

Those results reopened the question of whether the homologous response in urodeles might occur because of selective peripheral connections (Mark, 1969). Studies of the reinnervation of muscles that move the eyes of fish also show that there is a specific selection process involved in the formation of neuromuscular junctions. Marotte and Mark (1970a,b) concluded that the correct motor nerve terminals take command of the muscle previously innervated by an incorrect nerve by suppressing the function of the incorrect neuromuscular junctions without altering their morphology. After random regeneration of motor axons from the IIIrd and IVth cranial nerves to the inferior oblique muscle, the normal action of the muscle is restored. Although incorrect or foreign axons enter the muscle, and their electrical impulses can be recorded there, the foreign nerves have no detectable effect on the muscle, which contracts only in response to impulses in the correct nerve. From this evidence, Mark *et al.* (1970) concluded that *"a subtle but strong selectivity must operate to block transmission of excitation from foreign nerves as long as the correctly matched nerves are present."* This conclusion appears to be in conflict with other evidence that foreign motor nerves remain functionally effective after a muscle is reinnervated by its normal motor nerves. This has been reported in goldfish extraocular muscles (S. A. Scott, 1975), perch gill muscles (Frank and Jansen, 1976), frog skeletal muscle (Miledi, 1963), and mammalian skeletal muscle (Tonge, 1974a–c; Frank *et al.*, 1974). The very phenomenon of functional inactivation or repression at the synapse and the theoretical edifice of modifiable neuronal networks that has been raised upon it (Mark, 1974b) are no longer a *chose jugée*, they are now an open question.

11.5. Expression of Neuronal Specificity in the Development of Neuronal Projection Maps

A neuronal projection map develops when one set of neurons projects its axons to form connections with one or more neuronal sets so that the spatial order of the elements of one set is preserved in the spatial order of the connections to the other set or sets. Such orderly and continuous neuronal projection maps are found ubiquitously (Werner, 1970), for example, in the projection from the sensory receptors from lower to higher levels of the neuraxis. The topographical representation of the distribution of sensory neurons is preserved in such maps. but neurons with different functional properties at different levels introduce qualitative changes in the functional operations that are performed at successive levels of the projection. These anamorphic changes are well illustrated by the vertebrate visual system but also occur in all other sensory systems. The spatial order of the visual image is preserved, although processing of visual information occurs as the information passes from the receptors, through retinal interneurons, to retinal ganglion

cells, and then to visual centers which include the optic tectum in submammalian vertebrates and the superior colliculus, lateral geniculate nucleus, and cerebral cortex in mammals. Although the retinotopic organization of the visual projection is preserved at all levels in the brain, new kinds of functional organization, of increasing complexity, are created at higher levels of the projection by convergence and synthesis of inputs from the lower levels.

It is obvious that a rank order of complexity exists in the nervous system—the higher orders corresponding with higher levels in the sense introduced by John Hughlings Jackson and Charles Sherrington. The possibilities exist for combining inputs from one level to the next, and for introducing entirely new functional classes of neurons at each level. Hierarchical structures of this kind can be analyzed, according to Weyl (1949), in three steps of increasing resolution: (1) *morphology*, which describes the form as a whole; (2) *topology*, which deals with the combinatorial relationships of the elements; and (3) *geometry*, which deals with the metrics of the system. This structural analysis has to be associated with a functional analysis, and both have to be integrated into the analysis of the changes that occur during development. It is obvious that such an analysis is far from being achieved.

Development of projection maps requires at least four stages: (1) Differentiation of the types of neurons that are proper to each set, that is, expression of their phenotypic specificity. (2) Development of locus specificities in each neuronal set. These are defined as the position-dependent properties acquired by each element in the neuronal set which predispose it to connect selectively with an element at the corresponding position in other sets. (3) Expression of the specificities in the selection of the pathway along which axons from one set grow to another. (4) Expression of the locus specificity of each neuron of one set in selecting, as a synaptic target, a neuron at a corresponding position in another set. In addition, there may be a 5th stage involving competition, especially, but not necessarily only, if there is a numerical disparity between the two sets.

Neuronal sets develop in different places in the neural tube, and the question arises how each set develops the appropriate phenotypic specificities

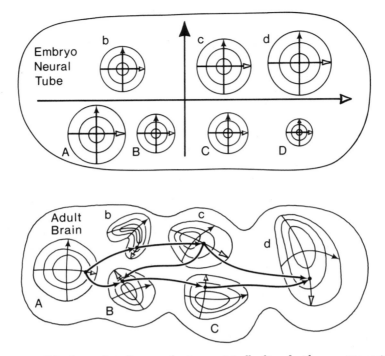

Figure 11.6. Illustration of the theory that all neuronal sets are originally aligned with respect to positional information in the embryo as a whole. In the upper diagram seven neuronal sets are shown in various places in the embryonic neural tube. They are aligned with one another because they all derive their positional information from the same source. The lower diagram shows a later stage of development. Cells originating after that time acquire locus specificities with reference to their own neuronal set, regardless of changes in size, shape, or position of the set as a whole. According to this theory, connections between sets may be made preferentially between neurons having the same locus specificities. From M. Jacobson, Neuronal recognition in the retinotectal system, pp. 3–23, in *Neuronal Recognition,* S. Barondes, (ed.), Plenum, New York.

and how all the necessary locus specificities become deployed throughout the neuronal population of each set so that the polarity of each set is aligned with other neuronal sets and with the polarity of the embryo as a whole (Fig. 11.6).

Number, order, and position are the three attributes of all things arranged in spatial patterns. One should beware of attaching special significance to the purely formal resemblance between patterns in different structures that have developed by different mechanisms, for example, comparing segments in insects with zebra's stripes and with cerebral cortical ocular dominance bands. Richard Feynman, in discussing the *"underlying unity"* of nature, observes that *". . . the thing which is common to all the phenomena is the space. . . . As long as things are reasonably smooth in space, then the important things that will be involved will be the rates of change of quantities with position in space. That is*

why we always get an equation with a gradient. . . ." (Feynman *et al.,* 1964).

It has been conjectured that the locus specificities in neuronal populations are stable cytochemical properties of nerve cells that develop as a result of the cells' interpretation of *positional information* (Wolpert, 1969). The nature of the positional information is not known: it might be a gradient of a morphogenetic agent arising from a restricted source, distributed through the cell population by diffusion, and determining cell fates by means of a concentration-dependent mechanism (Crick, 1970, 1971; Eichele and Thaller, 1987); it might be a gradient of a substance that is actively transported through the cell population; it might be information provided by the time delay between the arrival of two signals propagated at different velocities through the cell population (Goodwin and Cohen, 1969); or it might be a metabolic gradient based on many complex physiological processes rather than a gradient of a single agent (Child, 1941; Needham, 1942).

In all theories of the origin of position-dependent cellular properties, regardless of the nature of the developmental signal or its mode of propagation in the cell population, the cellular response to the signal depends on its amplitude, and this varies according to the positions of the cells in the population. According to Wolpert (1969, 1971, 1974), the cells "interpret" the positional information. This may mean that a developmental program is triggered or initiated that results in development of stable cellular position-dependent properties. In all discussions of this topic it is assumed that the propagated signal is free of noise and that a significant difference in the amplitude of the signal or level of the gradient across a single cell can be detected and interpreted as a difference in positional information at those cells' positions, thus giving each cell a unique cellular address.

The hypothesis that cells are able to use positional information in the differentiation of position-dependent properties has proved of considerable heuristic value in studies of the origins and expression of locus specificity in the retinotectal system (M. Jacobson and Hunt, 1973; Fraser and Hunt, 1980, reviews). However, in those experiments, as well as in other studies of neuronal connectivity, it is clear that neurons rarely form one-to-one connections, as might be expected if they are able to express unique cellular position-dependent properties. On the contrary, locus specificity is usually expressed by groups of cells in one neuronal set, such as a thalamic nucleus, connecting with groups of cells in other neuronal sets, such as the cerebral cortex. These cell groups have been defined as an element of a neuronal set (see Section 10.2). In different neuronal sets these cell groupings take the form of columns, blobs, patches, and other discrete, localized configurations.

Turing (1952) proposed a *"chemical theory of morphogenesis"* which can account for the development of patterns consisting of stripes or discrete patches or spots. He shows how cells that are coupled through permeable junctions or are able to interact by diffusion, starting with uniform chemical conditions in all cells, can develop marked nonuniform conditions that are initiated by small fluctuations that are always present in the system. Tur-

ing coined the term *"morphogen"* to describe a molecule produced in the embryo, whose concentration at various loci in the field is interpreted by the cells to develop in a particular way. The spatial pattern generated by a morphogen may be a monotonic gradient, with a maximum at one side and a minimum at the opposite side over a tissue no larger than about 60 cells or 1 mm wide (Wolpert, 1969; Crick, 1970). However, Turing's model and other similar models in which more than one morphogen interact or in which there are inhibitory as well as excitatory interactions between cells (Gmitro and Scriven, 1966; Gierer and Meinhardt, 1972; Meinhardt and Gierer, 1974) can result in the formation of repeating patterns such as bands (e.g., cerebral cortical ocular dominance stripes) or peaks and valleys (e.g., cerebral cortical barrels, columns, and blobs). Turing's model, unlike that of Crick (1970), is not limited to a small number of cells, but is size invariant and can form a pattern over an unlimited area within a few hours (Bard and Lauder, 1974). Although the maximum wavelength that can be generated by Turing systems is about 1 mm, or about 60 cells 15 μm in diameter, the wave can be repeated, so that the size of the system is unlimited. According to Bard and Lauder (1974), Turing systems generate periodic patterns that are *"characterized by a general regularity rather than absolute precision,"* like the zebra's stripes and the hair follicles on the skin. Turing systems might well be responsible for generating the patterns of neuronal projection from the sensory receptors to the CNS, for example, the ocular dominance columns, the thalamocortical somatosensory projections, and the retinotectal projection. The element of such a system would be the group of cells that forms a discrete band or patch.

In theory there are at least three possible modes of assembly of neuronal projection maps. (1) **The presynaptic neurons alone develop locus specificities. The axons carrying those locus specificities interact to preserve nearest-neighbor relationships as they grow to and form connections with the postsynaptic neurons. (2) The postsynaptic neurons as well as presynaptic neurons develop complementary locus specificities. Axons do not need to remain close to neighbors as they grow but they branch extensively until they find a matching postsynaptic cell, form synaptic connections with that cell, and retract all other branches. (3). Alter-**

natively, the axons may have extensive branches and even form an excessive number of synapses, but survival of synapses is determined by some functional rule, such as correlated activity. Other synapses in which activity is not correlated are eliminated or functionally masked (see Section 6.9).

At least five main stages in the formation of specific neuronal connections must be considered: firstly, the initial acquisition of locus specificities by the presynaptic neurons and possibly also by the postsynaptic neurons; secondly, the selection of pathways by axons growing to the postsynaptic neurons and selection of synaptic sites on those neurons; thirdly, the axon-to-axon interactions; fourthly, the interactions between axons and postsynaptic neurons; fifthly, the role of impulse traffic and function in modifying the map.

Recognition of the postsynaptic neuron by the presynaptic axons can occur without any interaction between the axons to maintain topographical order. This occurs in the sympathetic ganglia where the postsynaptic neurons of different types are randomly arranged. Nevertheless the preganglionic axons from different levels of the spinal cord form connections with the correct neurons in the ganglion during development as well as during regeneration (Langley, 1895, 1897; Guth and Bernstein, 1961; Landmesser and Pilar, 1970; McLachlan, 1974; Nja and Purves, 1977; Lichtman *et al.*, 1979, 1980). Axon–axon interactions that operate in formation of retinotopic maps are considered in Section 11.9.

11.6. Specification of Somatosensory Projections in Amphibians

Having questioned the validity of the theory of specification of motoneurons by muscles, it is now necessary to critically reevaluate the theory of specification of sensory neurons by sense organs. The evidence given in Section 9.12 shows that interaction between sensory nerve terminals and cutaneous cells is necessary for the differentiation of cutaneous sensory organelles. The question now being considered is whether the interaction between the skin and nerve also affects the differentiation of the neuron so that the central connections of the sensory neuron are specified according to the function and position of the receptor.

The problem was posed by Paul Weiss (1942) as follows: "*Is the biochemical diversification of the nerve fibers of central or peripheral origin? Logically, both possibilities exist: Either each nerve fiber receives its biochemical characteristics from its center, and then makes selective connections with a peripheral receptor of the appropriate type, or the fibers become specialized only after connecting with the receptors, each fiber assuming the distinctive character of its terminal organ.*" An experimental strategy for distinguishing between these two alternatives has been to graft an eye (Weiss, 1942) or skin (Miner, 1956; M. Jacobson and Baker, 1969; Sklar and Hunt, 1973; E. M. Bloom and Tompkins, 1976) to a different position, cutting the sensory nerves during the operation, and then to determine the central connections of the sensory nerves that reinnervate the grafts. As we shall see, all these studies show changes in reflexes that result from the operations but they fall far short of demonstrating whether the reflex changes are due to changes in the pattern of central connections or whether they are due to changes in the sensory nerves supplying the grafts.

Weiss (1942) and Kollros (1943b) transplanted an additional eye of the larval newt to other parts of the head and then observed the reflexes elicited by stimulating the cornea of the grafted eye. In normal newts, retraction of the eye (lid closure reflex) can be elicited by stimulating the cornea, but only after metamorphosis. The reflexogenic zone for this reflex is restricted to the cornea and the skin close to the eye, and is mediated by branches of the trigeminal nerve. Stimulation of the rest of the head, innervated by other branches of the trigeminal nerve, does not elicit a lid closure reflex but stimulates only reflex withdrawal of the head. Weiss (1942) showed that gentle tactile stimulation of the cornea of an extra eye grafted to the nose or ear region results in a lid closure reflex of the normal eye on the same side (Fig. 11.7). Weiss interpreted this observation in terms of his "modulation" theory, namely, that the cornea of the grafted eye transfers its local specificity to the branches of the trigeminal nerve in the nose or ear regions, causing them to connect selectively with the motoneurons to the retractor muscle of the eye. The same result is obtained when an additional eye grafted to the gill region is innervated by the vagus nerve; stimulating the cornea of the grafted eye results in reflex retraction of the normal

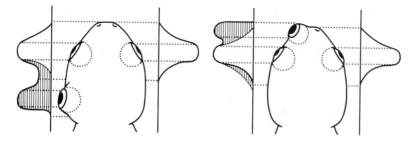

Figure 11.7. Tactile stimulation of the cornea of a grafted eye causes reflex retraction of the normal eye. Sensitivity profiles for that reflex are shown in newts with eye-to-ear or eye-to-nose grafts. The ordinates of the profiles represent sensitivity; shaded areas under the curves indicate increases in sensitivity caused by the grafts. From P. Weiss, *J. Comp. Neurol.* 77:131–169 (1942).

eye on the same side (Kollros, 1943b). The experiment was repeated and the result was confirmed by Székely (1959a). He observed that before metamorphosis, tactile stimulation of an eye grafted to the gill region results in gill movements, but the response changes after metamorphosis, when the corneal reflex normally develops in the newt; stimulation of the cornea of the grafted eye results in retraction of the normal eye.

Interpreting these experiments on grafted eyes is made even more difficult by the results of other experiments of Székely (1959a) in which he grafted a limb to the gill region in larval newts and salamanders. Neither corneal reflexes nor gill reflexes can be elicited by stimulating the grafted limb. However, after amputation of the terminal part of the grafted limb, a regeneration blastema is formed, and when this is stimulated a reflex retraction of the normal eye on the same side occurs. Székely inferred that the patterns of nerve impulses originating in the naked nerve endings of the regeneration blastema and of the cornea are so similar that the CNS responds to them in the same way. This is a version of the theory of impulse selectivity, according to which the origin and modality of a sensation are encoded in a pattern of nerve impulses. Székely (1966, 1968) has invented a formal model for this theory, which is implausible because there is no evidence from electrophysiological experiments to support it.

A general critique of all the experiments that have been described here is that they merely show changes in reflexes but infer the anatomical pathways and patterns of connectivity. There may be several alternative explanations of the changes in reflexes in terms of patterns of connections, as the

discussion of myotypic specification has shown. One of the alternative explanations—that the cutaneous nerves grow selectively to the correct places in the graft—was examined more carefully in some experiments on the effects of translocating skin between the back and belly of frog tadpoles (Miner, 1956; M. Jacobson and Baker, 1968, 1969; R. E. Baker and Jacobson, 1970).

Miner (1956) removed a piece of skin on one side of the body of a frog tadpole and replaced the skin with its dorsoventral and anteroposterior axes inverted. The skin undergoes self-differentiation so that, after metamorphoses, dark dorsal skin develops on the belly and light ventral skin on the back. Tactile stimulation of the skin graft elicits a reflex movement of the leg aimed at the original position of the skin and not at the point of stimulation: when the back is tickled, the frog scratches its belly, and *vice versa*. These misdirected reflexes persist permanently and are not modified as a result of experience. These observations were confirmed by M. Jacobson and Baker (1968, 1969). The misdirected reflexes indicate that the skin, after being grafted to a new position, is able to signal its original position to the CNS. There are three possible explanations of the mechanisms of this phenomenon. First, the cutaneous nerves might grow back to their original places in the skin as the results of a selective attraction of the nerves by the skin; or, merely as a result of trial and error, the nerves might selectively reconnect with a place in the skin for which they have a specific affinity. The second possibility is that the nerves connect at random with the skin and are then respecified by the skin. As a result of the respecification, the central connections of the skin might undergo compensatory changes so that the central and peripheral sensory connections become congruent. Finally, the localization of the stimulus on the skin might be due to different patterns of impulses in sensory nerves connected to different places in the skin.

In order to distinguish among these possibilities in a more direct way, we mapped the peripheral connections of cutaneous nerves originating in normal and grafted skin of the frog. This was done by electrophysiological recording of action potentials evoked in cutaneous nerve fibers by stimulating the skin gently with a fine hair (M. Jacobson and Baker, 1968, 1969). This experiment revealed no differences in the pattern of nerve impulses in nerve fibers originating from different places in the skin. Each nerve fiber connects with a small area of skin;

action potentials can be evoked in the nerve fiber only by stimulating within this receptive field, as Fig. 11.8 shows. There is no evidence that nerve fibers grow a long distance in the subcutaneous tissues or in the skin in order to connect selectively with their original places in the skin graft.

These experiments also show that reversal of reflexes occurs only when skin grafts are inverted before larval Stage XV in *Rana pipiens* (M. Jacobson and Baker, 1969). In *R. pipiens*, normal and correctly localized reflexes develop when the inverted skin grafts are made after larval Stage XV, during metamorphosis, or in adult frogs. Stage XV occurs several days before metamorphosis, which starts at Stage XX and ends at Stage XXV (A. C. Taylor and Kollros, 1946).

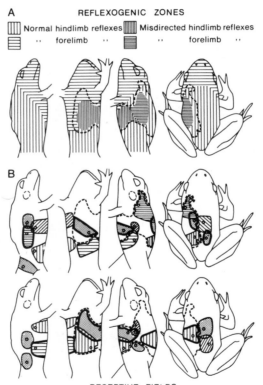

Figure 11.8. Maladaptive cutaneous reflexes develop in frogs with translocated skin grafts. (A) Grafting back skin to the belly and *vice versa* in the tadpole (after section of the cutaneous nerves) results, after metamorphosis, in misdirection of reflexes aimed at the original site of the stimulated skin, not at the site of stimulation. (B) The reflexogenic zones, mapped electrophysiologically 280 days after skin grafting, do not cross the graft margins. Each nerve enters the skin at the position shown by the small circle in its receptive field. Therefore, peripheral nerves do not appear to regenerate selectively to the skin, but central reflex connections appear to be determined by the original position occupied by the skin grafts. From M. Jacobson and R. E. Baker, *J. Comp. Neurol.* 137:121–142 (1969).

Regardless of the stage of development at which inverted skin grafts are made in larval frogs, reflex movements of the limbs, evoked by stimulating the graft, commence at the normal time during metamorphosis (M. Jacobson and Baker, 1969). The reflexes are normal at first, either from the whole graft or from most of the graft. In some cases, misdirected reflex movements of the leg are elicited from a small area of the graft; in others, normally localized reflexes are evoked from the entire graft. In the cases that show only normal reflexes, the origin of the grafted skin does not affect the reflex connections of its sensory nerves. The peripheral receptive fields of cutaneous nerves, mapped electrophysiologically, are normal in size, shape, and distribution.

These results show that the cutaneous nerves, which are cut close to the skin, initially regenerate nonselectively into the nearest skin regardless of their origin, with the result that normal cutaneous sensory localization is restored. After a period of normal behavior lasting several days or weeks, misdirected reflexes first appear on stimulation of a small region of the graft, while normal reflexes are elicited from the rest of the graft. In the majority of cases, the region of each graft giving rise to misdirected reflexes gradually increases in diameter at a rate of about 1 mm/day, until misdirected reflexes can be elicited from almost the entire graft. These misdirected reflexes persist indefinitely. The change from normal to maladaptive behavior is the reverse of that expected to result from learning. Whatever the mechanism of the change of behavior, it is not influenced by the animal's experience.

Because we could not detect any changes in the receptive fields of cutaneous sensory nerves during the period when reflexes changed from normal to misdirected, we inferred that the changes must have occurred in the CNS. We did not assert that this mechanism had been demonstrated, merely that it is considered probable pending further verification. Such rearrangements of connections in the spinal cord are conceivably possible in frogs because of extensive rostrocaudal spread of motoneuron dendrities for up to 2 mm (Stensaas and Stensaas, 1971), as well as rostral and caudal extension of dorsal root axons for several spinal cord segments (C. N. Liu and Chambers, 1958; B. Joseph and Whitlock, 1968). Filling the entire dorsal root ganglion cells with cobaltous lysine shows that in the dorsal horn

of the spinal cord there is extensive overlap of the terminals of nerves originating in back and belly skin of normal frogs, and no changes can be detected in frogs with back-to-belly skin grafts (Székely *et al.*, 1979). Therefore, it is conceivable that the reflex changes may result from unmasking of synapses that are already present rather than sprouting of terminals and formation of new synaptic connections (see Section 11.7).

The possibility of peripheral selection of connections has not been conclusively eliminated, and some evidence, also not conclusive, has recently been adduced in favor of selective reconnection of nerves with translocated skin grafts (Sklar and Hunt, 1973; E. M. Bloom and Tompkins, 1976). By contrast, J. Diamond *et al.* (1976) rotated large pieces of skin (up to 100 mm² rotated 180°) on the hindlimb of the salamander and found that ingrowing nerves show no preference for the skin to which they originally were connected. The nerves pay no regard to the axes of the skin but occupy a peripheral field that is the same, in relation to the entire limb, as they had previously occupied (Fig. 11.9). The formation of connections of sensory nerves with specific cutaneous domains and with sensory end-organs is considered in Section 9.10.

The circuit from muscle spindles to their homonymous motoneurons is an extremely favorable situation in which to study the development of specific connections. Therefore, efforts have been made to use this system to find solutions to the problems of the development of reflex circuits, and to resolve the antithesis between central and peripheral selectivity. Group 1a afferent nerve fibers from muscle spindles make monosynaptic connections only with alpha-motoneurons of the same muscle and its synergists. Each spindle afferent nerve fiber branches to terminate on a large percentage of the motoneurons of its muscle, and, conversely, a single motoneuron receives branches of afferent fibers from almost all the spindles in its muscle (Mendell and Henneman, 1968, 1971). How these specific connections develop in the embryo is an unsolved problem. Because of the high degree of specificity with which spindle afferents connect with motoneurons, any aberrant connections can be detected by microelectrode recording from single motoneurons while stimulating the group 1a afferents from individual muscles.

To study the specificity of the connections be-

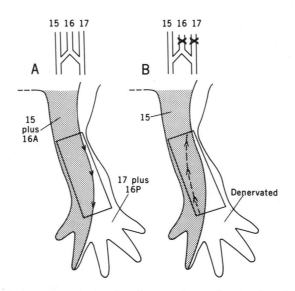

Figure 11.9. In the salamander leg, nerves that invade a denervated part of a rotated patch of skin (B) pay no heed to the original position of the skin but form a boundary at the same position in body space as that formed in the control leg (A). In some experiments of this kind, the original boundary is not re-formed, but there is an unusually large extenion of the remaining field into the denervated skin, both within the patch and outside it, without respect to the orientation of the patch. It is likely that the patch is innervated by regenerating nerve fibers in the latter case, while in the former case the graft is innervated by collaterals of intact nerves adjacent to the border of the grafted patch. Regenerating axons appear to ignore the spatial constraints which operate so effectively on sprouting axons of intact nerves. From J. Diamond, E. Cooper, C. Turner, and L. Macintyre, *Science* 193:371–377 (1976).

tween muscle spindle afferent nerves and their homonymous motoneurons, Eccles *et al.* (1960, 1962a,b) cross-united the nerves to antagonistic muscles of the hindlimb of the newborn kitten (medial gastrocnemius and peroneus muscles, or lateral gastrocnemius and plantaris). Some months after such nerve crosses, the Group 1a monosynaptic input from muscle spindles was recorded intracellularly from alpha-motoneurons. As a result of the nerve crosses, the peroneal motoneurons acquire a statistically significant increase in group 1a input from the synergistic muscles, lateral gastrocnemius, and plantaris. There is also a significant decrease in the group 1a inputs which have become functionally inappropriate as a result of crossing the nerves. No such rearrangements are found after cutting and self-union of the nerves to medial gastrocnemius and peroneal muscles (Eccles *et al.,* 1962a). The results indicate that new monosynaptic reflex pathways form, to a limited extent, and tend to reverse the effects of cross-union of nerves to antagonistic muscles. Such slight changes cannot be detected by

testing the reflex activity of the whole limb or by naked-eye studies of limb movements.

Cross-union of nerves involves axotomy and results in degeneration of up to two-thirds of the spinal ganglion cells. It is likely that the surviving group 1a afferent neurons sprout new terminal branches to occupy the synaptic sites left vacant by the degenerating group 1a afferents. Under such conditions, it is conceivable that only those synapses that are functionally effective are selected and that inappropriate synaptic connections are eliminated. Eccles *et al.* (1960, 1962a,b) were cautious in their interpretation of the results and were unwilling to distinguish between the latter hypothesis and that of myotypic specification.

Experiments similar to those described, but involving cross-union of nerves to agonistic muscles, were done by Mendell and Scott (1975). They cross-united the nerves to synergistic muscles (ankle extensors) in the kitten 5–8 days after birth and studied the effects on the connections of 1a fibers to the cross-united motoneurons. Under those conditions, they observed no rearrangement of synaptic connections. This evidence, showing lack of myotypic specification following nerve regeneration in newborn kittens, does not exclude the possibility that myotypic specification may occur during development. There clearly is some retrograde transsynaptic effect of muscle on motoneurons shown by the changes that occur in the motoneuron after it is disconnected from the muscle (see Sections 5.16, 6.14, and 9.5). In addition, reconnection of the motoneuron with the muscle can result in a recovery but not in a change in the functional properties of the motoneurons, which retain their original properties regardless of the type of muscle with which they reconnect (Kuno *et al.*, 1974a,b).

Afferent axons from muscle spindles project on motoneurons in developing frogs and adult frogs (Frank and Westerfield, 1983). Lichtman and Frank (1984) showed that sensory axons from triceps muscle of the adult frog form monosynaptic connections with homonymous triceps motoneurons but do not form connections with neighboring heteronymous motoneurons of the subscapularis and pectoralis muscles. Retrograde labeling of these three types of motoneurons by injections of horseradish peroxidase (HRP) into their muscles show that their cell bodies have overlapping distributions in lateral motor column and their dendrites overlap in the dorsal horn of the spinal cord (Lichtman *et al.*, 1984). In addition, the sensory afferents from triceps muscle arborize widely throughout the dorsal horn of the brachial spinal cord. But the sensory afferents make many more contacts with homonynous than with heteronymous motoneuron dendrites.

Axons regenerate from dorsal root ganglion (DRG) neurons to restore connections with the appropriate motoneurons in frog tadpoles (Sah and Frank, 1984). How does the sensory axon find its appropriate motoneuron? The sensory neurons are not prespecified but can change specificity to match the motoneuron. This is shown by grafting a thoracic DRG in place of a cervical one in bullfrog tadpoles with the result that some of the thoracic DRG neurons innervate limb muscles and make specific monosynaptic connections with the corresponding spinal motoneurons (Smith and Frank, 1987). This result shows that DRG neurons are specified through contact with muscle spindles. The ability for DRG neurons to be respecified by the periphery

is present in early tadpoles (before Stage 9) and is lost after the limb muscles normally become innervated (Frank and Westerfield, 1982).

In the frog, during normal development, muscle spindle afferents grow into the correct levels of spinal cord and terminate in the correct region, the ventral neuropil, even before the development of motoneuron dendrites with which they later form monosynaptic connections (P. C. Jackson and Frank, 1987). Regenerated spinal sensory axons also grow to their specific terminal zones: muscle afferents terminate in the ventral neuropil and cutaneous afferents in the dorsal neuropil of the spinal cord just as in normal frogs (Sah and Frank, 1984; Liuzzi and Lasek, 1985). Although they often take an abnormal pathway to reach the correct place the regenerating fibers rarely form aberrant collaterals (Peng and Frank, 1988). This is consistent with other evidence that collateral sprouting in the CNS after injury is specifically localized (Goldberger and Murray, 1982). No regeneration of sensory fibers occurs in the dorsal funiculi of the frog's spinal cord. The possible significance of the failure of axon regeneration in the white matter while good regeneration occurs in the gray matter should be considered in relation to evidence that oligodendrocytes inhibit axonal regeneration in the CNS (Schwab and Caroni, 1988; Caroni and Schwab, 1989).

11.7. Specification of Somatosensory Maps in Mammals

Somatosensory maps are specified by a combination of programs intrinsic to the developing neocortex, for example, the generation of microcolumns of neurons positioned in the characteristic six layers, and by extrinsic influences exerted by the activities of afferent nerve fibers (see Section 10.9).

A significant determinative role of the peripheral target tissue and of anterograde transneuronal trophic stimulation can be illustrated by the development of the organization known as barrels in the somatosensory cerebral cortex. The projection from the entire body to the primary somatosensory cortex (SMI) is organized in the form of cellular barrels, consisting of a core of afferent fibers surrounded by nerve cells in layer

IV of somatosensory cortex, demonstrable by Nissl staining or succinic dehydrogenase or cytochrome oxidase histochemistry. Single unit recording or 2-deoxyglucose studies show that stimulation of the appropriate peripheral field, such as a vibrissa, activates the corresponding barrel. Each barrel receives input from a specific region of the periphery on which the barrel depends for its normal development and survival. The barrels develop in rodents and carnivors during the early postnatal period. Thalamocortical afferents enter the cortical plate on P2–P3 and clustering of nerve fibers and cells to form barrels occurs on P3–P4 in rats. Development of individual barrels and of their somatotopic layout is greatly altered by peripheral injuries made before P5 in rodents.

In the mouse there are five rows of barrels representing the facial vibrissae in an area of the somatosensory cortex known as the barrel field, as shown in Fig. 11.10 (Lorente de Nó, 1922; Woolsey, 1967; Woolsey and Van der Loos, 1970). They are arranged in a pattern that mirrors the pattern of arrangement of the whiskers, known as mystacial vibrissae on the contralateral face (Woolsey and Van der Loos, 1970; Welker, 1971, 1976). Similar patterns of barrels, corresponding with the pattern of vibrissae, are found in other rodents (Welker and Woolsey, 1974; Woolsey et al., 1975b; Killacky and Belford, 1979) and the cat (Nomura, et al., 1986).

Each vibrissa is innervated by a bundle of 100–200 sensory nerve fibers with their cell bodies in the trigeminal ganglion (Renehan and Munger, 1986). Each ganglion cell innervates a single vibrissa (Zucker and Welker, 1969). The trigeminal ganglion cells project to the ipsilateral brainstem trigeminal nuclei in a somatotopic arrangement which mirrors the layout of the vibrissae (Belford and Killacky, 1979a,b; Erzurumlu et al., 1980; Erzurumlu and Killacky, 1983; Durham and Woolsey, 1984; Bates and Killacky, 1985; Nomura et al., 1986). From the trigeminal nuclei the neurons project to the contralateral ventrobasal complex of the thalamus where they end in a somatotopic representation called "barreloids" (Van der Loos, 1976). The ventrobasal neurons project in somatotopic order to the barrels in the ipsilateral somatosensory cortex. The barrel field is functionally organized in the form of vertical columns extending through the entire thickness of the cortex in which the barrels in layer IV are a morphological manifestation (Simons, 1978;

Simons and Woolsey, 1979; Simons et al., 1984; Kossut, 1988).

Barrels are separated from one another by septa with low cell density consisting of glial cells, some dendrites, and afferent fibers. The expression of astrocyte markers in the septa as early as P5 in the mouse is an indication of the role of glial cells in morphogenesis of barrels (Cooper and Steindler, 1986a,b). During the period of barrel morphogenesis in the mouse, the compaction of cells to form barrels is a complex process which is associated with expression of cell adhesion molecules, especially in the septa between barrels (Steindler et al., 1989).

The largest barrel (C1) in the mouse is composed of about 2000 neurons (Pasternak and Woolsey, 1975; Curcio and Coleman, 1982). In chimeric mice each barrel is formed of a mixture of cells from both genotypes, showing that the barrel is not the product of a unique founder cell population (Goldowitz, 1987). In rats the barrels are compact aggregates of cells except for the afferent fibers which enter the deep part and occupy the inside of the barrel (Welker and Woolsey, 1974; Patel-Vaidyu, 1985). In mice the sides of the barrel consist of densely packed neurons, mainly smooth and spiny stellate cells, including star pyramidal cells, with their dendrites predominantly directed toward the inside, but with the apical dendrite of the star pyramidal cells projecting to layer III. Only 15–25 percent of neurons have dendrites extending to neighboring barrels (Woolsey et al., 1975a; Simons and Woolsey, 1984). In the mouse the cells are less densely packed in the inside of the barrel but the density of synapses is higher inside than in the sides (White, 1976). Bundles of afferents from the thalamus enter the center or hollow of each barrel whereas the callosal and intracortical afferents end in the septa or outside the barrel field (Wise and Jones, 1976, 1978; Ollavaria et al., 1984).

There is a critical period during which development of barrels is affected by inputs from the periphery (Van der Loos and Woolsey, 1973; Weller and Johnson, 1975; Woolsey and Wann, 1976; Jeanmonod et al., 1981; Killacky, 1983; Kossut, 1988). Destruction of the vibrissal follicle at birth results in failure of development of the corresponding barrels, as shown in Figs. 11.10 and 11.11 (Van der Loos and Woolsey, 1973), whereas a similar lesion 5 days after birth has no effect (Weller and Johnson, 1975). The time at which a lesion of the vibrissal follicle no

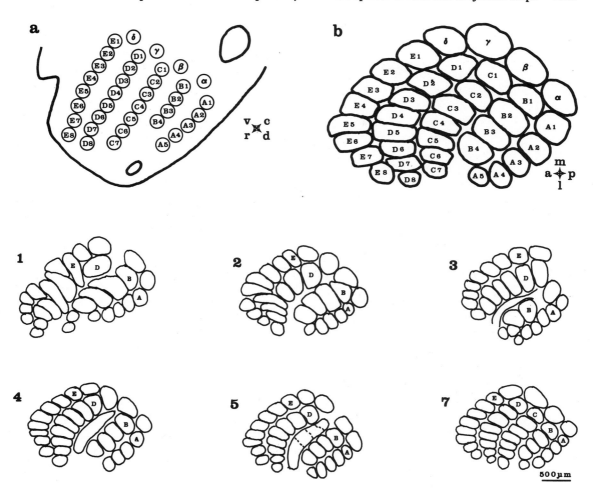

Figure 11.10. The barrel field of the mouse. Mystacial vibrissae of the mouse on the right side of the face (a) project to the posteromedial barrel subfield (b) of the left cerebral cortex. Barrels are arranged in five rows labeled A–E, corresponding with the arrangement of the vibrissae. Barrels are numbered within each row. Posteromedially, four barrels, designated α to δ, straddle the rows. The effect of cauterizing vibrissal follicles of row C on the right side on different days after birth is shown in the lower set of diagrams. There is progressively less disruption of the pattern of barrels after lesions made on postnatal days 1, 2, 3, 4, 5, and 7. From T. A. Woolsey and J. R. Wann, *J. Comp. Neurol.* 170:53–66 (1976).

longer results in failure of development of the barrel is correlated with the earliest appearance of the barrels on the 3rd or early 4th day after birth (Rice and Van der Loos, 1977). At that time, all the barrels first appear simultaneously in presumptive layer IV of the cortex, in the deepest layer of the cortical plate. Deafferented barrels are shrunken, while neighboring barrels, connected with normal vibrissae, are enlarged. This is associated with reorientation of dendrites from the deafferented to normal barrels (Harris and Woolsey, 1981) and by loss of the normal orientation of dendrites into the center of the barrel

(Steffen and Van der Loos, 1980). These changes do not occur after simple removal of vibrissae but damage to the follicle is required to produce anatomical changes in the thalamus and cortex (Verley and Axelrod, 1977; Killackey, 1980a,b). Section of a bundle of nerve fibers to a row of vibrissae or section of the trigeminal nerve results in more severe damage to the barrels than follicle lesions (Killacky and Shinder, 1981; Killácky and Erzurumlu, 1982).

The failure of development of the barrel after destruction of the vibrissal follicle is a transneuronal effect on the cortical neurons involving the thalamic

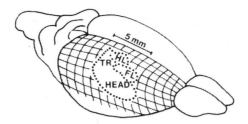

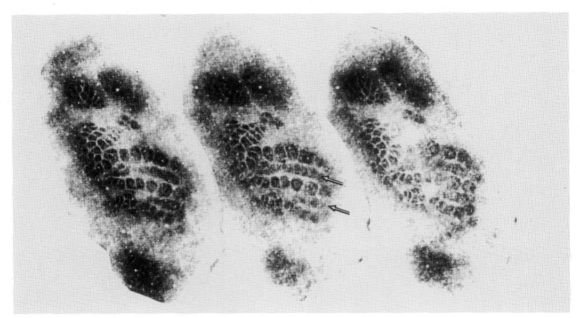

Figure 11.11. Mapping the thalamocortical somatosensory projection in the rat by means of the histochemical stain for succinic dehydrogenase, which is mainly localized in mitochondria, shows the barrel-like organization of the projection extending beyond the projection from the face to the projection from the trunk and limbs (see Fig. 11.12). The tangential histological sections, from left to right, are at progressively deeper levels in layer IV of the cerebral cortex. In this case, the vibrissal follicles of rows B and D (*cf.* Fig. 11.10) were destroyed at birth and the corresponding cortical barrels are disrupted (arrows: distance apart approximately 1 mm). The brain shows the primary somatosensory representation mapped electrophysiologically, superimposed on a 1-mm grid drawn on the surface of the cerebral hemisphere. The cortical projection zones are shown of the head, trunk (TR), hindlimb (HL), and forelimb (FL). Histological sections courtesy of G. Belford and H. P. Killackey.

relay neurons as well as their cortical targets. The time course of these effects has not been reported as all the studies were done several months after the vibrissal damage. However, studies of the plasticity of the somatosensory cortical map after peripheral nerve injuries show that there is a rapid phase of cortical reorganization within hours of the peripheral lesion, which does not involve growth processes in the cortex, and a slow phase lasting weeks to months involving growth processes (Kaas *et al.*, 1983, review). Sensory stimulation of the vibrissae may play a role in the development of the barrel. However,

such an effect may be expected to be on the final phase of development of synaptic connections rather than on the morphogenetic mechanisms that result in formation of the barrels. Chronic deprivation of sensory input results in reduction of the mitochondrial enzyme cytochrome oxidase, in the deprived barrels (Wong-Riley and Welt, 1980). By means of 2-deoxyglucose mapping, it has been shown that stimulation of single vibrissae always activates the corresponding barrels in layer IV of the somatosensory cortex (Durham and Woolsey, 1977, 1985; Durham *et al.*, 1981) and changes the pattern

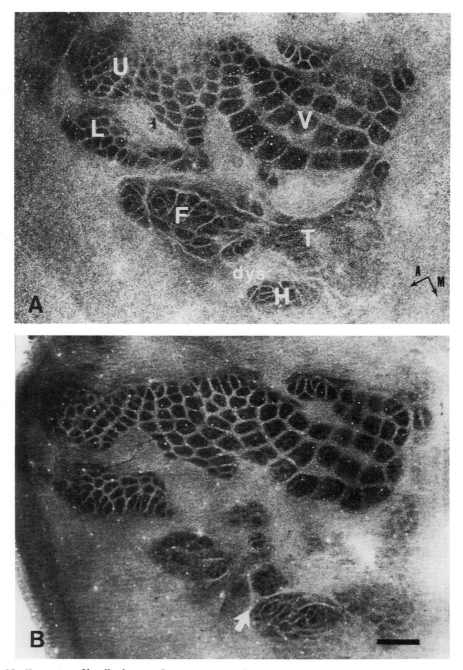

Figure 11.12. Expansion of hindlimb cortical representation after amputation of the forelimb in the rat fetus. (A) Normal pattern of succinic dehydrogenase activity in a tangential section through layer IV of the right primary somatosensory cortex of the rat. The representation is shown of the vibrissae (V), buccal pad in the upper jaw (U), lower jaw (L), forepaw (F), hindpaw (H), trunk (T), and the dysgranular cortex (dys) between forepaw and hindpaw representations. (B) Similar pattern after amputation of the contralateral forelimb on E16. Note the increase in size of the hindlimb region and loss of the dysgranular region (arrow). A = anterior; M = medial; magnification bar = 1 mm. From H. P. Killacky and D. R. Dawson, *Europ. J. Neurosci.* 1:210–221 (1989).

of activity between barrels in a manner that suggests that stimulation may determine the strength of intracortical connections (McCasland and Woolsey, 1988). Effects of sensory stimulation and the failure of development that can result from sensory deprivation are discussed in Sections 6.14, 11.15, and 11.21.

Reorganization of the somatosensory projection to the dorsal column nuclei, thalamus, and cerebral cortex has been reported after amputation of parts of the limbs, or section of a peripheral nerve or dorsal spinal root (reviewed by Kaas *et al.*, 1983; Devor, 1987). For example, after removal of a forelimb in the rat fetus on E16, reorganization of the somatosensory cortex occurs that normally receives afferents from the missing forepaw, and the somatosensory projection from the neighboring hindpaw enlarges to twice its normal size (Dawson and Killackey, 1987; Killacky and Dawson, 1989) as shown in Fig. 11.12. Reorganization of connections in the CNS after partial deafferentation could, in principle, occur by any of three different mechanisms separately or in combination: collateral sprouting of uninjured afferents and formation of new synaptic connections; strengthening of synaptic connections that previously existed in a weak form; change in the strength of inhibition (reviewed by Kaas *et al.*, 1983; Devor, 1987; J. T. Wall, 1988). There is evidence that collateral sprouting from intact afferents is responsible for recovery of function after partial deafferentation of of cat limb (Pubols and Goldberger, 1980; Pubols and Benowitz, 1982). Severe deafferentations resulting from dorsal rhizotomy are followed by gross reorganization of the somatotopic projections to the spinal cord (Mendell, 1984, review): dorsal column nuclei, thalamic nuclei, and cerebral cortex (reviewed by Devor, 1987; J. T. Wall, 1988). Changes in the spinal cord take days to weeks and probably involve collateral sprouting of intact axons and growth changes of existing synapses, but the changes in the nucleus gracilis occur immediately after dorsal rhizotomy and therefore result from unmasking of previously inactive or weakly active synapses (Dostrovsky *et al.*, 1976; Millar *et al.*, 1976; P. D. Wall and Devor, 1981; Devor, 1987, review).

Central reorganization after peripheral nerve damage has been demonstrated in adult monkeys (Schoppmann *et al.*, 1981; Merzenich *et al.*, 1983a,b), cats (Kalaska and Pomeranz, 1979; Franck, 1980), raccoons (Carson *et al.*, 1981; Kelahan and Doetsch, 1981; Rasmusson, 1982), and rats (P. D. Wall *et al.*, 1981). The deafferented cortex becomes reactivated by adjacent parts of the periphery, usually in a somatotopically organized projection, but there is some variability depending on species, site, and size of the operation (Kaas *et al.*, 1983, review).

There are rapid and slow components of this recovery. In the somatosensory cortex of the adult monkey the cortex is unresponsive to cutaneous stimulation immediately after median nerve section, but parts of the deprived cortex became responsive within hours and after several weeks the entire cortex became responsive to peripheral stimulation (Merzenich *et al.*, 1983b). Neurons in the somatosensory cortex of the cat change the location of their receptive fields after anesthetic block of dorsal roots but the original receptive fields return after recovery from the nerve block (Metzler and Marks, 1979). This shows that the rapid phase of the plasticity is not caused by nerve sprouting but must be due to unmasking of existing connections. Formation of new synapses is thought to take days (Cotman *et al.*, 1982, review). Increased formation of synapses in the rat somatosensory cortex occurs after spinal dorsal column lesions (Ganchrow and Bernstein, 1981).

There is evidence showing that use may increase central representation. For example, the somatosensory projection of the forepaw is greatly increased in size in kittens reared with daily avoidance training of shock to the forepaw (Spinelli and Jensen, 1979).

11.8. Development of Polarity and Position-Dependent Properties in the Retina

To investigate how retinal and tectal cells acquire locus specificities it is necessary to know the pattern of their histogenesis and whether they acquire locus specificities from their progenitors by a cell lineage mechanism or by interaction with neighboring cells. These experiments involve grafting the whole or parts of the retina or tectum into new positions or orientations in *Xenopus* embryos. Some time later, after metamorphosis, the retinotectal projection is mapped to see whether it reflects the alterations in positions or orientations of the cells or

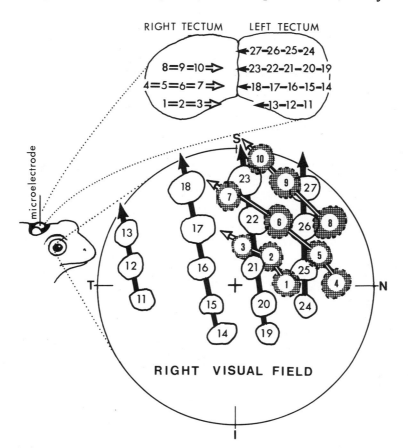

Figure 11.13. Map of the ipsilateral and contralateral visuotectal projections in the frog, *R. pipiens*. Each number in the right visual field is located in a small receptive field area from which a visual stimulus evokes action potentials recorded with a microelectrode at the position indicated by the same number in the optic tectum. Tectal electrode positions are 250 μm apart. The projection from the right eye to the left tectum is denoted by black arrows; the projection from the right eye to the right tectum is denoted by white arrows. The nasosuperior, binocular, region of the visual field projects to both sides of the optic tectum. The inferior part of the visual field projects to the lateroventral aspect of the tectum (not shown). The visual field extends 100° from the center and its poles are designated I (inferior or ventral), N (nasal or anterior), S (superior or dorsal), T (temporal or posterior).

whether it is normal (Fig. 11.13). If the map reflects the cellular alterations, it can be concluded that the cells have autonomously expressed stable locus specificities. If the map is normal, it may be concluded that the locus specificities have changed to conform with the final positions of the cells or that the graft has been replaced by new cells.

Many changes in the frog's visual system normally occur during the period between retinal or tectal surgery in the tadpole and mapping of the retinotectal projection in the postmetamorphic frog. During metamorphosis of the frog major changes in the visual system occur as adaptations to life on the land. There are changes in visual pigment (Wilt, 1959); pattern of cell division at the retinal margin (D. H. Beach and Jacobson, 1978a–c); an ipsilateral retinothalamic projection develops (Hoskins and Grobstein, 1984, 1985; Hoskins, 1986); the inner plexiform layer of the retina increases in complexity and number of synapses (L. J. Fisher, 1972); growth and increased branching of retinal ganglion cells occur (Pomeranz and Chung, 1970; Frank and Hollyfield, 1987); and there are changes in the receptive fields of retinal ganglion cells (Pomeranz and Chung, 1970; Pomeranz, 1972). Regulation of the retinotectal map may also result from cell migration and cell death during the period of weeks to months between the surgical rearrangements on the embryo and the mapping of the retinotectal projection. Failure to take cell migration and cell death into account led me to conclude that new retinal locus specificities can be acquired after eye rotation before but not after Stage 30 in *Xenopus* embryos (Jacobson, 1967, 1968). From those results I concluded incorrectly that the retina acquires locus specificities by interaction with neighboring tissues before Stage 30 but the locus specificities become stable or refractory to interactions after Stage 30. The error was corrected by Hollyfield and Sharma (1974), who showed that the retina, rotated before Stage 30, can express locus specificities autonomously.[7]

Those experiments were done before the extent of cell death in the retina was fully understood (see Section 8.3) and before Holt (1980) had demonstrated that neuronal progenitors can migrate from the optic stalk into the eye cup and re-form a normal retina after a retinal graft or rotation has been made. Extensive cell migration may occur within a surgically altered retina in *Xenopus* embryos (Ide *et al.*, 1984). Those new findings force a reconsideration of the experiments which show that regulation may occur in surgically altered embryonic eyes (Jacobson, 1967, 1968a; Hunt and Jacobson, 1973, 1974; Cooke and Gaze, 1983; Willshaw *et al.*, 1983; O'Rourke and Fraser, 1986a,b).

The eye of the *Xenopus* embryo at Stage 31 contains only a few hundred retinal ganglion cells and retinal axons have not yet grown out of the eye, yet rotation of the eye at Stage 31 results in corresponding rotation of the entire retinotectal map of the adult eye, which contains about 50,000 retinal ganglion cells (M. Jacobson, 1968a,b, 1976a). Apparently a developmental program has been established in the embryo that affects the entire set of specificities that will arise in the adult retina, and the unsolved problem is how the retinal ganglion cells that continue to be formed throughout life in amphibians and fish acquire their locus specificities. The retina grows by addition of new cells at its margin (Glücksmann, 1940; Hollyfield, 1971; Straznicky and Gaze, 1971; M. Jacobson, 1976a, 1977; D. H.

[7]I agree with Samuel Johnson when he says: *"As all error is meanness, it is incumbent on every man who consults his own dignity, to retract as soon as he discovers it, without fearing any censure so much as that of his own mind."*

Beach and Jacobson, 1978a–c) where a population of retinal stem cells persists throughout development. The retinal cells that are produced at the circumference of the retina must obtain their positional information from other cells in the eye and not from extraocular cues, because rotation of the eye results in a completely rotated retinotectal map (M. Jacobson, 1967, 1968a; Sharma and Hollyfield, 1974). The newly produced retinal ganglion cells may derive their locus specificities by cell lineage, by cellular interactions, or by a combination of both mechanisms.

In the cellular interaction mechanism the stem cells *(M)* at the retinal circumference do not possess locus specificities themselves and do not participate in the specification of their daughter cells, but serve merely to produce cells of the correct cellular phenotype; the daugher cell *(x)* is initially without locus specificity, but then interacts with the nearest specified neuron *(n)* and so acquires the locus specificity appropriate to its position in the array $(n + 1)$. This process is then repeated as follows:

$$1.2.3 \ldots\ldots n. \, (M)$$
$$\downarrow \quad \text{mitosis}$$
$$1.2.3 \ldots\ldots n. \, (x). \, (M)$$
$$\downarrow \quad \text{interaction} \ (x \xrightarrow{n} n + 1)$$
$$1.2.3 \ldots\ldots n.n + 1. \, (M)$$

In this cellular interaction model, all the stem cells *(M)* that produce ganglion cells at the retinal circumference are qualitatively identical in space and time, as are the newly produced neurons *(x)* that lack locus specificity initially. Random destruction of some stem cells and *(x)* cells or inhibition of DNA synthesis or mitosis in some stem cells would not alter the normal pattern of deployment of locus specificities, although the total number of cells would be reduced. However, inhibition of cell communication would be expected to alter the spatial pattern of locus specificities.

In a cell lineage mechanism locus specificities are inherited directly by retinal ganglion cells from the stem cells:

$$1.2.3 \ldots\ldots n.(M^n)$$
$$\downarrow \quad \text{mitosis}$$
$$1.2.3 \ldots\ldots n.n + 1.(M^{n-1})$$
$$\downarrow \quad \text{mitosis}$$
$$1.2.3 \ldots\ldots n.n + 1.n + 2.(M^{n-2})$$

The stem cell line changes its specificity with each cell division, and the positional information is not communicated from cell to cell except at mitosis, from stem cell to daughter cell. If this is the case, destruction of stem cells will result in a deficit in the set of locus specificities.

According to the cell lineage model, alterations of the orderly schedule of cell proliferation in the retina would result in a derangement of the normal pattern of deployment of locus specificities. Translocation of stem cells (such as are produced by combining parts of the eye rudiment in abnormal locations) would, according to the cell lineage model, give rise to predictable changes in the pattern of retinal locus specificities.

Clues to a solution of those problems are certain correlations between retinal histogenesis and the genesis of locus specificities in the retinal ganglion cell population. First, the retinal ganglion cells that are born in the central region of the retina cease DNA synthesis at Stages 29–31 in *Xenopus* (M. Jacobson, 1967, 1968b), as shown in Figs. 11.14 and 11.15, and it seems likely that changes in their developmental programs accompanying their with-

drawal from DNA synthesis and from the mitotic cycle initiate the transition, which is called "specification" or "determination." This change of state, according to one hypothesis, occurs in many different neuronal populations as nerve cells become postmitotic (M. Jacobson, 1968b, 1969, 1970b). A similar close correlation between cessation of DNA synthesis at Stages 12.5–13, withdrawal from the cell cycle, and histogenetic determination is seen in Mauthner neurons of *Xenopus* (Vargas-Lizardi and Lyser, 1974). Similarly, in the retina of the chick embryo, ganglion cell specification occurs at about the same time as the first ganglion cells withdraw from the cell cycle. Cessation of DNA synthesis in chick retinal ganglion cells is seen in Stages 12–13, at 45–52 hours of development (Kahn, 1973, 1974), and some of these ganglion cells can be seen to have sprouted an axon by Stage 15, at 50–55 hours of development (K. T. Rogers, 1957; Goldberg and Coulombre, 1972). Crossland *et al.* (1974a) have shown that these retinal events are correlated with a change in the response of the chick retinotectal system to removal of part of the retina. They observed that removal of 15–75 percent of the retina before

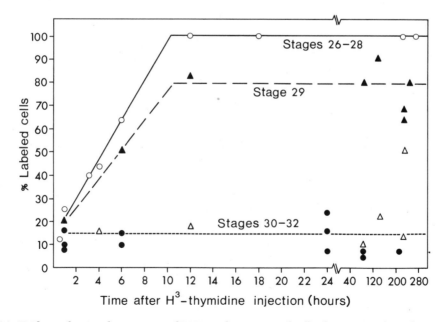

Figure 11.14. Evidence showing that cessation of DNA synthesis in retinal cells of *Xenopus* embryos begins at Stages 26–28 and is completed in more than 80 percent of retinal cells by Stage 32. Percentages of labeled cell nuclei after [³H]thymidine injections started at Stages 27–28 (open circles); Stage 29 (filled triangles); Stage 30 (open triangles); Stages 31 and 32 (filled circles). From M. Jacobson, *Dev. Biol.* 17:219–232 (1968), copyright Academic Press, Inc.

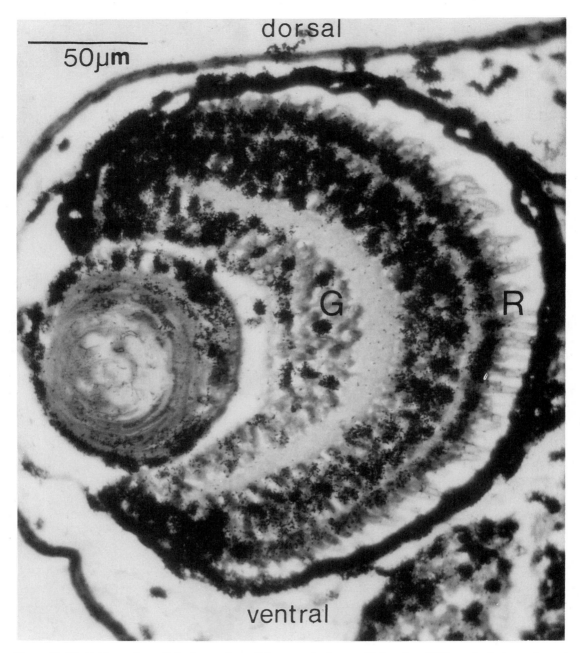

Figure 11.15. Evidence that cells in the ganglion cell layer are the first to withdraw from DNA synthesis. Autoradiograph of a vertical (coronal) section through the eye of a Stage 43 (*Xenopus*) embryo labeled cumulatively with [³H]thymidine, beginning at embryonic Stage 29. The unlabeled cells in the retinal ganglion cell layer (G) ceased DNA synthesis before Stage 29. Note the gradients of labeling from receptor cells (R) to ganglion cells (G), and from dorsal to ventral. From M. Jacobson, *Dev. Biol.* 17:219–232 (1968), copyright Academic Press, Inc.

Stage 11 (40–45 hours of development) results in development of retinal connections to all parts of the tectum, whereas removal of part of the retina after Stages 12–13 leaves the corresponding part of the tectum free of retinal connections. This change in the capacity of the reduced retina to send axons to occupy the entire tectum is correlated with the time of origin of the first retinal ganglion cells at Stage 11. In *Xenopus*, the capacity of a part of the retina to fill the entire tectum with its axons persists for a few stages after Stage 31 (R. K. Hunt and Jacobson, 1974a; R. K. Hunt and Frank, 1975). In the adult frog, this capacity is considerably slowed (Udin, 1975, 1976) or lost (Meyer and Sperry, 1973). By contrast, in the adult goldfish, the retinotectal map can form between a fragment of retina and the entire tectum (Yoon, 1972a) or between an entire retina and a residual fragment of the tectum (Yoon, 1971). This is discussed more amply in Section 11.13.

The change of state of the retina in its response to partial removal of the retina may involve a change in the intercellular communication between retinal cells themselves. According to this hypothesis, developing nerve cells, when grafted to another position, can acquire new position-dependent properties only if they can communicate with neighboring cells. The locus specificities of the grafted cells then develop in accord with their new positions. However, it seems that if the graft itself cannot communicate with neighboring cells, its locus specificities are derived from the preoperative position. Similarly, after surgical reduction in the size of the retina, the residual cells may be able to develop a complete range of position-dependent properties only as a result of cellular interactions. Such interactions probably require cell contact and may involve intercellular communication through specialized intercellular junctions (Loewenstein, 1968a,b, 1970, 1973, 1975; Dorresteijn *et al.*, 1983; Caveney, 1985, review; S. E. Fraser *et al.*, 1987; C. R. Green, 1988; S. C. Guthrie *et al.*, 1988; Nagajski *et al.*, 1989; S. C. Guthrie and Gilula, 1989, review) that provide intercellular pathways for ions and small molecules (Loewenstein, 1968a,b, 1973, 1987; Warner, 1970; I. Simpson *et al.*, 1977; A. Warner, 1988). Evidence in support of this hypothesis is the observation that gap junctions have been found ubiquitously between the cells of the embryonic retina of *Xenopus* before Stage 29 (while the retina is composed of mitotically active stem cells), but gap junctions disappear from the first retinal cells to withdraw from mitosis, and at later stages persist only between the cells at the retinal margins, which remain mitotically active (Dixon and Cronly-Dillon, 1972; Hayes, 1976).

Specification may involve withdrawal of retinal cells from the mitotic cycle and concomitant uncoupling of the postmitotic nerve cells from the rest of the retinal cell population. After uncoupling from the retinal population the nerve cell is characterized by a stable and irreversible program leading to development of a locus specificity. Development of this position-dependent specificity enables the young nerve cell to extend its outgrowing axon on the proper pathway and predisposes that axon to terminate at a specific position in the brain and to form synaptic connections selectively with particular nerve cells. It must be emphasized that the arguments associating specification with the terminal cell cycle are based on no more than circumstantial evidence, and the association with cellular uncoupling rests on a mere shred of evidence. We have yet to devise an experiment aimed at showing the neuron *in flagrante delicto* of specification.

11.9. Development of Polarity and Position-Dependent Properties in the Optic Tectum

The tectum must play an essential role in the formation of an orderly, continuous, and properly aligned retinotectal map, but whether the tectum merely aligns the map or whether it controls or directly influences the positions of individual elements of the map cannot be decided *a priori*. The problem can be generalized to include other orderly neuronal projections: either the entire presynaptic population may be deployed with reference to the polarity of the postsynaptic population as a whole, or individual presynaptic elements may position themselves with reference to the corresponding individual postsynaptic elements.

Polarity of the tectum as a whole, or at least two reference points giving the tectal axes, is the minimal condition for setting up a map of the retinal axon population properly aligned with the tectal axes or reference points, which are themselves aligned with the axes of the embryo as a whole. In that case, positions of individual retinal axons in the map would require interactions between the axons themselves in which they would express their retinal position-dependent properties (locus specificities) in selecting a place in the retinotectal map. Alternatively, or in addition to the expression of tectal polarity, individual tectal elements may have properties that depend on their positions in the tectum, and these positional markers may serve as targets for corresponding retinal elements.

The role of axon-to-axon interactions in establishing order in the optic nerve and optic tract has been the subject of numerous studies. These show that side-to-side adhesion between optic nerve fibers as well as competitive interactions between their terminals are only two among many factors involved in the formation and maintenance of orderly projections to the visual centers. There is a very large variation, according to species, in the amount of retinotopic order in the optic nerve: considerable retinotopic order is maintained from retina to tectum in fish (Scholes, 1979; Rusoff and Easter, 1980; Bodick and Levinthal, 1980; Bunt, 1982) and the chick (Rager and Rager, 1978; Rager, 1980; Thanos and Bonhoeffer, 1983). However, the optic nerve fibers do not maintain retinal nearest-neighbor relationships in the optic nerves of frogs (Maturana, 1959; Lettvin *et al.*, 1959, Bunt and Horder, 1983), rats (Bunt and Lund, 1982), cats (Horton *et al.*, 1979), or monkeys (Naito, 1989). Therefore, the orderly projection of the retina on the tectum and lateral geniculate can develop despite considerable disorder of axons in the optic nerve. In the optic tract, retinotopic order is found in all vertebrates that have been examined. The disorderly arrangement of optic nerve fibers becomes progressively more organized retinotopically after entering the optic tracts but it is not known how the sorting out occurs (Scalia and Fite, 1974; Fujisawa *et al.*, 1981a,b; Fawcett and Gaze, 1982). But retinotopic order in the optic nerve and tract is not an absolute requirement for mapping to the tectum: optic nerve fibers can take aberrant pathways from the retina to tectum and form an orderly map (Gaze, 1959; Harris, 1982). Optic nerve fibers from a 3rd eye or heterotopic eye grafted on the head can form an orderly retinotectal map (M. Jacobson and Hunt, 1973; Sharma, 1972b; Constantine-Paton, 1981). Optic nerve fibers are scrambled after regeneration, yet form an orderly retinotectal projection in the frog (Gaze and Jacobson, 1963). Those findings also rule out precise timing as a factor in formation of an orderly map.

We conjectured that there must be tectal locus specificities that are recognized by retinal axons carrying the complementary specificities. Strong experimental evidence showing the existence of tectal locus specificities in goldfish and *Xenopus* is that pieces of tectum exchanged between rostral and caudal positions in the tectum act as targets for the retinal axons that previously mapped to them (R. Levine and Jacobson, 1974; M. Jacobson and Levine, 1975a,b; Yoon, 1975a,b, 1977, 1980; Gaze and Hope, 1983). Additional evidence is that fibers growing out of embryonic retinal grafts on chick tectum show directional specificity (Thanos and Dütting, 1987).

Rotation of the tectum (rostrocaudal inversion), in part or whole, followed by assay of the retinotectal map, behaviorally or electrophysiologically, has shown that the tectal polarity becomes irreversible (i.e., refractory to tectal rotation) only after the retinal axons enter the tectum. The experiments do not indicate whether tectal polarity is present before that stage, but they show that polarity is stable thereafter. In the first experiments of this sort, Crelin (1952) excised the tectum in salamander embryos at various stages and replaced it back-to-front. When the operation is done before the stage at which the tectum is invaded by retinal axons, the animals develop normal vision. However, inversion of the tectum at later stages, while retinal axons are invading it, results in the development of confused visually guided behavior. These results are not easy to interpret because it cannot be shown how the altered behavior is related to the retinotectal map, and it is not demonstrated that the inverted tectum receives retinal inputs.

The possibility that the rotated tectum retains its original polarity if a "polarizing zone" is included in the rotated graft, but not if it is excluded, was suggested by R. Levine and Jacobson (1974). Evidence that the polarity of the tectum is determined by the diencephalon has been put forward by Chung and Cooke (1975). They showed that rotation of the mesencephalic anlage without including the diencephalon in *Xenopus* embryos at Stages 21–24 or at Stage 37 results in development of a retinotectal map that is normally aligned with the embryonic axes. This demonstrates that tectal polarity either is absent or can be reversed up to Stage 37. However, if the anlage of the diencephalon is included with the rotated mesencephalon, even at Stages 21–24, the resulting retinotectal map is inverted. In some cases, two retinotectal projections with opposed polarities develop in the same tissue, apparently showing that there are two sets of intermingled tectal cells which express their polarity independently (Fig. 11.16). These important experiments raise in an acute form the problem posed by rotation of the embryonic eye, namely, how the information about polarity (or possibly about position) is transmitted from the few stem cells present at Stage 21 to the hundreds of thousands of tectal cells that do not come into existence until later stages. The first cells of the tectum originate as postmitotic neurons at Stages 39–40, and by Stage 46 the tectum contains less than 5 percent of the neurons that are present at Stage 66. The population of tectal cells in the frog is built up over a period of more than 2 months

(Straznicky and Gaze, 1972; Currie and Cowan, 1974b, 1975; M. Jacobson, 1977).

Whether individual tectal elements have acquired position-dependent properties cannot be adduced from the results that have been discussed above. Therefore, we performed the additional experiment of rotating or translocating a small patch of tectum in larval and adult frogs (*Xenopus and Rana catesbeiana*) to see whether the patch expresses its original position-dependent properties independently or whether it expresses properties appropriate to its new location (R. Levine and Jacobson, 1974; M. Jacobson and Levine, 1975a,b). Rotation of a patch alters both the polarity and position of the patch relative to the surrounding tectum, whereas translocation without rotation changes the position but not the polarity of the piece of tissue. Both operations result in sharp discontinuities in the retinotectal map corresponding with the margins of the patch. This shows that the position-dependent en-

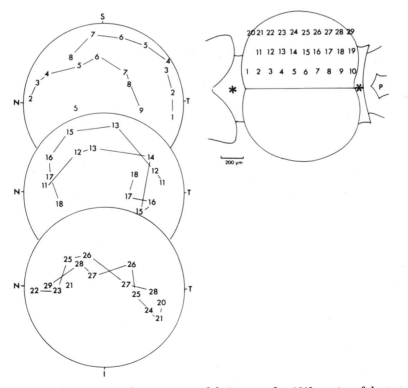

Figure 11.16. Duplication of the visuotectal projection in adult *Xenopus* after 180° rotation of the tectum at embryonic Stage 28. Either only half of the tectum had been rotated or a second tectum regenerated, or partial pattern regulation occurred in the rotated tectum. Asterisks show the positions of the duplicated diencephalon. With permission from S. H. Chung and J. Cooke.

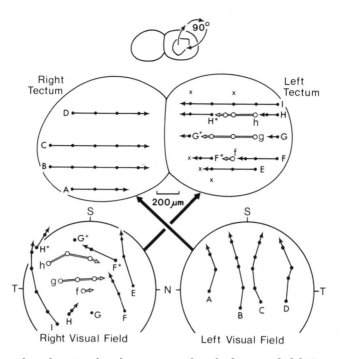

Figure 11.17. Expression of tectal positional markers in a rotated patch of tectum of adult *Xenopus* occurs independently of the expression of tectal positional markers in the tectum surrounding the patch. Visuotectal map made 195 days after surgical excision, 90° rotation, and reimplantation of a tectal patch. This shows that optic axons recognize their original positional markers in the tectal patch and surrounding tectum. The conventions are the same as in Figure 11.13. From R. Levine and M. Jacobson, *Exp. Neurol.* **43**:527–538 (1974).

tities in the tectum serve as targets for retinal elements (Fig. 11.17). That these tectal entities, named positional markers by R. Levine and Jacobson (1974), are expressed independently of the tectal polarity is shown by the discontinuity of the retinotectal map produced by moving a patch from anterior tectum to posterior tectum without rotation (M. Jacobson and Levine, 1975b). This also shows that positional information used in setting up an orderly map in the tectum is vectorial and not merely scalar. Rotation of patches of tectum in the goldfish (Sharma and Gaze, 1971; Yoon, 1975a,b, 1977, 1980) has also shown that the tectal patch behaves autonomously in serving as a target for retinal axons.

Additional evidence of the active role of the tectum in establishing the polarity of the map is provided by experiments in which surgical removal of the caudal half of the tectum, which results in rostrocaudal compression of the entire retinal projection to the residual half of the tectum, also results in compression of the projection to a rotated

patch in the residual half-tectum (Yoon, 1977). In such cases, the patch and the surrounding tectum each express their polarity independently in aligning the retinotectal projection to the patch and to the surrounding tectum, respectively (Fig. 11.18). In all cases, regardless of the orientation of the patch, including turning the grafted patch upside down, thus producing inversion in only one axis (Yoon, 1975b), the reestablished projection respects the original polarity of the patch, and a sharp discontinuity of the retinotectal projection occurs at the patch margin.

Such evidence in both the goldfish and the frog shows that the tectum as a whole, as well as a small tectal patch, has a strong effect in determining the polarity of the retinotectal projection, and that the interaction between retinal axons and tectal cells is stronger than the tendency of optic axons, interacting only with one another, to assemble themselves in a continuous map. The question of the relative strengths of axon–axon and axon–target interactions will be asked again whenever

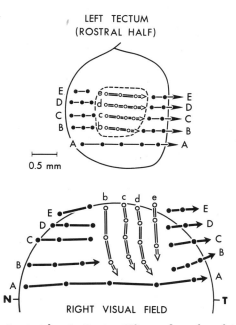

Figure 11.18. Compression of the visuotectal projection to a 90° rotated tectal patch in the goldfish with retention of the orginal polarity of the projection to the patch. The map was made 184 days after rotation of the tectal patch in the rostral half-tectum. the arrows on the tectum point to the caudal part of the tectum that had been removed. N = Nasal visual field; T = temporal visual field. From M. G. Yoon, *J. Physiol.* **264**:379–410 (1977).

we consider the mechanism of formation of topographic neuronal maps.

11.10. Expression of Locus Specificity in the Assembly of the Retinotectal Map

Several methods have been used for studying the expression of neuronal locus specificity during development of the retinotectal map. First, the normal appearances of the map during normal development can be observed; second, the map can be studied during and after regeneration of the optic nerve in fish and amphibians; third, the response of the map to removal of neurons in the retina and/or tectum can be determined; and, fourth, the effects of drugs can be determined that destroy retinal and tectal cells or inhibit their proliferation or differentiation.

As the destructive effects of these methods increase from first to fourth, their results become increasingly more difficult to interpret in terms of normal development. In each case, the retinotectal map

that develops after experimental perturbation must be assayed and compared with the normal map, and the normal maps obtained at various stages of assembly must be compared with one another and with the adult map.

Several methods of assaying the retinotectal map are available: (1) tests of visually guided behavior, (2) histological methods of tracing the optic axons from the retina to the tectum and other visual centers, and (3) electrophysiological mapping. Each of these techniques has its advantages and its limitations. Thus the tests of visually guided behavior show whether there are functional connections between the retina and visual centers but do not localize the function to any particular visual centers or to any synapses in those centers. The anatomical methods do not show whether the demonstrated structures are functional. Electrophysiological mapping can show whether the pattern of the map is normal and orderly, and functional synapses can be demonstrated by recording postsynaptically.

Normally, a ganglion cell at a particular retinal position always projects its axon to a particular position in the map of axon endings in the tectum. Thus the axon terminals originating in the retina are deployed in the tectum in a spatial pattern or map which reduplicates the pattern of deployment of the ganglion cells in the retina. To demonstrate this electrophysiologically, a microelectrode is lowered into the tectum at a succession of positions farther and farther back on the tectum, and nerve action potentials are recorded at each of these successive positions only by providing the animal with a visual stimulus at appropriate and successively temporal positions in the visual field. In this manner, we can map the visuotectal projection (M. Jacobson, 1962; M. Jacobson and Gaze, 1964) as shown in Fig. 11.13. This procedure has become the standard method of assaying the effects of experimental surgery to the retina, optic nerve and tract, or tectum (references on this topic include Gaze *et al.*, 1963, 1965; M. Jacobson and Gaze, 1965; Sharma, 1972a–d; Yoon, 1971, 1972a,b, 1976). In normal adult animals the visuotectal projection and the retinotectal projection can be regarded as equivalent, but they cannot be assumed to be equivalent in experimental animals with retinal lesions or during development when the intraretinal circuits and visual optics are changing. Because the map is obtained extracellularly from presynaptic terminals of retinal axons in the tectum, it does not show whether those terminals have formed functional synaptic connections in the tectum, and it should not be misused to make inferences about such connections. The retinotectal projection provides a convenient assay of the locus specificities of the retinal ganglion cells, but does not provide an assay of functional connectivity between them and tectal neurons. Such as assay can be obtained only by recording beyond the synapse, that is, by assaying the postsynaptic potentials arising in tectal neurons when retinal neurons are stimulated appropriately. This can be done by recording intracellularly from single tectal neurons (Witpaard, 1976), by recording extracellularly from individual tectal neurons (Lettvin *et al.*, 1961; Grüsser and Grüsser-Cornehls, 1968, 1973; Fite, 1969; Skarf, 1973; Skarf and Jacobson, 1974), or by recording extracellular field potentials in the tectum (J. A. Freeman and Stone, 1969; Chung *et al.*, 1974a,b), to cite only those who first introduced those techniques which have since been widely used.

The map is also limited with respect to the information that can be obtained from it. It provides no more than relative information about the disposition of the position-dependent properties across the retinal cell population. The map does not show which locus specificities are present; it only shows that the order of their spatial deployment in a retinal population occurs in a particular direction and across a population of cells within defined spatial boundaries. Thus it is extremely risky to try to correlate discontinuities or continuities in the retinal fiber projection to the tectum with a history of surgical manipulation of the retinotectal system. The main limitation of the mapping technique is that after experimental surgery to either the eye or the tectum, it cannot assay the range of the position-dependent properties in the retinal cell population or tell whether the set of properties that is finally expressed is complete, reduced, or augmented.

Exponents of retinotectal mapping with microelectrodes have a tendency to confuse the retinotectal map with the developmental mechanisms that produce it. There is some danger in this kind of confusion of levels because each level has unique concepts and research methods that are not applicable to other levels. Thus, on an abstract level, the expression of the developmental program of retinal ganglion cells can be represented as a series of retinotectal maps, but the latter do not indicate morphogenetic or biochemical mechanisms. The physicochemical level, which cannot be adduced from the maps, includes the program of synthesis and assembly of molecules in the retinal ganglion cells and tectal cells, which results in the acquisition of position-dependent cellular properties. The histogenesis and morphogenesis of the retina and tectum and formation of synaptic connection between retina and tectum are on yet another level, which cannot at present be adduced from either the maps or the biochemical assays.

Morphogenesis of the system can be assayed in terms of outgrowth of axons from retinal ganglion cells, selection of axonal pathways, tentative or permanent contacts between optic axons and tectal cells, growth of tectal cell dendrites, selection of synaptic sites, and formation of functional synapses. The role of glial cells in all those neuronal developments remains largely unexplored, although a start has been made (R. Levine, 1990). It is fair to believe that the mapping phenomena will eventually be explained in terms of morphogenesis and that the latter will be explicable in biochemical terms. Because we are so far from reducing one level to another and because different concepts and methods are used at the different levels, we have to respect the independence of the three levels of description of development of the retinotectal system. In order to avoid confusion we have to be very cautious in transferring data from one level to the others. Rarely, in developmental neurobiology has it become possible to grasp all the levels of description in a coherent synthesis.

11.11. Assembly of the Retinotectal Map during Normal Development

There are several ways in which the population of retinal ganglion cells can form connections with the tectal cell population during development. First, both retina and tectum may develop independently without forming connections until the development of both neuronal populations is complete. This occurs in the chick retinotectal system, in which retinal axons enter the tectum during the period of tectal histogenesis, but synapse formation is delayed until both retinal and tectal sets have been completed (LaVail and Cowan, 1971a,b; J. P. Kelly and Cowan, 1972; Crossland et al., 1974a,b; Rager, 1976b; Nakamura and O'Leary, 1989). Second, synaptic connection between retinal axons and tectal cells commences before the entire populations of retinal and tectal neurons have been produced. This occurs in the frog (Gaze et al., 1974; T. M. Scott, 1974; T. M. Scott and Lázár, 1976; M. Jacobson, 1977; D. H. Beach and Jacobson, 1978a–c) and in fish (Raymond and Easter, 1983; Easter and Stuermer, 1984; Stuermer, 1988a,b), in which the number of retinal and tectal neurons increases throughout life. In both the 1st and 2nd cases, an individual retinal axon may form a connection only once with the "correct" tectal neurons (Holt and Harris, 1983; Fujisawa, 1984, 1987; Sakaguchi and Murphey, 1985) or the axon may grow to "incorrect" positions from which it later retracts to connect with the "correct" position (Fujisawa, 1981, 1987; Fujisawa et al., 1981, 1982a,b; Nakamura and O'Leary, 1989); or, alternatively, the retinal axon may form a succession of temporary "correct" connections before finally making permanent connections with the "correct" neurons (Gaze et al., 1974, 1979; Reh and Constantine-Paton, 1984; Easter and Stuermer, 1984).

In 1974, Gaze et al. put forward their hypoth-

esis of shifting retinotectal connections (Fig. 11.19). They proposed that each retinal axon in Xenopus forms a succession of temporary synaptic connections with different tectal cells as the axon adjusts its position in the retinotectal map to accommodate newly produced retinal axons and tectal neurons. This adjustment is required, they argued, because the patterns of growth of retinal and tectal cell populations appear to be grossly mismatched—circumferential rings of cells are apparently added to the retina (Straznicky and Gaze, 1971), while lines of cells are added at the caudomedial margin of the tectum (Straznicky and Gaze, 1972)—and because synaptic connections develop during this period of retinal and tectal growth starting at tadpole Stage 46 and continuing through metamorphosis (T. M. Scott, 1974; Chung et al., 1974b). In postulating a shift of the retinal projection to the tectum on these grounds, they assumed that all retinal ganglion cells project to the tectum, in spite of evidence that the retina projects to several other visual centers (Muntz, 1962a,b; Székely, 1971; R. J. Mark and Feldman, 1974; Scalia and Fite, 1974). Even if retinal growth does not match tectal growth, it may match growth of the visual centers as a whole. Nevertheless, the theory of shifting retinotectal connections has had great heuristic value, stimulating efforts to test it by different techniques as they have become available.

While the tectal pattern of histogenesis has been confirmed (Currie and Cowan, 1974b; M. Jacobson, 1977), the original observations of Straznicky and Gaze (1971) showing that retinal histogenesis in Xenopus is radially symmetrical have been shown to be incorrect. The pattern of retinal histogenesis in Xenopus is markedly asymmetrical from tadpole Stage 53 through metamorphosis, with about 10 times as many cells added at the ventral as at the dorsal margin of the retina (M. Jacobson, 1976a; D. H. Beach and Jacobson, 1979a–c). This means, of course, that a succession of different retinal ganglion cells occupy the center of the retina, which by convention is taken to be the center of the retinotectal map. Thus the patterns of retinal histogenesis and tectal histogenesis are not as grossly mismatched in Xenopus as had been supposed when the theory of the shifting connections was first proposed. Also, the extensive death of retinal ganglion cells that occurs during normal development in Xenopus, and that may eliminate mismatched neurons, was not known when the theory of shifting connections was first

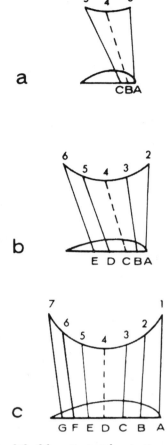

Figure 11.19. Diagrams representing the shift of the retinotectal projection across the tectum, which occurs with development. The numbers represent positions on sections through the retina and the letters indicate positions along the rostrocaudal axis of the tectum. The retina grows by the addition of new cells at the retinal margin, while the tectum grows in a curvilinear fashion, from rostrolateral to caudomedial. Eye and brain connect up early in development and both keep growing thereafter. Throughout development, the most temporal part of the retina at any time projects to the most rostral part of the tectum. (a) Early in development, only central retina has yet developed, and only rostral tectum. These interconnect, as shown, with most-temporal retina (3) sending fibers to most-rostral tectum (A). (b) Later in larval life, the retina has added more cells at the margin, indicated in this section by 2 and 6. The tectum has also added cells caudally, shown as D and E. Retina and tectum connect as shown, with most-temporal retina (now 2) sending fibers to most-rostral tectum (E), with intermediate bits of the retinal projection having to shift backward on the tectum to fit in. (c) Eventually, yet more retina appears at the margins (1 and 7) and more tectum is added caudally (F, G). Most-temporal retina (now 1) connects to most-rostral tectum (still A), with fibers from the original central retina now displaced to position D on the tectum. From R. M. Gaze, *Br. Med. Bull.* 30:116–121 (1974).

proposed. Retinal cell death may be a mechanism of matching retina with tectum in the chick embryo (Rager and Rager, 1978) and cell death probably performs a similar function in the frog. In *Xenopus*, retinal ganglion cell death occurs during the period when the disparity between retina and tectum is greatest and during the period when the retinotectal connections would shift according to the theory.

The number of ganglion cells is reduced by 20 percent from about 17,000 at Stage 53, shortly before metamorphosis, to about 13,000 by 6 months after metamorphosis in *Xenopus* (Jenkins and Straznicky, 1986). The loss of ganglion cells is much greater than these figures show because ganglion cells are added to the retina during the same period (D. H. Beach and Jacobson, 1978c). Moreover, many retinal ganglion cells initially project two or more axons to the tectum in *Xenopus* embryos (Holt, 1989), but the supernumerary axons and possibly the entire neuron bearing them are lost at later stages (Fig. 11.20).

Evidence which is consistent with the theory of shifting retinotectal connections has been reported in *Xenopus* (Gaze *et al.*, 1979; Fraser, 1983), *Rana* (Reh and Constantine-Paton, 1984; Fraser and Hunt, 1986), and fish (Easter and Stuermer, 1984; Rusoff, 1984). Those results imply that all the retinal axons are continually shifting their synaptic connections to

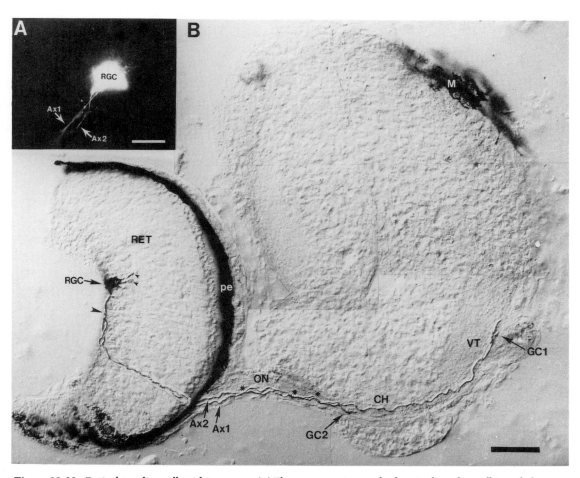

Figure 11.20. Retinal ganglion cells with two axons. (A) Fluorescence micrograph of a retinal ganglion cell in a whole-mount preparation soon after intracellular Lucifer yellow injection. Two axons (Ax1, Ax2) emerge from two different points on the cell body and cross over approximately 10 μm from the cell body. (B) Composite photomicrograph of a cell with two axons (six sections, 12 different focal planes of a Stage 37/38 embryo). The preparation was immunolabeled with HRP following Lucifer yellow injection. A single axon bifurcates (large arrowhead) some 20 μm from the cell body. The 2 axons (Ax1, Ax2) cross over one another 3 times (asterisks) in the optic nerve (ON) and are of different lengths, with one ending in a growth cone (GC2) soon after entering the ventral diencephalon and the other (GC1) in the contralateral ventral optic tract (VT). Both growth cones are fairly complex, having several filopodia. Two dendrites (small arrowheads) emerge from the cell body. The pigment on the upper-right surface of the brain is from melanocytes (M) inadvertently left in place through the dissection. RET = retina; pe = pigment epithelium; CH = chiasm. Scale bars: A = 20 μm; B = 50 μm. From C. E. Holt, *J. Neurosci.* 9:3123–3145 (1989), copyright Society for Neuroscience.

progressively more caudally located tectal cells, and that this extraordinary process continues throughout life without interfering with normal visual experience, or with visually guided behavior and learning. We do not know how sensory input to the tectum is converted into motor commands, but continual changes made in the input connections would require corresponding changes in connections with the output neurons.

The relationship between retinal axons growing into the tectum and the timetable of tectal histogenesis has been studied in *Xenopus* by labeling the retinal axons with [³H]proline injected into one eye, and at the same time injecting [³H]thymidine to label the retinal and tectal cells originating at that time (T. M. Scott and Lázár, 1976; M. Jacobson, 1977). Using that technique, T. M. Scott and Lázár (1976) reported that when both labels were injected at Stage 50 in *Xenopus* and the animals were killed 3 days later, the labeled retinal axons and tectal cells were congruent. However, if the animals were killed 2 or 4 weeks after the injections, the proline-labeled axons spread about 150 μm caudal to the rostral limit of the band of labeled tectal cells. From these observations it was concluded that a shift of optic nerve terminals had occurred relative to newly formed tectal cells. However, those observations were made before the completion of retinal ganglion cell death, and therefore it can be argued that the retinal axons that spread too far caudal would eventually be eliminated.

Using the same technique of intraocular injection of [³H]thymidine, but in larger series of animals injected at various stages from 46 to 66, I have shown that proline-labeled axons remain juxtaposed with cells in the rostral part of the tectum that were present before the time of the injection of label and that successively later contingents of ingrowing retinal axons grow to more caudal positions in the tectum (M. Jacobson, 1977). Measurements of the surface area of the tectum containing labeled retinal axons at various times up to 37 days after the injection of the label show no increase in the area occupied by labeled retinal axon terminals, although the total surface area of the tectum increases continuously, as shown in Fig. 11.21. Limitations of those experiments arise from the very small size of the tectum in *Xenopus* tadpoles relative to the size of individual retinal axon terminal arbors, and from their inability to reveal individual retinal axons. Oth-

er experiments in which pieces of the eye are labeled and reimplanted before outgrowth of optic axons (Holt and Harris, 1983; Holt, 1984; O'Rourke and Fraser, 1986) show large contingents of axons growing into the tectum and are also subject to errors which arise from the small size of the tectum relative to imprecision and variability of the grafting methods, and from inability to label individual retinal axons.

Observations made by Sakaguchi and Murphey (1985) on individually labeled retinal axons in *Xenopus* show that the axons form a topographically orderly map from the beginning but that the map is imprecise because of the large size of the retinal axon terminal arbors relative to the size of the tectum. At Stages 40–45 the arbors of a single retinal axon cover 33–50 percent of the medial-to-lateral extent of the tectum. *Xenopus* retinal ganglion cell axons individually labeled at Stage 50 grow accurately to their appropriate tectal targets (Fujisawa, 1987). In the zebrafish, individually labeled axons enter the tectum at the rostral edge, grow over the rostral part of the tectum that had earlier been occupied by retinal axons, and reach the correct targets in the caudal part of the tectum (Stuermer, 1988a).

Tectal histogenesis is completed rapidly in the chick, from E4 to E9 (La Vail and Cowan, 1971b). In the chick embryo, retinal axons from the central retina are the first to arrive in the tectum on E6 (Crossland *et al.*, 1975). These axons branch in the central tectum by E9 (Rager and Von Oeynhausen, 1979; Thanos and Bonhoefer, 1987). Axons from the temporal retina grow into the tectum by E9 and form branches along their length (Nakamura and O'Leary, 1989). Although many axons grow to the appropriate tectal targets, some make targeting errors and form excessive branches as seen after labeling individual axons (Nakamura and O'Leary, 1989). However, from E13 to E15, remodeling of the retinal axons occurs by elimination of redundant branches and by correction of the course of the axons (Nakamura and O'Leary, 1989). Refinement of the retinotectal map in the chick embryo also occurs as a result of cell death. The period of retinal axon remodeling coincides with the period of retinal ganglion cell death in the chick embryo (Rager and Rager, 1978; Hughes and McLoon, 1979). Retinal ganglion cell death also eliminates axons that have projected aberrantly to the ipsilateral tectum of the

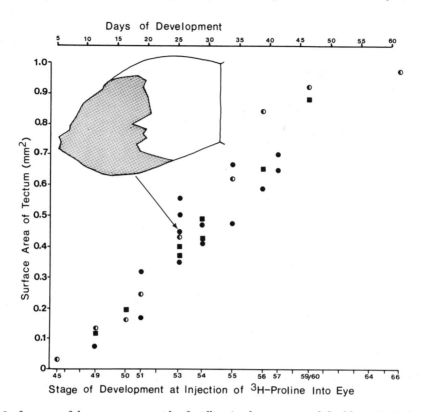

Figure 11.21. Surface area of the tectum to one side of midline (as shown at upper left of figure) in 21 frog tadpoles that each received a single injection of [^{3}H]proline at various stages of development. The tectal surface area over the labeled retinal axons in the superficial layers of tectum (stippled) was measured in autoradiographic serial sections in animals killed 1–2 days (squares) or 16–37 days (circles) after the injection, compared with the tectal surface area of uninjected normal controls (half-circles, each point the mean of four tecta). Regardless of the period of development after the injection, the labeled retinal axons occupy an area of tectum that correlates with the total tectal area of normal controls at the same stage of injection. The surface of the tectum shown at the upper left is from an animal that had received intraocular [^{3}H]proline at Stage 53, and was killed 33 days later, at Stage 66. The stippled area is the part of the tectum labeled with [^{3}H]proline. From M. Jacobson, *Brain Res.* **127**:55–67 (1977).

chick embryo (McLoon and Land, 1982; O'Leary *et al.*, 1983; Thanos and Bonhoefer, 1984).

In summary, the retinotectal map in fish and frogs is arranged in retinotopic order from the beginning of development and is built up over a long time by addition of new retinal axons growing to the caudomedial edge of the tectum where new tectal cells are added. This suggests that the mitotically active zone of the tectum is a source of some factor which promotes retinal axonal growth. The initial overlap between terminal arbors of retinal ganglion cells results in a less precise retinotectal map at first but this is refined at later stages. The refinement of the map occurs as a result of growth of the tectum relative to the size

of individual retinal axon terminals, degeneration of aberrant axonal branches, and death of aberrant retinal ganglion cells. The role of visual function on refinement of the retinotectal map is considered in Section 11.15.

11.12. Assembly of the Retinotectal Map during Regeneration of the Optic Nerve

Adult fish and amphibians can regain vision as a result of optic nerve regeneration, and this phenomenon has provided a means of studying the mechanisms of regeneration of optic nerve fibers and of the formation of connections between optic axons and their targets in the visual centers. Regeneration does not exactly recapitulate ontogeny; therefore, regeneration of the optic nerve may not be a reliable model of development of the retinotectal projection. Important results that emerge from all the investigations are that optic axons have a strong tendency to regain their positions in the retinotectal map; that functional connections are formed after regeneration on the basis of the inherent specificities of the optic axons and tectal neurons; and that, after surgical inversion of an eye or after size disparities between retina and tectum, anatomical recovery tends to occur without respect to the functional effects. The optic axons branch to project to widespread regions when they first regenerate into the tectum but later adjust their endings to the correct tectal loci, even during blockade of action potentials with tetrodotoxin.

A series of studies by Sperry (1943, 1944, 1945b, 1948, reviewed in 1951a,b) show that visuomotor coordination recovers completely after regeneration of the optic nerve in adult amphibians. These observations of behavior led him to infer that the optic nerve fibers regenerate to the correct positions in the visual centers, especially in the optic tectum. This has been confirmed more directly by recording the electrical activity in the optic tectum when stimulatiing the retina with a small spot of light or other suitable visual stimulus (Gaze, 1959; M. Jacobson, 1960b, 1961a,b; Gaze and M. Jacobson, 1963a; M. Jacobson and Gaze, 1965). Not only is an orderly, continuous, and properly aligned retinotectal map restored in many cases, but also the different functional classes of optic nerve fibers end at approximately normal depths in the tectum after regeneration of the optic nerve in adult frogs (Maturana *et al.*, 1959; Gaze and Keating, 1969).

Recovery of vision has been reported following a variety of surgical rearrangements of connections between the eye and brain in adult amphibians. Optic nerve section has been combined with inversion of the eye (Sperry, 1944, 1951a; L. S. Stone, 1944, 1948, 1953, 1960); an eye has been transplanted to the opposite orbit (L. S. Stone, 1930, 1941; L. S. Stone and Cole, 1943); the left and right eyes have been transposed (Sperry, 1945b); and the optic chiasm has been excised and each optic nerve deflected into the ipsilateral optic tract (Sperry,

1945b). Visual recovery also occurs in urodeles after transplantation of an eye to the orbit of another salamander of the same species (L. S. Stone, 1930; L. S. Stone and Cole, 1943) and after exchanges of eyes between different species of salamanders (Harrison, 1929; L. S. Stone, 1930; Twitty, 1932; L. S. Stone and Ellison, 1940). These observations on the formation of connections of optic axons in the wrong side of the brain show that optic nerve fibers treat the left and right sides of the brain as mirror-image replicas, and the capacity of an eye from one species of urodele to form a retinotectal map in the brain of another species shows that the same mechanisms operate in different species of urodeles and might thus be of greater universality.

In all cases, when the operation results in inversion of one or both axes of the retina, visuomotor reflexes are correspondingly inverted. For example, after 180° rotation of the eye, the animal's attempts to capture a fly in the nasosuperior quadrant of the visual field are misdirected toward the temporo–inferior visual field. Optokinetic reflexes are also inverted: after 180° rotation of the eye, the frog or salamander follows vertical bars moving in a naso-temporal direction across the visual field, whereas normal amphibians respond only to temporonasal movement of the stimulus. The surgical operations result in inversion of spatial localization and movement detection, both of which depend for their realization on orderly connections of the eye with the brain, although not necessarily with the tectum. Some visuomotor behavior is mediated by the diencephalon (Muntz, 1962a,b). Optokinetic responses are mediated by pretectal nuclei and are unaffected by removal of the tectum (Székely, 1971; R. J. Mark and Feldman, 1972).

The inverted visuomotor reflexes are permanent and are not corrected by experience or learning (Sperry, 1944, 1951a,b; L.S. Stone, 1944, 1953). In one newt, inverted visuomotor reflexes were observed for 4½ years after inversion of the eye, but recovery of normal optokinetic reflexes and accurate localization of a lure occurred immediately after the eye was returned to its normal orientation (L. S. Stone, 1953). All these experiments show that the optic nerve fibers in adult amphibians regenerate to form a continuous map properly aligned in the optic tectum irrespective of the alignment of the eye from which they originate or the side of the brain with which they connect, and regardless of the functional effect. The observations that optic nerve fibers show a very strong tendency to regenerate to the tectum and to re-form a functional retinotectal map pose a number of questions, none of which can yet be answered fully.

First, there are several questions relating to the routes taken by optic axons to the visual centers. How do the fibers select the correct pathway? Does pathway selection require interactions between axons and cells along the pathway? Do regenerated axons make use of vestiges of the degenerated axons? Are the mechanisms of selective regeneration the same as those of selection of a pathway in the embryo? How do the fibers select the proper side of the brain to enter at the optic chiasm, and how do fibers diverge from the main visual tract to enter branches to various visual centers?

Second, there are several questions about interactions between fibers during their growth. If interactions between axons occur, do they take place all along their length or only close to or at their growing tips? Do the interactions occur only during outgrowth of the axon, or are they maintained after the system has reached a steady state in the adult? Are interactions only positive (i.e., affinities resulting in fasciculation), or are there inhibitory interactions or disaffinities between axons? What are the mechanisms of such interactions? What are their strengths and the ranges of their actions?

Third, there are several questions relating to the control of axonal elongation and axonal branching. It is known that axons growing from eyes transplanted to the nose, ear, or flank will continue growing indefinitely unless they arrive at one of the visual centers of the brain (R. M. May and Detwiler, 1925; R. M. May and Capranica, 1975, 1976a,b). So the question arises, what determines that the axon stops elongating when it arrives at a target? Does the axon approach the target by random branching, or is it attracted by a neurotropic stimulus released from the target?

There must be a sorting-out process to ensure that optic nerve fibers arising from different places in the retina will terminate in the correct places in the brain. Some sorting out must occur even before the optic axons enter the tectum, since the optic axons enter the correct branches of the optic tract. When they arrive in the pretectal region, the axons destined for the dorsomedial part of the tectum may enter the medial brachium of the optic tract, while fibers destined for the ventrolateral part of the tectum may enter the lateral brachium (M. Jacobson, 1960a, 1961a,b, 1966; Arora and Sperry, 1962; Attardi and Sperry, 1963). The problem that is posed here is the general problem of how growing nerve fibers select the proper pathway, and especially how fibers that have grown along the same pathways are able to diverge into separate pathways at the proper branching points. Evidence of branching and of guidance is indirect and inadequate. Attempts to discover intermediate stages in the regeneration of the optic nerve in adult frogs showed that the earliest retinotectal projection map is random in both axes, that some cases also show a map that is organized in the nasotemporal retinal (caudal–rostral tectal axis) axis but random in the dorsoventral retinal axis (lateral–medial tectal axis), and finally, that the order of the map is restored in both axes (M. Jacobson, 1960a, 1961a,b; Gaze and Jacobson, 1963a).

Attardi and Sperry (1963) tried to determine the route taken by regenerating optic axons in the tectum of adult goldfish by examining serial sections of the tectum. They observed that optic axons grow through deafferented regions of the tectum to reach their correct destinations and concluded that the optic axons *"appear to be not only rather specifically destination bound, but also definitely inclined to follow particular routes to their respective destinations."* This conclusion, which was given by Sperry (1963) in support of his chemoaffinity theory, has been shown to be wrong by many other observations which show that retinal axons reach their tectal targets by a process of trial and error (see below). Such observations might lead one to suspect that the nerve fibers are guided by preformed chemical markers along their routes or are attracted by specific chemicals emanating from their final destinations. The observations of DeLong and Coulombre (1968) showing that optic axons appear to grow preferentially toward their correct destinations from retinal grafts placed on the surface of the tectum of the chick embryo have been shown by S. Goldberg (1974) to be the result of passive displacement of the grafts relative to the underlying tectum rather than of selective growth of optic axons toward their correct tectal targets, as was first supposed.

The investigations that have been reviewed to this point were all limited by their inability to trace individual retinal fibers regenerating into the tectum.

This has become possible recently by means of ante-rograde tracers such as HRP, wheat germ agglutinin, and fluorescent molecules. Such studies have shown that regenerating retinal axons in goldfish grow along abnormal routes (J. E. Cook, 1983; Stuermer and Easter, 1984a; Stuermer, 1986, 1988a,b). At first the individual retinal axons branch and are distributed over a far wider extent of tectum than normal, but they gradually adjust their positions over a period of several months until a near-normal retinotectal map is restored (Meyer *et al.*, 1985; Rankin and Cook, 1986; Stuermer, 1988a,b). This process of withdrawal or degeneration of aberrant axons and correction of the growth of axons to their appropriate tectal loci does not require nerve impulses, as it occurs in gold-fish treated with repeated introcular injections of tetrodotoxin as well as in controls (Stuermer, 1989). Blockade of impulses does not prevent correct choice of a brachium of the optic tract by which regenerating fibers enter the tectum (J. E. Cook and Becker, 1988) nor does it prevent targeting of retinal axons de-flected into the ipsilateral tectum (Meyer, 1987). However, nerve impulse activity is required for the physiological recovery of normal receptive field properties of regenerated optic axons: receptive fields of regenerated retinal axons remain several times larger than normal in goldfish treated chroni-cally with intraocular tetrodotoxin (Schmidt and Ed-wards, 1983). This is discussed further in Section 11.15.

11.13. Assembly of the Retinotectal Map after Surgical Removal of Parts of the Retinotectal System

The question posed by the finding that removal of brain tissue results in a reorganization of the re-sidual structures is "What is changing or being reor-ganized?" Are the structures themselves replaced? If not, are the properties or specificities of the re-sidual cells replaced or changed so that new cellular associations can form on the basis of the new specif-icities, for example, by nerve sprouting and forma-tion of new synaptic connections? Alternatively, do none of the above occur, but instead do the residual structures merely make different associations on the basis of their original properties and specificities, for example, by unmasking or disinhibiting preexisting synatic connections? The reader will realize that

these questions once again pose the problem of what components of the system are sensitive to changes in their context: are cell deployment, cellu-lar properties, or operations of cells sensitive to the change in context produced by such surgical opera-tions? Unambiguous answers to those questions have been very difficult to obtain.

When we consider the experimental strategies that have been used to study specificity and plas-ticity, in the nervous system, we are struck by the lack of critical appreciation of the limitations of the methodology. For example, a classical strategy is to make size disparities between neuron set A and set B, by removing parts, for example, of retina or tec-tum during embryonic development and ultimately mapping the final configuration of connections or projections between the two sets (Fig. 11.22). "Spec-ificity" in the system is assayed by determining whether the final map is normal or compressed, expanded or distorted in any other way. Unfortu-nately, this strategy is intrinsically limited because the result can never be interpreted unambiguously without additional evidence. One cannot ever tell, without other controls, whether the set of elements present in the altered map is the same as the set that would have developed without surgical interference. Thus the cells in set A (retina) and/or set B (tectum) might have been replaced by new cells. Or the cells might have changed their properties; or, if their properties were retained, their expression might have been altered in the novel context produced by the experimental situation. Attempts to force such maps to reveal the rules governing connectivity be-tween two sets of nerve cells lead inevitably to circu-lar arguments: the map is an operational indication of the relatively orderly expression of position-dependent properties in a set of elements, but after experimental surgery neither the identity of the set nor the expression of its properties can be deter-mined from the map. It is not known whether the same elements are present or the same properties persist, nor whether the expression of the properties has been altered under the experimental conditions. Realization of these limitations of the experimental methods reduces confidence in many of the conclu-sions that have been reached about neuronal speci-ficity and the mechanism of formation of synaptic connections in the retinotectal system or in other neural systems in which uncontrolled changes may result from ablation of part of the nervous system.

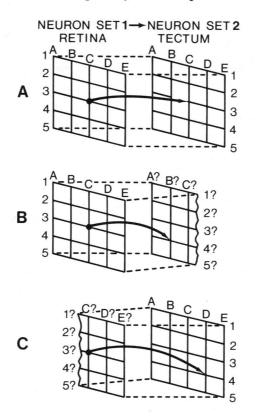

Figure 11.22. Relations between partial and complete neuronal sets. (A) Mapping of neuronal set 1 (retina) into set 2 (tectum), with elements connected at position C3 in both sets. Some time after removal of part of the tectum (B) or retina (C) compression or expansion of the map occurs. However, one cannot simply deduce the mechanisms from the map because the presynaptic or postsynaptic elements, or both, may have changed their positional values (locus specificities), or new elements may have been added, substracted, or substituted. From M. Jacobson, Neuronal recognition in the retinotectal system, pp. 3–23, in *Neuronal Recognition,* S. Barondes (ed.), Plenum, New York (1976).

The main experimental results of producing size disparities in the retinotectal system can now be reviewed in the light of these considerations of the limitations of the methodology. In the initial study of the effects of making size disparities in the retinotectal system, Attardi and Sperry (1963) removed part of the retina and cut the optic nerve in the goldfish. They showed histologically that after 3–67 days the optic nerve fibers grow back only to the appropriate parts of the tectum. They concluded that the regenerating optic nerve fibers are "destination bound" and that the optic nerve fibers grow by the most direct pathway to their proper synaptic sites in the tectum, bypassing inappropriate sites on the way. In such studies, each animal is studied at only one postoperative stage, and whether the system has arrived at a steady state or is at an inter-

mediate state cannot be known. A similar criticism can be leveled at the study of retinotectal size disparities in the goldfish by M. Jacobson and Gaze (1965). We did two kinds of experiments; in the first, the entire population of optic nerve fibers were allowed to regenerate into a residual lateral or medial part of the tectum; in the second, we studied the regeneration of about half the normal number of optic nerve fibers to the intact tectum. In both experiments, it seemed as if, by 139 days, the optic fibers had returned only to the appropriate positions in the tectum, and the assumption was made that the system had reached its final state.

The first strong suggestion of plasticity in the retinotectal system of the goldfish appeared after regeneration of the optic nerve into a residual rostral half-tectum (Gaze and Sharma, 1970). In such studies on goldfish, the entire retina is found to send its fibers into the residual part of the tectum: the optic fibers are deployed in the correct order, but are compressed by a factor of about 2 into the rostrocaudal axis of the tectum (Yoon, 1971; Sharma, 1972a). Yoon (1972a,b) showed that such compression of the optic nerve fibers into the residual part of the tectum can occur into either the mediolateral or rostrocaudal axis of the tectum, and is reversible (Fig. 11.23).

There is some evidence that the result of removing a part of the tectum may depend on the time after the operation. Thus Sharma (1972b) found that a few weeks after removing the central part of the goldfish tectum and crushing the optic nerve, the regenerated optic nerve fibers return to their correct places in the tectum, leaving a large central

scotoma in the visual field. In other fish, examined months after removal of the central part of the tectum, the scotoma is not present and the fibers from the entire retina seem to be compressed into the residual tectum. These results suggest that the optic nerve fibers initially return to their proper places in the tectum (as shown by Attardi and Sperry in 1963 and by M. Jacobson and Gaze in 1965), but later the optic nerve terminals are repositioned in order to accommodate all the regenerating optic fibers into the residual part of the tectum, as found by Yoon (1971, 1972a,b).

Two different mechanisms have been invoked to explain the phenomena of compression and expansion of the retinotectal map after removal of part of the tectum or part of the retina. The first type of mechanism invokes regulation of tectal or

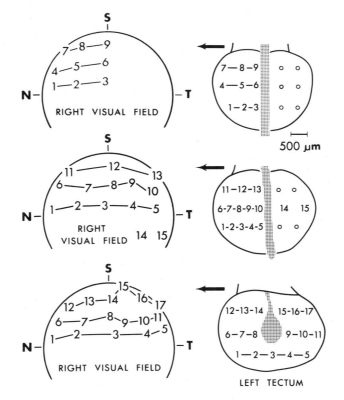

Figure 11.23. Reversible compression of the retinotectal map in goldfish. The top map was made immediately after insertion of a gelatin film in a mediolateral cut bisecting the tectum. The middle map, made 67 days later, shows the compression of the entire visual field into the rostral half–tectum. The bottom map, obtained 184 days postoperatively, after resorption of the gelatin film, shows expansion of the projection to the caudal half-tectum. The arrow points rostrally in the midsagittal plane of the tectum. N, S, T = nasal, superior, and temporal visual fields, respectively. From M. G. Yoon, *Exp. Neurol.* 35:565–577 (1972).

retinal position-dependent properties of the reduced set of retinal and tectal elements—after surgical reduction of the set, the residual elements assume the full range of properties of an entire set. The second type of hypothesis invokes interaction between the optic axons which results in their orderly deployment to form a map in the available tectal space. Neither mechanism alone can account for all the observations.

There is evidence for and against tectal regulation, and the conflict is unlikely to be resolved before the cellular mechanisms of regulation are better understood. Evidence for regulation is provided by Yoon (1976), who showed that when the map reforms rapidly, within a few weeks after removal of the caudal half-tectum plus section of the optic nerve, a partial map forms initially, appropriate to the residual part of the tectum, and compression of the entire map into the residual tectum occurs later, at 40–90 days postoperative. However, when optic nerve regeneration is delayed for more than 40 days after removal of the caudal half-tectum, an entire but compressed map forms from the start. Yoon concludes that tectal regulation is delayed for about 3–6 weeks after removal of part of the tectum.

In conflict with Yoon's conclusion is the evidence that when the optic nerve is cut after compression or expansion of the map has occurred, regeneration of the optic nerve results at first in assembly of a partial map appropriate to the residual part of the retinotectal system, and only later does the map compress or expand, as appropriate (J. E. Cook and Horder, 1974). It seems impossible to conceive of a single variable, namely regulation, that could be responsible for such widely divergent results. The conclusion seems inescapable that regulation (however broadly the term is defined) is not the only means of altering the spatial dimensions of the retinotectal map without altering its topological pattern. However, it also seems that axon–axon interactions cannot be the only mechanism of setting up the retinotectal map. This is not to imply that axonal interactions have no role to play, as they certainly do, but that they are insufficient to account for the evidence, for example, of mapping to grafted patches of tectum (see Section 11.9). Those experiments show that the optic axons grow to their correct destinations in a grafted patch of tectum, and therefore the axon-tectum interactions are stronger than the axon–axon interactions.

The notion that optic axons can assemble themselves in retinotopic order as a result of their affinities and disaffinities has frequently been proposed, largely as a theoretical possibility, for there is little direct evidence to support the notion. The possibility that axonal interactions play a role in assembly of the retinotectal map has been advanced in several forms, ranging from little more than a statement of that possibility (M. Jacobson, 1966, p. 371; Gaze and Keating, 1972; R. E. Cook and Horder, 1974; R. Levine and Jacobson, 1974, 1975) to more detailed models replete with computer simulations (Prestige and Willshaw, 1975; Willshaw and von der Malsberg, 1976; Hope *et al.*, 1976; Meinhardt, 1982). These models are considerably weakened by the evidence that fragments of tectum rotated or transplanted to different positions in the tectum of frogs and fish serve as targets for optic axons independently of the surrounding tectum (R. Levine and Jacobson, 1974; M. Jacobson and Levine, 1975b), and that compression of part of the map onto a rotated fragment of the tectum occurs independently of compression of the map to the surrounding part of the tectum of the goldfish (Yoon, 1977). Interactions between optic axons alone are insufficient to explain such results, and interactions between axons and tectal targets must also be invoked. **The final configuration of the retinotectal map may depend on the relative strengths of axon–axon and axon–tectum interactions. If axon–axon interactions are stronger than axon–tectum interactions, a retinal map will form on any part of the tectum that is available—a compressed map will form from a whole retina projecting to a reduced tectum and an expanded map will form from a reduced retina projecting to a whole tectum. By contrast, if axon–tectum interactions are strongest, the retinal axons will connect only with the appropriate tectal positions, and reduction of either retina or tectum will result in a correspondingly reduced retinotectal map. In both cases the possibility of selective death of retinal axons and tectal cells has to be taken into account. And, of course, the anatomical form of the topographical map does not necessarily reflect the functional states of the system.**

The phenomena of compression and expansion of the retinotectal map that occur easily and rapidly in adult goldfish occur very slowly, if at all, in amphibians and in the chick embryo. Removal of part of the tectum and section of the optic nerve in frogs are followed by regeneration of the optic nerve fibers only to the correct positions in the tectum (Straznicky, 1973; Meyer and Sperry, 1973). No compression occurs after removal of the caudal part of the tectum without section of the optic nerve in frogs, but if the optic nerve is cut, compression of the entire retinal projection to the residual half-tectum occurs in 260–414 days in frogs (Udin, 1975, 1976, 1977). Because of the long postoperative interval before any compression of the map is seen, it is unlikely that the compression results from tectal regulation or from interactions between the fibers themselves. Rather, slow reorganization of the retinotectal map in the frog probably involves death of the disconnected retinal ganglion cells whose tectal targets have been removed and their replacement by new retinal and tectal cells. No expansion of the retinotectal projection occurs in the chick embryo after the 3rd day of incubation. Removal of a retinal quadrant after the 3rd day of incubation results in permanent deafferentation of the corresponding area of the tectum (DeLong and Coulombre, 1965; Crossland *et al.*, 1974a).

Another serious limitation of all the experiments in which the retinal projection is mapped electrophysiologically by recording from presynaptic terminals of optic axons is that they do not show whether the regenerated optic nerve fibers form functional synaptic connections in the tectum either at the correct positions or at anomalous positions. Doubts about the formation of functional synaptic connections by optic fibers at anomalous positions in the tectum are increased by a report that, in the rabbit, optic nerve fibers which can be seen sprouting into tectal locations that they do not normally occupy do not activate tectal cells at anomalous positions, but drive tectal neurons only at the normal positions (Chow *et al.*, 1973). In the retinal mapping assay (as used in the goldfish, e.g., by M. Jacobson and Gaze, 1965; Yoon, 1971, 1972a,b; Sharma, 1972a,b), the presynaptic potentials, indicating the positions of optic fibers in the tectum, may originate from a sessile nerve terminal that has arrived at its final position or from one that is moving about; or the presynaptic potentials may come from a fiber that ends in a nonfunctional synapse, or as we usually assume, from a fiber that terminates in a functional synapse at the position at which we record the potentials.

Whatever the final configuration of connec-

tions, we want to know whether it was produced from the beginning or only after a period of trial and error—and, if so, whether malconnections were eliminated by error elimination, error correction, or, error neutralization. To study the kinetics of regrowth of the optic nerve fibers in the tectum will require repeated mapping of the retinotectal projection in the same animal at close intervals during the process of regeneration of the optic nerve or use of methods that allow continuous visualization of optic nerve terminals. To determine whether the regenerated optic nerve fibers have formed functional connections in the tectum will require postsynaptic recording (Skarf and Jacobson, 1974). Tests of visual behavior are of limited value in this regard for a number of reasons: First, there are other visual centers besides the tectum that might mediate the behavior in the absence of functional retinotectal connections. Second, abnormal behavior might occur even if the optic axons form functional synaptic connections in the tectum, either because the sensory map has expanded or contracted and is not congruent with the motor map or because malconnections have been made in other visual centers. Finally, although tests of visual function in fish and amphibians are relatively crude, the presence of visually guided behavior shows that at least some reflex circuits function normally, and a loss of visual function after a tectal lesion, followed by recovery of vision, shows that either the reflex circuits through the tectum have been restored or an alternative reflex pathway has developed. For example, M. Y. Scott (1977) has shown that the blind region produced in the goldfish immediately after removal of the caudal half of the tectum is gradually filled in as the entire retinal projection compresses onto the residual rostral half of the tectum.

Removal of part of a neuronal population during the time of histogenesis of that population may produce results that are difficult to interpret. The difficulty arises because "regulation" of the residual part may involve changes in nerve cell production and cell migration as well as changes in the genesis and expression of neuronal specificity. Therefore, whenever an experiment requires removal of part of a proliferating nerve cell population, adequate control experiments are required to determine the changes that occur in cell production. These controls have often been omitted or have been inadequate in experiments in which retinotectal size disparities have been produced by removing part of the retina and/or tectum in fish and amphibians at stages of development before cell proliferation has ceased. Surgical operations on such cell populations may result in changes in the rate of cell production, in the spatial pattern of cell proliferation, and in the rate and spatial pattern of cell death. Thus, after removal of the nasal or the temporal half of an eye rudiment in the tailbud frog embryo, and replacement with a temporal or nasal half-eye, respectively, double-nasal (NN) or double-temporal (TT) eyes can be constructed—so-called compound eyes

(Gaze *et al.*, 1963, 1965). Similarly, double-ventral (VV) and double-dorsal (DD) compound eyes can be made, but only the former project to the tectum (Straznicky et al., 1974), the DD eyes failing to form an optic nerve. When the projection of the compound eye to the tectum is mapped in the adult frog, each half-eye projects to the entire tectum (Fig. 11.24). When the optic nerve from a compound eye is cut and allowed to regenerate, each half again projects to the entire contralateral tectum. If the compound eye is made to project to the ipsilateral tectum which also carries the projection from the

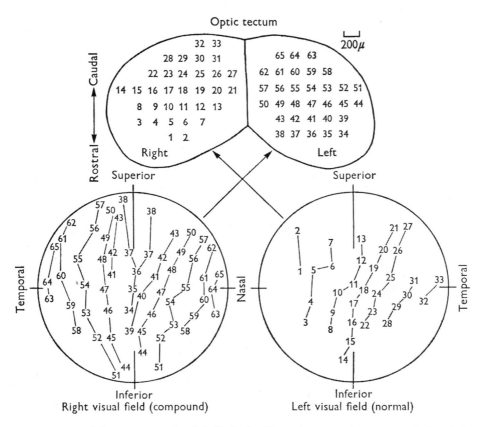

Figure 11.24. Expansion of the projection of each half of a double-nasal compound eye to occupy the whole tectum in *Xenopus*. A double-nasal compound eye is made at embryonic Stage 32 before retinal axons reach the tectum. The temporal half of the right eye is removed and replaced with the nasal half of a left eye (thus preserving the dorsoventral relationships). After metamorphosis the visuotectal projection from the double-nasal eye to the left tectum is mapped electrophysiologically. The normal projection from the left eye to the right tectum is also shown. Each number on the tectum represents an electrode position at which an optimal response was evoked when the stimulus was at the position (two positions in the case of the compound eye) indicated by the same number in the visual field. Because of the camera inversion of the visual field on the retina the superior field corresponds to ventral retina, nasal field to temporal retina, etc. The normal left eye projects across the whole of the right tectum. Each half of the double-nasal right eye spreads its projection across the whole of the left tectum (in an order appropriate to the nature of the half-retinas making up the compound eye). From R. M. Gaze, M. Jacobson, and G. Székely, *J. Physiol.* **165**:484–499 (1963).

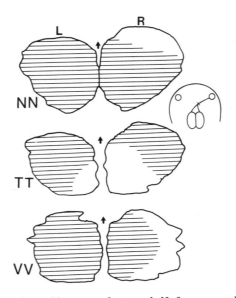

Figure 11.25. Evidence that the set of retinal locus specificities in half of a compound eye is the same as the set present in half of a normal eye. Double-nasal (NN), double-temporal (TT), and double-ventral (VV) compound eyes were made in *Xenopus* embryos after metamorphosis. The optic nerve was cut and allowed to regenerate to both sides of the tectum. The projection of the compound eye to the tectum was mapped autoradiographically after injection of [³H]proline into the compound eye. NN and VV compound eyes innervated the entire contralateral tectum. The TT compound eye innervated the entire contralateral tectum except for the caudomedial part, which is normally innervated by the nasal–ventral retinal quadrant. The projection of the compound retina to the ipsilateral (right) tectum competed with the normal projection from the left eye, and was in each case confined to the part of the tectum normally occupied by that half of the retina: NN projection was confined to caudal tectum; TT retina was confined to rostral tectum; VV retina was confined to medial tectum. The arrows are in the midline pointing rostrally. From R. M. Gaze and C. Straznicky, *J. Embryol. Exp. Morph.* **60:**125-140 (1980).

normal eye, each half of the compound eye projects only to the part of the tectum with which it normally connects, as shown in Fig. 11.25 (Gaze and Straznicky, 1980). These results indicate that each half-retina expresses the specific properties normally present in that half in a complete eye.

J. D. Feldman and Gaze (1972) reported that the pattern of histogenesis is not altered in compound eyes, but their observations were limited to embryonic and early larval stages. Studies of histogenesis of the retina from the embryo to the adult show that the pattern of retinal histogenesis of normal and compound eyes is markedly asymmetrical (M. Jacobson, 1976a; D. H. Beach and Jacobson, 1978a–c; Straznicky and Tay, 1978). In the compound eye, the pattern of histogenesis in each half-retina conforms to the pattern of that half in the intact eye (D. H. Beach and Jacobson, 1978a; Straznicky and Tay, 1977). Although the rates of retinal cell production and death and the final total number of ganglion cells in the compound eye have

not been measured, rough estimates suggest that they are within the normal limits.

Postsynaptic recording from tectal cells that are visually driven from both eyes assays the specificity of functional retinotectal synaptic connections. If two neurons with different locations of their cell bodies and different presynaptic trajectories converge to form synaptic connections on the same postsynaptic element, the presynaptic neurons must share the same specificity as regards the selection of a specific synaptic locus. The normal development of such converging inputs is in itself evidence of a shared specificity, but the evidence of a common specificity is much more compelling if the convergence onto a specific target occurs experimentally, for example, after eye rotation and optic nerve regeneration (Skarf and Jacobson, 1974) or after growth of both optic nerves into the same tectum.

Because there is no absolute measure of the specific properties of the elements that compose a neuronal set—the set of ganglion cells in the retina, for example—we are compelled to use some form of comparative or relative measure. The retinotectal map, for example, gives only a relative measure of some parameters within a set and permits us to map the relative order of elements within the set, but provides no information about the identity of individual elements. Inversions or translocations may be detected directly, but deletions or additions that do not alter the relative order of the elements in the map can be detected only by comparing the unknown set directly with a neuron set of known composition. Thus we lose information about the completeness of the set of nerve fibers projecting from the retina to the tectum because there is nothing in the tectum to compare with an unknown set of optic nerve fibers. One method of avoiding this theoretical impasse is to project two sets of optic nerve fibers into the same tectum, one from a test eye and another from a normal or reference eye grafted into the same socket. However, this strategy is foiled by the tendency of the optic nerve fibers to segregate into eye-specific domains in the tectum (see Section 11.14).

Sperry (1945b) showed that vision recovered in frogs after he uncrossed the optic nerves, thus demonstrating that the set of tectal locus specificities on left and right sides are equivalent but mirror-imaged across the midline. More recently, M. Jacobson and Hirsch (1973) found that removal of one eye in frog tadpoles frequently results in formation of complete retinotectal maps to both sides of the tectum, apparently as a result of branching of the optic axons at the chiasm.

The way in which the optic nerve fibers from two eyes mingle in the same tectum may provide a measure of their shared locus specificities, while the regions of tectum in which the two sets of optic fibers do not mingle may show which specificities are not common to both sets (M. Jacobson, 1973; M. Jacobson and Hunt, 1973; R. K. Hunt and Jacobson, 1974c). This can be done either by grafting an additional eye into the same socket as a normal eye in the frog embryo so that both sets of optic nerve fibers grow into the tectum at the same time or, alternatively, by deflecting one optic nerve at the chiasm so that both eyes innervate the tectum on the same side. Removal of the tectum on one side often results in projection of both eyes to the remaining tectum in adult goldfish (Sharma, 1972a,d). The surprising result is that the retinal fibers from

the two eyes sort themselves out into alternating stripes or patches in the shared optic tectum (R. Levine and Jacobson, 1975; Law and Constantine-Paton, 1980; Straznicky, 1980). This phenomenon is discussed in the following section.

11.14. Formation of Ocular Dominance Domains in the Tectum

R. Levine and Jacobson (1975) found that that after removal of the tectum on one side in adult goldfish both retinae innervate the remaining tectum. Microelectrode recording as well as autoradiographic tracing of the pathways from retina to tectum shows that when both eyes project directly to the same tectum, their optic nerve fibers form a series of tectal stripes or patches occupied by the retinal axons from one or the other eye, as shown in Fig. 11.26 (R. Levine and Jacobson, 1975). The retinotectal map is complete and orderly and no part of the map is duplicated, but instead of intermingling, the axons from the two eyes segregate into ocular dominance domains. This shows that the orderly deployment of optic axons must be under tectal control, for if it were not so there would be cases of duplication or absence of parts of the map, and those do not occur. Exclusion from parts of the tectum of retinal axons originating from the *normal* eye indicates that interaction and competition between the two sets of retinal axons results in elimination of some axons from the normal set. This was the first good evidence of competition between retinal axons for tectal space.

Development of ocular dominance domains in doubly innervated tectum has been confirmed in goldfish (Lo and Levine, 1980; R. L. Meyer, 1983), frogs (Constantine-Paton and Law, 1978; Law and Constantine-Paton, 1980; Straznicky *et al.*, 1980), and chicks (Fawcett and Cowan, 1985). The optic axons from the two halves of a compound eye may also segregate into different domains in the same tectum in *Xenopus* (Fawcett and Willshaw, 1982; Ide *et al.*, 1983). The formation of tectal ocular dominance domains can be prevented by blockade of electrical activity in the retinal axons with tetrodotoxin injected into one eye in the frog and goldfish (R. L. Meyer, 1982; Boss and Schmidt, 1984; Reh and Constantine-Paton, 1985). The role of impulse traffic in refinement of the retinotectal map is dis-

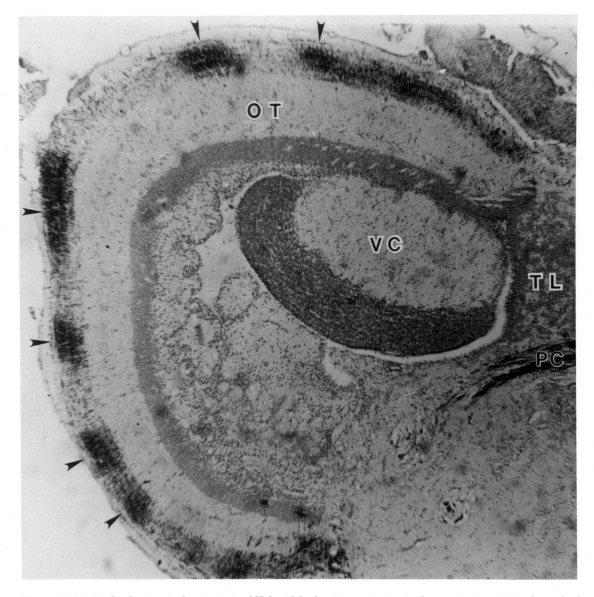

Figure 11.26. Ocular dominance domains in a goldfish with both retinae projecting to the same tectum. Autoradiograph of a coronal section through the right tectum after injection of [³H]proline into the right eye 3 days earlier. The left tectum had been removed 113 days before the fish was fixed. Each retina projects exclusively to alternating patches or stripes of the optic tectum (arrowheads). OT = optic tectum; PC = posterior commissure; TL = torus longitudinalis; VC = valvulae cerebellae. From R. L. Levine and M. Jacobson, *Brain Res.* 98:172–176 (1975), copyright Elsevier Scientific Publishing Company, Amsterdam.

cussed in the next section. However, the problem posed by the ocular dominance domains in fish and frogs is why the optic fibers mingle initially and later segregate into separate tectal domains. How can this be regulated by impulse traffic in the optic axons?

Mathematical models to account for development of ocular dominance domains have been formulated (von der Malsburg and Willshaw, 1976; K. D. Miller *et al.*, 1989).

The questions raised by these findings are: "For

what do the optic axons compete and why do they segregate into stripes or patches?" The interactions may be both *cooperative* (e.g., synchronous or correlated firing; synchronous release of a trophic factor) and *competitive* (e.g., competition for space on the dendrites of tectal neurons; competition for a trophic factor released by tectal cells). In theory, correlated firing of a group of axons coming from the same retinal region will have a greater effect on the postsynaptic neuron than firing of individual axons. The effect may be either to repress or to promote production of postsynaptic trophic factors. If such a factor exerted its effect by release from postsynaptic cells, followed by diffusion and uptake by retinal axons, the arrangement of sources and sinks could lead to a periodic pattern of concentrations of the trophic factor. The precise pattern of the periodicity (stripes or patches) could also depend on the geometries of the arbors of retinal axonal terminals and dendritic trees of tectal neurons.

There is a fairly strict segregation of dendritic trees of tectal neurons in neighboring ocular dominance stripes in three-eyed frogs (Katz and Constantine-Paton, 1988). A similar sharp restriction of dendritic trees occurs at the borders of ocular dominance columns in the monkey striate cortex (Katz *et al.*, 1989). It seems as if the dendrites retract or grow a certain length so as to maximize or optimize the amount of correlated synaptic input they receive from one eye. This evidence suggests that dendritic morphology can be altered as a result of local interactions between presynaptic terminals and dendrites.

11.15. Role of Nerve Activity in Development of the Retinotectal Projection

Blockade of action potentials with tetrodotoxin (TTX) does not prevent formation of the retinotectal projection in zebrafish embryos (Stuermer, 1988d), goldfish (Cook and Becker, 1988), salamanders (W. A. Harris, 1980), and *Xenopus* embryos (W. A. Harris, 1984). Those observations show that action potentials do not play an essential part in the outgrowth of optic axons, their choice of pathways and their selection of positions at which to terminate in the tectum.

In goldfish with retinotectal size disparities

treated with TTX , expansion or compression of the retinotectal map occurs as in untreated animals (Meyer and Wolcott, 1984).

TTX prevents or diminishes naturally occurring retinal ganglion cell death in the rat (Fawcett and O'Leary, 1985; O'Leary *et al.*, 1986). Because retinal ganglion cell death is one means of refining the retinotectal and retinogeniculate maps (O'Leary *et al.*, 1986), treatment with TTX might be expected to interfere with elimination of misrouted axons. However, recovery of the gross topography of the retinotectal projection after optic nerve regeneration in goldfish treated with TTX is as good as recovery of the topography in untreated controls (Meyer, 1982, 1983; Schmidt and Edwards, 1983; Schmidt, 1985; Stuermer, 1989). However, regenerated optic axons make transient but functional connections in the wrong positions in the tectum before becoming reorganized into refined retinotopic order, and this refinement is not affected by blocking action potentials with TTX (Stuermer, 1989). Some other aspects of refinement of the retinotectal projection, such as reduction in size of retinal receptive fields, are prevented by blocking nerve activity with intraocularly injected TTX (Meyer, 1983; Schmidt and Edwards, 1983; J. E. Cook and Becker, 1988) or by imposing an abnormal pattern of activity with stroboscopic light stimulation (Schmidt and Eisele, 1983; J. E. Cook and Rankin, 1986; J. E. Cook, 1987, 1988; J. E. Cook and Becker, 1988).

TTX blockade of action potentials in retinal ganglion cells does prevent the segregation of left and right retinal nerve fibers in an optic tectum doubly innervated by both eyes in the goldfish (Boss and Schmidt, 1984), frog (Constantine-Paton, 1982), and chick (Fawcett and Cowan, 1985). This is discussed in Section 11.14 (see Section 11.18 for the analogous effect on segregation of retinal fibers from left and right eye in the mammalian lateral geniculate nucleus). Because segregation of retinal axons occurs in the dark, it must be based on spontaneous discharge of retinal ganglion cells. This indicates that there is a greater correlation of discharge of different ganglion cells in the same retina than between ganglion cells belonging to different eyes. The effect of blocking impulses is, therefore, more marked in preventing segregation of left and right retinal axons in the tectum than in affecting the order of retinal axons projecting from one eye to the tectum.

11.16. Formation of Binocular Retinotectal Maps

In vertebrates with overlapping visual fields there are corresponding points on the two retinae which receive light stimulation from the same point in the binocular visual field. The projections from corresponding retinal positions both converge to one position on the ipsilateral tectum and both converge to another position on the contralateral tectum. Thus, when a frog looks at an object in the binocular visual field, nerve impulses in both eyes traverse separate pathways which converge onto binocularly driven tectal neurons (Gaze and Jacobson, 1962, 1963a; Fite, 1969; Keating and Gaze, 1970b; Skarf, 1973; Skarf and Jacobson, 1974). The contralateral retinotectal map starts developing at about embryonic Stage 46 in *Xenopus* (Gaze *et al.*, 1974), whereas the ipsilateral retinotectal map starts developing during metamorphosis (Beazley *et al.*, 1972). The contralateral map can form in the absence of visual stimulation and the initial formation of the ipsilateral map can occur in the absence of visual input (Keating and Kennard, 1987). Binocular visual experience is required for bringing the ipsilateral and contralateral maps into correspondence in *Xenopus* (Keating and Feldman, 1975) but not in the frog, *R. pipiens* (M. Jacobson and Hirsch, 1973; Skarf and Jacobson, 1974).

The binocular retinotectal projection is relayed to the contralateral tectum (or superior colliculus in mammals) via a midbrain nucleus known as the nucleus isthmi in amphibians (Grobstein *et al.*, 1978; Gruberg and Udin, 1978), the nucleus isthmi pars parvocellularis in birds (S. P. Hunt and Künzle, 1976) and the parabigeminal nucleus in mammals (Graybiel, 1978; Sherk, 1978). Retinotopic order is preserved in the projections to and from these nuclei. The retinotectal and isthmotectal pathways for binocular vision are as follows: The retina projects to the contralateral optic tectum, which then projects to the nucleus isthmi on the same side. The nucleus isthmi then sends a projection back to the tectum on the same side in frogs, birds, and mammals and a crossed projection to the contralateral tectum (in frogs and mammals but not birds). The crossed isthmotectal axons cross in the dorsal posterior part of the optic chiasm and then run with the retinotectal axons in the optic tract.

The uncrossed isthmotectal projection develops in the absence of visual stimulation and even after removal of both eyes in frogs (Constantine-Paton and Ferrari-Eastman, 1981) and birds (O'Leary and Cowan, 1983). Retinotectal axons and isthmotectal axons both project to the superficial layers of the tectum (Gruberg and Udin, 1978; Gruberg *et al.*, 1989). Electron microscopic evidence shows that the isthmotectal and retinotectal axons both synapse on tectal cell dendrites (Székely and Lazar, 1976; Udin and Fisher, 1986; Udin *et al.*, 1990). Therefore, it is most likely that interactions between isthmotectal axons and retinotectal axons are mediated by tectal cell dendrites. It may be significant that retinotectal axons probably release glutamate whereas isthmotectal axons probably are cholinergic (Roberts and Yates, 1976; Ricciuti and Gruberg, 1985; Desan *et al.*, 1987; Scherer and Udin, 1989).

The crossed isthmotectal projection develops in frogs (*Rana*) with one eye rotated: although corresponding retinal points receive different patterns of visual stimulation, they still project to the same position in the binocular retinotectal map and no compensation occurs (Skarf, 1973; M. Jacobson and Hirsch, 1973; Skarf and Jacobson, 1974; Beazley, 1979; Kennard and Keating, 1985). However, in the frog, *R. pipiens*, reared through metamorphosis with one eye occluded with a skin graft which permits light but not pattern stimulation of the retina, the binocularly driven tectal units have much larger receptive fields than normal (M. Jacobson and Hirsch, 1973). This effect may be due to functional competition between the eyes, perhaps analogous to the effect in mammals after monocular visual deprivation.

The effect of eye rotation on the isthmotectal projections is quite different in *Xenopus* than in *Rana*. In *Xenopus* the isthmotectal maps undergo reorientation to compensate for the disparity between the two eyes, as shown in Fig. 11.27 (Keating, 1968, 1974; Gaze *et al.*, 1970b). The reorientation requires visual stimulation as it does not occur in *Xenopus* reared in the dark (Keating and Feldman, 1975). Reorientation of the isthmotectal map is prevented by chronic application of NMDA antagonists to the tectum in *Xenopus* shortly after metamorphosis (Scherer and Udin, 1989).

Tracing the isthmotectal axons with HRP in *Xenopus* with one eye rotated shows that the axons take abnormal pathways to reorient the isthmotectal map (Udin and Keating, 1981; Udin, 1983). After rotation of an eye in *Xenopus* tadpoles, compensa-

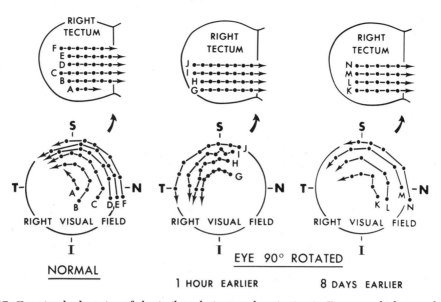

Figure 11.27. Functional adaptation of the ipsilateral visuotectal projection in *Xenopus*, which is mediated through isthmotectal connections. Shown are the normal ipsilateral visuotectal map in a young frog (left diagram), the map made immediately after 90° anticlockwise rotation of the right eye at Stage 63 (middle diagram), and the map 8 days postoperative (right diagram). From M. J. Keating, *Proc. Roy. Soc. (London) B Ser.* 189:603–610 (1975).

tion or reorientation occurs either in the direct ipsilateral retinothalamic projection (Kennard, 1981) or in the direct contralateral retinotectal projection (M. Jacobson, 1968a). Visual behavior continues to be maladaptive in *Xenopus* with an inverted eye in spite of reorientation of the isthmotectal projection, showing that the motor output does not undergo compensation. Observations of the visuomotor behavior of amphibians in which one eye has been inverted have established that these animals consistently misdirect their motor responses to visual stimuli, and that this maladaptive behavior is never corrected by visual experience (Sperry, 1943, 1944; Stone, 1953). The purpose of reorientation of the isthmotectal projection is not to compensate for the surgical inversion of an eye but may be an adaptation to changes of position of the eyes during normal growth of the head.

A brief digression to consider the effects of visual experience on development of the visual system of birds is required here. Like mammals, birds have separate mesencephalic and telencephalic visual projections. The tectofugal projections are strictly homologous, meaning that they evolved from a common ancestral form, in all vertebrates. It is debatable whether thalamotelencephalic projections are strictly homologous in birds and mammals. More-

over, there are considerable variations in the relative importance of these two visual projections between different species of birds depending, among other factors, on the extent of binocularity. In birds the thalamotelencephalic visual projection terminates in the visual *wulst*, a cortical structure (Pettigrew and Konishi, 1976; Watanabe *et al.*, 1983). Another visual projection extends from retina to optic tectum, nucleus rotundus, and ectostriatum, the telencephalic visual end-station of the tectofugal pathway (Benowitz and Karten, 1976). There are also direct connections between the optic tectum and visual *wulst* (Bagnoli *et al.*, 1980). Monocular visual deprivation of newly hatched birds results in changes in the visual *wulst* (Pettigrew and Konishi, 1976; Bagnoli *et al.*, 1983, 1983; Burkhalter, 1982), in the nucleus rotundus (Nixdorf and Bischof, 1987), and in the ectostriatum (Herrmann and Bischof, 1988).

11.17. Development of the Mammalian Visual System

The retina projects to several visual centers in mammals, but there are considerable variations in the number of retinal fibers going to the different brain structures in different classes of mammals (reviewed by Rodieck, 1979; Stone *et al.*, 1979; Lennie, 1980). The largest retinal projection goes to the dorsal lateral geniculate nucleus (LGNd); a large projection terminates in the superior colliculus; and there are smaller projections to the pretectal nuclei, the ventral lateral geniculate nucleus, the suprachiasmatic nucleus, and to cell groups in the tegmentum. There are reciprocal projections between the superior colliculus and visual cortex and between the LGNd and visual cortex. In addition to the striate visual cortex (area 17) and the adjacent area 18, there are other cortical representations of the visual field. Areas 17 and 18 have two main extrastriate targets in the cat: area 19 and a large region of suprasylvian cortex. For details of the functional organization of the mammalian visual system the reader may refer to recent reviews (J. S. Lund, 1988; Casagrande and Norton, 1991; Stein and Meredith, 1991). The effects of visual deprivation on the functional organization of the visual system have been reviewed by Sherman and Spear (1982) and by Wiesel (1988).

Any discussion of the development of the **mammalian visual system has to take into account the fact that there are three main types of retinal ganglion cells, named alpha, beta, and gamma on the basis of morphological differences, and Y, X, and W on the basis of functional differences.** They have different sizes, different dendritic tree branching patterns and dimensions, different distributions in the retina, different behavior in decussating at the chiasm and also in selecting targets in the visual centers (Boycott and Wässle, 1974; Rodieck, 1979, 1988; Stone *et al.*, 1979; Lennie, 1980; Stone, 1983). These form the anatomical basis for the physiological classification of three functional classes of retinal ganglion cells: Y, X, and W (reviewed by Levick and Thibos, 1983; Stone, 1983, Sherman, 1985). These three types of ganglion cells have been most thoroughly studied in the cat (Levick and Thibos, 1983; Sur *et al.*, 1984, 1987; Dann *et al.*, 1988), but similar classes of cells have been found in the monkey (Leventhal, 1981; Perry *et al.*, 1984) and they probably occur in most, if not all, mammals. The following description of these ganglion cell types reflects the nomenclature and results commonly accepted in the cat.

The alpha cells (functional Y cells) have the largest cell body (about 30 μm), large dendritic fields, larger in the retinal periphery, and the great-

est-caliber axons. They project to the largest cells of the A laminae of the LGNd, to the medial interlaminar nucleus, and to the superior colliculus (Kelly and Gilbert, 1975; Illing and Wässle, 1981; Wässle *et al.*, 1981c; Leventhal, 1982). Alpha cells can be specifically stained with a monoclonal antibody (Hockfield *et al.*, 1985; Sur *et al.*, 1988; Hockfield and Sur, 1990). Beta cells (which include most functional X cells) have medium-sized cell bodies (about 20 μm), compact dendritic fields, and medium-caliber axons. They project mainly to the smaller cells of the A layers of the cat's LGNd (Rodieck, 1979; Wässle *et al.*, 1981a; Leventhal, 1982). Gamma retinal ganglion cells (which include most functional W cells) have small to medium cell bodies, large dendritic fields, and fine-caliber axons. They project to the superior colliculus and pretectum. A small proportion also project to the C layers of the cats' LGNd (Leventhal, 1982). The dendritic fields of alpha and beta ganglion cells, but not gamma cells, increase in size with increasing distance from the fovea. Analogous classes of ganglion cells have been found in primates (Leventhal *et al.*, 1981; Perry *et al.*, 1984). Finally, the different ganglion cell types in all species studied have different retinal distributions as well as different functions.

These three classes of ganglion cells can be recognized at birth in cats (Maslim *et al.*, 1986; Dann *et al.*, 1988; Ramoa *et al.*, 1988) and monkeys (Leventhal *et al.*, 1989). During postnatal development of the cat, these ganglion cells undergo considerable morphological changes in dendritic axonal branching patterns (Fig. 11.28). Dendrites of alpha cells continue to grow until 3 weeks postnatally, whereas beta-cell dendritic growth occurs mainly after 3 weeks of age, as shown by intracellular injection of Lucifer yellow (Dann *et al.*, 1988). Axonal terminals of alpha (Y) cells and beta (X) cells behave differently during postnatal development of the cat. Axonal terminal arborizations of X cells grow profusely and are subsequently retracted, whereas axon terminal arborizations of Y cells grow steadily to reach their mature form without retraction or pruning (Friedlander *et al.*, 1985; Garraghty and Sur, 1988, review).

The functional properties of the three types of ganglion cells can be summarized briefly as follows (reviewed in Hirsch and Leventhal, 1978; Rodieck, 1979; Stone *et al.*, 1979; Lennie, 1980; Sherman and Spear, 1982; Saito, 1983; Stone, 1983): X cells have

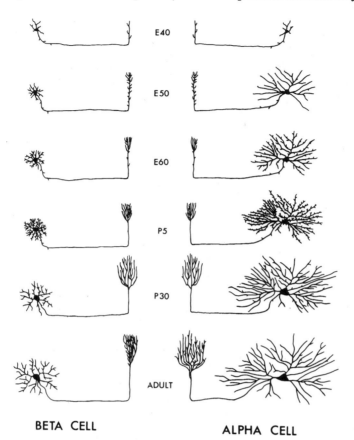

BETA CELL   ALPHA CELL

Figure 11.28. Scheme of stages of morphological development of typical alpha and beta retinal ganglion cells in the cat. The entire cell in the retina, its axon, and its terminals in the LGNd are shown (cells are not to scale; possible collaterals to the midbrain are omitted). This figure illustrates: (1) development of cell class-specific dendritic morphology occurs weeks before the development of morphological differences between their axonal terminal arbors; (2) the period of remodeling of ganglion cells in the retina (E60–P30) differs from the period of remodeling of their axon terminals in the LGNd (E40–E60, and P30– adult). Data from C. A. Mason (1982), Bowling and Michael (1984), Sur *et al.* (1984), Stretavan and Shatz (1986). From A. S. Ramoa, G. Campbell, and C. J. Shatz, *J. Neurosci.* 8:4239–4261 (1988). Copyright Society for Neuroscience.

axons with moderately fast conduction (20–25 m/second); they have a high rate of maintained discharge, have small receptive fields, sum the excitation of different parts of their receptive field linearly, and respond best to slowly moving stimuli. Y cells have the most rapidly conducting (35–45 m/second) axons; they have a low rate of maintained discharge, have large receptive fields, have a transient response to stimulation, sum excitation in different regions of the receptive field nonlinearly, and respond to a wider range of stimulus velocities. W cells have axons with the slowest conduction velocity (3–15 m/second); some of them lack the antagonistic center-surround organization found in other gan-

glion cells and they have large receptive fields. W cells are heterogeneous: tonic W cells have sustained discharges, while phasic W cells have transient discharges in response to appropriate stimulation; some are selectively sensitive to stimuli moving in a particular direction or orientation; others respond best to edges; and yet others are suppressed by stimulus contrast.

The neurons in the LGNd that receive direct inputs from X, Y, and W ganglion cells have response characteristics similar to those of the homonymous retinal ganglion cells. The response properties of the cells in the visual cortex also, in many respects, reflect the characteristics of their afferents from the LGNd (Hoffmann and Stone, 1971; J. Stone and Dreher, 1973; W. Singer *et al.*, 1975; J. R. Wilson and Sherman, 1976; Dreher *et al.*, 1980).

It has been shown that the W, X, and Y retinal ganglion cells behave differently in their tendency to cross at the optic chiasm (Fukuda and Stone, 1974; J. Stone and Fukuda, 1974a,b). X cells project to both sides of the brain; those on the nasal side of the vertical median project contralaterally, while those on the temporal side of the retinal vertical meridian project ipsilaterally. The region of nasotemporal overlap for X cells is only 300–400 μm wide. Y cells also project into both sides, but the region of nasotemporal overlap is 1.0–2.0 mm wide. However, about 5 percent of Y cells in the temporal retina project contralaterally. Finally, W cells as a group do not exhibit a sharp nasotemporal division. Most phasic W cells throughout the retina project contralaterally, while most tonic W cells in the temporal retina project ipsilaterally.

Evidence is provided in Section 11.20 showing that the different classes of retinal ganglion cells and the cells to which they project are affected differently by visual stimulation during development (Sherman and Spear, 1982, review; Sur *et al.*, 1982, 1985; Garraghty *et al.*, 1986a,b, 1987, 1989). The development of Y cells and their central projections appears to be more sensitive to visual stimulation during a critical period shortly after birth, while the development of X and W cells and their projections appears to be less sensitive (for reviews see Movshon and Von Sluyters, 1981; Sherman and Spear, 1982).

11.18. Development of Retinogeniculate Projections

The LGNd of the mammalian thalamus receives a retinotopically arranged projection from the retinal ganglion cells. In mammals with binocular vision the overwhelming majority of cells in the nasal part of each retina projects to the contralateral LGNd, while most optic nerve fibers from the temporal (binocular) part of the retina project to the same side of the brain. In mature animals the crossed and uncrossed retinal axons from the two eyes are completely segregated in different layers of the LGNd (Rodieck, 1979; Casagrande and Norton, 1991, review). In the cat

the LGNd has five cellular layers (A, A1, C, C1, and C2; Guillery, 1969). Contralateral optic axons terminate in layers A, C, and C2 whereas ipsilateral optic axons terminate in layer A1 and C1. In the higher primates the LGNd has six layers in which contralateral optic axons terminate in layers 1, 4 and 6 and ipsilateral optic axons end in layers 2, 3, and 5.

Although the projections of left and right eyes are segregated in adults, intermingling between branches of retinal axons from the two eyes in the visual centers has been reported as a transient phase of normal development in a wide variety of mammals: Australian marsupials (Wye-Dvorak, 1984; Coleman and Beazely, 1989; Harman and Beazely, 1989), opossum (Sanderson, 1982), mouse (Godement *et al.*, 1984), rat (Bunt *et al.*, 1983), hamster (Frost and Schneider, 1976, 1979; So *et al.*, 1978, 1984), cat (Williams and Chalupa, 1982; Shatz, 1983; Shatz and Stretavan, 1986), ferret (Linden *et al.*, 1981), and monkey (Rakic, 1976, 1977b, 1986, review).

During development there is an overproduction of retinal ganglion cells and, in fact, most retinal ganglion cells die prior to maturity, as we have discussed in Section 8.3. Segregation of optic axons from the two eyes appears to be one, but clearly not the only, function of retinal ganglion cell death. Specifically, the number of ganglion cells and optic axons is several times more during development than in adults, yet removal of one eye in the fetus results in saving of only 35 percent of ganglion cells in monkeys (Rakic and Riley, 1983). No saving at all has been reported in the wallaby (Coleman and Beazely, 1989) which has an extensive binocular visual field, or rat (Sefton and Lam, 1984; Crespo *et al.*, 1985), which has little binocular overlap. This shows that cell death in the developing retina is not strictly related to the amount of binocularity. In the cat, the period of ganglion cell death occurs between E47 and birth, and there is an eightfold decrease in the number of cells in the ganglion cell layer (Stone *et al.*, 1982). Segregation of retinal axons terminals in the LGNd also occurs from E47 to birth (Sretavan and Shatz, 1986). In the monkey, elimination of more than 500,000 optic nerve fibers occurs well after completion of segregation of their terminals in the LGNd (Rakic and Riley, 1983a,b; Rakic, 1986), as shown in Figure 11.29.

Tracing the retinogeniculate axons by means of

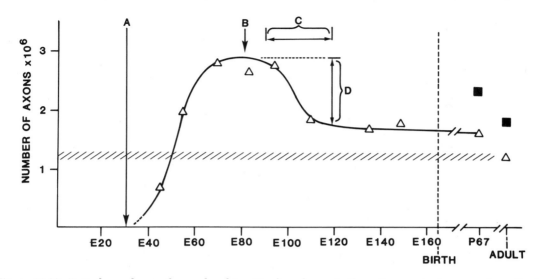

Figure 11.29. Retinal axon loss in the monkey fetus. Number of axons in the optic nerve in rhesus monkeys of various embryonic (E) and postnatal (P) ages. The thick striped line indicates the number of optic axons in adult monkeys. Arrow A points to the fetal age when, according to [³H]thymidine autoradiographic analysis, the genesis of retinal ganglion cells begins; arrow B indicates when it stops. Line C denotes the period when retinal input from the two eyes becomes segregated in the LGNd, which coincides with the period when more than 1 million optic axons are eliminated (vector D). The black squares indicate the number of optic axons in postnatal animals that had one eye removed around the 65th day of gestation. Adapted from P. Rakic and R. P. Riley, *Nature* 305:135–137 (1983).

radioactive tracers injected into one eye of the rhesus monkey fetus during midgestation results in diffuse labeling throughout both LGNd's (Rakic, 1976). Segregation of the fibers originating from left and right eyes occurs during the third quarter of gestation (E90–E120) in the rhesus monkey (Rakic, 1977b). Optic axon segregation occurs after completion of histogenesis of LGNd neurons, which takes place from E30 to E80 in the rhesus monkey.

Injection of HRP or radioactive amino acids into one eye of the cat fetus, resulting in anterograde labeling of optic axons, shows that retinal axons arrive at the LGNd before E32, early in its histogenesis, before any layers form in the LGNd (Shatz, 1983). Neurons originate and migrate into the LGNd until E46. The retinal axons segregate into layers in the LGNd from about E46 to E60. By E60, 5 days before birth, LGNd layering is like that of the adult cat. The distribution of optic axons in different layers of the LGNd during prenatal development in the cat has been studied by Sretavan and Shatz (1986), after injection of different labels into the two eyes (Fig. 11.30). From E40 to E46 the axon terminals from the contralateral eye are the sole occupants of the innermost layers of the LGNd but

the outermost layer is shared by axon terminal branches from both eyes. The intermingling of axon terminal branches diminishes over the following 3 weeks of fetal development. The fibers from the two eyes segregate totally before birth, with the contralateral fibers ending in layers A, C, and C2 and the ipsilateral fibers in layers A1 and C1.

The shapes of terminal arbors of single optic axons can be visualized by labeling the axons in the optic tract with HRP in a fetal LGNd maintained *in vitro* (Sretavan and Shatz, 1986). Those experiments show that during the period of segregation (E46–E53) numerous lateral axonal branches from both eyes mingle in the same layer but the lateral branches are eliminated by the time of birth (E65). At that time the axons of each eye terminate by branches restricted to a small region of one layer of the LGNd. Many geniculate neurons are functionally driven by both eyes during the period of overlap of the projections from the two eyes (Shatz and Kirkwood, 1984), as discussed later.

The retinogeniculate axons of both eyes form synaptic junctions with LGNd neurons during the process of segregation into separate layers and therefore interactions are possible at the postsynap-

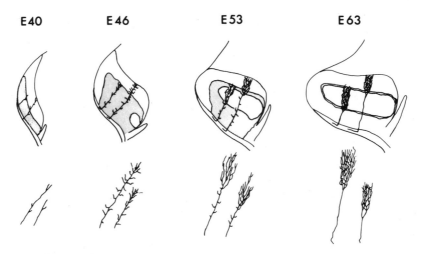

Figure 11.30. Segregation of afferents from the two eyes during development of the retinogeniculate projection in the cat fetus. The zone of intermingling (stippled) of retinogeniculate axon terminals in different layers of the LGNd diminishes from prenatal days 40 to 63 (E40–E63). Representative axon terminal arborizations from the ipsilateral retina (shorter axon in each case) and contralateral retina are shown. From D. W. Sretavan and C. J. Shatz, *J. Neurosci.* 6:234–251 (1986), copyright Society for Neuroscience.

tic cells of the LGNd. Synapses from retinal ganglion cell axons form on LGNd neurons in inappropriate layers during the fetal period of intermingling of retinogeniculate axons but are eliminated during segregation of the axons into layers in the cat (Shatz *et al.*, 1982; Campbell *et al.*, 1984; Campbell and Shatz, 1986). These anomalous synapses are functional, as shown by the finding that during the period of axonal intermingling about 90 percent of LGNd neurons studied electrophysiologically could be activated by inputs from both eyes, whereas in the adult the majority of LGNd neurons in the cat receive excitatory input from one eye only (Bowling and Michael, 1980; Sur and Sherman, 1982; Shatz and Kirkwood, 1984).

Retinal ganglion cell death and loss of optic axons projecting to the LGNd overlaps with the period of eye-specific segregation of optic axons in the LGNd of the cat (Williams *et al.*, 1983; Chalupa and Williams, 1984; Chalupa *et al.*, 1985) and monkey (Rakic and Riley, 1983a,b). This indicates that optic axon segregation occurs as a result of loss of entire retinal ganglion cells and not merely as the result of retraction of axonal branches. There is good evidence that retinal ganglion cell death is caused by competition between optic axons of the two eyes at their terminals in the LGNd. Firstly, removal of one eye before the period of optic axon

segregation results in about 30 percent reduction of retinal ganglion cell death in the monkey (Rakic and Riley, 1983b) and about 20 percent reduction in the cat (Williams *et al.*, 1983; Chalupa *et al.*, 1984) and 19 percent in the hamster (Sengelaud *et al.*, 1983). The possible significance of these differences is discussed later and in Section 8.3. Secondly, removal of one eye of the monkey fetus at E65 results in failure of segregation and expansion of terminals of the other eye in the LGNd and superior colliculus in a variety of different mammals (Chow *et al.*, 1973; Lund *et al.*, 1973; Frost and Schneider, 1976; Rakic, 1981, 1986; Godemont *et al.*, 1984; Jeffery, 1984; Jen *et al.*, 1984; So *et al.*, 1984; Woo *et al.*, 1982; Coleman and Beazely, 1989a). Thirdly, evidence showing that nerve activity is required for segregation of optic axons in different LGNd layers is summarized later.

Synapse elimination and segregation of anomalous connections in the cat LGNd require nerve impulses, as is shown by the fact that those changes do not occur in cat fetuses chronically infused with TTX (Shatz and Stryker, 1986). The nerve activity required for refinement of the retinogeniculate projection must be spontaneous since it occurs *in utero*, and starts before retinal receptors are fully developed and could not be due to visual stimulation. Changes in the retinogeniculate projection produced by intraocular injection of TTX in newborn kittens show that action potentials are required for refinement of the projections postnatally (Archer *et al.*, 1982; Dubin *et al.*, 1986). Blockade of retinal ganglion cell discharges during the first 2 postnatal weeks in the cat results in failure of development of binocular segregation of retinogeniculate nerve endings; prevents normal specific projection of on-center and off-center ganglion cells to different geniculate neurons; and also prevents the normal segregation of X and Y ganglion cell axons in the LGNd (Archer *et al.*, 1982). Prevention of binocular segregation of retinogeniculate nerve terminals is maximal when the blockade of retinal ganglion cell discharge occurs during the first 2 weeks after birth and is considerably less when blockade is started at P11–P15 and is absent when blockade starts later than P15 (Archer *et al.*, 1982; Dubin and Stark, 1983). Mastronarde (1983a,b) has shown that spontaneous activity occurs in retinal ganglion cells of the cat and that the discharge of neighboring cells is correlated in the absence of patterned visual stimulation. It is very likely that spontaneous discharge of retinal ganglion cells is necessary for segregation of retinogeniculate nerve endings in separate layers of the LGNd and for segregation of the geniculostriate terminals in ocular dominance bands in the striate cortex (see Section 11.20).

The evidence shows that nerve impulses are required for normal segregation of inputs from the two eyes to different layers of the mammalian LGNd and for subsequent refinement of the retinogeniculate map. The mechanism of the necessary interaction is unknown, but the best theory is that axonal and dendritic branches are supported if they receive correlated synaptic activity from neighboring ganglion cells in the same eye but are eliminated if they receive uncorrelated input from different eyes. Survival or elimination of presynaptic terminals could be dependent on trophic factors produced by postsynaptic cells, whose production or availability is regulated by correlation of nerve activity. But it should be remembered that the retinotopic order of retinogeniculate axons develops initially independently of action potentials in cats (Archer *et al.*, 1982). Interaction between retinogeniculate axons from the two eyes occurs in the binocular segment of the LGNd, but in the monocular segment the axons from one eye may interact and compete with one another for synaptic space or trophic factors. Evidence that this competition may be ganglion cell-class-specific has also been obtained (Leventhal *et al.*, 1988).

11.19. Expression of Neuronal Specificity of Retinal Ganglion Cells in Albino Mammals

Many of the retinal ganglion cells in the temporal retina in albino mammals project their axons across the optic chiasm to the opposite side of the brain, whereas in normal animals those axons do not cross at the chiasm but grow into the same side of the brain, as shown in Fig. 11.31 (Lund, 1965; Guillery, 1969, 1974; Guillery *et al.*, 1984; Leventhal and Creel, 1985). The congenital defect in the routing of optic nerve fibers has been found in all species albino mammals that have been examined but is most marked in species that have an extensive binocular visual field and thus a large percentage of optic axons that do not cross at the chiasm. The exact relation of the albino gene to the defect found in the visual pathways is not known.

In the mink, a number of different mutants that result in deficient retinal pigmentation are also associated with misrouting of optic axons. The more severe the retinal pigment defect, the greater the anomalous visual projection (Sanderson *et al.*, 1974). This shows that the retinal pigment deficiency is in some way related to the misrouting of optic axons. It is tempting to suggest that the pigment epithelium of the retina is the source of the positional information obtained by retinal ganglion cells, a suggestion that appears to be reasonable because the entire neural retina can regenerate from the pigment epithelium in amphibians (R. Levine, 1975) and in the chick embryo (Coulombre and Coulombre, 1965). However, in flecked mice, in which the pigment epithelium consists of unpigmented and normally pigmented patches, the spatial pattern of deficient retinal pigment does not coincide with the abnormal visual projection (Guillery *et al.*, 1973). Therefore, it is most likely that the deficient pigmentation and the abnormal visual pathways result from the same defect rather than that the pathway abnormality is the direct result of the lack of pigment. However, it remains possible that a pigment abnormality at the chiasm is responsible for the ab-

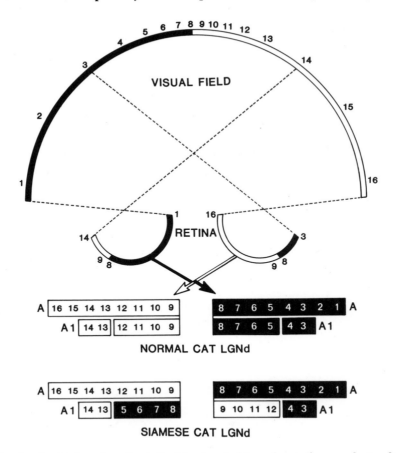

Figure 11.31. Visual projection from the retina to the lateral geniculate nucleus in the normal cat and in the Siamese cat.

normality or is associated with it. In albino rodents an absence of pigment in the developing optic stalk may be a factor resulting in disarrangement of outgrowing retinal axons (Silver and Sapiro, 1981). Siamese cats lack pigmentation in the optic stalk and at the chiasm (Kliot and Schatz, 1985; M. J. Webster *et al.*, 1988).

In normal cats, the nasal part of the retina sends its axons across the chiasm to end in laminae A, C, and C2 of the LGNd on the opposite side of the brain. The temporal part of the retina sends its axons into laminae A1 and C1 of the LGNd on the same side. In the Siamese cat, the nasal retinal fibers cross normally to end in lamina A and apparently also in C1 and C2 (Hickey and Guillery, 1974). However, a segment of temporal retina, representing some part of the first 20° of the ipsilateral projection, projects its axons aberrantly across the chiasm to end in lamina A1, in reversed retinotopic

order. Thus the retinal axons projecting anomalously to the wrong side of the brain of the Siamese cat simply insert themselves into the positions that are left vacant by the nerve fibers that would normally have come from the ipsilateral retina. The resulting projection is as one would expect on the basis of a strict specificity relationship between retinal ganglion cells and LGNd cells (Guillery and Kaas, 1971).

In albino mammals, although the misrouted optic nerve fibers end in the wrong side of the brain, they terminate in the proper part of the LGNd. As this occurs bilaterally, the result is a left-to-right exchange of some optic nerve fibers and a left-to-right reversal of the order of their projection to the LGNd (Guillery and Kaas, 1971), as shown in Fig. 11.31. This shows that there is no error made by the retinal fiber in selection of a terminal locus, and that the locus specificity of the retinal ganglion cells is normal in albinos. The initial abnormality of development is in the selection of the side of the brain into which optic nerve fibers are routed at the optic chiasm, and the anomalous projections to the visual centers probably arise secondarily during development (Kliot and Shatz, 1985). Evidence that the abnormal retinogeniculate projection in albinos is caused by misrouting of optic axons at the chiasm and not caused primarily by albinism is that albinolike visual projections can be produced experimentally in normally pigmented cats (Schall *et al.*, 1988) and ferrets (Guillery, 1989).

In the normal cat many ganglion cells in the temporal retina project to the contralateral LGNd in the embryo, but most of those cells die postnatally. If one eye is removed or if the optic tract is sectioned at birth, those cells persist and form visual projections like those in Boston siamese cats or heterozygous albino cats (Schall *et al.*, 1988). Removal of one eye of the normally pigmented ferret on E29 (gestation = 41 days) results in albino-like retinogeniculate projections whereas this does not occur after postnatal removal of one eye. Nor does any change occur after prenatal removal of one eye of the albino ferret. From these results Guillery (1989) concludes that removal of one eye eliminates binocular competition which is necessary for ipsilateral routing of retinal axons during normal development, and this competition is lacking in albinos.

The projection from the lateral geniculate nucleus to the striate cortex also forms a continuous and orderly map in which the projection from the anomalous geniculate laminae can be dealt with in three different ways (Fig. 11.32). In "midwestern" Siamese cats the anomalous inputs from lamina A1 tend to be suppressed (Kaas and Guillery, 1973; Shatz, 1977) or are relatively small (Cooper and Blasdel, 1980), while in "Boston" Siamese cats (Hubel and Wiesel, 1971; Shatz, 1977; Cooper and Blasdel, 1980) and in heterozygous albino cats (Leventhal *et al.*, 1985b) the input from lamina A1 is reversed and inserted as a separate projection at the border between areas 17 and 18 of the cortex (Fig. 11.32). There is some evidence showing that "Boston" and "midwestern" patterns can both exist in the same animal and this may mean that, rather than two separate types, these patterns represent ends of a continuum (Cooper and Blasdel, 1980). The patterns of geniculostriate projections in Siamese cats are relatively unaffected by postnatal binocular visual deprivation (Hubel and Wiesel, 1971).

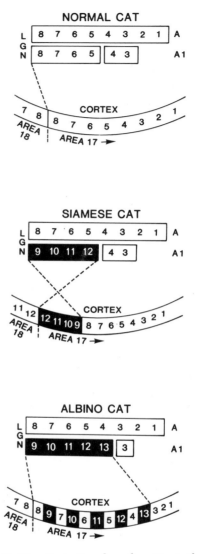

Figure 11.32. Projections from the retina to the LGNd and visual cortex of normal, Siamese, and albino cats.

However, the fact that monocular visual deprivation can unmask the anomalous projection to the cortex from the experienced eye in midwestern Siamese cats shows that the suppression of this projection to the cortex is due to competition between the inputs from the two eyes (Guillery and Casagrande, 1975a,b).

In albino (tyrosinase negative) cats the visual projection anomalies are different from those in Siamese cats, as shown in Fig. 11.32 (Leventhal and Creel, 1985). Less than 5 percent of ganglion cells in the temporal retina project to the ipsilateral LGNd in albino cats, and in the visual cortex (areas 17 and 18) the contralateral and ipsilateral projections are often segregated in alternating bands, representing nasal and temporal retina, respectively, of the same eye in area 17 and are always segregated into bands in area 18 (Leventhal and Creel, 1985). This suggests that nasal–temporal segregation may occur because in albino cats nearly all axons from the temporal retina project contralaterally and thus compete successfully with axons from the nasal retina.

The anomalous retinal projection to the lateral geniculate nucleus shows that misrouted optic axons express their locus specificities in selecting targets in lamina A1 independently of the neighboring normal axons. By contrast, the projection to the cerebral cortex in Boston Siamese cats may reflect a contextual form of mapping, in which interactions between geniculostriate axons themselves as well as between the axons and their postsynaptic targets determine that the order and continuity of the map are re-established at the visual cortex. These anomalous projections illustrate the principle that even a detailed knowledge of the final product gives little insight into the processes of its development. To obtain that insight requires much more information about the intermediate stages of development of the anomalous visual projections as well as information about the corresponding stages of development of the visual system in normal mammals.

Analysis of this anomaly, whether by anatomical tracing of fibers or by electrical recording, is severely limited by inadequate knowledge of the normal mechanisms that control the routes taken by growing axons and of the factors that determine whether optic axons cross or do not cross over at the optic chiasm. In mammals in which some optic axons do not cross at the chiasm, there is a boundary (line of decussation) between the temporal region of the retina, which projects its optic fibers ipsilaterally, and the more nasal retinal region, which projects contralaterally. One can conceive of the anomaly in albinos resulting from a temporal shift in the position of the boundary between ganglion cells that project to the same side and those that project to the opposite side of the brain. The problem is complicated by the fact that the line of decussation for each type of retinal ganglion cell (W, X, Y) is different. Thus, in normal cats, the X cells and the tonic W cells more or less faithfully respect the ver-

tical meridian of the retina as the line of decussation, which the Y cells and the phasic W cells do not respect. This class-related difference also applies to albinos but the nasotemporal division for all cell types is shifted into the temporal retina. At present, it is not possible to say whether the misrouting of optic nerve fibers in albino mammals is a primary defect of the optic axon's growth mechanism or whether the primary defect is in the specification of the retinal ganglion cells. Conceivably, both mechanisms contribute.

11.20. Formation of Geniculocortical Projections

Geniculocortical axon terminals are normally segregated into alternating eye-specific bands or patches in layer IV of the visual cortex (areas 17 and 18). This has been observed in cats (Shatz et al., 1977; LeVay et al., 1978), ferrets (Law and Stryker, 1983), monkeys (Hubel and Wiesel, 1972; LeVay et al., 1975; Hubel et al., 1977), and humans (Hitchcock and Hickey, 1980; Horton and Hedley-White, 1984). These ocular dominance bands have a periodicity of about 1 mm in layer IV of area 17 and a 2-mm periodicity in area 18 (Shatz et al., 1977; Cynader et al., 1987; Swindale, 1988). **The ocular dominance patches or bands are the anatomical substrate for the physiological ocular dominance columns which span all layers of the visual cortex of the cat (LeVay et al., 1978) and monkeys (Hubel and Wiesel, 1968; Rakic, 1976, 1977; Hubel et al., 1977; LeVay et al., 1980; Blasdel and Lund, 1983; Blasdel and Fitzpatrick, 1984). Neurons in layer IVc receive monocular input but they converge on binocular neurons in the supragranular layers of the striate cortex (Fitzpatrick et al., 1985). This is the first stage in the retinogeniculostriate projection at which inputs from the two eyes converge on binocular neurons.**

The evidence showing clustering of cells into ocular dominance columns was first obtained by microelectrode recording (Hubel and Wiesel, 1962, 1965, as shown in Fig. 11.33). Anatomical evidence was then obtained by making lesions confined to a single geniculate layer and tracing degenerating geniculostriate nerve terminals in the cortex (Hubel and Wiesel, 1969, 1972). The columnar arrangement in the visual cortex was demonstrated by trans-

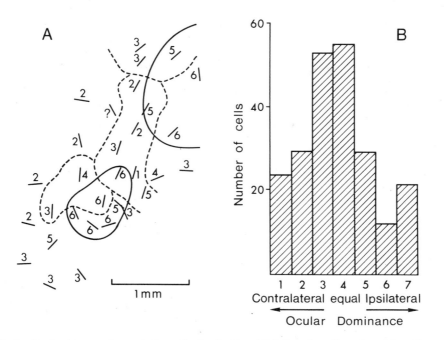

Figure 11.33. Ocular dominance columns in the cat's visual cortex. (A) Suface view of a region of the right striate cortex in normal adult cat, showing receptive field orientations and ocular dominance of the first cells, encountered near the surface, in 31 microelectrode penetrations. Dashed lines separate regions of relatively constant receptive field orientation. The numbers refer to ocular dominance groups. Continuous lines separate areas of strong ipsilateral dominance from areas of mixed or contralateral dominance. From D. H. Hubel and T. N. Wiesel, *J. Neurophysiol* 28:1041–1059 (1965). (B) Ocular dominance distribution of 223 cells recorded from striate cortex of normal adult cats in a series of 45 penetrations. Cells in group 1 receive input only from the contralateral eye; cells in group 7 receive input only from the ipsilateral eye; and cells in groups 2–6 receive input in different proportions from both eyes. From D. H. Hubel and T. N. Wiesel, *J. Physiol. (London)* 160:106–154 (1962).

neuronal labeling after intraocular injection of radio-active tracers (Wiesel *et al.,* 1974; Shatz *et al.,* 1977), or of wheat germ agglutinin conjugated to HRP (Il-aya and van Huesen, 1982). Physiologically charac-terized single geniculocortical axons have been la-beled with HRP, and their terminal arbors mapped anatomically in layer IV of the striate cortex (Gilbert and Wiesel, 1979; Humphrey *et al.,* 1984). Finally, ocular dominance columns extending through all cortical layers have been mapped functionally by showing differences in cortical metabolism resulting from stimulating one eye, either using cytochrome oxidase histochemistry (Wong-Riley, 1979; Horton and Hubel, 1981; Wong-Riley and Riley, 1983) or 2-deoxyglucose autoradiography (Kennedy *et al.,* 1975, 1976; Hubel *et al.,* 1978; Humphrey *et al.,* 1980; Schoppmann and Stryker, 1981; Tootell *et al.,* 1982, 1983, 1988a-e; Redies *et al.,* 1990), as shown in Fig. 11.34. The microelectrode technique has also been extended by optical recording techniques

using voltage-sensitive dyes (Orbach *et al.,* 1985; Blasdel and Salama, 1986; Grinvald *et al.,* 1986).

Ocular dominance bands develop from an ini-tial state of intermingled geniculocortical nerve terminals from the two eyes. Starting before birth in the monkey and 2 weeks after birth in the cat, geniculocortical nerve endings from the left and right eyes segregate slowly until they form alter-nating bands.

Segregation of the geniculostriate terminals into alternating bands can be demonstrated by auto-radiography after injection of [³H]proline into one eye in a series of newborn kittens at different ages (Fig. 11.35). Ocular dominance bands in the striate cortex of the cat develop gradually starting at 2 weeks after birth, but they appear to be fully formed at the time of birth in the superior colliculus. In the cat the segregation of geniculocortical terminals from the two eyes occurs gradually over a period of 4 to 8 weeks so that the separation is completed by

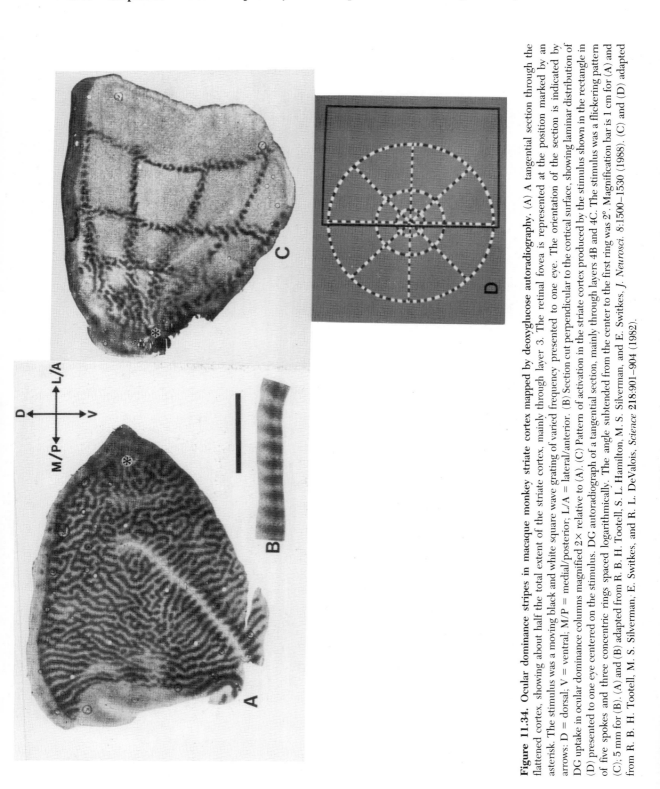

Figure 11.34. Ocular dominance stripes in macaque monkey striate cortex mapped by deoxyglucose autoradiography. (A) A tangential section through the flattened cortex, showing about half the total extent of the striate cortex, mainly through layer 3. The retinal fovea is represented at the position marked by an asterisk. The stimulus was a moving black and white square wave grating of varied frequency presented to one eye. The orientation of the section is indicated by arrows: D = dorsal; V = ventral; M/P = medial/posterior; L/A = lateral/anterior. (B) Section cut perpendicular to the cortical surface, showing laminar distribution of DG uptake in ocular dominance columns magnified 2× relative to (A). (C) Pattern of activation in the striate cortex produced by the stimulus shown in the rectangle in (D) presented to one eye centered on the stimulus. DG autoradiograph of a tangential section, mainly through layers 4B and 4C. The stimulus was a flickering pattern of five spokes and three concentric rings spaced logarithmically. The angle subtended from the center to the first ring was 2°. Magnification bar is 1 cm for (A) and (C); 5 mm for (B). (A) and (B) adapted from R. B. H. Tootell, S. L. Hamilton, M. S. Silverman, and E. Switkes, *J. Neurosci.* 8:1500–1530 (1988). (C) and (D) adapted from R. B. H. Tootell, M. S. Silverman, E. Switkes, and R. L. DeValois, *Science* 218:901–904 (1982).

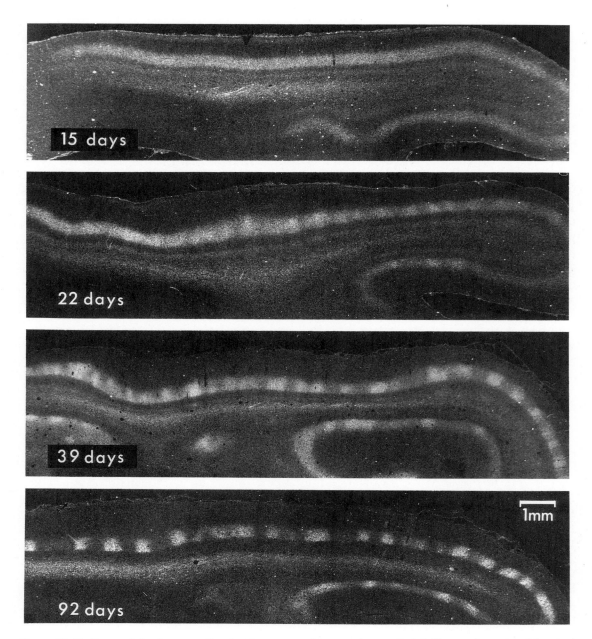

Figure 11.35. Postnatal development of ocular dominance columns in the cat. Dark-field autoradiographs of the visual cortex at four different ages, ipsilateral to an eye which was injected with [³H]proline. Horizontal sections, midline at the top in each figure, anterior to the left. The geniculocortical afferents serving the ipsilateral eye are labeled by transneuronal transport. At 15 days of age the afferents are spread uniformly along layer IV, completely intermingled with the (unlabeled) afferents serving the contralateral eye. At later ages the afferents progressively aggregate into clumps—the anatomical basis for the physiologically described ocular dominance columns. The gaps are occupied by unlabeled afferents serving the other eye. Physiological recordings show that in young kittens neurons in layer IV may be influenced readily by stimulation of either eye, but at later ages they come to be strongly dominated by one eye or the other. Courtesy of S. LeVay, M. P. Stryker, and C. J. Shatz.

10 weeks of age (Le Vày et al., 1978; LeVay and Stryker, 1979).

In the rhesus monkey, ocular dominance columns start appearing more than 3 weeks before birth in the superior colliculus and striate cortex (Rakic, 1977). Those in the superior colliculus of the rhesus monkey appear to be fully developed at birth (Rakic, 1977). Geniculocortical terminals start segregating into ocular dominance bands 3–6 weeks before birth in the monkey (Rakic, 1976, 1977) and segregation is well advanced at the time of birth, as evidenced by anatomical, physiological, and metabolic studies (Wiesel and Hubel, 1974; Hubel et al., 1977; De Rosiers et al., 1978; Le Vay et al., 1980). Ocular dominance bands continue developing after birth in the monkey and are then vulnerable to monocular visual deprivation. If one eye is misaligned or occluded during a critical period, then that eye loses its effectiveness in driving cortical neurons (Hubel and Wiesel, 1963), and its geniculostriate terminals contract while those from the normal eye expand their territory in layer IVc of the striate cortex (Hubel et al., 1977; Shatz et al., 1977; Shatz and Stryker, 1978; LeVay et al., 1980).

11.21. Role of Visual Activity in Development of Mammalian Visual Centers

Reviews of the role of visual stimulation on development of the visual system have appeared at regular intervals (C. Blakemore, 1974; Barlow, 1975; Hirsch and Jacobson, 1975; P. Grobstein and Chow, 1975, 1976; Daniels and Pettigrew, 1976; Rakic, 1977, 1986; Hirsch and Leventhal, 1978; Movshon and Van Sluyters, 1981; Sherman and Spear, 1982; Sherman, 1985). The effects of visual deprivation on the lateral geniculate nucleus depend on whether the deprivation is monocular or binocular. Binocular deprivation appears to affect the Y cells selectively in all parts of the LGNd (Sherman et al., 1972; Kratz et al., 1979; Sherman and Spear, 1982). The effect is clearly less severe than the effects of monocular deprivation, and there have been several reports of failure to find any effects of binocular deprivation (Chow and Stewart, 1972; Guillery, 1973a,b; Hendrickson and Boothe, 1976). By contrast, monocular deprivation results in severe shrinking of the affected segments of the LGNd (Wiesel and Hubel,

1965a). Because these effects of monocular deprivation are confined to the binocular segments of the LGNd while the monocular segment to which the deprived eye projects is virtually unaffected (except after prolonged deprivation, lasting more than 6 months), the effects must be due to interaction between the two eyes (Wiesel and Hubel, 1963a, 1965a; Guillery, 1972a, 1973a,b, 1974). Guillery (1972a) demonstrated this very elegantly by showing that no apparent effects of visual deprivation occur in an artificial monocular segment of the LGNd made by destroying a small area of temporal retina in one eye shortly after birth and then occluding the intact eye (Fig. 11.36). Because interactions between laminae of the LGNd are very weak, the interactions between LGNd cells must occur at their endings in the visual cortex. The shrinkage of LGNd cell bodies is a retrograde effect, originating in the striate cortex.

Earlier reports that visual deprivation has no effect on the functions of LGNd neurons (Wiesel and Hubel, 1963a, 1965; Chow and Stewart, 1972) have been contradicted by the reports that considerable reduction in the number of Y cells but not X cells in the cat LGNd results from binocular as well as monocular deprivation, and that Y-cell reponses can be recorded from an artificial monocular segment but not from the binocular segment of the LGNd of the cat after monocular deprivation (Sherman et al., 1972, 1975; Hoffmann and Cynader, 1975). Monoclonal antibodies specifically stain mature Y cells in the LGNd (Hockfield et al., 1983; Hendry et al., 1984; Sur et al., 1988; Hockfield and Sur, 1990) and cells in the visual cortex (Guimarïes et al., 1990). Staining with these antibodies, which recognize epitopes on a cell-surface proteoglycan, is reduced by monocular lid suture (Fig. 11.37) or rearing cats from birth in the dark, but is unaffected by visual deprivation in adult cats (Sur et al., 1988; Guiomarïes et al., 1990).

The effect of visual deprivation on the superior colliculus in newborn cats, first shown by Wickelgren and Sterling (1969), has been shown to be mediated by the indirect Y-cell projection from the complex cells of the visual cortex to the superior colliculus. These cells respond to fast-moving stimuli, and are directionally selective and binocular. Reduction of their activity after visual deprivation is due to absence of Y cells in the LGNd (Hoffmann and Sherman, 1974, 1975). The bin-

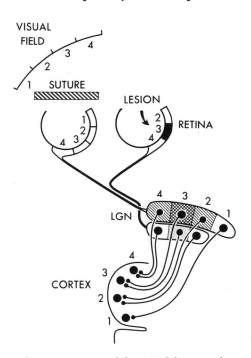

Figure 11.36. Binocular competition between neurons of the LGNd for cortical synaptic space is shown in this experiment. Left eyelid closure (shown by oblique shading) produces cell shrinkage in segments 2, 3, and 4 of lamina A of the right LGNd. When an additional lesion is made in the right temporal retina, resulting in atrophy of cells in segment 3 of lamina A₁, the cells in the corresponding segment (segment 3) of lamina A grow more than the cells in segments 2 and 4. From R. W. Guillery, *J. Comp. Neurol.* **144**:117–130 (1972).

ocularly driven cells in the superior colliculus require visual stimulation for their normal development: they cannot be recorded in newborn kittens. Their activity normally increases during the first few weeks after birth, but this is prevented by visual deprivation (Hoffmann and Sherman, 1974, 1975).

The roles of visual stimulation and deprivation in the development of the visual cortex vary according to species, according to the type of neuron in question, and according to whether the deprivation is monocular or binocular. Some types of neurons develop largely or entirely under intrinsic control, while others require sensory stimulation. These may be termed "invariant" and "variable" components, and their proportions vary in different species, so that results cannot be freely generalized from one species to others. Thus, in the mouse, rat, and rabbit, development of the visual cortex is completed in the absence of visual stimulation, although the rate of development is slowed by binocular visual deprivation. In these species, after a short period

of visual deprivation the striate cortex is found to be less mature structurally and functionally than in normal controls, but after about 6–8 months in the dark the structure and function of the visual cortex are virtually indistinguishable from normal (Boas *et al.*, 1969; Vrensen and de Groot, 1974; P. Grobstein and Chow, 1975; P. Grobstein *et al.*, 1975). This is considered at greater length in Section 11.20.

Almost normal ocular dominance and orientation columns, or moderately reduced proportions of binocularly driven cells, have been reported to develop in cats reared from birth in the dark or with the eyelids of both eyes sutured closed (Wiesel and Hubel, 1965a; Hubel and Wiesel, 1974c; Blakemore and van Sluyters, 1975; Buisseret and Imbert, 1976; Cynader *et al.*, 1976; Kratz and Spear, 1976; Sherk and Stryker, 1976; Leventhal and Hirsch, 1977, 1980; Fregnac and Imbert, 1978; Le Vay *et al.*, 1980; Mower, 1981; Sherman and Spear, 1982, review). In partial disagreement with those authors Swindale (1981, 1988), using transneuronal autoradiography,

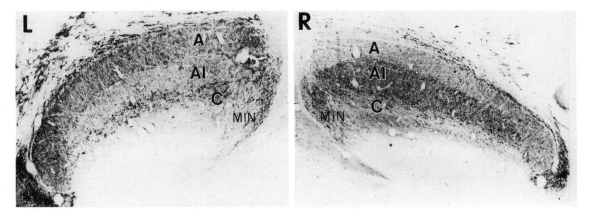

Figure 11.37. Monocular visual deprivation from birth results in an irreversible reduction of Y cells in the cat's LGNd stained with monoclonal antibody Cat-301. Antibody Cat-301 recognizes Y cells in layers A, A1, and C of the LGNd of the normal cat. Suture of the eyelids of the left eye from birth to P100 results in reduced Cat-301 immunoreactivity in layer A1 in the left (L) LGNd and in layer A and C in the right (R) LGNd. This reduction is permanent, as reverse lid suture after P100 does not change the pattern of antibody staining (Sur *et al.*, 1988). Figure kindly provided by S. Hockfield.

found total absence of ocular dominance patches in area 17 of the cat's visual cortex after binocular lid suture or rearing in total darkness from shortly after birth. Normal ocular dominance bands were present in area 18 of dark-reared cats. The minimum amount of binocular visual experience sufficient for segregation of ocular dominance bands to occur is between 48 and 128 hours, given before 8 weeks of age. No recovery occurs after more than 30 weeks of rearing kittens in the dark (Swindale, 1988).

The effects of monocular deprivation are significantly different from those of binocular deprivation. Monocular lid suture for 2–3 months after birth results in a significant reduction, although not complete absence of cells in the striate cortex that can be driven by the deprived eye (Fig. 11.38). Those that can be driven by the deprived eye have very abnormal receptive fields. The reduction of binocularly driven cortical neurons that occurs after monocular visual deprivation during the neonatal period has been found in the cat, monkey, rabbit, rat, and mouse (Wiesel and Hubel, 1963b, 1965; Hubel and Wiesel, 1970; Shaw *et al.*, 1974; Van Sluyters and Stewart, 1974; Drager, 1976; Pettigrew and Konishi, 1976; Movshon and Van Sluyters, 1981; Sherman and Spear, 1982, review), and in the visual *wulst* of some birds (Pettigrew and Konishi, 1976; Bagnoli *et al.*, 1982, 1983; Burkhalter, 1982).

Monocular visual deprivation of monkeys and cats from birth results in an increase in width of the cortical ocular dominance columns of the normal eye and a commensurate decrease in width of the ocular dominance columns of the deprived eye, as shown by transneuronal autoradiography (Hubel *et al.*, 1975, 1977; Shatz and Stryker, 1978; Le Vay *et al.*, 1980), illustrated in Fig. 11.39. Similar abnormalities in the ocular dominance columns after monocular deprivation are revealed by the deoxyglucose method (Des Rosiers *et al.*, 1978) and by staining for cytochrome oxidase (Wong-Riley, 1979).

The loss of binocularity can occur after a few days of monocular deprivation during a critical period. The critical period for plasticity of ocular dominance begins as early as the 2nd week after birth in the cat (Van Sluyters and Freeman, 1977), and the effects are most marked during the 5th week (Blakemore and Van Sluyters, 1974). After this time the effects diminish until deprivation has little or no effect by 8–20 weeks of age (Hubel and Wiesel, 1970; Cynader *et al.*, 1980). During the critical period a brief exposure of the binocularly deprived cat to a short period (6–20 hours) of monocular stimulation is sufficient to reduce the number of binocularly driven cortical neurons (Peck and Blakemore, 1975; C. R. Olson and Freeman, 1975). The critical period can be extended for as long as 11 months by rearing cats in the dark from the time of eye opening (Cynader and Mitchel, 1980; Cynader, 1983; Mower *et al.*, 1985).

Considerable reduction in the number of binocularly driven cortical neurons without any reduction in orientation selectivity is found in kittens 3 months after strabismus is produced by cutting the medial rectus muscle shortly after birth (Hubel and Wiesel, 1965b). A similar effect can be produced by placing an opaque shield over the left or right eye on alternate days (Hubel and Wiesel, 1965b; Blake and Hirsch, 1975). It seems that, for each neuron, the dominant eye has taken over. Thus, strabismus accentuates segregation into ocular dominance bands. The effect is not due to visual deprivation but to lack of correspondence or cooperation between the two eyes. Neurons in the visual cortex appear to require congruent inputs from corresponding points on the two retinae: if the inputs are made incongruent by producing strabismus or by alternating monocular occlusion, the neurons that were binocularly connected at birth lose the ability to respond to stimulation of one eye but retain the input from the other eye.

The physiological basis of this shift in ocular dominance appears to be an inhibition of the input from the deprived eye. This can be inferred from the evidence that the binocularity can be partially restored in monocularity deprived cats immediately after intravenously injected or iontophoretically applied bicuculline, a drug which blocks the action of the inhibitory synaptic transmitter gamma-aminobutyric acid (GABA) (Sillito, 1975a,b; Duffy *et al.*, 1976, 1978; Burchfiel and Duffy, 1981; see Section 6.11 for the effects of stimulation on cortical GABAergic synapses). A similar rapid restoration of function of the deprived eye occurs after removal of the experienced eye (Kratz and Spear, 1976; Kratz *et al.*, 1976; Smith *et al.*, 1978).

The effect of monocular deprivation in cats can be prevented by depletion of norepinephrine in the brain by infusion of 6-hydroxydopamine into the lateral ventricle (Kasamatsu and Pettigrew, 1976, 1979) or by continuous infusion directly into the visual

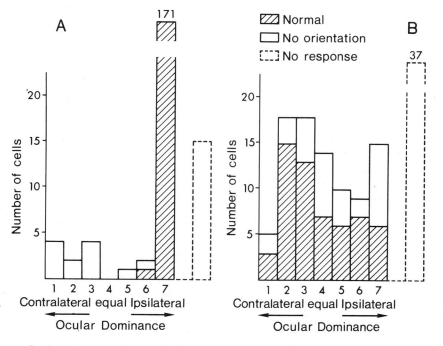

Figure 11.38. Ocular dominance distribution of cells in the striate cortex of kittens deprived of pattern vision in one eye (A) compared with kittens deprived of pattern vision in both eyes (B) by suturing the eyelids of one or both eyes from about 4 weeks to 8–14 weeks of age. (A) The ocular dominance distribution of 199 cells recorded in the striate cortex of five monocularly deprived kittens. (B) The ocular dominance distribution of 126 striate cortical cells recorded in four binocularly deprived kittens. Shading indicates that cells had normal specific responses to visual stimulation; absence of shading indicates that cells lacked orientation specificity; dashed lines indicate that cells did not respond to visual stimulation of either eye. From T. N. Wiesel and D. H. Hubel, *J. Neurophysiol.* 28:1029–1040 (1965).

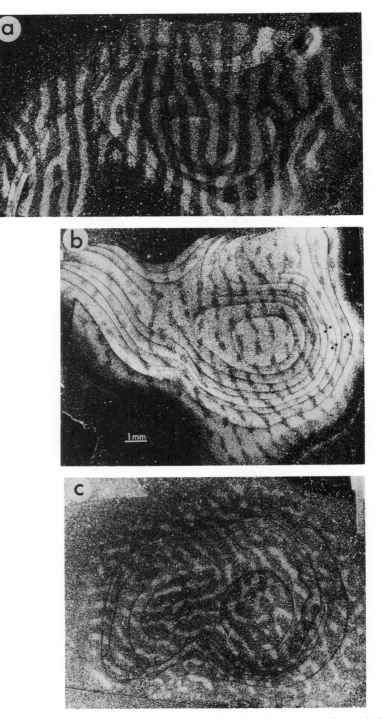

Figure 11.39. Ocular dominance columns in a normal rhesus monkey (a) and in monkeys deprived of vision in one eye from shortly after birth (b, c). Montages made from serial tangential sections through layer IV of primary visual cortex (area 17), processed for autoradiography, and photographed with dark-field illumination. Each monkey had one eye injected with tritiated proline 10 days prior to death: the bright bands correspond to the terminal fields of transneuronally labeled geniculocortical afferents serving the injected eye. In (b) the injection was made into the eye which was left open; in (c) it was made into the closed eye. The autoradiographs show that in monkeys raised with one eye closed the ocular dominance columns for the open eye are wider than normal, while those for the closed eye are narrowed. The combined width of a left- and right-eye pair is the same as normal. From D. H. Hubel, T. N. Wiesel, and S. LeVay, *Phil. Trans. Roy. Soc. London Ser. B* **278**:377–409 (1977).

cortex during the period of monocular deprivation (Kasamatsu *et al.*, 1979). Treatment with 6-hydroxydopamine does not reverse the effect of an established monocular deprivation but prevents the effect from occurring. The effect has been attributed to selective depletion of cortical norepinephrine (reviewed by Kasamatsu, 1983). But other methods of depletion of cortical norepinephrine have not prevented the ocular dominance plasticity (Bear *et al.*, 1983; Daw *et al.*, 1984, 1985a–c; Adrien, 1985). However, depletion of cortical norepinephrine in addition to acetylcholine (by lesioning the basal forebrain cholinergic neurons projecting to the cortex) reduces the response to monocular deprivation, although lesions to either the norepinephrine or the acetylcholine system are ineffective (Bear and Singer, 1986). Evidence that norepinephrine alters plasticity in the visual cortex by binding selectively to beta-adrenergic receptors is that the effect of monocular deprivation is decreased by the beta-receptor antagonists but not alpha-receptor antagonists (Kasamatsu and Shirokawa, 1985a,b). There is also evidence that the effect is mediated by cyclic nucleotides (Kasamatsu, 1980) and it is plausible that the effect involves phosphorylation of proteins that modify synaptic transmission in the cortical cells.

Normal development of orientation-selective neurons in the visual cortex requires congruent inputs from the two eyes. The effects of selective visual stimulation on orientation-selective neurons can be studied by fitting kittens with goggles which allow one eye to view vertical lines and the other to view horizontal lines (Hirsch, 1970; Hirsch and Spinelli, 1970, 1971; Leventhal and Hirsch, 1975; Stryker *et al.*, 1976). Kittens that have worn these goggles for the first 12 weeks after birth have a majority of cortical neurons whose orientation selectivity matches the orientation of the stimulus to which the eye was exposed. However, some neurons respond best to orientations at right angles to the lines to which the eye was exposed (Leventhal and Hirsch, 1975). After selective exposure of kittens to diagonal lines, cortical cells are found that respond selectively to horizontal or vertical as well as other cells that respond best to the diagonal orientation to which the eye was exposed (Leventhal and Hirsch, 1975). These observations suggest that some neurons are inherently predisposed to develop vertical or horizontal orientation selectivity, while others require appropriate visual stimulation. Another method of selective visual exposure, by raising kittens in

cylinders decorated inside with either vertical or horizontal stripes, results in development of visual cortical cells whose orientation selectivity matches the orientation of the stripes which the animal was allowed to see (C. Blakemore and Cooper, 1970; C. Blakemore, 1974). Failure to confirm these results shows that the striped cylinder is a less reliable method of restricting visual experience than goggles attached to the head (Stryker and Sherk, 1975; Daw and Wyatt, 1976).

The embryo and fetus are buffered against the effects of the external environment. Although susceptibility of the fetus to normal environmental conditions starts, to a limited extent, shortly before birth, it reaches a peak only after birth. The period during which development of the nervous system is sensitive to external conditions is termed the *sensitive period*, or the *vulnerable period*, if the effect of external conditions or agents is harmful. If a specific condition or stimulus is required for the normal development of the system, the condition or stimulus is termed *critical*, and the period during which its action is required is termed the *critical period*. The times when various critical conditions or stimuli are effective are concentrated in the same relatively short period, shortly after birth in birds and mammals, the animals in which critical periods have been studied extensively. A number of effects or events occur only during the relatively brief critical period. For example, the effect of monocular deprivation on the ocular dominance of visual cortical neurons in cats and monkeys (Wiesel and Hubel, 1963), imprinting in birds (Ewert, 1980, review), and the learning of song in some species of birds (Marler, 1981; Nottebohm, 1981; DeVoogd and Nottebohm, 1981).

Although the critical periods for various systems and conditions overlap in time, it is unlikely that they all share the same underlying mechanism. For example, the vulnerability of the nervous system to nutritional deficiency affects cellular differentiation and growth, synaptogenesis, and myelination, depending on the time and duration of the deprivation. Quite different effects are produced by sensory deprivation, depending on the quality and quantity, time, and duration of the deprivation. In general, however, the critical period is fairly specific for each form of deprivation in a particular species. Thus, in the cat, the critical period for development of binocular vision, for which congruent input from both eyes is required, extends from 3 to 16 weeks of age, after which the vulnerability to monocular visual deprivation or to strabismus is greatly diminished. The comparable critical period in the human infant, during which both eyes must work together to ensure development of binocularity, can be determined from studies of the effect of strabismus originating in children at different ages (Boothe *et al.*, 1985, review). The maximal deleterious effect is produced if the strabismus starts before the age of 2 $1/2$ years (Hofmann and Creutzfeldt, 1975), and the effect is greatly diminished thereafter, although some deleterious effects may be produced by strabismus starting at up to 6 years of age (Banks *et al.*, 1975).

The ability of the system to recover from deprivation diminishes with age: the capacity for recovery falls off sharply after the critical period. This may be a reflection of the progressive loss with age of the capacity for growth and differentiation of nerve cells. An apparently similar loss of functional recovery occurs after brain injury sustained at later ages. For example, the cerebral lateralization of functions such as language is already present at birth in humans (see Section 2.13), but recovery of function occurs after removal of or damage to the dominant cerebral hemisphere provided that the damage occurs before the age of 3 or 4 years. The importance of age on the capacity to recover, whether from sensory deprivation, undernutrition, or loss of brain tissue, is well known, but the reasons for this age dependence are still open to conjecture. The resemblances between recovery from brain damage and recovery from sensory deprivation may be only formal, and there is no reason, *a priori*, for the same mechanisms to operate in both types of recovery. There is also so little evidence regarding the neuronal and developmental mechanisms underlying critical periods that it is impossible to determine whether different critical periods have the same or different underlying mechanisms.

At present, virtually nothing is known about the molecular and cellular mechanisms by which the critical conditions produce changes in the development of nerve cells that result in permanent changes in neuronal function and behavior. The mechanisms are also unknown by means of which neuronal modifiability increases during the critical period and later diminishes or disappears. In those neurons in which the final stage of development is contingent on adequate sensory stimulation, there must be a mechanism by which the activity evoked in the neuron by sensory stimulation may control the synthesis or assembly of materials required for neuronal differentiation and growth. Either the effect may be simply proportional to the total quantity of nervous activity, or qualitative differences in the effect on the neuron may be produced by different spatiotemporal patterns of neuronal activity. The latter is implied in all theories of the formation or stabilization of neuronal connections as a result of "association," "concomitance," "correspondence," or "functional interaction" of nerve impulses (see Section 11.1). Whatever the mechanism of stimulation of the final differentiation of the neuron by functional activity, the last is not regarded as the primary formative agent in the development of nerve connections and circuits, but the stimulation is believed to constitute a functional validation or modification, either progressive or regressive, of preexisting neuronal structures. The initial development of those structures is determined by genetic and developmental mechanisms that are relatively unaffected by the normal range of environmental conditions. To understand how an appropriate combination of genetic determination and sensory stimulation interacts to control the final stages of development of some types of neurons is one of the most important tasks for the future.

The importance of early experience for the development of normal behavior has been repeatedly confirmed in many species from birds to humans, but the underlying mechanisms are unknown. The effects of early experience are greatest in those species in which the large-scale development of the brain continues after birth. While imprinting occurs even in precocial animals, the altricial animals are far more susceptible to a larger range of environmental conditions. This reaction range is greatest in humans, less in other mammals, and least in submammals (Fig. 11.40). The increased reaction range is gained at the risk of increased vulnerability of the brain to unfavorable conditions during the neonatal period. The concept of reaction norm or range was introduced by Richard Woltereck in the first decade of this century (see Dunn, 1965, p. 96). This concept emphasized the sovereignty of the genotype. As one of the greatest of geneticists has put it: *"One hears frequently that the organism is a product of heredity and environment. I cannot agree with this. Environ-*

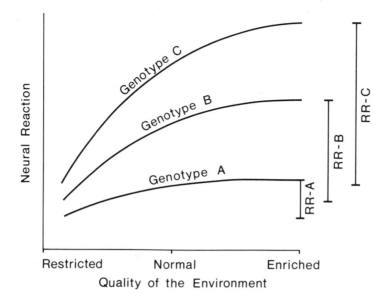

Figure 11.40. Reaction ranges for three hypothetical genotypes. RR denotes the range of neural reaction to the quality of the environment. Neural reactions may include biochemical changes, changes of the numbers and sizes of neurons and glial cells, changes in synaptic connections, and variations of behavior.

ment can affect the organism only within the limits set by its hereditary constitution. Beyond these limits there is no reaction or no organism. . . . This idea, a basic one, I think, is expressed best in Woltereck's definition of the genotype as a norm of reaction" (Richard B. Goldschmidt, 1951).

This book is only a preliminary reconnaissance along the trail leading to an understanding of the development of the human brain and mind. Although all the problems that have been considered here have relevance for human development, we are far from understanding why the duration and final extent of development of the human brain, particuarly in the postnatal period, so greatly exceed that of the other mammals. Why do no residues remain in later life of the experiences of infancy? Psychoanalysis notwithstanding, this period of life seems to be totally beyond recall. As Tolstoy described in his *Recollections*, jotted down between the ages of 74 and 80, "From the day I was born until I was three years old, all the time I was nursing and being weaned, beginning to crawl and walk and talk, however I rack my brains, I can remember

nothing. . . . From the child of five to me is only a step. From the newborn babe to the child of five is a great leap. From the embryo to the newborn child is an abyss." Why are the memories of infancy beyond recall? Are they obliterated by the growth and regression of dendrites and by development and elimination of synapses that occur in the cerebral cortex during the first years after birth? Or are they suppressed by inhibitory mechanisms from which they may be released by the appropriate treatment? What part do those early experiences play in the postnatal development of the human brain and behavior? I believe that research on the development of the nervous system will eventually provide answers to such questions and that these answers will be the means of arriving at a deeper understanding of the nature of humans.

> We shall not cease from exploration
> And the end of all our exploring
> Will be to arrive where we started
> And to know the place for the first time.
>   T. S. Eliot (1888–1965), "Little Gidding"

References

Aakre, B., D. A. Strobel, R. R. Zimmerman, and C. R. Geist (1973). *Percept. Mot. Skills* 36:787–790. Reactions to intrinsic and extrinsic reward in protein malnourished monkeys.

Abbott, J., and H. Holtzer (1968). *Proc. Natl. Acad. Sci. U.S.A.* 59:1144–1151. The loss of phenotypic traits by differentiated cells. V. The effect of 5-bromodeoxyuridine on cloned chondrocytes.

Abbott, N. J., and A. M. Butt (1986). *J. Physiol. (London)* 377:103P. Permeability of the dogfish glial blood-brain barrier to ions and small molecules.

Abbott, N. J., N. J. Lane, and M. Bundegaard (1986). *Ann. N.Y. Acad. Sci.* 481:20–41. The blood-brain interface in invertebrates.

Abe, T., T. Miyatake, W. T. Norton, and K. Suzuki (1979). *Brain Res.* 161:179–182. Activities of glycolipid hydrolases in neurons and astroglia from rat and calf brains and in oligodendroglia from calf brain.

Abeles, M., and M. H. Goldstein, Jr. (1970). *J. Neurophysiol.* 33:172–187. Functional architecture in cat primary auditory cortex. Columnar organization and organization according to depth.

Abercrombie, M. (1946). *Anat. Rec.* 94: 239–247. Estimation of nuclear population from microtome sections.

Abercrombie, M. (1950). *Phil. Trans. Roy. Soc. (London) Ser. B.* 234:317–338. The effects of anteroposterior reversal of lengths of the primitive streak in the chick.

Abercrombie, M. (1967). *Natl. Cancer Inst. Monograph* 26:249–277. Contact inhibition: The phenomenon and its biological implications.

Abercrombie, M. (1970). *In vitro* 6: 128–142. Contact inhibition in tissue culture.

Abercrombie, M. (1980). *Proc. Roy. Soc. (London) Ser. B.* 207:129–147. The crawling movement of metazoan cells.

Abercrombie, M., and R. Bellairs (1954). *J. Embryol. Exp. Morphol.* 2:55–72. The effects in chick blastoderms of replacing the primitive node by a graft of the posterior primitive streak.

Abercrombie, M., and J. Heaysman (1954). *Exp. Cell Res.* 6:293–306. Observations on the social behavior of cells in tissue culture. II. "Monolayering" of fibroblasts.

Abercrombie, M., and M. L. Johnson (1942). *J. Exp. Biol.* 19:266–278. The outwandering of cells in tissue cultures of nerves undergoing Wallerian degeneration.

Abercrombie, M., and M. L. Johnson (1946). *J. Anat. (London)* 80:37–47. Quantitative histology of Wallerian degeneration. I. Nuclear population in rabbit sciatic nerve.

Abercrombie, M., and J. E. Santler (1957). *J. Cell. Comp. Physiol.* 50:429–450. An analysis of growth in nuclear population during Wallerian degeneration.

Abercrombie, M., M. L. Johnson, and G. A. Thomas (1949). *Proc. Roy. Soc. (London) Ser. B.* 136:448–460. The influence of nerve fibres on Schwann cell migration investigated in tissue culture.

Acheson, A., W. Vogl, W. B. Huttner, and H. Thoenen (1986). *Eur. Mol. Biol. Org. J.* 5:2799–2803. Methyltransferase inhibitors block NGF-regulated survival and protein phosphorylation in sympathetic neurons.

Acheson, G., and J. Remolina (1955). *J. Physiol. (London)* 127:602–616. The temporal course of the effects of postganglionic axotomy on the inferior mesenteric ganglion of the cat.

Achúcarro, N. (1915). *Trav. Lab. Rech. Biol. Univ. Madrid* 13:169–212. De l'evolution de la névroglie et spécialment de ses relations avec l'appareil vasculaire. English transl. *J. Nerv. Ment. Dis.* 48:333–342 (1918).

Ackerknecht, E. (1953). *Rudolf Virchow: Doctor, Statesman, Anthropologist.* Univ. Wisconsin Press, Madison.

Adams, J. C. (1977). *Neuroscience* 2:141–145. Technical considerations on the use of horseradish peroxidase as a neuronal marker.

Adams, R. D., and J. M. Foley (1953). *Res. Pub. Assoc. Res. Nerv. Ment. Dis.* 32: 198–237. The neurological disorder associated with liver disease.

Adams-Smith, W. N. (1967). *J. Embryol. Exp. Morphol.* 17: 1–10. The ovary and sexual maturation of the brain.

Addison, W. H. F. (1911). *J. Comp. Neurol.* 21:459–485. The development of the Purkinje cells and of the cortical layers in the cerebellum of the albino rat.

Adelmann, H. B. (1966). *Marcello Malpighi and the Evolution of Embryology*, 5 Vols. Cornell University Press, Ithaca, New York.

Adelmann, H. B. (1925). *J. Comp. Neurol.* 39:19–171. The development of the neural folds and cranial ganglia of the rat.

Adinolfi, A. M. (1972a). *Exp. Neurol.* 34:372–382. Morphogenesis of synaptic junctions in layers I and II of the somatic sensory cortex.

Adinolfi, A. M. (1972b). *Exp. Neurol.* 34:383–393. The organization of paramembranous densities during postnatal maturation of synaptic junctions in the cerebral cortex.

Adinolfi, M. (1985). *Dev. Med. Child Neurol.* 27:532–537. The development of the human blood-CSF barrier.

Adkins-Regan, E. (1987). *Trends Neurosci.* 10:517–522. Sexual differentiation in birds.

Adler, A. J., and K. M. Klucznik (1982). *J. Neurochem.* 38:909–915. Glycerol phosphate dehydrogenase in developing chick retina and brain.

Adler, J. (1966). *Science* 153:708–716. Chemotaxis in bacteria.

Adler, J., and W. W. Tso (1974). *Science* 184:1292–1294. "Decision"-making in bacteria: Chemotactic response of *Escherichia coli* to conflicting stimuli.

Adler, R., J. Jerdan, and A. T. Hewitt (1985). *Dev. Biol.* 112:100–114. Responses of cultured neural retinal cells to substratum-bound laminin and other extracellular matrix molecules.

Adolph, E. E. (1949). *Science* 109:579–585. Quantitative relations in the physiological constitution of mammals.

Adrian, E. A. (1941). *J. Physiol. (London)* 100:159–191. Afferent discharges to the cerebral cortex from peripheral sense organs.

Adrian, E. D. (1924). *Brain* 47:399–416. Some recent work on inhibition.

Adrian, E. K., and R. L. Schelper (1981). Microglia, monocytes and macrophages, pp. 113–124. In *Glial and Neuronal Cell Biology*, (Fedoroff, ed.), Liss, New York.

Adrian, E. K., Jr., and R. D. Smothermon (1970). *Anat. Rec.* 166:99–116. Leukocytic infiltration into the hypoglossal nucleus following injury to the hypoglossal nerve.

Adrian, E. K., Jr., and B. E. Walker (1962). *J. Neuropathol. Exp. Neurol.* 21:597–609. Incorporation of thymidine-³H by cells in normal and injured mouse spinal cord.

Adrian, E. K., Jr., and M. G. Williams (1973a). *Anat. Rec.* 175:261–262. An electron microscopic study of reactive cells in the spinal cord labeled with ³H-thymidine before spinal cord injury.

Adrian, E. K., Jr., and M. G. Williams (1973b). *J. Comp. Neurol.* 151:1–24. Cell proliferation in injured spinal cord. An electron microscopic study.

Adrian, E. K., Jr., M. G. Williams, and F. C. George (1978). *J. Comp. Neurol.* 180:815–840. Fine structure of reactive cells in injured nervous tissue labelled with ³H-thymidine injected before injury.

Adrien, J., G. Blanc, P. Buisseret, Y. Fregnac, E. Gary-Bobo, M Imbert, J. P. Tassin, and Y. Trotter (1985). *J. Physiol. (London)* 367:73–98. Noradrenaline and functional plasticity in kitten visual cortex: A re-examination.

Aebischer, P., A. N. Salessiotis, and S. R. Winn (1989). *J. Neurosci. Res.* 23:282–289. Basic fibroblast growth factor released from synthetic guidance channels facilitates peripheral nerve regeneration across long nerve gaps.

Aggerwal, A. S., and W. J. Hendelman (1980). *J. Comp. Neurol.* 193:1081–1096. The Purkinje neuron: II. Electron microscopic analysis of the mature Purkinje neuron in organotypic culture.

Aghajanian, G. K., and F. E. Bloom (1967). *Brain Res.* 6:716–727. The formation of synaptic junctions in developing rat brain: A quantitative electron microscopic study.

Aguayo, A. J. (1985). Axonal regeneration from injured neurons in the adult mammalian central nervous system, pp. 457–484. In *Synaptic Plasticity* (C. W. Cotman, ed.), Guilford, New York.

Aguayo, A. J., J. Epps, J. Charton, and G. M. Bray (1976a). *Brain Res.* 104:1–20. Multipotentiality of Schwann cells in cross-anastomosed and grafted unmyelinated nerves—Quantitative microscopy and radiography.

Aguayo, A. J., L. Charron, and G. M. Bray (1976b). *J. Neurocytol.* 5:565–573. Potential of Schwann cells from unmyelineated nerves to produce myelin: A quantitative ultrastructural and radiographic study.

Aguayo, A. J., M. Attiwell, J. Trecarten, C. S. Perkins, and C. M. Bray (1976c). *Clin. Res.* 24:688A. Schwann cell transplantation: Evidence for a primary disorder of myelination in trembler mouse nerves.

Aguayo, A. J., M. Attiwell, J. Trecarten, S. Perkins, and G. M. Bray (1977). *Nature* 265:73–75. Abnormal myelination in transplanted Trembler mouse Schwann cells.

Aguayo, A. J., S. David, P. Richardson, and G. Bray (1982). Axonal elongation studied in peripheral and central nervous system transplants, pp. 215–234. In *Advances in Cellular Neurobiology*, Vol. 3 (S. Fedoroff, and L. Hertz, eds.), Academic, New York.

Aguayo, A. J., M. Benfey, and S. David (1983). A potential for axonal regeneration in neurons of the adult mammalian nervous system, pp. 327–340. In *Nervous System Regeneration*, (B. Haber, J. R. Perez-Polo, G. A. Hashim, and A. M. G. Stella, eds.), Liss, New York.

Aguilar, C. E., M. A. Bisby, E. Cooper, and J. Diamond (1973). *J. Physiol. (London)* 234:449–464. Evidence that axoplasmic transport of trophic factors is involved in the regulation of peripheral nerve fields in salamanders.

Aitken, J. T. (1950). *J. Anat. (London)* 84:38–49. Growth of nerve implants in voluntary muscle.

Aitken, J. T., M. Sharman, and J. Z. Young (1947). *J. Anat. (London)* 81:1–22. Maturation of regenerating nerve fibers with various peripheral connexions.

Akam, M. (1983). *EMBO J.* 2:2075–2084. The location of *ultrabithorax* transcripts in *Drosophila* tissue sections.

Akam, M. (1987). *Development* 101:1–22. The molecular basis for metameric pattern in the *Drosophila* embryo.

Akam, M. (1989). *Cell* 57:347–349. Hox and *HOM*: Homologous gene clusters in insects and vertebrates.

Akam, M. E., I. Dawson, and G. Tear (1988). *Development* 104:Suppl.123–133. Homeotic genes and the control of segment diversity.

Akers, R. F., and A. Routtenberg (1985). *Brain Res.* 334:147–151. Kinase C phosphorylates a protein involved in synaptic plasticity.

Akers, R. M., C. R. Phillips and N. K. Wessells (1986). *Science* 231:613–616. Expression of an epidermal antigen is controlled by tissue interactions in the *Xenopus laevis* embryo.

Akert, K., K. Pfenninger, C. Sandri, and H. Moor (1972). Freeze-etching and cytochemistry of vesicles and membrane complexes in synapses of the CNS. In *Structure and Function of Synapse* (G. D. Pappas, and D. P. Purpura, eds.), Raven Press, New York.

Albarracin, A. (1982). *Santiago Ramón y Cajal o la Passion de España*. Editorial Labor, Barcelona.

Alberch, P., and P. Alberch (1981). *J. Morphol.* 167:249–264.

Heterochronic mechanisms of morphological deversification and evolutionary change in the neotropical salamander, *Bolitoglossa occidentalis* (Amphibia: Plethodontidae).

Alberch, P., S. J. Gould, G. F. Oster, and D. B. Wake (1979). *Paleobiology* 5:296–317. Size and shape in ontogeny and phylogeny.

Albers, B. (1987). *Dev., Growth and Diff.* 29:535–545. Competence as the main factor determining the size of the neural plate.

Alberts, B. M. (1989). *Amer. Zool.* 29:483–486. Introduction: On the great excitement in cell biology.

Albuquerque, E. X., and S. Thesleff (1968). *Acta Physiol. Scand.* 73:471–480. A comparative study of membrane properties of innervated and chronically denervated fast and slow skeletal muscles of the rat.

Albuquerque, E. X., J. E. Warnick, J. R. Tasse, and F. M. Sansone (1972). *Exp. Neurol.* 37:607–634. Effects of vinblastine and colchicine on neural regulation of the fast and slow skeletal muscles of the rat.

Alderman, A. L. (1935). *J. Exp. Zool.* 70:205–232. The determination of the eye in the anuran *Hyla regilla*.

Aldskogius, H. (1974). *Neurobiology* 4:132–150. Indirect Wallerian degeneration in intramedullary root fibres of the kitten hypoglossal nerve. Light and electron microscopical observations on silver impregnated sections.

Aldskogius, H. (1982). *J. Neuropathol. Appl. Neurobiol.* 8:341–349. Glial cell responses in the adult rabbit dorsal motor vagal nucleus during axon reaction.

Aldskogius, H., and L. Thomander (1986). *Brain Res.* 375:126–134. Selective reinnervation of somatotopically appropriate muscles after facial nerve transection and regeneration in the neonatal rat.

Aldskogius, H., K. D. Barron, and R. Regal (1980). *J. Comp. Neurol.* 193:165–177. Axon reaction in dorsal motor vagal and hypoglossal neurons of the adult rat. Light microscopy and RNA-cytochemistry.

Aletta, J. M., and L. A. Greene (1988). *J. Neurosci.* 8:1425–1435. Growth cone configuration and advance: A time-lapse study using video-enhanced differential interference contrast microscopy.

Aletta, J. M., S. A. Lewis, N. J. Cowan, and L. A. Greene (1988). *J. Cell Biol.* 106:1573–1581. Nerve growth factor regulates both the phosphorylation and steady-state levels of microtubule-associated protein 1.2 (MAP1.2).

Alfert, M. (1950). *J. Cell. Comp. Physiol.* 36:381–409. A cytochemical study of oogenesis and cleavage in the mouse.

Alitalo, K., M. Kurkinen, I. Virtanen, K. Mellstrom, and A. Vaheri (1982). *J. Cell Biochem.* 18:25–35. Deposition of basement membrane proteins in attachment and neurite formation of cultured murine C-1300 neuroblastoma cells.

Allan, I. J., and D. F. Newgreen (1980). *Am. J. Anat.* 157:137–154. The origin and differentiation of enteric neurons of the intestine of the fowl embryo.

Allara, E. (1952). *Riv. Biol.* 44:209–229. Sull' influenza esercitata dagli ormoni sulla stattura dell formazioni gustative di mus rattus albinus.

Allbrook, D. B., and J. T. Aitken (1951). *J. Anat. (London)* 85:376–390. Reinnervation of striated muscle after acute ischaemia.

Allcutt, D., M. Berry, and J. Sievers (1984a). *Dev. Brain Res.* 16:219–230. A quantitative comparison of the reactions of retinal ganlion cells to optic nerve crush in neonatal and adult mice.

Allcutt, D., M. Berry, and J. Sievers (1984b). *Dev. Brain Res.* 16:231–240. A qualitative comparison of the reactions of retinal ganglion cell axons to optic nerve crush in neonatal and adult mice.

Allen, B. M. (1924). *Endocrinology* 8:639–651. Brain development in anuran larvae after thyroid or pituitary gland removal.

Allen, F. (1912). *J. Comp. Neurol.* 22:547–568. The cessation of mitosis in the central nervous system of the rat.

Allen, L. S., M. Hines, J. E. Shryne, and R. A. Gorski (1989). *J. Neurosci.* 9:497–506. Two sexually dimorphic cell groups in the human brain.

Allen, R. D., and N. S. Allen (1983). *J. Microsc.* 129:3–17. Video-enhanced microscopy with a computer frame memory.

Allen, R. D., N. S. Allen, and J. L. Travis (1981). *Cell Motil.* 1:291–302. Video-enhanced contrast, differential interference contrast (AVEC-DIC) microscopy: A new method capable of analyzing microtubule related motility in the reticulopodial network of *Allogromia laticollaris*.

Allen, R. D., J. Metuzals, I. Tasaki, S. T. Brady, and S. Gilbert (1982). *Science* 218:1127–1129. Fast axonal transport in squid giant axon.

Allen, R. D., D. T. Brown, S. P. Gilbert, and H. Fujiwaka (1983). *Biol. Bull.* 165:523. Transport of vesicles along filaments dissociated from squid axoplasm.

Alley, K. E. (1973). *Anat. Rec.* 177:49–60. Quantitative analysis of the synaptogenic period in the trigeminal mesencephalic nucleus.

Alley, K. E. (1974). *J. Embryol. Exp. Morphol.* 31:99–121. Morphogenesis of the trigeminal mesencephalic nucleus in the hamster: Cytogenesis and neurone death.

Allsopp, G., and H. J. Gamble (1979). *J. Anat. (London)* 128:461–477. Light and electron microscopic observations on the development of the blood vascular system of the human brain.

Aloe, L., and Levi-Montalcini (1980). *Exp. Cell Res.* 125:15–22. Comparative studies on testosterone and L-thyroxine effects on the synthesis of nerve growth factor in mouse submaxillary salivary glands.

Alouf, J. (1929). *J. Psychol. Neurol.* 38:5–41. Die vergleichende Cytoarchitektonik der Area striata.

Alpers, B. J., and W. Haymaker (1934). *Brain* 57:195–205. The participation of the neuroglia in the formation of myelin in prenatal infantile brain.

Altman, J. (1962). *J. Comp. Neurol.* 119:77–96. Some fiber projections to the superior colliculus in the cat.

Altman, J. (1963). *Anat. Rec.* 145:573–591. Autoradiographic investigation of cell proliferation in the brains of rats and cats.

Altman, J. (1966a). *Exp. Neurol.* 16:263–278. Proliferation and migration of undifferentiated precursor cells in the rat during postnatal gliogenesis.

Altman, J. (1966b). *J. Comp. Neurol.* 128:431–474. Autoradiographic and histological studies of postnatal neurogenesis. II. A longitudinal investigation of the kinetics, migration and transformation of cells incorporating tritiated thymidine in infant rats, with special reference to postnatal neurogenesis in some brain regions.

Altman, J. (1967). Postnatal growth and differentiation of the mammalian brain, with implications for a morphological theory of memory. In *The Neurosciences: A Study Pro-*

gram (G. Quarton, T. Melnechuk, and F. O. Schmitt, eds.), Rockefeller University Press, New York.

Altman, J. (1969). *J. Comp. Neurol.* 136:269–294. Autoradiographic and histological studies of postnatal neurogenesis. III. Dating the time of production and onset of differentiation of cerebellar microneurons in rats.

Altman, J. (1971). *Brain Res.* 30:311–322. Coated vesicles and synaptogenesis. A developmental study in the cerebellar cortex of the rat.

Altman, J. (1972a). *J. Comp. Neurol* 145:353–398. Postnatal development of the cerebellar cortex in the rat. I. The external germinal layer and the transitional molecular layer.

Altman, J. (1972b). *J. Comp. Neurol.* 145:399–464. Postnatal development of the cerebellar cortex in the rat. II. Phases in the maturation of Purkinje cells and of the molecular layer.

Altman, J. (1972c). *J. Comp. Neurol.* 145:465–514. Postnatal development of the cerebellar cortex in the rat. III. Maturation of the components of the granular layer.

Altman, J. (1982). *Exp. Brain Res. (Suppl.)* 6:8–46. Morphological development of the rat cerebellum and some of its mechanisms.

Altman, J., and W. J. Anderson (1972). *J. Comp. Neurol.* 146:355–406. Experimental reorganization of the cerebellar cortex. I. Morphological effects of elimination of all microneurons with prolonged x-irradiation started at birth.

Altman, J., and S. A. Bayer (1978a). *J. Comp. Neurol.* 179:23–48. Prenatal development of the cerebellar system in the rat. I. Cytogenesis and histogenesis of the deep nuclei and the cortex of the cerebellum.

Altman, J., and S. A. Bayer (1978b). *J. Comp. Neurol.* 179:49–76. Prenatal development of the cerebellar system in the rat. II. Cytogenesis and histogenesis of the inferior olive, pontine gray, and the precerebellar reticular nuclei.

Altman, J., and S. A. Bayer (1979a). *J. Comp. Neurol.* 188:455–472. Development of the diencephalon in the rat. IV. Quantitative study of the time of origin of neurons and the internuclear chronological gradients in the thalamus.

Altman, J., and S. A. Bayer (1979b). *J. Comp. Neurol.* 188:473–500. Development of the diencephalon in the rat. V. Thymidine-radiographic observations on internuclear and intranuclear gradients in the thalamus.

Altman, J., and S. A. Bayer (1979c). *J. Comp. Neurol.* 188:501–524. Development of the diencephalon in the rat. VI. Re-evaluation of the embryonic development of the thalamus on the basis of thymidine-radiographic datings.

Altman, J., and S. A. Bayer (1980a). *J. Comp. Neurol.* 194:1–35. Development of the brain stem in the rat. I. Thymidine-radiographic study of the time of origin of neurons of the lower medulla.

Altman, J., and S. A. Bayer (1980b). *J. Comp. Neurol.* 194:37–56. Development of the brain stem in the rat. II. Thymidine-radiographic study of the time of origin of neurons of the upper medulla, excluding the vestibular and auditory nuclei.

Altman, J., and S. A. Bayer (1980c). *J. Comp. Neurol.* 194:877–904. Development of the brain stem in the rat. III. Thymidine-radiographic study of the time of origin of neurons of the vestibular and auditory nuclei of the upper medulla.

Altman, J., and S. A. Bayer (1980d). *J. Comp. Neurol.* 194:905–929. Development of the brain stem in the rat. IV. Thymidine-radiographic study of the time of origin of neurons in the pontine region.

Altman, J., and S. A. Bayer (1981). *Exp. Brain Res.* 42:411–423. Time of origin of neurons of the rat inferior colliculus and the relations between cytogenesis and tonotopic order in the auditory pathway.

Altman, J., and S. A. Bayer (1982). *Adv. Anat. Embryol. Cell Biol.* 74:1–90. Development of the cranial nerve ganglia and related nuclei in the rat.

Altman, J., and S. A. Bayer (1984). *Adv. Anat. Embryol. Cell Biol.* 85:1–166. The development of the rat spinal cord.

Altman, J., and S. A. Bayer (1985a). *J. Comp. Neurol.* 231:1–26. Embryonic development of the rat cerebellum. I. Delineation of the cerebellar primordium and early cell movements.

Altman, J., and S. A. Bayer (1985b). *J. Comp. Neurol.* 231:27–41. Embryonic development of the rat cerebellum. II. Translocation and regional distribution of the deep neurons.

Altman, J., and S. A. Bayer (1985c). *J. Comp. Neurol.* 231:42–65. Embryonic development of the rat cerebellum. III. Regional differences in the time of origin, migration, and settling of Purkinje cells.

Altman, J., and S. A. Bayer (1988a). *J. Comp. Neurol.* 275:346–377. Development of the rat thalamus: I. Mosaic organization of the thalamic neuroepithelium.

Altman, J., and S. A. Bayer (1988b). *J. Comp. Neurol.* 275:378–405. Development of the rat thalamus: II. Time and site of origin and settling pattern of neurons derived from the anterior lobule of the thalamic neuroepithelium.

Altman, J., and S. A. Bayer (1988c). *J. Comp. Neurol.* 275:406–428. Development of the rat thalamus: III. Time and site of origin and settling pattern of neurons of the reticular nucleus.

Altman, J., and S. L. Chorover (1963). *J. Physiol. (London)* 169:770–779. Autoradiographic investigation of the distribution and utilization in intraventricularly injected adenine-^{3}H, uracil-^{3}H and thymidine-^{3}H in the brains of cats.

Altman, J., and G. D. Das (1964). *Nature* 204:1161–1165. Autoradiographic examination of the effects of enriched environment on the rate of glial multiplication in the adult rat brain.

Altman, J., and G. D. Das (1965a). *Nature* 207:953–956. Postnatal origin of microneurones in the rat brain.

Altman, J., and G. D. Das (1965b). *J. Comp. Neurol.* 124:319–336. Autoradiographic and histological evidence of postnatal hippocampal neurogenesis in rats.

Altman, J., and G. D. Das (1966). *J. Comp. Neurol.* 126:337–390. Autoradiographic and histological studies of postnatal neurogenesis. I.

Altman, J., and G. D. Das (1967). *Nature* 214: 1098–1101. Postnatal neurogenesis in the guinea-pig.

Altman, J., and A. T. Winfree (1977). *J. Comp. Neurol.* 171:1–16. Postnatal development of the cerebellar cortex in the rat. V. Spatial organization of Purkinje cell perikarya.

Altman, J., W. J. Anderson, and K. A. Wright (1968a). *Exp. Neurol.* 22:52–74. Differential radiosensitivity of stationary and migratory primitive cells in the brains of infant rats.

Altman, J., G. D. Das, and W. J. Anderson (1968b). *Dev. Psychobiol.* 1:10–20. Effects of infantile handling on morphological development of rat brain: An exploratory study.

Altman, J., R. B. Wallace, W. J. Anderson, and G. D. Das (1968c). *Dev. Psychobiol.* 1:112–117. Behaviourally induced changes in length of cerebrum in rats.

Altman, J., W. J. Anderson, and K. A. Wright (1969). *Exp. Neurol.* 24:196–216. Early effects of X-irradiation of the cerebellum in infant rats: Decimation and reconstitution of the external granular layer.

Alvarez-Buylla, A., M. Theelen, and F. Nottebohm (1988). *Proc. Natl. Acad. Sci. U.S.A* 85:8722–8726. Birth of projection neurons in the higher vocal center of the canary forebrain before, during, and after song learning.

Alvarez, J., and M. Puschel (1972). *Brain Res.* 37:265–278. Transfer of material from efferent axons to sensory epithelium in goldfish vestibular system.

Alvarez, J., and J. Zarour (1983). *Exp. Neurol.* 79:283–286. Microtubules in short and in long axons of the same caliber: Implications for the maintenance of the neuron.

Alvarez, J., F. Arredondo, F. Espejo, and V. Williams (1982). *Neuroscience* 7:2551–2559. Regulation of axonal microtubules: Effect of sympathetic hyperactivity elicited by reserpine.

Alzheimer, A. (1910). *Hist. u. Histopath. Arb. Nissl-Alzheimer* 3:401. Beiträge zur Kenntniss der pathalogischen Neuroglia und ihrer Beziehungen zu den Abbauvorgangen im Nervengewebe.

Ambronn, H. (1890). *Ber. Verh. königl. sächs. Ges. Wissensch. Leipzig* 42:419–429. Das optische Verhalten markhaltiger und markloser Nervenfasern.

Amprino, R. (1943). *Arch. Ital. Anat. Embriol.* 49:261–300. Correlazioni quantitative fra centri nervosi e territori d'innervazione peritevica durante lo sviluppo.

Ancel, P., and P. Vintemberger (1948). *Bull. Biol. Fr. Belg. Suppl.* 31:1–182. Recherches sur le déterminisme de la symétrie bilatérale dans l'oeuf des amphibiens.

Anders, H. E. (1921). *Arch. Entw.-Mech. Organ.* 114:272–363. Die entwicklungsmechanische Bedeutung der Doppelbildungen nebst Untersuchungen über den Einfluss des Zentralnervensystems auf die quergestreifte Muskulatur des Embryo.

Andersen, P., J. C. Eccles, and Y. Loyning (1963a). *Nature* 198:541–542. Recurrent inhibition in the hippocampus with identification of the inhibitory cell and its synapses.

Andersen, P., J. Eccles, and P. E. Voorhoeve (1963b). *Nature* 199:655–656. Inhibitory synapses on somas of Purkinje cells in the cerebellum.

Andersen, P., T. W. Blackstad, and T. Lomo (1966). *Exp. Brain Res.* 1:236–248. Location and identification of excitatory synapses on hippocampal pyramidal cells.

Andersen, P., S. H. Sundberg, O. Sveen, and H. Wigstrom (1977). *Nature* 266:736–737. Specific long-lasting potentiation of synaptic transmission in hippocampal slices.

Andersen, R. A., C. Asanuma, and W. M. Cowan (1985). *J. Comp. Neurol.* 232:443–455. Callosal and prefrontal associational projecting cell populations in area 7A of the macaque monkey: A study using retrogradely transported fluorescent dyes.

Anderson, C. B., and S. Meier (1982). *J. Exp. Zool.* 221:329–335. Effect of hyaluronidase treatment on the distribution of cranial neural crest cells in the chick embryo.

Anderson, D. J. (1989). *Trends Neurosci.* 12:83–85. New roles for PDGF and CNTF in controlling the timing of glial cell differentiation in the optic nerve.

Anderson, D. J., and R. Axel (1985). *Cell* 42:649–662. Molecular probes for the development and plasticity of neural crest derivatives.

Anderson, D. J., and R. A. Axel (1986). *Cell* 47:1079–1090. Bipotential neuroendocrine precursor whose choice of cell fate is determined by NGF and glucocorticoids.

Anderson, D. J., R. Stein, and R. Axel (1985). *Cold Spring Harbor Symp. Quant. Biol.* 50:855–863. Gene expression in differentiating and transdifferentiating neural crest cells.

Anderson, K. E., A. Edstrom, and M. Hanson (1972). *Brain Res.* 43:299–302. Heavy water reversibly inhibits fast axonal transport of proteins in frog sciatic nerves.

Anderson, K. J., D. Dam, S. Lee, and C. W. Cotman (1988). *Nature* 332:360–361. Basic fibroblast growth factor prevents death of lesioned cholinergic neurons *in vivo*.

Anderson, M. J., and M. W. Cohen (1977). *J. Physiol. (London)* 268:757–773. Nerve-induced and spontaneous redistribution of acetylcholine receptors on cultured muscle cells.

Anderson, M. J., and D. M. Fambrough (1983). *J. Cell Biol.* 97:1396–1411. Aggregates of acetylcholine receptors are associated with plaques of a basal lamina heparan sulfate proteoglycan on the surface of skeletal muscle fibers.

Anderson, M. J., Y. Kidokoro, and R. Gruener (1979). *Brain Res.* 166:185–190. Correlation between acetylcholine receptor localization and spontaneous synaptic potentials in cultures of nerve and muscle.

Anderson, P. N., A. R. Medlen, J. Mitchell, and D. Mayor (1981). *J. Neurophysiol.* 10:19–26. The uptake and retrogade transport of horseradish peroxidase-polylysine conjugate by ligated postganglionic sympathetic nerves *in vitro*.

Ando, S. (1983). *Neurochem. Int.* 5:507–537. Gangliosides in the nervous system.

Andres, G. (1953). *J. Exp. Zool.* 122:507–540. Experiments on the fate of dissociated embryonic cells (chick) disseminated by the vascular route. Part II. Teratomas.

Andres, K. H. (1964). *Z. Zellforsch.* 64:63–73. Mikropinozytose im Zentralnervensystem.

Andres, K. H., and M. Von During (1966). *Naturwissenschaften* 23:615–616. Mikropinozytose im motorische Endplatten.

Andrew, A. (1971). *J. Anat. (London)* 108:169–184. The origin of intramural ganglia. IV. The origin of enteric ganglia: A critical review and discussion of the present state of the problem.

Andrew, W., and C. T. Ashworth (1945). *J. Comp. Neurol.* 82:101–127. The adendroglia.

Andriezen, W. L. (1893a). *Br. Med. J.* 2:227–230. The neuroglia elements of the brain.

Andriezen, W. L. (1893b). *Inter. Monatschr. Anat. Physiol.* 10:533. On a system of fibre-cells surrounding the blood-vessels of the brain of man and its physiological significance.

Andy, O. J., and H. Stephan (1966). *J. Comp. Neurol.* 126:157–171. Septal nuclei in primate phylogeny; a quantitative investigation.

Angant-Petit, D., A. Mallart, and L. Faille (1982). *Biol. Cell* 46:277–290. Role of denervated sheaths and end-plates in muscle reinnervation by collateral sprouting in the mouse.

Angaut, P., and J.-P. Raffin (1981). *Dev. Neurosci.* 4:1–14. Embryonic development of the nucleus isthmo-opticus in the chick: A Golgi and electron microscopic study.

Angeletti, P. U., and R. Levi-Montalcini (1970). *Proc. Natl. Acad. Sci. U.S.A.* 65:114–121. Sympathetic nerve cell destruction in newborn mammals by 6-hydroxydopamine.

Angeletti, P. U., A. Liuzzi, and R. Levi-Montalcini (1964a). *Biochim. Biophys. Acta* 84:778–781. Stimulation of lipid biosynthesis in sympathetic and sensory ganglia by a specific nerve growth factor.

Angeletti, P. U., A. Liuzzi, R. Levi-Montalcini, and D. G. Gandini-Attardi (1964b). *Biochim. Biophys. Acta* 90:445–450. Effect of a nerve growth factor on glucose metabolism by sympathetic and sensory nerve cells.

Angeletti, P. U., D. Gandini-Attardi, G. Toschi, M. L. Salvi, and R. Levi-Montalcini (1965). *Biochim. Biophys. Acta* 95: 111–120. Metabolic aspects of the effect of nerve growth factor on sympathetic and sensory ganglia: Protein and ribonucleic acid synthesis.

Angeletti, P. U., R. Levi-Montalcini, and P. Calissano (1968). *Adv. Enzymol.* 31:51–75. The nerve growth factor: Chemical properties and metabolic effects.

Angeletti, P. U., L. Levi-Montalcini, and F. Caramia (1971a). *Brain Res.* 27:343–355. Analysis of the effects of the antiserum to the nerve growth factor in adult mice.

Angeletti, P. U., R. Levi-Montalcini, and F. Caramia (1971b). *J. Ultrastruct. Res.* 36:24–36. Ultrastructural changes in sympathetic neurons of newborn and adult mice treated with nerve growth factor.

Angeletti, P. U., R. Levi-Montalcini, R. Kettler, and H. Thoenen (1972). *Brain Res.* 44:197–206. Comparative studies on the effect of the nerve growth factor on sympathetic ganglia and adrenal medulla in newborn rats.

Angeletti, R. H., and R. A. Bradshaw (1971). *Proc. Natl. Acad. Sci. U.S.A.* 68:2417–2420. Nerve growth factor from mouse submaxillary gland: Amino acid sequence.

Angell, J. R. (1903). *Philos. Rev.* 12:243–271. The relations of structural and functional psychology to philosophy.

Angell, J. R. (1909). *Psychol. Rev.* 16:152–169. The influence of Dawin on psychology.

Angevine, J. B. (1965). *Exp. Neurol. Suppl.* 2:1–70. Time of neuron origin in the hippocampal region: An autoradiographic study in the mouse.

Angevine, J. B., Jr. (1968). *Anat. Rec.* 160:308. Autoradiographic study of neuronal proliferation gradients in the diencephalon of the mouse.

Angevine, J. B., Jr. (1970a). *J. Comp. Neurol.* 139:129–187. Time of neuron origin in the diencephalon of the mouse.

Angevine, J. B., Jr. (1970b). Critical cellular events in the shaping of the neural centers. In *The Neurosciences*, Vol. II (F. O. Schmitt and T. Melnechuck, eds.), Rockefeller University Press, New York.

Angevine, J. B., Jr., and R. L. Sidman (1961). *Nature* 192:766–768. Autoradiographic study of the cell migration during histogenesis of cerebral cortex in the mouse.

Angevine, J. B., Jr., and R. L. Sidman (1962). *Anat. Rec.* 142:210. Autoradiographic study of histogenesis in the cerebral cortex of the mouse.

Angevine, J. B., Jr., D. Bodian, A. J. Coulombre, M. V. Edds, Jr., V. hamburger, M. Jacobson, K. M. Lyser, M. C. Prestige, R. L. Sidman, S. Varon, and P. A Weiss (1970). *Anat. Rec.* 166:257–262. Embryonic vertebrate central nervous system: Revised terminology.

Anglister, L., and U. J. McMahan (1985). *J. Cell Biol.* 101:735–743. Basal lamina directs acetylcholinesterase accumulation at synaptic sites in regenerating muscle.

Angulewitsch, A., M. F. Utset, C. P. Hart, W. McGinnis, and F. H. Ruddle (1986). *Nature* 320:328–335. Spatial restriction in expression of a mouse homoeo box locus within the central nervous system.

Angulo y Gonzalez, A. W. (1929). *J. Comp. Neurol.* 48:459–464. Is myelogeny an absolute index of behavioral capacity?

Angulo y Gonzalez, A. W. (1932). *J. Comp. Neurol.* 55:395–442. The prenatal development of behavior in the albino rat.

Anokhin, P. K. (1968). *The Biology and Neurophysiology of the Conditional Reflex* (in Russian). Meditsina, Moscow.

Antal, M. (1984). *J. Neurosci. Meth.* 12:69–77. The application of cobalt labelling to electron microscopic investigations of serial sections.

Antal, M., R. Kraftsik, G. Székely, and H. Van der Loos (1986). *J. Neurocytol.* 15:303–310. Distal dendrites of frog motor neurons: A computer-aided electron microscopic study of cobalt-filled cells.

Apáthy, S. (1889). *Biol. Zbl.* 9:625–648. Nach welcher Richtung hin soll die Nervenlehre reformiert werden?

Apáthy, S. (1897). *Mittheil. aus der zool. Station zur Neapal* 12:495–748. Das leitende Element des Nervensystems und seine topographischen Beziehungen zu den Zellen.

Appelhauser, G. S. L., C. Benech, A. Levitas, and C. M. Franchi (1965). *Exp. Neurol.* 12:215–229. Uptake of C^{14}-L-Lysine into segments of normal rat sciatic nerve.

Archer, S. M., M. W. Dubin, and L. A. Stark (1982). *Science* 217:743–745. Abnormal development of kitten retinogeniculate connectivity in the absence of action potentials.

Ardeleanu, A., and N. Sterescu (1978). *Psychoneuroendocrinology* 3:93–101. RNA and DNA synthesis in developing rat brain: Hormonal influences.

Arees, E. A., and K. E. Åström (1977). *Anat. Embryol.* 151:29–34. Cell death in the optic tectum of the developing rat.

Arens, M., and C. Straznicky (1985). *Neurosci. Letts. Suppl.* 19:37. The development of the neurons of the motor trigeminal nucleus in normal and in curare treated chick embryos..

Arens, M., and C. Straznicky (1986). *Anat. Embryol.* 174:67–72. The development of the trigeminal (V) motor nucleus in normal and tubocurare treated chick embryos.

Arey, L. B., M. J. Tremaine, and F. L. Monzingo (1935). *Anat. Rec.* 64:9–25. The numerical and topographical relations of taste buds to human circumvallate papillae throughout the life span.

Argiro, V., M. B. Bunge, and M. I. Johnson (1985). *J. Neurosci.* 13:149–162. A quantitative study of growth cone filopodial extension.

Ariëns Kappers, C. U. (1907). *Folia Neurobiol.* 1:507–534. Weitere Mitteilungen über Neurobiotaxis. Die Selektivität der Zellwanderung: Die Bedeutung synchronischer Reizwandschaft.

Ariëns Kappers, C. U. (1909). *Arch. Neurol. Psych.* 4:161–173. The phylogenesis of the palaeocortex and archicortex compared with the evolution of the visual neocortex.Ariëns Kappers, C. U. (1917). *J. Comp. Neurol.*

Ariëns Kappers, C. U. (1917). *J. Comp. Neurol.* 27:261–298. Further contributions on neurobiotaxis. IX. An attempt to compare the phenomenon of neurobiotaxis with other phenomena of taxis and tropism. The dynamic polarization of the neuron.

Ariëns Kappers, C. U. (1921). *Brain* 44:125–149. On the structural laws in the nervous system: The principles of neurobiotaxis.

Ariëns Kappers, C. U. (1932). Principles of development of the nervous system (neurobiotaxis), pp. 43–89. In *Cytology and Cellular Pathology of the Nervous System*, Vol. I (W. Penfield, ed.), Hoeber, New York.

Ariëns Kappers, C. U., G. C. Huber, and E. C. Crosby (1936). *The Comparative Anatomy of the Nervous System of Vertebrates Including Man.* 2 vols., 1845 pp., Macmillan, New York.

Arimatsu, Y., and A. Seto (1982). *Brain Res.* 234:27–39. Ontogeny of sexual difference in alpha-bungarotoxin binding capacity in the mouse amygdala.

Armson, P. F., and M. R. Bennett (1983). *Neurosci. Lett.* 38:181–186. Neonatal retinal ganglion cell cultures of high purity: Effect of superior colliculus on their survival.

Armstrong, R. C., and P. G. H. Clarke (1979). *Neuroscience* 4:1635–1647. Neuronal death and the development of the pontine nuclei and inferior olive in the chick.

Arnett, D. W. (1978). *Exp. Brain Res.* 32:49–53. Statistical dependence between neighbouring retinal ganglion cells in goldfish.

Arnold, A. P., and R. A. Gorski (1984). *Ann. Rev. Neurosci.* 7:413–442. Gonadal steroid induction of structural sex differences in the central nervous system.

Arnold, J. (1867). *Virchow's Archiv.* 41:178–220. Ein Beitrag zu der feineren Structur der Ganglienzellen.

Arora, H. L., and R. W. Sperry (1957). *J. Embryol. Exp. Morphol.* 5:256–263. Myotypic respecification of regenerated nerve fibres in cichlid fishes.

Arora, H. L., and R. W. Sperry (1962). *Am. Zool.* 2:61. Optic nerve regeneration after surgical cross-union of medial and lateral optic tracts.

Arquint, M., J. Roder, L.-S. Chia, J. Down, D. Wilkinson, H. Bayley, P. Braun, and R. Dunn (1987). *Proc. Natl. Acad. Sci. U.S.A* 84:600–604. Molecular cloning and primary structure of myelin-associated glycoprotein.

Asanuma, H., and I. Rosén (1973). *Exp. Brain Res.* 16:507–520. Spread of monosynaptic and polysynaptic connexions within cat's motor cortex.

Asanuma, H., and H. Sakata (1967). *J. Neurophysiol.* 30:35–54. Functional organization of a cortical efferent system examined with focal depth stimulation in cats.

Asbury, A. L. (1967). *J. Cell Biol.* 34:735–743. Schwann cell proliferation in developing mouse sciatic nerve.

Aschoff, P. (1924). Reticulo-endothelial system. In *Lectures on Pathology.* Hoeber, New York.

Ashby, W. R. (1936–1937). *J. Neurol. Psychiat.* 17:322–327. Tissue culture methods in the study of the nervous system: Review.

Ashwell, K. (1989). *J. Comp. Neurol.* 287:286–301. Development of microglia in the albino rabbit retina.

Assouline, J. G., P. Bosch, R. Lim, S. N. Kim, R. Jensen, and N. J. Pantazis (1987). *Dev. Brain Res.* 31:103–108. Rat astrocytes and schwann cells in cluture synthesize nerve growth factor-like neurite-promoting factors.

Athias, M. (1897a). *J. Anat. Physiol. (Paris)* 33:372–404. L'histogénese de l'ecorce du cervelet.

Athias, M. (1897b). *Bibl. Anat.* 5:58–89. Structure histologique de la moelle épinière du têtard de la grenouille.

Atlas, M., and V. P. Bond (1965). *J. Cell Biol.* 26:19–24. The cell generation cycle of the eleven-day mouse embryo.

Atsumi, S. (1971). *Acta Anat.* 80:161–182. The histogenesis of motor neurons with special reference to the correlation of their endplate formation. I. The development of endplates in the intercostal muscle in the chick embryo.

Atsumi, S. (1977). *J. Neurocytol.* 6:691–709. Development of neuromuscular junctions of fast and slow muscles in the chick embryo: A light and electron microscopic study.

Atsumi, S. (1981). *Dev. Biol.* 86:122–135. Localization of surface and internal acetylcholine receptors in developing fast and slow muscles of the chick embryo.

Attardi, B., and E. Ruoslahti (1976). *Nature* 263:685–687. Foetoneonatal oestradiol-binding protein in mouse brain cytosol is a foetoprotein.

Attardi, D. G., and R. W. Sperry (1963). *Exp. Neurol.* 7:46–64. Preferential selection of central pathways by regenerating optic fibers.

Attardi, G., P. Borst, and P. P. Slonimski (1982). *Mitochondrial Genes*, Cold Spring Harbor Lab., New York.

Auburger, G., Heumann, R., R. Hellweg, S. Korsching, and H. Thoenen (1987). *Dev. Biol.* 120:322–328. Developmental changes of nerve growth factor and its mRNA in the rat hippocampus: Comparison with choline acetyltransferase.

Auerbach, L. (1898). *Neurol. Zbl.* 17:445–454. Nervenendigung in den Centralorganen.

Auerbach, R. (1960). *Dev. Bio.* 2:271–284. Morphogenetic interactions in the development of the mouse thymus gland.

Aufsess, A. von (1941). *Arch. Entw.-Mech. Organ.* 141:248–339. Defeckt und Isolationsversuche an der Medullarplatte und ihrer Unterlagerung an Triton alpestris- und Amblystoma-Keimen, mit besonderer Berücksichtigung der Rumpf- und Schwantzregion.

Ausoni, S., L. Gorza, S. Schiaffino, K. Gundersen, and T. Lømo (1990). *J. Neurosci.* 10:153–160. Expression of myosin heavy chain isoforms in stimulated fast and slow rat muscles.

Austin, L., and I. Morgan (1967). *J. Neurochem.* 14: 377–387. Incorporation of radioactively labelled leucine into synaptosomes from rat cerebral cortex *in vitro*.

Autilio-Gambetti, L., P. Gambetti, and B. Shafer (1973). *Brain Res.* 53:387–398. RNA and axonal flow, biochemical and autoradiographic study in the rabbit optic system.

Autillo-Touati, A., B. Chamak, D. Araud, J. Vuillet, R. Seite, and A. Prochiantz (1988). *J. Neurosci. Res.* 19:326–342. Region-specific neuro-astroglial interactions: Ultrastructural study of the *in vitro* expression of neuronal polarity.

Awgulewitsch, A., and D. Jacobs (1990). *Development* 108:411–420. Differential expression of *Hox 3.1* protein in subregions of the embryonic and adult spinal cord.

Awgulewitsch, A., M. F. Utset, C. P. Hart, W. McGinnis, and F. H. Ruddle (1986). *Nature* 320:328–335. Spatial restriction in expression of a mouse homoeobox locus within the central nervous system.

Axelsson, J., and S. Thesleff (1959). *J. Physiol. (London)* 149:178–193. A study of supersensitivity in denervated mammalian skeletal muscle.

Ayala, F. J. (1970). *Phil. Sci.* 37:1–15. Teleological explanations in evolutionary biology.

Ayer-LeLievre, C., L. Olson, T. Ebendahl, A. Seiger, and H. Persson (1988). *Science* 240:1339–1341. Expression of the β-nerve growth factor gene in hippocampal neurons.

Ayer-Le Lièvre, C. S. and N. M. Le Douarin (1982). *Dev. Biol.* 94:291–310. The early development of cranial sensory ganglia and the potentialities of their component cells studied in quail-chick chimeras.

Baack, J., C. de Lacoste-Utamsing, and D. J. Woodward (1982). *Neuroscience* 8:18. Sexual dimorphism in human fetal corpora callosa.

Baas, P. W., J. S. Deitch, M. M. Black, and G. A. Banker (1988). *Proc. Natl. Acad. Sci. U.S.A.* 85:8335–8339. Polarity orientation of microtubules in hippocampal neurons: Uniformity in the axon and nonuniformity in the dendrite.

Bacher, B. E. (1973). *J. Exp. Zool.* 185:209–216. The peripheral dependency of Rohon-Beard cells.

Baden, V. (1936). *J. Morphol.* 60:159–190. Embryology of the nervous system in the grasshopper, *Melanoplus differentialis.*

Baffoni, G. M. (1953). *Rend. Accad. Nazl. Lincei, Ser. 8,* 14:138–144. Azione dell' attività mitotica e modificazioni cellulari nel prosencefalo e nel mesencefalo di Anfibi.

Baffoni, G. M. (1957a). *Rend. Acade. Nazl. Lincei, Ser. 8,* 23:90–96. Tardiva determinazione numerica di cellule nervose nel rombencefalo di Anfibi.

Baffoni, G. M. (1957b). *Rend. Accad. Nazl. Linci, Ser. 8,* 23:495–503. Influena dell' ormone tiroideo sull' attivita mitotica del rombencephalo di un Anfibio anuro.

Baffoni, G. M. (1959). *Rend. Accad. Nazl. Lincei, Ser. 8,* 27:427–435. Effetti del' ormone tiroidea sul midollo spinale di larve di Anfibi anuri.

Baffoni, G. M. (1960). *Rend. Accad. Nazl. Lincei, Ser. 8,* 28:102–108. Variazioni dell' attività mitotica e modificazioni cellulari nel prosencefalo e nel mesencefalo di larve di Anfibi anuri trattate con ormone tiroideo.

Baffoni, G. M., and G. Catte (1950). *Rend. Acad. Nazl. Lincei. Ser. 8,* 9:282–287. Il comportamento della cellula di' Mauthner di raganella nella metamorfosi accelerata con somministrazione di tiroide.

Baffoni, G. M., and G. Catte (1951). *Riv. Biol.* 43:373–397. La citomorfosi della cellula di Mauthner in *Hyla arborea savignyi* (nello sviluppo normale e nella metamorfosi sperimentalmente anticipata).

Baffoni, G. M., and E. Elia (1957). *Rend. Accad. Nazl. Lincei, Ser. 8,* 22:109–114. L'attivitata mitotica durante la morfogenesi cerebellare in un Anfibio anuro.

Bagnall, K. M., S. J. Higgins, and E. J. Sanders (1989). *Development* 107:931–943. The contribution made by cells from a single somite to tissues within a body segment and assessment of the integration with similar cells from adjacent segments.

Bagnoli, P., S. Grassi, and F. Magni (1980). *Arch. Ital. Biol.* 118:72–88. A direct connection between the visual wulst and the tectum opticum in the pigeon *(Columbia livia)* demonstrated by horseradish peroxidase.

Bagnoli, P., A. Burkhalter, A. Visher, H. Henke, and M. Cuenod (1982). *Brain Res.* 247:289–302. Effects of monocular deprivation in choline acetyltransferase and glutamic acid decarboxylase in the pigeon visual wulst.

Bagnoli, P., R. Barselotti, M. Pellegrini, and R. Alesci (1983). *Dev. Brain Res.* 10:243–250. Norepinephrine levels in developing pigeon brain: Effect of monocular deprivation on the wulst noradrenergic system.

Bagust, J., D. M. Lewis, and R. A. Westerman (1973). *J. Physiol. (London)* 229: 241–255. Polyneuronal innervation of kitten skeletal muscle.

Bahler, M., and P. Greengard (1987). *Nature* 326:704–707. Synapsin I bundles F-actin in a phosphorylation-dependent manner.

Bailey, C. H., and M. Chen (1983). *Science* 220:91–93. Morphological basis of long-term habituation and sensitization in *Aplysia.*

Bailey, C. H., and M. Chen (1988). *Proc. Natl. Acad. Sci. U.S.A.* 85:2373–2377. Long-term memory in *Aplysia* modulates the total number of varicosities of single identified sensory neurons.

Bailey, P., and G. von Bonin (1951). *The Isocortex of Man.* University of Illinois Press, Urbana.

Baimbridge, K. G., and J. J. Miller (1982). *Brain Res.* 245:223–229. Immunohistochemical localization of calcium-binding protein in the cerebellum, hippocampal formation and olfactory bulb of the rat.

Bain, A. (1901). Association of ideas, pp. 511–513. In *Chamber's Encyclopedia,* Vol. 1, Chambers, London.

Baird, H. W., III, M. Chavez, J. Adams, H. T. Wycis, and E. A. Spiegel (1957). *Confin. Neurol.* 17:288–299. Studies in stereoencephalotomy. VII. Variations in the position of the globus pallidus.

Baitinger, C., J. Levine, T. Lorenz, C. Simon, P. Skene, and M. Willard (1982). Characteristics of axonally transported proteins, pp. 111–120. In *Axoplasmic Transport* (D. G. Weiss, ed.) Springer-Verlag, Berlin; Heidelberg, New York.

Baker, F. H., P. Grigg, and G. K. von Noorden (1974). *Brain Res.* 66:185–208. Effects of visual deprivation and strabismus on the response of neurons in the visual cortex of the monkey, including studies on the striate and prestriate cortex in the normal animal.

Baker, J. R. (1955). *Quart. J. microsc. sci.* 96:449–481. The cell-theory: a restatement, history and critique: V. The multiplication of nuclei.

Baker, P. C., and T. E. Schroeder (1967). *Dev. Biol.* 15:432–450. Cytoplasmic filaments and morphogenetic movement in the amphibian neural tube.

Baker, R. C., and G. O. Graves (1939). *J. Comp. Neurol.* 71:389–415. The behavior of the neural crest in the forebrain region of *Amblystoma.*

Baker, R. E. and M. Jacobson (1970). *Dev. Biol.* 22:476–494. Development of reflexes from skin grafts in *Rana pipiens:* Influence of size and position of grafts.

Baker, R. E., A. P. J. Richter, and N. Piller (1976). *Neuroscience* 1:367–370. A light and electron microscopic examination of dorsal root afferent development in three species of anurans.

Balak, K., M. Jacobson, J. Sunshine, and U. Rutishauser (1987). *Dev. Biol.* 119:540–550. Neural cell adhesion molecule expression in *Xenopus* embryos.

Balakier, H., and R.A. Pedersen (1982) *Dev. Biol.* 90: 352–352. Allocation of cells to inner cell mass and trophectoderm lineages in preimphantation mouse embryos.

Balázs, R. (1974). *Br. Med. Bull.* 30:126–134. Influence of metabolic factors on brain development.

Balázs, R., and W. A. Cocks (1967). *J. Neurochem.* 14:1035–1055. RNA metabolism in subcellular fractions of brain tissue.

Balázs, R., S. Kovács, P. Teichgraber, W. A. Cocks, and J. T. Eayrs (1968). *J. Neurochem.* 15:1335–1349. Biochemical effects of thyroid deficiency on the developing brain.

Balázs, R., B. W. L. Brooksbank, A. N. Davison, J. T. Eayrs, and D. A. Wilson (1969). *Brain Res.* 15:219–232. The effect of neonatal thyroidectomy on myelination in the rat brain.

Balázs, R., S. Kovács, W. A. Cocks, A. L. Johnson, and J. T. Eayrs (1971). *Brain Res.* 25:555–570. Effect of thyroid hormone on the biochemical maturation of rat brain: Postnatal cell formation.

Balázs, R., T. Jordan, P. D. Lewis, and A. J. Patel (1986). Undernutrition and brain development, pp.415–473. In *Human Growth*, Vol. 3, 2nd edn., (F. Falkner, and J. M. Tanner, eds.) Plenum Publishing, New York.

Baldwin, J. M. (1901). *Dictionary of Philosophy and Psychology*, 3 vols. in 4, Macmillan, New York.

Baldwin, J. M. (1905). *Psychol. Rev.* 12:144–165. Sketch of the history of psychology.

Baldwin, J. M. (1913). *History of Psychology: A sketch and an Interpretation*, 2 Vols., Watts, London.

Balfour, F. M. (1876). *J. Anat. Physiol. London* 11:128–172. The development of elasmobranch fishes. Development of the trunk.

Balfour, F. M. (1881). *A Treatise on Comparative Embryology*, 2 vols., Macmillan, London.

Balice-Gordon, R. J., and J. W. Lichtman (1990). *J. Neurosci.* 10:894–908. *In vivo* visualization of the growth of pre- and postsynaptic elements of neuromuscular junctions in the mouse.

Balice-Gordon, R. J., and W. J. Thompson (1988). *J. Physiol. (London)* 398:211–231. The organization and development of compartmentalized innervation in rat extensor digitorum longus muscle.

Balinsky, B. I. (1935). *Anat. Anz.* 80:136–142. Experimentelle Extremitateinduktion und die Theorien des phylogenetischen Ursprungs der paarigen Extremitäten der Wirbeltiere.

Balinsky, B. I. (1974). *J. Exp. Zool.* 188:195–201. Supernumerary limb induction in the Anura.

Ballard, K. J., and S. J. Holt (1968). *J. Cell Sci.* 3:245–262. Cytological and cytochemical studies on cell death and digestion in foetal rat foot; the role of macrophages and hydrolytic enzymes.

Ballotti, R., F. C. Nielsen, N. Pringle, A. Kowalski, W. D. Richardson, E. Van Obberghen, and S. Gammeltoft (1987). *EMBO J.* 6:3633–3639. Insulin-like growth factor I in cultured rat astrocytes: Expression of the gene, and receptor tyrosine kinase.

Bamburg, J. R., E. M. Shooter, and L. Wilson (1973). *Biochemistry* 12:1476–1482. Developmental changes in microtubule protein of chick brain.

Bamburg, J. R., D. Bray, and K. Chapman (1986). *Nature* 321:788–790. Assembly of microtubules at the tip of growing axons.

Banerjee, S. P., S. H. Snyder, P. Cuatrecasas, and L. A. Greene (1973). *Proc. Natl. Acad. Sci. U.S.A.* 70:2519–2523. Binding of nerve growth factor receptor in sympathetic ganglia.

Banks, M. S., R. N. Aslin, and R. D. Letson (1975). *Science* 190:675–677. Sensitive period for the development of human binocular vision.

Banks, P., D. Mangnall, and D. Mayor (1969). *J. Physiol. (London)* 200:745–762. The re-distribution of cytochrome oxidase, noradrenaline and adenosine triphosphate in adrenergic nerves constricted at two points.

Banks, P., D. Mayor, and T. Owen (1975). *Brain Res.* 83:277–292. Effects of low temperatures on microtubules in the non-myelinated axons of post-ganglionic sympathetic nerves.

Bantle, J. A., and W. E. Hahn (1976). *Cell* 8:139–150. Complexity and characterization of polyadenylated RNA in mouse brain.

Bär, T. (1978). Morphometric evaluation of capillaries in different laminae of rat cerebral cortex by automatic image analysis: changes during development and aging, pp. 1–9. In *Advances in Neurology* Vol. 20, Raven, New York.

Bär, T., and J. R. Wolff (1972). *Z. Zellforsch.* 133:231–248. The formation of capillary basement membranes during internal vascularization of the rat's cerebral cortex.

Bär, T., and J. R. Wolff (1973). *Z. Anat. Entwickl.-Gesch.* 141:207–221. Quantitative Beziehungen zwischen der Verzweigungsdichte und Länge von Capillaren im Neocortex der Ratte während der postnatalen Entwicklung.

Bar-Sagi, D., and J. R. Feramisco (1985). *Cell* 42:841–848. Microinjection of the *ras* oncogene protein into PC12 cells induces morphological differentiation.

Barald, K. F. (1982). Monoclonal antibodies to embryonic neurons: Cell-specific markers for chick ciliary ganglion, pp.101–119. In *Neuronal Development* (N. C. Spitzer, ed.), Plenum Press, New York.

Barald, K. F. (1988a). *J. Neurosci. Res.* 21:107–118. Monoclonal antibodies made to chick mesencephalic neural crest cells and to ciliary ganglion neurons identify a common antigen on the neurons and a neural crest subpopulation.

Barald, K. F. (1988b). *J. Neurosci. Res.* 21:119–134. Antigen recognized by monoclonal antibodies to mesencephalic neural crest and to ciliary ganglion neurons is involved in the high affinity choline uptake mechanism in these cells.

Barber, P. C., and R. M. Lindsay (1982). *Neuroscience* 7:3077–3099. Schwann cells of the olfactory nerves contain GFAP and resemble astrocytes.

Barber, R. P., J. E. Vaughn, R. E. Wimer, and C. C. Wimer (1974). *J. Comp. Neurol.* 156:417–434. Genetically associated variations in the distribution of dentate granule cell synapses upon the pyramidal cell dendrites in mouse hippocampus.

Barbera, A. J. (1975). *Dev. Biol.* 46:167–191. Adhesive recognition between developing retinal cells and optic tecta of the chick embryo.

Barbera, A. J., R. B. Marchase, and S. Roth (1973) *Proc. Natl. Acad. Sci. U.S.A.* 70:2482–2486. Adhesive recognition and retinotectal specificity.

Barbin, G., M. Manthorpe, and S. Varon (1984). *J. Neurochem.* 43:1468–1478. Purification of the chick eye ciliary neurotrophic factor.

Barbin, G., D. M. Katz, B. Chamak, J. Glowinski, and A. Prochiantz (1988). *GLIA* 1:96–103. Brain astrocytes express region-specific surface glycoproteins in culture.

Barbu, M., C. Ziller, P. M. Rong, and N. M. LeDourain (1986). *J. Neurosci.* 6:2215–2225. Heterogeneity in migrating neural crest cells revealed by a monoclonal antibody.

Bard, J., and I. Lauder (1974). *J. Theor. Biol.* 45:501–531. How well does Turing's theory of morphogenesis work?

Barde, Y.-A. (1989). *Neuron* 2:1525–1534. Trophic factors and neuronal survival.

Barde, Y.-A., R. M. Lilndsay, D. Monard, and H. Thoenen (1978). *Nature* 274:818. A new factor released by cultured glioma cells supporting survival and growth of sensory neurones.

Barde, Y.-A., D. Edgar and H. Thoenen (1982). *EMBO J.*

1:549–553. Purification of a new neurotrophic factor from mammalian brain.

Barde, Y.-A., A. M. Davies, J. E. Johnson, R. M. Lindsay, and H. Thoenen (1987). *Prog. Brain Res.* 71:185–189. Brain derived neurotrophic factor.

Bardin, C. W., L. P. Bullock, R. J. Sherins, I. Mowszowicz, and W. R. Blackburn (1973). *Recent Progr. Horm. Res.* 29:65–109. Androgen metabolism and mechanism of action in male pseudohermaphroditism: A study of testicular feminization.

Barker, D. (1974). The morphology of muscle receptors, pp. 1–190. In *Handbook of Sensory Physiology*, Vol. III, part 2, (C. C. Hunt, ed.), Springer-Verlag, New York.

Barker, D., and M. C. Ip (1966). *Proc. Roy. Soc. (London) Ser. B.* 163:538–554. Sprouting and degeneration of mammalian motor axons in normal and deafferented skeletal muscle.

Barker, D., and A. Milburn (1972). *J. Physiol. (London)* 222:159–168. Increase in number of intrafusal muscle fibres during the development of muscle spindles in the rat.

Barker, D., and A. Milburn (1984). *Sci. Prog. Oxf.* 69:45–64. Development and regeneration of mammalian muscle spindles.

Barker, R. (1988). *Trends Neurosci.* 11:533–534. Trophic role of neurotransmitters.

Barlow, H. B. (1975). *Nature* 258:199–204. Visual experience and cortical development.

Barlow, H. B., and J. D. Pettigrew (1971). *J. Physiol. (London)* 218:98–100. Lack of specificity of neurones in the visual cortex of young kittens.

Barlow, R. M. (1969). *J. Comp. Neurol.* 135:249–262. The foetal sheep: Morphogenesis of the nervous system and histochemical aspects of myelination.

Barnard, E. A., J. Wieckowski, and T. H. Chiu (1974). *Nature* 234:207. Cholinergic receptor molecules and cholinesterase molecules at mouse skeletal junctions.

Barnard, R. I. (1940). *J. Comp. Neurol.* 73:235–264. Experimental changes in end-feet of Held-Auerbach changes in the spinal cord of the cat.

Barnes, B. G. (1961). *J. Ultrastruct. Res.* 5:453–467. Ciliated secretory cells in the pars distalis of the mouse hypophysis.

Barnes, R. H., S. R. Cunnold, R. R. Zimmerman, H. Simmons, R. B. MacCleod, and L. Krook (1966). *J. Nutr.* 89:399–410. Influence of nutritional deprivation in early life on learning behavior as measured by performance in a water maze.

Barnes, R. H., U. A. Moore, and W. G. Pond (1970). *J. Nutr.* 100:149–155. Behavioral abnormalities in young adult pigs caused by malnutrition in early life.

Barnett, S. A., J. L. Smart, and E. M. Widdowson (1971). *Dev. Psychobiol.* 4:1–15. Early nutrition and the activity and feeding of rats in an artificial environment.

Barnicot, N. A. (1964). Biological variation in modern populations. In *Human Biology* (G. A. Harrison, J. S. Weiner, J. M. Tanner, and N. A. Barnicot, eds.), Clarendon, Oxford.

Barnstable, C. J. (1980). *Nature* 286:231–235. Monoclonal antibodies which recognize different cell types in the rat retina.

Baroffio, A., E. Dupin, and N. M. Le Douarin (1988). *Proc. Natl. Acad. Sci. U.S.A.* 85:5325–5329. Clone-forming ability and differentiation potential of migratory neural crest cells.

Baron, M., and A. Gallego (1972). *Z. Zellforsch. mikrosk. Anat.* 128:42–57. The relation of the microglia with the pericytes in the cat cerebral cortex.

Barondes, S. H. (1966). *J. Neurochem.* 13:221–227. On the site of synthesis of the mitochondrial protein of nerve endings.

Baron-van Evercooren, A., H. D. Kleinman, S. Ohno, P. Marangos, J. P. Schwartz, and M. E. Dubois-Dalcq (1982). *J. Neurosci. Res.* 8:179–183. Nerve growth factor, laminin and fibronectin promote nerve growth in human fetal sensory ganglia cultures.

Barr, M. L. (1939). *J. Anat. (London)* 74:1–11. Some observations on the morphology of the synapse in the cat's spinal cord.

Barr, M. L. (1940). *Anat. Rec.* 77:367–374. Axon reaction in motoneurones and its effect upon the endbulbs of Held-Auerbach.

Barr, M. L., and E. G. Bertram (1951). *J. Anat. (London)* 85:171–181. The behaviour of nuclear structures during depletion and restoration of Nissl material in motor neurons.

Barrera-Moncada, G. (1963). *Estudios sobre alteraciones del crecimiento y del desarrollo psicológico del sindrome pluricarencial (kwashiorkor)*. Editora Grafos, Caracas.

Barres, B. A., L. L. Y. Chun, and D. P. Corey (1988). *GLIA* 1:10–30. Ion channel expression by white matter glia: I. Type 2 astrocytes and oligodendrocytes.

Barrett, D. E., and D. A. Frank (1987). *The Effects of Undernutrition on Children's Behavior*. Gordon and Breach, New York.

Barron, D. H. (1943). *J. Comp. Neurol.* 78:1–26. The early development of the motor cells and columns in the spinal cord of the sheep.

Barron, D. H. (1946). *J. Comp. Neurol.* 85:149–169. Observations on the early differentiation of the motor neuroblasts in the spinal cord of the chick.

Barron, D. H. (1948). *J. Comp. Neurol.* 88:93–127. Some effects of amputation of the chick wing bud on the early differentiation of the motor neuroblasts in the associated segments of the spinal cord.

Barron, D. H. (1950). *J. Exp. Zool.* 113:553–573. An experimental analysis of some factors involved in the development of the fissure pattern of the cerebral cortex.

Barron, D. H., and J. Barcroft (1938). *J. Physiol. (London)* 93:29P. A case of amputation of leg, 90 days before birth.

Barron, K. D. (1983). Comparative observations on the cytologic reactions of central and peripheral nerve cells to axotomy, pp. 7–40. In *Spinal Cord Reconstruction* (C. C. Kao, R. P. Bunge, and P. J. Reier, eds.), Raven, New York.

Barron, K. D., and T. O. Tuncbay (1962). *Am. J. Pathol.* 40:637–652. Histochemistry of acid phosphatase and thiamine pyrophosphatase during axon reaction.

Barron, K. D., and T. O. Tuncbay (1964). *J. Neuropathol. Exp. Neurol.* 23:368–386. Phosphatase histochemistry of feline cervical spinal cord after brachial plexectomy.

Barron, K. D., C. M. McGuiness, L. J. Misantone, M. F. Zanakis, B. Grafstein, and M. Murray (1985). *J. Comp. Neurol.* 236:265–273. RNA content of normal and axotomized retinal ganglion cells of rat and goldfish.

Bartelmez, G. (1962). *Contr. Embryol. Carnegie Inst. Washington* 37:1–12. The proliferation of neural crest from forebrain levels in the rat.

Bartelmez, G., and A. S. Dekaban (1962). *Contr. Embryol.*

Carnegie Inst. Washington 37:13–32. The early development of the human brain.

Bartelmez, G. W. (1915). *J. Comp. Neurol.* 25:87–128. Mauthner's cell and the nucleus motorius tegmenti.

Bartelmez, G. W. (1962). *Contr. Embryol. Carnegie Inst. Publ.* 621:1–12. The proliferation of neural crest from forebrain levels in the rat.

Bartelmez, G. W., and N. L. Hoerr (1933). *J. Comp. Neurol.* 57:401–428. The vestibular club endings in Ameiurus. Further evidence on the morphology of the synapse.

Barth, E.-M, S. Korsching, and H. Thoenen (1984). *J. Cell Biol.* 99:839–843. Regulation of nerve growth factor synthesis and release in organ cultures of rat iris.

Barth, L. G. (1965). *Biol. Bull.* 129:471–481. The nature of the action of ions as inductors.

Barth, L. G., and L. J. Barth (1969). *Dev. Biol.* 20:236–262. The sodium dependence of embryonic induction.

Barth, L. G., and L. J. Barth (1972). *Dev. Biol.* 28:18–34. ^{22}Sodium and ^{45}calcium uptake during embryonic induction in *Rana pipiens*.

Bartlett, W. P., and R. P. Skoff (1989). *Dev. Brain Res.* 47:1–11. Expression of the jimpy gene in the spinal cords of heterozygous female mice. II. Oligodendroglial and endothelial cell hyperplasia.

Bartlett, W. P., P. E. Knapp, and R. P. Skoff (1988). *GLIA* 1:253–259. Glial conditioned medium enables jimpy oligodendrocytes to express properties of normal oligodendrocytes: Production of myelin antigens and membranes.

Barton, P. J. R., A. J. Harris, and M. E. Buckingham (1989). *Development* 107:819–824. Myosin light chain gene expression in developing and denervated fetal muscle in the mouse.

Barylko, B., P. J. Tooth, and J. Kendrick-Jones (1986). *Eur. J. Biochem.* 158:271–282. Proteolytic fragmentation of brain myosin and localization of the heavy chain phosphorylation site.

Basbaum, A. I., and P. D. Wall (1976). *Brain Res.* 116:181–204. Chronic changes in the response of cells in adult cat dorsal horn following partial deafferentation. The appearance of responding cells in a previously non-responsive region.

Basco, E., P. L. Woodhams, F. Hajos, and R. Balazs (1981). *Anat. Embryol.* 162:217–223. Immunocytochemical demonstration of glial fibrillary acidic protein in mouse tanycytes.

Baskin, D. G., B. J. Wilcox, D. P. Figlewicz, and D. M. Dorsa (1988). *Trends Neurosci.* 11:107–111. Insulin and insulin-like growth factors in the CNS.

Bass, N. H., M. G. Netsky, and E. Young (1970a). *Archs Neurol.* 23:289–302. Effect of neonatal malnutrition on developing cerebrum. I. Microchemical and histologic study of cellular differentiation in the rat.

Bass, N. H., M. G. Netsky, and E. Young (1970b). *Archs Neurol.* 23:303–313. Effect of neonatal malnutrition on developing cerebrum. II. Microchemical and histologic study of myelin formation in the rat.

Bastian, H. C. (1887). *Brain* 10:1–137. 'The muscular sense', its nature and cortical localization.

Bastiani, M. J., S. du Lac, and C. S. Goodman (1985). The first neuronal growth cones in insect embryos: Model system for studying the development of neuronal specificity, pp. 149–175. In *Model Neural Networks and Behavior* (A. I. Selverston, ed.), Plenum Publishing Corporation.

Bate, C. M. (1976a). *J. Embryol. Exp. Morphol.* 35:107–123. Embryogenesis of an insect nervous system. I. A map of the thoracic and abdominal neuroblasts in *Locusta migratoria*.

Bate, C. M. (1976b). *Nature* 260:54–56. Pioneer neurons in an insect embryo.

Bate, C. M. (1978). The development of sensory systems in arthropods. In *Handbook of Sensory Physiology*, Vol. 9: *Development of Sensory Systems* (M. Jacobson, ed.), Springer-Verlag, New York.

Bate, C. M. (1982). *NRP Bull.* 20:803–813. Proliferation and pattern formation in the embryonic nervous system of the grasshopper.

Bate, C. M., and E. B. Grunewald (1981). *J. Embryol. Exp. Morphol.* 61:317–330. Embryogenesis of an insect nervous sytem. II. A second class of neuron precursor cells and the origin of the intersegment connectives.

Bates, C. A., and H. Killackey (1984). *Dev. Brain Res.* 13:265–273. The emergence of a discretely distributed pattern of corticospinal projection neurons.

Bates, C. A., and H. P. Killackey (1985). *J. Comp. Neurol.* 240:265–287. The organization of the neonatal rat's brainstem trigeminal complex and its role in the formation of central trigeminal pathways.

Bate, C. M., C. S. Goodman, N. C. Spitzer (1981). *J. Neurosci.* 1:103–106. Embryonic development of identified neurons: Segment specific differences in H cell homologues.

Bateson, W. (1894). *Materials for the Study of Variation.* Macmillan, London.

Batten, E. H. (1958). *J. Embryol. Exp. Morphol.* 6:597–615. The origin of the acoustic ganglion in the sheep.

Battisti, O., A. Bach, and P. Gerard (1986). *Early Human Dev.* 13:13–20. Brain growth in sick newborn infants: A clinical and real-time ultrasound analysis.

Bauchot, R. (1978). *Brain Behav. Evol.* 15:1–18. Encephalization in vertebrates.

Bauer, K. F. (1953). *Organisation des Nervengewebe und Neurencytiumtheorie.* Urban & Schwarzenberg, Berlin.

Bauer, V. (1904). *Zool. Jahrb. Abt. Anat. Ontog. Tiere* 20:123–150. Zur inneren Metamorphose des Zentralnervensystems der Insekten.

Baumann, L., and W. Landauer (1943). *J. Comp. Neurol.* 79:153–163. Polydactyly and anterior horn cells in fowl.

Bautzmann, H. (1933). *Arch. Entw.-Mech. Organ.* 128:666–765. Über Determinationsgrad und Wirkungsbeziechungen der Randzonenteilanlagen (Chorda, Ursegmente, Seitenplatte und Kopfdarmanlage) bei Urodelen und Anuren.

Bautzmann, H. (1955). *Naturwissenschaften* 42: 286–294. Die Problemlage des Spemannschen Organisators.

Bayer, S. A. (1979a). *J. Comp. Neurol.* 183:89–106. The development of the septal region in the rat. I. Neurogenesis examined with ^{3}H-thymidine autoradiography.

Bayer, S. A. (1979b). *J. Comp. Neurol.* 183:107–120. The development of the septal region in the rat. II. Morphogenesis in normal and X-irradiated embryos.

Bayer, S. A. (1980a). *J. Comp. Neurol.* 190:87–114. Development of the hippocampal region in the rat. I. Neurogenesis examined with ^{3}H-thymidine autoradiography.

Bayer, S. A. (1980b). *J. Comp. Neurol.* 190:115–134. Development of the hippocampal region in the rat. II. Morphogenesis during embryonic and early postnatal life.

Bayer, S. A. (1980c). *J. Comp. Neurol.* 194:845–875. Quantitative ³H-thymidine radiographic analyses of neurogenesis in the rat amygdala.

Bayer, S. A. (1983). *Exp. Brain Res.* **50**:329–340. [³H]-Thymidine radiographic studies of neurogenesis in the rat olfactory bulb.

Bayer, S. A., and J. Altman (1987). *Prog. Neurobiol.* **29**:57–106. Directions in neurogenetic gradients and patterns of anatomical connections in the telencephalon.

Bayley, N. (1956). *J. Pediat.* **48**:187–194. Growth curves of height and weight by age for boys and girls, scaled according to physical maturity.

Baylor, D. A., and J. G. Nicholls (1971). *Nature* **237**:268–270. Patterns of regeneration between individual nerve cells in the central nervous system of the leech.

Beach, D., B. Durkacz, and P. Nurse (1982). *Nature* **300**:706–709. Functionally homologous cell cycle control genes in fission yeast and budding yeast.

Beach, D. H., and M. Jacobson (1978a). *J. Comp. Neurol.* **183**:603–614. Patterns of cell proliferation in the developing retina of the clawed frog in relation to blood supply and position of choroidal fissure.

Beach, D. H., and M. Jacobson (1978b). *J. Comp. Neurol.* **183**:615–623. Influences of thyroxine on cell proliferation in the retina of the clawed frog at different ages.

Beach, D. H., and M. Jacobson (1978c). *J. Comp. Neurol.* **183**:625–632. Patterns of cell proliferation in the retina of the clawed frog during development.

Beach, F. A. (1975). *Psychoneuroendocrinology* **1**:3–23. Hormonal modification of sexually dimorphic behavior.

Beale, L. S. (1860). *Phil. Trans. Roy. Soc. (London) Ser. B.* **1860**:611–618. On the distribution of nerves to the elementary fibres of striped muscle.

Beale, L. S. (1862). *Phil. Trans. Roy. Soc. (London) Ser. B.* **1862**:889–910. Further observations on the distribution of nerves to the elementary fibres of striped muscles.

Beams, H. W., and R. G. Kessel (1968). *Int. Rev. Cytol.* **23**:209–267. The Golgi apparatus: Structure and function.

Bear, M. F., and W. Singer (1986). *Nature* **320**:172–176. Modulation of visual cortical plasticity by acetylcholine and noradrenaline.

Bear, M. F., M. A. Paradiso, M. Schwartz, S. B. Nelson, K. M. Carnes, and J. D. Daniels (1983). *Nature* **302**:245–247. Two methods of catecholamine depletion in kitten visual cortex yield different effects on plasticity.

Bear, M. F., K. M. Carnes, and F. F. Ebner (1985). *J. Comp. Neurol.* **237**:519–532. Postnatal changes in the distribution of acetylcholinesterase in kitten striate cortex.

Bear, R. S., and F. O. Schmitt (1936). *J. Opt. Soc. Am.* **26**:206–212. The optics of nerve myelin.

Bear, R. S., K. J. Palmer, and F. O. Schmitt (1941). *J. Cell Comp. Physiol.* **17**:355–367. X-ray diffraction studies of nerve lipides.

Beard, J. (1889). *Proc. Roy. Soc. (London) Ser. B.* **46**:108–118. The early development of Lepidosteus osseus.

Beard, J. (1892). *Anat. Anz.* **7**:191–206. The transient ganglion-cells and their nerves in Raja batis.

Beard, J. (1896a). *Zool. Jahrbücher Abt. morphol.* **9**:1–106. The history of a transient nervous apparatus in certain Ichthyopsida. An account of the development and degeneration of ganglion-cells and nerve fibres.

Beard, J. (1896b). *On Certain Problems of Vertebrate Embryology.* Gustav Fischer, Jena.

Beaudoin, A. R. (1955). *Anat. Rec.* **121**:81–96. The development of lateral motor column cells in the lumbo-sacral cord in *Rana pipiens.* I. Normal development and development following unilateral limb ablation.

Beaudoin, A. R. (1956). *Anat. Rec.* **125**:247–259. The development of lateral motor column cells in the lumbo-sacral cord in *Rana pipiens.* II. Development under the influence of thyroxine.

Beaulaton, J., and R. A. Lockshin (1982). *Int. Rev. Cytol.* **79**:215–235. The relation of programmed cell death to development and reproduction; comparative studies and an attempt at classification.

Beaulieu, C., and M. Colonnier (1987). *J. Comp. Neurol.* **266**:478–494. The effect of the richness of the environment on cat visual cortex.

Beaulieu, C., and M. Colonnier (1988). *J. Comp. Neurol.* **274**:347–356. Richness of environment affects the number of contacts formed by boutons containing flat vesicles but does not alter the number of these boutons per neuron.

Beazley, L., M. J. Keating, and R. M. Gaze (1972). *Vision Res.* **12**:407–410. The appearance, during development, of responses in the optic tectum following stimulation of the ipsilateral eye in *Xenopus laevis.*

Beazley, L. D. (1979). *Exp. Neurol.* **63**:411–419. Intertectal connections are not modified by visual experience in developing *Hyla moorei.*

Beazley, L. D. (1981). *Dev. Biol.* **85**:164–170. Retinal ganglion cell death and regeneration of abnormal retinotectal projections after removal of a segment of optic nerve in *Xenopus* tadpoles.

Beazley, L. D., J. E. Darby, and V. H. Perry (1986). *Vision Res.* **26**:543–556. Cell death in the retinal ganglion cell layer during optic nerve regeneration for the frog *Rana pipiens.*

Beccari, N. (1907). *Arch. Ital. Anat. e Embr.* **6**:660–708. Ricerche sulle cellule e sullle fibre di Mauthner e sulle loro connessioni in pesci e anfibi.

Bechterew, W. von (1894). *Die Leitungsbahnen im Gehirn und Rückenmark,* Translated from the Russian by R. Weinberg. Verlag von Arthur Georgi, Leipzig.

Bechterew, W. (1899). Die Leitungsbahnen. In *Gehirn Und Ruckenmark,* 2 Aufl. Verlag von Arthur Georgi, Leipzig.

Beck, D. W., R. L. Roberts, and J. J. Olson (1986). *Brain Res.* **381**:131–137. Glial cells influence membrane-associated enzyme activity at the blood-brain barrier.

Becker, D. L., and J. E. Cook (1987). *Development* **301**:323–337. Initial disorder and secondary retinotopic refinement of regenerating axons in the optic tract of the goldfish: Signs of a new role for axon collateral loss.

Beckner, M. (1969). *J. Hist. Biol.* **2**:151–164. Function and teleology.

Bedi, K. S., Y. M. Thomas, C. A. Davies, and J. Dobbing (1980a). *J. Comp. Neurol.* **193**:49–56. Synapse-to-neuron ratios of the frontal and cerebellar cortex of 30-day-old and adult rats undernourished during early postnatal life.

Bedi, K. S., R. Hall, C. A. Davies, and J. Dobbing (1980b). *J. Comp. Neurol.* **193**:863–870. A steriological analysis of the cerebellar granule and Purkinje cells of 30-day-old and adult rats undernourished during early postnatal life.

Bedi, K. S., R. F. Massey, and J. L. Smart (1989). *J. Comp. Neurol.* **289**:89–98. Neuronal and synaptic measurements in the visual cortex of adult rats after undernutrition during normal or artificial rearing.

Beesley, P. W., T. Paladino, C. Gravel, R. A. Hawkes, and J. W. Gurd (1987). *Brain Res.* 408:65–78. Characterization of gp50, a major glycoprotein present in rat brain synaptic membranes with a monoclonal antibody.

Behnke, O. (1975). *Nature* 257:709–710. An outer component of microtubules.

Beidler, L. M. (1963) Dynamics of taste cells, pp. 133–148. In *Olfaction and Taste* (Y. Zotterman, ed.), Pergamon, Oxford.

Beidler, L. M., and R. L. Smallman (1965). *J. Cell Biol.* 27:263–272. Renewal of cells within taste buds.

Bekoff, A. (1976). *Brain Res.* 106: 271–291. Ontogeny of leg motor output in the chick embryo: A neural analysis.

Belecky, T. L., and D. V. Smith (1990). *J. Comp. Neurol.* 293:646–654. Postnatal development of palatal and laryngeal taste buds in the hamster.

Belford, G. R., and H. P. Killackey (1979a). *J. Comp. Neurol.* 183:305–322. Vibrissae representation in subcortical trigeminal centers of the neonatal rat.

Belford, G. R., and H. P. Killackey (1979b). *J. Comp. Neurol.* 188:63–74. The development of vibrissae representation in subcortical trigeminal centers of the neonatal rat.

Bell, C (1811). *Idea of a new anatomy of the brain submitted for observations of his friends.* Strahan and Preston, London. Reprinted in Cranefield (1974).

Bellairs, R. (1959). *J. Embryol. Exp. Morphol.* 7:94–115. The development of the nervous system in chick embryos studied by electron microscopy.

Bellairs, R. (1979). *J. Embryol. Exp. Morph.* 51:227–243. The mechanism of somite segmentation in the chick embryo.

Benedict, F. F. (1919). *Carnegie Inst. of Washington,* Pub. No. 20. Human vitality and efficiency under prolonged restricted diet.

Benes, F. M., T. N. Parks, and F. W. Rubel (1975). *Neurosci. Abstr.* 1:669. Dendritic atrophy following deafferentation in nucleus laminaris of the chicken: An E. M. morphometric analysis.

Benes, F. M., T. N. Parks, and E. W. Rubel (1977). *Brain Res.* 122:1–13. Rapid dendritic atrophy following deafferentation: An EM morphometric analysis.

Benfey, M., and A. J. Aguayo (1982). *Nature* 296:150–152. Extensive elongation of axons from rat brain into peripheral nerve grafts.

Ben Hamida, C., J. C. Bisconte, and S. Margules (1983). *J. Anat. (London)* 137:371–385. Postnatal maturation of the vascularisation of the suprasylvian gyrus of the cat.

Benjamin, P. R. (1976). *Nature* 260:338–340. Interganglionic variation in cell body location of snail neurones does not affect synaptic connections or central axonal projections.

Benjamins, J. A., and M. E. Smith (1984). Metabolism of myelin, pp. 225–258. In *Myelin* (P. Morell, ed.), Plenum, New York.

Benjelloun-Touini, S., C. M. Jacque, P. Dever, F. DeVitry, R. Maunoury, and P. Dupouey (1985). *J. Neuroimmunol.* 9:7–97. Evidence that mouse astrocytes may be derived from radial glia.

Bennett, E. L., M. L. Diamond, D. Krech, and M. R. Rosenzweig (1964). *Science* 146:610–619. Chemical and anatomical plasticity of brain.

Bennett, G., L. DiGiamberardino, H. L. Koenig, and B. Droz (1973). *Brain Res.* 60:129–146. Axonal migration of protein and glycoprotein to nerve endings. II. Radioautographic analysis of the renewal of glycoproteins in nerve endings of chicken ciliary ganglion after intracerebral injection of [^{3}H] fucose and [^{3}H] gluscosamine.

Bennett, G. S. (1987). *Curr. Top. Dev. Biol.* 21:151–184. Changes in intermediate filament composition during neurogenesis.

Bennett, G. S., and C. DiLullo (1985). *J. Cell Biol.* 100:1799–1804. Slow posttranslational modification of a neurofilament protein.

Bennett, M. R. (1972). *Autonomic Neuromuscular Transmission,* Cambridge University Press, London.

Bennett, M. R. (1983). *Physiolog. Rev.* 63:915–1048. Development of neuromuscular synapses.

Bennett, M. R., and N. A. Lavidis (1984). *J. Neurosci.* 4:2204–2212. Development of the topographical projection of motor neurons to a rat muscle accompanies loss of polyneuronal innervation.

Bennett, M. R., and A. G. Pettigrew (1974a). *J. Physiol. (London)* 241:515–545. The formation of synapses in striated muscle during development.

Bennett, M. R., and A. G. Pettigrew (1974b). *J. Physiol. (London)* 241:547–573. The formation of synapses in reinnervated and cross-reinnervated striated muscle during development.

Bennett, M. R., and A. G. Pettigrew (1975). *J. Physiol. (London)* 252:203–239. The formation of synapses in amphibian striated muscle during development.

Bennett, M. R., and A. G. Pettigrew (1976). *Cold Spring Harbor Symp. Quant. Biol.* 40:409–424. The formation of neuromuscular synapses.

Bennett, M. R., and J. Raftos (1977). *J. Physiol. (London)* 265:261–295. The formation and regression of synapses during the reinnervation of axolotl striated muscles.

Bennett, M. R., E. M. McLachlan, and R. S. Taylor (1973a). *J. Physiol. (London)* 233:481–500. The formation of synapses in reinnervated mammalian striated muscle.

Bennett, M. R., E. M. McLachlan, and R. S. Taylor (1973b). *J. Physiol. (London)* 233:501–508. The formation of synapses in mammalian striated muscle reinnervated with autonomic preganglionic nerves.

Bennett, M. R., A. G. Pettigrew, and R. S. Taylor (1973c). *J. Physiol. (London)* 230:331–357. The formation of synapses in reinnervated and cross-reinnervated adult avian muscle.

Bennett, M. R., R. Lindeman, and A. G. Pettigrew (1979). *J. Embryol. Exp. Morphol.* 54:141–154. Segmental innervation of the chick forelimb following embryonic manipulation.

Bennett, M. R., D. F. Davey, and K. E. Uebel (1980). *J. Comp. Neurol.* 189:335–357. The growth of segmental nerves from the brachial myotomes into the proximal muscles of the chick forelimb during development.

Bennett, M. R., D. F. Davey, and J. Marshall (1983). *J. Comp. Neurol.* 215:217–227. The growth of nerves in relation to the formation of pre-muscle cell masses in the developing chick forelimb.

Benoit, P., and J.-P. Changeux (1975). *Brain Res.* 99:354–358. Consequences of tenotomy on the evolution of multiinnervation in developing rat soleus muscle.

Benowitz, L., and H. J. Karten (1976). *J. Comp. Neurol.* 167:503–520. Organization of the tectofugal pathway in the pigeon: A retrograde transport study.

Benowitz, L. I., and A. Routtenberg (1987). *Trends Neurosci.* 10:527–532. A membrane phosphoprotein associated with neural development, axonal regeneration, phospholipid metabolism, and synaptic plasticity.

Benowitz, L. I., M. G. Yoon, and E. R. Lewis (1983). *Science* 222:185–188. Transported proteins in the regenerating optic nerve: Regulation by interactions with the optic tectum.

Benson, T. E., D. K. Ryugo, and J. W. Hinds (1984). *J. Neurosci.* 4:638–653. Effects of sensory deprivation on the developing mouse olfactory system: A light and electron microscopic, morphometric analysis.

Bensted, J. P. M., J. Dobbing, R. S. Morgan, R. T. W. Reid, and G. P. Wright (1957). *J. Embryol. Exp. Morphol.* 5:428–437. Neuroglial development and myelination in the spinal cord of the chick embryo.

Bentley, D., and H. Keshishian (1982). *Trends Neurosci.* 5:364–367. Pioneer neurons and pathways in insect appendages.

Bentley, D. R., and R. R. Hoy (1970). *Science* 170:1409–1411. Postembryonic development of adult motor patterns in crickets: A neural analysis.

Benton, J. W., H. W. Moser, P. R. Dodge, and S. Carr (1966). *Pediatrics* 38:801–807. Modification of the schedule of myelination in the rat by early nutritional deprivation.

Benzer, S. (1973). *Sci. Am.* 229:24–37. Genetic dissection of behavior.

Berg, D. K., R. B. Kelly, P. B. Sargent, P. Williamson, and Z. Hall (1972). *Proc. Natl. Acad. Sci. U.S.A.* 69:147. Binding of a a-bungarotoxin to acetylcholine receptor in mammalian muscle.

Bergen, L. A., and G. G. Borisy (1980). *J. Cell Biol.* 84:141–150. Head to tail polymerization of microtubules *in vitro.* Electron microscopic analysis of seeded assembly.

Berger, B., A. M. Thierry, J. P. Tassin, and M. A. Moyne (1976). *Brain Res.* 106:133–145. Dopaminergic innervation of the rat prefrontal cortex: A fluorescence histochemical study.

Berger, H. (1921). *Z. Ges. Neurol. Psychiat.* 69:46–59. Untersuchungen uber den Zellgehalt der menschlichen Grosshirnrinde.

Bergey, G. K., R. K. Hunt, and H. Holtzer (1973). *Anat. Rec.* 175:271. Selective effects of bromodeoxy-uridine on developing *Xenopus laevis* retina.

Bergh, R. S. (1900). *Anat. Hefte* 14:379–407. Beiträge zur vergleichenden Histologie.

Bergquist, H. (1952). *Acta Zool. Stockholm* :117–187. Studies on the cerebral tube in vertebrates. The neuromeres.

Bergquist, H. (1960). *J. Embryol. Exp. Morphol.* 8:69–72. Volumetric investigation on overgrowth (hypermorphosis) in chick embryo brains.

Bergson, H. (1911). *Creative Evolution,* A. Mitchell, transl. Henry Holt, New York.

Beritoff, J. S. (1969). *Structure and Functions of the Cerebral Cortex* (in Russian), Nauka, Moscow.

Berkley, H. J. (1897). *Johns Hopkins Hosp. Rep.* 6:1–88. Studies on the lesions produced by the action of certain poisons on the cortical nerve cell.

Berl, S., S. Puszkin, and W. K. Nicklas (1973). *Science* 179:441–446. Actomyosin-like protein in brain.

Berland, M., J. Bullier, C. Dehay, Z. Jaffar-Bandjee, and H. Kennedy (1987). *J. Physiol. (London)* 382:95P. Callosal connexions and cytochrome oxidase staining of visual areas V1 and V2 in the prenatal monkey.

Berlin, R. (1858). *Beiträge zur Strukturlehre der Grosshirnwindungen,* Junge, Erlangen.

Berlinrood, M., S. M. McGee-Russell, and R. D. Allen (1972). *J. Cell Sci.* 11:875–886. Patterns of particle movement in nerve fibres *in vitro* - An analysis by photokymography and microscopy.

Berman, N., and P. Sterling (1976). *J. Physiol. (London)* 255:263–274. Cortical suppression of retinocollicular pathway in the monocularly deprived cat.

Bernal, J., and F. Pekonen (1984). *Endocrinology* 114:677–679. Ontogenesis of the nuclear T$_3$ receptor in the human fetal brain.

Bernard, C. (1852). *Mém. Soc. de biol.* 5:77–107. De l'influence du système nerveux grand sympathetique et spécialement sur l'influence que section de ce nerf exerce sur la chaleur animale.

Bernard, C. (1878). Le curare, pp. 237–315. In *La Science expérimentale.* Baillière, Paris.

Bernd, P. (1985). *Dev. Biol.* 112:145–156. Appearance of nerve growth factor receptors on cultured neural crest cells.

Bernd, P., and L. A. Greene (1984). *J. Biol. Chem.* 259:15509–15514. Association of ^{125}I nerve growth factor with PC12 pheochromocytoma cells: Evidence for internalization via high-affinity receptors only and for long term regulation by nerve growth factor of both high and low affinity receptors.

Bernd, P., H. J. Martinez, C. F. Dreyfus, and I. B. Black (1988). *Neuroscience* 26:121–129. Localization of high-affinity and low-affinity nerve growth factor with PC12 pheochromocytoma cells.

Bernfield, M. R. (1981). Organization and remodeling of the extracellular matrix in morphogenesis, pp. 139–162. In *Morphogenesis and Pattern Formation* (T. C. Connelly, L. L. Brinkley, and B. M. Carlson, eds.), Raven Press, New York.

Bernfield, M. R., and N. K. Wessells (1970). *Dev. Biol. Suppl.* 4:195–249. Intra- and extracellular control of epithelial morphogenesis.

Bernhardt, R., and A. Matus (1984). *J. Comp. Neurol.* 226:203–221. Light and electron microscopic studies of the distribution of microtubule-associated protein 2 in rat brain: A difference between the dendritic and axonal cytoskeletons.

Bernhardt, R., G. Huber, A. Matus (1985). *J. Neurosci.* 5:977–991. Differences in the developmental patterns of three microtubule-associated proteins in brain.

Bernier, L., F. Alverez, E. M. Norgard, D. W. Raible, A. Mentaberry, J. G. Schembri, D. D. Sabatini, and D. R. Colman (1987). *J. Neurosci.* 7:2703–2710. Molecular cloning of a 2',3-cyclic nucleotide 3'-phosphodiesterase: mRNAs with different 5' ends encode the same set of proteins in nervous and lymphoid tissues.

Bernstein, B. W., and J. R. Bamburg (1989). *Neuron* 3:257–265. Cycling of actin assembly in synaptosomes and neurotransmitter release.

Bernstein, J. (1912). *Elektrobiologie,* Vieweg, Braunschweig.

Bernstein, J. J., and L. Guth (1961). *Exp. Neurol.* 4:262–275. Nonselectivity in establishment of neuromuscular connections following nerve regeneration in the rat.

Berrill, N. J. (1955). *The Origin of the Vertebrates,* Clarendon Press, Oxford.

Berry, M., and P. M. Bradley (1976a). *Brain Res.* 109:111–132. The application of network analysis to the study of branching patterns of large dendritic fields.

Berry, M., and P. Bradley (1976b). *Brain Res.* 112:1–35. The growth of dendritic trees of Purkinje cells in the cerebellum of the rat.

Berry, M., and J. T. Eayrs (1963). *Nature* 197:884–885. Histogenesis of the cerebral cortex.

Berry, M., and J. T. Eayrs (1966). *J. Anat. (London)* 100:707–722. The effects of X-irradiation on the development of the cerebral cortex.

Berry, M., and R. Flinn (1984). *Proc. R. Soc. (London) Ser. B.* 221:321–348. Vertex analysis of Purkinje cell dendritic trees in the cerebellum of the rat.

Berry, M., and A. C. Riches (1974). *Br. Med. Bull.* 30:135–140. An immunological approach to regeneration in the central nervous system.

Berry, M., and A. W. Rogers (1965). *J. Anat. (London)* 99:691–709. The migration of neuroblasts in the developing cerebral cortex.

Berry, M., and A. W. Rogers (1966). Histogenesis of mammalian neocortex, pp. 197–205. In *Evolution of the Forebrain* (R. Hassler and H. Stephan, eds.), Plenum, New York.

Berry, M., A. W. Rogers, and J. T. Eayrs (1964a). *Nature* 203:591–593. Pattern of cell migration during cortical histogenesis.

Berry, M., A. W. Rogers, and J. T. Eayrs (1964b). *J. Anat. (London)* 98:291–292. The pattern and mechanism of migration of the neuroblasts of the developing cerebral cortex.

Berry, M., P. Bradley, and S. Borges (1978). *Prog. Brain Res.* 48:133–146. Environmental and genetic determinants of connectivity in the central nervous system. An approach through dendritic field analysis.

Berry, M., P. McConnell, and J. Sievers (1980). Dendritic growth and the control of neuronal form, pp. 67–101. In *current topics in development biology*, Vol. 15, (K. Hunt, ed.), Academic Press, New York.

Berry, M., S. Hall, R. Follows, L. Rees, N. Gregson, and J. Sievers (1988a). *J. Neurocytol.* 17:727–744. Response of axons and glia at the site of anastomosis between the optic nerve and cellular or acellular sciatic nerve grafts.

Berry, M., L. Rees, S. Hall, P. Yiu, and J. Sievers (1988b). *Brain Res. Bull.* 20:223–231. Optic axons regenerate into sciatic nerve isografts only in the presence of Schwann cells.

Bershadsky, A. D., and J. M. Vasiliev (1988). *Cytoskeleton.* Plenum, New York.

Berthold, C.-H., and I. Nilsson (1987). *J. Neurocytol.* 16:811–828. Schwann cells in developing feline L7 ventral spinal roots.

Berthold, C.-H., and S. Skoglund (1968). *Acta Societatis Medicorum Upsaliensis* 73:127–144. Postnatal development of felin paranodal myelin sheath segments. II. Electron microscopy.

Bethe, A. (1900). *Archiv Mikroskop. Anat.* 55:513–558. Ueber die Neurofibrillen in den Ganglienzellen von Wirbelthieren und ihre Beziehungen zu den Golginetzen.

Bethe, A. (1903). *Allgemeine Anatomie und Physiologie des Nervensystems.* Verlag von Georg Thieme, Leipzig.

Bethe, A. (1904). *Deutsche Med. Woch.* 30:1201–1204. Der heutige Stand der Neurontheorie.

Betz, W., and B. J. Sakmann (1973). *J. Physiol. (London)* 230:673–688. Effects of proteolytic enzymes on function and structure of frog neuromuscular junctions.

Betz, W. J. (1987). Motoneuron death and synapse elimination in vertebrates, pp. 117–162. In *The Vertebrate Neuromuscular Junction* (M. M. Salpeter, ed.), Alan Liss, New York.

Betz, W. J., J. H. Caldwell, and R. R. Ribchester (1979). *J. Physiol. (London)* 297:463–478. The size of motor units during post-natal development of rat lumbrical muscle.

Beuche, W., and R. L. Friede (1984). *J. Neurocytol.* 13:767–796. The role of non-resident cells in Wallerian degeneration.

Bevan, S., and J. H. Steinbach (1977). *J. Physiol. (London)* 267:195–213. The distribution of alpha-bungarotoxin binding sites on mammalian skeletal muscle developing *in vivo.*

Beyer, C., and H. H. Feder (1987). *Ann. Rev. Physiol.* 49:349–364. Sex steroids and afferent input: Their roles in brain sexual differentiation.

Bhide, P. G., and K. S. Bedi (1982). *J. Comp. Neurol.* 207:403–409. The effects of environmental diversity on well-fed and previously undernourished rats: I. Body and brain measurements.

Bhide, P. G., and K. S. Bedi (1984a). *J. Comp. Neurol.* 227:296–304. The effects of a lengthy period of environmental diversity on well-fed and previously undernourished rats. I. Neurons and glial cells.

Bhide, P. G., and K. S. Bedi (1984b). *J. Comp. Neurol.* 227:305–310. The effects of a lengthy period of environmental diversity on well-fed and previously undernourished rats. II. Synapse-to-neuron ratios.

Bichat, X. (1801). *Anatomie générale appliquée à la physiologie et à la médecine.* Paris. English transl. by G. Hayward, *General Anatomy Applied to Physiology and Medicine,* 2 Vols. Boston, 1822.

Bidder, F., and C. Kupffer (1857). *Untersuchungen über die Textur des Rückenmarks und die Entwickelung seine Formelemente,* 121 pp. Leipzig.

Bidder, F. H., and A. W. Volkmann (1842). *Die Selbständigkeit des sympathischen Nervensystems durch anatomische Untersuchungen nachgewiesen.* Breitkopf & Härtel, Leipzig.

Bielschowsky, M. (1904). *J. Psychol. Neurol.* 3:169–189. Die silberimprägnation der Neurofibrillen.

Bielschowsky, M. (1923). *J. Psychol. Neurol.* 30:29–76. Über die Oberflächengestaltung des Grosshirnmantels bei Mikrogyrie und bei normaler Entwicklung.

Bignami, A. (1984). *Brain Res.* 300:175–178. Glial fibrillary acidic (GFA) protein in Müller glia. Immunofluorescence study of the goldfish retina.

Bignami, A., and D. Dahl (1973). *Brain Res.* 49:393–402. Differentiation of astrocytes in the cerebellar cortex and the pyramidal tracts of the newborn rat: An immunofluorescence study with antibodies to a protein specific to astrocytes.

Bignami, A., and D. Dahl (1974a). *Nature* 252:55–56. Astrocyte specific protein and radial glia in the cerebral cortex of newborn rat.

Bignami, A., and D. Dahl (1974b). *J. Comp. Neurol.* 153:27–38. Astrocyte-specific protein and neuroglial differentiation: An immunofluorescence study with antibodies to the glial fibrillary acidic protein.

Bignami, A., and D. Dahl (1974c). *J. Comp. Neurol.* 155:219–230. The development of Bergmann glia in mutant mice with cerebellar malformations: Reeler, staggerer and weaver. Immunofluorescence study with antibodies to the glial fibrillary acidic protein.

Bignami, A., and D. Dahl (1975). *Dev. Biol.* **44**: 204–209. Astroglial protein in the developing spinal cord of the chick embryo.

Bignami, A., and D. Dahl (1979). *Exp. Eye Res.* **28**:63–69. The radial glia of Müller in the rat retina and their response to injury. An immunofluorescence study with antibodies to the glial fibrillary acidic protein.

Bignami, A., L. F. Eng, D. Dahl, C. T. Uyeda (1972). *Brain Res.* **43**:429–435. Localization of the glial fibrillary acidic protein in astrocytes by immunofluorescence.

Bignami, A., T. Raju, and D. Dahl (1982). *Dev. Biol.* **91**:286–295. Localization of vimentin, the non-specific intermediate filament protein, in embryonal glia and in early differentiating neurons.

Bijlenga, G., and T. Heaney (1978). *J. Gen. Virol.* **39**:381–385. Post-exposure local treatment of mice infected with rabies with two axonal flow inhibitors, colchicine and vinblastine.

Bijtel, H. (1931). *Roux' Arch. EntwMech* **125**:448–486. Über die Entwicklung des Schwanzes bei Amphibien.

Billings-Gagliardi, S. (1977). *Am. J. Anat.* **150**:73–88. Mode of locomotion of Schwann cells migrating *in vivo*.

Billings-Gagliardi, S., H. deF. Webster, and M. F. O'Connell (1974). *Am. J. Anat.* **141**:375–392. *In vivo* and electron microscopic observations on Schwann cells in developing tadpole nerve fibers.

Billings, S. M. (1972). *Z. Anat. Entwickl.-Gesch.* **136**:168–191. Development of the Mauthner cell in *Xenopus laevis*: A light and electron microscopic study of the perikaryon.

Billings, S. M., and F. J. Swartz (1969). *Z. Anat. Entwicklungsgeschichte* **129**:14–23. DNA content of Mauthner cell nuclei in *Xenopus laevis*: A spectrophotometric study.

Bilozur, M. E., and E. D. Hay (1987). *Dev. Biol.* **125**:19–33. Neural crest migration in 3D extracellular matrix utilizes laminin, fibronectin and collagen.

Binder, L. I., W. L. Dentler, and J. L. Rosenbaum (1975). *Proc. Natl. Acad. Sci. U.S.A.* **72**:1122–1126. Assembly of chick brain tubulin onto flagellar microtubules from *Chlamydomonas* and sea urchin sperm.

Binder, L. I., A. Frankfurter, H. Kim, A. Carceres, M. R. Payne, L. I. Rebhun (1984). *Proc. Natl. Acad. Sci. U.S.A.* **81**:5613–5617. Heterogeneity of microtubule-associated protein 2 during rat brain development.

Binder, L. I., A. Frankfurter, and L. I. Rebhun (1985). *J. Cell Biol.* **101**:1371–1378. The distribution of tau in the mammalian central nervous system.

Binder, M. D., J. C. Houk, T. R. Nichols, W. Z. Rymer, and D. G. Stuart (1982). *Fed. Proc.* **41**:2907–2918. Properties and segmental actions of mammalian muscle receptors: An update.

Biondi, R. J., M. J. Levy, and P. A. Weiss (1972). *Proc. Natl. Acad. Sci. U.S.A.* **69**:1732–1736. An engineering study of the peristaltic drive of axonal flow.

Birch, H. G. (1972). *Am. J. Publ. Hlth* **62**:773–784. Malnutrition, learning and intelligence.

Birch, H. G., and L. Belmont (1964). *Am. J. Orthopsychiat.* **44**:852–861. Auditory-visual integration in normal and retarded readers.

Birks, R. I. (1966). *Ann. N.Y. Acad. Sci.* **135**:8–19. The fine structure of motor nerve endings at frog myoneural junctions.

Birks, R. I., M. C. Mackey, and P. R. Weldon (1972). *J. Neurocytol.* **I**:311–340. Organelle formation from pinocytotic elements in neurites of cultured sympathetic ganglia.

Birmingham, M. K, W. E. Stumpf, and M. Sar (1979). *Experientia* **35**:1240–1241. Nuclear localization of aldosterone in rat brain cells assessed by autoradiography.

Birmingham, M. K., M. Sar, and W. E. Stumpf (1984). *Neurochem. Res.* **9**:333–350. Localization of aldosterone and corticosterone in the central nervous system, assessed by quantiative autoradiography.

Birnstiel, M. L., M. I. H. Chipchase, and B. B. Hyde (1963). *Biochim. Biophys. Acta* **76**:454–462. The nucleolus, a source of ribosomes.

Birren, J. E., and P. D. Wall (1956). *J. Comp. Neurol.* **104**:1–16. Age changes in conduction velocity, refractory period, number of fibers, connective tissue space and blood vessels in sciatic nerve of rats.

Birse, S. C., and G. D. Bittner (1976). *Brain Res.* **113**:575–581. Regeneration of giant axons in earthworms.

Bisby, M. A. (1975). *Exp. Neurol.* **47**:481–489. Inhibition of axonal transport in nerves chronically treated with local anesthetics.

Bisby, M. A. (1982a). Ligature techniques, pp. 193–199. In *Axonal Transport* (D. G. Weiss, ed.), Springer-Verlag, Berlin.

Bisby, M. A. (1982b). *Fed. Proc.* **41**:2307–2311. Functions of retrograde transport.

Bischoff, T. L. W. (1880). *Das Hirngewicht des Menschen*, Bonn, Neusser.

Bisconte, J. C., and R. Marty (1975). *Exp. Brain Res.* **22**:37–56. Etude quantitative du marquage radiographique dans le système nerveux du Rat. II. Caractéristiques finales dans le cerveau de l'animal adulte: Lois d'interprétation et concept de chronoarchitectonic corticale.

Bishop, G. H. (1959). *J. Nerv. Ment. Dis.* **128**:89–114. The relation between nerve fiber size and sensory modality: Phylogenetic implications of the afferent innervation of cortex.

Bishop, G. H., P. Heinbecker, and J. L. O'Leary (1933). *Am. J. Physiol.* **106**:647–669. The function of the non-myelinated fibers of the dorsal roots.

Bishop, J. M. (1983). *Ann. Rev. Biochem.* **52**:301–354. Cellular oncogenes and retroviruses.

Bittner, G. D. (1973). *Am. Zool.* **13**:379–408. Degeneration and regeneration in crustacean neuromuscular systems.

Bjerre, B., A. Bjorklund, and U. Stenevi (1973). *Brain Res.* **60**:161–176. Stimulation of growth of new axonal sprouts from lesioned monoamine neurones in adult rat brain by nerve growth factor.

Bjerre, B., A. Bjorklund, and U. Stenevi (1974a). *Brain Res.* **74**:1–18. Inhibition of the regenerative growth of central noradrenergic neurons by intracerebrally administered anti-NGF serum.

Bjerre, B., A. Bjorklund, and D. C. Edwards (1974b). *Cell Tissue Res.* **148**:441–476. Axonal regeneration of peripheral adrenergic neurons. Effects of antiserum to nerve growth factor in mouse.

Bjerre, B., L. Wiklund, and D. C. Edwards (1975a). *Brain Res.* **92**:257–278. A study of the de- and regenerative changes in the sympathetic nervous system of the adult mouse after treatment with the antiserum to nerve growth factor.

Bjerre, B., A. Bjorklund, W. Mobley, and E. Rosengren (1975b). *Brain Res.* 94:263–277. Short- and long-term effects of nerve growth factor on the sympathetic nervous system in the adult mouse.

Björklund, A., and U. Stenevi (1972). *Science* 175:1251–1253. Nerve growth factor: Stimulation of regenerative growth of central noradrenergic neurons.

Björklund, A., and U. Stenevi (1981). *Brain Res.* 229:403–428. *In vivo* evidence for a hippocampal adrenergic neuronotrophic factor specifically released on septal deafferentation.

Black, I. B. (1978). *Ann. Rev. Neurosci.* 1:183–214. Regulation of autonomic development.

Black, I. B., and S. C. Green (1973). *Brain Res.* 63:291–302. Transsynaptic regulation of adrenergic neuron development: Inhibition of ganglionic blockade.

Black, I. B., and C. Mytilineou (1976a). *Brain Res.* 101:503–521. Trans-synaptic regulation of the development of end organ innervation by sympathetic neurons.

Black, I. B., and C. Mytilineou (1976b). *Brain Res.* 108:199–204. The interaction of nerve growth factor and transsynaptic regulation in the development of target organ innervation by sympathetic neurons.

Black, I. B., E. M. Bloom, and R. W. Hamill (1976). *Proc. Natl. Acad. Sci. U.S.A.* 73:3575–3578. Central regulation of sympathetic neuron development.

Black, M. M., and R. J. Lasek (1979a). *Brain Res.* 171:401–413. Axonal transport of actin: Slow component b is the principal source of actin for the axon.

Black, M. M, and R. J. Lasek (1979b). *Exp. Neurol.* 63:108–119. Slowing of the rate of axonal regeneration during growth and maturation.

Black, M. M, and R. J. Lasek (1980). *J. Cell. Biol.* 86:616–623. Slow components of axonal transport: Two cytoskeletal networks.

Black, M. M., J. M. Aletta, and L. A. Greene (1986). 103:545–557. Regulation of microtubule composition and stability during nerve growth factor-promoted neurite outgrowth.

Black, S. D, and J.-P. Vincent (1988). *Dev. Biol.* 128:65–71. The first cleavage plane and the embryonic axis are determined by separate mechanisms in *Xenopus laevis*.

Blackshaw, S. E., and A. E. Warner (1976a). *J. Physiol. (London)* 255:231–247. Alterations in resting membrane properties during neural plate stages of development of the nervous system.

Blackshaw, S. E., and A. Warner (1976b). *Nature* 262:217–218. Onset of acetylcholine sensitivity and endplate activity in developing myotome muscles of *Xenopus*.

Blackshaw, T. W. (1956). *J. Comp. Neurol.* 105:417–538. Commissural connections of the hippocampal region in the rat, with special reference to their mode of termination.

Blackstad, T. W., and P. R. Flood (1963). *Nature* 198:542–543. Ultrastructure of hippocampal axosomatic synapses.

Blake, R., and H. V. B. Hirsch (1975). *Science* 190:1114–1116. Deficits in binocular depth perception in cats after alternating monocular deprivation.

Blakemore, C. (1974) *Br. Med. Bull.* 30:152–157. Development of functional connexions in the mammalian visual system.

Blakemore, C., and G. F. Cooper (1970). *Nature* 228: 477–478. Development of the brain depends on visual experience.

Blakemore, C., and R. C. Van Sluyters (1974). *J. Physiol. (London)* 237:195–216. Reversal of the physiological effects of monocular deprivation in kittens. Further evidence for a sensitive period.

Blakemore, C., and R. C. Van Sluyters (1975). *J. Physiol. (London)* 248:663–716. Innate and environmental factors in the development of the kitten's visual cortex.

Blakemore, C., R. C. Van Sluyters, and J. A. Movshon (1975). *Cold Spring Harbor Symp. Quant. Biol.* 40:601–609. Synaptic competition in the kitten's visual cortex.

Blakemore, L., and R. Van Sluyters (1975). *J. Physiol. (London)* 248:663–716. Innate and environmental factors in the development of the kitten's visual cortex.

Blakemore, W. F. (1969). *J. Anat. (London)* 104:423–433. The ultrastructure of the subependymal plate in the rat.

Blakemore, W. F. (1975). *Acta neuropathologica* 6:Suppl. 273–278. The ultrastructure of normal and reactive microglia.

Blakemore, W. F., and R. D. Jolly (1972). *J. Neurocytol.* 1:69–84. The subependymal plate and associated ependyma in the dog: An ultrastructural study.

Blakemore, W. F., and R. C. Patterson (1975). *J. Neurocytol.* 4:573–585. Observations on the interaction of Schwann cells and astrocytes following X-irradiation of neonatal spinal cord.

Blam, S. B., R. Michell, E. Tischer, J. S. Rubin, M. Silva, S. Silver, J. C. Fiddes, J. A. Abraham, and S. A. Aaronson (1988). *Oncogene* 3:129–136. Addition of growth hormone secretion signal to basic fibroblast growth factor results in cell transformation and secretion of aberrant forms of the protein.

Blanks, J. C., R. J. Mullen, and M. M. LaVail (1982). *J. Comp. Neurol.* 212:231–246. Retinal degeneration in the *pcd* cerebellar mutant mouse. II. Electron microscopic analysis.

Blanton, S. (1919). *Ment. Hyg. N.Y.* 3:343–386. Mental and nervous changes in the children of the Volksschulen of Trier, Germany, caused by malnutrition. Reprinted in part in Brozek (1985).

Blasdel, G. G., and D. Fitzpatrick (1984). *J. Neurosci.* 4:880–895. Physiological organization of layer 4 in macaque striate cortex.

Blasdel, G. G., and J. S. Lund (1983). *J. Neurosci.* 3:1389–1413. Termination of afferent axons in macaque striate cortex.

Blasdel, G. G., and G. Salama (1986). *Nature* 321:579–585. Voltage-sensitive dyes reveal a modular organization in monkey striate cortex.

Blatt, G. J., and L. M. Eisenman (1985). *J. Neurogenet.* 2:51–66. A qualitative and quantitative light microscopic study of the inferior olivary complex in the adult staggerer mutant mouse.

Blatt, G. J., and L. M. Eisenman (1988). *J. Comp. Neurol.* 267:603–615. Topographic and zonal organization of the olivocerebellar projection in the reeler mutant mouse.

Blaurock, A. E. (1976). *Biophys. J.* 16:491–501. Myelin x-ray patterns reconciled.

Blenkinsopp, W. K. (1967). *J. Cell Sci.* 2:305–308. Effect of tritiated thymidine on cell proliferation.

Blinkov, S. M., and I. Glezer (1968). *The Human Brain in Figures and Tables*, Plenum, New York.

Blinzinger, K. H., and G. W. Kreutzberg (1968). *Z. Zellforsch. Mikrosk. Anat.* 85:145–147. Displacement of synaptic terminals from regenerating motoneurons by microglial cells.

Bliss, T. V. P., and S. H. Chung (1974). *Nature* 252:153–155.

An electrophysiological study of the hippocampus of the "reeler" mutant mouse.

Bliss, T. V. P., and T. Lomo (1973a). *J. Physiol. (London)* **232**:331–356. Long-lasting potentiation of synaptic transmission in the dentate area of the anesthetized rabbit following stimulation of the perforant path.

Bliss, T. V. P., and T. Lomo (1973b). *J. Physiol. (London)* **232**:357–374. Long-lasting potentiation of synaptic transmission in the dentate area of the anesthetized rabbit following stimulation of the perforant path.

Block, J. B., and W. B. Essman (1965). *Nature* **205**:1136–1137. Growth hormone administration during pregnancy: A behavioral difference in offspring rats.

Bloom, B. S. (1964). *Stability and Change in Human Characteristics*, Wiley, New York.

Bloom, E. M., and R. Tompkins (1976). *J. Exp. Zool.* **195**:237–246. Selective reinnervation in skin rotation grafts in *Rana pipiens*.

Bloom, F. E. (1972). The formation of synaptic junctions in developing rat brain, pp. 101–120. In *Structure and Function of Synapses* (G. D. Pappas, and D. P. Purpura, eds.), Raven Press, New York.

Bloom, F. E., and G. K. Aghajanian (1968). *J. Ultrastruct. Res.* **22**:361–375. Fine structural and cytochemical analysis of the staining of synaptic junctions with phosphotungstic acid.

Bloom, G. S., T. A. Schoenfield, and R. B. Vallee (1984). *J. Cell Biol.* **98**:320–330. Widespread distribution of the major polypeptide component of MAP1 (Microtubule-associated protein 1) in the nervous system.

Bloom, G. S., F. C. Luca, and R. B. Vallee (1985). *Proc. Natl. Acad. Sci. U.S.A.* **82**:5404–5408. Microtubule associated protein 1B: Identification of a major component of the neuronal cytoskeleton.

Bloom, W. (1938). *Physiol. Rev.* **17**:589–617. Cellular differentiation and tissue culture.

Blottner, D., W. Brüggemann, and K. Unsicker (1989). *Neurosci. Let.* **105**:316–320. Ciliary neurotrophic factor supports target-deprived preganglionic sympathetic spinal cord neurons.

Blue, M. E., and J. G. Parnavelas (1983). *J. Neurocytol.* **12**:697–712. The formation and maturation of synapses in the visual cortex of the rat. II. Quantitative analysis.

Bluemink, J. G., J. Faber, and K. A. Lawson (1984). *Nature* **312**:107. Basement membranes and epithelia.

Blum, P. (1893). *Z. wiss. Med.* **10**:314–315. Der Formaldehyd als Härtungsmittel. Vorläufige Mittheilung.

Blumenbach, J. F. (1792). *An Essay On Generation.* Translated from the German by Alexander Crichton. T. Cadell, London.

Blumenbach, J. F. (1817). *The Institutions of Physiology.* Translated from the Latin of the third and last edition [1810] by J. Elliotson. 2nd Edn. Bensley and Son, for E. Cox and Son, London.

Blunt, M. J., C. P. Wendell-Smith, P. B. Paisley, and F. Baldwin (1967). *J. Anat. (London)* **101**:13–26. Oxidative enzyme activity in macroglia and axons of cat optic nerve.

Blunt, M. J., F. Baldwin, and C. P. Wendell-Smith (1972) *Z. Zellforsch. Mikrosk. Anat.* **124**:293–310. Gliogenesis and myelination in kitten optic nerve.

Boas, J. A. R., R. L. Ramsey, A. J. Riesen, and J. P. Walker (1969). *Psychon. Sci.* **15**:251–252. Absence of change in some measures of cortical morphology in dark-reared adult rats.

Bockman, D. E., M. E. Redmond, K. Waldo, H. Davis and M. L. Kirby (1987). *Amer. J. Anat.* **180**:332–341. Effect of neural crest ablation on development of the heart and arch arteries in the chick.

Bodenstein, D. (1957). *J. Exp. Zool.* **136**:89–115. Studies on nerve regeneration in *Periplaneta americana*.

Bodian, D. (1936). *Anat. Rec.* **65**:89–97. A new method for staining nerve fibers and nerve endings in mounted paraffin sections.

Bodian, D. (1937). *J. Comp. Neurol.* **68**:117–159. The structure of the vertebrate synapse. A study of the axon endings on Mauthner's cell and neighboring centers in the goldfish.

Bodian, D. (1947). *Symp. Soc. Exp. Biol.* **1**:163–178. Nucleic acid in nerve-cell regeneration.

Bodian, D. (1948). *Bull. Johns Hopkins Hosp.* **83**:1–108. The virus, the nerve cell and paralysis. A study, of experimental poliomyelitis in the spinal cord.

Bodian, D. (1952). *Cold Spring Harbor Symp. Quant. Biol.* **17**:1–13. Introductory survey of neurons.

Bodian, D. (1964). *Bull. Johns Hopkins Hosp.* **114**:13–40. An electron-microscopic study of the monkey spinal cord. I. Fine structure of normal motor column. II. Effects of retrograde chromatolysis. III. Cytologic effects of mild and virulent poliovirus infection.

Bodian, D. (1966a). *Bull. Johns Hopkins Hosp.* **119**:129–149. Development of fine structure of spinal cord in monkey foetuses. I. Motoneuron neuropil at time of onset of reflex activity.

Bodian, D. (1966b). *Bull. Johns Hopkins Hosp.* **119**:217–234. Spontaneous degeneration in the spinal cord of monkey foetuses.

Bodian, D. (1968). *J. Comp. Neurol.* **133**:113–166. Development of fine structure of spinal cord in monkey fetuses. II. Pre-reflex period to period of long intersegmental reflexes.

Bodian, D., and H. A. Howe (1941a). *Bull. Johns Hopkins Hosp.* **68**:248–267. Experimental studies on intraneural spread of poliomyelitis virus.

Bodian, D., and H. A. Howe (1941b). *Bull. Johns Hopkins Hosp.* **69**:79–85. The rate of progression of poliomyelitis virus in nerves.

Bodian, D., and R. C. Mellors (1945). *J. Exp. Med.* **81**:469–488. The regeneration cycle of motoneurons, with special reference to phosphatase activity.

Bodick, N., and C. Levinthal (1980). *Proc. Natl. Acad. Sci. U.S.A.* **77**:4374–4378. Growing optic nerve fibers follow neighbors during embryogenesis.

Boeke, J. (1932). Nerve endings, motor and sensory, pp. 243–315. In *Cytology and Cellular Pathology of the Nervous System*, Vol. 1, (W. Penfield, ed.), Hoeber, New York.

Boeke, J. (1942). *Schweiz Arch. Neurol. Psychiat.* **49**:9–32. Sur les synapses à distance. Les glomerules cérébelleux, leur structure et leur développement.

Boerema, I. (1929). *Arch. Entw.-Mech. Organ.* **115**:601–615. Die Dynamik des Medullarrohrschlusses.

Bogarad, L. D., M. F. Utset, A. Awgulewitsch, T. Miki, C. P. Hart, and F. H. Ruddle (1989). *Dev. Biol.* **133**:537–549. The developmental expression pattern of a new murine homeo box gene: *Hox-2*.

Bohn, M. C. (1979). *Effect of Hydrocortisone on Neurogenesis in the Neonatal Rat Brain: a Morphological and Autoradiographic Study* (PhD dissertation). Storrs: Univ. of Connecticut.

Bohn, M. C. (1980). *Neuroscience* 5:2003–2012. Granule cell genesis in the hippocampus of rats treated neonatally with hydrocortisone.

Bohn, M. C., and V. L. Friedrich, Jr. (1982). *J. Neurosci.* 2:1292–1298. Recovery of myelination in rat optic nerve after developmental retardation by cortisol.

Bohn, M. C., and J. M. Lauder (1978). *Dev. Neurosci.* 1:250–266. The effects of neonatal hydrocortisone on rat cerebellar development. An autoradiographic and light-microscopic study.

Bohn, M. C., and J. M. Lauder (1980). *Dev. Neurosci.* 3:81–89. Cerebellar granule cell genesis in the hydrocortisone-treated rat.

Bohn, M. C., M. Goldstein, and I. B. Black (1982). *Dev. Biol.* 89:299–308. Expression of phenylethanolamine N-methyltransferase in rat sympathetic ganglia and extra-adrenal chromaffin tissue.

Bohn, M. C., E. Bloom, M. Goldstein, and I. B. Black (1984). *Dev. Biol.* 105:130–136. Glucocorticoid regulation of phenylethanolamine N-methyltransferase (PNMT) in organ culture of superior cervical ganglion.

Bok, S. T. (1915). *Folia Neurobiol.* 9:475–565. Die Entwicklung der Hirnnerven und ihrer zentralen Bahnen. Die stimulogene Fibrillation.

Bok, S. T. (1929). *Z. ges. Neurol. Psychiat.* 121:682–750. Der Einfluss in den Furchen und Windungen auftretenden Krummungen der Grosshirnrinde auf die Rindenarchitektur.

Bok, S. T. (1959). *Histonomy of the Cerebral Cortex.* Elsevier, Amsterdam.

Bolin, L. M., and R. V. Rouse (1986). *J. Neurocytol.* 15:29–36. Localization of *Thy-1* expression during postnatal development of the mouse cerebellar cortex.

Boll, F. (1874). *Arch. f. Psychiatr. u. Nervenkr.* 4:71. Die histologie und histogenese der nervösen Centralorgane.

Boller, K., D. Vestweber, and R. Kemler (1985). *J. Cell Biol.* 100:327–332. Cell adhesion molecule uvomorulin is localized in the intermediate junctions of adult intestinal epithelial cells.

Boncinelli, E., R. Somma, D. Acampora, M. Pannese, M. D'Esposito, and A. Simeone (1988). *Hum. Reprod.* 3:880–886. Organization of human homeobox genes.

Bondareff, W. (1965). *Anat. Rec.* 152:119–128. The extracellular compartment of the cerebral cortex.

Bondareff, W. (1966). *Z. Zellforsch. Mikrosk. Anat.* 72:487–495. Electron microscopic evidence for the existence of an intercellular substance in rat cerebral cortex.

Bondareff, W. (1967a). *Anat. Rec.* 157:527–536. An intercellular substance in rat cerebral cortex: Submicroscopic distribution of ruthenium red.

Bondareff, W. (1967b). *Z. Zellforsch. Mikrosk. Anat.* 81:366–373. Demonstration of an intercellular substance in mouse cerebral cortex.

Bondareff, W., and J. J. Pysh (1968). *Anat. Rec.* 160:773–780. Distribution of the extracellular space during postnatal maturation of rat cerebral cortex.

Bondy, S. C. (1972). *J. Neurochem.* 19:1769–1776. Axonal migration of various ribonucleic acid species along the optic tract of the chick.

Bondy, S. C., and C. J. Madsen (1971). *J. Neurobiol.* 2:279–286. Development of rapid axonal flow in the chick embryo.

Bondy, S. C., and C. J. Madsen (1973). *J. Neurobiol.* 4:535–542. Axoplasmic transport of RNA.

Bondy, S. C., and C. J. Madsen (1974). *J. Neurochem.* 23:905–910. The extent of axoplasmic transport during development, determined by migration of various radioactively-labelled materials.

Bondy, S. C., and P. C. Marchisio (1973). *Exp. Neurol.* 41:29–37. Development of axonal transport of RNA and its precursors in the optic pathway of the chick embryo.

Bone, Q. (1964). *Int. Rev. Neurobiol.* 6:99–147. Patterns of muscular innervation in the lower chordates.

Bonhoeffer, F., and A. Gierer (1984). *Trends Neurosci.* 1:378–381. How do retinal axons find their targets on the tectum?

Bonhoeffer, F., and J. Huf (1982). *EMBO J.* 1:427–431. *In vitro* experiments on axon guidance demonstrating an anterior-posterior gradient on the tectum.

Bonhoeffer, F., and J. Huf (1985). *Nature* 315:409–410. Position-dependent properties of retinal axons and their growth cones.

Bonin, G. von (1960). *Some Paper on the Cerebral Cortex.* Springfield: Thomas.

Bonner, J. T. (1947). *J. Exp. Zool.* 106:1–26. Evidence for the formation of cell aggregates by chemotaxis in the development of slime mould *Dictyostelium discoideum.*

Bonner, J. T. (1959). *The Cellular Slime Molds*, Princeton University Press, Princeton, N.J.

Bonner, P. H. (1978). *Dev. Biol.* 66:207–219. Nerve dependent changes in clonable myoblast populations.

Bonner, P. H. (1980). *Dev. Biol.* 76:79–86. Differentiation of chick embryo myoblast is transiently sensitive to functional denervation.

Bonnet, R. (1878). *Morphol. Jahrb. Leipzig* 4:329–398. Studien ueber die Innervation der Haarbälge der Hausthiere.

Boothe, R. G., V. Dobson, and D. Y. Teller (1985). *Ann. Rev. Neurosci.* 8:495–545. Postnatal development of vision in human and nonhuman primates.

Borasio, G. D., J. John, A. Wittinghofer, Y.-A. Barde, M. Sendtner, and R. Heumann (1989). *Neuron* 2:1087–1096. *ras* p21 protein promotes survival and fiber outgrowth of cultured embryonic neurons.

Bordeu, T. (1775). *Recherches sur les maladies chroniques.* In *Oeuvres complètes de Bordeu.* Paris, 1818.

Borgens, R. B., L. F. Jaffe, and M. J. Cohen (1980). *Proc. Natl. Acad. Sci. U.S.A.* 77:1209–1213. Large and persistent electrical currents enter the transected lamprey spinal cord.

Borgens, R. B., E. Roederer, and M. J. Cohen (1981). *Science* 213:611–617. Enhanced spinal cord regeneration in lamprey by applied electric fields.

Boring, E. G. (1942). *Sensation and Perception in the History of Experimental Psychology.* Appleton-Century-Crofts, New York.

Boring, E. G. (1950). *A History of Experimental Psychology,* 2nd edn. Appleton-Century-Crofts, New York.

Boring, E. G. (1963). *History of Psychology, and Science: Selected Papers,* (R. I. Watson, and D. T. Campbell, eds.), Wiley, New York.

Borisy, G. G., and E. W. Taylor (1967a). *J. Cell Biol.* 34:525–533. The mechanism of action of colchicine: Binding of colchicine-^{3}H to cellular protein.

Borisy, G. G., J. B. Olmsted, J. M. Marcum, and C. Allen (1974). *Fed. Proc.* 33:167–174. Microtubule assembly *in vitro.*

Borit, A., and G. C. McIntosh (1981). *Neuropathol. Appl. Neu-*

robiol. 7:279–287. Myelin basic protein and glial fibrillary acidic protein in human fetal brain.

Born, D. E., and E. W. Rubel (1985). *J. Comp. Neurol.* 231:435–445. Afferent influences on brain stem auditory nuclei of the chicken: neuron number and size following cochlea removal.

Born, D. E., and E. W. Rubel (1988). *J. Neurosci.* 8:901–919. Afferent influences on brain stem auditory nuclei of the chicken: Presynaptic action potentials regulate protein sythesis in nucleus magnocellularis neurons.

Born, G. (1896). *Arch. Entw. Mech. Organ.* 4:349–465, 517–623. Ueber Verwachsungversuche mit Amphibienlarven.

Bornstein, M. B., and M. R. Murray (1958). *J. Biophys. Biochem. Cytol.* 4:499–504. Serial observations on patterns of growth, myelin formation, maintenance and degeneration in cultures of newborn rat and kitten cerebellum.

Bornstein, M. B., H. Iwanami, G. M. Lehrer, and L. Breitbart (1968). *Z. Zellforsch. Mikrosk. Anat. Abt. Histochem.* 92:197–206. Observations on the appearance of neuromuscular relationships in cultured mouse tissues.

Borst, P., L. A. Grivell, and G. S. P. Groot (1984). *Trends Biochem. Sci.* 9:128–130. Organelle DNA.

Bosch, E. P., J. G. Assouline, J. F. Miller, and R. Lim (1984). *Brain Res.* 304:311–319. Glia maturation factor promotes proliferation and morphologic expression of rat Schwann cells.

Bosch, E. P., W. Zhong, and R. Lim (1989). *J. Neurosci.* 9:3690–3698. Axonal signals regulate expression of glia maturation factor-beta in Schwann cells: An immunohistochemical study of injured sciatic nerves and cultured Schwann cells.

Boss, V. C., and J. T. Schmidt (1984). *J. Neurosci.* 4:2891–2905. Activity and the formation of ocular dominance patches in dually innervated tectum of goldfish.

Botha-Antoun, E., S. Babayan, and J. K. Harfouche (1968). *J. Trop. Pediat.* 14:112–115. Intellectual development relating to nutritional status.

Bothwell, M. A., and E. M. Shooter (1977). *J. Biol. Chem.* 252:8532–8536. Dissociation equilibrium constant of β-nerve growth factor.

Bottjer, S. W. (1987). *J. Neurobiol.* 18:125–139. Ontogenetic changes in the pattern of androgen accumulation in song-control nuclei of male zebra finches.

Bottjer, S. W., S. L. Glaessner, and A. P. Arnold (1985). *J. Neurosci.* 5:1556–1562. Ontogeny of brain nuclei controlling song learning and behavior in zebra finches.

Boulder Committee: Angevine, J. B., Jr., D. Bodian, A. J. Coulombre, M. V. Edds, Jr., V. Hamburger, M. Jacobson, K. M. Lyser, M. C. Prestige, R. L. Sidman, S. Varon, and P. Weiss (1970). *Anat. Rec.* 166:257–262. Embryonic vertebrate central nervous system: Revised terminology.

Bourgeois, J.-P., P. J. Jastreboff, and P. Rakic (1989). *Proc. Natl. Acad. Sci. U.S.A.* 86:4297–4301. Synaptogenesis in visual cortex of normal and preterm monkeys: Evidence for intrinsic regulation of synaptic overproduction.

Bouvet, J., Y. Usson, and J. Legrand (1987). *Int. J. Dev. Neurosci.* 5:345–355. Morphometric analysis of the cerebellar Purkinje cell in the developing normal and hypothyroid chick.

Bovolenta, P., and C. Mason (1987). *J. Neurosci.* 7:1447–1460. Growth cone morphology varies with position in the developing mouse visual pathway from retina to first targets.

Bovolenta, P., R. K. L. Liem, and C. A. Mason (1984). *Dev. Biol.* 102:248–259. Development of cerebellar astroglia: Transitions in form and cytoskeletal content.

Bovolenta, P., R. K. H. Liem, and C. A. Mason (1987). *Dev. Brain Res.* 33:113–126. Glial filament protein expression in astroglia in the mouse visual pathway.

Bowers, J. Z. (1970). *Western Medical Pioneers in Feudal Japan.* Johns Hopkins, Baltimore.

Bowling, D. B., and C. R. Michael (1980). *Nature* 286:899–902. Projection patterns of single physiologically characterized optic tract fibers in cat.

Bowling, D. R., and C. R. Michael (1984). *J. Neurosci.* 4:198–216. Terminal patterns of single, physiologically characterized optic trait fibers in the cat's lateral geniculate nucleus.

Bowman, W. C., and M. W. Nott (1969). *Pharmacol. Rev.* 21:27–72. Actions of sympathomimetic amines and their antagonists on skeletal muscle.

Boya, J. (1976). *Acta anat.* 95:598–608. An ultrastructural study of the relationship between pericytes and cerebral macrophages.

Boya, J., J. Calvo, and A. Prado. (1979). *J. Anat. (London)* 129:177–186. The origin of microglial cells.

Boya, J., J. Calvo, A. L. Carbonell, and E. Garcia-Mauriño (1986). *Acta anat.* 127:142–145. Nature of macrophages in rat brain. A histochemical study.

Boya, J., A. L. Carbonell, J. Calvo, and A. Borregón (1987). *Acta anat.* 130:329–335. Ultrastructural study on the origin of rat microglia cells.

Boycott, B. B., and H. Wässle (1974). *J. Physiol. (London)* 240:397–419. The morphological types of ganglion cells of the domestic cat's retina.

Boyd, I. A., and M. H. Gladden (1985). Morphology of mammalian muscle spindles, a review, pp. 3–22. In *The muscle spindle* (I. A. Boyd, and M. H. Gladden, eds.), Macmillan, London.

Boyd, J. D. (1960). Development of striated muscle, pp. 63–85. In *Structure and Functions of Muscle*, Vol. 1 (G. H. Bourne, ed.), Academic Press, New York.

Boyd, W. C. (1974). *Science* 186:846. How specific is specific?

Boydston, W. R., and G. S. Sohal (1979). *Brain Res.* 178:403–410. Grafting of additional periphery reduces embryonic loss of neurons.

Boyle, R. (1772). *The Works of the Honourable Robert Boyle. A New Edition.* 6 vols. J. & F. Rivington, London.

Bozyczko, D., and A. F. Horwitz (1986). *J. Neurosci.* 6:1241–1251. The participation of a putative cell surface receptor for laminin and fibronectin in peripheral neurite extension.

Braak, H. (1976). *J. Comp. Neurol.* 166:341–363. On the striate area of the human isocortex. A Golgi- and pigmentarchitectonic study.

Braak, H. (1980). *Architectonics of the Human Telencephalic Cortex.* Springer-Verlag, Berlin.

Braak, H., and E. Braak (1985). *Prog. In Neurobiol.* 25:93–139. Golgi preparations as a tool in neuropathology with particular reference to investigations of the human telencephalic cortex.

Bracegirdle, B. (1978). *A History of Microtechnique.* Cornell University Press, Ithaca, New York.

Brackenbury, R., U. Rutishauser, and G. M. Edelman (1981). *Proc. Natl. Acad. Sci. U.S.A.* 78:387–391. Distinct calcium-independent and calcium-dependent adhesion systems of chicken embryo cells.

Bradley, P. B., J. T. Eayrs, and K. Schmalbach (1960a). *Electroencephalog. Clin. Neurophysiol.* 12:467–477. The electroencephalogram of normal and hypothyroid rats.

Bradley, P. B., J. T. Eayrs, A. Glass, and R. W. Heath (1960b). *Electroencephalog. Clin. Neurophysiol.* 12:759–760. The recruiting response in neonatal hypothyroidism.

Bradley, R. M. (1972). Development of the taste bud and gustatory papillae in human fetuses, pp. 137–162. In *Third Symposium on Oral Sensation and Perception. The Mouth of the Infant* (J. F. Bosma ed.), Thomas, Springfield, Ill.

Bradley, R. M. (1975). *Physiol. Rev.* 55:352–382. Fetal sensory receptors.

Bradley, R. M., and C. M. Mistretta (1973). *J. Physiol. (London)* 231:271–282. The gustatory sense in foetal sheep during the last third of gestation.

Bradley, R. M., and C. M. Mistretta (1975). *Physiol. Rev.* 55:352–382. Fetal sensory receptors.

Bradley, R. M., and C M. Mistretta (1979). *Neurosci. Abstr.* 5:125. Changes in taste reponses from sheep chorda tympani nerve during development.

Bradley, R. M., and I. B. Stern (1967). *J. Anat. (London)* 101:743–752. The development of the human taste bud during the foetal period.

Bradley, W. G., and M. Jenkison (1973). *J. Neurol. Sci.* 18:227–247. Abnormalities of peripheral nerve in murine muscular dystrophy.

Bradley, W. G., E. Jaros, and M. Jenkison (1977). *J. Neuropathol. Exp. Neurol.* 36:797–806. The nodes of Ranvier in the nerves of mice with muscular dystrophy.

Bradom, W. F. (1960). *J. Exp. Zool.* 143:323–345. Genedosage studies in polyploid hybrids of California newts.

Bradom, W. F. (1962). *Biol. Bull.* 123:253–263. Karyoplasmic studies in haploid, androgenetic hybrids of California newts.

Bradshaw, J. L., and N. C. Nettleton (1981). *Behav. Brain Sci.* 4:51–92. The nature of hemispheric specialization in man.

Brady, S. T. (1981). *J. Cell Biol.* 91:333a. Biochemical and solubility properties of axonal tubulin.

Brady, S. T., and R. J. Lasek (1981). *Cell* 23:515–523. Nerve specific enolase and creatine phosphokinase in axonal transport: Soluable proteins and the axoplasmic matrix.

Brady, S. T., and R. J. Lasek (1982). The slow components of axonal transport: movements, composition and organization, pp. 207–217. In *Axoplasmic Transport* (D. G. Weiss, ed.), Springer-Verlag, Berlin.

Brady, S. T., S. D. Crothers, C. Nosal, and W. O. McClure (1980a). *Proc. Natl. Acad. Sci. U.S.A.* 77:5909–5913. Fast axoplasmic transport in the presence of high Ca^{2+}: Evidence that microtubules are not required.

Brady, S. T., M. Tytell, and R. J. Lasek (1980b). *Trans. Amer. Soc. Neurochem.* 11:80. Calmodulin is axonally transported in slow component b.

Brady, S. T., M. Tytell, and R. J. Lasek (1984). *J Cell Biol.* 99:1716–1724. Axonal tubulin and axonal microtubules: Biochemical evidence for cold stability.

Braekevelt, C. R., and M. J. Hollenberg (1970). *Am. J. Anat.* 102:281–302. The development of the retina of the albino rat.

Braekevelt, C. R., L. D. Beazley, S. A. Dunlop, and J. E. Darby (1986). *Dev. Brain Res.* 25:117–125. Numbers of axons in the optic nerve and of retinal ganglion cells during development in the marsupial *Setonix brachyurus.*

Brœndgaard, H., and H. J. G. Gundersen (1986). *J. Neurosci. Meth.* 18:39–78. The impact of recent stereological advances on quantitative studies of the nervous system.

Brœndgaard, H., S. M. Evans, C. V. Howard, and H. J. G. Gundersen (1990). *J. Microsc.* 157:285–304. Total number of neurons in human neocortex unbiasedly estimated using optical disectors.

Braitenberg, V., and M. Kemali (1970). *J. Comp. Neurol.* 138:137–146. Exceptions to bilateral symmetry in the epithalamus of lower vertebrates.

Braithwaite, R. B. (1953). *Scientific Explanation.* Cambridge Univ. Press, Cambridge.

Brand, S., and P. Rakic (1984). *Anat. Embryol.* 169:21–34. Cytodifferentiation and synaptogenesis in the neostriatum of fetal and neonatal rhesus monkeys.

Brandon, J. G., and R. G. Coss (1982). *Brain Res.* 252:51–61. Rapid dendritic spine stem, shortening during one-trial learning: The honeybee's first orientation flight.

Brattgard, S.-O., J. E. Edstrom, and H. Hyden. (1957). *J. Neurochem.* 1:316–325. The chemical changes in regenerating neurons.

Brauer, A. (1904). *Zool. Jahrb. Suppl.* 7:409–428. Beiträge zur Kenntnis der Entwicklung und Anatomie der Gymnophionen, IV.

Brauer, P. R., and R. R. Markwald (1987). *Anat. Rec.* 219:275–285. Attachment of neural crest cells to endogenous extracellular matrices.

Brauer, P. R., and R. R. Markwald (1988). *Anat. Rec.* 222:69–82. Specific configurations of fibronectin-containing particles correlate with pathways taken by neural crest cells at two axial levels.

Brauer, P. R., D. L. Bolender, and R. R. Markwald (1985). *Anat. Rec.* 211:57–68. The distribution and spatial organization of the extracellular matrix encountered by mesencephalic neural crest cells.

Braus, H. (1905). *Anat.Anz.* 26:433–479. Experimentelle Beiträge zur Frage nach der Entwicklung peripherer Nerven.

Bray, D. (1970). *Proc. Natl. Acad. Sci. U.S.A.* 65:905–910. Surface movements during the growth of single explanted neurons.

Bray, D. (1973a). *Nature* 244:93–96. Model for membrane movements in the neural growth cone.

Bray, D. (1973b). *J. Cell. Biol.* 56:702–712. Branching patterns of individual sympathetic neurons in culture.

Bray, D. (1974). *Endeavour* 33:131–136. The fibrillar proteins of nerve cells.

Bray, D. (1979). *J. Cell Sci.* 37:391–410. Mechanical tension produced by nerve cells in tissue culture.

Bray, D. (1982). Filopodial contraction and growth cone guidance, pp. 299–317. In *Cell Behavior* (R. Bellairs, A. Curtis, G. Dunn, eds.), Cambridge University Press.

Bray, D. (1987). *Trends Neurosci.* 10:431–434. Growth cones: Do they pull or are they pushed?

Bray, D., and M. B. Bunge (1973). The growth cone in neurite extension, pp. 195–209. In *Locomotion of Tissue Cells*, Ciba Foundation Symposium 14 (new series), Elsevier, Amsterdam.

Bray, D., and K. Chapman (1985). *J. Neurosci.* 5:3204–3213.

Analysis of microspike movements on the neuronal growth cone.

Bray, D., and P. J. Hollenbeck (1988). *Ann. Rev. Cell Biol.* 4:43–61. Growth cone motility and guidance.

Bray, D., C. Thomas, and G. Shaw (1978). *Proc. Natl. Acad. Sci. U.S.A.* 81:5626–5629. Growth cone formation in cultures of sensory neurons.

Bray, D., J. Heath, and D. Moss (1986). *J. Cell Sci.* Suppl. 4:71–88. The membrane-associated "cortex" of animal cells: Its structure and mechanical properties.

Bray, G. M., M. Rasminsky, and A. J. Aguayo (1981). *Ann. Rev. Neurosci.* 4:127–162. Interactions between axons and their sheath cells.

Bray, J. J., and L. Austin (1966). *J. Neurochem.* 13:731–740. Flow of protein and ribonucleic acid in peripheral nerve.

Bray, J. J., and L. Austin (1969). *Brain Res.* 12:230–233. Axoplasmic flow of ^{14}C proteins at two rates in chicken sciatic nerve.

Brazier, M. (1959). The historical development of neurophysiology. In *Handbook of Physiology, Section 1: Neurophysiology* (J. F. Field, H. W. Magoun, and V. E. Hall, eds.), American Physiol. Society, Washington, D. C.

Brazier, M. B. (1984). *A History of Neurophysiology in the 17th and 18th Centuries.* Raven Press, New York.

Breathnach, A. S. (1977). *J. Invest. Dermatol.* 69:8–26. Electron microscopy of cutaneous nerves and receptors.

Breathnach, A. S. (1980). The mammalian and avian Merkel cell, pp. 283–291. In *The Skin of Vertebrates,* Linnean Society Symposium Series no. 9 (R. I. C. Spearman and P. A. Riley, eds.), Academic Press, London.

Breathnach, A. S., and E. Robins (1970). *J. Anat. (London)* 106:411. Ultrastructural observations on Merkel cells in human foetal skin.

Breedlove, S. M., and A. P. Arnold (1981). *Brain Res.* 225:297–307. Sexually dimorphic motor nucleus in rat spinal cord: Response to adult hormone manipulation, absence in androgen-insensitive rats.

Breedlove, S. M., and A. P. Arnold (1983a). *J. Neurosci.* 3:417–423. Hormonal control of a developing neuromuscular system: I. Complete demasculinization of the male rat spinal nucleus of the bulbocavernosus using the antiandrogen flutamide.

Breedlove, S. M., and A. P. Arnold (1983b). *J. Neurosci.* 3:424–432. Hormonal control of a developing neuromuscular system: II. Sensitive periods for the androgen-induced masculinization of the rat spinal nucleus of the bulbocavernosus.

Breedlove, S. M., C. D. Jacobson, R. A. Gorski, and A. P. Arnold (1982). *Brain Res.* 237:173–181. Masculinization of the female rat spinal cord following a single neonatal injection of testosterone propionate but not estradiol benzoate.

Bremermann, H. J. (1963). *IEEE Trans.* MIL7:200–205. Limits of genetic control.

Brenner, S. (1974). *Genetics* 77:71–94. The genetics of *Caenorhabditis elegans.*

Bretscher, M. S. (1987). *Sci. Am.* 257:72–90. How animal cells move.

Brett, G. S. (1953). *Brett's History of Psychology* (R. S. Peters, ed.), Allen and Unwin, London.

Breuer, A. C., M. P. Lynn, M. B. Atkinson, S. M. Chou, A. J. Wilbourn, K. E. Marks, J. E. Culver, and E. J. Fleegler (1987). *Neurology* 37:738–748. Fast axonal transport in amyotrophic lateral sclerosis: An intra-axonal organelle traffic analysis.

Breur, A. C., C. M. Christian, M. Henkart, and P. G. Nelson (1975). *J. Cell Biol.* 65:562–576. Computer analyses of organelle translocation in primary neuronal cultures and continuous cell lines.

Brierley, J. B., and A. W. Brown (1982). *J. Comp. Neurol.* 211:397–406. The origin of lipid phagocytes in the central nervous system. I. The intrinsic microglia.

Brightman, M. W. (1965). *J. Cell Biol.* 26:99–123. The distribution within the brain of ferritin injected into cerebrospinal fluid compartments. I. Ependymal distribution.

Brightman, M. W., and S. L. Palay (1963). *J. Cell Biol.* 19:415–439. The fine structure of ependyma in the brain of the rat.

Brightman, M. W., and T. S. Reese (1969). *J. Cell Biol.* 40:648–677. Junctions between intimately aposed cell membranes in the vertebrate brain.

Britten, R. J., and E. H. Davidson (1969). *Science* 165:349–357. Gene regulation for higher cells: A theory.

Britten, R. J., and E. H. Davidson (1971). *Quart. Rev. Biol.* 46:111–138. Repetitive and non-repetitive DNA sequences and a speculation on the origins of evolutionary novelty.

Brizzee, K. R. (1949). *J. Comp. Neurol.* 91:129–146. Histogenesis of the supporting tissue in the spinal and sympathetic trunk ganglia in the chick.

Brizzee, K. R. (1987). *Neurobiol. Aging* 8:579–580. Neuron numbers and dendritic extent in normal aging and Alzheimer's disease.

Brizzee, K. R., and L. A. Jacobs (1959). *Growth* 23:337–347. Early postnatal changes in neuron packing density and volumetric relationships in the cerebral cortex of the white rat.

Brizzee, K. R., J. Vogt, and X. Kharetheko (1964). *Prog. Brain Res.* 4:136–149. Postnatal changes in glia neuron index with a comparison of methods of cell enumeration in the white rat.

Brizzee, K. R., N. Sherwood, and P. S. Timiras (1968). *J. Gerontol.* 23:289–291. A comparison of cell populations at various depth levels in cerebral cortex of young adult and aged Long-Evans rats.

Broadwell, R. D., and M. W. Brightman (1979). *J. Comp. Neurol.* 185:31–74. Cytochemistry of undamaged neurons transporting exogenous protein *in vivo.*

Broadwell, R. D., H. M. Charlton, B. J. Balin, and M. Salcman (1987). *J. Comp. Neurol.* 260:47–62. Angioarchtecture of the CNS, pituitary gland and intracerebral grafts revealed with peroxidase cytochemistry.

Broca, P. P. (1878). *Rev. Anthrop.* 1:385–498. Anatomie comparée des circonvolutions cérébrales. Le grand lobe limbique et la scissure limbique dans la série mammifères.

Brochu, G., L. Maler, and R. Hawkes (1990). *J. Comp. Neurol.* 291:538–552. Zebrin II: A polypeptide antigen expressed selectively by Purkinje cells reveals compartments in rat and fish cerebellum.

Brock, L. G., J. S. Coombs, and J. C. Eccles (1952). *J. Physiol. (London)* 117:431–460. The recording of potentials from motoneurones with an intracellular electrode.

Brockes, J. P. and Z. W. Hall (1975). *Proc. Natl. Acad. Sci. U.S.A.* 72:1368–1372. Synthesis of acetylcholine receptor by denervated rat diaphragm muscle.

Brockes, J. P., M. C. Raff, D. J. Nishiguchi, and J. Winter

(1979). *J. Neurocytol.* 9:67–77. Studies on cultured rat Schwann cells. III. Assays for peripheral myelin proteins.

Brockes, J. P., K. J. Fryxell, and G. E. Lemke (1981). *J. Exp. Biol.* 95:215–230. Studies on cultured Schwann cells: The induction of myelin synthesis, and the control of their proliferation by a new growth factor.

Brockes, J. P., X. O. Breakefield, and R. L. Martuza (1986). *Ann. Neurol.* 20:317–322. Glial growth factor-like activity in Schwann cell tumours.

Brockman, L. M., and H. N. Ricciuti (1971). *Dev. Psychobiol.* 4:312–319. Severe protein-calorie malnutrition and cognitive development in infancy and early childhood.

Brodal, A. (1940a). *Arch. Neurol. Psychiat. (Chicago)* 43:45–58. Modification of Gudden method for study of cerebral localization.

Brodal, A. (1940b). *Z. Ges. Neurol. Psychiat.* 169:1–153. Experimenteller Untersuchungen über die olivo-cerebellare Lokalisation.

Brodmann, K. (1905). *J. für Psychologie und Neurologie* 6:108–120. Beiträge zur histologischen Lokalisation der Grosshirnrinde. 4, Mitteilung: Der Riesenpyramidentypus und sein Verhalten zu den Furchen bei den Karnivoren.

Brodmann, K. (1908). *Vergleichende Lokalisationslehre der Grosshirnrinde.* Barth, Leipzig.

Brody, H. (1955). *J. Comp. Neurol.* 102:511–556. Organization of the cerebral cortex. III. A study of aging in the human cerbral cortex.

Bronfenbrenner, U. (1968). Early deprivation in mammals: A cross-species analysis, pp. 627–764. In *Early experience and behavior* (Newton, and Levine, eds.), Thomas, Springfield.

Bronner-Fraser, M. (1985a). *Dev. Biol.* 108:131–145. Effects of different fragments of the fibronectin molecule on latex bead translocation along neural crest migratory pathways.

Bronner-Fraser, M. (1985b). *J. Cell Biol.* 101:610–617. Alteration of neural crest cell migration by a monoclonal antibody that affects cell adhesion.

Bronner-Fraser, M. (1986a). *Amer. Zool.* 26:555–558. On the guidance of neural crest migration: Latex beads as probes of surface-substratum interactions.

Bronner-Fraser, M. (1986b). *Dev. Biol.* 117:528–536. An antibody to a receptor for fibronectin and laminin perturbs cranial neural crest development *in vivo.*

Bronner-Fraser, M., and T. Lallier (1988). *J. Cell Biol.* 106:1321–1329. A monoclonal antibody against a laminin-heparan sulfate proteoglycan complex perturbs cranial neural crest migration *in vivo.*

Bronstein, P. M., H. Neiman, F. D. Wolkoff, and M. J. Levine (1974). *Anim. Learning Behav.* 2:92–96. The development of habituation in the rat.

Brown, A. G., and A. Iggo (1962). *J. Physiol. (London)* 165:28–29. The structure and function of cutaneous "touch corpuscles" after nerve crush.

Brown, D. L., and W. L. Salinger (1975). *Science* 189:1011–1012. Loss of X-cells in lateral geniculate nucleus with monocular paralysis: Neural plasticity in the adult cat.

Brown, D. R, and A. W. Everett (1990). *J. Comp. Neurol.* 292:363–372. Compartmental and topographical specificity of reinnervation in the glutaeus muscle in the adult toad *(Bufo marinus).*

Brown, D. R., A. W. Everett, and M. R. Bennett (1989). *J.* Comp. Neurol. 284:231–241. Compartmental and topographical distributions of axons in nerves to the amphibian *(Bufo marinus)* glutaeus muscle.

Brown-Séquard, C.-E. (1866). *Arch. physiol. norm. et path.* 2:211–220, 422–438, 496–503. Nouvelles recherches sur l'épilepsie due à certaines lésions de la moelle épinière et des nerfs rachidiens.

Brown Séquard, C.-E. (1871–1872). *Arch. physiol. norm. et path.* 4:116–120. Quelques faits nouveaux relatifs à l'épilepsie qu'on observe à la suite de diverses lésions du système nerveux, chez les cobayes.

Brown-Séquard, E. (1853). *Experimental Researches Applied to Physiology and Pathology,* H. Ballière, New York.

Brown, G. L., and J. E. Pascoe (1954). *J. Physiol. (London)* 123:565–573. The effect of degenerative section of ganglionic axons on transmission through the ganglion.

Brown, I. R., and R. B. Church (1972). *Dev. Biol.* 29:73–84. Transcription of nonrepeated DNA during mouse and rabbit development.

Brown, J. W. (1980). *Anat. Rec.* 196:23–35. Developmental history of nervus terminalis in embryos of insectivorous bats.

Brown, M. C., and C. M. Booth (1983). *Nature* 304:741–742. Postnatal development of the adult pattern of motor axon distribution in rat muscle.

Brown, M. C., and R. L. Holland (1979). *Nature* 282:724–726. A central role of denervated tissues in causing nerve sprouting.

Brown, M. C., and R. Ironton (1976). *J. Physiol. (London)* 263:181–182. The fate of motor axon sprouts in a partially denervated mouse muscle when regenerating nerve fibers return.

Brown, M. C., and R. Ironton (1977a). *Nature* 265:459–461. Motor neurone sprouting induced by prolonged tetrodotoxin block of nerve action potentials.

Brown, M. C., and R. Ironton (1977b). *J. Physiol. (London)* 272:70–71. Suppression of motor nerve terminal sprouting in partially denervated mouse muscles.

Brown, M. C., and R. Ironton (1978). *J. Physiol. (London)* 278:325–348. Sprouting and regression of neuromuscular synapses in partially denervated mammalian muscles.

Brown, M. C., J. K. S. Jansen, and D. Van Essen (1976). *J. Physiol. (London)* 261:387–422. Polyneuronal innervation of skeletal muscle in new-born rats and its elimination during maturation.

Brown, M. C., G. M. Goodwin, and R. Ironton (1977). *J. Physiol. (London)* 267:42–43. Prevention of motor sprouting in botulinum poisoned mouse soleus muscle by direct stimulation of the muscle.

Brown, M. C., R. L. Holland, W. G. Hopkins, and R. J. Keynes (1980). *Brain Res.* 219:145–151. An assessment of the spread of the signal for terminal sprouting within and between muscles.

Brown, M. C., R. L. Holland, and W. G. Hopkins (1981). *Ann. Rev. Neurosci.* 4:17–42. Motor nerve sprouting.

Brown, M. E. (1946). *Am. J. Anat.* 78:79–113. The histology of the tadpole tail during metamorphosis, with special reference to the nervous system.

Brown, N. A., and L. Wolpert (1990). *Development* 109:1–9. The development of handedness in left/right asymmetry.

Brown, T. H., V. C. Chang, A. H. Ganong, C. L. Keenan, and S. R. Kelso (1988). *Neurol. Neurobiol.* 35:201–264. Biophysical properties of dendrites and spines that may control the induction and expression of long-term synaptic potentiation.

Browne, K. M. (1950). *J. Comp. Neurol.* 93:441–455. The spatial distribution of segmental nerve to striate musculature of the hindlimb of the rat.

Brozek, J. (1979). Behavioral effects of energy and protein deficits. *US Department of Health, Education and Welfare,* NIH Publ. No. (NIH) 79–1906.

Brozek, J., ed. (1985). *Malnutrition and Human Behavior.* Van Nostrand Reinhold, New York.

Bruckenstein, D. A., and D. Higgins (1988a). *Dev. Biol.* 128:324–336. Morphological differentiation of embryonic rat sympathetic neurons in tissue culture. I. Conditions under which neurons form axons but not dendrites.

Bruckenstein, D. A., and D. Higgins (1988b). *Dev. Biol.* 128:337–348. Morphological differentiation of embryonic rat sympathetic neurons in tissue cultures. II. Serum promotes dendritic growth.

Brugal, G. (1971). *Arch. Entw.-Mech. Organ.* 168:205–225. Etude autoradiographique de l'influence de la température sur la prolifération cellulaire ches les embryones âgés de *Pleurodeles waltlii Michah.*

Brummelkamp, R. (1939). *Acta Morphol. Neerl. Scand.* 2:268–271. Das Wachstum der Gehirnmasse mit kleinen Cephalisierungssprungen (sog. 2-Sprungen) bei Amphibien und Fischen.

Brun, R. B., and J. A. Garson (1983). *J. Embryol. Exp. Morph.* 74:275–295. Neurulation in the Mexican salamander *(Ambystoma mexicanum):* A drug study and cell shape analysis of the epidermis and the neural plate.

Brunden, K. R., and J. F. Poduslo (1987). *J. Cell Biol.* 104:661–669. Lysosomal delivery of the major myelin glycoprotein in the absence of myelin assembly: Post-translational regulation of the level of expression by Schwann cells.

Brunder, D. G., and E. M. Lieberman (1988). *J. Neurosci.* 25:951–959. Studies of axon-glia interactions and periaxonal K homeostasis: I. The influence of Na, K, Cl and cholinergic agents on the membrane potential of the adaxonal glia of the crayfish medial giant axon.

Brunjes, P. C., and L. L. Frazier (1986). *Brain Res. Rev.* 11:1–45. Maturation and plasticity in the olfactory system.

Brushart, T. M., and M.-M. Mesulam (1980). *Science* 208:603–605. Alteration in connections between muscle and anterior horn motoneurons after peripheral nerve repair.

Brustowicz, R. J., and J. W. Kernohan (1952). *Arch. Neurol. Psychiat.* 67:592. Cell rests in the region of the 4th ventricle.

Bryan, J. (1974). *Fed. Proc.* 33:152–157 Biochemical properties of microtubules.

Bryans, W. A. (1959). *Anat. Rec.* 133:65–71. Mitotic activity in the brain of the adult rat.

Bryant, P. J., and H. A. Schneiderman (1969). *Dev. Biol.* 20:263–290. Cell lineage, growth, and determination in the imaginal leg discs of *Drosophila melanogaster.*

Bucher, V. M., and S. M. Burgi (1950). *J. Comp. Neurol.* 93:139–172. Some observations on the fiber connections of the di- and mesencephalon in the rat.

Buck, C. A., and A. F. Horwitz (1987). *Ann. Rev. Cell Biol.* 3:179–205. Cell surface receptors for extracellular matrix molecules.

Buck, C. R., H. J. Humberto, I. B. Black, and M. V. Chao (1987). *Proc. Natl. Acad. Sci. U.S.A.* 84:3060–3063. De-velopmentally regulated expression of the nerve growth factor receptor gene in the periphery and brain.

Buck, C. R., H. J. Martinez, M. V. Chao, and I. B. Black (1988). *Dev. Brain Res.* 44:259–268. Differential expression of the nerve growth factor receptor gene in multiple brain areas.

Bueker, E. D. (1943). *J. Exp. Zool.* 93:99–129. Intracentral and peripheral factors in the differentiation of motor neurons in transplanted lumbo-sacral cords of chick embryos.

Bueker, E. D. (1944). *Science* 100:169. Differentiation of the lateral motor column in the avian spinal cord.

Bueker, E. D. (1945a). *J. Comp. Neurol.* 82:335–361. The influence of a growing limb on the differentiation of somatic motor neurons in transplanted avian spinal cord segments.

Bueker, E. D. (1945b). *Anat. Rec.* 93:323–331. Hyperplastic changes in the nervous system of a frog *(Rana)* as associated with multiple functional limbs.

Bueker, E. D. (1948). *Anat. Rec.* 102:369–390. Implantation of tumors in the hindlimb field of the embryonic chick and developmental response of the lumbosacral nervous system.

Bueker, E. D., I. Schenkein, and J. L. Bane (1960). *Cancer Res.* 20:1220–1228. The problem of distribution of a nerve growth factor specific for spinal and sympathetic ganglia.

Buettner-Ennever, J. A., P. Grob, and K. Akert (1981). A transsynaptic autoradiographic study of the pathways controlling the extra ocular eye muscles using (1251) B-IIb tetanus toxin fragment, pp. 157–170. In *Vestibular and Oculomotor Physiology* (B. Cohen, ed.), New York Academy of Science, New York.

Bugbee, N. M., and P. S. Goldman-Rakic (1983). *J. Comp. Neurol.* 220:355–364. Columnar organization of corticocortical projections in squirrel and rhesus monkeys: Similarity of column width in species differing in cortical volume.

Buisseret, P., and P. Imbert (1976). *J. Physiol. (London)* 255:511–525. Visual cortical cells: Their developmental properties in normal and dark-reared kittens.

Buller, A. J. (1966). *Br. Med. Bull.* 22:45–48. Developmental physiology of the neuronmuscular system.

Buller, A. J., and D. M. Lewis (1946). *J. Physiol. (London)* 176:355–370. Further observations on the differentiation of skeletal muscles in the kitten hindlimb.

Buller, A. J., and D. M. Lewis (1965). *J. Physiol. (London)* 178:343–358. Further observations on mammalian cross-innervated skeletal muscle.

Buller, A. J., J. C. Eccles, and R. M. Eccles (1960a). *J. Physiol. (London)* 150:399–416. Differentiation of fast and slow muscles in the cat hindlimb.

Buller, A. J., J. C. Eccles, and R. M. Eccles (1960b). *J. Physiol. (London)* 150:417–439. Interactions between motoneurons and muscles in respect of the characteristic speeds of their responses.

Bullock, T. H., and G. A. Horridge (1965). *Structure and Function in the Nervous Systems of Invertebrates,* 2 vols., Freeman, San Francisco.

Bullough, W. S. (1962). *Biol. Rev.* 37:307. The control of mitotic activity in adult mammalian tissues.

Bunge, M. (1959). *Causality.* Harvard Univ. Press, Cambridge, Mass.

Bunge, M. B. (1973a). *Anat. Rec.* 175:280. Uptake of peroxidase by growth cones of cultured neurons.

Bunge, M. B. (1973b). *J. Cell Biol.* 56:713–735. Fine structure of nerve fibers and growth cones of isolated sympathetic neurons in culture.

Bunge, M. B., R. P. Bunge, and H. Ris (1961). *J. Biophys. Biochem. Cytol.* 10:67–94. Ultastructural study of remyelination in an experimental lesion in adult cat spinal cord.

Bunge, M. B., R. P. Bunge, and G. D. Pappas (1962). *J. Cell Biol.* 12:448–453. Electron microscopic demonstration of connections between glia and myelin sheaths in the developing mammalian nervous system.

Bunge, M. B., R. P. Bunge, and E. R. Peterson (1967). *Brain Res.* 6:728–749. The onset of synapse formation in spinal cord cultures as studied by electron microscopy.

Bunge, M. B., A. K. Williams, and P. M. Wood (1982). *Dev. Biol.* 92:449–460. Neuron-Schwann cell interaction in basal lamina formation.

Bunge, R. P. (1968). *Physiol. Rev.* 48:197–251. Glial cells and the central myelin sheath.

Bunge, R. P. (1973). *J. Cell Biol.* 56:713–735. Fine structure of nerve fibers and growth cones of isolated sympathetic neurons in culture.

Bunge, R. P., and M. B. Bunge (1981). Cues and constraints in Schwann cell development, pp. 322–353. In *Studies in Developmental Neurobiology* (W. M. Cowan, ed.), Oxford Univ. Press, New York.

Bunge, R. P., M. B. Bunge, and C. F. Eldridge (1986). *Ann. Rev. Neurosci.* 9:305–328. Linkage between axonal ensheathment and basal lamina production by Schwann cells.

Bunge, R. P., M. B. Bunge, and M. Bates (1989). *J. Cell Biol.* 109:273–284. Movements of the Schwann cell nucleus implicate progression of the inner (axon-related) Schwann cell process during myelination.

Bunt, A. H., R. D. Lund, and J. S. Lund (1974). *Brain Res.* 73:215–228. Retrograde axonal transport of horseradish peroxidase by ganglion cells of the albino rat retina.

Bunt, S. M. (1982). *J. Comp. Neurol.* 206:209–266. Retinotopic and temporal organization of the optic nerve and tracts in the adult goldfish.

Bunt, S. M., and T. J. Horder (1983). *J. Comp. Neurol.* 213:94–114. Evidence for an orderly arrangement of optic axons within the optic nerves of the major nonmammalian verterbrate classes.

Bunt, S. M., and R. D. Lund (1981). *Brain Res.* 211:399–404. Development of a transient retino-retinal pathway in hooded and albino rats.

Bunt, S. M., R. D. Lund, and P. W. Land (1983). *Dev. Brain Res.* 6:149–168. Prenatal development of the optic projection in albino and hooded rats.

Buonanno, A., and J. P. Merlie (1986). *J. Biol. Chem.* 261:11452–11455. Transcriptional regulation of nicotinic acetylcholine receptor genes during muscle development.

Burchfiel, J. L., and F. H. Duffy (1981). *Brain Res.* 206:479–484. Role of intracortical inhibition in deprivation amblyopia: Reversal by microiontophoretic bicuculline.

Burden, S. (1977). *Dev. Biol.* 57:317–329. Development of the neuromuscular junction of the chick embryo: The number, distribution and stability of acetylcholine receptors.

Burden, S. J., P. B. Sargent, and U. J. McMahan (1979). *J. Cell Biol.* 82:412–425. Acetylcholine receptors in regenerating muscle accumulate at original synaptic sites in the absence of the nerve.

Burdick, M. L. (1968). *J. Exp. Zool.* 167:1–20. A test of the capacity of chick embryo cells to home after vascular dissemination.

Burdman, J. A. (1967). *J. Neurochem.* 14:367–371. Early effects of a nerve growth factor on the RNA content and base ratios of isolated chick embryo sensory ganglia neuroblasts in tissue culture.

Burdman, J. A., G. A. Jahn, and I. Szijan (1975). *J. Neurochem.* 24:663–666. Early events in the effect of hydrocortisone acetate on DNA replication in the rat brain.

Burdwood, W. O. (1965). *J. Cell Biol.* 27:115A. Rapid bidirectional particle movement in neurons.

Burger, M. M. (1974). Role of the cell surface in growth and transformation, pp. 3–24. In *Macromolecules Regulating Growth and Development* (E. D. Hay, T. J. King, and J. Papaconstantinou, eds.), Academic Press, New York.

Burger, M. M., R. S. Turner, W. J. Kuhns, and G. Weinbaum (1975). *Phil. Trans. Roy. Soc. (London) Ser. B.* 271:379–393. A possible model for cell-cell recognition via surface macromolecules.

Burgess, J. W., and R. G. Coss (1983). *Brain Res.* 265:217–223. Rapid effect of biologically relevant stimulation on tectal neurons: Changes in dendritic spine morphology after nine minutes are retained for twenty-four hours.

Burgess, P. R., and K. W. Horch (1973). *J. Neurophysiol.* 36:101–114. Specific regeneration of cutaneous fibers in the cat.

Burgess, P. R., K. B. English, K. W. Horch, and L. J. Stensaas (1974). *J. Physiol. (London)* 236:57–82. Patterning in the regeneration of type I cutaneous receptors.

Burgess, S. K., S. Jacobs, P. Cuatrecasas, and N. Sayhoun (1987). *J. Biol. Chem.* 262:1618–1622. Characterization of a neuronal subtype of insulin-like growth factor I receptor.

Burgess, W. H., and T. Maciag (1989). *Ann. Rev. Biochem.* 58:575–606. The heparin-binding (fibroblast) growth factor family of proteins.

Bürgi, S. (1957). *Deutsch. Z. Nervenheilk.* 176:701–729. Das Tectum opticum. Seine Verbindungen bei der Katze und seine Bedeutung beim Menschen.

Burgin, K. E., M. N. Waxham, S. Rickling, S. A. Westgate, W. C. Mobley, and P. T. Kelly (1990). *J. Neurosci.* 10:1788–1798. *In situ* hybridization histochemistry of $Ca^{2+}/$ calmodulin-dependent protein kinase in developing rat brain.

Burgoyne, R. D., and R. Cumming (1984). *Neurosci.* 11:156–167. Ontogeny of microtubule-associated protein 2 in rat cerebellum: Differential expression of the doublet polypeptides.

Burke, R. E., and P. Tsairis (1973). *J. Physiol. (London)* 234:749–765. Anatomy and innervation ratios in motor units of cat gastrocnemius.

Burke, R. E., P. L. Strick, K. Kanda, C. C. Kim, and B. Walmsley (1977). *J. Neurophysiol.* 40:667–680. Anatomy of medial gastrocnemius and soleus motor nuclei in cat spinal cord.

Burke, W., and W. R. Hayhow (1968). *J. Physiol. (London)* 194:495–519. Disuse in the lateral geniculate nucleus of the cat.

Burkhalter, A., P. Streit, P. Bagnoli, A. Visher, H. Henke, and M. Cuenod (1982). Deprivation induced functional modification in the pigeon visual system, pp. 477–485. In *Neuronal Plasticity and Memory Formation* (C. A. Marsand, and H. Mathies, eds.), Raven Press, New York.

Burleigh, I. G. (1974). *Biol. Rev.* 49:267–320. On the cellular regulation of growth and development in skeletal muscle.

Burmeister, D. W., and B. Grafstein (1985). *Brain Res.* 327:45–51. Removal of optic tectum prolongs the cell body reaction to axotomy in goldfish retinal ganglion cells.

Burmeister, D. W., M. Chen, C. H. Bailey, and D. J. Goldberg (1988). *J. Neurocytol.* 17:783–795. The distribution and movement of organelles in maturing growth cones: Correlated video-enhanced and electron microscopic studies.

Burnette, W. N. (1981). *Anal. Biochem.* 112:195–203. Western blotting: Electrophoretic transfer of proteins from sodium dodecyl sulfate polyacrylamide gels to unmodified nitrocellulose and radiographic detection with antibody and radioiodinate protein A.

Burnham, P., and S. Varon (1973). *Neurobiology* 3:232–245. *In vitro* uptake of active nerve growth factor by dorsal root ganglia of embryonic chick.

Burnham, P., and S. Varon (1974). *Neurobiology* 4:57–70. Biosynthetic activities of dorsal root ganglia *in vitro* and the influence of nerve growth factor.

Burnham, P., C. Raiborn, and S. Varon (1972). *Proc. Natl. Acad. Sci. U.S.A.* 69:3556–3560. Replacement of nerve growth factor by ganglionic non-neuronal cells for the survival *in vitro* of dissociated ganglionic neurons.

Burnside, B. (1971). *Dev. Biol.* 26:416–441. Microtubules and microfilaments in newt neurulation.

Burnside, B. (1973). *Am. Zool.* 13:989–1006. Microtubules and microfilaments in amphibian neurulation.

Burnside, B. (1975). *Ann. N.Y. Acad. Sci.* 253:14–26. The form and arrangement of microtubules: An historical, primarily morphological, review.

Burnside, B., and A. G. Jacobson (1968). *Dev. Biol.* 18:537–552. Analysis of morphogenetic movements in the neural plate of the newt *Taricha torosa*.

Burr, H. S. (1916). *J. Exp. Zool.* 20:27–57. The effects of the removal of the nasal pits in *Amblystoma* embryos.

Burr, H. S. (1920). *J. Exp. Zool.* 30:159–169. The transplantation of the cerebral hemispheres of *Amblystoma*.

Burr, H. S. (1924). *J. Comp. Neurol.* 37:455–479. Some experiments on the transplantation of the olfactory placode in *Amblystoma*. I. An experimentally produced aberrant cranial nerve.

Burr, H. S. (1930). *J. Exp. Zool.* 55:171–191. Hyperplasia in the brain of *Amblystoma*.

Burr, H. S. (1932). *J. Comp. Neurol.* 56:347–371. An electrodynamic theory of development suggested by studies of proliferation rates in the brain of *Amblystoma*.

Burr, H. S. (1947). *Sci. Month.* 64:217–225. Field theory in biology.

Burrows, M. T. (1911). *J. Exper. Zool.* 10:63–84. The growth of tissues of the chick embryo outside the animal body, with special reference to the nervous system.

Burry, R. W. (1980). *Brain Res.* 184:85–98. Formation of apparent presynaptic elements in response to poly-basic compounds.

Burry, R. W., D. A. Kniss, and L. R. Scribner (1984). *Current Topics Res. Synapses* 1:1–51. Mechanisms of synapse formation and maturation.

Burt, A. M., and C. H. Narayanan (1970). *Exp. Neurol.* 29:201–210. Effect of extrinsic neuronal connections on development of acetylcholinesterase and choline acetyltransferase activity in the ventral half of the chick spinal cord.

Burton, H., and R. M. Benjamin (1971). Central projections of the gustatory system, pp. 148–164. In *Handbook of Sensory Physiology*, Vol. IV, Part 2: *Chemical Senses*, 2. *Taste* (L. M. Beidler, ed.), Springer-Verlag, New York.

Burton, P. R. and H. L. Fernandez (1973). *J. Cell Sci.* 12:567–583. Delineation by lanthanum staining of filamentous elements associated with the surfaces of axonal microtubules.

Burton, R. R., and J. L. Paige (1981). *Proc. Natl. Acad. Sci. U.S.A.* 78:3269–3273. Polarity of axoplasmic microtubules in the olfactory nerve of the frog.

Buskirk, D. R., J.-P. Thiery, U. Rutishauser, and G. M. Edelman (1980). *Nature* 285:488–489. Antibodies to a neural cell adhesion molecule disrupt histogenesis in cultured chick retinae.

Butler, J., E. Cosmos, and J. Brierley (1982). *J. Exp. Zool.* 224:65–80. Differentiation of muscle fiber types in aneurogenic brachial muscles of the chick embryo.

Butterfield, H. (1931). *The Whig Interpretation of History*. London.

Buxser, S. E., L. Watson, and G. L. Johnson (1983). *J. Cell. Biochem.* 2:219–233. A comparison of binding properties and structure of NGF receptor on PC12 pheochromocytoma and A875 melanoma cells.

Byers, M. R. (1974). *Brain Res.* 75:97–113. Structural correlates of rapid axonal transport: Evidence that microtubules may not be directly involved.

Byne, W., and R. Bleier (1987). *J. Neurosci.* 7:2688–2696. Medial preoptic sexual dimorphisms in the guinea pig. I. An investigation of their hormonal dependence.

Cabak, V., and R. Najdanyic (1965). *Arch. Dis. Child.* 40:532–534. Effect of undernutrition in early life on physical and mental development.

Cabak, V., R. Najdanvic, B. Curcic, E. Serstney, and L. Skoric (1967). The long-term prognosis of infantile malnutrition, pp. 521–532. In *Proceedings of the First Congress of the International Association for Scientific Study of Mental Deficiency* (B. W. Richards, ed.), Michael Jackson, Montpellier, France.

Caceres, A., and O. Steward (1983). *J. Comp. Neurol.* 214:387–403. Dendritic reorganization in the denervated dentate gyrus of the rat following entorhinal cortical lesions: A Golgi and electron microscopic analysis.

Caceres, A., M. R. Payne, L. I. Binder, and O. Steward (1983). *Proc. Natl. Acad. Sci. U.S.A.* 80:1738–1742. Immunocytochemical localization of actin and microtubule associated protein (MAP 2) in dendritic spines.

Caceres, A., G. A. Banker, O. Steward, L. Binder, and M. Payne (1984). *Dev. Brain Res.* 13:314–318. MAP2 is localized to the dendrites of hippocampal neurons which develop in culture.

Caddy, K. W. T., and T. J. Biscoe (1975). *Brain Res.* 91:276–280. Preliminary observations on the cerebellum in the mutant mouse lurcher.

Caddy, K. W. T., and T. J. Biscoe (1979). *Phil. Trans. Roy. Soc. B* 287:167–201. Structural and quantitative studies on the normal C3H and lurcher mutant mouse.

Cajal, S. R. See Ramón y Cajal, S.

Calaresu, F. R., and J. L. Henry (1971). *Science* 173:343–344. Sex difference in the number of sympathetic neurons in the spinal cord of the cat.

Caldani, M., B. Rolland, C. Fages, and M. Tardy (1982). *Experientia* 38:1199–1202. Glutamine synthetase activity during mouse brain development.

Calder, W. A. (1984). *Size, Function and Life History.* Harvard Univ. Press, Cambridge, Mass.

Caley, D. W., and D. S. Maxwell (1968). *J. Comp. Neurol.* 138:31–48. Development of the blood vessels and extracellular spaces during postnatal maturation of rat cerebral cortex.

Caley, D. W., and D. S. Maxwell (1970). *J. Comp. Neurol.* 128:31–48. Development of the blood vessels and extracellular spaces during postnatal maturation of rat cerebral cortex.

Calleja, C. (1892). *La región olfactorio del cerebro. Moya,* Madrid.

Calvert, R., and B. H. Anderton (1985). *EMBO J.* 4:1171–1176. A microtubule-associated protein (MAP1) which is expressed at elevated levels during development of the rat cerebellum.

Calvet, M.-C., J. Calvet, and R. Camacho-Garcia (1985). *Brain Res.* 331:235–250. The Purkinje cell dendritic tree: A computer-aided study of its development in the cat and in culture.

Cameron, I. L. (1964). *J. Cell Biol.* 20:185–188. Is the duration of DNA synthesis in somatic cells of mammals and birds a constant?

Cameron, J., N. Livson, and N. Bayley (1967). *Science* 157:331–332. Infant vocalizations and their relationship to mature intelligence.

Cameron, J. A., and J. F. Fallon (1977). *Dev. Biol.* 55:331–338. The absence of cell death during development of free digits in amphibians.

Cameron-Curry, P., C. Dulac, and N. M. LeDouarin (1989). *Development* 107:825–833. Expression of the SMP antigen by oligodendrocytes in the developing avian central nervous system.

Cameron, W. D., D. B. Averill, and A. J. Berger (1983). *J. Comp. Neurol.* 219:70–80. Morphology of cat phrenic motoneurons as revealed by intracellular injection of horseradish peroxidase.

Cameron, W. D., D. B. Averill, and A. J. Berger (1985). *J. Comp. Neurol.* 230:91–101. Quantitative analysis of the dendrites of cat phrenic motoneurons stained intracellularly with horseradish peroxidase.

Caminiti, R., and G. M. Innocenti (1981). *Exp. Brain Res.* 42:53–62. The postnatal development of somatosensory callosal connections after partial lesions of somatosensory areas.

Cammer, W. (1984). *Ann. N.Y. Acad. Sci.* 429:494–497. Carbonic anhydrase in oligodendrocytes and myelin in the central nervous system.

Cammer, W., and F. A. Tansey (1988). *J. Neurochem.* 50:319–322. Carbonic anhydrase immunostaining in astrocytes in the rat cerebral cortex.

Cammer, W., and T. R. Zimmerman, Jr. (1982). *Brain Res.* 282:21–26. Glycerol-phosphate dehydrogenase, glucose–6-phosphate dehydrogenase, lactate dehydrogenase and carbonic anhydrase activities in oligodendrocytes and myelin: Comparisons between species and CNS regions.

Cammer, W., D. S. Snyder, T. R. Zimmerman, Jr., M. Farooq, and W. T. Norton (1982). *J. Neurochem.* 38:360–367. Glycerol phosphate dehydrogenase, glucose–6-phosphate dehydrogenase, and lactate dehydrogenase: activities in oligodendrocytes, neurons, astrocytes, and myelin isolated from developing rat brains.

Cammer, W., R. Sarchi, S. Kahn, and V. Sapirstein (1985). *J. Neurosci. Res.* 14:303–316. Oligodendroglial structures and distribution shown by carbonic anhydrase immunostaining in the spinal cords of developing normal and Shiverer mice.

Cammermeyer, J. (1963). *J. Neuropathol. Exp. Neurol.* 12:594–616. Differential response of two neuron types to facial nerve transection in young and old rabbits.

Cammermeyer, J. (1965a). *Ergeb. Anat. Entwicklungsgesch.* 38:1–22. Juxtavascular karyokinesis and microglia cell proliferation during retrograde reaction in the mouse facial nucleus.

Cammermeyer, J. (1965b). *Ergeb. Anat. Entwicklungsgesch.* 38:195–229. Histiocytes, juxtavascular mitotic cells and microglia cells during retrograde changes in the facial nucleus of rabbits of various age.

Cammermeyer, J. (1965c). *Z. Anat. Entwicklungsgeschichte* 124:543–561. The hypo-ependymal microglial cell.

Cammermeyer, J. (1970). The life history of the microglial cell: A light microscopic study, pp. 43–129. In *Neurosciences Research*, Vol. 3, (S. Ehrenpreis, and O. Z. Solnitzky, eds.), Academic Press, New York.

Campagnoni, A. T., C. W. Campagnoni, J. M. Bourre, C. Jacque, and N. Baumann (1984). *J. Neurochem.* 42:733–739. Cell-free synthesis of myelin basic proteins in normal and dysmyelinating mutant mice.

Campbell, A. C. P. (1939). *Arch. Neurol. Psychiat.* 41:223–242. Variation in vascularity and oxidase content in different regions of the brain of the cat.

Campbell, G., and D. O. Frost (1987). *Proc. Natl. Acad. Sci. U.S.A.* 84:6929–6933. Target-controlled differentiation of axon terminals and synaptic organization.

Campbell, G., and D. O. Frost (1988). *J. Comp. Neurol.* 272:383–408. Synaptic organization of anomalous retinal projections to the somatosensory and auditory thalamus: Target-controlled morphogenesis of axon terminals and synaptic glomeruli.

Campbell, G., and C. J. Shatz (1986). *Soc. Neurosci. Abstr.* 12:589. Synapses formed by individual retinogeniculate axons in inappropriate LGN territory during formation of eye-specific layers.

Campbell, G., K. F. So, and A. R. Lieberman (1984). *Neuroscience* 13:743–759. Normal postnatal development of retinogeniculated axons and terminals and identification of inappropriately located transient synapses.

Campenot, R. B. (1977). *Proc. Natl. Acad. Sci. U.S.A.* 74:4516–4519. Local control of neurite development by nerve growth factor.

Campenot, R. B. (1981). *Science* 214:579–581. Regeneration of Neurites in long-term cultures of sympathetic neurons deprived of nerve growth factor.

Campenot, R. B. (1982a). *Dev. Biol.* 93:1–12. Development of sympathetic neurons in compartementalized cultures: I. Local control of neurite growth by nerve growth factor.

Campenot, R. B. (1982b). *Dev. Biol.* 93:13–21. Development of sympathetic neurons in compartementalized cultures: II. Local control of neurite survival by nerve growth factor.

Campos-Ortega, J. A., and A. Hofbauer (1977). *Wilhelm Roux's Arch. Dev. Biol.* 181:227–245. Cell clones and pattern formation in the lineage of photoreceptor cells in the compound eye of *Drosophila*.

Campos-Ortega, J. A., G. Jurgens, and A. Hofbauer (1978). *Nature* 274:584–586. Clonal segregation and positional information in late ommatidial development in *Drosophila*.

Cancalon, P. (1983a). *Brain Res.* 285:265–278. Regeneration of three populations of olfactory axons as a function of temperature.

Cancalon, P. (1983b). *Brain Res.* 285:279–289. Influence of temperature on slow flow in populations of regenerating axons with different elongation velocities.

Cancilla, P. A., R. N. Baker, P. S. Pollock, and S. P. Frommes (1972). *Lab. Invest.* 26:376–383. The reaction of pericytes of the central nervous system to exogenous protein.

Cannon, H. G. (1955). *Proc. Linn. Soc. London* 168:70–87. What Lamarck really said.

Cannon, H. G. (1958). *Lamarck and Modern Genetics.* Manchester Univ. Press, Manchester.

Cantino, D., and L. S. Daneo (1972). *Brain Res.* 38:13–25. Cell death in the developing chick optic tectum.

Cantor, G. N. (1975). *Ann. Sci.* 32:195–218. The Edinburgh phrenology debate: 1803–1828.

Cantor, G. N. (1975). *Ann. Sci.* 32:245–256. A critique of Shapin's social interpretation of the Edinburgh phrenological debate.

Capps-Covey, P., and D. L. McIlwain (1975). *J. Neurochem.* Bulk isolation of large ventral spinal neurons.

Cardasis, C. A., and H. Padykula (1979). *Anat. Rec.* 193:497. Ultrastructural evidence of reorganization at the neuromuscular junction.

Carden, M. J., W. W. Schlaepfer, and V. M.-Y. Lee (1985). *J. Bio. Chem.* 260:9805–9817. The structure, biochemical properties and immunogenicity of neurofilament peripheral regions are determined by phosphorylation.

Carden, M. J., J. Q. Trojanowski, W. W. Schlaepfer, and V. M.-Y. Lee (1987). *J. Neurosci.* 7:3489–3504. Two-stage expression of neurofilament polypeptides during rat neurogenesis with early establishment of adult phosphorylation patterns.

Carey, D. J., and R. P. Bunge (1981). *J. Cell Biol.* 91:666–672. Factors influencing the release of proteins in cultured Schwann cells.

Carey, D. J., C. F. Eldridge, C. J. Cornbrooks, R. Timpl, and R. P. Bunge (1983). *J. Cell Biol.* 97:473–479. Biosynthesis of type IV collagen by cultured rat Schwann cells.

Carlson, B. M. (1973). *Am. J. Anat.* 137:119–150. The regeneration of skeletal muscle. A review.

Carlson, E. A. (1966). *The Gene: A Critical History.* Saunders, Philadelphia.

Carmel, P. W., and B. M. Stein (1969). *J. Comp. Neurol.* 135:145–166. Cell changes in sensory ganglia following proximal and distal nerve section in the monkey.

Carmichael, L. (1926). *Psychol. Rev.* 33:51–58. The development of behavior in vertebrates experimentally removed from the influence of external stimulation.

Carmichael, L. (1927). *Psychol. Rev.* 34:34–47. A further study of the development of behavior in vertebrates experimentally removed from the influence of external stimuli.

Carmignoto, G., L. Maffei, P. Candeo, R. Canella, and C. Comelli (1989). *J. Neurosci.* 9:1263–1272. Effect of NGF on the survival of rat retinal ganglion cells following optic nerve section.

Carnop, R. (1932–33). *Erkenntnis* 3:215–228. Über Protokollsätze.

Caroni, P., and M. E. Schwab (1988a). *J. Cell Biol.* 106:1281–1288. Two membrane protein fractions from rat central myelin with inhibitory properties for neurite growth and fibroblast spreading.

Caroni, P., and M. E. Schwab (1988b). *Neuron* 1:85–96. Antibody against myelin-associated inhibitor of neurite growth neutralizes non-permissive substrate properties of CNS white matter.

Caroni, P., and M. E. Schwab (1989). *Dev. Biol.* 136:287–295. Codistribution of neurite growth inhibitors and oligodendrocytes in rat CNS: Appearance follows nerve fiber growth and precedes myelination.

Carpenter, E. M., and M. Hollyday (1986). *Soc. Neurosci. Abstr.* 12:1210. Defective innervation of chick limbs in the absence of presumptive Schwann cells.

Carpenter, F. G., and R. M. Bergland (1957). *Am. J. Physiol.* 190:371–376. Excitation and conduction in immature nerve fibers of the developing chick.

Carpenter, P. M., A. J. Sefton, B. Dreher, and W.-L. Lim (1986). *J. Comp. Neurol.* 251:240–259. The role of target tissue in regulating the development of retinal ganglion cells in the albino rat: Effects of kainase lesions in the superior colliculus.

Carr, F. E., L. R. Need, and W. W. Chin (1987). *J. Biol. Chem.* 262:981–987. Isolation and characterization of the rat thyrotropin β-subunit gene. Differential regulation of two transcriptional start sites by thyroid hormone.

Carr, V. M. (1975). *Neurosci. Abstr.* 1:749. Peripheral effects on early development of chick spinal ganglia.

Carr, V. M. (1976). Ph.D. Thesis, Northwestern Univ., Evanston, Ill.

Carr, V. M. (1984). *J. Neurosci.* 4:2434–2444. Dorsal root ganglia development in chicks following partial ablation of the neural crest.

Carr, V. M., and S. Simpson (1975). *Neurosci. Abstr.* 1:749. Peripheral effects on early development of chick spinal ganglia.

Carr, V. M., and S. B. Simpson (1978). *J. Comp. Neurol.* 182:727–740. Proliferative and degenerative events in the early development of chick dorsal root ganglia.

Carr, V. M., and S. B. Simpson (1982). *Dev. Brain Res.* 2:157–162. Rapid appearance of labeled degenerating cells in the dorsal root ganglia after exposure of chick embryos to tritiated thymidine.

Carson, L. V., A. M. Kelahan, R. H. Ray, C. E. Massey, and G. S. Doetsch (1981). *Clin. Neurosurg.* 28:532–546. Effects of early peripheral lesions on the somatotopic organization of the cerebral cortex.

Carter, S. B. (1972). *Endeavour* 3:77–82. The cytochalasins as research tools in cytology.

Casagrande, V. A., and T. T. Norton (1990). Lateral geniculate nucleus: A review of its physiology and function, pp. 41–84. In *The Neural Bases of Visual Function* (A. G. Leventhal, ed.), MacMillan, London.

Casola, L., G. A. Davis, and R. E. Davis (1969). *J. Neurochem.* 16:1037–1041. Evidence for RNA transport in rat optic nerve.

Caspar, D. L. D., and D. A. Kirschner (1971). *Nature (New Biol.)* 231:46–52. Myelin membrane structure at 10 A resolution.

Caspersson, T. (1940). *J. Roy. Microscop. Soc.* 60:8–25. Methods for the determination of the absorption spectra of cell structures.

Caspersson, T. (1950). *Cell Growth and Cell Function*, Norton, New York, 185 pp.

Cass, D. T., T. J. Sutton, and R. F. Mark (1973). *Nature* 243:201–203. Competition between nerves for functional connections with axolotl muscles.

Cassimeris, L. U., R. A. Walker, N. K. Pryer, and E. D. Salmon (1987). *BioEssays* 7:149–154. Dynamic instability of microtubules.

Castillo, J. del, and B. Katz (1956). *Prog. Biophys. Biophys. Chem.* 6:121–170. Biophysical aspects of neuro-muscular transmission.

Catsicas, S., and P. G. H. Clarke (1987a). *J. Comp. Neurol.* 262:512–522. Spatiotemporal gradients of kainate-sensitivity in the developing chicken retina.

Catsicas, S., and P. G. H. Clarke (1987b). *J. Comp. Neurol.* 262:523–534. Abrupt loss of dependence of retinopetal neurons on their target cells, as shown by intraocular injections of kainate in chick embryos.

Caudy, M., and D. Bentley (1986). *J. Neurosci.* 6:1781–1795. Pioneer growth cone steering along a series of neuronal and non-neuronal cues of different affinites.

Causey, G. (1960). *The Cell of Schwann.* Livingston, Edinburgh.

Cavalieri, R. R., L. A. Gavin, R. Cole, and J. de Vellis (1986). *Brain Res.* 364:382–385. Thyroid hormone deiodinases in purified primary glial cell cultures.

Cavanagh, J. B. (1970). *J. Anat. (London)* 106:471–487. The proliferation of astrocytes around a needle wound in the rat brain.

Cavanagh, J. B. (1974). *Res. Publ. Assoc. Nerv. Ment Dis.* 53:13–38. Liver bypass and the glia.

Cavanagh, J. B., and M. H. Kyu (1971). *J. Neurol. Sci.* 12:241–261. On the mechanism of Type I Alzheimer abnormality in the nuclei of astrocytes.

Cavanagh, J. B., and P. D. Lewis (1969). *J. Anat. (London)* 104:341–350. Perfusion-fixation, colchicine and mitotic activity in the adult rat brain.

Cavanaugh, M. W. (1951). *J. Comp. Neurol.* 94:181–219. Quantitative effects of the peripheral innervation area on nerves and spinal ganglion cells.

Caveney, S. (1985). *Ann. Rev. Physiol.* 47:319–335. The role of gap junctions in development.

Caviness, V. S., Jr. (1973). *J. Comp. Neurol.* 151:113–120. Time of neuron origin in the hippocampus and dentate gyrus of normal and reeler mutant mice: An autoradiographic analysis.

Caviness, V. S., Jr. (1976). *J. Comp. Neurol.* 170:435–448. Patterns of cell and fiber distribution in the neocortex of the reeler mutant mouse.

Caviness, V. S., Jr. (1977). *Neurosci. Symp.* 2:27–46. Reeler mutant mouse: A genetic experiment in developing mammalian cortex.

Caviness, V. S., Jr. (1982). *Dev. Brain Res.* 4:293–302. Neocortical histogenesis in normal and reeler mice: A developmental study based upon ^{3}H-thymidine autoradiography.

Caviness, V. S., Jr., and M. G. Korde (1981). *Brain Res.* 209:1–9. Monoaminergic afferents to the neocortex: A developmental histofluorescence study in normal and reeler mouse embryos.

Caviness, V. S., Jr., and P. Rakic (1978). *Ann. Rev. Neurosci.* 1:297–326. Mechanisms of cortical development: A view from mutations in mice.

Caviness, V. S., Jr., and R. L. Sidman (1972). *J. Comp. Neurol.* 145:85–104. Olfactory structures of the forebrain in the reeler mutant mouse.

Caviness, V. S., Jr., and R. L. Sidman (1973). *J. Comp. Neurol.* 148:141–152. Time of origin of corresponding cell classes in the cerebral cortex of normal and reeler mutant mice: An autoradiographic analysis.

Caviness, V. S., Jr., and C. H. Yorke, Jr. (1976). *J. Comp. Neurol.* 170:449–460. Interhemispheric neocortical connections of the corpus callosum in the reeler mutant mouse: A study based on anterograde and retrograde methods.

Ceccarelli, B., F. Clementi, and P. Mantegazza (1971). *J. Physiol. (London)* 216:87–98. Synaptic transmission in the superior cervical ganglion of the cat after reinnervation by vagus fibres.

Ceccarelli B., W. P. Hurlbut and A. Mauro (1973). *J. Cell Biol.* 57:499–524. Turnover of transmitter and synaptic vesicles at the frog neuromuscular junction.

Celestino da Costa, A. (1931). *Arch. biol. (Liége)* 42:71–105. Sur la constitution et le développement des ébauches ganglionnaires craniens chez les mammifères.

Celio, M. R., E. G. Gray, and G. M. Yasargil (1979). *J. Neurocytol.* 8:19–29. Ultrastructure of the Mauthner axon collateral and its synapses in the goldfish spinal cord.

Ceni, C. (1896–1897). *Arch. Ital. Biol.* 26:97–111. Sur les fines altérations histologiques de la moelle épinière dans le dégénérescences secondaires ascendantes et descendantes.

Cerf, J. A., and L. W. Chacko (1958). *J. Comp. Neurol.* 109:205–216. Retrograde reaction in motoneuron dendrites following ventral root section in the frog.

Cervos-Navarro, J., and F. Matakas (1974). *Neurol.* 24:282–286. Electron microscopic evidence for innervation of intracerebral arterioles in the cat.

Chader, G. J. (1973). *J. Neurochem.* 21:1525–1532. Some factors affecting the uptake, binding and retention of (^{3}H)cortisol by the chick embryo retina as related to enzyme induction.

Chalfie, M., H. R. Horwitz, and J. E. Sulston (1981). *Cell* 24:59–69. Mutations that lead to reiterations of cell lineages of *C. elegans.*

Chalupa, L. M., and H. P. Killackey (1989). *Proc. Natl. Acad. Sci. U.S.A.* 86:1076–1079. Process elimination underlies ontogenetic change in the distribution of callosal projection neurons in the postcentral gyrus of the fetal rhesus monkey.

Chalupa, L. M., R. W. Williams, and Z. Henderson (1984). *Neuroscience* 12:1139–1146. Binocular interaction of the fetal cat regulates the size of ganglion cell population.

Chamak, B., and A. Prochiantz (1989a). *C. R. Acad. Sci. Paris* 308:353–358. Axones, dendrites et adhesion.

Chamak, B., and A. Prochiantz (1989b). *Development* 106: 483–491. Influence of extracellular matrix proteins on the expression of neuronal polarity.

Chamak, B., A. Fellous, J. Glowinski, and A. Prochiantz (1987). *J. Neurosci.* 7:3163–3170. MAP2 expression and neuritic outgrowth and branching are co-regulated through region-specific neuroastroglial interactions.

Chamberlain, J. G. (1973). *Dev. Biol.* 31:22–30. Analysis of developing ependymal and choroidal surfaces in rat brains using scanning electron microscopy.

Chambers, W. W., C. N. Liu, and G. P. McCouch (1973). *Brain, Behav. Evol.* 8:5–26. Anatomical and physiological correlates of plasticity in the central nervous system.

Chamley, J. H., I. Goller, and G. Burnstock (1973). *Dev. Biol.* 31:362–379. Selective growth of sympathetic nerve fibers to explants of normally densely innervated autonomic effector organs in tissue culture.

Champakam, S., S. G. Srikantia, C. Gopalan (1968). *Am. J. Clin. Nutr.* 21:844–855. Kwashiorkor and mental development.

Chan, K. Y., and M. R. Byers (1985). *J. Comp. Neurol.* 234:201–217. Anterograde axonal transport and intercellular transfer of WGA-HRP in trigeminal-innervated sensory receptors of rat incisive papilla.

Chan-Palay, V. (1971). *Z. Anat. Entwickl-Gesch.* 134:200–234. The recurrent collaterals of Purkinje cell axons: A correlated study of the rat's cerebellar cortex with electron microscopy and the Golgi method.

Chan-Palay, V. (1973a). *Z. Anat. Entw. Gesch.* 139:115–117. A brief note on the chemical nature of the precipitate within nerve fibres after the rapid Golgi reaction: Selected area diffraction in high voltage electron microscopy.

Chan-Palay, V. (1973b). *Z. Anat. Entwicklungsgesch.* 142:23–35. Neuronal plasticity in the cerebellar cortex and lateral nucleus.

Chan-Palay, V., and S. L. Palay (1972). *Z. Anat. Entw. Gesch.* 137:125–152. High voltage electron microscopy of rapid Golgi preparations. Neurons and their processes in the cerebellar cortex of monkey and rat.

Chan-Palay, V., G. Nilaver, S. L. Palay, M. C. Beinfeld, E. A. Zimmerman, J.-Y. Wu, and T. L. O'Donohue (1981). *Proc. Natl. Acad. Sci. U.S.A.* 78:7787–7791. Chemical heterogeneity in cerebellar PCs: Existence and coexistence of glutamic acid decarboxylase-like and motilin-like immunoreactivities.

Chan-Palay, V., S. L. Palay, and J.-Y. Wu (1982). *Proc. Natl. Acad. Sci. U.S.A.* 79:4221–4225. Sagittal cerebellar microbands of taurine neurons: Immunocytochemical demonstration by using antibodies against the taurine synthesizing enzyme cystein sulfinic acid decarboxylase.

Chan, W. Y. and P. P. L. Tam (1988). *Development* 102:427–442. A morphological and experimental study of the mesencephalic neural crest cells in the mouse embryo using wheat germ agglutinin-gold conjugate as the cell marker.

Chanda, R., D. J. Woodward, and S. Griffin (1973). *J. Neurochem.* 21:547–555. Cerebellar development in the rat after early postnatal damage by methylazoxymethanol: DNA, RNA and protein during recovery.

Chandler, C. E., L. M. Parsons, M. Hosang, and E. M. Shooter (1984). *J. Biol. Chem.* 259:6882–6889. A monoclonal antibody modulates the interaction of nerve growth factor with PC12 cells.

Chang, C. (1972). *J. Cell Biol.* 55:37. Effect of colchicine and cytochalasin B on axonal particle movement and outgrowth *in vitro*.

Chang, C. C., and M. C. Huang (1975). *Nature* 253:643–644. Turnover of junctional and extrajunctional acetylcholine receptors of the rat diaphragm.

Chang, H. T. (1952). *Cold Spring Harbor Symp. Quant. Biol.* 17:189–202. Cortical neurons with particular reference to the apical dendrites.

Chang, H.-T., T. C. Ruch, and A. A. Ward (1947). *J. Neurophysiol.* 10:39–56. Topographic representation of muscles in the motor cortex of monkeys.

Changeux, J.-P., and A. Danchin (1976). *Nature* 264:705–711. Selective stabilization of developing synapses as a mechanism for the specification of neuronal networks.

Changeux, J.-P., A. Devillers-Thiéry, and P. Chemouilli (1984). *Science* 225:1335–1345. Acetylcholine receptor: An allosteric protein.

Chapula, L. M., and H. P. Killackey (1989). *Proc. Natl. Acad. Sci. U.S.A.* 86:1076–1079. Process elimination underlies ontogenetic change in the distribution of callosal projection neurons in the postcentral gyrus of the fetal rhesus monkey.

Charp, P. A., R. J. Kinders, and T. C. Johnson (1983). *J. Cell Biol.* 97:311–316. G_2 cell cycle arrest induced by glycopeptides isolated from the bovine cerebral cortex.

Chase, H. B. (1945). *J. Comp. Neurol.* 83:121–140. Studies on an anophthalmic strain of mice. V. Associated cranial nerve and brain centers.

Chase, H. P., and H. P. Martin (1970). *New Engl. J. Med.* 282:933–976. Undernutrition and child development.

Chase, H. P., J. Dorsey, and G. M. McKhann (1967). *Pediatrics* 40:551–559. The effect of malnutrition on the synthesis of a myelin lipid.

Chase, H. P., C. A. Canosa, C. S. Dabiere, N. N. Welch, and D. O'Brien (1974). *J. Ment. Defic. Res.* 18:355–366. Postnatal undernutrition and human brain development.

Chaube, S. (1959). *J. Exp. Zool.* 140:29–78. On axiation and symmetry in transplanted wing of the chick.

Chaudhury, S., and P. K. Sarkar (1983). *Biochim. Biophys. Acta* 763:93–98. Stimulation of tubulin synthesis by thyroid hormone in the developing rat brain.

Chavéz, A., C. Martínez, and T. Yaschine (1974). *Symp. Swedish Nutr. Found.* 12:211. The importance of nutrition and stimuli on child mental and social development. In *Early Nutrition and Mental Development*, pp. 255–269, (Cravioto, Hambraeus, Vahlquist, eds.).

Cheal, M., and B. Oakley (1977). *J. Comp. Neurol.* 200:609–626. Regeneration of fungiform taste buds: Temporal and spatial characteristics.

Chen, D. H., W. W. Chambers, and C. N. Liu (1977). *Exp. Neurol.* 57:1026–1041. Synaptic displacement in intracellular neurons of Clarke's nucleus following axotomy in the cat.

Chen, F. D. H. (1977). *Anat. Rec.* 187:550. Qualitative and quantitative study of synaptic displacement in chromatolyzed spinal motoneurons of the cat.

Chen, S., and D. E. Hillman (1982a). *Brain Res.* 240:205–220. Plasticity of the parallel fiber-Purkinje cell synapse by spine takeover and new synapse formation in the adult rat.

Chen, S., and D. E. Hillman (1982b). *Brain Res.* **245**:131–135. Marked reorganization of Purkinje cell dendrites and spines in adult rat following vacating of synapse due to deafferentation.

Chen, S., and D. E. Hillman (1985). *Brain Res.* **333**:369–373. Plasticity of cerebellar parallel fibers following developmental deficits in synaptic number.

Chen, S., and D. E. Hillman (1989). *Dev. Brain Res.* **45**:137–147. Regulation of granule cell number by a predetermined number of Purkinje cells in development.

Cheng, H., and M. Bjerknes (1982). *Anat. Rec.* **203**:251–264. Whole population cell kinetics of mouse duodenal, jejunal, ileal, and colonic epithelia as determined by radioautography and flow cytometry.

Cheng, T. P. O., and T. S. Reese (1985). *J. Cell Biol.* **101**:1473–1480. Polarized compartmentalization of organelles in growth cones from developing optic tectum.

Cheng, T. P. O., and T. S. Reese (1987). *J. Neurosci.* **7**:1752–1759. Recycling of plasmalemma in chick tectal growth cones.

Cheng, T. P. O., and T. S. Reese (1988). *J. Neurosci.* **8**:3190–3199. Compartmentalization of anterogradely and retrogradely transported organelles in axons and growth cones from chick optic tectum.

Chernenko, G. A., and R. W. West (1976). *J. Comp. Neurol.* **167**:49–62. A re-examination of anatomical plasticity in the rat retina.

Chevallier, A. (1978). *Wilhelm Roux Entwicklungsmech. Org. Arch.* **184**:57–73. Etude de la migration des cellules somitiques dans le mesoderme somatopleural de l'ébauche de l'aile.

Chevallier, A. (1979). *J. Embryol. Exp. Morphol.* **49**:73–88. Role of the somitic mesoderm in the development of the thorax in bird embryos. II. Origin of thoracic and appendicular musculature.

Chevallier, A., M. Kieny, and A. Mauger (1977). *J. Embryol. Exp. Morphol.* **41**:243–258. Limb-somite relationship: Origin of the limb musculature.

Chiakulas, J. J., and J. E. Pauly (1965). *Anat. Rec.* **152**:55–61. A study of postnatal growth of skeletal muscle in the rat.

Chiarugi, G. (1894). *Contribuzioni allo studio dello sviluppo dei nervi encefalici nei mammiferi.* Firenze.

Chibon, P. (1966). *Mém. Soc. Fr. Zool.* **36**:1–107. Analyse expérimentale de la régionalisation et des capacités morphogénétiques de la crête neurale chez l'Amphibien Urodèle *Pleurodeles waltlii* Michah.

Chibon, P. (1967). *J. Embryol. Exp. Morphol.* **18**:343–358. Marquage nucléaire par la thymidine tritiée des dérivés de la crête neurale chez l'Amphibien urodéle *Pleurodeles waltlii* Michah.

Chikaraishi, D. M. (1979). *Biochemistry* **18**:3250–3256. Complexity of cytoplasmic polyadenylated and nonadenylated rat brain ribonucleic acids.

Chikaraishi, D. M., S. S. Deeb, and N. Sueoka (1978). *Cell* **13**:111–120. Sequence complexity of nuclear RNAs in adult rat tissues.

Chikaraishi, D. M., M. H. Brilliant, and E. J. Lewis (1983). *Cold Spring Harbor Symp. Quant. Biol.* **48**:309–318. Cloning and characterization of rat-brain-specific transcripts: Rare, brain-specific transcripts and tyrosine hydroxylase.

Child, C. M. (1911). *Science* **39**:73–76. Susceptibility gradients in animals.

Child, C. M. (1921). *The origin and development of the nervous system, from a physiological viewpoint.* The University of Chicago Press, Chicago.

Child, C. M. (1928). *Protoplasma* **5**:447–476. The physiological gradients.

Child, C. M. (1936). *Arch. Entw.-Mech. Organ.* **135**:426–451. Differential reduction of vital dyes in the early development of echinoderms.

Child, C. M. (1941). *Patterns and Problems of Development,* Univ. Chicago Press, Chicago, Ill. 811 pp.

Child, C. M. (1946). *Physiol. Zool.* **19**:89–148. Organizers in development and the organizer concept.

Child, C. M. (1947). *J. Exp. Zool.* **104**:153–193. Oxidation and reduction of indicators by Hydra.

Chiquet, M. (1989). *Trends Neurosci.* **12**:1–3. Neurite growth inhibition by CNS myelin proteins: A mechanism to confine fiber tracts?

Chiquet-Ehrismann, R. (1990). *FASEB J.* **4**:2598–2604. What distinguishes tenascin from fibronectin?

Chiquet-Ehrismann, R., E. J. Mackie, C. A. Pearson, and T. Sakarura. *Cell* **47**:131–139. Tenascin: An extracellular matrix protein involved in tissue interactions during fetal development and oncogenesis.

Chiu, S. Y. (1987). *J. Physiol. (London)* **386**:181–203. Sodium currents in axon-associated Schwann cells from adult rabbits.

Chiu, S. Y. (1988). *J. Physiol. (London)* **396**:173–188. Changes in excitable membrane properties in Schwann cells of adult rabbit sciatic nerves following nerve transection.

Chiu, S. Y., and G. F. Wilson (1989). *J. Physiol. (London)* **408**:199–222. The role of potassium channels in Schwann cell proliferation in Wallerian degeneration of explant rabbit sciatic nerves.

Chiu, S. Y., P. Shrager, and J. M. Ritchie (1984). *Nature* **311**:156–157. Neuronal-type Na^+ and K^+ channels in rabbit cultured Schwann cells.

Choi, B. H. (1981). *Dev. Brain Res.* **1**:249–267. Radial glia of developing human fetal spinal cord: Golgi, immunohistochemical and electron microscopic study.

Choi, B. H., and R. C. Kim (1984). *Science* **223**:407–409. Expression of glial fibrillary acidic protein in immature oligodendroglia.

Choi, B. H., and R. C. Kim (1985). *J. Neuroimmunol.* **8**:215–235. Expression of glial fibrillary acidic protein by immature oligodendroglia and its implications.

Choi, B. H., and L. W. Lapham (1978). *Brain Res.* **148**:295–311. Radial glia in the human fetal cerebrum: A combined Golgi, immunofluorescence and electron microscope study.

Choi, B. H., R. C. Kim, and L. Lapham (1983). *Dev. Brain Res.* **8**:119–130. Do radial glia give rise to both astroglia and oligodendroglial cells?

Choi, D. W. (1988). *Trends Neurosci.* **11**:465–469. Calcium-mediated neurotoxicity: Relationship to specific channel types and role in ischemic damage.

Choinowski, H. (1958). *Zool. Anz.* **161**:259–279. Vergleichende Messungen an Gehirnen von Wild- und Hauskaninchen.

Chouchkov, H. N. (1971). *Z. Mikrosk. Anat. Forsch.* **86**:33–46. Ultrastructure of Pacinian corpuscle after the section of nerve fibres.

Chow, I., and M. W. Cohen (1983). *J. Physiol. (London)* **339**:553–571. Developmental changes in the distribution of acetylocholine receptors in the myotomes of *Xenopus laevis*.

Chow, K. L., and J. H. Dewson (1966). *J. Comp. Neurol.* 128:63–74. Numerical estimates of neurons and glia in lateral geniculate body during retrograde degeneration.

Chow, K. L., and N. Randall (1964). *Psychon. Sci.* 1:259–260. Learning and retention in cats with lesions in reticular formation.

Chow, K. L., and P. D. Spear (1974). *Exp. Neurol.* 42: Morphological and functional effects of visual deprivation on the rabbit visual system.

Chow, K. L., and D. L. Stewart (1972). *Exp. Neurol.* 34:409–433. Reversal of structural and functional effects of long-term visual deprivation in cats.

Chow, K. L., L. H. Mathers, and P. D. Spear (1973). *J. Comp. Neurol.* 151: 307–322. Spreading of uncrossed retinal projection in superior colliculus of neonatally enucleated rabbits.

Christensen, B. N. (1973). *Science* 182:1255–1256. Procion brown: An intracellular dye for light and electron microscopy.

Christiansen, M., L. Vuori, J. O Mora, and M. Wagner (1974). *Symp. Swedish Nutr. Found.* 12:186–199. Social environment as it relates to malnutrition and mental development.

Chronwall, B. M., and J. R. Wolff (1981). *Biblthca anat.* 19:147–151. Non-pyramidal neurons in early developmental stages of the rat neocortex.

Chu-Wang, I.-W., and R. W. Oppenheim (1978). *J. Comp. Neurol.* 177:59–86. Cell death of motor neurons in the chick embryo spinal cord. II. A quantitative and qualitative analysis of degeneration in the ventral root, including evidence for axon outgrowth and limb innervation prior to cell death.

Chun, J. J. M, M. J. Nakamura, and C. J. Shatz (1986). *Soc. Neurosci. Abstr.* 12:502. Transient fibronectin-like immunoreactivity in the subplate during development of the cat's telencephelon.

Chun, J. J. M, M. J. Nakamura, and C. J. Shatz (1987). *Nature* 325:617–620. Transient cells of the developing mammalian telencephalon are peptide-immunoreactive neurons.

Chung, S. H., and J. Cooke (1975). *Nature* 258:126–132. Polarity of structure and of ordered nerve connections in the developing amphibian brain.

Chung, S. H., R. V. P. Bliss, and M. J. Keating (1974a). *Proc. Roy. Soc. (London) Ser. B.* 187:421–447. The synaptic organization of optic afferents in the amphibian tectum.

Chung, S. H., M. J. Keating, and T. V. P. Bliss (1974b). *Proc. Roy. Soc. (London) B.* 187:449–459. Functional synaptic relations during the development of the retino-tectal projection in amphibians.

Chuong, C.-M., and G. M. Edelman (1985a). *J. Cell Biol.* 101:1009–1026. Expression of cell-adhesion molecules in embryonic induction. I. Morphogenesis of nestling feathers.

Chuong, C.-M., and G. M. Edelman (1985b). *J. Cell Biol.* 101:1027–1043. Expression of cell-adhesion molecules in embryonic induction. II. Morphogenesis of adult feathers.

Chuong, C.-M., D. A. McClain, P. Streit, and G. M. Edelman (1982). *Proc. Natl. Acad. Sci. U.S.A.* 79:4234–4238. Neural cell adhesion molecules in rodent brains isolated by monoclonal antibodies with cross-species reactivity.

Church, J. C. T. (1969). *J. Anat. (London)* 105:419–438. Satellite cells and myogenesis: A study in the fruit bat web.

Church, J. C. T. (1970). *J. Embryol. Exp. Morphol.* 23:531–537. Cell populations in skeletal muscle after regeneration.

Churchill, F. (1969). *J. Hist. Biol.* 2:165–185. From machine theory to entelechy: Two studies in developmental teleology.

Churchill, J. A., J. W. Neff, and D. F. Caldwell (1966). *Obstet. Gynecol.* 28: 425–429. Birth weight and intelligence.

Chytil, F., and D. E. Ong (1984). Cellular retinoid-binding proteins, pp. 89–123, Vol. 2. In *The Retinoids* (M. B. Sporn, A. B. Roberts, and D. S. Goodman, eds.), Academic Press, Orlando, FL.

Ciaranello, R. D., and J. Axelrod (1975). *J. Neurochem.* 24:775–778. Effects of dexamethasone on neurotransmitter enzymes in chromaffin tissue of the newborn rat.

Ciaranello, R. D., D Jacobowitz, and J. Axelrod (1973). *J. Neurochem.* 20:799–805. Effect of dexamethasone on phenylethanolamine N-methyltransferase in chromaffin tissue of the neonatal rat.

Cicero, T. J., and R. R. Provine (1972). *Brain Res.* 44:294–298. The levels of the brain-specific proteins, S-100 and 14-3-2, in the developing chick spinal cord.

Ciment, G., and J. De Vellis (1982). *J. Neurosci. Res.* 7:371–386. Cell surface-mediated cellular interactions: Effects of B104 neuroblastoma surface determinants on C6 glioma cellular properties.

Ciment, G., and J. A. Weston (1982). *Dev. Biol.* 93:355–367. Early appearance in neural crest and crest-derived cells of an antigenic determinant present in avian neurons.

Ciment, G., and J. A. Weston (1983). *Nature* 305:424–427. Enteric neurogenesis by neural crest-derived branchial arch mesenchymal cells.

Citi, S., and J. Kendrick-Jones (1986). *J. Mol. Biol.* 188:369–382. Regulation *in vitro* of brush border myosin by light chain phosphorylation.

Citi, S., and J. Kendrick-Jones (1987). *BioEssays* 7:155–159. Regulation of non-muscle myosin structure and function.

Clark, D. A. (1931). *Amer. J. Physiol.* 96:296–304. Muscle counts of motor units: A study in innervation ratios.

Clark, M. B., and M. B. Bunge (1989). *Dev. Biol.*133:393–404. Cultured schwann cells assemble normal-appearing basal lamina only when they ensheathe axons.

Clark, S. C., and R. Kamens (1987). *Science* 236:1229–1237. The human hematopoietic colony-stimulating factors.

Clark, W. G. (1937a). *Plant Physiol.* 12:409–440. Electrical polarity and auxin transport.

Clark, W. G. (1937b). *Plant Physiol.* 13:529–552. Polar transport of auxin and electrical polarity in the coleoptile of Avena.

Clark, W. G. (1938). *Plant Physiol.* 13:529–552. Electrical polarity and auxin transport.

Clarke, D. M. (1989). *Occult Powers and Hypotheses: Cartesian Natural Philosophy under Louis XIV*. Clarendon Press, Oxford.

Clarke, E. (1968). The doctrine of the hollow nerve in the seventeenth and eighteenth centuries, pp. 123–141. In *Medicine, Science and Culture,* (Stevenson, and Multhauf, eds.), Johns Hopkins Press, Baltimore.

Clarke, E., and C. D. O'Malley (1968). *The Human Brain and Spinal Cord. A Historical Study Illustrated by Writings from Antiquity to the Twentieth Century*. Univ. Calif. Press, Berkeley and Los Angeles.

Clarke, M., and J. A. Spudich (1977). *Ann. Rev. Biochem.*

46:797–822. Nonmuscle contractile proteins: The role of actin and myosin in cell motility and shape determination.

Clarke, P. G. (1985). *J. Comp. Neurol.* 234:365–379. Neuronal death during development in the isthmo-optic nucleus of the chick: Sustaining role of afferents from the tectum.

Clarke, P. G. H. (1975). *J. Physiol. (London)* 256:44–45P. Neuronal death as an error-correcting mechanism in the development of the chick's isthmo-optic nucleus.

Clarke, P. G. H. (1981). *Perspec. Biol. Med.* 25:2–19. Chance, repetition and error in the development of normal nervous system.

Clarke, P. G. H. (1982a). *Neurosci. Lett.* 30:223–228. Labelling of dying neurons by peroxidase injected intravascularly in chick embryos.

Clarke, P. G. H. (1982b). *Anat. Embryol.* 165:389–404. The genuineness of isthmo-optic neuronal death in chick embryos.

Clarke, P. G. H. (1984). *Histochem. J.* 16:955–969. Identical populations of phagocytes and dying neurons revealed by intravascularly injected horseradish peroxidase, and by endogenous glutaraldehyde-resistant acid phosphatase, in the brains of chick embryos.

Clarke, P. G. H. (1985a). *Trends Neurosci.* 8:345–349. Neuronal death in the development of the vertebrate nervous system.

Clarke, P. G. H. (1985b). *J. Comp. Neurol.* 234:365–379. Neuronal death during development in the isthmo-optic nucleus of the chick: Sustaining role of afferents from the tectum.

Clarke, P. G. H., and W. M. Cowan (1975). *Proc. Natl. Acad. Sci.* 72:4455–4458. Ectopic neurons and aberrant connections during neural development.

Clarke, P. G. H., and W. M. Cowan (1976). *J. Comp. Neurol.* 167:143–164. The development of the isthmo-optic tract in the chick, with special reference to the occurrence and correction of developmental errors in the location and connections of isthmo-optic neurons.

Clarke, P. G. H., and M. Egloff (1988). *Anat. Embryol. (Berl.)* 179:103–108. Combined effects of deafferentation and de-efferentation on isthmo-optic neurons during the period of their naturally occurring cell death.

Clarke, P. G. H., and J. P. Hornung (1989). *J. Comp. Neurol.* 283:438–449. Changes in the nuclei of dying neurons as studied with thymidine autoradiography.

Clarke, P. G. H., L. A. Rogers, and W. M. Cowan (1976). *J. Comp. Neurol.* 167: 125–142. The time of origin and the pattern of survival of neurons in the isthmo-optic nucleus of the chick.

Clarke, S., and Innocenti, G. M. (1986). *J. Comp. Neurol.* 251:1–22. Organization of the immature intrahemispheric connections.

Clavert, J. (1960a). *Arch. Anat. Micro. Morph. Exp.* 49:1–22. Déterminisme de la symétrie bilatérale chez les oiseaux. II. Influence de la "présentation" de l'oeuf dans l'utérus sur l'orientation de l'embryon.

Clavert, J. (1960b). *Arch. Anat. Micro. Morph. Exp.* 49:207–227. Déterminisme de la symétrie bilatérale chez les oiseaux. III. Influence de la position de l'axe de l'oeuf dans l'utérus sur l'orientation de l'embryon.

Claxton, J. H. (1964). *J. Theoret. Biol.* 7:302–317. The determination of patterns with special reference to the of the central primary skin follicles in sheep.

Clay, R. S., and T. H. Court (1975). *The History of the Microscope.* Holland Press, London (reprint of 1932 first edn.).

Clayton, C. J., R. I. Grosser, and W. Stevens (1977). *Brain Res.* 134:445–453. The ontogeny of corticosterone and dexamethasone receptors in rat brain.

Cleaver, J. E. (1967). In *Thymidine Metabolism and Cell Kinetics.* Vol. 6, p. 45. In *Frontiers of Biology.* North Holland Publ., Amsterdam.

Cleaver, J. E., G. H. Thomas, and H. J. Burki (1972). *Science* 177:996–998. Biological damage from intranuclear tritium: DNA strand breaks and their repair.

Clemente, C. (1964). *Int. Rev. Neurobiol.* 6:257–301. Regeneration in the vertebrate central nervous system.

Clendinnen, B. G., and J. T. Eayrs (1961). *J. Endocrinol.* 22:183–193. The anatomical and physiological effects of prenatally administered somatotrophin on cerebral development.

Cleveland, D. W., S. Hwo, and M. W. Kirschner (1977a). *J. Mol. Biol.* 116:207–225. Purification of tau, a microtubule-associated protein that induces assembly of microtubules from purified tubulin.

Cleveland, D. W., S. Hwo, and M. W. Kirschner (1977b). *J. Mol. Biol.* 116:227–247. Physical and chemical properties of purified tau factor and the role of tau in microtubule assembly.

Cliff, W. J. (1963). *Philos. Trans. Roy. Soc. (London) Ser. B.* 246:305–325. Observations on healing tissue: A combined light and electron microscopic investigation.

Clos, J., and J. Legrand (1969). *Arch. Anat. Mikr. Morph. Exp.* 58:339–354. Influence de la déficience thyroidienne et de la sous-alimentation sur la croissance et la myélinisation des fibres nerveuses de la moelle cervicale et du nerf sciatique chez le jeune rat blanc.

Clos, J., and J. Legrand (1970). *Brain Res.* 22:285–297. Influence de la déficience thyroïdienne et de la sous-alimentation sur la croissance et la myélinisation des fibres nerveuses du nerf sciatique chez le jeune rat blanc. Étude au microscope électronique.

Clos, J., and J. Legrand (1973). *Brain Res.* 63:450–455. Effects of thyroid deficiency on the different cell populations of the cerebellum in the young rat.

Clos, J., F. Crépel, C. Legrand, J. Legrand, J. Rabié, and E. Vigouroux (1974). *Gen. Comp. Endocrinol.* 23:178–192. Thyroid physiology during the postnatal period in the rat: A study of the development of thyroid function and of the morphogenetic effects of thyroxine with special references to cerebellar maturation.

Clos, J., C. Legrand, and J. Legrand (1979). *Ann. Biol. Anim. Biochem. Biophys.* 19:167–172. Early effects of undernutrition on the development of cerebellar Bergmann glia cells.

Clos, J., J. Legrand, N. Limozin, C. Dalmasso, and G. Laurent (1982a). *Dev. Neurosci.* 5:243–251. Effects of abnormal thyroid state and undernutrition on carbonic anhydrase and oligodendroglia development in the rat cerebellum.

Clos, J., C. Legrand, J. Legrand, M. S. Ghandour, G. Labourdette, G. Vincendon, and G. Gombos (1982b). *Dev. Neurosci.* 5:285–292. Effects of thyroid state and undernutrition on S100 protein and astroglia development in rat cerebellum.

Close, R. (1964). *J. Physiol. (London)* 173:74–95. Dynamic properties of fast and slow skeletal muscles of the rat during development.

Close, R. (1965). *Nature* 206:831–832. Effects of cross-union of motor nerves to fast and slow skeletal muscles.

Close, R. (1967). *J. Physiol. (London)* 193: 45–55. Properties of motor units in fast and slow skeletal muscles of the rat.

Cochard, P., and P. Coltey (1983). 98:221–238. Cholinergic traits in the neural crest: Acetylcholinesterase in crest cells of the chick embryo.

Cochard, P., and D. Paulin (1984). *J. Neurosci.* 4:2080–2094. Initial expression of neurofilaments and vimentin in the central and peripheral nervous system of the mouse embryo *in vivo.*

Cochran, S. L., J. T. Hackett, and D. L. Brown (1980). *Neuroscience* 5:1629–1646. The anuran mauthner cell and its synaptic bed.

Coërs, C. (1967). *Int. Rev. Cytol.* 22:239–267. Structure and organization of the myoneural junction.

Coërs, C., and A. L. Woolf (1959). *The Innervation of Muscle.* Blackwell, Oxford.

Coffin, J. D., and T. J. Poole (1988). *Development* 102:735–748. Embryonic vascular development: Immunohistochemical identification of the origin and subsequent morphogenesis of the major vessel primordia in quail embryos.

Coggeshall, R. E. (1967). *J. Neurophysiol.* 30:1263–1287. A light and electron microscopic study of the abdominal ganglion of *Aplysia californica.*

Coghill, G. E. (1924). *J. Comp. Neurol.* 37:71–120. Correlated anatomical and physiological studies of the growth of the nervous system of *Amphibia.* IV. Rates of proliferation and differentiation in the central nervous system of *Amblystoma.*

Coghill, G. E. (1933). *J. Comp. Neurol.* 57:327–358. Correlated anatomical and physiological studies of the growth of the nervous system of *Amphibia.* XI. The prolifertion of cells in the spinal cord as a factor in the individuation of the hind leg of *Amblystoma punctatum.*

Cohan, C. S., and S. B. Kater (1986). *Science* 232:1638–1640. Suppression of neurite elongation and growth cone dynamics by electrical activity.

Cohan, C. S., J. A. Connor, and S. B. Kater (1987). *J. Neurosci.* 7:3588–3599. Electrically and chemically mediated increases in intracellular calcium in neuronal growth cones.

Cohen, A. M. (1972). *J. Exp. Zool.* 179:167–182. Factors directing the expression of sympathetic nerve traits in cells of neural crest origin.

Cohen, A. M., and I. R. Konigsberg (1975). *Dev. Biol.* 46:262–280. A clonal approach to the problem of neural crest determination.

Cohen, J., V. Mares, and Z. Lodin (1973). *J. Neurochem.* 20:651–657. DNA content of purified preparations of mouse Purkinje neurons isolated by a velocity sedimentation technique.

Cohen, J., J. F. Burne, J. Winter, and P. Bartlett (1986). *Nature* 322:465–467. Retinal ganglion cells lose response to laminin with maturation.

Cohen, J., J. F. Burne, C. McKinley, and J. Winter (1987). *Dev. Biol.* 122:407–418. The role of laminin and the laminin/fibronectin receptor complex in the outgrowth of retinal ganglion cell axons.

Cohen, M. H., and A. Robertson (1971). *J. Theor. Biol.* 31:119–130. Chemotaxis and the early stages of aggregation in cellular slime molds.

Cohen, M. J. (1967). Correlations between structure function and RNA metabolism in central neurons of insects, pp. 65–78. In *Invertebrate Nervous Systems* (C. A. G. Wiersma, ed.), Univ. Chicago Press, Chicago.

Cohen, M. J., and J. W. Jacklet (1965). *Science* 148:1237–1239. Neurons of insects: RNA changes during injury and regeneration.

Cohen, M. J., and J. W. Jacklet (1967). *Phil. Trans. Roy. Soc. (London) Ser. B.* 781:561–572. The functional organization of motor neurons in an insect ganglion.

Cohen, M. W. (1972). *Brain Res.* 41:457–463. The development of neuromuscular connexions in the presence of D-tubocurarine.

Cohen, M. W. (1980). *J. Exp. Biol.* 89:43–56. Development of an amphibian neuromuscular junction *in vivo* and in culture.

Cohen, R. S., H. C. Pant, S. House, and H. Gainer (1987). *J. Neurosci.* 7:2056–2074. Biochemical and immunocytochemical characterization and distribution of phosphorylated and nonphosphorylated subunits of neurofilaments in squid giant axon and stellate ganglion.

Cohen, S. (1958). A nerve growth-promoting protein, pp. 665–679. In *The Chemical Basis of Development* (W. D. McElroy, and B. Glass, eds.), Johns Hopkins Press, Baltimore.

Cohen, S. (1959). *J. Biol. Chem.* 234:1129–1137. Purification and metabolic effects of a nerve growth-promoting protein from snake venom.

Cohen, S. (1960). *Proc. Natl. Acad. Sci. U.S.* 46:302–311. Purification of a nerve-growth promoting protein from the mouse salivary gland and its neurocytotoxic antiserum.

Cohen, S. (1964). *Nat. Cancer Inst. Monogr.* 13:14–37. Isolation and biological effects of an epidermal growth-stimulating protein.

Cohen, S. (1965). *Dev. Biol.* 12:394–407. The stimulation of epidermal proliferations by a specific protein (EGF).

Cohen, S., and R. Levi-Montalcini (1956). *Proc. Natl. Acad. Sci. U.S.* 42:571–574. A nerve growth stimulating factor isolated from snake venom.

Cohen, S., and M. Stastny (1968). *Biochim. Biophys. Acta* 166:427–437. Epidermal growth factor. III. Stimulation of polysome formation in chick embryo epidermis.

Cohen, S., and J. M. Taylor (1974). Epidermal growth factor: Chemical and biological characterisation, pp. 25–42. In *Macromolecules Regulating Growth and Development* (E. D. Hay, T. J. Kind, and J. Papaconstantinous, eds.), Academic Press, New York.

Cohen, S., R. Levi-Montalcini, and V. Hamburger (1954). *Proc. Natl. Acad. Sci. U.S.* 40:1014–1018. A nerve growth-stimulating factor isolated from sarcomas 37 and 180.

Cohnheim, J. (1866). *Virchow's Archiv.* 38:343–386. Über die Endigung der sensiblen Nerven in der Hornhaut.

Cole, F. J. (1930). *Early Theories of Sexual Generation.* Clarendon Press, Oxford.

Cole, F. J. (1944). *A History of Comparative Anatomy.* Macmillan, London.

Cole, M. (1968). Retrograde degeneration of axon and soma in the central nervous system, pp. 269–300. In *The Structure and Function of Nervous Tissue,* (G. H. Bourne, ed.), Academic Press, New York.

Coleman, L.-A., and L. D. Beazley (1989a). *Dev. Brain Res.* 48:273–291. Expanded retinofugal projections to the dorsal lateral geniculate nucleus and superior colliculus after unilateral enucleation in the wallaby *Setonix brachyurus,* quokka.

Coleman, L.-A., and L. D. Beazley (1989b). *Dev. Brain Res.* 48:293–307. Retinal ganglion cell number is unchanged in the remaining eye following early unilateral eye removal in the wallaby *Setonix brachyurus,* quokka.

Coleman, P. D., and D. G. Flood (1987). *Neurobiol. Aging* 8:521–545. Neuron numbers and dendritic extent in normal aging and Alzheimer's disease.

Coleman, P. D., and A. H. Riesen (1968). *J. Anat. (London)* 102:363–374. Environmental effects on cortical dendritic fields: I. Rearing in the dark.

Coleman, R. W., and S. Provence (1957). *J. Pediat.* 19:285. Environmental retardation (hospitalism) in infants living in families.

Collin, C. D., and C. M. Cone (1976). *Science* 192:155–158. Induction of mitosis in mature neurons in central nervous system by sustained depolarization.

Collins, F., and K. A. Crutcher (1985). *J. Neurosci.* 5:2809–2814. Neurotrophic activity in the adult rat hippocampal formation: Regional distribution and increase after septal lesion.

Collins, F., and J. Garrett (1980). *Proc. Natl. Acad. Sci. U.S.A.* 77:6226–6228. Elongating nerve fibers are guided by a pathway of material released from nonneuronal cells.

Collins, R. (1906). *Névraxe* 8:181–308. Recherches cytologiques sur le développement de la cellule nerveuse.

Colman, D. R., G. Kreibich, A. B. Frey, and D. D. Sabatini (1982). *J. Cell Biol.* 95:598–608. Synthesis and incorporation of myelin polypeptides into CNS myelin.

Colonnier, M. (1964). *J. Anat. (London)* 98:327–344. The tangential organization of the visual cortex.

Colonnier, M. (1966). The structural design of the neocortex, pp. 1–23. In *Brain and Conscious Experience* (J. C. Eccles, ed.), Springer-Verlag, Berlin.

Colonnier, M. (1968). *Brain Res.* 9:268–287. Synaptic patterns on different cell types in the different laminae of the cat visual cortex. An electron microscope study.

Commins, D., and P. Yahr (1984). *J. Comp. Neurol.* 224:132–140. Adult testosterone levels influence the morphology of a sexually dimorphic area in the Mongolian gerbil brain.

Comte, A. (1864). *Cours de Philosophie Positive,* 2nd edn. Ballière, Paris.

Concalon, P., and L. M. Beidler (1975). *Brain Res.* 89:225–244. Distribution along the axon and into various subcellular fractions of molecules labeled with (^{3}H) leucine and rapidly transported in the garfish olfactory nerve.

Condie, B. G., and R. M. Harland (1987). *Development* 101:93–105. Posterior expression of a homeobox gene in early *Xenopus* embryos.

Conel, J. L. (1939–1963). *The Postnatal Development of the Human Cerebral Cortex,* 6 vols. Harvard Univ. Press, Cambridge, Mass.

Conger, A. D., and M. A. Wells (1969). *Radiat. Res.* 37:31–49. Radiation and aging effect on taste structure and function.

Conlee, J. W., and T. N. Parks (1981). *J. Comp. Neurol.* 202:373–384. Age- and position-dependent effects of monaural acoustic deprivation in nucleus magnocellularis of the chicken.

Conlee, J. W., and T. N. Parks (1983). *J. Comp. Neurol.* 217:216–226. Late appearance and deprivation-sensitive growth of permanent dendrites in the avian cochlear nucleus (nuc. magnocellularis).

Conn, H. J. (1928). *Stain Technology* 3:1–12. The history of staining. The pioneers.

Conn, H. J. (1930). *Stain Technology* 5:3–10. The history of staining. Anilin dyes in histology.

Connold, A. L., J. V. Evers, and G. Vrbova (1986). *Dev. Brain Res.* 28:99–107. Effect of low calcium and protease inhibitors on synapse elimination during postnatal development in the rat soleus muscle.

Connolly, C. J. (1950). *External Morphology of the Primate Brain,* 378 pp., Thomas, Springfield, Ill.

Connolly, J. L., P. J. Seeley, and L. A. Greene (1985). *J. Neurosci. Res.* 13:183–198. Regulation of growth cone morphology by nerve growth factor: A comparative study by scanning electron microscopy.

Conradi, S., and L.-O. Ronnevi (1975). *Brain Res.* 92:505–510. Spontaneous elimination of synapses on cat spinal motoneurons after birth: Do half of the synapses on the cell bodies disappear?

Constantine-Paton, M. (1981). Induced ocular-dominace zones in tectal cortex, pp. 47–67. In *Organization of the Cerebral Cortex* (F. O. Schmidt, F. G. Worden, G. Adelman, and S. G. Dennis, eds.), MIT Press, Cambridge.

Constantine-Paton, M., and R. R. Capranica (1975). *Science* 189:480–482. Central projection of optic tract from translocated eyes in the leopard frog *(Rana pipiens).*

Constantine-Paton, M., and R. R. Capranica (1976a). *J. Comp. Neurol.* 170:17–31. Axonal guidance of developing optic nerves in the frog. I. Anatomy of the projection from transplanted eye primordia.

Constantine-Paton, M., and R. R. Capranica (1976b). *J. Comp. Neurol.* 170:33–51. Axonal guidance of developing optic nerves in the frog. II. Electrophysiological studies of the projection from transplanted eye primorida.

Constantine-Paton, M., and P. Ferrari-Eastman (1981). *J. Comp. Neurol.* 196:645–661. Topographic and morphometric effects of bilateral embryonic eye removal on the optic tectum and nucleus isthmus of the leopard frog.

Constantine-Paton, M., A. S. Blum, R. Mendez-Otero, and C. J. Barnstable (1986). *Nature* 324:459–462. A cell surface molecule distributed in a dorsoventral gradient in the perinatal rat retina.

Conti-Tronconi, B. M., and M. A. Raftery (1982). *Ann. Rev. Biochem.* 51:491–530. The nicotinic cholinergic receptor: Correlation of molecular structure with functional properties.

Contopoulos, A. M., M. E. Simpson, and A. A. Koneff (1958). *Endocrinology* 63:642–653. Pituitary function in the thyroidectomized rat.

Cook, J. E. (1983). *Exp. Brain Res.* 51:433–442. Tectal paths of regenerating optic axons in the goldfish: Evidence from retrograde labelling with horseradish peroxidase.

Cook, J. E. (1987). *Exp. Brain Res.* 68:319–328. A sharp retinal image increases the topographic precision of the goldfish retinotectal projection during optic nerve regeneration in stroboscopic light.

Cook, J. E. (1988). *Exp. Brain Res.* 70:109–116. Topographic refinement of the goldfish retinotectal projection: Sensitivity to stroboscopic light at different periods during optic nerve regeneration.

Cook, J. E., and D. L. Becker (1988). *Development* 104:321–329. Retinotopic refinement of the regenerating goldfish optic tract is not linked to activity-dependent refinement of the retinotectal map.

Cook, J. E., and T. J. Horder (1974). *J. Physiol. (London)* 241:89–90. Interactions between optic fibres in their regeneration to specific sites in the goldfish tectum.

Cook, J. E., and E. C. C. Rankin (1986). *Exp. Brain Res.* 63:421–430. Impaired refinement of the regenerated retinotectal projection of the goldfish in stroboscopic light: A quantitative WGA-HRP study.

Cook, L. M. (1971). *Coefficients of Natural Selection*, Hutchinson and Co., London.

Cook, W. H., J. H. Walker, and M. L. Barr (1951). *J. Comp. Neurol.* 94:267–292. A cytological study of transneuronal atrophy in the cat and the rabbit.

Cooke, J. (1973a). *J. Embryol. Exp. Morphol.* 30:49–62. Properties of the primary organization field in the embryo of *Xenopus laevis* IV. Pattern formation and regulation following early inhibition of mitosis.

Cooke, J. (1973b). *J. Embryol. Exp. Morphol.* 30:283–300. Properties of the primary organization field in the embryo of *Xenopus laevis* V. Regulation after removal of the head organizer, in normal early gastrulae and in those already possessing a second implanted organizer.

Cooke, J. (1973c). *Nature* 242:55–57. Morphogenesis and regulation in spite of continued mitotic inhibition in *Xenopus* embryos.

Cooke, J. (1985). *J. Embryol. Exp. Morphol.* 89:Suppl. 68–87. The system specifying body position in the early development of *Xenopus*, and its response to early perturbations.

Cooke, J. (1989). *Development* 107:229–241. Mesoderm-inducing factors and Spemann's organiser phenomenon in amphibian development.

Cooke, J., and R. M. Gaze (1983). *J. Embryol. Exp. Morphol.* 77:53–71. The positional coding system in the early eye rudiment of *Xenopus laevis*, and its modification after grafting operations.

Cooke, J., J. C. Smith, E. J. Smith, and M. Yaqoob (1987). *Development* 101:893–908. The organization of mesodermal pattern in *Xenopus laevis:* Experiments using a *Xenopus* mesoderm-inducing factor.

Coomber, B. L., and S. R. Scadding (1983). *Cell Tiss. Kinet.* 16:77–83. Evidence for a chalone control mechanism in the limb regeneration blastema of the newt, *Notophthalmus viridescens.*

Cooper, E., and J. Diamond (1977). *J. Physiol. (London)* 264:695–723. A quantitative study of the mechanosensory innervation of the salamander skin.

Cooper, G. W. (1965). *Dev. Biol.* 12:185–212. Induction of somite chondrogenesis by cartilage and notochord: A correlation between inductive activity and specific stages of cytodifferentiation.

Cooper, J. A. (1987). *J. Cell Biol.* 105:1473–1478. Effects of cytochalasin and phalloidin on actin.

Cooper, M. L., and G. G. Blasdel (1980). *J. Comp. Neurol.* 193:237–254. Regional variation in the representation of the visual field in the visual cortex of the Siamese cat.

Cooper, M. S., and R. E. Keller (1984). *Proc. Natl. Acad. Sci. U.S.A.* 81:160–164. Perpendicular orientation and directional migration of amphibian neural crest cells in DC electrical fields.

Cooper, M. S., and M. Schliwa (1985). *J. Neurosci. Res.* 13:223–244. Electrical and ioinic control of tissue cell locomotion in DC electric fields.

Cooper, N. G. F. and D. A. Steindler (1986a). *J. Comp. Neurol.* 249:157–169. Lectins demarcate the barrel subfield in the somatosensory cortex of the early postnatal mouse.

Cooper, N. G. F., and D. A. Steindler (1986b). *Brain Res.* 380:341–348. Monoclonal antibody to glial fibrillary acidic protein reveals a parcellation of individual barrels in the early postnatal mouse somatosensory cortex.

Cooper, P. D., and R. S. Smith (1974). *J. Physiol. (London)* 242:77–97. The movement of optically detectable organelles in myelinated axons of *Xenopus laevis.*

Copp, A. J., and M. Bernfield (1988). *Dev. Biol.* 130:573–582. Glycosaminoglycans vary in accumulation along the neuraxis during spinal neurulation in the mouse embryo.

Corliss, C. E., and G. C. Robertson (1963). *J. Exp. Zool.* 153:125–140. The pattern of mitotic density in the early chick neural epithelium.

Cornbrooks, C. J., D. J. Cary, J. A. McDonald, R. Timpl, and R. P. Bunge (1983). *Proc. Natl. Acad. Sci. U.S.A.* 80:3850–3854. *In vivo* and *in vitro* observations on laminin production by Schwann cells.

Cornell-Bell, A. H., S. M. Finkbeiner, M. S. Cooper, and S. J. Smith (1990). *Science* 247:470–473. Glutamate induces calcium waves in cultured astrocytes: Long-range glial signaling.

Corner, M. A. (1963). *J. Exp. Zool.* 153:301–311. Development of the brain of *Xenopus laevis* after removal of parts of the neural plate.

Corner, M. A. (1964). *J. Comp. Neurol.* 123: 243–256. Localization of capacities for functional development in the neural plate of *Xenopus laevis.*

Corner, M. A., and S. M. Crain (1964). *Experientia* 21:1–7. Spontaneous contractions and bioelectric activity after differentiation in culture of presumptive neuromuscular tissues in the early frog embryo.

Corner, M. A., J. P. Schade, J. Sedlacek, and A. P. C. Bot (1967). *Prog. Brain Res.* 26:145–192. Developmental patterns in the central nervous system of birds. I. Electrical activity in the cerebral hemisphere, optic lobe and cerebellum.

Cornwall, J., and O. T. Phillipson (1988). *J. Neurosci. Meth.* 24:1–9. Quantitative analysis of axonal branching using the retrograde transport of fluorescent latex microspheres.

Corpechot, C., E. E. Baulieu, and P. Robel (1981). *Acta Endocrinol.* 96:127–135. Testosterone, dihydrotestosterone, and androstanediols in plasma, testes, and prostates of rats during development.

Coss, R. G. (1985). *Behav. Neural Biol.* 44:151–185. The function of dendritic spines: A review of theoretical issues.

Costantino-Ceccarini, E., and P. Morell (1971). *Brain Res.* 29:75–84. Quaking mouse: *In vitro* studies of brain sphingolipid biosynthesis.

Costanzo, R., R. L. Watterson, and G. C. Schoenwolf (1982). *J. Exp. Zool.* 219:233–240. Evidence that secondary neurulation occurs autonomously in the chick embryo.

Cotman, C. W., and L. L. Iversen (1987). *Trends Neurosci.* 10:263–265. Excitatory amino acids in the brain focus on NMDA receptors.

Cotman, C. W., and D. T. Monaghan (1988). *Ann. Rev. Neurosci.* 11:61–80. Excitatory amino acid neurotransmission: NMDA receptors and Hebb-type synaptic plasticity.

Cotman, C. W., D. Taylor, and G. Lynch (1973a). *Brain Res.* 63:205–213. Ultrastructural changes in synapses in the dentate gyrus of the rat during development.

Cotman, C. W., M. Nieto-Sampedro, and E. W. Harris (1982). *Physiol Rev.* 61:684–784. Synapse turnover in adult vertebrates.

Cotterrell, M., R. Balázs, and A. L. Johnson (1972). *J. Neurochem.* 19:2151–2167. Effects of corticosteroids on the biochemical maturation of rat brain: Postnatal cell formation.

Couchie, D., and J. Nunez (1985). *FEBS Lett.* 188:331–335. Immunological characterization of microtubule-associated proteins specific for the immature brain.

Couchie, D., C. Fages, A. M. Bridoux, B. Rolland, M. Tardy, and J. Nunez (1985). *J. Cell Biol.* 101:2095–2103. Microtubule-associated proteins and *in vitro* astrocyte differentiation.

Couchman, J. R., D. A. Rees, M. R. Green, and C. G. Smith (1982). *J. Cell Biol.* 93:402–410. Fibronectin has a dual role in locomotion and anchorage of primary chick fibroblasts and can promote entry into the divison cycle.

Coughlin, M. D. (1975). *Dev. Biol.* 43:140–158. Target organ stimulation of parasympathetic nerve growth in the developing mouse submandibular gland.

Coulombre, J. L., and A. J. Coulombre (1965). *Dev. Biol.* 12:79–92. Regeneration of neural retina from the pigmented epithelium in the chick embryo.

Couly, G., and N. M. LeDouarin (1987). *Dev. Biol.* 120:198–214. Mapping of the early neural primordium in quail-chick chimaeras. II. The prosencephalic neural plate and neural folds: Implications for the genesis of cephalic human congenital abnormalities.

Couly, G. F., and N. M. LeDouarin (1985). *Dev. Biol.* 110:422–439. Mapping of the neural early primordium in quail-chick chimaeras. I. Developmental relationship between placodes facial ectoderm and prosencephalon.

Count, E. W. (1947). *Ann. N.Y. Acad. Sci.* 46:993–1122. Brain and body weight in man: Their antecedents in growth and evolution.

Couraud, J. Y., and L. Di Giamberardino (1980). *J. Neurochem.* 35:1053–1066. Axonal transport of the molecular forms of Acetylcholinesterase in chick sciatic nerve.

Coursin, D. B. (1967). *Fed. Proc.* 26:134–138. Relationship of nutrition to central nervous system development and function.

Coutard, M., and M. J. Osborne-Pellegrin (1979). *Cell Tissue Res.* 197:531–538. Autoradiographic studies of a glucocorticoid agonist and antagonist: Localization of ^{3}H-corticosterone and ^{3}H-cortexolone in mouse brain.

Couteaux, R. (1963). *Proc. Roy. Soc. (London) Ser. B.* 158:457–480. The differentiation of synaptic areas.

Cowan, W. M. (1970). Anterograde and retrograde transneuronal degeneration in the central and peripheral nervous system, pp. 217–251. In *Contemporary Research Methods in Neuroanatomy* (W. J. H. Nauta, and S. O. E. Ebbesson, eds.), Springer Verlag, New York, Heidelberg, Berlin.

Cowan, W. M. (1973). Neuronal death as a regulative mechanism in the control of cell number in the nervous system, pp. 19–41. In *Development and Aging in the Nervous System* (M. Rockstein, ed.), Academic Press, New York.

Cowan, W. M., and P. G. H. Clarke (1976). *Brain Behav. Evol.* 13:345–375. The development of the isthmo-optic nucleus.

Cowan, W. M., and E. Wenger (1967). *J. Exp. Zool.* 164:267–280. Cell loss in the trochlear nucleus of the chick during

normal development and after radical extirpation of the optic vesicle.

Cowan, W. M., and E. Wenger (1968a). *J. Comp. Neurol.* 133:207–239. The development of the nucleus of origin of centrifugal fibers to the retina in the chick.

Cowan, W. M., and E. Wenger (1968b). *J. Exp. Zool.* 168:105–124. Degeneration in the nucleus of origin of the preganglionic fibers to the chick ciliary ganglion following early removal of the optic vesicle.

Cowan, W. M., A. H. Martin, and E. Wenger (1968). *J. Exp. Zool.* 169:71–92. Mitotic patterns in the optic tectum of the chick during normal development and after early removal of the optic vesicle.

Cowan, W. M., D. I. Gottlieb, A. E. Hendrickson, J. L. Price, and T. A. Woolsey (1972). *Brain Res.* 37:21–51. The autoradiographic demonstration of axonal connections in the central nervous system.

Cowan, W. M., J. W. Fawcett, D. D. M. O'Leary, and B. B Stanfield (1984). *Science* 225:1258–1265. Regressive events in neurogenesis.

Cowdry, E. V. (1914). *Am. J. Anat.* 15: 389–429. The development of the cytoplasmic constituents of the nerve cells of the chick. I. Mitochondria and neurofibrils.

Cowdry, E. V. (1932). *Special Cytology*, 2nd ed., 3 vols. Hoeber, New York.

Cowley, J. J., and R. D. Griesel (1963) *J. Genet. Psychol.* 103:233–242. Development of second generation low protein rats.

Coyle, J. T., and M. E. Moliver (1977). *Science* 196:444–447. Major innervation of new born rat cortex by monoaminergic neurons.

Cozzens, S. E. (1989). *Social Control and Multiple Discovery in Science. The Opiate Receptor Case.* State Univ. New York Press, Albany.

Cragg, B. G. (1967). *J. Anat. (London)* 101:639–654. The density of synapses and neurons in the motor and visual areas of the cerebral cortex.

Cragg, B. G. (1969). *Brain Res.* 13:53–67. The effects of vision and dark- rearing on the size and density of synapses in the lateral geniculate nucleus measured by electron microscopy.

Cragg, B. G. (1970). *Brain Res.* 23:1–21. What is the signal for chromatolysis?

Cragg, B. G. (1972a). *Brain* 95:143–150. The development of cortical synapses during starvation in the rat

Cragg, B. G. (1972b). *Invest. Ophthalmol.* 11:377–385. The development of synapses in cat visual cortex.

Cragg, B. G. (1972c). Plasticity of synapses, pp. 1–66. In *Structure and Function of Nervous Tissue*, Vol 4, (G. H. Bourne, ed.), Academic Press, New York.

Cragg, B. G. (1975a). *Exp. Neurol.* 46:445–451. The development of synapses in kitten visual cortex during visual deprivation.

Cragg, B. G. (1975b). *Exp. Neurol.* 49:858–862. Absence of barrels and disorganization of thalamic afferent distribution in the sensory cortex of reeler mice.

Cragg, B. G. (1975c). *J. Comp. Neurol.* 160:147–166. The development of synapses in the visual system of the cat.

Craig, R., R. Smith, and J. Kendrick-Jones (1983). *Nature* 302:435–439. Light chain phosphorylation controls the conformation of vertebrate nonmuscle and smooth muscle myosin molecules.

Craigie, E. H. (1925). *J. Comp. Neurol.* 39: 301–324. Postnatal changes in vascularity in the cerebral cortex of the male albino rat.

Craigie, E. H. (1938). *Res. Publ. Assoc. Res. Nerv. Men. Dis.* 18:3–28. The comparative anatomy and embryology of the capillary bed of the central nervous system.

Crain, B., C. Cotman, D. Taylor, and G. Lynch (1973). *Brain Res.* 63:195–204. A quantitative electron microscopic study of synaptogenesis in the dentate gyrus of the rat.

Crain, S. M. (1964). *Anat. Rec.* 148:273–274. Electrophysiological studies of cord-innervated skeletal muscle in long-term tissue cultures of mouse embryo myotomes.

Crain, S. M. (1966). *Int. Rev. Neurobiol.* 9:1–43. Development of "organotypic" bioelectric activities in central nervous tissues during maturation in culture.

Crain, S. M. (1968). *Anat. Rec.* 160:466. Development of functional neuromuscular connections between separate explants of fetal mammalian tissues after maturation in culture.

Crain, S. M. (1974). Tissue culture models of developing brain functions, pp. 69–114. In *Studies on the Development of Behavior and the Nervous System*, Vol. 2, Aspects of Neurogenesis, (G. Gottlieb, ed.), Academic Press, New York.

Crain, S. M. (1976). *Neurophysiologic Studies in Tissue Culture*, Raven Press, New York.

Crain, S. M., and E. R. Peterson (1967). *Brain Res.* 6:750–762. Onset and development of functional interneuronal connections in explants of rat spinal cord ganglia during maturation in culture.

Crain, S. M., and E. R. Peterson (1974). *Ann. N.Y. Acad. Sci.* 228:6–34. Development of neural connections in culture.

Crain, S. M., H. Benitez, and A. E. Vatter (1964a). *Ann. N.Y. Acad. Sci.* 118:206–231. Some cytologic effects of salivary nerve-growth factor on tissue cultures of peripheral ganglia.

Crain, S. M., R. P. Bunge, M. B. Bunge, and E. R. Peterson (1964b). *J. Cell Biol.* 23:114A–115A. Bioelectric and electron microscope evidence for development of synapses in spinal cord cultures.

Crain, S. M., M. B. Bornstein, and E. R. Peterson (1968). *Brain Res.* 8:363–372. Maturation of cultured embryonic CNS tissues during chronic exposure to agents which prevent bioelectrical activity.

Crain, S. M., L. Alfei, and E. Peterson (1970). *J. Neurobiol.* 1:471–489. Neuromuscular transmission in cultures of adult human and rodent skeletal muscle after innervation *in vitro* by fetal rodent spinal cord.

Crandall, J. E., J. M. Whitcomb, and V. S. Caviness, Jr. (1985). *J. Comp. Neurol.* 239:205–215. Development of the spino-medullary projection from the mouse barrel field.

Cranefield, P. F. (1951). *J. Hist. Med.* 12:407–423. The organic physics of 1844 and the biophysics of today.

Cranefield, P. F. (1974). *The Way In and The Way Out.* Rockefeller Univ. Press, New York.

Cravioto, J. (1966). Malnutrition and behavioral development in the preschool child. In *Preschool Child Malnutrition*, National Health Science Publ. No. 128.

Cravioto, J. (1970). *Biblthca Nutr. Dieta* 14:7–22. Complexity of factors involved in protein-calorie malnutrition.

Cravioto, J., and E. R. DeLicardie (1970). *Amer. J. Dis. Child.* 120:404–410. Mental performance in school age children. Findings, after recovery from early severe malnutrition.

Cravioto, J., and E. R. DeLicardie (1972). *Environmental Correlates of Severe Clinical Malnutrition, and Language Development in Survivors from Kwashiorkor and Marasmus*, Pan American Health Organization, Scientific Publ. No. 251, Washington, D.C.

Cravioto, J., and E. M. DeLicardie (1975). Neurointegrative development and intelligence in children rehabilitated from severe malnutrition, pp. 53–72. In *Brain function and malnutrition: neuropsychological methods of assessment* (Prescott, and Read, eds.), Wiley & Sons, New York.

Cravioto, J., E. R. De Licardi, and H. G. Birch (1966). *Pediatrics* 38:319–372. Nutrition, growth and neurointegrative development: An experimental and ecologic study.

Cravioto, J., L. Hambraeus, and B. Vahlquist, eds. (1974). *Symp. Swedish Nutr. Found. XII.* Early malnutrition and mental development. Uppsala.

Creasey, W. A. (1968). *Cancer Chemother. Rep.* 52:501–507. Modifications in biochemical pathways produced by the vinca alkaloids.

Creazzo, T. L., and G. S. Sohal (1979). *Exp. Neurol.* 66:135–145. Effects of chronic injections of alpha-bungarotoxin on embryonic cell death.

Crelin, E. S. (1952). *J. Exp. Zool.* 120:547–578. Excision and rotation of the developing Amblystoma optic tectum and subsequent visual recovery.

Crepel, F. (1974). *Exp. Brain Res.* 20:403–420. Excitatory and inhibitory processes acting upon cerebellar Purkinje cell during maturation in the rat: Influence of hypothyroidism.

Crepel, F. (1982). *Trends Neurosci.* 5:266–270. Regression of functional synapses in the immature mammalian cerebellum.

Crepel, F., and N. Delhaye-Bouchaud (1979). *J. Physiol. (London)* 290:97–112. Distribution of climbing fibers on cerebellar Purkinje cells in X-irradiated rats.

Crepel, F., and J. Mariani (1976). *J. Neurobiol.* 7:579–582. Multiple innervation of Purkinje cells by climbing fibres in the cerebellum of the weaver mutant mouse.

Crepel, F., N. Delhaye-Bouchaud, and J. Legrand (1976a). *Arch. Ital. Biol.* 114:49–74. Electrophysiological analysis of the circuitry and of the corticonuclear relationships in the agranular cerebellum of irradiated rats.

Crepel, F., J. Mariani, and N. Delhaye-Bouchard (1976b). *J. Neurobiol.* 7:567–578. Evidence for a multiple innervation of Purkinje cells by climbing fibres in the immature rat cerebellum.

Crepel, F., N. Delhaye-Bouchaud, J. M. Guastavino, and I. Sampaio (1980). *Nature* 283:483–484. Multiple innervation of cerebellar Purkinje cells by climbing fibres in *staggerer* mutant mouse.

Crepel, F., N. Delhaye-Bouchaud, and J. L. Dupont (1981). *Dev. Brain Res.* 1:59–71. Fate of the multiple innervation of cerebellar Purkinje cells by climbing fibers in immature control, X-irradiated and hypothyroid rats.

Creps, E. S. (1974a). *J. Comp. Neurol.* 157:139–160. Time of neuron origin in the anterior olfactory nucleus and nucleus of the lateral olfactory tract of the mouse: An autoradiographic study.

Creps, E. S. (1974b). *J. Comp. Neurol.* 157:161–244. Time of neuron origin in preoptic and septal areas of the mouse: An autoradiographic study.

Crespo, D., D. D. M. O'Leary, and W. M. Cowan (1985). *Dev. Brain Res.* 19:129–134. Changes in the number of optic nerve fibers during late prenatal and postnatal development in the albino rat.

Creutzfeldt, O. D. (1975). Neurophysiological correlates of different functional states of the brain, pp. 21–46. In *Brain Work. Alfred Benzon Symposium VIII* (D. H. Ingvar and N. A. Lassen, eds.), Academic Press, New York.

Crick, F. (1970). *Nature* 225:420–422. Diffusion in embryogenesis.

Crick, F. (1982). *Trends Neurosci.* 5:44–46. Dendritic spines twitch?

Crick, F. H. C. (1971). *Symp. Soc. Exp. Biol.* 25:429–438. The scale of pattern formation.

Crile, G. W., and D. P. Quiring (1940). *Ohio J. Sci.* 40:219–259. A record of body weight and certain organ and gland weights of 3,690 animals.

Criley, B. B. (1969). *J. Morphol.* 128:465–501. Analysis of the embryonic sources and mechanisms of development of posterior levels of chick neural tubes.

Crissman, H. and J. Steinkamp (1986). Multivariate cell analysis: Techniques for correlated measurements of DNA and other cellular constituents. In *Techniques in Cell Cycle Analysis.* (J. Gray, and Z. Darzynkiewicz, eds.), Humana, New Jersey.

Crome, L., and J. Stern (1972). *Pathology of Mental Retardation*, 2nd Ed., Churchill, Livingstone, Edinburgh.

Crome, L., V. Tymms, and L. I. Woolf (1962). *J. Neurol. Neurosurg. Psychiat.* 25:143–153. A chemical investigation of the defects of myelination in phenylketonuria.

Cronkite, E. P., T. M. Fliedner, S. A. Killmann, and J. R. Rubini (1962). Tritium-labelled thymidine (H³-TdR): Its somatic toxicity and use in the study of growth rates and potentials in normal and malignant tissue of man and animals. pp. 189–206. In *Tritium in the Physical and Biological Sciences,* Vol. 2. International Atomic Energy Agency, Vienna.

Croskerry, P. G., and G. K. Smith (1975). *Science* 189:648–650. Prolongation of gestation by growth hormone: A confounding factor in the assessment of its prenatal action.

Croskerry, P. G., G. K. Smith, G. J. Shepard, and K. B. Freeman (1973). *Brain Res.* 52:413–418. Perinatal brain DNA in the normal and end growth hormone treated rat.

Crossin, K. L., Chuong, C-M., and Edelman, G. M. (1985). *Proc. Natl. Acad. Sci. USA* 82:6942–6946. Expression sequences of cell adhesion molecules.

Crossland, W. J., and C. P. Hughes (1978). *Brain Res.* 145:239–256. Observations on the afferent and efferent connections of the avian isthmo-optic nucleus.

Crossland, W. J., W. M. Cowan, and J. P. Kelly (1973). *Brain Res.* 56:77–105. Observations on the transport of radioactively labeled proteins in the visual system of the chick.

Crossland, W. J., W. M. Cowan, L. A. Rogers, and J. P. Kelly (1974a). *J. Comp. Neurol.* 155:127–164. The specification of the retino-tectal projection in the chick.

Crossland, W. J., J. R. Currie, L. A. Rogers, and W. M. Cowan (1974b). *Brain Res.* 78:483–489. Evidence for a rapid phase of axoplasmic transport at early stages in the development of the visual system of the chick and frog.

Crowder, C. M., and J. P. Merlie (1986). *Proc. Natl. Acad. Sci. U.S.A.* 83:8405–8409. DNase I-hypersensitive sites surround the mouse acetylcholine receptor delta-subunit gene.

Crowther, J. G. (1940). *British Scientists of the Nineteenth Century*, 2 Vols., Penguin Books, London.

Cruce, W. L. R. (1974). *J. Comp. Neurol.* 153:59–76. The anatomical organization of hindlimb motoneurons in the lumbar spinal cord of the frog., *Rana catesbiana*.

Crutcher, K. A., and C. F. Marfurt (1988). *J. Neurosci.* 8:2289–2302. Nonregenerative axonal growth within the mature mammallian brain: Ultrastructural identification of sympathohippocampal sprouts.

Cserr, H. F., and M. Bundegaard (1984). *Ann. J. Physiol.* 246:R277–R288. Blood-brain interface in vertebrates: A comparative approach.

Cuadros, M. A., and A. Rios (1988). *Anat. Embryol.* 178:543–551. Spatial and temporal correlation between early nerve fiber growth and neuroepithelial cell death in the chick embryo retina.

Cuajunco, F. (1927a). *Anat. Rec.* 35:8–9. The embryology of the neuromuscular spindles.

Cuajunco, F. (1927b). *Contrib. Embryol. Carnegie Inst.* 19:45–72. Embryology of the neuromuscular spindle.

Cuatrecasas, P. (1969). *Proc. Natl. Acad. Sci. U.S.A.* 63:450–457. Interaction of insulin with the cell membrane: The primary action of insulin.

Cuenod, M., and J. Schonbach (1971). *J. Neurochem.* 18:809–816. Synaptic proteins and axonal flow in the pigeon visual pathway.

Culican, S. M., N. L. Baumrind, M. Yamamoto, and A. L. Pearlman (1990). *J. Neurosci.* 10:684–692. Cortical radial glia: Identification in tissue culture and evidence for their transformation to astrocytes.

Cull, R. E. (1974). *Exp. Brain Res.* 20:307–310. Role of nerve-muscle contact in maintaining synaptic connection.

Culley, W. J., and E. T. Mertz (1965). *Proc. Soc. Exp. Biol. N.Y.* 118:233–235 . Effect of restricted food intake on growth and composition of preweaning rat brain.

Cullheim, S., and J. O. Kellerth (1976). *Neurosci. Lett.* 2:307–313. Combined light and electron microscopic tracing of neurons, including axons and synaptic terminals, after intracellular injection of horseradish peroxidase.

Cullheim, S., R. E. Burke, J. W. Fleshman, and I. Segev (1983). *Neurosci. Abstr.* 9:340. Spatial analysis of the dendritic trees of triceps surae alpha-motoneurons.

Cullheim, S., J. W. Fleshman, L. L. Glenn, and R. E. Burke (1987b). *J. Comp. Neurol.* 255:68–81. Membrane area and dendritic structure in type-identified triceps surae alpha motoneurons.

Cullheim, S., J. W. Fleshman, L. L. Glenn, and R. E. Burke (1987a). *J. Comp. Neurol.* 255:82–96. Three-dimensional architecture of dendritic trees in type-identified alpha-motoneurons.

Cullheim, S., T. Carlstedt, H. Linda, M. Risling, and B. Ulfhake (1989). *Neuroscience* 29:725–733. Motoneurons reinnervate skeletal muscle after ventral root implantation into the spinal cord of the cat.

Cummins, R. A., and P. Livesey (1979). *Brain Res.* 178:88–98. Enrichment-isolation, cortex length, and the rank order effect.

Cunningham, B. A., S. Hoffman, U. Rutishauser, J. J. Hemperly and G. M. Edelman (1983). *Proc. Natl. Acad. Sci. U.S.A.* 80:3116–3120. Molecular topography of N-CAM: Surface orientation and the location of sialic acid-rich and binding regions.

Cunningham, B. A., J. J. Hemperly, B. A. Murray, E. A. Prediger, R. Brackenbury, and G. M. Edelman (1987). *Science* 236:799–806. Neural cell adhesion molecule: Structure, immunoglobulin-like domains, cell surface modulation, and alternative RNA splicing.

Cunningham, T. J. (1976). *Science* 194:857–859. Early eye removal produces excessive bilateral branching in the rat; application of cobalt filling method.

Cunningham, T. J. (1982). *Int. Rev. Cytol.* 74:163–186. Naturally-occurring neuron death and its regulation by developing neural pathways.

Cunningham, T. J., C. Huddleston, and M. Murray (1979). *J. Comp. Neurol.* 184:423–434. Modification of neuron numbers in the visual system of the rat.

Cunningham, T. J., I. M. Mohler, and D. L. Giordano (1982). *Dev. Brain Res.* 2:203–215. Naturally occurring neuronal death in the ganglion cell layer of the neonatal rat: Morphology and evidence for regional correspondence with neuron death in the superior colliculus.

Curcio, C. A., and P. D. Coleman (1982). *J. Comp. Neurol.* 212:158–172. Stability of neuron number in cortical barrels of aging mice.

Currie, J., and W. M. Cowan (1974a). *Brain Res.* 71:133–139. Evidence for the late development of the uncrossed retinothalamic projections in the frog, *Rana pipiens.*

Currie, J., and W. M. Cowan (1974b). *J. Comp. Neurol.* 156:123–142. Some observations on the eary development of the optic tectum in the frog *(Rana pipiens),* with special reference to the effects of early eye removal on mitotic activity in the larval tectum.

Currie, J., and W. M. Cowan (1975). *Dev. Biol.* 46:103–119. The development of the retinotectal projection in *Rana pipiens.*

Currie, J. R., M.-F. Pfenninger, and K. H. Pfenninger (1984). *Dev. Biol. 106:*109–120. Developmentally regulated plasmalemmal glycoconjugates of the surface and neural ectoderm.

Curtis, A. S. G. (1960). *J. Embryol. Exp. Morphol.* 8:163–173. Cortical grafting in *Xenopus laevis.*

Curtis, A. S. G. (1962). *Biol. Rev.* 37:82–129. Cell contact and adhesion.

Curtis, A. S. G. (1967). *The Cell Surface: Its Molecular Role in Morphogenesis.* Logos, London.

Curtis, A. S. G. (1973). Cell adhesion, pp. 315–383. In *Progress in Biophysics and Molecular Biology,* Vol. 27, (J. A. V. Butler, and D. Noble, eds.), Pergamon Press, Oxford.

Cuzner, M. L., and A. N. Davision (1968). *Biochem. J.* 106:29–34. The lipid composition of rat brain myelin and subcellular fractions during development.

Cyert, M. S., and M. W. Kirschner (1988). *Cell* 53:185–195. Regulation of MPF activity *in vitro.*

Cynader, M. (1983). *Dev. Brain Res.* 8:155–164. Prolonged sensitivity to monocular deprivation in dark-reared cats: Effects of age and visual exposure.

Cynader, M., and D. E. Mitchell (1980). *J. Neurophysiol.* 43:1026–1040. Prolonged sensitivity to monocular deprivation in dark reared cats.

Cynader, M., N. Berman, and A. Hein (1976). *Exp. Brain Res.* 25:139–156. Recovery of function in cat visual cortex following prolonged deprivation.

Cynader, M., B. N. Timney, and D. E. Mitchell (1980). *Brain Res.* 191:545–550. Period of susceptibility of kitten visual cortex to the effects of monocular deprivation extends beyond six months of age.

Cynader, M., N. V. Swindale, and J. A. Matsubara (1987). *J. Neurosci.* 7:1401–1413. Functional topography in cat area 18.

Czéh, G., and G. Szekely (1971). *Acta Physiol. Acad. Scient. Hung.* 40:287–302. Muscle activities recorded simultaneously from normal and supernumerary forelimbs in *Ambystoma.*

Czosnek, H., D. Soifer, and H. M. Wisniewski (1980). *J. Cell Biol.* 85:726–734. Studies on the biosynthesis of neurofilament proteins.

Dahl, D. (1981). *J. Neurosci. Res.* 6:741–748. The vimentin-GFA protein transition in rat neuroglia cytoskeleton occurs at the time of myelination.

Dahl, D., and A. Bignami (1973). *Brain Res.* 63:279–293. Immunochemical and immunofluorescence studies of the glial fibrillary acidic protein in vertebrates.

Dahl, D., and A. Bignami (1983). The glial fibrillary acidic protein and astrocytic 10-nanometer filaments, pp. 127–152. In *Handbook of Neurochemistry,* Vol. 5 (A. Lajtha, ed.), Plenum Press, New York.

Dahl, D., D. C. Rueger, A. Bignami, K. Weber, and M. Osborn (1981). *Eur. J. Cell Biol.* 24:191–196. Vimentin, the 57,000 molecular weight protein of fibroblast filaments is the major cytoskeletal component in immature glia.

Dahl, D., N. H. Chi, L. E. Miles, B. T. Nguyen, and A. Bignami (1982). *J. Histochem. Cytochem.* 30:912–918. GFA protein in Schwann cells: Fact or artifact.

Dahl, D. R., and F. E. Samson, Jr., (1959). *Am. J. Physiol.* 196:470–472. Metabolism of rat brain mitochondria during postnatal development.

Dahl, H. A. (1963). *Z. Zellforsch. Mikrokop Anat. Abt. Histochem.* 60:369–386. Fine structure of cilia in rat cerebral cortex.

Dahlback, K., H. Lofberg, and B. Dahlback (1986). *Acta Dermato-Venereol.* 66:461–467. Localization of vitronectin (s-protein of complement) in normal human skin.

Dahlström, A. (1967a). *Acta Physio. Scand.* 69:158–166. The transport of noradrenaline between two simultaneously performed ligations of the sciatic nerves of rat and cat.

Dahlström, A. (1967b). *Acta Physiol. Scand.* 69:167–179. The effect of reserpine and tetrabenazine on the accumulation of noradrenaline in the rat sciatic nerve after ligation.

Dahlström, A. (1968). *Europ. J. Pharmacol.* 5:111–113. Effect of colchicine on transport of amine storage granules in sympathetic nerves of rat.

Dahlström, A., and J. Haggendal (1966). *Acta Physio. Scand.* 67:278–288. Transport and life-span of amine storage granules in peripheral adrenergic neuron system.

Dahlström, A., and J. Haggendal (1967). *Acta Physio. Scand.* 69:153–157. Studies on the transport and life-span of amine storage granules in the adrenergic neuron system of the rabbit sciatic nerve.

Dahm, L., and L. Landmesser (1988). *Dev. Biol.* 130:621–644. The regulation of intramuscular nerve branching during normal development and following activity blockade.

Daitz, H. M., and T. P. S. Powell (1954). *J. Neurol. Neurosurg. Psychiat.* 17:75–82. Studies on the connexions of the fornix system.

Dale, H. H. (1935). *Proc. Roy. Soc. Med.* 28:319–332. Pharmacology and nerve-endings.

Dale, L., J. C. Smith and J. M. W. Slack (1985). *J. Embryol. Exp. Morphol.* 89:289–312. Mesoderm induction in *Xenopus laevis:* A quantitative study using a cell lineage label and tissue-specific antibodies.

Dalton, M. M., O. R. Hommes, and C. P. Leblond (1968). *J.*

Comp. Neurol. 134:397–400. Correlation of glial proliferation with age in the mouse brain.

D'Amato, R. J., M. E. Blue, B. L. Largent, D. R. Lynch, D. J. Ledbetter, M. E. Molliver, and S. H. Snyder (1987). *Proc. Natl. Acad. Sci. U.S.A.* 84:4322–4326. Ontogeny of the serotonergic projection to rat neocortex: Transient expression of a dense innervation to primary sensory areas.

D'Amico-Martel, A. and D. M. Noden (1983). *Am. J. Anat.* 166:445–468. Contributions of placodal and neural crest cells to avian cranial peripheral ganglia.

Damjanov, I., A. Damjanov, and C. H. Damsky (1986). *Dev. Biol.* 116:194–202. Developmentally regulated expression of the cell-cell adhesion glycoprotein cell-CAM 120/80 in peri-implantation mouse embryos and extraembryonic membranes.

Damsky, C. H., J. Richa, D. Solter, K. Knudsen, and C. A. Buck (1983). *Cell* 34:455–466. Identification and purification of a cell surface glycoprotein mediating intercellular adhesion in embryonic and adult tisue.

Daneo, L. S., and G. Filogamo (1974). *J. Submicros. Cytol.* 6:219–228. Ultrastructure of developing myo-neural junctions. Evidence for two patterns of synaptic area differentiation.

Daniels, J. D., and J. D. Pettigrew (1976). Development of neuronal responses in the visual system of cats, pp. 195–232. In *Studies on the Development of Behavior and the Nervous System*, Vol. 3, *Neuronal and Behavioral Specificity*, (G. Gottlieb, ed.), Academic Press, New York.

Daniels, M. (1975). *Ann. N.Y. Acad. Sci.* 253:535–544. The role of microtubules in the growth and stabilization of nerve fibers.

Daniels, M. P. (1972). *J. Cell Biol.* 53:164–176. Colchicine inhibition of nerve fiber formation *in vitro*.

Daniels, M. P. (1973). *J. Cell Biol.* 58:463–470. Ultrastructural changes in neurons and nerve fibers associated with colchicine inhibition of nerve fiber formation *in vitro*.

Daniel, P. M., and D. Whitteridge (1961). *J. Physiol. (London)* 159:203–221. The representation of the visual field on the cerebral cortex in monkeys.

Danilchik, M. V., and S. D. Black (1988). *Dev. Biol.* 128:58–64. The first cleavage plane and the embryonic axis are determined by separate mechanisms in *Xenopus laevis*. I. Independence in undisturbed embryos.

Dann, J. F., E. H. Buhl, and L. Peichl (1987). *Neurosci. Lett.* 80:21–26. Dendritic maturation in cat retinal ganglion cells: A lucifer yellow study.

Dann, J. F., E. H. Buhl, and L. Peichl (1988). *J. Neurosci.* 8:1485–1499. Postnatal dendritic maturation of alpha and beta ganglion cells in cat retina.

D'Arcy Thompson, W. (1942). *On Growth and Form*, 2nd ed., 1116 pp., Cambridge Univ. Press. London.

Darkschewitsch, L. (1892). *Neurol. Centralbl. Leipzig* 11:658–668. Ueber die Veränderungen in dem centralen Abschnitt eines motorischen Nerven bei Verletzung des peripheren Abschnittes.

Darwin, C. (1868). *The Variations of Animals and Plants under Domestication*, 2 vols., John Murray, London.

Darwin, C. (1871). *The Descent of Man*, 2 Vols., Appleton, New York.

Darwin, C. (1888). *The Life and Letters of Charles Darwin Including an Autobiographical Chapter*, 3 vols., (F. Darwin, ed.), John Murray, London.

David, J. B., and T. D. Sargent. (1988). *Science.* 240:1443–1448. *Xenopus laevis* in developmental and molecular biology.

David, S., and A. J. Aguayo (1981). *Science* 214:931–933. Axonal elongation into peripheral nervous system "bridges" after central nervous system injury in adult rats.

David, S., and A. J. Aguayo (1985). *J. Neurocytol.* 14:1–12. Axonal regeneration after crush injury of rat central nervous system fibres innervating peripheral nerve grafts.

David, S., R. H. Miller, R. Patel, and M. C. Raff (1984). *J. Neurocytol.* 13:961–974. Efffects of neonatal transection on glial cell development in the rat optic nerve: Evidence that the oligodendrocyte-type-2 astrocyte cell lineage depends on axons for its survival.

Davidoff, M. (1973). *Z. Zellforsch.* 141:427–442. Über die Glia in Hypoglossuskern der Ratte nach Axotomie.

Davidson, E. H. (1989). *Development* 105:421–445. Lineage-specific gene expresion and the regulative capacities of the sea urchin embryo: A proposed mechanism.

Davidson, E. H. (1990). *Development* 108:365–389. How embryos work: A comparative view of diverse modes of cell fate specification.

Davidson, E. H., and R. J. Britten (1973). *Quart. Rev. Biol.* 48:565–613. Organization, transcription, and regulation in the animal genome.

Davidson, J. M., and S. Levine (1972). *Ann. Rev. Physiol.* 34:375–408. Endocrine regulation of behavior.

Davidson, R. L. (1973). Control of the differentiated state in somatic cell hybrids, pp. 295–328. In *Genetic Mechanisms of Development*, (F. H. Ruddle, ed.), Academic Press, New York.

Davies, A. M. (1988). *Trends Neurosci.* 11:243–244. The emerging generality of the neurotrophic hypothesis.

Davies, A. M., H. Thoenen, and Y.-A. Barde (1986a). *Nature* 319:497–499. Different factors from the central nervous system and periphery regulate the survival of sensory neurons.

Davies, A. M., H. Thoenen, and Y.-A. Barde (1986b). *J. Neurosci.* 6:1897–1904. The response of chick sensory neurons to brain-derived neurotrophic factor.

Davies, A. M., C. Bandtlow, R. Heumann, S. Korsching, H. Rohrer, and H. Thoenen (1987). *Nature* 326:353–363. The site and timing of nerve growth factor (NGF) synthesis in developing skin in relation to its innervation by sensory neurons and their expression of NGF receptors.

Davies, P. A., and A. L. Stewart (1975). *Br. Med. Bull.* 31:85–91. Low-birth-weight infants: Neurological sequelae and later intelligence.

Davis, C. A., S. E. Noble-Topham, J. Rossant, and A. L. Joyner (1988). *Genes Dev.* 2:361–371. Expression of the homeobox-containing gene *En-2* delineates a specific region of the developing mouse brain.

Davis, C. J. F. (1970). Prolonged nembutal narcosis of the cat and its effects upon the isometric contraction characteristics of fast twitch and slow twitch skeletal muscle. Ph.D. Thesis, Univ. of Bristol.

Davis, J. B. (1868). *Phil. Trans. Roy. Soc. (London) Ser. B.* 158:505–527. Contributions towards determining the weight of the brain in different races of man.

Davis, L., B. Burger, G. A. Banker, and O. Steward (1990). *J. Neurosci.* 10:3056–3068. Dendritic transport: Quantitative analysis of the time course of somatodendritic transport of recently synthesized RNA.

Davis, M. R., and M. Constantine-Paton (1983a). *J. Comp. Neurol.* 221:444–452. Hyperplasia in the spinal sensory system of the frog. I. Plasticity in the most caudal dorsal root ganglion.

Davis, M. R., and M. Constantine-Paton (1983b). *J. Comp. Neurol.* 221:453–465. Hyperplasia in the spinal sensory system of the frog. II. Central and peripheral connectivity patterns.

Davison, A. N., and J. Dobbing (1960a). *Biochem. J.* 75:565–570. Phospholipid metabolism in nervous tissue. II. Metabolic stability.

Davison, A. N., and J. Dobbin (1960b). *Biochem. J.* 75:571–574. Phospholipid metabolism in nervous tissue. III. The anatomical distribution of metabolically inert phospholipid in the central nervous system.

Davison, A., N., and M. B. Dobbing (1966). *Br. Med. Bull.* 22:40–44. Myelination as a vulnerable period in brain development.

Davison, A. N., M. L. Cuzner, N. L. Banik, and J. Oxberry (1966). *Nature* 212: 1373–1374. Myelinogenesis in the rat brain.

Davison, P. F., and B. Winslow (1974). *J. Neurobiol.* 5:119–133. The protein subunit of calf brain neurofilament.

Davson, H., K. Welch, and M. B. Segal (1987). *Physiology and Pathophysiology of the Cerebrospinal Fluid.* Churchill and Livingstone, Edinburgh.

Daw, N. W., and H. J. Wyatt (1976). *J. Physiol. (London)* 257:155–170. Kittens reared in a unidirectional environment: Evidence for a critical period.

Daw, N. W., T. W. Robertson, R. W. Rader, T. O. Videen, and C. J. Coscia (1984). *J. Neurosci.* 4:1354–1360. Effects of lesions of the dorsal noradrenergic bundle on visual deprivation in the kitten striate cortex.

Daw, N. W., T. O. Videen, R. K. Rader, T. W. Robertson, and C. J. Coscia (1985a). *Exp. Brain Res.* 59:30–35. Substantial reduction of noradrenaline in kitten visual cortex by intraventricular injections of 6-hydroxydopamine does not always prevent ocular dominance shifts after monocular deprivation.

Daw, N. W., T. O. Videen, T. W. Robertson, and R. K. Rader (1985b). An evaluation of the hypothesis that noradrenaline affects plasticity in the developing visual cortex, pp. 133–144. In *The Visual System* (A. Fein, and J. S Levine, eds.), Alan Liss, New York.

Daw, N. W., T. O. Videen, D. Parkinson, and R. K. Rader (1985c). *J. Neurosci.* 5:1925–1933. DSP-4 (N-(2-Chloroethyl)-N-ethyl-2-bromobenzylamine) depletes noradrenaline in kitten visual cortex without altering the effects of monocular deprivation.

Dawid, I. B. and T. D. Sargent (1988). *Science* 240:1443. *Xenopus laevis* in developmental and molecular biology.

Dawson, D. R., and H. P. Killackey (1987). *J. Comp. Neurol.* 256:246–256. The organization and mutability of the forepaw and hindpaw representations in the somatosensory cortex of the neonatal rat.

Dawydoff, C. (1928). *Traité D'Embryologie Comparée des Invertébrés.* Masson, Paris, 930 pp.

Dayton, D. H., L. J. Filer, and C. Canosa (1969). *Fed. Proc.* 28:488. Cellular changes in placentas of undernourished mothers in Guatamala.

Deadwyler, S. A., T. Dunwiddie, and G. Lynch (1987). *Synapse* 1:90–95. A critical level of protein synthesis is required for long-term potentiation.

Dean, P. N., F. Dolbeare, H. Gratzner, G. Rice and J. W. Gray (1984). *Cell Tissue Kinet.* 17:427–436. Cell-cycle analysis using a monoclonal antibody to BrdUrd.

De Anda, G., M. A. Rebollo, and M. Achaval (1963). *Acta Neurol. Latinoam.* 9:93–101. Differentiation of the skeletal muscle in the chicken. II. Development of the myoneural synapse.

DeBault, L. E., and P. A. Cancilla (1980). *Science* 207:653–655. Glutamyl transpeptidase in isolated brain endothelial cells: Induction by glial cells *in vitro.*

Debbage, P. L. (1986). *J. Neurol. Sci.* 72:319–336. The generation and regeneration of oligodendroglia.

De Beer, G. R. (1937). *The Development of the Vertebrate Skull.* Clarendon Press, Oxford.

De Beer, G. R. (1947). *Proc. Roy. Soc. (London) Ser. B.* 134:377–398. The differentiation of neural crest cells into visceral cartilages and odontoblasts in *Amblystoma,* and a re-examination of the germ-layer theory.

De Beer, G. R. (1951). *Embryos and Ancestors.* Revised Edition. Clarendon Press, Oxford.

De Brabander, M., F. Aerts, R. Van de Veire, and M. Borgers (1975). *Nature* 253:119–120. Evidence against interconversion of microtubules and filaments.

De Camilli, P., R. Cameron, and P. Greengard (1983). *J. Cell Biol.* 96:1337–1354. Synapsin-1 (protein-1), a nerve terminal-specific phosphoprotein. I. Its general distribution in synapses of the central and peripheral nervous-system demonstrated by immunofluorescence in frozen and plastic sections.

De Camilli, P., P. E. Miller, P. Levitt, U. Walter, and P. Greengard (1984a). *Neuroscience* 11:761–817. Anatomy of cerebellar Purkinje cells in the rat determined by a specific immunohistochemical marker.

De Camilli, P., P. E. Miller, F. Navone, W. E. Theurkauf, and R. B. Vallee (1984b). *Neuroscience* 11:817–846. Distribution of microtubule-associated protein 2 in the nervous system of the rat studied by immunofluorescence.

Decker, R. S. (1976). *Dev. Biol.* 49:101–118. Influence of thyroid hormones on neuronal death and differentiation in larval *Rana pipiens.*

Decker, R. S. (1978). *J. Comp. Neurol.* 180:635–660. Retrograde repsonses of developing lateral motor column neurons.

DeFelipe, J., and E. G. Jones (1988). *Cajal on the Cerebral Cortex.* Oxford Univ. Press, New York.

Defendi, V., and L. A. Manson (1963). *Nature* 198:359–361. Analysis of the life cycle in mammalian cells.

de Ferra, F., H. Engh, L. Hudson, J. Kamholz, S. Puckett, S. Molineaux, and R. A. Lazzarini (1985). *Cell* 43:721–727. Alternative splicing accounts for the four forms of myelin basic protein.

de Groot, D. M. G., and E. P. B. Bierman (1986). *J. Neurosci. Meth.* 18:79–101. A critical evaluation of methods of estimating the numerical density of synapses.

DeHan, R. S., and P. Graziadei (1973). *Life Sci.* 13:1435–1449. The innervation of frog's taste organ. "A histochemical study".

Dehay, C., J. Bullier, and H. Kennedy (1984). *Exp. Brain Res.* 57:208–212. Transient projections from the frontoparietal and temporal cortex to areas 17, 18 and 19 in the kitten.

Dehay, C., J. Bullier, and H. Kennedy (1988). *J. Comp. Neurol.* 272:68–89. Characterization of transient cortical projections from auditory, somatosensory and motor cortices to visual areas 17, 18 and 19 in the kitten.

Dehay, C., G. Horsburgh, M. Berland, H. Killackey, and H. Kennedy (1989). *Nature* 337:265–267. Maturation and connectivity of the visual cortex in monkey is altered by prenatal removal of retinal input.

Deitch, A. D., and M. R. Murray (1956). *J. Biophys. Biochem. Cytol.* 2:433–444. The Nissl substance of living and fixed spinal ganglion cells.

Deitch, J. S., and E. W. Rubel (1984). *J. Comp. Neurol.* 229:66–79. Afferent influences on brain stem auditory nuclei of the chicken: The course and specificity of dendritic atrophy following deafferentation.

Deiters, O. (1865). *Untersuchungen über Gehirn und Rückenmark des Menschen und der Säugethiere,* (M. Schultze, ed.), F. Vieweg u. Sohn, Braunschweig.

Dekaban, A. (1956). *Anat. Rec.* 126:111–122. Oligodendroglia and axis cylinders in rabbits before, during, and after myelination.

Dekaban, A. S., and D. Sadowsky (1978). *Ann. Neurol.* 4:345–356. Changes in brain weights during the span of human life: Relation of brain weights to body heights and body weights.

de Lacoste, M. C., R. L. Holloway, and D. J. Woodward (1986). *Human Neurobiol.* 5:92–96. Sex differences in the fetal human corpus callosum.

de Lacoste-Utamsing, M. C., and R. L. Holloway (1982). *Science* 216:1431–1432. Sexual dimorphism in the human corpus callosum.

Delage, Y. (1903). *L'Hérédité et les grandes problèmes de la biologie générale.* Dixième Édition. Libraire C. Reinwald, Paris.

Delay, R. J., and S. D. Roper (1988). *J. Comp. Neurol.* 277:268–280. Ultrastructure of taste cells and synapses in the mudpuppy *Necturus maculosus.*

Delay, R. J., J. C. Kinnamon, and S. D. Roper (1986). *J. Comp. Neurol.* 253:242–252. Ultrastructure of mouse vallate taste buds. II. Cell types and cell lineage.

Del Castillo, J., and A. D. Vizoso (1953). *J. Physiol. (London)* 122:33–34. The electrical activity of embryonic nerves.

Del Cerro, M. (1974). *J. Comp. Neurol.* 157:245–280. Uptake of tracer proteins in the developing cerebellum, particularly by the growth cones and blood vessels.

Del Cerro, M., and A. A. Monjan (1979). *Neuroscience* 4:1399–1404. Unequivocal demonstration of the hematogenous origin of brain macrophages in a stab wound by a double-label technique.

Del Cerro, M. P., and R. S. Snider (1967). *Microscop.* 133:515–518. Cilia in the cerebellum of immature and adult rats.

Del Cerro, M. P., and R. S. Snider (1968). *J. Comp. Neurol.* 133:341–362. Studies on the developing cerebellum. Ultrastructure of the growth cones.

Del Cerro, M. P., and R. S. Snider (1969). *Anat. Rec.* 165:127–140. The Purkinje cell cilium.

Del Cerro, M. P., R. S. Snider, and M. L. Oster (1968). *Experientia* 24:929–930. Evolution of the extracellular space in immature neurons.

Dellon, A. L. (1976). *J. Hand Surg.* 1:98–109. Reinnervation of denervated Meissner corpuscles: A sequential histologic study in the monkey following fascicular nerve repair.

De Long, G. R., and A. J. Coulombre (1965). *Exp. Neurol.* 13:351–363. Development of the retinotectal topographic projection in the chick embryo.

De Long, G. R., and A. J. Coulombre (1968). *Dev. Biol.* 16:513–531. The specificity of retino-tectal connections studied by retinal grafts onto the optic tectum in chick embryos.

De Long, G. R., and R. L. Sidman (1962). *J. Comp. Neurol.* 118:205–224. Effects of eye removal at birth on histogenesis of the mouse superior colliculus. An autoradiographic analysis with tritiated thymidine.

de Lorenzo, A. J. (1963). Studies on the ultrastructure and histophysiology of cell membranes, nerve fibers and synaptic junctions in chemoreceptors, pp. 5–17. In *Olfaction and Taste* (Y. Zotterman, ed.), Macmillan, New York.

Delorme, P. G. Grignon, and J. Gayet (1968). *Z. Zellforsch.* 87:592–601. Ultrastructure des capillaires dans le télencéphale du poulet au cours de l'embryogenèse et de la croissance postnatale.

Del Rio-Hortega, P. See Rio-Hortega, P. del.

Delsman, H. C. (1922). *The Ancestry of Vertebrates,* Valkoff, Amersfoort (Holland).

Denburg, J. L., R. L. Seecof, and G. A. Horridge (1976). *Brain Res.* 125:213–226. The path and rate of growth of regenerating motor neurons in the cockroach.

Denenberg, V. H. (1981). *Behav. Brain Sci.* 4:1–9. Hemispheric laterality in animals and the effects of early experience.

Denham, S. (1967). *J. Embryol. Exp. Morph.* 18:53–66. A cell proliferation study of the neural retina in the two-day rat.

Denis-Donini, S., J. Glowinski, and A. Prochiantz (1984). *Nature* 307:641–643. Glial heterogeneity may define the three dimensional shape of mouse mesencephalic dopaminergic neurons.

Dennis, M. J. (1981). *Ann. Rev. Neurosci.* 4:43–68. Development of the neuromuscular junction: Inductive interactions between cells.

Dennis, M. J., L. Ziskind-Conhaim, and A. J. Harris (1980). *Dev. Biol.* 81:266–279. Development of neuromuscular junctions in rat embryos.

Dennis, W. (1948). *Readings in the History of Psychology.* Appleton-Century-Crofts, New York.

Denny-Brown, D. (1929a). *Proc. Roy. Soc. (London) Ser. B.* 104:252–301. On the nature of postural reflexes.

Denny-Brown, D. (1929b). *Proc. Roy. Soc. (London) Ser. B.* 104:371–411. The histological features of striped muscle in relation to its functional activity.

Denny-Brown, D. (1970). Augustus Volney Waller (1816–1870), pp. 88–91. In *The Founders of Neurology,* 2nd edn., (W. Haymaker, and F. Schiller, eds.), Thomas, Springfield, Illinois.

Dent, J. A., A. G. Polson, and M. W. Klymkowsky (1989). *Development* 105:61–74. A whole-mount immunocytochemical analysis of the expression of the intermediate filament protein vimentin in *Xenopus.*

Dentler, W. L., S. Granett, G. B. Witman, and J. L. Rosenbaum (1974). *Proc. Natl. Acad. Sci. U.S.A.* 71:1710–1714. Directionality of brain microtubule assembly *in vitro.*

Denton, G. B. (1921). *Am. J. Psychol.* 32:5–15. Early psychological theories of Herbert Spencer.

Deol, M. S. (1967). *J. Embryol. Exp. Morphol.* 17:533–541. The neural crest and the acoustic ganglion.

Deol, M. S. (1970). *J. Embryol. Exp. Morphol.* 23:773–784. The origin of the acoustic ganglion and effects of the gene dominant spotting (W^v) in the mouse.

Derby, M. A. (1978). *Dev. Biol.* 66:321–336. Analysis of glycosaminoglycans within the extracellular environments encountered by migrating neural crest cells.

De Robertis, E., and H. S. Bennett (1954). *Federation*

Proc. 13:35. Submicroscopic vesicular component in the synapse.

De Robertis, E., and H. S. Bennett (1955). *J. Biophys. Biochem. Cytol.* 1:47–58. Some features of the submicroscopic morphology of synapses in frog and earthworm.

De Robertis, E. D. P. (1956). *J. Biophys. Biochem. Cytol.* 2:503–512. Submicroscopic changes in the synapse after nerve section in the acoustic ganglion of the guinea pig. An electron microscope study.

De Robertis, E. D. P., and H. M. Gershenfeld (1961). *Int. Rev. Neurobiol.* 3:1–65. Submicroscopic morphology and function of glial cells.

Derrick, G. E. (1937). *J. Morphol.* 61:257–284. An analysis of the early development of the chick by means of the mitotic index.

Desan, P. H., E. R. Gruberg, K. M. Grewell, and F. Eckenstein (1987). *Brain Res.* 413:344–349. Cholinergic innervation of the optic tectum in the frog *Rana pipiens*.

Descarries, L., and Y. Lapierre (1973). *Brain Res.* 51:141–160. Noradrenergic axon terminals in the cerebral cortex of rat. I. Radioautographic visualization after topical application of DL-[^{3}H] norepinephrine.

Descarries, L., K. C. Watkins, and Y. Lapierre (1977). *Brain Res.* 133:197–222. Noradrenergic axon terminals in the cerebral cortex of rat. III. topometric ultrastructural analysis.

Desmond, M. E. (1982). *Anat. Rec.* 204:89–93. A description of the occlusion of the lumen of the spinal cord in early human embryos.

Desmond, M. E., and A. G. Jacobson (1977). *Dev. Biol.* 66:321–336. Embryonic brain enlargement requires cerebrospinal fluid pressure.

Desmond, M. E., and G. C. Schoenwolf (1985). *J. Comp. Neurol.* 235:479–487. Timing and positioning of occlusion of the spinal neurocele in the chick embryo.

Desmond, M. E. and G. C. Schoenwolf (1986). *J. Embryol. Exp. Morphol.* 97:25–46. Evaluation of the roles of intrinsic and extrinsic forces in occlusion of the spinal neurocoel during rapid brain enlargement in the chick embryo.

Desmond, N. L., and W. B. Levy (1983). *Brain Res.* 265:21–30. Synaptic correlates of associative potentiation/depression: An ultrastructural study in the hippocampus.

Desmond, N. L., and W. B. Levy (1986a). *J. Comp. Neurol.* 253:466–475. Changes in numerical density of synaptic contacts with long term potentiation in the hippocampal dentate gyrus.

Desmond, N. L., and W. B. Levy (1986b). *J. Comp. Neurol.* 253:476–482. Changes in the postsynaptic density with long term potentiation in the dentate gyrus.

Desmond, N. L., and W. B. Levy (1988). Anatomy of associative long term synaptic modification, pp. 265–305. In *Long-term Potentiation: From Biophysics to Behavior* (P. W. Lanfield, and S. A. Deadwyler, eds.), Liss, New York.

de Solla Price, D. J. (1964). *Tech. Cult.* 5:9–23. Automata and the origins of mechanism and mechanistic philosophy.

Des Rosiers, M. H., O. Sakurada, J. Jehle, M. Shinohara, C. Kennedy, and L. Sokoloff (1978). *Science* 200:447–449. Demonstration of functional plasticity in the immature striate cortex of the monkey by means of the [^{14}C] deoxyglucose method.

Dessoir, M. (1912). *Outlines of the History of Psychology*, Macmillan, New York.

Detwiler, S. R. (1920a). *J. Exp. Zool.* 31:117–169. Experi-ments on the transplantation of limbs in *Amblystoma*. The formation of nerve plexuses and the function of the limbs.

Detwiler, S. R. (1920b). *Proc. Natl. Acad. Sci. U.S.A.* 6:96–101. On the hyperplasia of nerve centers resulting from excessive peripheral loading.

Detwiler, S. R. (1923). *J. Exp. Zool.* 37:339–393. Experiments on the transplantation of the spinal cord in *Amblystoma* and their bearing upon the stimuli involved in differentiation of nerve cells.

Detwiler, S. R. (1924). *J. Comp. Neurol.* 37:1–14. The effects of bilateral extirpation of the anterior limb rudiments in *Amblystoma* embryos.

Detwiler, S. R. (1925). *J. Comp. Neurol.* 38:461–490. Coordinated movements in supernumerary transplanted limbs.

Detwiler, S. R. (1930a). *J. Exp. Zool.* 55:319–379. Observations upon the growth, function and nerve supply of limbs when grafted to the head of salamander embryos.

Detwiler, S. R. (1930b). *J. Exp. Zool.* 57:183–203. Some observations upon the growth, innervation, and function of heteroplastic limbs.

Detwiler, S. R. (1933a). *Biol. Rev.* 8:269–310. Experimental studies upon the development of the amphibian nervous system.

Detwiler, S. R. (1933b). *J. Exp. Zool.* 64:405–414. On the time of determination of the antero-posterior axis of the forelimb in *Amblystoma*.

Detwiler, S. R. (1933c). *Anat. Rec.* 57:81–98. Growth and cell proliferation in heterotopic spinal cord grafts.

Detwiler, S. R. (1934). *J. Exp. Zool.* 67:395–441. An experimental study of the spinal nerve segmentation in *Ambystoma* with reference to the plurisegmental contribution to the brachial plexus.

Detwiler, S. R. (1936) *Neuroembryology: An experimental Study*. Macmillan, New York.

Detwiler, S. R. (1937a). *Am. J. Anat.* 61:63–94. Observations upon the migration of neural crest cells, and upon the development of the spinal ganglia and vertebral arches in *Amblystoma*.

Detwiler, S. R. (1937b). *J. Exp. Zool.* 77:109–122. Does the developing medulla influence cellular proliferation within the spinal cord?

Detwiler, S. R. (1937c). *J. Exp. Zool.* 77:395–441. An experimental study of spinal nerve segmentation in amblystoma with reference to the plurisegmental contribution to the brachial plexus.

Detwiler, S. R. (1940). *J. Exp. Zool.* 84:13–22. Unilateral reversal of the anteroposterior axis of the medulla in *Amblystoma*.

Detwiler, S. R. (1943). *J. Exp. Zool.* 94:169–179. Reversal of the medulla in *Amblystoma* embryos.

Detwiler, S. R. (1944). *J. Exp. Zool.* 96:129–142. Restitution of the medulla following unilateral excision in the embryo.

Detwiler, S. R. (1947). *J. Exp. Zool.* 104:53–68. Restitution of the brachial region of the cord following unilateral excision in the embryo.

Detwiler, S. R. (1949). *J. Exp. Zool.* 111:79–93. The swimming capacity of *Amblystoma* larvae following reversal of the embryonic hind brain.

Detwiler, S. R. (1951). *J. Exp. Zool.* 116:431–446. Structural and functional adjustments following reversal of the embryonic medulla in *Amblystoma*.

Detwiler, S. R., and R. L. Carpenter (1929). *J. Comp. Neurol.*

47:427–447. An experimental study of the mechanism of coordinated movements in heterotopic limbs.

Detwiler, S. R., and K. Kehoe (1939). *J. Exp. Zool.* 81:415–435. Further observations on the origin of the sheath cells of Schwann.

Deuel, T. F. (1987). *Ann. Rev. Biol.* 3:443–492. Polypeptide growth factors: Roles in normal and abnormal cell growth.

de Vellis, J. (1973). Mechanisms of enzymatic differentiation in the brain and in cultured cells, pp. 171–198. In *Development and Aging in the Nervous System*, (M. Rockstein, ed.), Academic Press, New York.

de Vellis, J., and D. Inglish (1968). *J. Neurochem.* 15:1061–1070. Hormonal control of glycerolphosphate dehydrogenase in the rat brain.

de Vellis, J., and D. Inglish (1973). Age-dependent changes in the regulation of glycerolphosphate dehydrogenase in the rat brain and in a glial cell line. In *Neurobiological Aspects of Maturation and Aging* (D. H. Ford, ed.), Elsevier, Amsterdam.

de Vellis, J., and G. Kukes (1973). *Tex. Rep. Biol. Med.* 31:271–293. Regulation of glial cell functions by hormones and ions: A review.

de Vellis, J., and O. A. Schjeide (1968). *Biochem. J.* 107:259–264. Time-dependence of the effect of X-irradiation on the formation of glycerol phosphate dehydrogenase and other dehydrogenases in the developing rat brain.

Devine, C. E., and F. O. Simpson (1968). *J. Cell Biol.* 38:184–192. Localization of tritiated norepinephrine in vascular sympathetic axons of the rat intestine and mesentery by electron microscope radioautography.

De Vito, J. L., K. W. Clausing, and O. A. Smith (1974). *Brain Res.* 82:269–271. Uptake and transport of horseradish peroxidase by cut end of the vagus nerve.

DeVoogd, T., and F. Nottebohm (1981). *Science* 214:202–204. Gonadal hormones induce dendritic growth in the adult avian brain.

Devor, M. (1975). *Science* 190:998–1000. Neuroplasticity in the sparing or deterioration of function after early olfactory tract lesions.

Devor, M. (1983). *Birth Defects* 19:287–314. Plasticity of spinal cord somatotopy in adult mammals: Involvement of relatively ineffective synapses.

Devor, M. (1987). *Effects of Injury on Trigeminal and Spinal Somatosensory Systems* (Pubols, L. M., and B. J. Sessle, eds.), pp. 215–225, Alan R Liss.

Devor, M., and G. E. Schneider (1975). *Inserm* 43:191–200. Neuroanatomical plasticity: The principle of conservation of total axonal arborization.

Devor, M., and P. D. Wall (1978). *Nature* 276:75–76. Reorganization of spinal cord sensory map after peripheral nerve injury.

Devor, M., and P. D. Wall (1981a). *J. Comp. Neurol.* 199:277–291. Effect of peripheral nerve injury on receptive fields of cells in the cat spinal cord.

Devor, M., and P. D. Wall (1981b). *J. Neurosci.* 1:679–684. Plasticity in the spinal cord sensory map following peripheral nerve injury in rats.

Devor, M., V. S. Caviness, Jr., and P. Derer (1975). *J. Comp. Neurol.* 164:471–482. A normally laminated afferent projection to an abnormally laminated cortex: Some olfactory connections in the reeler mouse.

Devreotes, P., and S. Zigmond (1988). *Ann. Rev. Cell Biol.* 4:649–686. Chemotaxis in eucaryotic cells.

Devreotes, P. N., and D. M. Fambrough (1976a). *Proc. Natl.* *Acad. Sci. U.S.A.* 73:161–164. Synthesis of acetylcholine receptors by cultured chick myotubes and denervated mouse extensor digitorum longus muscles.

Devreotes, P. N., and D. M. Fambrough (1976b). *Cold Spring Harbor Symp. Quant. Biol.* 40:237–251. Turnover of acetylcholine receptors in skeletal muscle.

DeVries, G. H., J. L. Salzer, and R. P. Bunge (1982). *Dev. Brain Res.* 3:295–299. Axonlemma-enriched fractions isolated from PNS and CNS are mitogenic for Schwann cells.

De Vries, G. J., R. M. Buijs, and D. F. Swaab (1981). *Brain Res.* 218:67–78. Ontogeny of the vasopressinergic neurons of the suprachiasmatic nucleus and their extrahypothalamic projections in the rat brain — presence of a sex difference in the lateral septum.

De Vries, G. J., W. Best, and A. A. Sluiter (1983). *Brain Res.* 8:377–380. The influence of androgens on the development of a sex difference in the vasopressinergic innervation of the rat lateral septum.

Dewey, M. J., A. G. Gervais, and B. Mintz (1976). *Dev. Biol.* 50:68–81. Brain and ganglion development from two genotype classes of cells in allophenic mice.

Deysson, G. (1968). *Int. Rev. Cytol.* 24:99–148. Antimitotic substances.

Dezeimeris, J. E. (1828–1839). *Dictionnaire historique de la médecine ancienne et moderne,* 4 vols. Chez Béchet Jeune, Paris.

Diamant, A., M. Eshel, and S. Ben-Or (1975). *Cell Differ.* 4:101–112. Interaction of cortisol with the neural retina of the chick embryo in culture.

Diamond, J. (1971). The Mauthner cell, pp. 265–346. In *Fish Physiology* (W. S. Hoar, and D. J. Randall, eds.), Academic Press, New York.

Diamond, J. (1982a). *Curr. Top. Dev. Biol.* 17:147–205. Modeling and competition in the nervous system: Clues from the sensory innervation of the skin.

Diamond, J. (1982b). *Amer. Zool.* 22:153–172. The patterning of neuronal connections.

Diamond, J., and R. Miledi (1962). *J. Physiol. (London)* 162:393–408. A study of foetal and new-born rat muscle fibres.

Diamond, J., E. G. Gray, and G. M. Yasargil (1970). The function of dendritic spines: An hypothesis, pp. 213–222. In *Excitatory Synaptic Mechanisms, Proceedings of the 5th International Meeting of Neurobiologists* (P. Andersen, and J. Jensen, eds.), Universitets Forlaget, Oslo.

Diamond, J., E. Cooper, C. Turner, and L. Macintyre (1976). *Science* 193:371–377. Trophic regulation of nerve sprouting.

Diamond, J., M. Holmes, and C. A. Nurse (1986). *J. Physiol. (London)* 376:101–120. Are Merkel cell-neurite reciprocal synapses involved in the initiation of tactile responses in salamander skin.

Diamond, J., M. Coughlin, L. Macintyre, M. Holmes, and B. Visheau (1987). *Proc. Natl. Acad. Sci. U.S.A.* 84:6596–6600. Evidence that endogenous β nerve growth factor is responsible for the collateral sprouting, but not the regeneration, of nociceptive axons in adult rats.

Diamond, M. C., D. Krech, and M. R. Rosenweig (1964). *J. Comp. Neurol.* 123:111–119. The effects of an enriched environment on the histology of the rat cerebral cortex.

Diamond, M. C., F. Law, H. Rhodes, B. Lindner, M. R. Rosenzweig, D. Krech, and E. L. Bennett (1966). *J. Comp. Neurol.* 128:117–126. Increases in cortical depth and glia numbers in rats subjected to enriched environment.

Diamond, M. C., R. E. Johnson, C. Ingham, and B. Stone (1969). *Exp. Neurol.* 23:51–57. Lack of direct effect of hypophysectomy and growth hormone on postnatal rat brain morphology.

Diamond, M. C., G. A. Dowling, and R. E. Johnson (1981). *Exp. Neurol.* 71:261–268. Morphological cerebral cortical asymmetry in male and female rats.

Diamond, M. C., R. E. Johnson, D. Young, and S. S. Singh (1983). *Exp. Neurol.* 81:1–13. Age related morphological differences in the rat cerebral cortex and hippocampus: Male-female; right-left.

Diaz, P. C. (1972). *Una contribución a la ciencia histológica: la obra de don Pío del Rio-Hortega.* Doctoral Thesis, Univ. Madrid.

Dibner, M. D., and I. B. Black (1976). *J. Neurochem.* 30:1479–1483. Biochemical and morphological effects of testosterone treatment on developing sympathetic neurons.

Diehl, H.-J., M. Schaich, R.-M. Budzinski, and W. Stoffel (1986). *Proc. Natl. Acad. Sci. U.S.A.* 83:9807–9811. Individual exons encode the integral membrane domains of human myelin proteolipid protein.

DiGiamberardino (1973). *Brain Res.* 60:93–127. Axonal migration of protein and glycoprotein to nerve endings. I. Radioautographic analysis of the renewal of protein in nerve endings of chicken ciliary ganglion after intracerebral injection of (^{3}H) lysine.

DiGiamberardino, L., G. Bennett, H. L. Koenig, and B. Droz (1973). *Brain Res.* 60:147–159. Axonal migration of protein and glycoprotein to nerve endings. III. Cell fraction analysis of chicken ciliary ganglion after intracerebral injection of labelled precursors of proteins and glycoproteins.

Dijksterhuis, E. J. (1950). *The Mechanization of the World Picture.* English transl. by C. Dikshoorn, (1961), Clarendon Press, Oxford.

Dijkstra, C. (1933). *Z. Mikrop. Anat. Forsch.* 34:75–158. Die De- und Regeneration der sensiblen Endkörperchen des Entenschnabels (Grandry- und Herbst-Körperchen) nach Durchschneidung des Nerven, nach Fortnahme der ganzen Haut und nach Transplantation des Hautstückchens.

Di Liegro, I., G. Savettieri, and A. Cestelli (1987). *Differentiation* 35:165–175. Cellular mechanism of action of thyroid hormones.

Diller, D. A., R. H. Brownson, and D. B. Suter (1964). *J. Neuropathol. Exp. Neurol.* 23:446–456. X-irradiation induced acute brain damage as a function of age.

Dinarello, C. A. (1984). *Rev. Infect. Dis.* 6:51–95. Interleukin–1.

Ding, R., J. K. S. Jansen, N. G. Laing, and H. Tonnesen (1983). *J. Neurocytol.* 12:887–919. The innervation of skeletal muscles in chickens curarized during early development.

Dinger, B., S. Fidone, and L. J. Stensaas (1985). *Exp. Neurol.* 89:189–203. Regeneration of taste buds by nongustatory nerve fibers.

DiStefano, P. S., and E. M. Johnson, Jr. (1988a). *J. Neurosci.* 8:231–241. Nerve growth factor receptors on cultured rat Schwann cells.

DiStefano, P. S., and E. M. Johnson, Jr. (1988b). *Proc. Natl.* *Acad. Sci. U.S.A.* 85:270–274. Identification of a truncated form of the nerve growth factor receptor.

Dixon, J. E., and C. R. Kintner (1989). *Development* 106:749–757. Cellular contacts required for neural induction in *Xenopus* embryos: Evidence for two signals.

Dixon, J. S., and J. R. Cronly-Dillon (1972). *J. Embryol. Exp. Morphol.* 28:659–666. The fine structure of the developing retina in *Xenopus laevis*.

Dixon, R. G., and L. G. Eng (1981). *J. Comp. Neurol.* 195:305–322. Glial fibrillary acidic protein in the retina of the developing albino rat: An immunoperoxidase study of paraffin-embedded tissue.

Dobbing, J. (1963). *Proc. Roy. Soc. (London) Ser. B.* 159:503–509. The influence of early nutrition on the development and myelination of the brain.

Dobbing, J. (1968a). *Prog. Brain Res.* 29:417–425. The development of the blood-brain barrier.

Dobbing, J. (1968b). Vulnerable periods in developing brain, pp. 287–316. In *Applied Neurochemistry.* Blackwell, Oxford.

Dobbing, J. (1970). *Am. J. Dis. Child.* 120:411–415. Undernutrition and the developing brain. The relevance of animal models to the human problem.

Dobbing, J. (1971). *Psychiatr. Neurol. Neruochir.* 74:433–442. Undernutrition and the developing brain: The use of animal models to elucidate the human problem.

Dobbing, J. (1973). *Nutr. Rep. Int.* 7:401–406. The developing brain: A plea for more critical interspecies extrapolation.

Dobbing, J. (1976). Vulnerable periods in brain growth and somatic growth, pp. 137–147. In *The Biology of Human Fetal Growth*, (D. F. Roberts, and A. M. Thomson eds.), Taylor and Francis, London.

Dobbing, J., and J. Sands (1970a). *Nature* 226:639–640. Timing of neuroblast multiplication in developing human brain.

Dobbing, J., and J. Sands (1970b). *Brain Res.* 17:115–123. Growth and development of the brain and spinal cord of the guinea pig.

Dobbing, J., and J. Sands (1971). *Biol. Neonate* 19:363–378. Vulnerability of the developing brain. IX. The effect of nutritional growth retardation on the timing of the brain growth spurt.

Dobbing, J., and J. Sands (1979). *Early Hum. Dev.* 3:79–83. Comparative aspects of the brain growth spurt.

Dobbing, J., and J. L. Smart (1974). *Br. Med. Bull.* 30:164–168. Vulnerability of developing brain and behaviour.

Dobbing, J., J. W. Hopewell, and A. Lynch (1971). *Exp. Neurol.* 32:439–447. Vulnerability of developing Brain: VII. Permanent deficit of neurons in cerebral and cerebellar cortex following early mild undernutrition.

Dobzhansky, T. (1951). *Genetics and the Origin of Species*, 3rd edn. Columbia Univ. Press, New York.

Dodd, J., D. Solter, and T. M. Jessell (1984). *Nature* 311:469–472. Monoclonal antibodies against carbohydrate differentiation antigens identify subsets of primary sensory neurons.

Dodds, W. J. (1878). *J. Anat. Physiol.* 12:340–363, 454–494, 636–660. On the localisation of the functions of the brain: Being an historical and critical analysis of the question.

Dodt, E., and M. Jacobson (1963). *J. Neurophysiol.* 26:752–

758. Photosensitivity of a localized region of the frog diencephalon.

Doe, C. Q., and C. S. Goodman (1985). *Dev. Biol.* 111:193–205. Early events in insect neurogenesis. I. Development and segmental differences in the pattern of neuronal precursor cells.

Doe, C. Q., and M. P. Scott (1988). *Trends Neurosci.* 11:101–106. Segmentation and homeotic gene function in the developing nervous system of *Drosophila*.

Dogial, A. S. (1890). *Arch. mikr. Anat. Bonn* 35:305–320. Methylenblautinktion der motorischen Nervenendigungen in den Muskeln der Amphibien und Reptilien.

Döhler, K.-D., and R. A. Gorski (1981). *Br. Bull.* 5:5–9. Sexual differentiation of the brain: Past, present and future.

Dohrmann, U., D. Edgar, M. Sendtner, and H. Thoenen (1986). *Dev. Biol.* 118:209–221. Muscle-derived factors that support survival and promote fiber outgrowth from embryonic chick spinal motor neurons in culture.

Dohrmann, U., D. Edgar, and H. Thoenen (1987). *Dev. Biol.* 124:145–152. Distinct neurotrophic factors from skeletal muscle and the central nervous system interact synergistically to support the survival of cultured embryonic spinal motor neurons.

Dohrn, A. (1902). *Mitt. Zool. Sta. Neapel.* 15:555–654. Weiterer Beiträge zur Beurteilung der Occipitalregion und der Ganglienleiste der Selachier.

Dolbeare, F. H. Gratzner, M. Pallavicini, and J. W. Gray (1983). *Proc. Natl. Acad. Sci. U.S.A.* 80:5573–5577. Flow cytometric measurement of total DNA content and incorporated bromodeoxyuridine.

Dollinger, I. (1814). *Beyträge zur Entwicklungsgeschichte des menschlichen Gehirns.* Heinrich Ludwig Brönner, Frankfurt am Main.

Donahue, S., and C. D. Pappas (1961). *Am. J. Anat.* 115:17–26. The fine structure of capillaries in the cerebral cortex of the rat at various stages of development.

Donahue, S. P., and A. W. English (1987). *Dev. Biol.* 124:481–489. The role of synapse elimination in the establishment of neuromuscular compartments.

Donahue, S. P., and A. W. English (1989). *J. Neurosci.* 9:1621–1627. Selective elimination of cross-compartmental innervation in rat lateral gastrocnemius muscle.

Donaldson, H. H. (1925). *Arch. Neurol. Psychiat.* 13:385–386. The significance of brain weight.

Donaldson, H. H., and G. Nagasaka (1918). *J. Comp. Neurol.* 29:529–552. On the increase in the diameter of nerve cell bodies and of the fibers arising from them during the later phases of growth (albino rat).

Donegani, G., and G. Gabella (1967). *Boll. Soc. Ital. Biol. Sper.* 43:1165–1167. Effetto della sezione intracranica del nervo glosso-faringeo sui corpuscoli gustativi nel coniglio.

Donkelaar, H. J., ten, and P. J. W. Dederen (1979). *Anat. Embryol.* 156:331–348. Neurogenesis in the basal forebrain of the Chinese hamster *(Cricetulus griseus)*.

Dony, C., and P. Gruss (1987). *EMBO J.* 6:2965–2975. Specific expression of the Hox 1.3 homeobox gene in murine embryonic structures originating from or induced by the mesoderm.

Dorgan, W. J., and R. L. Schultz (1971). *J. Exp. Zool.* 178 497–512. An *in vitro* study of programmed death in rat placental giant cells.

Dörner, G. (1976). *Hormones and Brain Differentiation.* Elsevier, Amsterdam.

Dörner, G. (1980). *Vitam. Horm. N.Y.* 38:325–381. Sexual differentiation of the brain.

Dörner, G., and J. Staudt (1969). *Neuroendocrinol.* 5:103–106. Perinatal structural sex differentiation of the hypothalamus in rats.

Dorresteijn, A. W. C., H. A. Wagemaker, S. W. de Laat, and J. A. M. van den Biggelaar (1983). *Roux's Arch. Dev. Biol.* 192:262–269. Dye-coupling between blastomeres in early embryos of *patella vulgata* (mollusca, gastropoda): Its relevance for cell determination.

Dorris, F. (1939). *J. Exp. Zool.* 86:315–345. The production of pigment by chick neural crest in grafts to the 3-day limb bud.

Dostrovsky, J. O, J. Millar, and P. D. Wall (1976). *Exp. Neurol.* 52:480–495. The immediate shift of afferent drive of dorsal column nucleus cells following deafferentation in gracile nucleus and spinal cord.

Dostrovsky, J. O, G. J. Ball, J. N. Hu, and B. J. Sessle (1982). Functional changes associated with partial tooth pulp removal in neurons of the trigeminal spinal tract nucleus, and their clinical implications. In *Anatomical, Physiological and Pharmacological Aspects of Trigeminal Pain* (R. G. Hill and B. Matthews, eds.), Excerpta Medica, Amsterdam.

Dotti, C. G., and G. A. Banker (1987). *Nature* 330:254–256. Experimentally induced alteration in the polarity of developing neurons.

Dotti, C. G., C. A. Sullivan, and G. A. Banker (1988). *J. Neurosci.* 8:1454–1468. The establishment of polarity by hippocampal neurons in culture.

Doucette, R., and J. Diamond (1987). *J. Comp. Neurol.* 261:592–603. The normal and precocious sprouting of heat nociceptors in the skin of adult rats.

Dougherty, T. F. (1944). *Am. J. Anat.* 74:61–95. Studies on the cytogenesis of microglia and their relation to cells of the reticulo-endothelial system.

Doupe, A. J., S. C. Landis and P. H. Patterson (1985). *J. Neurosci.* 5:2119–2142. Environmental influences in the development of neural crest derivatives: Glucocorticoids, growth factors and chromaffin cell plasticity.

Doupe, A. J., P. H. Patterson and S. C. Landis (1985). *J. Neurosci.* 5:2143–2160. Small intensely fluorescent (SIF) cells in culture: Role of glucocorticoids and growth factors in their development and phenotypic interconversions with other neural crest derivatives.

Dow, K. E., S. E. L. Mirski, J. C. Roder and R. J. Riopelle (1988). *J. Neurosci.* 8:3278–3289. Neuronal proteoglycans: Biosynthesis and functional interaction with neurons *in vitro*.

Dow, R. S., and G. Moruzzi (1958). *The Physiology and Pathology of the Cerebellum.* Univ. Minnesota Press, Minneapolis.

Dowling, J. E., and W. M. Cowan (1966). *Z. Zellforsch.* 71:14–28. An electron microscope study of normal and degenerating centrifugal fiber terminals in the pigeon retina.

Doyère (1840). *Ann des Sciences nat.* Serie 2. Memoire sur les Tardigrades. Cited in Kühne, W. (1870).

Drabkin, D. L. (1958). *Thudichum. Chemist of the Brain.* Univ. Pennsylv. Press, Philadelphia.

Drachman, D. B. (1967). *Arch. Neurol.* 17:206–218. Is acetylcholine the trophic neuromuscular transmitter?

Drachman, D. B. (1972). *J. Physiol. (London)* 226:619–627.

Neurotrophic regulation of muscle cholinesterase: Effects of botulinum toxin and denervation.

Drachman, D. B. (1976). Trophic interactions between nerves and muscles: The role of cholinergic transmission (including usage) and other factors, pp. 161–186. In *Biology of Cholinergic Function* (A. M. Goldberg, and I. Hanin eds.), Raven Press, New York.

Drachman, D. B. (1981). *Ann. Rev. Neurosci.* 4:195–225. The biology of Myasthenia Gravis.

Drachman, D. B., and F. Witzke (1972). *Science* 176:514–516. Trophic regulation of acetylcholine sensitivity of muscle: Effect of electrical stimulation.

Draeger, A., A. G. Weeds, and R. B. Fitzsimons (1987). *J. Neurol. Sci.* 81:19–43. Primary, secondary, and tertiary myotubes in developing skeletal muscle: A new approach to the analysis of human myogenesis.

Draetta, G., and D. Beach (1988). *Cell* 54:17–26. Activation of cdc2 protein kinase during mitosis in human cells; cell cycle-dependent phosphorylation and subunit rearrangement.

Dräger, U. C. (1976). The effects of monocular deprivation on mouse striate cortex. Paper presented at the Society for Neuroscience, Toronto.

Dräger, U. C. (1981). *J. Comp. Neurol.* 201:555–570. Observations on the organization of the visual cortex in the reeler mouse.

Dratman, M. B., Y. Futaesaku, F. L. Crutchfield, N. Berman, B. Payne, M. Sar, and W. E. Stumpf (1982). *Science* 215:309–312. Iodine–125-labeled triiodothyronine in rat brain: Evidence for localization in discrete neural systems.

Dreher, B., R. A. Potts, and M. R. Bennett (1983). *Neurosci. Lett.* 36:255–260. Evidence that the early postnatal reduction in number of rat retinal ganglion cells is due to a wave of ganglion cell death.

Drejer, J., O. M. Larsson, and A. Schousboe (1982). *Exp. Brain Res.* 47:259–269. Characterization of 1-glutamate uptake into and release from astrocytes and neurons cultured from different brain regions.

Dressler, G. R., and P.Gruss (1988). *Trends Genet.* 4:214–219. Do multigene families regulate vertebrate development?

Dreyer, D., A. Lagrange, C. Grothe, and K. Unsicker (1989). *Neurosci. Lett.* 99:35–38. Basic fibroblast growth factor prevents ontogenetic neuron death *in vivo*.

Dribin, L., and M. Jacobson (1978). *Exp. Brain Res.* 150:543–557. Effects of 5-bromodeoxyuridine on development of Mauthner's neuron and neural retina of *Xenopus laevis* embryos.

Driesch, H. (1896). *Arch. Entw.-Mech.* 3. Die tactische Reizbarkeit der Mesenchymzellen von Echinus microtuberculatus.

Driesch, H. (1908). *The Science and Philosophy of the Organism*, 2 Vols. Adam and Charles Black, London.

Driesch, H. (1914). *The History and Theory of Vitalism*. Macmillan, London.

Driever, W., and C. Nüsslein-Volhard (1988). *Cell* 54:83–93. A gradient of *bicoid* protein in *Drosophila* embryos.

Driever, W., and C. Nüsslein-Volhard (1989). *Nature* 337:138–143. The bicoid protein is a positive regulator of hunchback transcription in the early *Drosophila* embryo.

Drillien, C. M. (1958). *Archs. Dis. Childh.* 33:10–18. Growth and development in a group of very low birth weight.

Droz, B. (1973). *Brain Res.* 62:383–394. Renewal of synaptic proteins.

Droz, B., A. Rambourg, and H. L. Koenig (1975). *Brain Res.* 93:1–13. The smooth endoplasmic reticulum: Structure and role in the renewal of axonal membrane and synaptic vesicles by fast axonal transport.

Drubin, D. G., S. C. Feinstein, E. M. Shooter, and M. W. Kirschner (1985). *J. Cell Biol.* 101:1799–1807. Nerve growth factor-induced neurite outgrowth in PC12 cells involves the coordinate induction of microtubule assembly and assembly-promoting factors.

Drubin, D. G., S. Kobayashi, and M. Kirschner (1986). *Ann. N.Y. Acad. Sci.* 466:257–268. Association of tau protein with microtubules in living cells.

Drubin, D. G., S. Kobayashi, D. Kellogg, and M. Kirschner (1988). *J. Cell Biol.* 106:1583–1591. Regulation of microtubule protein levels during cellular morphogenesis in nerve growth factor-treated PC12 cells.

Duband, J.-L., and J. P. Thiery (1982) *Dev. Biol.* 93:308–323. Distribution of fibronectin in the early phase of avian cephalic neural crest cell migration.

Duband, J.-L., and J. P. Thiery (1987). *Development* 101:461–478. Distribution of laminin and collagens during avian neural crest development.

Duband, J.-L., and J. P. Thiery (1990). *Development* 108:421–433. Spatial and temporal distribution of vinculin and talin in migrating avian neural crest cells and their derivatives.

Duband, J.-L., T. J. Tucker, T. J. Poole, M. Vincent, H. Aoyama, and J. P. Thiery (1985). *J. Cell. Biochem.* 27:189–203. How do the migratory and adhesive properties of the neural crest govern ganglia formation in the avian peripheral nervous system?

Duband, J.-L., S. Rocher, W.-T. Chen, K. M. Yamada, and J. P. Thiery (1986). *J. Cell Biol.* 102:160–178. Cell adhesion and migration in the early vertebrate embryo: Location and possible role of the putative fibronectin receptor complex.

Duband, J.-L., S. Dufour, K. Hatta, M. Takeichi, G. M. Edelman, and J. P. Thiery (1987). *J. Cell Biol.* 104:1361–1374. Adhesion molecules during somitogenesis in the avian embryo.

Duband, J.-L., T. Volberg, I. Sabanay, J. P. Thiery, and B. Geiger (1988). *Development* 103:325–344. Spatial and temporal distribution of adherens-junction associated adhesion molecule A-CAM during avian embryogenesis.

Dubey, P. N., D. K. Kadasne, and V. S. Gosavi (1968). *J. Anat. (London)* 102:407–414. The influence of the peripheral field on the morphogenesis of Hofmann's nucleus major of chick spinal cord.

Dubin, M., and L. Stark (1983). *Invest. Ophthalmol. Suppl.* 24:138. Time-course of effects of action potential blockade on development of retino-geniculate connections in kittens.

Dubin, M. W., L. A. Stark, and S. M. Archer (1986). *J. Neurosci.* 6:1021–1036. A role for action-potential activity in the development of neuronal connections in the kitten retinogeniculate pathway.

Dubois, E. (1923). *Proc. Koninkl. Med. Akad. Wetenschap (Amsterdam)* 25:230–255. Phylogenetic and ontogenetic increase of the volume of the brain in vertebrata.

Du Bois-Reymond, E. (1848). *Über die Lebenskraft. Aus der Vorrede zu den "Untersuchungen über tierische Elektrizität."* Veit, Leipzig.

Du Bois-Reymond, E. (1877). *d. Allgem. Muskel-und Nervenphysik* 2:700. Gesammelte Abhandl.

Dubois-Dalcq, M., T. Behar, L. Hudson, and R. A. Lazzarini (1986). *J. Cell Biol.* 102:384–392. Emergence of three myelin proteins in oligodendrocytes cultured without neurons.

Dubowitz, V. and A. G. E. Pearse. (1960). *Histochimie* 2:105–117. A comparative histochemical study of oxidative enzyme and phosphorylase activity in skeletal muscle.

Duchen, L. W. (1971). *J. Neurol. Sci.* 14:47–60. An electron microscopic study of the changes induced by botulinum toxin in the motor end-plate of slow and fast skeletal muscle fibres of the mouse.

Duchen, L. W. (1972). *Proc. Roy. Soc. Med.* 65:10–11. Motor nerve growth induced by botulinum toxin as regenerative phenomenon.

Duchen, L. W., and S. J. Strich (1968). *Quart. J. Exp. Physiol.* 53:84–89. The effects of botulinum toxin on the pattern of innervation of skeletal muscle in the mouse.

Duckett, S., and A. G. E. Pearse (1968). *J. Anat. (London)* 102:183–187. The cells of Cajal-Retzius in the developing human brain.

Duffy, C., T. J. Teyler, and E. Shashoua (1981). *Science* 212:1148–1151. Long-term potentiation in the hippocampal slice: Evidence for stimulated secretion of newly synthesized proteins.

Duffy, F. H., S. R. Snodgrass, J. L. Burchfiel, and J. L. Conway (1976). *Nature* 260:256–257. Bicuculline reversal of deprivation amblyopia in the cat.

Duffy, F. H., J. L. Burchfiel, and J. R. Snodgrass (1978). *Ophthalmology* 85:489–495. The pharmacology of amblyopia.

Duffy, P. E. (1983). *Astrocytes: Normal, Reactive and Neoplastic.* Raven Press, New York.

Duffy, P. E., K. I. Huang, and M. M. Rapport (1982). *Exp. Cell Res.* 139:145–157. The relationship of GFAP to the shape, motility, and differentiation of human astrocytoma cells.

Dufour, S., J.-L. Duband, A. R. Kornblihtt, and J. P. Thiery (1988). *Trends Genet.* 4:198–204. The role of fibronectins in embryonic cell migrations.

Duncan, D. (1934a). *J. Comp. Neurol.* 60:437–472. A relation between axon diameter and myelination determined by measurement of myelinated spinal root fibers.

Duncan, D. (1934b). *Science* 79:363. The importance of axon diameter as a factor in myelination.

Duncan, D. (1957). *Texas Rep. Biol. Med.* 15:367–377. Electron microscope study of the embryonic neural tube and notochord.

Duncan, I. D., J. P. Hammang, and K. F. Jackson (1987a). *Soc. Neurosci. Abstr.* 13:118. Jimpy myelin lacks PLP and has a defect in the intraperiod line.

Duncan, I. D., J. P. Hammang, and B. D. Trapp (1987b). *Proc. Natl. Acad. Sci. U.S.A.* 84:6287–6291. Abnormal compact myelin in the myelin deficient rat: Absence of proteolipid protein correlates with a defect in the intraperiod line.

Dunglison, R. (1833). *A New Dictionary of Medical Science and Literature,* 2 vols., Charles Bowen, Boston.

Dunlop, D. S. (1983). Protein turnover in brain: Synthesis and degradation, pp. 25–63. In *Handbook in Neurochemistry* 5 (A. Lajtha, ed.), Plenum, New York.

Dunlop, S. A., and L. D. Beazley (1985). *Dev. Brain Res.* 23:81–90. Changing distribution of retinal ganglion cells during area centralis and visual streak formation in the marsupial *Setonix brachyurus.*

Dunlop, S. A., and L. D. Beazley (1987). *J. Comp. Neurol.* 264:14–23. Cell death in the retinal ganglion cell layer of the wallaby *Setonix brachyurus.*

Dunlop, S. A., W. A. Langley, and L. D. Beazley (1987). *Vision Res.* 27:151–164. Development of area centralis and visual streak in the grey kangaroo *Macropus fuliginosus.*

Dunn, G. A. (1971). *J. Comp. Neurol.* 143:491–508. Mutual contact inhibition of extension of chick snesory nerve fibres *in vitro.*

Dunn, L. C. (1965). *A Short History of Genetics.* McGraw Hill, New York.

Dunnebacke, T. H. (1953). *J. Comp. Neurol.* 98:155–177. The effects of the extirpation of the superior oblique muscle on the trochlear nucleus in the chick embryo.

Dunning, H. S., and J. Furth (1935). *Am. J. Path.* 11:895–914. Studies on the relation between microglia, histiocytes and monocytes.

Dunning, H. S., and H. G. Wolff (1937). *J. Comp. Neurol.* 67:433–450. The relative vascularity of various parts of the central and peripheral nervous system of the cat and its relation to function.

Dupouey, P., S. Benjelloun-Touini, and D. Gomes (1985). *Dev. Neurosci.* 7:81–93. Histochemical demonstration of an organized cytoarchitecture of the radial glia in the CNS of the embryonic mouse.

Durham, D., and E. W. Rubel (1985). *J. Comp. Neurol.* 231:446–456. Afferent influences on brain stem auditory nuclei of the chicken: Changes in succinate dehydrogenase activity following cochlea removal.

Durham, D., and T. A. Woolsey (1977). *Brain Res.* 137:169–174. Barrels and columnar cortical organization: Evidence from 2-deoxyglucose (2-DG) experiments.

Durham, D., and T. A. Woolsey (1984). *J. Comp. Neurol.* 223:424–447. Effects of neonatal whisker lesions on mouse central trigeminal pathways.

Durham, D., and T. A. Woolsey (1985). *J. Comp. Neurol.* 235:97–110. Functional organization in cortical barrels of normal and vibrissae-damaged mice: A (3H)2-deoxyglucose study.

Durham, D., T. A. Woolsey, and L. Kruger (1981). *J. Neurosci.* 1:519–526. Cellular localization of 2-[(3)]deoxy-D-glucose from paraffin-embedded brains.

Dürken, B. (1911). *Z. Wiss. Zool.* 99:189–355. Über frühzeitige Extirpation von Extremitätenanlagen beim Frosch.

Dürken, B. (1913). *Z. Wiss. Zool. Abt. A* 105:192–242. Über einseitige Augenextirpation bei jungen Froschlarven.

Dürken, B. (1930). *Biol. Generalis* 6:511–552. Zur Frage nach der Wirkung einseitiger Augenextirpation bei Froschlarven.

Durston, A. J., J. P. M. Timmermans, W. J. Hage, H. F. J. Hendriks, N. J. de Vries, M. Heideveld, and P. D. Nieuwkoop (1989). *Nature* 340:140–144. Retinoic acid causes an anteroposterior transformation in the developing central nervous system.

Dusart, I., F. Nothias, F. Roudier, and M. Peschanski (1987). *C. R. Acad. Sci.* 305:277–283. Role possible de l'environment neuronal dans la vascularisation d'une greffe intracerebrale.

Du Shane, G. P. (1935). *J. Exp. Zool.* 72:1–31. An experimental study of the origin of pigment cells in Amphibia.

Du Shane, G. (1938). *J. Exp. Zool.* 78:485–503. Neural fold derivatives in the Amphibia: Pigment cells, spinal ganglia and Rohon-Beard cells.

Dussault, J. H., and J. Ruel (1987). *Ann. Rev. Physiol.* 49:321–334. Thyroid hormones and brain development.

Dustin, A. P. (1910). *Arch. Biol. Liége* 25: 269–388. Le rôle des tropismes et de l'odogenés dans la régéneration du systéme nerveux.

Dustin, P. (1984). *Microtubules,* 2nd ed. Springer Verlag, New York.

Duval, M. (1895). *Compts Rend. Soc. Biol. Paris* 10:74–77. Hypothèse sur la physiologie des centre nerveux; théorie histologique du sommeil.

Duval, M. (1897). *Précis d'Histologie.* Masson, Paris.

Duval, M. (1900). *Rev. d. l'École d'Anthropologie de Paris* 10. Les neurones, l'amiboïdisme nerveux et la Théorie histologique du sommeil.

Duxon, M. J., and Y. Usson (1989). *Development* 107:243–251. Cellular insertion of primary and secondary myotubes in embryonic rat muscles.

Duxon, M. J., Y. Usson, and A. J. Harris (1989). *Development* 107:743–750. The origin of secondary myotubes in mammalian skeletal muscles: Ultrastructural studies.

Dyson, S. E., and D. G. Jones (1976a). *Brain Res.* 114:365–378. Some effects of undernutrition on synaptic development—a quantitative ultrastructural study.

Dyson, S. E., and D. G. Jones (1976b). *Prog. Neurobiol.* 7:171–196. Undernutrition and the developing nervous system.

Dyson, S. E., and D. G. Jones (1980). *Brain Res.* 183:43–59. Quantitation of terminal parameters and their interrelationships in maturing central synapses: A perspective for experimental studies.

Eagles, P. A. M., H. C. Pant, and H. Gainer (1988). Neurofilaments. In *Intermediate Filaments* (P. M. Steinert, and R. D. Goldman, eds.), Plenum, New York.

Eagleson, K. L., and M. R. Bennett (1986). *Dev. Brain Res.* 29:161–172. Motoneuron survival requirements during development: The change from immature astrocyte dependence to myotube dependence.

Easter, S. S. Jr., and C. A. O. Stuermer (1984). *J. Neurosci.* 4:1052–1063. An evaluation of the hypothesis of shifting terminals in the goldfish optic tectum.

Easter, S. S., Jr., and J. S. H. Taylor (1989). *Development* 107:553–573. The development of the *Xenopus* retinofugal pathway: Optic fibers join a pre-existing tract.

Eastlick, H. L. (1943). *J. Exp. Zool.* 93:27–49. Studies on transplanted embryonic limbs of the chick. I. The development of muscle in nerveless and in innervated grafts.

Eastlick, H. L., and R. A. Wortham (1947). *J. Morphol.* 80:369–389. Studies on transplanted embryonic limbs of the chick. III. The replacement of muscle by adipose tissue.

Eayers, J. T. (1952). *Br. J. Ophthal. Mol.* 36:453–459. Relationship between the ganglion cell layer of the retina and the optic nerve in the rat.

Eayrs, J. T. (1955). *Acta Anat.* 25:160–183. The cerebral cortex of normal and hypothyroid rats.

Eayrs, J. T. (1960). *Brit. Med. Bull.* 16:122–126. Influence of the thyroid on the central nervous system.

Eayrs, J. T. (1961). *Growth* 25:175–189. Protein anabolism as a factor ameliorating the effects of early thyroid deficiency.

Eayrs, J. T., and B. Goodhead (1959). *J. Anat. (London)* 93:385–402. Postnatal development of the cerebral cortex in the rat.

Eayrs, J. T., and W. A. Lishman (1953). *Brit. J. Animal Behav.* 3:17–24. The maturation of behaviour in hypothyroidism and starvation.

Ebbott, S., and I. Hendry (1978). *Brain Res.* 139:160–163. Retrograde transport of nerve growth factor in the rat central nervous system.

Ebendal, T. (1976a). *Exp. Cell Res.* 98:159–169. The relative roles of contact inhibition and contact guidance in orientation of axons extending on aligned collagen fibrils *in vitro.*

Ebendal, T. (1976b). Experiments *in vitro* on neuron development and axon orientation in the chick embryo. Doctoral Thesis, Uppsala University, Sweden.

Ebendal, T. (1977). *Cell Tiss. Res.* 175:439–458. Extracellular matrix fibrils and cell contacts in the chick embryo.

Ebendal, T., and K.-O. Hedlund (1975). *Zoon* 3:33–47. Effects of nerve growth factor on the chick embryo trigeminal ganglion in culture.

Ebendal, T. and C.-O. Jacobson (1975). *Zoon* 3:169–172. Human glial cells stimulating outgrowth of axons in cultured chick embryo ganglia.

Ebendal, T., and C.-O, Jacobson (1976) *Exp. Cell Res.* 105:379–387. Tissue explants affecting extension and orientation of axons in cultured chick embryo ganglia.

Ebendal, T., and H. Persson (1988). *Development* 102:101–106. Detection of nerve growth factor mRNA in the developing chicken embryo.

Ebendal, T., D. Larhammar, and H. Persson (1986). *EMBO J.* 5:1483–1487. Structure and expression of the chicken β nerve growth factor gene.

Eberhardt, N. L., T. Valcana, and P. S. Timiras (1978). *Endocrinology* 102:556–561. Triiodothyronine nuclear receptors: An *in vitro* comparison of the binding of triiodothyronine to nuclei of adult rat liver, cerebral hemisphere, and anterior pituitary.

Ebinger, P. (1974). *Z. Anat. Entwicklungsgesch.* 144:267–302. A cytoarchitectonic volumetric comparison of brains in wild and domestic sheep.

Ebner, F. F., and M. Colonnier (1975). *J. Comp. Neurol.* 160:51–80. Synaptic patterns in the visual cortex of turtle: An electron microscopic study.

Eccles, J. C. (1959). The Development of Ideas on the Synapse. In *The Historical Development of Physiological Thought* (C. M. Brooks, and P. F. Cranefield, eds.), Hafner, New York.

Eccles, J. C. (1964). *The Physiology of Synapses.* Springer-Verlag, Berlin.

Eccles, J. C. (1989). *Evolution of The Brain: Creation of The Self.* Routledge, London.

Eccles, J. C., and C. S. Sherrington (1930). *Proc. Roy. Soc. (London) Ser. B.* 106:326–357. Numbers and contraction-values of individual motor-units examined in some muscles of the limb.

Eccles, J. C., R. M. Eccles, and A. Lundberg (1958a). *J. Physiol. (London)* 142:275–291. The action potentials of the alpha motoneurones supplying fast and slow muscles.

Eccles, J. C., B. Libet, and R. R. Young (1958b). *J. Physiol. (London)* 143: 11–40. The behavior of chromatolyzed motoneurones studied by intracellular recording.

Eccles, J. C., R. M. Eccles, and F. Magni (1960). *J. Physiol.*

(London) 154:68–88. Monosynaptic excitatory action on motoneurones regenerated to antagonistic muscles.

Eccles, J. C., R. M. Eccles, and C. N. Shealy (1962a). *J. Neurophysiol.* 25: 544–558. An investigation into the effect of degenerating primary afferent fibers on the monosynaptic innervation of motoneurons.

Eccles, J. C., R. M. Eccles, C. N. Shealy, and W. D. Willis (1962b). *J. Neurophysiol.* 25:559–580. Experiments utilizing monosynaptic excitatory action on motoneurons for testing hypotheses relating to specificity of neuronal connections.

Eccles, J. C., M. Ito, and J. Szentágothai (1967). *The Cerebellum as a Neuronal Machine.* Springer, New York.

Eccleston, P. A., P. G. C. Bannerman, D. E. Pleasure, J. Winter, R. Mirsky, and K. R. Jessen (1989). *Development* 107:107–112. Control of peripheral glial cell proliferation: Enteric neurons exert an inhibitory influence on Schwann cell and enteric glial cell DNA synthesis in culture.

Ecker, A. (1869). *Die Hirnwindung des Menschen nach eigenen Untersuchungen insbesondere über die Entwicklung derselben beim Fötus.* Vieweg, Braunschweig. (English transl. 1873, by J. C. Galton, On the convolutions of the human brain, Smith and Elder, London).

Ecker, A. (1873). *The Cerebral Convolutions of Man Represented According to Original Observations, Especially Upon Their Development in the Foetus.* Transl. by R. T. Edes from the 1870 German edn. Appleton, New York.

Eckholm, R., and H. Hyden (1965). *Ultrastruct. Res.* 13:269–280. Polysomes from microdissected fresh neurons.

Edds, M. V., Jr. (1950a). *J. Exp. Zool.* 113:517–552. Collateral regeneration of residual motor axons in partially denervated muscles.

Edds, M. V., Jr. (1950b). *J. Comp. Neurol.* 93:258–276. Hypertrophy of nerve fibers to functionally overloaded muscles.

Edds, M. V., Jr. (1953). *Quart. Rev. Biol.* 28:260–276. Collateral nerve regeneration.

Edelman, G. M. (1983a). *Proc. Natl. Acad. Sci. U.S.A.* 81: 1460–1464. Cell adhesion and morphogenesis: The regulator hypothesis.

Edelman, G. M. (1983b). *Science* 219:450–457. Cell adhesion molecules.

Edelman, G. M. (1984). *Ann. Rev. Neurosci.* 7:339–377. Modulation of cell adhesion during induction, histogenesis and perinatal development of the nervous system.

Edelman, G. M. (1988a). *Biochemistry* 27:3533–3543. Morphoregulatory molecules.

Edelman, G. M. (1988b). *Neural Darwinism.* Basic Books, New York.

Edelman, G. M. (1988c). *Topobiology.* Basic Books, New York.

Edelman, G. M., and C.-M. Chuong (1982). *Proc. Natl. Acad. Sci. U.S.A.* 79:7036–7040. Embryonic to adult conversion of neural cell adhesion molecules in normal and staggerer mice.

Edelman, G. M., W. J. Gallin, A. Delouvée, B. A. Cunningham, and J.-P. Thiery (1982). *Proc. Natl. Acad. Sci. U.S.A.* 80:4384–4388. Early epochal maps of two different cell adhesion molecules.

Edelman, G. M., B. A. Murray, R.-M. Mege, B. A. Cunningham, and W. J. Gallin (1987). *Proc. Natl. Acad. Sci. U.S.A.* 84:8502–8506. Cellular expression of liver and neural cell adhesion molecules after transfection with their cDNA's results in specific cell-cell binding.

Edgar, D. (1985). *J. Cell Sci.* 3:Supp.107–113. Nerve growth factors and molecules of the extracellular matrix in neuronal development.

Edgar, D. (1989). *Trends Neurosci.* 12:248–251. Neuronal laminin receptors.

Edgar, D., R. Timpl, and H. Thoenen (1984). *EMBO J.* 3:1463–1468. The heparin binding domain of laminin is responsible for its effects on neurite outgrowth and neuronal survival.

Edgar, D. H., and H. Thoenen (1978). *Brain Res.* 154:186–190. Selective enzyme induction in a nerve growth factor-responsive pheochromocytoma cell line (PC 12).

Edinger, L. (1908a). *J. Comp. Neurol. Psychol.* 18:437–457. The relations of comparative anatomy to comparative psychology.

Edinger, L. (1908b). *Vorlesungen über den Bau der Nervösen Zentralorgane des Menschen und der Tiere. II. Vergleichende Anatomie des Gehirns.* F. C. W. Vogel, Leipzig.

Edmunds, S. M., and J. G. Parnavelas (1982). *J. Neurocytol.* 11:427–446. Retzius-Cajal cells: an ultrastructural study in the developing visual cortex of the rat.

Edström, A. (1964a). *J. Neurochem.* 11:309–314. The ribonucleic acid in the Mauthner neuron of the goldfish.

Edström, A. (1964b). *J. Neurochem.* 11:557–559. The effect of spinal cord transection on the base composition and content of RNA in the Mauthner nerve fibre of the goldfish.

Edström, A. (1966). *J. Neurochem.* 13:315–321. Amino acid incorporation in isolated Mauthner nerve fibre components.

Edström, A. (1967). *J. Neurochem.* 14:239–243. Inhibition of protein synthesis in Mauthner nerve fibre components by Actinomycin-D.

Edström, A., and J. Sjöstrand (1969). *J. Neurochem.* 16:67–82. Protein synthesis in the isolated Mauthner nerve fibre of the goldfish.

Edström, J.-E., D. Eichner, and A. Edström (1962). *Biochim. Biophys. Acta* 61: 178–184. The ribonucleic acid of axons and myelin sheaths from Mauthner neurons.

Edström, A., J.-E. Edström, and T. Hökfelt (1969). *J. Neurochem.* 16:53–66. Sedimentation analysis of ribonucleic acid extracted from isolated Mauthner nerve fiber components.

Edvinsson, L., A. Degueurce, D. Duverger, E. T. MacKenzie, and B. Scatton (1983). *Nature* 306:55–57. Central serotonergic nerves project to the pial vessels of the brain.

Edwards, J. S., and J. Palka (1973). Neural specificity as a game of cricket: Some rules for sensory regeneration in *Acheta domesticus*, pp. 131–146. In *Developmental Neurobiology of Arthropods* (D. Young, ed.), Cambridge Univ. Press, London.

Edwards, M. A., and M. Jacobson (1984). *J. Comp. Neurol.* 226:141–153. Effects of permeability of midtectal barriers in goldfish on compression of the visuotectal projection rostrally and regenerative escape caudally.

Edwards, M. J. (1981). Clinical disorders of fetal brain development: Defects due to hyperthermia, pp. 335–364. In *Fetal Brain Disorders-Recent approaches to the Problem of Mental Deficiency* (B. S. Hetzel, and R. M. Smith, eds.), Elsevier/North Holland Biomedical Press, Amsterdam.

Edwards, M. J., J. G. Lyle, K. M. Jonson, and R. H. C. Penny (1973). *Dev. Psychobiol.* 7:579–584. Prenatal retardation of brain growth by hyperthermia and the learning capacity of mature guinea-pigs.

Edwards, M. J., R. A. Wanner, and R. C. Mulley (1976). *Neuropathol. Appl. Neurobiol.* 2:439–450. Growth and development of the brain in normal and heat-retarded guinea-pigs.

Edwards, M. J., C. H. Gray, and J. Beatson (1984). *Teratology* 29:305–312. Retardation of brain growth of guinea pigs by hyperthermia: Effect of varying intervals between successive exposures.

Edwards, R. H., M. J. Selby, P. D. Garcia, and W.J. Rutter (1988). *J. Biol. Chem.* 263:6810–6815. Processing of the native nerve growth factor precursor to form biologically active nerve growth factor.

Egan, D. A., B. A. Flumerfelt, and D. G. Gwyn (1977a). *Acta Neuropathol.* 37:13–19. Axon reaction in the red nucleus of the rat. Perikaryal volume changes and the time course of chromatolysis following cervical and thoracic lesions.

Egan, D. A., B. A. Flumerfelt, and D. G. Gwyn (1977b). *Neuropathol. Appl. Neurobiol.* 3:423–439. A light and electron microscopic study of axon reaction in the red nucleus of the rat following cervical and thoracic lesions.

Egger, M. D. (1989). *Trends Neurosci.* 12:11. The development of confocal microscopy.

Egger, M. D., and L. D. Egger (1982). *Brain Res.* 253:19–30. Quantitative morphological analysis of spinal motoneurons.

Eglmeier, W. (1987). *Anat. Embryol.* 176:493–500. The development of the Merkel cells in the tentacles of *Xenopus laevis* larvae.

Ehrenberg, C. G. (1833). *Annalen der Physik und Chemie (Poggendorf's)* 28:449–465. Nothwendigkeit einer feineren mechanischen Zerlegung des Gehirns und der Nerven vor der chemischen, dargestellt aus Beobachtungen von C. G. Ehrenberg.

Ehrenberg, C. G. (1836). *Beobachtung einer auffallenden bisher unerkannten Struktur des Seelenorgans bei Menschen und Thieren.* Berlin: Königlichen Akademie der Wissenschaften. English trans. in *Edin. Med. Surg. J.* 48:258–304.

Ehrlich, P. (1885). *Sauerstoffbedürfnis des Organismus.* Springer, Berlin.

Ehrlich, P. (1886). *Deutsche Med. Wochnschr.* 12:49–52. Ueber die Methylenblaureaktion der lebenden Nervensubstanz.

Ehrlich, P., R. Krause, M. Mosse, H. Rosin, and C. Weigert (1903). *Encyklopädie der mikroskopischen Technik mit besonder Berücksichtigung der Farbenlehre.* Urban & Schwarzenberg, Berlin.

Eichele, G. (1989). *Trends Genetics* 5:246–251. Retinoids and vertebrate limb pattern formation.

Eichele, G., and C. Thaller (1987). *J. Cell Biol.* 105:1917–1923. Characterization of concentration gradients of a morphogenetically active retinoid in the chick limb bud.

Eichler, V. (1971). *J. Comp. Neurol.* 141:375–396. Neurogenesis in the optic tectum of larval *Rana pipiens* following unilateral enucleation.

Eichorn, D. H., and N. Bayley (1962). *Child Dev.* 33:257–271. Growth in head circumference from birth through young adulthood.

Eisele, L. E., and J. T. Schmidt (1988). *J. Neurobiol.* 19:395–411. Activity sharpens the regenerating retinotectal projection in goldfish: Sensitive period for strobe illumination and lack of effect on synaptogenesis and on ganglion cell receptive field properties.

Eisenfeld, A. J., and J. Axelrod (1965). *J. Pharmacol. Exp. Therap.* 150:469–475. Selectivity of estrogen distribution in tissues.

Eken, T., and K. Gundersen (1988). *J. Physiol. (London)* 402:651–669. Chronic electrical stimulation resembling normal motor-unit activity: Effects on denervated fast and slow rat muscles.

Elam, J. S., and B. W. Agranoff (1971). *J. Neurobiol.* 2:379–390. Transport of proteins and sulfated mucopolysaccharides in the goldfish visual system.

Eldridge, C. F., M. B. Bunge, R. P. Bunge, and P. M. Wood (1987). *J. Cell Biol.* 105:1023–1034. Differentiation of axon-related Schwann cells *in vitro*. I. Ascorbic acid regulates basal lamina assembly and myelin formation.

Eldridge, C. F., M. B. Bunge, and R. P. Bunge (1989). *J. Neurosci.* 9:625–638. Differentiation of axon-related Schwann cells *in vitro*: II. Control of myelin formation by basal lamina.

Elias, H., and D. Schwartz (1971). *Z. Säugetierk* 36:147–163. Cerebrocortical surface areas, volumes, lengths of gyri and their intedependence in mammals, including man.

Elias, H., H. Haus, W. Lange, G. Schlenska, and D. Schwartz (1969). *Anat. Anz.* 63:461–463. Oberflächenmessungen der Grosshirnrinde von Säugern mit besonderer Berücksichtigung des Menschen, der Cetacea, des Elephanten und der Marsupialia.

Ellenberger, C., Jr., J. Hanaway, and M. G. Netsky (1969). *J. Comp. Neurol.* 137:71–88. Embryogenesis of the inferior olivary nucleus in the rat: A radioautographic study and re-evaluation of the rhombic lip.

Ellingson, R. J., and R. C. Wilcott (1960). *J. Neurophysiol.* 23:363–375. Development of evoked responses in visual and auditory cortices of kittens.

Elliott, B. J., and D. G. F. Harriman (1974). *Nature* 251:622–624. Growth of human muscle spindles *in vitro*.

Ellis, H. M., and H. R. Horvitz (1986). *Cell* 44:817–829. Genetic control of programmed cell death in the nematode C. elegans.

Ellis, R. S. (1919). *J. Comp. Neurol.* 30:229–252. A preliminary quantitative study of the Purkinje cells in normal, subnormal and senescent human cerebella.

Ellis, R. S. (1920). *J. Comp. Neurol.* 32:1–33. Norms for some structural changes in the human cerebellum from birth to old age.

Elsasser, W. M. (1989). *Reflections on a Theory of Organisms.* Orbis, Québec.

Elsberg, C. A. (1917). *Science* 45:318–320. Experiments on motor nerve regeneration and the direct neurotization of paralyzed muscles by their own and by foreign nerves.

Emmelin, N., and L. Malmfors (1965). *Quart. J. Exp. Physiol.* 50:142–145. Development of supersensitivity as dependent on the length of degenerating nerve fibers.

Engberg, I., and A. Lundberg (1962). *Experientia* 18:174–177. An electromyographic analysis of stepping in the cat.

Engel, A. K., and G. W. Kreutzberg (1988). *J. Comp. Neurol.* 275:181–200. neuronal surface changes in the dorsal vagal motor nucleus of the guinea pig in response to axotomy.

Engelmann, W. (1863). *Untersuchungen über die Zusammenhang von Nerven- und Muskelfasern.* Leipzig.

Engelmann, W. (1868). *Jenaische Zeitschr f. Med. u. Naturw.* 4:307. Zur Lehre von der Nervenendigung im Muskel.

English, A. W., and O. I. Weeks (1984). *Exp. Brain Res.* 56:361–368. Compartmentalization of single motor units in cat lateral gastrocnemius.

English, K. B., P. R. Burgess, and D. Kavka-van Norman (1980). *J. Comp. Neurol.* 194:475–496. Development of rat Merkel cells.

Epperlein, H. H., and J. Löfberg (1984). *Wilhelm Roux's Arch. Dev. Biol.* 193:357–369. Xanthophores in chromatophore groups of the premigratory neural crest initiate the pigment pattern of the axolotl larva.

Epperlein, H. H., W. Halfter, and R. P. Tucker (1988). *Development* 103:743–756. The distribution of fibronectin and tenascin along migratory pathways of neural crest in the trunk of amphibian embryos.

Eränkö, L., and O. Eränkö (1972). *Acta Physiol. Scand.* 84:125–133. Effect of hydrocortisone on histochemically demonstrable catecholamines in the sympathetic ganglia and extra-adrenal chromaffin tissue of the rat.

Eränkö, O, and S. Soinila (1981). *J. Neurocytol.* 10:1–18. Effect of early postnatal division of the postganglionic nerves on the development of principal cells and small intensely fluorescent cells in the rat superior cervical ganglion.

Eränkö, O., L. Eränkö, C. E. Hill, and G. Burnstock (1972). *Histochem. J.* 4:49–58. Hydrocortisone-induced increase in the number of small intensely fluorescent cells and their histochemically demonstrable catecholamine content in cultures of sympathetic ganglia of the newborn rat.

Eränkö, O, V. M. Pickel, M. Härkönen, L. Eränkö, T. H. Joh, and D. J. Reis (1982). 14:461–478. Effect of hydrocortisone on catecholamines and the enzymes sythesizing them in the developing sympathetic ganglion.

Ericcson, J. L. E. (1969). Mechanism of cellular autophagy, pp. 354–394. In *Lysosomes in Biology and Pathology,* Vol. 2, (J. T. Dingle, and H. B. Fell, eds.), North Holland Publishing Company, Amsterdam.

Erickson, C. A. (1985). *Expl. Biol. Med.* 10:194–208. Control of directional migration of avian and murine neural crest.

Erickson, C. A., and R. Nuccitelli (1982). *J. Cell Biol.* 95:314a. Embryonic cell motility can be guided by weak electric fields.

Erickson, C. A., and J. A. Weston (1983). *J. Embryol. Exp. Morphol.* 74:97–118. A SEM analysis of neural crest migration in the mouse.

Erickson, H. P., and M. A. Bourdon (1989). *Annu. Rev. Cell. Biol.* 5:71–92. Tenascin: an extracellular matrix protein prominent in specialized embryonic tissues and tumors.

Erickson, T. C., and C. N. Woolsey (1951). *Trans. Amer. Neurol. Assoc.* 76:50–52. Observations of the supplementary motor area of man.

Ernsberger, U., M. Sendtner, and H. Rohrer (1989). *Neuron* 2:1275–1284. Proliferation and differentiation of embryonic chick sympathetic neurons: Effects of ciliary neurotrophic factor.

Ernst, M. (1926). *Z. Anat. Entwicklungsgesch.* 79:228–262. Über Untergang von Zellen während der normalen Entwicklung bei Wirbeltieren.

Erzurumlu, R. S., and H. P. Killackey (1983). *J. Comp. Neurol.* 213:365–380. Development of order in the rat trigeminal system.

Erzurumlu, R. S., C. A. Bates, and H. P. Killackey (1980). *Brain Res.* 198:427–433. Differential organization of thalamic projection cells in the brainstem trigeminal complex of the rat.

Escurat, M., M. Gumpel, F. Lachapelle, F. Gros, and M.-M. Portier (1988). *C. R. Acad. Sci. Paris* 306:447–456. Expression comparée de deux protéines de filaments intermédiaires, la périphérine et la protéine de neurofilament 68 kDa, au cours du développement embryonnaire du rat.

Ettensohn, C. A. (1985). *Quart. Rev. Biol.* 60:289–307. Mechanisms of epithelial invagination.

Eurenius, L. (1977). *Anat. Embryol.* 152:89–108. An electron microscope study of the differentiating capillaries of the mouse neurohypophysis.

Euteneuer, U., and J. R. McIntosh (1980). *J. Cell Biol.* 87:509–515. Polarity of midbody and phragmoplast microtubules.

Evans, R. M. (1988). *Science* 240:889–895. The steroid and thyroid hormone receptor superfamily.

Evans, T., E. T. Rosenthal, J. Youngblom, D. Distel, and T. Hunt (1983). *Cell* 33:389–396. Cyclin: A protein specified by maternal mRNA in sea urchin eggs that is destroyed at each cleavage division.

Eveleth, D. D., and R. A. Bradshaw (1988). *Neuron* 1:929–936. Internalization and cycling of nerve growth factor in PC12 cells: interconversion of type II (fast) and type I (slow) nerve growth factor receptors.

Ewald, A. (1876). *Pflüg. Arch.* 12:529–549. Ueber die Endigung der motorische Nerven in den quergestreiften Muskel.

Ewald, A., and W. Kühne (1877). *Verhandl. naturhist.-med. Vereins, Heidelberg* 1:457–464. Uber einen neuen Bestandteil des Nervensystems.

Ewert, J.-P (1980). *Neuroethology.* Springer-Verlag, Berlin.

Exner, S. (1884). *Sitz. Ber. Akad. Wiss. Wien* 89:63–118. Die Innervation des Kehl-kopfes.

Exner, S. (1885). *Pflugers Arch.* 36:572–576. Notiz zu der frage von der faservertheilung mehrerer nerven in einem Muskel.

Eyal-Giladi, H. (1969). *J. Embryol. Exp. Morph.* 21:177–192. Differentiation potencies of the young chick blastoderm as revealed by different manipulations. I. Folding experiments and position effects of the culture medium.

Eyal-Giladi, H. (1984). *Cell Diff.* 14: 245–256. The gradual establishment of cell commitments during early stages of chick development.

Eysel, U. T., L. Peichl, and H. Wässle (1985). *J. Comp. Neurol.* 242:134–145. Dendritic plasticity in the early postnatal feline retina: Quantitative characteristics and sensitive period.

Faber, D. S., and H. Korn (1978). *Neurobiology of the Mauthner Cell.* Raven, New York.

Faber, D. S., and H. Korn (1989). *Physiol. Rev.* 69:821–863. Electrical field effects: Their relevance in central neural networks.

Fadic, R., J. Vergara, and J. Alvarez (1986). *J. Comp. Neurol.* 236:258–264. Microtubules and calibers of central and peripheral processes of sensory axons.

Faissner, A. (1989). *BioEssays* 10:79–81. Cell-cell adhesion in the nervous system—Structural groups emerge.

Faissner, A., J. Kruse, C. Goridis, E. Bock, and M. Schachner (1984a). *EMBO J.* 3:733–737. The neural cell adhesion molecule L1 is distinct from the N-CAM related group of surface antigens BSP-2 and D2.

Faissner, A., J. Kruse, J. Nieke, and M. Schachner (1984b). *Dev. Brain Res.* 15:69–82. Expression of neural cell adhesion molecule L1 during development, in neurological mutants and in the peripheral nervous system.

Faissner, A., D. B. Teplow, D. Kübler, G. Keilhauer, V. Kinzel, and M. Schachner (1985). *EMBO J.* 4:3105–3113. Biosynthesis and membrane topography of the neural cell adhesion molecule L1.

Faivre, C., C. Legrand, and A Rabié (1983). *Dev. Brain Res.* 8:21–30. Effects of thyroid deficiency and corrective effects of thyroxine on microtubules and mitochondria in cerebellar Purkinje cell dendrites of developing rats.

Falconer, D. S. (1951). *J. Genet.* 50:192–201. Two new mutations, trembler and reeler with neurological action in the house mouse.

Fallon, J. F., and J. W. Saunders, Jr. (1968). *Dev. Biol.* 18:553–570. *In vitro* analysis of the control of cell death in a zone of prospective necrosis from the chick wing bud.

Fallon, J. F., and B. K. Simandl (1978). *Am. J. Anat.* 152:111–130. Evidence of a role for cell death in the disappearance of the embryonic human tail.

Fallon, J. H., and R. Y. Moore (1978). *J. Comp. Neurol.* 180:545–580. Catecholamine innervation of the basal forebrain. IV. Topography of the dopamine projection to the basal forebrain and neostriatum.

Fallon, J. H., D. A. Koziell, and R. Y. Moore (1978). *J. Comp. Neurol.* 180:509–532. Catecholamine innervation of the basal forebrain. II. Amygdala, suprarhinal cortex and entorhinal cortex.

Fallon, J. R., R. M. Nitkin, N. E. Resit, B. G. Wallace, and U. J. McMahan (1985). *Nature* 315:571–574. Acetylcholine receptor-aggregating factor is similar to molecules concentrated at neuromuscular junctions.

Falzi, G., P. Perrone, and L. A. Vignolo (1982). *Arch. Neurol.* 39:239–240. Right-left asymmetry in the anterior speech region.

Fambrough, D. M. (1970). *Science* 168:372. Acetylcholine sensitivity of muscle fiber membranes: Mechanism of regulation by motoneurons.

Fambrough, D. M. (1974a). *J. Gen. Physiol.* 64:468–472. Revised estimates of extrajunctional receptor density in denervated rat diaphragm.

Fambrough, D. M. (1974b). Cullular and developmental biology of acetylcholine receptors in skeletal muscle, pp. 85–113. In *Neurochemistry of Cholinergic Receptors* (E. de Roberts, and J. Schact, eds.), Raven Press, New York.

Fambrough, D. M. (1979). *Physiol. Rev.* 59:165–227. Control of acetylcholine receptors in skeletal muscle.

Fambrough, D. M. (1983). *Met. Enzym.* 96:331–352. Biosynthesis and intracellular transport of acetylcholine receptors.

Fambrough, D. M., and J. E. Rash (1971). *Dev. Biol.* 26:55–68. Development of acetycholine sensitivity during myogenesis.

Fambrough, D. M., D. B. Drachman, and S. Satyamurti (1973). *Science* 182:293–295. Neuromuscular junction in myasthenia gravis: Decreased acetylcholine receptors.

Fangboner, R. F., and J. W. Vanable (1974). *J. Comp. Neurol.* 157:391–406. Formation and regression of inappropriate nerve sprouts during trochlear nerve regeneration in *Xenopus laevis*.

Fankhauser, G. (1941). *J. Morphol.* 68:161–177. Cell size, organ and body size in triploid newts *(Triturus viridescens)*.

Fankhauser, G. (1945a). *J. Exp. Zool.* 100:445–455. Maintenance of normal structure in heteroploid salamander larvae, through compensation of changes in cell size by adjustment of cell number and cell shape.

Fankhauser, G. (1945b). *Quart. Rev. Biol.* 20:20–78. The effects of changes in chromosome number on amphibian development.

Fankhauser, G., J. A. Vernon, W. H. Frank, and W. V. Slack (1955). *Science* 122:692–693. Effect of size and number of brain cells on learning in larvae of the salamander, *Triturus viridescens*.

Farbman, A. I. (1965). *Dev. Biol.* 11:110–135. Electron microscope study of the developing taste bud in rat fungiform papilla.

Farbman, A. I. (1971). Development of the taste bud, pp. 50–62. In *Handbook of Sensory Physiology*, Vol. 4, Part 2 *Chemical Senses: Taste* (L. M. Beidler, ed.), Springer Verlag, Heidelberg.

Farbman, A. I. (1972). *J. Cell. Biol.* 52:489–493. Differentiation of taste buds in organ culture.

Farbman, A. I. (1980). *Cell Tissue Kinet.* 13:349–357. Renewal of taste bud cells in rat circumvallate papillae.

Farbman, A. I., and M. Ziegner (1968). *Anat. Rec.* 160:347. Differentiation of fetal rat tongue grafts in the anterior chamber of the eye.

Farel, P. B. (1989). *J. Neurosci.* 9:2103–2113. Naturally occurring cell death and differentiation of developing spinal motoneurons following axotomy.

Farel, P. B., and S. E. Bemelmans (1985). *J. Comp. Neurol.* 238:128–134. Specificity of motoneuron projection patterns during development of the bullfrog tadpole *(Rana catesbiana)*.

Farel, P. B., and S. E. Bemelmans (1986). *J. Comp. Neurol.* 254:125–132. Restoration of neuromuscular specificity following ventral rhizotomy in the bullfrog tadpole, *Rana catesbeiana*.

Farquhar, M. G., and J. F. Hartmann (1957). *J. Neuropath. Exp. Neurol.* 16:18–39. Neuroglial structure and relationships as revealed by electron microscopy.

Fass, B., and O. Steward (1983). *Neuroscience* 9:653–664. Increases in protein-precursor incorporation in the denervated neuropil of the dentate gyrus during reinnervation.

Fatt, P. (1954). *Physiol. Rev.* 34:674–710. Biophysics of junctional transmission.

Fatt, P., and B. Katz (1951). *J. Physiol. (London)* 117:109–128. Spontaneous subthreshold activity at motor nerve endings.

Faúndez, V., and J. Alvarez (1986). *J. Comp. Neurol.* 250:73–80. Microtubules and caliber in developing axons.

Fautrez, J. (1942). *Acad. Roy. Belg. Bull. Classe Sci.* 28:391–403. La signification de la partie céphalique du bourrelet de la plaque médullaire chez les Urodéles. Localisation des ébauches présomptives des microplacodes des nerfs crâniens it de la crête ganglionnaire de la tête au stade neurula.

Fawcett, J. W., and W. M. Cowan (1985). *Dev. Brain Res.* 17:149–163. On the formation of eye dominance stripes and patches in the doubly innervated optic tectum of the chick.

Fawcett, J. W., and R. M. Gaze (1982). *J. Embryol. Exp. Morphol.* 72:19–37. The retinotectal fibre pathways from normal and compound eyes in *Xenopus*.

Fawcett, J. W., and D. D. M. O'Leary (1985). *Trends Neurosci.* 8:201–206. The role of electrical activity in the formation of topographic maps in the nervous system.

Fawcett, J. W., and D. J. Willshaw (1982). *Nature* 296:350–352. Compound eyes project stripes on the optic tectum in *Xenopus*.

Fawcett, J. W., D. D. M. O'Leary, and W. M. Cowan (1984). *Proc. Natl. Acad. Sci. U.S.A.* 81:5589–5593. Activity and the control of ganglion cell death in the rat retina.

Fearing, F. (1930). *Reflex Action: A Study in the History of Physiological Psychology.* Williams and Wilkins, Baltimore.

Feder, H. H. (1984). *Ann. Rev. Psychol.* 35:165–200. Hormones and sexual behavior.

Fedoroff, S. (1983). The development of glial cells in primary cultures, pp. 83–92. In *Dynamic Properties of Glial Cells* (G. Franck, L. Hertz, E. Schoffeniels, and D. B. Towers, eds.), Pergamon, Oxford.

Fedoroff, S. (1985). Macroglial cell lineages, pp. 91–117. In *Molecules Bases of Neural Development* (G. M. Edelman, W. E. Gall, and W. M. Cowan, eds.), Neuroscience Res. Found., New York.

Fedoroff, S. (1986). Prenatal ontogenesis of astrocytes, pp. 35–67. In *Cellular Neurobiology: A Series. Astrocytes, Development, Morphology and Regional Specialization of Astrocytes,* Vol 1 (S. Fedoroff, and A. Vernadakis, eds.), Academic Press, Orlando.

Feeney, J. F., and R. L. Watterson (1946). *J. Morphol.* 78:231–303. The development of the vascular pattern within the walls of the central nervous system of the chick embryo.

Feinberg, A. A., M. F. Utset, L. D. Bogarad, C. P. hart, A. Awgulewitsch, A. Ferguson-Smith, A. Fainsod, M. Rabin, and F. H. Ruddle (1987). *Curr. Top. Dev. Biol.* 23:233–256. Homeobox genes in murine development.

Feit, H., G. R. Dutton, S. H. Barondes, and M. L. Shelanski (1971). *J. Cell Biol.* 51:138–147. Microtubule protein. Identification in and transport to nerve endings.

Feldberg, W., and J. H. Gaddum (1934). *J. Physiol. (London)* 81:305–319. The chemical transmitter at synapses in a sympathetic ganglion.

Feldman, J. D., and R. M. Gaze (1972). *J. Embryol. Exp. Morphol.* 27:381–387. The growth of the retina in *Xenopus Laevis*. II. An autoradiographic study.

Feldman, J. D., and R. M. Gaze (1975). *J. Embryol. Exp. Morphol.* 33:775–787. The development of the retinotectal projection in *Xenopus* with one compound eye.

Feldman, J. D., R. M. Gaze, and M. J. Keating (1983). *Dev. Brain Res.* 6:269–277. Development of the orientation of the visuo-tectal map in *Xenopus*.

Feldman, M. L. (1984). Morphology of the neocortical pyramical neuron, pp. 123–200. In *the Cerebral Cortex,* Vol. 1, (A. Peters, and E. G. Jones, eds.), Plenum Press, New York.

Feldman, M. L., and J. M. Harrison (1969). *J. Comp. Neurol.* 137:267–294. The projection of the acoustic nerve to the ventral cochlear nucleus of the rat. A Golgi study.

Feldman, M. L., and A. Peters (1973). *Anat. Rec.* 175:318–319. The significance of barrels in the cerebral cortex.

Fellous, A., A. M. Lennon, J. Francon, and J. Nunez (1979). *Eur. J. Biochem.* 101:365–376. Thyroid hormone and neurotubule assembly *in vitro* during brain development.

Felten, D. L., H. Hallman, and G. Jonsson (1982). *J. Neurocytol.* 11:119–135. Evidence for a neurotrophic role of noradrenaline neurons in the postnatal development of rat cerebral cortex.

Feremutsch, K. (1952). *Bibliotheca Psychiat. Neurol. Suppl.* 91:33–73. Die Morphogenese des Paleocortex und des Archicortex.

Feremutsch, K. (1960). *Z. Anat. Entwicklungsgeschichte* 122:155–172. Die cytoarchitektonische Hetermorphie.

Ferguson, R. K., and D. M. Woodbury (1969). *Exp. Brain Res.* 7:181–194. Penetration of ^{14}C-inulin and ^{14}C-sucrose into brain, cerebrospinal fluid, and skeletal muscle of developing rat.

Ferguson, T. (1966). *Gen. Comp. Endocrinol.* 7:74–79. Thyroxine effects upon the mitotic activity of the medulla oblongata after unilateral excision in embryos of the frog.

Fernández-Morán, H. (1950a). *Exp. Cell Res.* 1:143–149. Electron microscope observations on the structure of the myelinated nerve fiber sheath.

Fernández-Morán, H. (1950b). *Exp. Cell Res.* 1:309–340. Sheath and axon structures in the internode portion of vertebrate myelinated nerve fibers, an electron microscope study of rat and frog sciatic nerves.

Fernández-Morán, H. (1952). *Exp. Cell Res.* 3:282–350. The submicroscopic organization of vertebrate nerve fibres. An electron microscope study of vertebrate nerve fibres. An electron microscopic study of myelinated and unmyelinated nerve fibres.

Fernández-Morán, H., and J. B. Finean (1957). *J. Biophys. Biochem. Cytol.* 3:725–748. Electron microscope and low-angle X-ray diffraction studies of the nerve myelin sheath.

Fernandez, H. L., F. C. Huneeus, and P. F. Davison (1970). *J. Neurobiol.* 1:395–409. Studies on the mechanism of axoplasmic transport in the crayfish cord.

Fernandez, H. L., P. R. Burton, and F. E. Samson (1971). *J. Cell Biol.* 53:258–263. Axoplasmic transport in the crayfish nerve cord.

Fernandez, V. (1969). *J. Comp. Neurol.* 136:423–452. An autoradiographic study of the development of the anterior thalamic group and limbic cortex in the rabbit.

Fernandez, V., and H. Bravo (1974). *Brain Behav. Evol.* 9:317–332. Autoradiographic study of development of the cerebral cortex in the rabbit.

Fernando, D. A. (1971). *Brain Res.* 27:365–368. A third glial cell seen in retrograde degeneration of the hypoglossal nerve.

Ferrara, N., F. Ousley, and D. Gospodarowicz (1988). *Brain Res.* 462:223–232. Bovine brain astrocytes express basic fibroblast growth factor, a neurotropic and angiogenic mitogen.

Ferrer, I., and J. Sarmiento (1980). *Acta Neuropathol.* 50:61–67. Nascent microglia in the developing brain.

Ferrier, D. (1875). *Proc. Roy. Soc. (London) Ser. B.* 23:409–430. Experiments in the brain of monkeys.

Ferrier, D. (1876). *The Function of the Brain.* Smith, Elder and Co., London.

Ferrier, D. (1886). *The Function of the Brain,* 2nd edition. Smith and Elder, London.

Ferrier, D. (1890). *The Croonian Lectures on Cerebral Localisation.* Smith and Elder, London.

Fertuck, H. C., and M. M. Salpeter (1976). *J. Cell. Biol.* 69:144–158. Quantitation of junctional and extrajunctional acetylcholine receptors by electron microscopy autoradiography after 125 I-alpha-bungarotoxin binding at mouse neuromuscular junctions.

Fetchko, J. R. (1987). *Brain Res. Rev.* 12:243–280. A review of the organization and evolution of motoneurons innervating the axial musculature of vertebrates.

Feulgen, R., and H. Rossenbeck (1924). *Hoppe Seylers Z. Physiol. Chem.* 135:203–248. Mikroskopisch-chemischer Nachweis einer Nucleinsäure vom Typus der Thymonucleinsäure und die darauf beruhrende elektive Färbung von Zellkernen in mikroskopischen Präperaten.

Fex, S., and S. Thesleff (1967). *Life Sci.* 6:635–639. The time required for innervation of denervated muscles by nerve implants.

Fex, S., B. Sonesson, S. Thesleff, and J. Zelená (1966). *J. Physiol. (London)* 184:872–882. Nerve implants in botulinum poisoned mammalian muscle.

Feyerabend, P. K. (1965, 1970). Problems of empiricism. In *Univ. Pittsburgh Series in Philosophy of Science,* Vols. 2, 4, (R. G. Colodny, ed.), Prentice-Hall, Englewood Cliffs, New Jersey.

Feyerabend, P. K. (1970). *Falsification and the Methodology of Scientific Research Programmes* (I. Lakatos, and A. Musgrave, eds.), Cambridge Univ. Press, Cambridge. Reprinted in Feyerabend, 1981, Vol. 2, pp. 131–161.

Feyerabend, P. K. (1981). *Philosophical papers. Vol. 1. Realism Rationalism and Scientific Method, Vol. 2. Problems of Empiricism.* Cambridge Univ. Press, Cambridge.

Feynman, R. P., R. B. Leighton, and M. Sands (1964). *The Feynman Lectures in Physics,* Vol. 2, p. 12, Addison-Wesley, Reading, Mass.

ffrench-Constant, C. and M. C. Raff (1986). *Nature* 323:335–338. The oligodendrocyte-type-2 astrocyte cell lineage is specialized for myelination.

ffrench-Constant, C., R. H. Miller, J. Kruse, M. Schachner, M. C. Raff (1986). *J. Cell Biol.* 102:844–852. Molecular specialization of astrocyte processes at nodes of Ranvier in rat optic nerve.

Field, E. J., D. Hughes, and C. S. Raine (1968a). *J. Neurol. Sci.* 8:49–60. Electron microscopic observations on the development of myelin in cultures of neonatal rat cerebellum.

Field, E. J., C. S. Raine, and D. Hughes (1968b). *J. Neurol. Sci.* 8:129–141. Failure to induce myelin sheath formation around artificial fibers with a note on the toxicity of polyester fibers for nervous tissue *in vitro.*

Fifková, E. (1972). *Exp. Neurol.* 35:458–469. Effect of visual deprivation on the retina.

Fifková, E. (1973). *Experientia* 29:851–854. Effect of light on the synaptic organization of the inner plexiform layer of the retina in albino rats.

Fifková, E. (1974). Plastic and degenerative changes in visual centers, pp. 59–131. In *Advances in Psychobiology* (G. Newton, and A. H. Riesen, eds.), Wiley, New York.

Fifková, E. (1985a). *Brain Res. Rev.* 9:187–215. Actin in the nervous system.

Fifková, E. (1985b). *Cell Mol. Neurobiol.* 5:47–63. A possible mechanism of morphometric changes in dendritic spines induced by stimulation.

Fifková, E., and C. L. Anderson (1981). *Exp. Neurol.* 74:621–627. Stimulation-induced changes in dimension of stalks of dendritic spines in the dentate molecular layer.

Fifková, E., C. A. Anderson, S. J. Young, and A. Van Harreveld (1982). *J. Neurocytol.* 11:183–210. Effect of anisomycin on stimulation-induced changes in dendritic spines of the dentate granule cells.

Figlewicz, D. A., F. Gremo, and G. M. Innocenti (1988). *Dev. Brain Res.* 42:181–189. Differential expression of neurofilament subunits in the developing corpus callosum.

Filogamo, G. (1950). *Riv. Biol. Coloniale (Rome)* 42:73–79. Conseguenze della demolizione dell'abbozzo dell' occhio sullo sviluppo del lobo ottico nell' embrione di pollo.

Filogamo, G. (1960). *Arch. Biol. (Liege)* 71:159–198. Recherches expérimentales sur l'activité des cholinestérases spécifique el non spécifique dans le développment du lobe optique du poulet.

Filogamo, G., and G. Gabella (1976). *Arch. Biol. Liège* 78:9–60. The development of neuromuscular correlations in vertebrates.

Fine, R. E., and D. Bray (1971). *Nature (New Biol.)* 234:115–118. Actin in growing nerve cell.

Finger, S., B. Walbran, and D. G. Stein (1973). *Brain Res.* 63:1–18. Brain damage and behavioral recovery: Serial lesion phenomena.

Fink, R. P., and L. Heimer (1967). *Brain Res.* 4:369–374. Two methods for selective silver impregnation of degenerating axons and their synaptic endings in the central nervous system.

Finkelstein, S. P., P. J. Apostolides, C. G. Caday, J. Prosser, M. F. Philips, and M. Klagsbrun (1988). *Brain Res.* 460:253–259. Increased basic fibroblast growth factor (bFGF) immunoreactivity at the site of local brain wounds.

Finlay, B. L., and M. Slattery (1983). *Science* 219:1349–1351. Local differences in the amount of early cell death in neocortex predict adult local specializations.

Finlay, B. L., K. G. Wilson, and G. E. Schneider (1979). *J. Comp. Neurol.* 183:721–740. Anomalous ipsilateral retinotectal projections in Syrian hamsters with early lesions: Topography and functional capacity.

Finlay, B. L., A. T. Berg, and D. R. Sengelaub (1982). *J. Comp. Neurol.* 204:318–324. Cell death in the mammalian visual system during normal development. II. Superior colliculus.

Finlay, B. L., D. R. Sengelaub, and R. P. Dolan (1984). *Neurosci. Abstr.* 9:135. Cell generation and death in the hamster retina: Changes in the spatial distribution of cells from the late postnatal period to adulthood.

Finne, J., U. Finne, H. Deagostini-Bazin, and C. Goridis (1983). *Biochem. Biophys. Res. Commun.* 112:482–487. Occurrence of alpha–2–8 linked polysialosyl units in a neural cell adhesion molecule.

Fish, H. S., D. D. Malone, and C. P. Richter (1944). *Anat. Rec.* 89:429–440. The anatomy of the tongue of the domestic Norway rat. I. The skin of the tongue, the various papillae, their number and distribution.

Fischbach, G. D. (1972). *Dev. Biol.* 28:407–429. Synapse formation between dissociated nerve and muscle cells in low density cell cultures.

Fischbach, G. D., and N. Robbins (1969). *J. Physiol. (London)* 201:305–320. Changes in contractile properties of disused soleus muscles.

Fischer, C. A., and P. Morell (1974). *Brain Res.* 74:51–65. Turnover of proteins in myelin and myelin-like material of mouse brain.

Fischer, G., V. Künemund, and M. Schachner (1986). *J. Neurosci.* 6:605–612. Neurite outgrowth patterns in cerebellar microexplant cultures are affected by antibodies to the cell surface glycoprotein L1.

Fischer, K. (1967). *Acta Neuropath.* 8:242–252. Subependymale Zellproliferation und Tumordisposition brachycephaler Hunderassen.

Fish, I., and M. Winick (1969). *Exp. Neurol.* 25:534–540. Effect of malnutrition on regional growth of the developing rat brain.

Fisher, L. J. (1972). *Nature* 235:391–393. Changes during maturation and metamorphosis in the synaptic organization of the tadpole retina inner plexiform layer.

Fisher, M. (1984). *Proc. Natl. Acad. Sci. U.S.A.* 81:4414–4418. Neuronal influence on glial enzyme expression: Evidence from mutant mouse cerebella.

Fisher, M., and R. J. Mullen (1988). *Neuron* 1:151–157. Neuronal influence on glial enzyme expression: Evidence from chimeric mouse cerebellum.

Fisher, M., D. A. Gapp, and L. P. Kozak (1981). *Dev. Brain Res.* 1:341–354. Immunohistochemical localization of *sn*-glycerol–3-phosphate dehydrogenase in Bergmann glia and oligodendroglia in the mouse cerebellum.

Fisher, S., and M. Jacobson (1970). *Z. Zellforsch. Mikroskop. Anat.* 104:165–177. Ultrastructural changes during early development of retinal ganglion cells in *Xenopus*.

Fisher, M., and M. Solursh (1979). *J. Embryol. Exp. Morph.* 49:295–306. The influence of local environments on the organization of mesenchyme cells.

Fisher, M. M., M. C. Killcross, M. Simonsson, and K. A. Elgie (1978). *Trans. R. Soc. Trop. Med. Hyg.* 66:471–478. Malnutrition and reasoning ability in Zambian school-children.

Fishman, M. A., A. L. Prensky, and P. R. Dodge (1969). *Nature* 221:552–553. Low content of cerebral lipids in infants suffering from malnutrition.

Fite, K. V. (1969). *Exp. Neurol.* 24:475–486. Single-unit analysis of binocular neurons in the frog optic tectum.

Fitzgerald, M. J. T. (1961). *J. Anat. (London)* 95:495–514. Developmental changes in epidermal innervation.

Fitzgerald, M. J. T. (1962). *J. Anat. (London)* 96:189–208. On the structure and life history of bulbous corpuscles (corpuscula nervorum terminalia bulboidea).

Fitzpatrick, D., J. S. Lund, and G. G. Blasdel (1985), *J. Neurosci.* 5:3329–3349. Intrinsic connections of Macaque striate cortex: Afferent and efferent connections of layer 4C.

Flamm, J. (1968). *Z. Anat. Entwicklungsgeschichte* 127:359–366. Über die Beziehung zwischen der Dicke motorischer Nervenfasern und der Grösse der Endplatter.

Flanagan, A. E. H. (1969). *J. Morphol.* 129:281–306. Differentiation and degeneration in the motor horn of the foetal mouse.

Flechsig, P. (1876). *Die Leitungsbahnen im Gehirn und Ruckenmark des Menschen auf Grund entwicklungsgeschichtlicher Untersuchungen.* Engelmann, Leipsig.

Flechsig, P. (1901). *Arch. Ital. Biol.* 36:30–39. Ueber die entwickelungsgeschichtliche (myelogenetische) Flächengliederung der Grosshirnrinde des Menschen.

Flechsig, P. (1920). *Anatomie des menschlichen Gehirns und Rückenmarks auf myelogenetischer Grundlage.* G. Thieme, Leipzig.

Flechsig, P. (1927). *Meine myelogenetische Hirnlehre. Mit biographischer Einleitung.* Springer, Berlin.

Fleischhauer, K., K. Zilles, and A. Schleicher (1980). *Anat. Embryol.* 161:121–143. A revised cytoarchitectonic map of the neocortex of the rabbit (*Oryctolagus cuniculus*).

Flood, D. G., and P. D. Coleman (1988). *Neurobiol. Aging* 9:453–463. Neuron numbers and sizes in aging brain: Comparisons of human, monkey, and rodent data.

Florkin, M. (1960). *Naissance et Déviation de la Théorie Cellulaire dans l'Oeuvre de Théodore Schwann.* Hermann, Paris.

Flourens, P. (1824). *Researches Expérimentales sur les Propriétés et les Fonctions du Systeme Nerveux dans les Animaux Vertébrés,* 2nd edi., Balliere, Paris.

Foelix, R. F., and R. Oppenheim (1974). *J. Neurocytol.* 3:277–294. The development of synapses in the cerebellar cortex of the chick embryo.

Foerster, O, O. Gagel, and D. Sheehan (1933). *Z. Anat. EntwGesch.* 101:553–565. Veränderungen an den Endösen im Rückenmark des Affen nach Hinterwurzeldurchschneidung.

Folkman, J. (1982). *Ann. N.Y. Acad. Sci.* 401:212–227. Angiogenesis: Initiation and control.

Folkman, J. (1985). *Adv. Cancer Res.* 43:175–203. Tumor angiogenesis.

Fontaine, B., A. Klarsfeld, T. Hökfelt, and J. P. Changeux (1986a). *J. Cell Biol.* 105:1337–1342. Calcitonin gene-related peptide and muscle activity regulate acetylcholine receptor alpha-subunit mRNA levels by distinct intracellular pathways.

Fontaine, B., A. Klarsfeld, T. Hökfelt, and J. P. Changeux (1986b). *Neurosci. Lett.* 71:59–65. Calcitonin gene-related peptide, a peptide present in spinal cord motoneurons, increases the number of acetylcholine receptors in primary cultures of chick embryo myotubes.

Fontaine, B., D. Sassoon, M. Buckingham, and J. P. Changeux (1988). *EMBO J.* 7:603–609. Detection of the nicotinic acetylcholine receptor α-subunit mRNA by in situ hybridization at neuromuscular junctions of 15-day old chick striated muscles.

Fontaine-Perus, J., M. Chanconie, and N. M. Le Douarin (1988). *Dev. Biol.* 128:359–375. Developmental potentialities in the nonneuronal population of quail sensory ganglia.

Ford, E. B. (1945). *Biol. Rev.* 20:73–88. Polymorphism.

Forel, A. (1887). *Arch. f. Psychiat. u. Nervenkr.* 18:162–198. Einige hirnanatomische Betrachtungen und Ergebnisse.

Forer, A. (1988). *J. Cell Sci.* 91:449–453. Do anaphase chromosomes chew their way to the pole or are they pulled by actin?

Forman, D. S., B. S. McEwen, and B. Grafstein (1971). *Brain Res.* 28:119–130. Rapid transport of radioactivity in goldfish optic nerve following injections of labeled glucosamine.

Forman, D. S. A. L. Padjen, and G. R. Siggins (1977). *Brain Res.* 136:197–213. Axonal transport of organelles visualized by light microscopy: Cinematographic and computer analysis.

Forssman, J. (1898). (*Ziegler's*) *Beitr. Pathol. Anat. Allgem. Pathol.* 24:56–100. Ueber die Ursachen, welche die Wachstumsrichtung der peripheren Nervenfasern bei der Regeneration bestimmen.

Forssman, J. (1900). (*Ziegler's*) *Beitr. Pathol. Anat. Allgem. Pathol.* 27:407–430. Zur Kenntnis des Neurotropismus.

Forströnen, P. F. (1963). *Acta Neurol. Scand.* 39:314–316. The origin and the morphogenetic significance of the external granular layer of the cerebellum as determined experimentally in chick embryos.

Foster, G. A., D. Dahl, and V. M.-Y. Lee (1987). *J. Neurosci.* 7:2651–2663. Temporal and topographic relationships between the phosphorylated and nonphosphorylated epitopes of the 200 kDa neurofilament protein during development *in vitro*.

Foster, M. assisted by C. S. Sherrington (1897). *A Text-Book of Physiology*, 7th edition, Part III. *The Central Nervous System*. London.

Foster, M. (1899). *Claude Bernard*, T. Fisher Unwin, London.

Foster, M. (1901). *Lectures on the History of Physiology*, Cambridge University Press, Cambridge.

Fouvet, P. B. (1973). *Arch. Anat. Microsc. Morphol. Exp.* 62:269–280. Innervation et morphogenèse de la patte chez l'embryon de poulet. I. Mise en place de l'innervation normale.

Fowler, I., and B. F. Sisken (1982). *J. Exp. Zool.* 221:49–59. Effect of augmentation of nerve supply upon limb regeneration in the chick embryo.

Fowler, J. A. (1970). *Quart. Rev. Biol.* 45:148–167. Control of vertebral number in teleosts—an embryological problem.

Fox, C. A., D. E. Hillman, K. A. Siegesmund, and C. R. Dutta (1967). *Prog. Brain Res.* 25:174–225. The primate cerebellar cortex: A Golgi and electron microscope study.

Fox, G. O., G. D. Pappas, and D. P. Purpura (1976). *Brain Res.* 101:411–425. Fine structure of growth cones in medullary raphe nuclei in the postnatal cat.

Fox, G. Q., G. D. Pappas, and D. P. Purpura (1976). *Brain Res.* 101:411–425. Fine structure of growth cones in medullary raphe nuclei in the postnatal cat.

Fox, H. (1970). *J. Embryol. Exp. Morph.* 24:139–157. Tissue degeneration: An electron microscopic study of the pronephros of *Rana temporaria*.

Fox, H. (1973). *J. Embryol. Exp. Morphol.* 30:377–396. Degeneration of the nerve cord in the tail of *Rana temporaria* during metamorphic climax: Study by electron microscopy.

Fox, H., and J. M. Moulton (1968). *Arch. Anat. Microscop. Morphol. Exp.* 57:107–120. Mauthner cells and the thyroid hormonal level in *larvae* of *Rana temporaria*.

Fox, J. H., and W. Wilczynski (1986). *Brain Behav. Evol.* 28:157–169. Allometry of major CNS divisions: Towards a reevaluation of somatic brain-body scaling.

Fox, J. H., M. A. Fishman, P. R. Dodge, and A. L. Prensky (1972). *Neurology* 22:1213–1216. The effect of malnutrition on human central nervous system myelin.

Fox, M. W., O. R. Inman, and W. A. Himwich (1966). *J. Comp. Neurol.* 127:199–206. The postnatal development of neocortical neurons in the dog.

Fox, M. W., O. Inman, and S. Glisson (1968). *Dev. Psychobiol.* 1:48–54. Age differences in central nervous effects of visual deprivation in the dog.

Fraher, J. P., G. F. Kaar, D. C. Bristol, and J. P. Rossiter (1988). *Prog. Neurobiol.* 31:199–239. Development of ventral spinal motoneurone fibres: A correlative study of the growth and maturation of central and peripheral segments of large and small fibre classes.

Francis-Williams, J., and P. A. Davies (1974). *Dev. Med. Child Neurol.* 16:709–728. Very low birthweight and later intelligence.

Franck, J. I. (1980). *Brain Res.* 186:458–462. Functional reor-

ganization of cat somatic sensory-motor cortex (SmI) after selective dorsal root rhizotomies.

Francon, J., A. Fellous, A. M. Lennon, and J. Nunez (1977). *Nature* 266:188–190. Is thyroxine a regulatory signal for neurotubule assembly during brain development?

Francon, J., A. M. Lennon, A. Fellous, A. Mareck, M. Pierre, and J. Nunez (1982). *Eur. J. Biochem.* 129:465–472. Heterogeneity of microtubule-associated proteins and brain development.

Frank, B. D., and J. G. Hollyfield (1987). *J. Comp. Neurol.* 266:435–444. Retina of the tadpole and frog: Delayed dendritic development in a subpopulation of ganglion cells coincident with metamorphosis.

Frank, E., and G. D. Fishbach (1979). *J. Cell Biol.* 83:143–158. Early events in neuromuscular junction formation *in vitro*: Induction of acetylcholine receptor clusters in the postsynaptic membrane and morphology of newly formed synapses.

Frank, E., and P. C. Jackson (1986). *Brain Res.* 378:147–151. Normal electrical activity is not required for the formation of specific sensory-motor synapses.

Frank, E., and J. K. S. Jansen (1976). *J. Neurophysiol.* 39:84–90. Interaction between foreign and original nerves innervating gill muscles in fish.

Frank, E., and M. Westerfield (1982). *J. Physiol. (London)* 324:495–505. The formation of appropriate central and peripheral connections by foreign sensory neurons of the bullfrog.

Frank, E., and M. Westerfield (1983). *J. Physiol. (London)* 343:593–610. Development of sensory-motor synapses in the spinal cord of the frog.

Frank, E., J. K. S. Jansen, T. Lomo, and R. Westgaard (1974). *Nature* 247:375–376. Maintained function of foreign synapses on hyperinnervated skeletal muscle fibres of the rat.

Frank, E., J. K. S. Jansen, T. Lomo, and R. H. Westgaard (1975). *J. Physiol. (London)* 247:725–743. The interaction between foreign and original motor nerves innervating the soleus muscle of rats.

Frank, E., K. Gautvik, and H. Sommerchild (1976). *Cold Spring Harbor Symp. Quant. Biol.* 40:275–281. Persistance of junctional acetylcholine receptors following denervation.

Frank, J. I. (1980). *Brain Res.* 186:458–462. Functional reorganization of cat somatic sensory-motor cortex (SMI) after selective dorsal root rhizotomies.

Franková, S. (1973). *Activitas Nerv. Sup.* 15:207–216. Interaction among the familiarity with the environment, avoidance learning and behaviour of early malnourished rats.

Franková, S. (1982). *Biblthca Nutr. Dieta* 31:40–54. Lasting effects of early malnutrition on children's behaviour.

Franková, S., and R. H. Barnes (1968). *J. Nutr.* 96:485–493. Effect of malnutrition in early life on avoidance conditioning and behavior of adult rat.

Franková, S., and R. Zemanová (1978). *Activitas nerv. sup.* 20:113–114. Development and long-term characteristics of habituation to novel environment in malnourished rats.

Franson, P., and C. Hildebrand (1975). *Neurobiol.* 5:8–22. Postnatal growth of nerve fibres in the pyramidal tract of the rabbit.

Franz, J. and J. Klienebrecht (1982). *Teratology* 26:195–202. Teratogenic and clastogen effects of BrdUrd in mice.

Franz, S. I. (1923). *Psychol. Rev.* 30:438–446. Conceptions of cerebral functions.

Fraser, S. E. (1983). *Dev. Biol.* 95:505–511. Fiber optic mapping of the *Xenopus* visual system: Shift in the retinotectal projection during development.

Fraser, S. E., and R. K. Hunt (1980). *Ann. Rev. Neurosci.* 3:319–352. Retinotectal specificity: Models and experiments in search of a mapping function.

Fraser, S. E., B. A. Murray, C. M. Chuong, and G. M. Edelman (1984). *Proc. Natl. Acad. Sci. U.S.A.* 81:4222–4226. Alteration of the retinotectal map in *Xenopus* by antibodies to neural cell adhesion molecules.

Fraser, S. E., C. R. Green, H. R. Bode, and N. B. Gilula (1987). *Science* 237:49–55. Selective disruption of gap junctional communication interferes with a patterning process in hydra.

Fraser, S. E., R. J. Keynes, and A. Lumsden (1990). *Nature* 344:431–435. Segmentation in the chick embryo hindbrain is defined by cell lineage restrictions.

Frazier, L. L., and P. C. Brunjes (1988). *J. Comp. Neurol.* 269:355–370. Unilateral odor deprivation: Early postnatal changes in olfactory bulb cell density and number.

Frazier, W. A., R. A. Angeletti, and R. A. Bradshaw (1972). *Science* 176:482–488. Nerve growth factor and insulin.

Frazier, W. A., L. F. Boyd, and R. A. Bradshaw (1973a). *Proc. Natl. Acad. Sci. U.S.A.* 70:2931–2935. Interaction of nerve growth factor with surface membranes: Biological competence of insolubilized nerve growth factor.

Frazier, W. A., C. E. Ohlendorf, L. F. Boyd, L. Aloe, E. M. Johnson, J. A. Ferrendelli, and R. A. Bradshaw (1973b). *Proc. Natl. Acad. Sci. U.S.A.* 70:2448–2452. Mechanism of action of nerve growth factor and cyclic AMP on neurite outgrowth in embryonic chick sensory ganglia: Demonstration of independent pathways of stimulation.

Fredens, K. (1981). *Anat. Embryol.* 161:265–281. Genetic variation in the histoarchitecture of the hippocampal region of mice.

Freeman, J. A., and J. Stone (1969). A technique for current density analysis of field potentials and its application to the frog cerebellum, pp. 421–430. In *Neurobiology of Cerebellar Evolution and Development* (R. R. Llinás, ed.), American Medical Association, Chicago.

Freeman, J. A., P. B. Manis, G. J. Snipes, B. N. Mayes, P. C. Samson, J. P. Wikswo, Jr., and D. B. Freeman (1985). *J. Neurosci. Res.* 13:257–283. Steady growth cone currents revealed by a novel circularly vibrating probe: A possible mechanism underlying neurite growth.

Freeman, R. D., and L. N. Thibos (1973). *Science* 180:876–878. Electrophysiological evidence that abnormal early visual experience can modify the human brain.

Freeman, R. D., D. E. Mitchell, and M. Millodot (1972). *Science* 175:1384–1386. A neural effect of partial visual deprivation in humans.

Freeman, S. S., A. G. Engel, and D. B. Drachman (1976) *Ann. N.Y. Acad. Sci.* 274:46–59. Experimental acetylcholine blockade of the neuromuscular junction. Effects on endplate and muscle fiber ultrastructure.

Fregnac, Y., and M. Imbert (1978). *J. Physiol. (London)* 278:27–44. Early development of visual cortical cells in normal and dark-reared kittens: Relationship between orientation selectivity and ocular dominance.

French, V. (1990). *Seminars Dev. Biol.* 1:9–100. The development of segments in the invertebrates.

Friauf, E., S. K. McConnell, and C. J. Shatz (1990). *J. Neurosci.* 10:2601–2613. Functional synaptic circuits in the subplate during fetal and early postnatal development of cat visual cortex.

Frick, H., and H. J. Nord (1963). *Anat. Anz.* 113:307–316. Domestikation und Hirngewicht.

Fried, K., C. Hildebrand, and G. Erdélyi (1982). *J. Neurolog. Sci.* 54:47–57. Myelin sheath thickness and internodal length of nerve fibres in the developing feline inferior alveolar nerve.

Friede, R. L. (1954). *Acta Anat.* 20:290–296. Der quantitative Anteil der Glia an der Cortexentwicklung.

Friede, R. L. (1961). *J. Neurochem.* 8:17–30. A histochemical study of DPN-diaphorase in human white matter, with some notes on myelination.

Friede, R. L. (1963). *Proc. Natl. Acad. Sci. U.S.A.* 49:187–193. The relationship of body size, nerve cell size, axon length and glial density in the cerebellum.

Friede, R. L. (1966). *Topographic Brain Chemistry*. Academic Press, New York.

Friede, R. L. (1972). *J. Comp. Neurol.* 144:233–252. Control of myelin formation by axon caliber (with a model of the control mechanism).

Friede, R. L. (1973a). *Z. Neurol.* 204:243–254. Principles of quantitative organization of peripheral nerve fibers and their relation to growth and pathologic changes.

Friede, R. L. (1973b). *Prog. Brain Res.* 40:425–436. Mechanics of myelin sheath expansion.

Friede, R. L., and R. Bischhausen (1982). *Brain Res.* 235:335–350. How are sheath dimensions affected by axon caliber and internodal length?

Friede, R. L., and K.-C. Ho (1977). *J. Physiol. (London)* 265:507–519. The relation of axonal transport of mitochondria with microtubules and other axoplasmic organelles.

Friede, R. L., and T. Samorajski (1968). *J. Neuropath. Exp. Neurol.* 27:546–570. Myelin formation in the sciatic nerve of the rat. A quantitative electron microscopic, histochemical and radioautographic study.

Friede, R. L., and T. Samorajski (1970). *Anat. Rec.* 167:379–388. Axon caliber related to neurofilaments and microtubules in sciatic nerve fibers of rats and mice.

Friede, R. L., and W. H. van Houten (1962). *Proc. Natl. Acad. Sci. U.S.A.* 48:817–821. Neuron extension and glial supply: Functional significance of glia.

Friede, R. L., T. Meier, and M. Diem (1981). *J. Neurolog. Sci.* 50:217–228. How is the exact length of an internode determined?

Friede, R. L., J. Brzoska, and U. Hartmann (1985). *J. Anat. (London)* 143:103–113. Changes in myelin sheath thickness and internode geometry in the rabbit phrenic nerve during growth.

Friedlander, M. J., K. A. C. Martin, and C. Vahle-Hinz (1985). *J. Physiol. (London)* 359:293–313. The structure of the terminal arborizations of physiologically identified retinal ganglion cell y axons in the kitten.

Friedrich, V. L., Jr. (1975). *Anat. Embryol.* 147:259–271. Hyperplasia of oligodendrocytes in quaking mice.

Frisch, R. E. (1971). *Psychiatr. Neurol. Neurochir.* 74:463–479. Does malnutrition cause permanent mental retardation in human beings?

Fritsch, G., and E. Hitzig (1870). *Arch. Anat. Physiol. Wiss. Med.* 37:300–332. Ueber die electrische Erregbarkeit des Grosshirns.

Fritz, A. F., K. W. Y. Cho, C. V. E. Wright, B. G. Jegalian, and E. M. De Robertis (1989). *Dev. Biol.* 131:584–588. Duplicated homeobox genes in *Xenopus*.

Froesch, E. R., C. Schmid, J. Schwander, and J. Zapf (1985). *Ann. Rev. Physiol.* 47:443–467.

Frost, D. O. (1981). *J. Comp. Neurol.* 203:227–256. Orderly anomalous retinal projections to the medial geniculate, ventrobusal, and lateral posterior nuclei of the hamster.

Frost, D. O. (1982). *Dev. Brain Res.* 3:627–635. Anomalous visual connections to somatosensory and auditory systems following brain lesions in early life.

Frost, D. O. (1984). *J. Comp. Neurol.* 230:576–592. Axonal growth and target selection during development: Retinal projections to the ventrobasal complex and other 'nonvisual' structures in neonatal Syrian hamster.

Frost, D. O., and C. Metin (1985). *Nature* 317:162–164. Induction of functional retinal projections to the somatosensory system.

Frost, D. O., and G. E. Schneider (1976). *Brain Res.* 142:223–235. Normal and abnormal uncrossed retinal projections to the superior colliculus in the golden hamster.

Frost, D. O., K.-F. So, and G. E. Schneider (1979). *Neuroscience* 4:1649–1677. Postnatal development of retinal projections in Syrian hamster: A study using autoradiographic and anterograde degeneration techniques.

Frost, D. O., V. S. Caviness, and G. M. Sachs (1982). *Soc. Neurosci. Abst.* 8:821. Fiber abnormalities of thalamus and midbrain in reeler mutant mice.

Fry, F. J., and W. M. Cowan (1972). *J. Comp. Neurol.* 144:1–24. A study of retrograde cell degeneration in the lateral mamillary nucleus of the cat, with special reference to the role of axonal branching in the preservation of the cell.

Fuchs, E., and I. Hanukoglu (1983). *Cell* 34:332–334. Unraveling the structure of the intermediate filaments.

Fujisawa, H. (1971). *Dev. Growth Diff.* 13:25–36. A complete reconstruction of the neural retina of chick embryo grafted onto the chorio-allantoic membrane.

Fujisawa, H. (1981). *Brain Res.* 206:27–37. Retinotopic analysis of fiber pathways in the regenerating retinotectal system of the adult newt *Cynops pyrrhogaster*.

Fujisawa, H. (1984). *Dev. Growth Differ.* 26:545–553. Pathways of retinotectal projection in developing *Xenopus* tadpoles revelaed by selective labeling of retinal axons with horseradish peroxidase (HRP).

Fujisawa, H. (1987). *J. Comp. Neurol.* 260:127–139. Mode of growth of retinal axons within the tectum of *Xenopus* tadpoles, and implications in the ordered neuronal connections between the retina and the tectum.

Fujisawa, H., and M. Jacobson (1980). *Brain Res.* 194:431–441. Transsynaptic labelling of neurons in the optic tectum of *Xenopus* after intraocular 3H-proline injection.

Fujisawa, H., H. Nakamura, and M. Chin (1974). *J. Embryol. Exp. Morphol.* 31:139–149. The fine structure of the reconstructed neural retina of chick embryos.

Fujisawa, H., H. Morioka, K. Watanabe, and H. Nakamura (1976). *J. Cell Sci.* 22:585–596. A decay of gap junctions in association with cell differentiation of neural retina in chick embryonic development.

Fujisawa, H., K. Watanabe, N. Tani, and Y. Ibata (1981a).

Brain Res. 206:9–20. Retinotopic analysis of fiber pathways in amphibians. I. The adult newt, *Cynops pynogaster*.

Fujisawa, H., N. Tani, K. Watanabe, and Y. Ibata (1981b). *Brain Res.* 206:21–26. Retinotopic analysis of fiber pathways in amphibians. II. The frog *Rana nigromaculata*.

Fujisawa, H., N. Tani, K. Watanabe, and Y. Ibata (1982). *Dev. Biol.* 90:43–57. Branching of regenerating retinal axons and preferential selection of appropriate branches for specific neuronal connection in the newt.

Fujita, H., and S. Fujita (1963). *Z. Zellforsch. Mikroskop. Anat.* 60:463–478. Electron microscopic studies on neuroblast differentiation in the central nervous system of domestic fowl.

Fujita, S. (1962). *Exp. Cell Res.* 28:52–60. Kinetics of cell proliferation.

Fujita, S. (1963). *J. Comp. Neurol.* 120:37–42. The matrix cell and cytogenesis in the developing central nervous system.

Fujita, S. (1964). *J. Comp. Neurol.* 122:311–328. Analysis of neuron differentiation in the central nervous system by tritiated thymidine autoradiography.

Fujita, S. (1965a). *Laval Med.* 36:125–130. The matrix cell and histogenesis of the nervous system.

Fujita, S. (1965b). *J. Comp. Neurol.* 124:51–60. An autoradiographic study on the origin and fate of the subpial glioblasts in the embryonic chick spinal cord.

Fujita, S. (1966). Application of light and electron microscopic autoradiography to the study of cytogenesis of the forebrain, pp. 180–196. In *Evolution of the Forebrain* (R. Hassler and H. Stephan, eds.), Plenum Press, New York.

Fujita, S. (1967). *J. Cell Biol.* 32:277–287. Quantitative analysis of cell proliferation and differentiation in the cortex of the postnatal mouse cerebellum.

Fujita. S. (1974). *J. Comp. Neurol.* 155:195–202. DNA constancy in neurons of the human cerebellum and spinal cord as revealed by Feulgen cytophotometry.

Fujita, S., and M. Horii (1963). *Arch. Histol. (Japan)* 23:359–366. Analysis of cytogenesis in chick retina by tritiated thymidine autoradiography.

Fujita, S., and T. Kitamura (1975). *Acta Neuropath. Suppl.* 6:291–296. Origin of Brain macrophages and the nature of the so-called microglia.

Fujita, S., M. Shimada, and T. Nakamura (1966). *J. Comp. Neurol.* 128:191–208. 3H-Thymidine autoradiographic studies on the cell proliferation and differentiation in the external and internal granular layers of the mouse cerebellum.

Fujita, S., S. Yoshida, and M. Fukuda (1971). *Acta Histochem. Cytochem.* 4:126–136. Improvement of technique to minimize non-specific absorption in microspectrophotometric measurement of nuclear DNA.

Fujita, S., M. Fukuda, T. Kitamura, and S. Yoshida (1972). *Acta Histochem. Cytochem.* 5:146–152. Two-wave-length-scanning method in Feulgen cytophotometry.

Fujita, S., T. Hattori, M. Fukuda, and T. Kitamura (1974). *Develop. Growth Differentiation* 16:205–211. DNA contents in Purkinje cells and inner granule neurons in the developing rat cerebellum.

Fujita, S., Y. Tsuchihashi, and T. Kitamura (1981). *Prog. Clin. Biol. Res.* 59:141–169. Origin, morphology and function of microglia. In *Glial and Neuronal Cell Biology*, S. Fedoroff, ed.

Fukuda, Y., and J. Stone (1974). *J. Neurophysiol.* 37:749–772. Retinal distribution and central projections of Y-, X-, and W-cells of the cat's retina.

Fulton, B. P., and K. Walton (1986). *J. Physiol. (London)* 370:651–678. Electrophysiological properties of neonatal rat motoneurones studied *in vitro*.

Fulton, B. P., R. Miledi, and T. Takahashi (1980). *Proc. Roy. Soc. (London) B.* 208:115–120. Electrical synapses between motoneurones in the spinal cord of the new born rat.

Fulton, J. F. (1926). *Muscular Contraction and the Reflex Control of Movement.* Wilkins, Baltimore.

Fulton, J. F. (1935). *Brain* 58:311–316. A note on the definition of 'motor' and 'premotor' areas.

Fulton, J. F. (1943). *Physiology of the Nervous System.* 2nd Edition, Revised and Reset. Oxford Univ. Press, London.

Fulton, J. F. (1959). Historical reflections on the backgrounds of neurophysiology, pp. 67–80. In *The Historical Development of Physiological Thought* (C. M. C. Brooks, and P. F. Cranefield, eds.), Hafner, New York.

Fulton, J. F., and A. D. Keller (1932). *The Sign of Babinski. A Study of the Evolution of Cortical Dominance In Primates.* Thomas, Springfield, Illinois.

Fulton, J. F., and M. A. Kennard (1934). *Res. Publ. Assoc. Nerv. Ment. Dis.* 13:158–210. A study of flaccid and spastic paralysis produced by lesions of the cerebral cortex.

Funder, J. W., and K. Sheppard (1987). *Ann. Rev. Physiol.* 49:397–411. Adrenocortical steroids and the brain.

Furbringer, M. (1896). *Festschrift fur Gegenbaur* 3:541–580. Ueber die spino-occipitalen Nerven der Selachier und Holocephalen und Ihre vergleichende Morphologie.

Furcht, L. T. (1986). *Lab. Invest.* 55:505–509. Critical factors controlling angiogenesis: Cell products, cell matrix, and growth factors. Editorial.

Furmanski, P., D. L. Silverman, and M. Lubin (1971). *Nature (New Biol.)* 233:413–415. Expression of differentiated functions in mouse neuroblastoma mediated by dibutyrylcyclic monophosphate.

Furshpan, E. J., and D. D. Potter (1957). *Nature* 180:342–343. Mechanism of nerve-impulse transmission at a crayfish synapse.

Furshpan, E. J., and D. D. Potter (1959). *J. Physiol. (London)* 145:289–325. Transmission at the giant motor synapses of the crayfish.

Furth, M. E., T. H. Aldrich, and C. Gordon-Carols (1987). *Oncogene* 1:47–58. Expression of *ras* proto-oncogene protein in normal human tissues.

Furthmayr, H. (1988a). Assembly of basement membrane macromolecules, pp. 43–59 In *Self-Assembling Architecture.* Alan R. Liss, New York.

Furthmayr, H. (1988b). Basement membrane, pp. 525–558. In *The Cellular and Molecular Basis of Wound Healing* (R. A. F. Clark, and P. M. Henson, eds.), Plenum Press, New York.

Furukawa, T. (1966). Synaptic interaction at the mauthner cell of goldfish, pp. 44–70. In *Progress In Brain Research* (T. Tokizane, and J. P. Schadé, eds.), Amsterdam, Elsevier.

Fuxe, K., B. Hamberger, and T. Hökfelt (1968). *Brain Res.* 8:125–131. Distribution of nerve terminals in the cortical areas of the rat.

Gabbott, P. L., and J. Somogyi (1984). *J. Neurosci. Methods* 11:221–230. The 'single' section Golgi-impregnation procedure: Methodological description.

Gabella, G. (1969). *J. Neurol. Sci.* 9:237–242. Taste buds and adrenergic fibres.

Gabella, G. (1981). *Neuroscience* 6:425–436. Ultrastructure of the nerve plexuses of the mammalian intestine: The enteric glial cells.

Gadamer, H.-G. (1975). *Truth and Method,* (G. Barden, and J. Cumming, eds.), Seabury Press, New York.

Gadamer, H.-G. (1976). *Philosophical Hermeneutics.* Univ. California Press.

Gadamer, H.-G. (1982). *Reason in the Age of Science.* F. G. Lawrence, transl. M.I.T. Press, Cambridge, Mass.

Gadamer, H.-G. (1989). *Truth and Method,* 2nd English edn., Translated from the 5th German edition by J. Weinsheimer and D. G. Marshall. Crossroads, New York.

Gadamer, H.-G., E. K. Specht, and W. Stegmüller (1988). *Hermeneutics Versus Science? Three German Views.* J. M. Connolly and T. Keutner, transl. and ed. Univ. Notre Dame Press, Notre Dame, Indiana.

Gadow, H. F. (1933). *The Evolution of the Vertebral Column. A Contribution to the Study of Vertebrate Phylogeny.* (J. F. Gaskell, and H. L. H. H. Green, eds.), Cambridge Univ. Press.

Gage, F. H., K. Wictorin, W. Fischer, L. R. Williams, S. Varon, and A. Bjorklund (1986). *Neuroscience* 19:241–256. Life and death of cholinergic neurons: In the septal and diagonal band region following complete fimbria fornix transection.

Gahwiler, B. H., and F. Hefti (1984). *Neuroscience* 13:681–689. Guidance of acetylcholinesterase-containing fibres by target tissue in co-cultured brain slices.

Gahwiler, B. H., A. Enz, and F. Hefti (1987). *Neurosci. Lett.* 75:6–10. Nerve growth factor promotes development of the rat septo-hippocampal cholinergic projection *in vitro*.

Gainer, H. (1978). *Trends Neurosci.* 1:93–96. Intercellular transfer of proteins from glial cells to axons.

Gajdusek, C., P. DiCortelo, R. Ross, and S. M. Schwartz (1980). *J. Cell Biol.* 85:467–472. An endothelial cell-derived growth factor.

Galaburda, A. M. (1980). *Revue Neurologique* 136:609–616. La région de Broca. Observations anatomiques faites un siecle apres de la mort de son découvreur.

Galaburda, A. M., and G. F. Sherman (1982). *Anat. Rec.* 202:60A. The cytoarchitectonic organization of the isocortex of the albino rat.

Galaburda, A. M., M. Lemay, T. L. Kemper, and N. Geschwind (1978). *Science* 199:852–856. Right-left asymmetries in the brain.

Galileo, D. S., G. E. Gray, G. C. Owens, J. Majors, and J. R. Sanes (1990). *Proc. Natl. Acad. Sci. U.S.A.* 87:458–462. Neurons and glia arise from a common progenitor in chicken optic tectum: Demonstration with two retroviruses and cell type-specific antibodies.

Gall, F. J. (1825). *Organologie ou exposition des instincts, des penchans, des sentimens et des talens, ou des qualités morales et des facultés intellectuelles fondamentales de l'homme et des animaux, et du siége de leurs organes,* J. B. Bailliere, Paris.

Gall, F. J., and J. C. Spurzheim (1835). *On the functions of the Brain and of Each of Its Parts: With Observations on the Possibility of Determining the Instincts, Propensities, and Talents, or the Moral and Intellectual Dispositions of Men and Animals, by the Configuration of the Brain and Head,* 6 vols., March, Capen and Lyon, Boston.

Gallera, J. (1967). *Experientia* 23:461. L'induction neurogene chez les oiseaux passage du flux inducteur par le filtre millipore.

Gallera, J., G. Nicolei, and M. Baumann (1968). *J. Embryol. Exp. Morph.* 19:439–450. Induction neurale chez les oiseaux à travers un filtre millipore: Étude au microscope optique et électronique.

Gallin, W. J., G. M. Edelman, and B. A. Cunningham (1983). *Proc. Natl. Acad. Sci. U.S.A.* 80:1038–1042. Characterization of L-CAM, a major cell adhesion molecule from embryonic liver cells.

Gallin, W. J., E. A. Prediger, G. M. Edelman, and B. A. Cunningham (1985). *Proc. Natl. Acad. Sci. U.S.A.* 82: 2809–2813. Isolation of a cDNA clone for the liver cell adhesion molecule (L-CAM).

Gallin, W. J., B. C. Sorkin, G. M. Edelman, and B. A. Cunningham (1987). *Proc. Natl. Acad. Sci. U.S.A.* 84:2808–2812. Sequence analysis of a cDNA clone encoding the liver cell adhesion molecule, L-CAM.

Gamble, E., and C. Koch (1987). *Science* 236:1311–1315. The dynamics of free calcium in dendritic spines in response to repetitive synaptic input.

Gamble, H. J. (1975). *J. Anat. (London)* 118:360. Preliminary observations on the vascularization of the embryonic human brain.

Ganchrow, D., and J. J. Bernstein (1981). *J. Neurosci. Res.* 6:525–537. Bouton renewal patterns in rat hindlimb cortex after thoracic dorsal funicular lesions.

Gans, C., and R. G. Northcutt (1983). *Science* 220:268–274. Neural crest and the origin of vertebrates: A new head.

Garber, B. B., and A. A. Moscona (1972a). *Dev. Biol.* 27:217–234. Reconstruction of brain tissue from cell suspensions. I. Aggregation patterns of cells dissociated from different regions of the developing brain.

Garber, B. B., and A. A. Moscona (1972b). *Dev. Biol.* 27:235–243. Reconstruction of brain tissue from cell suspensions. II. Specific enhancement of aggregation of embryonic cerebral cells by supernatant from homologous cell cultures.

Garcia-Bellido, A. (1975). Genetic control of wing disc development in *Drosophila*, pp. 161–178. In *Cell Patterning*, Ciba Foundation Symposium 29, Elsevier, New York.

Garcia-Bellido, A. (1985). *Phil. Trans. Roy. Soc. (London) Ser. B.* 312:101–128 Cell lineages and genes.

Garcia-Bellido, A., and J. R. Merriam (1969). *J. Exp. Zool.* 170:61–76. Cell lineage of the imaginal disk in *Drosophila* gynandromorphs.

Garcia-Bellido, A., P. Ripoll, and G. Morata (1973). *Nature (New Biol.)* 245:251–253. Developmental compartmentalisation of the wing disk of *Drosophila*.

Garcia-Porrero, J. A., E. Colvée, and J. L. Ojeda (1984). *J. Embryol. Exp. Morphol.* 80:241–249. Cell death in the dorsal part of the optic cup. Evidence for a new necrotic area.

Gard, A. L., and S. E. Pfeiffer (1989). *Development* 106:119–132. Oligodendrocyte progenitors isolated directly from developing telencephalon at a specific phenotypic stage: Myelinogenic potential in a defined environment.

Gardette, R., F. Crepel, R. M. Alvarado-Mallart, and C. Sotelo (1990). *J. Comp. Neurol.* 295:188–196. Fate of grafted embryonic Purkinje cells in the cerebellum of the adult "Purkinje cell degeneration" mutant mouse. II. Development of synaptic responses: An *in vitro* study.

Garey, L. J., and J. D. Pettigrew (1974). *Brain Res.* 66:165–172. Ultrastructural changes in kitten visual cortex after environmental modification.

Garner, C. C., and A. Matus (1988). *J. Cell Biol.* 106:779–783. Different forms of microtubule-associated protein 2 are encoded by separate mRNA transcripts.

Garner, C. C., A. Matus, B. Anderton, and R. Calvert (1989). *Mol. Brain Res.* 5:85–92. Microtubule-associated proteins MAP5 and MAP1x: Closely related components of the neuronal cytoskeleton with different cytoplasmic distributions in the developing brain.

Garland, D., and D. Teller (1973). *J. Cell Biol.* 59:107a. Mechanism of colchicine binding.

Garner, J., and R. J. Lasek (1981). *J. Cell Biol.* 88:172–178. Clathrin is axonally transported as part of slow component b: The microfilament complex.

Garner, J., and R. J. Lasek (1982). *J. Neurosci.* 2:1824–1835. Cohesive axonal transport of the slow component b complex of polypeptides.

Garraghty, P. E., and M. Sur (1988). Interactions between retinal axons during development of their terminal arbors in the cat's lateral geniculate nucleus, pp. 465–477. In *Cellular Thalamic Mechanisms* (M. Bentovoglio, and R. Spreafico, eds.), Elsevier, Amsterdam.

Garraghty, P. E., M. Sur, and S. M. Sherman (1986a). *J. Comp. Neurol.* 251:216–239. Role of competitive interactions in the postnatal development of X and Y retinogeniculate axons.

Garraghty, P. E., M. Sur, R. E. Weller, and S. M. Sherman (1986b). *J. Comp. Neurol.* 251:198–215. Morphology of retinogeniculate X and Y axon arbors in monocularly enucleated cats.

Garraghty, P. E., D. O. Frost, and M. Sur (1987). *Exp. Brain Res.* 66:115–127. The morphology of retinogeniculate X- and Y-cell axonal arbors in dark-reared cats.

Garraghty, P. E., A. W. Roe, Y. M. Chino, and M. Sur (1989). *J. Comp. Neurol.* 289:202–212. Effects of convergent strabismus on the development of physiologically identified retinogeniculate axons in cats.

Garson, J. A., P. C. L. Beverley, H. B. Coakham, and E. I. Harper (1982). *Nature* 298:375–377. Monoclonal antibodies against human T lymphocytes label Purkinje neurons of many species.

Gaskell, W. H. (1885). *J. Physiol. (London)* 7:1–56. On the structure, distribution, and function of the nerves which innervate the visceral and vascular systems.

Gaskell, W. H. (1889). *J. Physiol. (London)* 10:153–211. On the relation between the structure, function and origin of the cranial nerves, together with a theory on the origin of the nervous system of vertebrata.

Gaskell, W. H. (1908). *The Origin of Vertebrates*, Longmans, Green, London.

Gasser, H. S. (1958). Comparison of the structure, as revealed with the electron microscope, and the physiology of the unmedullated fibers in the skin nerves and in the olfactory nerves, pp. 3–17. In *The Submicroscopic Organization and Function of Nerve Cells* (H. Fernandez-Moran, ed.), Academic Press, New York.

Gasser, U. E., and M. E. Hatten (1990). *J. Neurosci.* 10:1276–1285. Neuron-glia interactions of rat hippocampal cells *in vitro*: Glial-guided neuronal migration and neuronal regulation of glial differentiation.

Gasser, U. E., G. Weskamp, U. Otten, and A. R. Dravid

(1986). *Brain Res.* **376**:351–356. Time course of the elevation of nerve growth factor (NGF) content in the hippocampus and septum following lesions of the septohippocampal pathway in rats.

Gaunt, S. J. (1988). *Development* **103**:135–144. Mouse homeobox gene transcripts occupy different but overlapping domains in embryonic germ layers and organs: A comparison of *Hox-3.1* and *Hox-1.5.*

Gaunt, S. J., P. T. Sharpe, and D. Duboule (1988). *Development* **104**:Suppl. 169–179. Spatially restricted domains of homeogene transcripts in mouse embryos: Relation to a segmented body plan.

Gause, G. (1932). *Quart. Rev. Biol.* **7**:27–46. Ecology of populations.

Gause, G. (1934). *The Struggle for Existence.* Williams and Wilkins, Baltimore (Reprinted, 1971, Dover Publ., New York).

Gautier, J., C. Norbury, M. Lohka, P. Nurse, and J. Maller (1988). *Cell* **54**:433–439. Purified maturation-promoting factor contains the product of a Xenopus homolog of the fission yeast cell cycle control gene cdc^{2+}.

Gaze, R. M. (1959). *Quart. J. Exp. Physiol.* **44**:209–308. Regeneration of the optic nerve in *Xenopus laevis.*

Gaze, R. M. (1960). *Int. Rev. Neurobiol.* **2**:1–40. Regeneration of the optic nerve in Amphibia.

Gaze, R. M. (1970). *Formation of Nerve Connections*, Academic Press, New York.

Gaze, R. M., and R. Hope (1983). *J. Physiol. (London)* **344**:257–275. The visuotectal projection following translocation of grafts within an optic tectum in the goldfish.

Gaze, R. M., and M. Jacobson (1959). *J. Physiol.* **148**:45–46. The response of the frog's optic lobe to stimulation of the eye to light, after section and regeneration of the optic nerve.

Gaze, R. M., and M. Jacobson (1962a). *Quart. J. Exp. Physiol.* **47**:273–280. The projection of the binocular visual field on the optic tecta of the frog.

Gaze, R. M., and M. Jacobson (1962b). *J. Physiol.* **163**:39–40P. Anomalous retino-tectal projection in frogs with regenerated optic nerves.

Gaze, R. M., and M. Jacobson (1963a). *J. Physiol. (London)* **165**:73–74. The path from the retina to the ipsilateral optic tectum of the frog.

Gaze, R. M., and M. Jacobson (1963b). *Proc. Roy. Soc. (London) Ser. B.* **157**:420–448. A study of the retino-tectal projection during regeneration of the optic nerve in the frog.

Gaze, R. M., and M. Jacobson (1963c). *J. Physiol. (London)* **169**:1–3. 'Convexity detectors' in the frog's visual system.

Gaze, R. M., and M. Jacobson (1963d). *J. Physiol. (London)* **169**:92–93. Types of single-unit responses from different depths in the optic tectum of the goldfish.

Gaze, R. M., and M. J. Keating (1969). *J. Physiol. (London)* **200**:128–129. The depth distribution of visual units in the tectum of the frog following regeneration of the optic nerve.

Gaze, R. M., and M. J. Keating (1972). *Nature* **237**:375–378. The visual system and "neuronal specificity"

Gaze, R. M., and A. Peters (1961). *Quart. J. Exp. Physiol.* **46**:299–309. The development, structure and composition of the optic nerve of *Xenopus laevis* (Daudin).

Gaze, R. M., and S. C. Sharma (1970). *Exp. Brain Res.* **10**:171–181. Axial differences in the reinnervation of the goldfish optic tectum by regenerating optic nerve fibres.

Gaze, R.M., and C. Straznicky (1980). *J. Embryol. Exp. Morphol.* **60**:125–140. Regenation of optic nerve fibres from a compound eye to both tecta in *Xenopus:* evidence relating to the state of specification of the eye and the tectum.

Gaze, R. M., M. Jacobson, and G. Székely (1963). *J. Physiol. (London)* **165**:484–499. The retinotectal projection in *Xenopus* with compound eyes.

Gaze, R. M., M. Jacobson, and G. Székely (1965). *J. Physiol. (London)* **176**:409–417. On the formation of connections by compound eyes in *Xenopus.*

Gaze, R. M., M. J. Keating, and K. Straznicky (1970a) *J. Physiol. (London)* **207**:51. The re-establishment of retinotectal projections after uncrossing the optic chiasma in *Xenopus laevis* with one compound eye.

Gaze, R. M., M. J. Keating, G. Székely, and L. Beazley (1970b). *Proc. Roy. Soc. (London) Ser. B.* **175**:107–147. Binocular interaction in the formation of specific intertectal neuronal connexions.

Gaze, R. M., S. H. Chung, and M. J. Keating (1972). *Nature (New Biol.)* **236**:133–135. Development of the retinotectal projection in *Xenopus.*

Gaze, R. M., M. J. Keating, and S. H. Chung (1974). *Proc. Roy. Soc. (London) Ser. B.* **185**:301–330. The evolution of the retinotectal map during development in *Xenopus.*

Gaze, R. M., M. J. Keating, A. Ostberg, and S.-H. Chung (1979). *J. Embryol. Exp. Morphol.* **53**:103–143. The relationship between retinal and tectal growth in larval *Xenopus.* Implications for the development of the retinotectal projection.

Gebhardt, D. O. E., and P. D. Nieuwkoop (1963). *J. Embryol. Exp. Morphol.* **12**:317–331. The influence of lithium on the competence of the ectoderm in *Ambystoma mexicanum.*

Geel, S., and P. S. Timiras (1967). *Brain Res.* **4**:135–142. The influence of neonatal hypothyroidism and of thyroxine on the ribonucleic acid and deoxyribonucleic acid concentrations of rat cerebral cortex.

Geel, S. E., and P. S. Timiras (1970). *Brain Res.* **22**:63–72. Influence of growth hormone on cerebral cortical RNA metabolism in immature hypothyroid rats.

Geffen, L. B. (1969). *J. Neurochem.* **16**:469–474. Is there bidirectional transport of noradrenaline in sympathetic nerves?

Gegenbaur, C. (1898). *Vergleichende Anatomie der Wirbelthiere mit Berucksichtigung der Wirbellosen*, 2 Vols. Wilhelm Engelmann, Leipzig.

Gehring, W. J., ed. (1978). *Genetics Mosaics and Cell Differentiation*, Spring-Verlag, New York.

Gehring, W. J. (1985). *Cell* **40**:3–5. The homeobox: A key to the understanding of development.

Gehring, W. J. (1987). *Science* **236**:1245–1252. Homeoboxes in the study of development.

Geiger, B. (1983). *Biochim. Biophys. Acta* **737**:305–341. Membrane-cytoskeleton interaction.

Geiger, B., Z. Avnur, T. E. Kreis and J. Schlessinger (1984). The dynamics of cytoskeletal organization in areas of cell contact, pp. 195–234. In *Cell and Muscle Motility*, Vol. 5, (J. W. Shay, ed.), Plenum, New York.

Geinitz, B. (1925). *Roux' Arch. EntwMech.* **106**:357–408. Embryonale Transplantation zwischen Urodelen und Anuren.

Geist, F. D. (1933). *Arch. Neurol. Psychiat.* 29:88–103. Chromatolysis of efferent neurons.

Gemund, J. J. van, and L. de Angulo (1971). The effects of early hypothyroidism on I.Q., school performance, and electroencephalogram pattern in children, pp. 299–313. In *Normal and Abnormal Development of Brain and Behaviour* (G. B. A. Stoelinga, and J. J. van der Werff ten Bosch, eds.), Leiden University Press.

Gentschev, T., and C. Sotelo (1973). *Brain Res.* 62:37–60. Degenerative patterns in the ventral cochlear nucleus of the rat after primary deafferentation. An ultrastructural study.

George, S. A., and W. B. Marks (1974). *Exp. Neurol.* 42:467–482. Optic nerve terminal arborizations in the frog: Shape and orientation inferred from electrophysiological measurements.

Gerard, R. W. (1932). *Physiol. Rev.* 12:469–592. Nerve metabolism.

Geraudie, J., and M. Singer (1977). *Exp. Neurol.* 57:1012–1025. Morphologic effects of denervation on the taste buds of the catfish barbel.

Gerding, R., N. Robbins, and J. Antosiak (1977). *Dev. Biol.* 61:177–183. Efficiency of reinnervation of neonatal rat muscle by original and foreign nerves.

Geren, B. B. (1954). *Exp. Cell Res.* 7:558–562. The formation from the Schwann cell surface of myelin in the peripheral nerves of chick embryos.

Geren, B. B., and J. Raskind (1953). *Proc. Natl. Acad. Sci. U.S.A.* 39:880–884. Development of the fine structure of the myelin sheath in sciatic nerves of chick embryos.

Geren, B. B., and F. O. Schmitt (1954). *Proc. Natl. Acad. Sci. U.S.A.* 40:863–870. The structure of the Schwann cell and its relation to the axon in certain invertebrate nerve fibers.

Gerhardt, J. D. and B. Mintz (1972). *Dev. Biol.* 29:27–37. Clonal origins of the somites and their muscle derivatives: Evidence from allophenic mice.

Gerhart, J. C. (1980). Mechanisms regulating pattern formation in the amphibian egg and early embryo, pp. 133–316. In *Biological Regulation and Development* Vol. 2. *Molecular Organization and Cell Function,* (R. F. Goldberger, ed.), Plenum Press, New York.

Gerisch, G. (1977). *Curr. Top. Dev. Biol.* 14:243–270. Univalent antibody fragments as tools for the analysis of cell interactions in *Dictyostelium.*

Gerisch, G., D. Hulser, D. Malchow, and U. Wick (1975). *Phil. Trans. Roy. Soc. (London) Ser. B.* 272:181–192. Cell communication by periodic cyclic-AMP pulses.

Gerlach, J. (1854). *Handbuch der allgemeinen und speciellen Gewebelehre des menschlichen Körpers,* 2nd edi., Mainz.

Gerlach, J. (1858). *Mikroskopische Studien aus dem Gebiete der menschlichen Morphologie.* Enke, Erlangen.

Gerlach, J. (1872a). Von dem Rückenmark, pp. 665–693. In *Stricker's Handbuch der Lehre von den Geweben,* Vol. 2. Engelmann, Leipzig. English transl. in Stricker, S. (1872). *Manual of Human and Comparative Histology,* Vol. 2. New Sydenham Society, London.

Gerlach, J. L., and B. S. McEwen (1972). *Science* 175:1133–1136. Rat brain binds adrenal steroid hormone: Radioautography of hippocampus with corticosterone.

Gershon, M. D. (1981). *Ann. Rev. Neurosci.* 4:227–272. The enteric nervous system.

Gershon, M. D., M. L. Epstein, and L. Hegstrand (1980).

Dev. Biol. 77:41–51. Colonization of the chick gut by progenitors of enteric serotonergic neurons: Distribution, differentiation, and maturation within the gut.

Gershon, M. D., T. P. Rothman, T. H. Joh, and G. N. Teitelman (1984). *J. Neurosci.* 4:2269–2280. Transient and differential expression of aspects of the catecholaminergic phenotype during development of the fetal bowel of rats and mice.

Geschwind, N. (1970). *Science* 170:940–944. The organization of language and the brain.

Geschwind, N. (1972). *Sci. Am.* 236:6–83. Language and the brain.

Geschwind, N., and W. Levitsky (1968). *Science* 161:186–187. Human brain: Left-right asymmetries in temporal speech region.

Ghandour, M. S., O. K. Langley, G. Vincendon, G. Gombos, D. Filippi, N. Limozin, C. Dalmasso, and G. Laurent (1980). *Neuroscience* 5:559–571. Immunochemical and immunohistochemical study of carbonic anhydrase II in adult rat cerebellum: A marker for oligodendrocytes.

Ghandour, M. S., O. K. Langley, G. Labourdette, G. Vincendon, and G. Gombos (1981a). *Dev. Neurosci.* 4:66–78. Specific and artefactual cellular localization of S100 protein: An astrocyte marker in rat cerebellum.

Ghandour, M. S., G. Labourdette, G. Vincendon, and G. Gombos (1981b). *Dev. Neurosci.* 4:98–109. A biochemical and immunohistological study of S100 protein in developing rat cerebellum.

Ghatak, N. R., A. Hirano, Y. Doron, H. M. Zimmerman (1973). *Arch. Neurol.* 29:262–267. Remyelination in multiple sclerosis with peripheral type myelin.

Ghetti, B., J. Norton, and L. C. Triarhou (1987). *J. Comp. Neurol.* 260:409–422. Nerve cell atrophy and loss in the inferior olivary complex of "Purkinje cell degeneration" mutant mice.

Ghosh, A., A. Antonini, S. K. McConnell, and C. J. Shatz (1990). *Nature* 347:179–181. Requirement for subplate neurons in the formation of thalamocortical connections.

Ghysen, A., and C. Dambly-Chaudiere (1989). *Trends Genet.* 5:251–255. Genesis of the *Drosophila* peripheral nervous system.

Giacobini, G., G. Filogamo, M. Weber, P. Bouquet, and J. P. Changeux (1973). *Proc. Natl. Acad. Sci. U.S.A.* 70:1708–1712. Effects of a snake a-neurotoxin on the development of innervated skeletal muscles in chick embryo.

Gibralter, D., and D. C. Turner (1985). *Dev. Biol.* 112:292–307. Dual adhesion systems of chick myoblasts.

Gierer, A., and H. Meinhardt (1972). *Kybernetik* 12:30–39. A theory of biological pattern formation.

Giguere, V., E. S. Ong, P. Segui, and R. M. Evans (1987). *Nature* 330:624–629. Identification of a receptor for the morphogen retinoic acid.

Gilbert, C. D. (1983). *Ann. Rev. Neurosci.* 6:217–247. Microcircuitry of the visual cortex.

Gilbert, C. D., and T. N. Wiesel (1979). *Nature* 280:120–125. Morphology and intracortical projections of functionally characterised neurones in the cat visual cortex.

Gilbert, C. D., and T. N. Wiesel (1989). *J. Neurosci.* 9:2432–2442. Columnar specificity of intrinsic horizontal and corticocortical connections in cat visual cortex.

Gillespie, M. J., T. Gordon, and P. R. Murphy (1986). *J. Physiol. (London)* 372:485–500. Reinnervation of the lateral gastrocnemius and soleus muscles by their common nerve.

Gillet, J. P., P. Derer, and H. Tsiang (1986). *J. Neuropathol. Exp. Neurol.* 45:619–634. Axonal transport of rabies virus in the central nervous system of the rat.

Gillette, R. (1944). *J. Exp. Zool.* 96:201–222. Cell number and cell size in the ectoderm during neurulation.

Gilliatt, R. W. (1961). *Proc. Roy. Soc. Med.* 54:324–326. Sensory nerve conduction in man.

Gillilan, L. A. (1958). *J. Comp. Neurol.* 110:75–103. The arterial blood supply of the human spinal cord.

Gilmore, S. A. (1971). *Anat. Rec.* 171:283–292. Neuroglial population in the spinal white matter of neonatal and early postnatal rats. An autoradiographic study on numbers of neuroglia and changes in their proliferative activity.

Gimenez-Gallego, G., J. Rodkey, C. Bennett, M. Rios-Candelore, J. DiSalvo, and K. Thomas (1985). *Science* 230:1385–1388. Brain-derived acidic fibroblast growth factor: Complete amino acid sequence and homologies.

Gimlich, R. L., and J. Braun (1985). *Dev. Biol.* 109:509–514. Improved fluorescent compounds for tracing cell lineage.

Gimlich, R. L., and J. Cooke (1983). *Nature* 306:471–473. Cell lineage and the induction of a second nervous system in amphibian development.

Ginsburg, M. H., J. Loftus, J.-J. Ryckwaert, M. D. Pierschbacher, R. Pytela, E. Ruoslahti, and E. F. Plow (1987). *J. Biol. Chem.* 262:5427–5440. Immunochemical and N-terminal sequence comparison of two cytoadhesins indicates they contain similar or identical beta subunits and distinct alpha subunits.

Giordano, D. L., M. Murray, and T. J. Cunningham (1980). *J. Neurocytol.* 9:603–614. Naturally occurring neuron death in the optic layers of superior colliculus of the postnatal rat.

Giraudat, J., and J.-P. Changeux (1980). *Trends Pharmacol. Sci.* 1:198–202. The acetylcholine receptor.

Girdlestone, J., and J. A. Weston (1985). *Dev. Biol.* 109:274–287. Identification of early neuronal subpopulations in avian neural crest cell cultures.

Gitlin, D., J. Kumate, and C. Morales (1965). *J. Clin. Endocrinol.* 25:1599–1608. Metabolism and maternotransfer of human growth hormone in the pregnant woman at term.

Giulian, D. (1987). *J. Neurosci. Res.* 18:155–171. Ameboid microglia as effectors of inflammation in the central nervous system.

Giulian, D., and T. J. Baker (1985). *J. Cell. Biol.* 101:2411–2415. Peptides released by ameboid microglia regulate astroglial proliferation.

Giulian, D., and T. J. Baker (1986). *J. Neurosci.* 6:2163–2178. Characterization of ameboid microglia isolated from developing mammalian brain.

Giulian, D., and J. E. Ingeman (1988). *J. Neurosci.* 8:4707–4717. Colony-stimulating factors as promoters of ameboid microglia.

Giulian, D., and L. B. Lachman (1985). *Science* 228:497–499. Interleukin-1 stimulates astroglial proliferation after brain injury.

Giulian, D., D. G. Young, J. Woodward, D. C. Brown, and L. B. Lachman (1988). *J. Neurosci.* 8:709–714. Interleukin-1 is an astroglial growth factor in the developing brain.

Gladue, B. A., and L. G. Clemens (1980). *Physiol. Behav.* 25:589–593. Masculinization diminished by disruption of prenatal estrogen biosynthesis in male rats.

Glaser, O. C. (1914). *Anat. Rec.* 8:525–551. On the mechanisms of morphological differentiation in the nervous system.

Glees, P. (1955). *Neuroglia Morphology and Function.* C. C. Thomas, Springfield, Illinois.

Glicksman, M. A., and J. R. Sanes (1983). *J. Neurocytol.* 12:661–671. Differentiation of motor nerve terminals formed in the absence of muscle fibres.

Glicksman, M. A., and M. Willard (1985). *Ann. N.Y. Acad. Sci.* 455:479–491. Differential expression of the three neurofilament polypeptides.

Globus, A. (1975). Brain morphology as a function of presynaptic morphology and activity, pp. 9–91. In *Developmental Neuropsychology of Sensory Deprivation* (A. H. Riesen, ed.), Academic Press, New York.

Globus, A., and A. B. Scheibel (1966). *Nature* 212:463–465. Loss of dendrite spines as an index of presynaptic terminal patterns.

Globus, A., and A. B. Scheibel (1967a). *Exp. Neurol.* 18:116–131. Synaptic loci on visual cortical neurons of rabbit: Specific afferent radiation.

Globus, A., and A. B. Scheibel (1967b). *Exp. Neurol.* 19:331–345. The effect of visual deprivation on cortical neurons: A Golgi study.

Globus, A., and A. B. Scheibel (1967c). *J. Comp. Neurol.* 131:155–172. Pattern and field in cortical structure: The rabbit.

Globus, A., and A. B. Scheibel (1967d). *Science* 156:1127–1129. Synaptic loci on parietal cortical neurons: Terminations of corpus callosum fibers.

Globus, A., M. R. Rosenzweig, E. L. Bennett, and M. C. Diamond (1973). *J. Comp. Physiol. Psychol.* 82:175–181. Effects of differential experience on dendritic spine counts in rat cerebral cortex.

Globus, J. H., and H. Kuhlenbeck (1944). *J. Neuropathol. Exp. Neurol.* 3:1–35. The subependymal cell plate. The subependymal cell plate (matrix) and its relationship to brain tumors of the ependymal type.

Gloor, S., K. Odink, J. Guenther, H. Nick, and D. Monard (1986). *Cell* 487:687–693. A glia-derived neurite promoting factor with protease inhibitory activity belongs to the protease nexins.

Glorieux, J., J. H. Dussault, J. Morissette, M. Desjardins, J. Letarte, and H. Guyda (1985). *J. Pediatr.* 107:913–915. Follow-up at ages 5 and 7 years on mental development in children with hypothyroidism detected by Quebec screening program.

Glücksmann, A. (1940). *Br. J. Ophthalmol.* 24:153–178. Development and differentiation of the tadpole eye.

Glücksmann, A. (1951). *Biol. Rev.* 26:59–86. Cell deaths in normal vertebrate ontogeny.

Glücksmann, A. (1965). *Arch. Biol. (Liége)* 76:419–437. Cell death in normal development.

Gmitro, J. I., and L. E. Scriven (1966). A physicochemical basis for pattern and rhythm, pp. 221. In *Intracellular Transport,* Academic Press, New York.

Gnahn, H., F. Hefti, R Heumann, M. E. Schwab, and H. Thoenen (1983). *Dev. Brain Res.* 9:45–52. NGF-mediated increase of choline acetyltransferase (ChAT) in the neonatal rat forebrain: Evidence for a physiological role of NGF in the brain.

Godement, P., and F. Bonhoeffer (1989). *Development* 106:313–320. Cross-species recognition of tectal cues by retinal fibers *in vitro*.

Godement, P., P. Saillour, and M. Imbert (1980). *J. Comp. Neurol.* 190:611–626. The ipsilateral optic pathway to the dorsal lateral geniculate nucleus and superior colliculus in mice with prenatal or postanatal loss of one eye.

Godement, P., J. Salaun, and M. Imbert (1984). *J. Comp. Neurol.* 230:552–575. Prenatal and postnatal development of retinogeniculate and retinocollicular projections in the mouse.

Goedert, M. (1986). *Biochem. Biophys. Res. Com.* 141:1116–1121. Molecular cloning of the chicken nerve growth factor gene: mRNA distribution in developing and adult tissues.

Goedert, M., U. Otten, S. P. Hunt, A. Bond, D. Chapman, M. Schlumpf, and W. Lichtensteiger (1984). *Proc. Natl. Acad. Sci. U.S.A.* 81:1580–1584. Biochemical and anatomical effects of antibodies against nerve growth factor on developing rat sensory ganglia.

Goedert, M., A. Fine, S. P. Hunt, and A. Ullrich (1986). *Mol. Brain Res.* 1:85–92. Nerve growth factor mRNA in peripheral and central rat tissues and in the human central nervous system: Lesion effects in the rat brain and levels in Alzheimer's disease.

Goedert, M., M. G. Spillantini, M. C. Potier, J. Ulrich, and R. A. Crowther (1989). *EMBO J.* 8:393–399. Cloning and sequencing of the cDNA encoding an isoform of microtubule-associated protein tau containing four tandem repeats: Differential expression of tau protein mRNA in human brain.

Goerke, H. (1973). *Linnaeus*, Charles Scribner's Sons, New York.

Goerttler, K. (1925). *Arch. Entw.-Mech. Organ.* 106:503–541. Die Formbildung der Medullaranlage bei Urodelen.

Goethe, J. W. von (1827). Homer noch einmal. Reprinted in *Goethes sämtliche Werke*, Vol. 38, p. 78. Cotta, Berlin.

Goetsch, W. (1957). *The Ants*, Univ. Michigan Press, Ann Arbor.

Goette, A. (1874). *Arch. microsk. Anat. EntwMech.* 15:139–200. Ueber die Entwicklung des Zentralnervensystems der Teleostier.

Goffinet, A. M. (1979). *Anat. Embryol.* 157:205–216. An early developmental defect in the cerebral cortex of the reeler mouse. A morphological study leading to a hypothesis concerning the action of the mutant gene.

Goffinet, A. M. (1981). *Neurosci. Lett.* 7:S122. Abnormal development of the inferior olivary complex in reeler mutant mice.

Goffinet, A. M. (1983). *J. Comp. Neurol.* 219:10–24. The embryonic development of the inferior olivary complex in normal and reeler (rl^{ORL}) mutant mice.

Goffinet, A. M. (1983). *J. Comp. Neurol.* 215:437–452. The embryonic development of the cortical plate in reptiles: A comparative study in *Emys orbicularis* and *Lacerta agilis*.

Goffinet, A. M. (1984a). *J. Anat. (London)* 138:207–215. Abnormal development of the facial nerve nucleus in reeler mutant mice.

Goffinet, A. M. (1984b). *Brain Res. Rev.* 7:261–296. Events governing organization of postmigratory neurons: Studies on brain development in normal and reeler mice.

Goffinet, A. M., and G. Lyon (1979). *Neurosci. Lett.* 14:61–66. Early histogenesis in the mouse cerebral cortex: A Golgi study.

Goffinet, A. M., K.-F. So, M. Yamamoto, M. Edwards, and V. S. Caviness, Jr. (1984). *Dev. Brain Res.* 16:263–276. Architectonic and hodological organization of the cerebellum in reeler mutant mice.

Goldberg, D. J. (1982). Actin and myosin in nerve cells, pp. 73–80. In *Axoplasmic Transport* (D. G. Weiss, ed.), Springer-Verlag, Berlin.

Goldberg, D. J. (1988). *J. Neurosci.* 8:2596–2605. Local Role of Ca^{2+} in formation of veils in growth cones.

Goldberg, D. J., and D. W. Burmeister (1986). *J. Cell Biol.* 103:1921–1932. Stages in axon formation: Observations of growth by *Aplysia* axons in culture using video-enhanced contrast-differential interference contrast microscopy.

Goldberg, D. J., and D. W. Burmeister (1988). *Trends Neurosci.* 11:257–258. Growth cone movement.

Goldberg, G. (1985). *Beh. Brain Sci.* 8:567–616. Supplementary motor area structure and function: Review and hypotheses.

Goldberg, S. (1974). *Dev. Biol.* 36:24–43. Studies on the mechanics of development of the visual pathways in the chick embryo.

Goldberg, S. (1976a). *Dev. Biol.* 53:126–127. Progressive fixation of morphological polarity in the developing retina.

Goldberg, S. (1976b). *J. Comp. Neurol.* 168:379–392. Polarization of the avian retina. Ocular transplantation studies.

Goldberg, S., and A. J. Coulombre (1972). *J. Comp. Neurol.* 146:507–518. Topographical development of the ganglion cell fiber layer in the chick retina. A whole mount study.

Goldberg, S., and M. Kotani (1967). *Anat. Rec.* 158:325–331. The projection of optic nerve fibers in the frog *Rana catesbiana* as studied by radioautography.

Goldberger, M. E., and M. Murray (1982). *Brain Res.* 241:227–239. Lack of sprouting and its presence after lesions of the cat spinal cord.

Goldfarb, J., C. Cantin, and M. W. Cohen (1990). *J. Neurosci.* 10:500–507. Intracellular and surface acetylcholine receptors during the normal development of a frog skeletal muscle.

Goldman, D., H. R. Brenner, and S. Heinemann (1988). *Neuron* 1:329–333. Acetylcholine receptor α-, β-, γ-, and δ-subunit mRNA levels are regulated by muscle activity.

Goldman, J. E., M. Hirano, R. K. Yu, and T. N. Seyfried (1984). *J. Neuroimmunol.* 7:179–192. GD$_3$ ganglioside is a glycolipid characteristic of immature neuroectodermal cells.

Goldman, P. S. (1974). An alternative to developmental plasticity: Heterology of CNS structures in infants and adults, pp. 149–174. In *Plasticity and Recovery of Function in the Central Nervous System* (D. G. Stein, J. J. Rosen, and N. Butters, eds.), Academic Press, New York.

Goldowitz, D. (1987). *Dev. Brain Res.* 35:1–9. Cell partitioning and mixing in the formation of the CNS: Analysis of the cortical somatosensory barrels in chimeric mice.

Goldowitz, D. (1989a). *Neuron* 2:1565–1575. The weaver granuloprival phenotype is due to intrinsic action of the mutant locus in granule cells: Evidence from homozygous weaver chimeras.

Goldowitz, D. (1989b). *Neuron* 3:705–713. Cell allocation in mammalian CNS formation: Evidence from murine interspecies aggregation chimeras.

Goldowitz, D., and C. W. Cotman (1980). *Brain Res.* 181:325–344. Do neurotrophic interactions control synapse formation in the adult rat brain?

Goldowitz, D., and R. J. Mullen (1982). *J. Neurosci.* 2:1474–

1485. Granule cell as a site of gene action in the weaver mouse cerebellum: Evidence from heterozygous mutant chimeras.

Goldscheider, A. (1898). *Die Bedeutung der Reize für Pathologie und Therapie im Lichte der Neuronlehre*. Leipzig.

Goldschmidt, R. G. (1951). The impact of genetics upon science, pp. 1–23. In *Genetics In the 20th Century* (L. C. Dunn, ed.), MacMillan, New York.

Goldstein, J. L., and J. D. Wilson (1975). *J. Cell. Physiol.* 85:365–378. Genetic and hormonal control of male sexual differentiation.

Goldstein, J. L., R. G. W. Anderson, and M. S. Brown (1979). *Nature* 279:679–685. Coated pits, coated vesicles, and receptor-mediated endocytosis.

Goldstein, J. L., M. S. Brown, R. G. W. Anderson, D. W. Russel, and W. J. Schneider (1985). *Ann. Rev. Cell Biol.* 1:1–39. Receptor-mediated endocytosis: Concepts emerging from the LDL receptor system.

Goldstein, L. A., E. M. Kurz, and D. R. Sengelaub (1990). *J. Neurosci.* 10:935–946. Androgen regulation of dendritic growth and retraction in the development of a sexually dimorphic spinal nucleus.

Goldstein, M. E., H. Cooper, J. Bruce, M. J. Carden, V. M.-Y. Lee, and W. W. Schlaepfer (1987). *J. Neurosci.* 7:1586–1594. Alterations in the phosphorylation of neurofilament proteins following transection of rat sciatic nerve and chromatolysis.

Goldstein, M. N., and J. A. Burdman (1965). *Anat. Rec.* 151:199–208. Studies of the nerve growth factor in submandibular glands of female mice treated with testosterone.

Golgi, C. (1873). *Gazz. Med. Ital. Lombardo* 6:41–56. Sulla struttura della sostanza grigia del cervello.

Golgi, C. (1874). Sulla fina anatomia del cervelleto umano. Lecture, Istituto Lombardo di Sci e Lett. 8 Jan. 1874. Chap. V in *Opera Omnia*, Vol. 1: Istologia normale, 1870–1883, pp. 99–111. Ulrico Hoepli, Milan, 1903.

Golgi, C. (1875a). *Riv. sper. freniat. Reggio-Emilia* 1:66–78. In *Opera Omnia* (1903).

Golgi, C. (1875b). *Riv. sper. freniat. Reggio-Emilia* 1:405–425. Sulla fina struttura dei bulbi olfattorii.

Golgi, C. (1879). *Ist. Lomb. Rendiconti* 12:206–212. Un nuovo processo tecnica microscopica.

Golgi, C. (1880a). Studi istologici sul midollo spinale. *Communicatione fatta al terzo congresso freniatrico italiano tenuto in Reggio-Emilia nel Sett. 1880*. Also in *Arch. ital. per le malattie nervose*, anno 18, 1881. In *Opera Omnia* 235–242 (1903).

Golgi, C. (1880b) *Giornale internaz. della Scienze mediche Anno III*. Sulla origine centrale dei nervi. Communicatione fatta alle sezione anatom. del III Congresso medico in Genova nel Sett 1880.

Golgi, C. (1880c). Archiv oper le scienze mediche, Sulla struttura delle fibre nervose midollate periferiche e centrali. In *Opera Omnia*, 149–170 (1903).

Golgi, C. (1880d). *Mem. Roy. Acad. Sci. Tor.* 32:359–385. Sui nervi nei tendini dell'uomo e di altri vertebrati e di un nuovo organo nervoso terminale musculo-tendineo.

Golgi, C. (1882–1885). *Rivista sperimentale di Freniatria* 8:165–195, 361–391 (1882); 9:1–17, 161–192, 385–402 (1883); 11:72–123, 193–220 (1885). Sulla fina anatomia degli organi centrali del sistema nervoso. Also in *Opera Omnia* 295–393, 397–536 (1903).

Golgi, C. (1883a). *Archives Ital. Biol.* 3:285–317; 4:92–123. Recherches sur l'histologie des centres nerveux.

Golgi, C. (1883b). *Atti del IV Congresso freniatrico ital. ten. in Voghera nel Sett. 1883*. La cellula nervosa motrice.

Golgi, C. (1886). *Archives Ital. Biol.* 7:15–47. Sur l'anatomie microscopique des organes centraux du système nerveux.

Golgi, C. (1891a). *Rendiconti R. Ist Lombardo Sci. Lett., Ser. 2* 24:595–656. La rete nervosa diffusa degli organi centrali del sistema nervosa: Suo significato fisiologico.

Golgi, C. (1891b). *Archives Ital. Biol.* 15:434–463. Le réseau nerveux diffus des centres du système nerveux; ses attributs physiologiques; méthode suivie dans les recherches histologiques.

Golgi, C. (1894). Das diffuse nervöse Netz der Centralorgane des Nervensystems. In *Untersuchungen über den feineren Bau des centralen und peripherischen Nevensystems*. A compilation of papers by C. Golgi, R. Teuscher, transl. Fisher, Jena.

Golgi, C. (1898a). *Archives Ital. Biol.* 30:60–71. Sur la structure des cellules nerveuses.

Golgi, C. (1898b). *Archives Ital. Biol.* 30:278–286. Sur la structure des cellules nerveuses des ganglions spinaux.

Golgi, C. (1898c). *Boll. Soc. Med. Pavia* 1:3–16. Intorno alla Struttura delle cellule nervose.

Golgi, C. (1898d). *Boll. Soc. Med. Pavia* 2:5–15. Sulla struttura delle cellule nervose dei gangli spinali.

Golgi, C. (1899a). *Arch. Ital. Biol.* 31:273–280. Di nuovo sulla struttura delle cellule nervose dei gangli spinali.

Golgi, C. (1900). *Verhandl. deutsch. Anat. Gesellsch.* 14:164–176. Intorno alla struttura delle cellule nervose della corteccia cerebrale.

Golgi, C. (1901). Sulla fina organizzazione del sistema nervoso. In L. Luciani, *Trattato di fisiologia dell'uomo*. Società editrice libraria, Milan. (Also in *Opera Omnia*, 721–733).

Golgi, C. (1903). *Opera Omnia*. Ulrico Hoepli, Milan.

Golgi, C. (1907). La Doctrine du Neurone. Théorie et Faits. In *Les Prix Nobel en 1906*. Imprimerie Royale, P.-A. Norstedt et Fils, Stockholm. The neuron doctrine—Theory and facts, pp. 189–217. In *Nobel Lectures: Physiology or Medicine, 1901–1921*, Amsterdam, Elsevier, 1967.

Goll, W. (1967). *Z. Morphol. Oekol Tiere* 59:143–210. Strukturuntersuchungen am Gehirn von *Formica*.

Golosow, N., and C. Grobstein (1962). *Dev. Biol.* 4:242–255. Epitheliomesenchymal interaction between embryonic mouse tissues separated by a transmembrane filter.

Gombos, G., W. Filipowicz, and G. Vincendon (1971). *Brain Res.* 26:475–479. Fast and slow components of S-100 protein fraction: Regional distribution in bovine central nervous system.

Gomez, C. J., N. E. Ghittoni, and J. M. Dellacha (1966). *Life Sci.* 5:243–246. Effects of L-thyroxine or somatotrophin on body growth and cerebral development in neo-natally thyroidectomized rats.

Gómez-Ramos, P., E. León-Felíu, and E. L. Rodríguez-Echandía (1979). *Anat. Embryol.* 156:217–224. Taste buds in vallate papillae grafted to the anterior chamber of the eye.

Gona, A. G. (1972). *J. Comp. Neurol.* 146:133–142. Morphogenesis of the cerebellum of the frog tadpole during spontaneous metamorphosis.

Gona, A. G. (1973). *Exp. Neurol.* 38:494–501. Effects of thyroxine, thyrotropin, prolactin, and growth hormone on the maturation of the frog cerebellum.

Gona, A. G. (1975). *Brain Res.* 95:132–136. Golgi studies of cerebellar maturation in frog tadpoles.

Gona, A. G. (1976). *J. Comp. Neurol.* 165:77–88. Autoradiographic studies of cerebellar histogenesis in the bullfrog tadpole during metamorphosis: The external granular layer.

Gonatas, N. K., and E. Robbins (1965). *Protoplasma* 59:377–391. The homology of spindle tubules and neuro-tubules in the chick embryo retina.

Gonatas, N. K., S. U. Kim, A. Stieber, and S. Avrameas (1977). *J. Cell Biol.* 73:1–13. Internalisation of lectins in neuronal GERL.

Gonatas, N. K., C. Harper, T. Mizutani, and J. O. Gonatas (1979). *J. Histochem. Cytochem.* 27:728–734. Superior sensitivity of conjugates of horseradish peroxidase with wheat germ agglutinin for studies of retrograde axonal transport.

Gonchoroff, N., P. Greipp, J. Katzman, and R. Kyle (1985). *Cytometry* 6:506–512. A monoclonal antibody reactive with 5-bromo-2-deoxyuridine that does not require DNA denaturation.

Goodman, C. (1974). *J. Comp. Physiol.* 95:185–201. Anatomy of locust ocellar interneurons: Constancy and variability.

Goodman, C. (1982). Embryonic development of identified neurons in the grasshopper, pp. 171–212. In *Neuronal Development* (N. C. Spitzer, ed.), Plenum, New York/London.

Goodman, C. S., J. A. Raper, R. K. Ho, and S. Chang (1982). Pathfinding by neuronal growth cones in grasshopper embryo, pp. 275–316. In *Developmental Order: Its Origin and Regulation*, Alan R. Liss, Inc., New York.

Goodman, D. C., and J. A. Horel (1966). *J. Comp. Neurol.* 127:71–88. Sprouting of optic tract projections in the brain stem of the rat.

Goodman, D. C., R. S. Bogdasarian, and J. A. Horel (1973). *Brain Behav. Evol.* 8:27–50. Axonal sprouting of ipsilateral optic tract following opposite eye removal.

Goodrich, E. S. (1913). *Quart. J. Micr. Sci.* 59:227–248. Metameric segmentation and homology.

Goodrich, E. S. (1918). *Quart. J. Micr. Sci.* 63:1–30. On the development of the segments of the head in Scyllium.

Goodrich, E. S. (1930). *Studies on the Structure and Development of Vertebrates*. Macmillan, London.

Goodrum, G. R., and A. G. Jacobson (1981). *J. Exp. Zool.* 216:399–408. Cephalic flexure formation in the chick embryo.

Goodwin, B. C., and M. H. Cohen (1969). *J. Theor. Biol.* 25:49–107. A phase-shift model for the spatial and temporal organization of developing systems.

Goosen, H. (1949). *Zool. Jahrb. Abt. Allgem. Zool. Physiol. Tiere* 62:1–64. Untersuchungen an Gehirnen verschieden grosser, jeweils verwandter Coleopteren-und Hymenopterenarten.

Gopinath, G., V. Bijlani, and M. G. Deo (1976). *Exp. Neurol.* 35:125–135. Undernutrition and the developing cerebellar cortex in the rat.

Görcs, T., M. Antal, É. Oláh, and G. Székely (1979). *Acta Biol. Acad. Sci. Hung.* 30:79–86. An improved colbalt labeling technique with complex compounds.

Gordon, B., E. E. Allen, and P. Q. Trombley (1988). *Prog. Neurol.* 30:171–191. The role of norepinephrine in plasticity of visual cortex.

Gordon-Taylor, G., and E. W. Walls (1958). *Sir Charles Bell. His Life and Times*. Livingstone, Edinburgh.

Gordon-Weeks, P. R. (1989). *Trends Neurosci.* 12:363–365. GAP-43: What does it do in the growth cone?

Gordon-Weeks, P. R., and R. O. Lockerbie (1984). *Neuroscience* 13:119–136. Isolation and partial characterization of neuronal growth cones from neonatal rat forebrain.

Gordon, T., R. Perry, A. R. Tuffery, and G. Vrbová (1974). *Cell Tiss. Res.* 155:13–25. Possible mechanisms determining synapse formation in developing skeletal muscles of the chick.

Goridis, C., M. Hirn, M.-J. Santoni, G. Gennarini, H. Deagostini-Bazin, B. R. Jordan, M. Kiefer, and M. Steinmetz (1985). *EMBO J.* 4:631–635. Isolation of mouse N-CAM-related cDNA: detection and cloning using monoclonal antibodies.

Gorski, R. A. (1966). *J. Reprod. Fertil. Suppl.* 1:67–88. Localization and sexual differentiation of the nervous structures which regulate ovulation.

Gorski, R. A., J. H. Gordon, J. E. Shryne, and A. M. Shoutam (1978). *Brain Res.* 148:333–346. Evidence for a morphological sex difference within the medial preoptic area of the rat brain.

Gorski, R. A., R. E. Harlan, C. D. Jacobson, J. E Shryne, and A. M. Southam (1980). *J. Comp. Neurol.* 193:529–539. Evidence for the existence of a sexually dimorphic nucleus in the preoptic area of the rat.

Gorza, L., K. Gundersen, T. Lømo, and S. Schiaffino (1988). *J. Physiol. (London)* 402:627–649. Slow-to-fast transformation of denervated soleus muscles by chronic high-frequency stimulation in the rat.

Goshgarian, H. G., and L. Guth (1977). *Exp. Neurol.* 57:613–621. Demonstration of functionally ineffective synapses in the guinea pig spinal cord.

Goshgarian, H. G., X.-J. Yu, and J. A. Rafols (1989). *J. Comp. Neurol.* 284:519–533. Neuronal and glial changes in the rat phrenic nucleus occurring within hours after spinal cord injury.

Goslin, K., and G. Banker (1989). *J. Cell Biol.* 108:1507–1516. Experimental observations on the development of polarity by hippocampal neurons in culture.

Goslin, K., D. J. Schreyer, J. H. P. Skene, and G. Banker (1988). *Nature* 336:672–674. Development of neuronal polarity: GAP-43 distinguishes axonal from dendritic growth cones.

Gospodarowicz, D. (1987). *Meth. Enzymol.* 147:107–119. Isolation and characterization of acidic and basic fibroblast growth factor.

Goto, T., P. MacDonald, and T. Maniatis (1989). *Cell* 57:413–422. Early and late periodic patterns of even skipped expression are controlled by distinct regulatory elements that respond to different spatial cues.

Gottlieb, D. I., and W. M. Cowan (1972). *Brain Res.* 41:452–456. Evidence for a temporal factor in the occupation of available synaptic sites during development of the dentate gyrus.

Gottlieb, D. I., and W. M. Cowan (1973). *J. Comp. Neurol.* 149:393–422. Autoradiographic studies of the commissural and ipsilateral associational connections of the hippocampus and dentate gyrus of the rat. I. The commissural connections.

Gottlieb, D. I., K. Rock, and L. Glaser (1976). *Proc. Natl. Acad. Sci. U.S.A.* 73:410–414. A gradient of adhesive specificity in developing avian retina.

Gottlieb, G. (1973). Introduction to behavioral embryology,

pp. 3–45. In *Studies on the Development of Behavior and the Nervous System: Behavioral Embryology*. Vol. 1, (G. Gottlieb, ed.), Academic Press, New York.

Gottlieb, G. (1976). The roles of experience in the development of behavior and the nervous system, pp. 25–54. In *Neural and Behavioral Specificity* (G. Gottlieb, ed.), Academic Press, New York.

Gottschaldt, K. M., and C. Vahle-Hinz (1982). *Exp. Brain Res.* 45:459–463. Evidence against transmitter function of Met-enkephalin and chemosynaptic impulse generation in "Merkel cell" mechanoreceptors.

Gould, E., and L. L. Butcher (1989). *J. Neurosci.* 9:3347–3358. Basal forebrain neurons are sensitive to thyroid hormone.

Gould, E., A. Westlind-Danielsson, M. Frankfurt, and B. S. McEwen (1990). *J. Neurosci.* 10:996–1003. Sex differences and thyroid hormone sensitivity of hippocampal pyramidal cells.

Gouin, F. J. (1965). *Fortschr. Zool.* 17:189–237. Morphologie, Histologie und Entwicklungsgeschichte der Myriapoden und Insekten III. Das Nervensystem und die neurocrinen Systeme.

Gould, B. B., and P. Rakic (1981). *Exp. Brain Res.* 44:195–206. The total number, time of origin and kinetics of proliferation of neurons comprising the deep cerebellar nuclei in the rhesus monkey.

Gould, S. J. (1966). *Biol. Rev.* 41:587–640. Allometry and size in ontogeny and phylogeny.

Gould, S. J. (1977). *Ontogeny and Phylogeny*. Belknap, Harvard Univ. Press, Cambridge, Mass.

Gould, S. J. (1981). *The Mismeasure of Man*. Norton, New York.

Gould, V. E., R. Moll, I. Moll, I. Lee, and W. W. Franke (1985). *Lab Invest.* 52:334–353. Biology of disease. Neuroendocrine (Merkel) cells of the skin: Hyperplasias, dysplasias, and neoplasms.

Gourdon, J., J. Clos, C. Coste, J. Dainat, and J. Legrand (1973). *J. Neurochem.* 21:861–871. Comparative effects of hypothyroidism, hyperthyroidism and undernutrition on the protein and nucleic acid contents of the cerebellum in the young rat.

Gower, D. J., and M. Tytell (1986). *J. Neurol. Sci.* 72:11–18. Slow axonal protein transport and axoplasmic organization.

Gower, D. J., and M. Tytell (1987). *Brain Res.* 407:1–8. Axonal transport of clathrin-associated proteins.

Goy, R. W., and B. S. McEwen (1980). *Sexual Differentiation of the Brain*. MIT Press, Cambridge, Mass.

Goz, B. (1978). *Pharmacol. Rev.* 19:249–272. The effects of incorporation of 5-halogenated deoxyuridines into the DNA of eukaryotic cells.

Gozes, I. (1982). *Neurochem. Int.* 4:101–120. Tubulin in the nervous system.

Gozzo, S., and M. Ammassari-Teule (1983). *Neurosci. Lett.* 36:111–116. Different mossy fiber patterns in two inbred strains of mice: A functional hypothesis.

Grabower, C. (1902). *Arch. mikr. Anat.* 60:1–16. Ueber Nervenendigungen im menschlichen Muskel.

Grady, K. L., C. H. Phoenix, and W. C. Young (1965). *J. Comp. Physiol. Psychol.* 59:176–182. Role of the developing rat testes in differentiation of the neural tissues mediating mating behavior.

Graeber, M. B., and G. W. Kreutzberg (1986). *J. Neurocytol.* 15:363–373. Astrocytes increase in glial fibrillary acidic

protein during retrograde changes of facial motor neurons.

Graeber, M. B., W. J. Streit, and G. W. Kreutzberg (1988). *J. Neurocytol.* 17:573–580. The microglial cytoskeleton: Vimentin is localized within activated cells *in situs*.

Graeber, M. B., W. Tetzlaff, W. J. Streit, and G. W. Kreutzberg (1988b). *Neurosci. Lett.* 85:317–321. Microglial cells but not astrocytes undergo mitosis following rat facial nerve axotomy.

Grafstein, B. (1975). Axonal transport: The intracellular traffic of the neuron. In *Handbook of the Nervous System*, Vol. 1, *Cellular Biology of Neurones* (E. R. Kandel, ed.), Amer. Physiol. Soc., Washington, D.C.

Grafstein, B., and D. S. Forman (1980). *Physiol. Rev.* 60:1167–1283. Intracellular transport in neurons.

Grafstein, B., and N. A. Ingoglia (1982). *Exp. Neurol.* 76:318–330. Intracranial transection of the optic nerve in adult mice: Preliminary observations.

Grafstein, R., and R. Laureno (1973). *Exp. Neurol.* 39:44–57. Transport of radioactivity from eye to visual cortex in the mouse.

Graham, A., N. Papalopulu, J. Lorimer, J. H. McVey, E. G. D. Tudenham, and R. Krumlauf (1988). *Genes Dev.* 2:1424–1438. Characterization of a murine homeobox gene, *Hox-2.6*, related to the *Drosophila Deformed* gene.

Graham, A., N. Papalopulu, and Robb Krumlauf (1989). *Cell* 57:367–378. The murine and drosophila homeobox gene complexes have common features of organization and expression.

Graham, C. F., and R. W. Morgan (1966). *Dev. Biol.* 14:439–460. Changes in the cell cycle during early amphibian development.

Graham, G. (1964). Diet and bodily constitution, p. 11. In *Ciba Foundation Study Group No. 17*. Churchill, London.

Graham, R. C., and M. J. Karnovsky (1966). *J. Histochem. Cytochem.* 14:271–302. The early stages of absorption of injected horseradish peroxidase in the proximal tubules of mouse kidney. Ultrastructural cytochemistry by a new technique.

Grampp, W., and J.-E. Edström (1963). *J. Neurochem.* 10:725–732. The effect of nervous activity on ribonucleic acid of the crustacean stretch receptor neuron.

Granato, D. A., B. W. Fulpius, and J. F. Moody (1976). *Proc. Natl. Acad. Sci. U.S.A.* 73:2872–2876. Experimental myasthenia in Balb/C mice immunized with rat acetylcholine receptor from rat denervated muscle.

Granick, S., and A. Gibor (1967). *Prog. Nucl. Acid Res. Molec. Biol.* 6:143–168. The DNA of chloroplasts, mitochondria, and centrioles.

Granit, R. (1972). *Ann. Rev. Physiol.* 34:1–12. Discovery and understanding.

Granit, R., H. D. Henatsch, and G. Steg (1956). *Acta Physiol. Scand.* 37:114–126. Tonic and phasic ventral horn cells differentiated by post-tetanic potentiation in cat extensors.

Grant, G. (1965). *Experientia* 21:1–4. Degenerative changes in dendrites following axonal transection.

Grant, G. (1970). Neuronal changes central to the site of axon transection. A method for the identification of retrograde changes in perikarya, dendrites and axons by silver impregnation, pp. 173–185. In *Contemporary Research Methods in Neuroanatomy* (W. J. H. Nauta, and S. O. E. Ebbesson eds.), Springer-Verlag, Berlin.

Grant, G., and J. Westman (1968). *Experientia* 24:169–170.

Degenerative changes in dendrites central to axonal transection. Electron microscopical observations.

Grant, P., E. Rubin, and C. Cima (1980). *J. Comp. Neurol.* 189:593–613. Ontogeny of the retina and optic nerve in *Xenopus laevis*. I. Stages in the early development of the retina.

Graper, L. (1913). *Arch. mikr. Anat.* 83:371–426. Die Rhombomeren und ihre Nervenbeziehungen.

Grasso, A., and R. Pirazzi (1975). *Brain Res.* 90:324–328. Changes in the concentration of the brain specific protein 14-3-2, during the development of the superior cervical ganglion of the rat and effects of surgical decentralization.

Gratzner, H. (1982). *Science* 218:474–475. Monoclonal antibody against 5-bromo- and 5-iododeoxyuridine: A new reagent for detection of DNA replication.

Gray, E. G. (1959). *J. Anat. (London)* 93:420–433. Axosomatic and axo-dendritic synapses of the cerebral cortex: An electron microscope study.

Gray, E. G. (1982). *Trends Neurosci.* 5:5–6. Rehabilitating the dendritic spine.

Gray, E. G., and R. W. Guillery (1961). *J. Physiol. (London)* 157:581–588. The basis for silver staining of synapses of the mammalian spinal cord: A light and electron microscope study.

Gray, E. G., and R. W. Guillery (1966). *Int. Rev. Cytol.* 19:111–182. Synaptic morphology in the normal and degenerating nervous system.

Gray, J. (1950). The role of peripheral sense organs during locomotion in the vertebrates, pp. 112–126. In *Physiological Mechanisms in Animal Behaviour* (J. F. Danielli, and J. Brown, eds.), Cambridge Univ. Press, Cambridge.

Gray, P. T. A., and J. M. Ritchie (1985). *Trends Neurosci.* 8:411–415. Ion channels in Schwann and glial cells.

Graybiel, A. M. (1976). *Brain Res.* 114:318–327. Evidence for banding of the cat's ipsilateral retinotectal connection.

Graybiel, A. M. (1978). *Brain Res.* 145:365–374. A satellite system of the superior colliculus: The parabigeminal nucleus and its projections to the superficial collicular layers.

Graybiel, A. M., K. Ohta, S. Roffler-Tarlov (1990). *J. Neurosci.* 10:720–733. Patterns of cell and fiber vulnerability in the mesostriatal system of the mutant mouse weaver. I. Gradients and compartments.

Graziadei, P. P. C. (1970). The ultrastructure of taste buds in mammals, pp. 5–35. In *2nd Symposium on Oral Sensation and Perception* (J. F. Bosma, ed.), Thomas, Springfield.

Graziadei, P. P. C. (1973). *Tiss. Cell* 5:113–131. Cell dynamics in the olfactory mucosa.

Graziadei, P. P. C. (1974). The olfactory organ of vertebrates: A survey, pp. 191–222. In *Essays on the Nervous System* (R. Bellairs, and E. G. Gray, eds.), Clarendon Press, Oxford.

Graziadei, P. P. C., and R. S. DeHan (1973). *J. Cell Biol.* 59:525–530. Neuronal regeneration in frog olfactory system.

Graziadei, P. P. C., and G. A. Monti Graziadei (1978). Continuous nerve cell renewal in the olfactory system. In *Handbook of Sensory Physiology*, Vol. 9, *Development of Sensory Systems* (M. Jacobson, ed.), Springer Verlag, New York.

Green, C. R. (1988). *BioEssays* 8:7–10. Evidence mounts for the role of gap junctions during development.

Green, J. B. A., G. Howes, K. Symes, J. Cooke, and J. C. Smith (1990). *Development* 108:173–183. The biological effects of XTC-MIF: Quantitative comparison with *Xenopus* bFGF.

Greenblatt, S. H. (1965). *Bull. Hist. Med.* 39:346–376. The major influences on the early life and work of John Hughlings Jackson.

Greene, L. A., and E. M. Shooter (1980). *Ann. Rev. Neurosci.* 3:353–402. The nerve growth factor: Biochemistry, synthesis, and mechanism of action.

Greene, L. A., S. Varon, A. Piltch, and E. M. Shooter (1971). *Neurobiol.* 1:37–48. Substructure of the p subunit of mouse 7S nerve growth factor.

Greene, L. S., and F. E. Johnston, eds. (1980). *Social and Biological Predictors of Nutritional Status, Physical Growth, and Neurological Development*. Academic Press, New York.

Greene, W. F. (1947). *Anat. Rec.* 97:389. Histogenesis of Mauthner's neurone in *Amblystoma*.

Greenough, W. T. (1984). *Trends. Biochem. Sci.* 7:229–233. Structural correlates of information storage in the mammalian brain. A review and hypothesis.

Greenough, W. T., and F. R. Volkmar (1973). *Exp. Neurol.* 40:491–504. Pattern of dendritic branching in occipital cortex of rats reared in complex environments.

Greenough, W. T., F. R. Volkmar, and J. M. Juraska (1973). *Exp. Neurol.* 41:371–378. Effects of rearing complexity on dendritic branching in frontolateral and temporal cortex of the rat.

Greenspan, R. J., and M. C. O'brien (1989). *J. Neurogen.* 5:25–36. Genetic evidence for the role of *Thy-1* in neurite outgrowth in the mouse.

Greenwald, I. S., P. W. Sternberg, and H. R. Horvitz (1983). *Cell* 34:435–444. The *lin-12* locus specifies cell fates in *Caenorhabditis elegans*.

Gregory, K. M., and M. C. Diamond (1968a). *Exp. Neurol.* 20:394–414. The effects of early hypophysectomy on brain morphogenesis in the rat.

Gregory, K. M., and M. C. Diamond (1968b). *Exp. Neurol.* 21:502–511. Acetylcholinesterase and cholinesterase activities, protein content and wet weight measures in the rat brain after early hypophysectomy.

Greiner, J. W., and T. A. Weidman (1980). *Exp. Eye Res.* 30:439–453. Histogenesis of the cat retina.

Grenell, R., and R. Scammon (1943). *J. Comp. Neurol.* 79:329–354. An iconometrographic representation of the growth of the central nervous system in man.

Griffin, C. G., and P. C. Letourneau (1980). *J. Cell Biol.* 86:156–161. Rapid retraction of neurites by sensory neurons in response to increased concentrations of nerve growth factor.

Griffin, J. W., P. N. Hoffman, A. W. Clark, P. T. Carrol, and D. L Price (1978). *Science* 202:633–635. Slow axonal transport of neurofilament proteins: Impairment by iminodipropionitrile administration.

Griffin, J. W., D. L. Price, D. B. Drachman, and J. Morris (1981). *J. Cell Biol.* 88:205–214. Incorporation of axonally transported glycoproteins into axolemma during nerve regeneration.

Griffin, J. W., P. N. Hoffman, and D. L. Price (1982). Axonal transport in iminodipropionitrile neuropathy, pp. 109–118. In *Axoplasmic Transport* (D. G. Weiss, ed.), Springer-Verlag, Berlin.

Griffin, W. S. T., D. J. Woodward, and R. Chanda (1977a).

Exp. Neurol. 56:298–311. Malnutrition-induced alterations of developing Purkinje cells.

Griffin, W. S. T., D. J. Woodward, and R. Chanda (1977b). *J. Neurochem.* 28:1269–1279. Malnutrition and brain development: Cerebellar weight, DNA, RNA, protein and histological correlations.

Griffiths, G., and K. Simons (1986). *Science* 234:438–443. The trans Golgi network: Sorting at the exit site of the Golgi complex.

Griffiths, I. R., L. S. Mitchell, K. McPhilemy, S. Morrison, E. Kyriakides, and J. A. Barrie (1989). *J. Neurocytol.* 18:345–352. Expression of myelin protein genes in Schwann cells.

Griglatti, T., D. T. Suzuki, and R. Williamson (1972). *Dev. Biol.* 28:352–371. Temperature-sensitive mutations in *Drosophila.* X. Developmental analysis of the paralytic mutation parats.

Grillner, S. (1981). Control of locomotion in bipeds, tetrapods, and fish, pp. 1179–1236. In *Handbook of Physiology* Sect. 1. *The Nervous System,* Vol 2, *Motor Control* (V. B. Brooks, ed.), American Physiological Society, Bethesda, MD.

Grillner, S., and P. Zangger (1974). *Acta Physiol. Scand.* 91:38A. Locomotor movements generated by the deafferented spinal cord.

Grillo, M. A., and S. L. Palay (1963). *J. Cell Biol.* 16:430–436. Ciliated Schwann cells in the autonomic nervous system of the adult rat.

Grim, M. (1970). *Z. Anat. Entwicklungsgesch.* 132:260–271. Differentiation of myoblasts and the relationship between somites and the wing bud of the chick embryo.

Grim, M., K. Nensa, B. Christ, H. J. Jacob, and K. W. Tosney (1989). *Anat. Embryol.* 180:179–189. A hierarchy of determining factors controls motoneuron innervation: Experimental studies on the development of the plantaris mucle (PL) in avian chimeras.

Grimes, G. J., and F. S. Barnes (1973). *Exp. Cell Res.* 79:375–385. A technique for studying chemotaxis of leucocytes in well-defined chemotactic fields.

Grimm, L. M. (1971). *J. Exp. Zool.* 178:479–496. An evaluation of myotypic respecification in Axolotls.

Grinvald, A. E., E. Lieke, R. D. Frostig, C. D. Gilbert, and T. N. Wiesel (1986). *Nature* 324:361–364. Functional architecture revealed by optical imaging of intrinsic signals.

Grivell, L. A. (1983). *Sci. Amer.* 248:60–73. Mitochondrial DNA.

Grobstein, C. (1953). *Nature* 172:869–871. Morphogenetic interaction between embryonic mouse tissues separated by a transmembrane filter.

Grobstein, C. (1957). *Exp. Cell Res.* 13:575–587. Some transmission characteristics of the tubule inducing influence on mouse metanephrogenic mesenchyme.

Grobstein, C. (1959). *J. Exp. Zool.* 142:203–213. Autoradiography of the interzone between tissues in inductive interaction.

Grobstein, C. (1967). *Natl. Cancer Inst. Monogr.* 26:279–299. Mechanisms of organogenetic tissue interaction.

Grobstein, P., and K. L. Chow (1975). *Science* 190:352–358. Receptive field development and individual experience.

Grobstein, P., and K. L. Chow (1976). Receptive field organization in the mammalian visual cortex: The role of individual experience in development, pp. 155–193. In *Studies on the Development of Behavior and the Nervous*

System, Vol. 3, (G. Gottlieb, ed.), Academic Press, New York.

Grobstein, P., and C. Comer (1976). *Neurosci. Abstr.* 2:278. Differences in development of adult relative eye position in *Xenopus* and *Rana.*

Grobstein, P., K. L. Chow, P. D. Spear, and L. H. Mathers (1973). *Science* 180:1185–1187. Development of rabbit visual cortex: Late appearance of a class of receptive fields.

Grobstein, R., K. L. Chow, P. C. Fox (1975). *Proc. Natl. Acad. Sci. U.S.A.* 72:1543–1545. Development of receptive fields in rabbit visual cortex: Changes in the course due to delayed eye-opening.

Grobstein, P., C. Comer, M. Hollyday, and S. M. Archer (1978). *Brain Res.* 156:117–123. A crossed isthmotectal projection in *Rana pipiens* and its involvement in the ipsilateral visuo-tectal projection.

Gross, G. W., and L. M. Beidler (1975). *J. Neurobiol.* 6:213–232. A quantitative analysis of istope concentration profiles and rapid axonal transport in the C-fibers of the garfish olfactory nerve.

Grossfeld, R. M., M. A. Klinge, E. M. Lieberman, and L. C. Stewart (1988). *GLIA* 1:292–300. Axon-glia transfer of a protein and a carbohydrate.

Grouse, L., M. D. Chilton, and B. J. McCarthy (1972). *Biochem.* 11:798–805. Hybridization of ribonucleic acid with unique sequences of mouse deoxyribonucleic acid.

Gruberg, E. R., and S. B. Udin (1978). *J. Comp. Neurol.* 179:487–500. Topographic projections between the nucleus isthmi and the tectum of the frog *Rana pipiens.*

Gruberg, E. R., M. T. Wallace, and R. F. Waldeck (1989). *J. Comp. Neurol.* 288:39–50. Relationship between isthmotectal fibers and other tectopetal systems in the leopard frog.

Grumet, M., and G. M. Edelman (1988). *J. Cell Biol.* 106:487–503. Neuron-glia cell adhesion molecule interacts with neurons and glia via different binding mechanisms.

Grumet, M., U. Rutishauser, and G. M. Edelman (1982). *Nature* 295:693–695. NCAM mediates adhesion between embryonic nerve and muscle *in vitro.*

Grumet, M., S. Hoffman, C. M. Chuong, and G. M. Edelman (1984). *Proc. Natl. Acad. Sci. U.S.A.* 81:7989–7993. Polypeptide components and binding function of neuron-glia cell adhesion molecules.

Grünbaum, A. S. F., and C. S. Sherrington (1902). *Proc. Royal Soc. (London) Ser. B.* 69:206–209. Observations on the physiology of the cerebral cortex of some of the higher apes.

Grünbaum, A. S. F., and C. S. Sherrington (1903). *Proc. Royal Soc. (London) Ser. B.* 72:152–155. Observations on the physiology of the cerebral cortex of the anthropoid apes.

Grundfest, H. (1963). *J. Hist. Med.* 18:125–129. The different careers of Gustav Fritsch (1838–1927).

Grüneberg, H. (1952). *The genetics of the mouse.* 2nd edn. Nijhof, The Hague.

Grüneberg, H. (1963). *The Pathology of Development. A Study of Inherited Skeletal Disorders in Animals.* Wiley, New York

Gruner, J. E., and J. P. Zahnd (1967). Sur la maturation synaptique dans le cortex visual du lapin, pp. 125–133. In *Regional development of the brain in early life* (A. Minkowski, ed.), Blackwells, Oxford.

Grunz, H., J. Born, M. Davids, P. Hoppe, B. Loppnow-Blinde, L. Tackle, H. Tiedemann, and H. Tiedemann

(1989). *Dev. Biol.* 198:8–13. A mesoderm-inducing factor from a *Xenopus laevis* cell line.

Grüsser, O.-J., and U. Grusser-Cornehls (1968). *Z. Vergl. Physiol.* 59:1–24. Neurophysiologische Grundlagen visueller angeborener Auslosemechanismen beim Frosch.

Grusser, O.-J., and U. Grusser-Cornehls (1973). Neuronal mechanisms of visual movement preception and some psychophysical and behavioral correlations, pp. 333–429. In *Handbook of Sensory Physiology*, Vol. 7, (H. Autrum, R. Jung, W. R. Loewenstein, D. M. MacKay, and H. L. Teuber, eds.), Springer-Verlag, Berlin.

Grynkiewicz, G., M. Poenie, and R. Y. Tsien (1985). *J. Biol. Chem.* 260:3440–3450. A new generation of Ca^{2+} indicators with greatly improved fluorescence properties.

Gudden, B. von (1870a). *Arch. Psychiat.* (Berlin) 2:364–366. Über einen bisher nicht beschriebenen Nervenfasernstrang im Gehirne der Säugethiere und des Menschen.

Gudden, B. von (1870b). *Arch. Psychiat.* (Berlin) 2:693–723. Experimentaluntersuchungen über das peripherische und centrale Nervensystem.

Gudden, B. von (1889). *Gesammelte und hinterlassene Abhandlungen.* H. Grashey, Wiesbaden.

Guenther, J., H. Nick, and D. Monard (1985). *EMBO J.* 4:1963–1966. A glia-derived neurite-promoting factor with protease inhibitor activity.

Guernsey, D. L., and I. S. Edelman (1983). Regulation of thyroid thermogenesis by thyroid hormones, p. 293. In *Molecular Basis of Thyroid Hormone Action* (J. H. Oppenheimer, and H. H. Samuels, eds.), Academic Press, New York.

Guerrero, I., H. Wong, A. Pellicer, and D. E. Burstein (1986). *J. Cell. Physiol.* 129:71–76. Activated N-*ras* gene induces neuronal differentiation of PC12 rat pheochromocytoma cells.

Guiditta, A., M. Libonati, A. Packard, and N. Prozzo (1971). *Brain. Res.* 25:55–62. Nuclear counts in the brain lobes of octopus vulgaris as a function of body size.

Guillery, R. W. (1965). *Prog. Brain Res.* 14:57–76. Some electron microscopical observations of degenerative changes in central nervous synapses.

Guillery, R. W. (1969). *Brain Res.* 14:739–741. An abnormal retinogeniculate projection in Siamese cats.

Guillery, R. W. (1970). Light- and electron-microscopical studies of normal and degenerating axons, pp. 77–105. In *Contemporary Research Methods in Neuroanatomy* (W. J. H. Nauta, and S. O. E. Ebbesson, eds.), Springer-Verlag, New York.

Guillery, R. W. (1972a). *J. Comp. Neurol.* 144:117–130. Binocular competition in the control of geniculate cell growth.

Guillery, R. W. (1972b). *J. Comp. Neurol.* 146:407–420. Experiments to determine whether retinogeniculate axons can form translaminar collateral sprouts in the dorsal lateral geniculate nucleus of the cat.

Guillery, R. W. (1973a). *J. Comp. Neurol.* 148:417–422. The effect of lid suture upon the growth of cells in the dorsal lateral geniculate nucleus of kittens.

Guillery, R. W. (1973b). *J. Comp. Neurol.* 149:423–438. Quantitative studies of transneuronal atrophy in the dorsal lateral geniculate nucleus of cats and kittens.

Guillery, R. W. (1974a). *Sci. Am.* 230:44–54. Visual pathways in albinos.

Guillery, R. W. (1974b). On structural changes that can be produced experimentally in the mammalian visual pathways, pp. 299–326. In *Essays on the Nervous System* (R. Bellairs, and E. G. Gray, eds.), Clarendon Press, Oxford.

Guillery, R. W. (1989). *J. Anat.* (London) 164:73–84. Early monocular enucleations in fetal ferrets produce a decrease of uncrossed and an increase of crossed retinofugal components: A possible model for the albino abnormality.

Guillery, R. W., and V. A. Cassagrande (1975a). *Cold Spring Harbor Symp. Quant. Biol.* 15:611–617. Adaptive synaptic connections formed in the visual pathways in response to congenitally aberrant inputs.

Guillery, R. W., and V. A. Cassagrande (1975b). *Anat. Rec.* 181:366. On restoring visual functions to the temporal retina of siamese cats.

Guillery, R. W., and J. H. Kaas (1971). *J. Comp. Neurol.* 143:73–100. A study of normal and congenitally abnormal retinogeniculate projections in cats.

Guillery, R. W., and D. J. Stelzner (1970). *J. Comp. Neurol.* 139:413–422. The differential effects of unilateral lid closure upon the monocular and binocular segments of the dorsal lateral geniculate nucleus in the cat.

Guillery, R. W., G. L. Scott, B. M. Cattanach, and M. S. Deol (1973). *Science* 179:1014–1016. Genetic mechanisms determining the central visual pathways of mice.

Guillery, R. W., T. L. Hickey, J. H. Kaas, D. J. Felleman, E. J. Debruyn, and D. L. Sparks (1984). *J. Comp. Neurol.* 226:165–183. Abnormal central visual pathways in the brain of an albino green monkey (*Cercopithecus aethiops*).

Guimariés, A., S. Zaremba, and S. Hockfield (1990). *J. Neurosci.* 10:3014–3024. Molecular and Morphological Changes in the Cat Lateral Geniculate Nucleus and Visual Cortex Induced by Visual Deprivation Are Revealed by Monoclonal Antibodies Cat-304 and Cat-301.

Gulley, R. L., R. J. Wenthold, and G. R. Neises (1977). *J. Cell Biol.* 75:837–850. Remodeling of neuronal membranes as an early response to deafferentation: A freeze-fracture study.

Gumbinas, M., M. Oda, and P. Huttenlocher (1973). *Biol. Neonate* 22:355–366. The effects of corticosteroids on myelination of the developing rat brain.

Gumpel, M., F. Lachapelle, M. Baulac, A. Baron van Evercooren, C. Lubetzki, A. Gansmuller, P. Lombrail, C. Jacque, and N. Baumann (1987). Myelination in the mouse by transplanted oligodendrocytes, pp. 819–830. In *Glial and Neuronal Communication in Development and Regeneration* (H. H. Althaus, and W. Seifert, eds.), Springer-Verlag, Berlin.

Gundersen, K., E. Leberer, T. Lømo, D. Pette, and R. S. Staron (1988). *J. Physiol.* (London) 398:177–189. Fibre types, calcium-sequestering proteins and metabolic enzymes in denervated and chronically stimulated muscles of the rat.

Gundersen, R. W. (1985). *J. Neurosci. Res.* 13:199–212. Sensory neurite growth cone guidance by substrate adsorbed nerve growth factor.

Gundersen, R. W. (1987). *Dev. Biol.* 121:423–431. Response of sensory neurites and growth cones to patterned substrata of lamin-in and fibronectin *in vitro*.

Gundersen, R. W., and J. N. Barrett (1979). *Science* 206:1079–1080. Neuronal chemotaxis; chick dorsal root axons turn towards high concentrations of nerve growth factor.

Gundersen, R. W., and J. N. Barrett (1980). *J. Cell Biol.*

87:546–554. Characterization of the turning repsonse of dorsal root neurites toward nerve growth factor.

Gurdon, J. B. (1959). *J. Exp. Zool.* 141:519–543. Tetraploid frogs.

Gurdon, J. B. (1970). *Proc. Roy. Soc. (London) Ser. B.* 176: 303–314. Nuclear transplantation and the control of gene activity in animal development.

Gurdon, J. B. (1974). *The Control of Gene Expression in Animal Development*, Harvard Univ. Press, Cambridge Mass.

Gurdon, J. B., and H. R. Woodland (1968). *Biol. Rev.* 43:233–267. The cytoplasmic control of nuclear activity in animal development.

Gurdon, J. B., S. Fairman, T. J. Mohun and S. Brennan (1985). *Cell* 41:913–922. Activation of muscle specific actin genes in *Xenopus* development by an induction between animal and vegetal cells of a blastula.

Gurney, M. (1981). *J. Neurosci.* 1:658–673. Hormonal control of cell form and number in the zebra finch song system.

Gurtrecht, J. A., and P. J. Dyck (1970). *J. Comp. Neurol.* 138:117–129. Quantitative teased-fiber and histologic studies of human sural nerve during postnatal development.

Guth, L. (1956a). *Am. J. Physiol.* 185:205–208. Functional recovery following vagosympathetic anastomosis in the cat.

Guth, L. (1956b). *Physiol. Rev.* 36:441–478. Regeneration in the mammalian peripheral nervous system.

Guth, L. (1958). *Anat. Rec.* 130:25–38. Taste buds on the cat's circumvallate papilla after reinnervation by glossopharyngeal, vagus, and hypoglossal nerves.

Guth, L. (1962). *Exp. Neurol.* 6:129–141. Neuromuscular function after regeneration of interrupted nerve fibers into partially denervated muscles.

Guth, L. (1963). *Exp. Neurol.* 8:336–349. Histological changes following partial denervation of circumvallate papilla of the rat.

Guth, L. (1968). *Physiol. Rev.* 48:645–687. "Trophic" influences of nerve on muscle.

Guth, L. (1971). Degeneration and regeneration of taste buds, pp. 63–74. In *Handbook of Sensory Physiology*, Vol. 4, *Chemical Senses*, Part 2, Springer Verlag, New York.

Guth, L. (1976). *Exp. Neurol.* 51:414–420. Functional plasticity in the respiratory pathway of the mammalian spinal cord.

Guth, L., and J. J. Bernstein (1961). *Exp. Neurol.* 4:59–69. Selectivity in the reestablishment of synapses in the superior cervical sympathetic ganglion of the cat.

Guth, L., and P. K. Watson (1967). *Exp. Neurol.* 17:107–117. The influence of innervation on the soluble proteins of slow and fast muscles of the rat.

Guth, L. R., W. Albers, and W. C. Brown (1964). *Exp. Neurol.* 10:236–250. Quantitative changes in cholinesterase activity of denervated muscle fibres and sole plates.

Guthrie, S. C., and N. B. Gilula (1989). *Trends Neurosci.* 12:12–16. Gap junctional communication and development.

Guthrie, S. C., L. Turin, and A. Warner (1988). *Development* 103:769–783. Patterns of junctional communication during development of the early amphibian embryo.

Gutman, E., and J. Z. Young (1944). *J. Anat. (London)* 78:15–43. The reinnervation of muscle after various periods of atrophy.

Habermas, J. (1971). *Knowledge and Human Interests.* Beacon Press, Boston.

Habermas, J, (1973). *Theory and Practice.* Beacon Press, Boston.

Habermas, J. (1977a). *Communication and the Evolution of Human Society.* Beacon Press, Boston.

Habermas, J. (1977b). A review of Gadamer's Truth and Method, pp. 335–363. In *Understanding and Social Inquiry* (F. R. Dallmeyr, and T. McCarthy, eds.), Notre Dame Univ. Press, Notre Dame.

Habermas, J. (1978). *Knowledge and Human Interests*, 2nd edn., J. J. Shapiro, transl. Heinemann, London.

Habermas, J. (1987). *The Theory of Cummunicative Action*, 2 Vols., T. McCarthy, transl. Beacon Press, Boston.

Hackett, J. T., S. L. Cochran, and D. L. Brown (1979). *Brain Res.* 176:148–152. Functional properties of afferents which synapse on the Mauthner neuron in the amphibian tadpole.

Haddara, M. (1956). *J. Anat. (London)* 90:494–501. A quantitative study of the postnatal changes in the packing density of the neurons in visual cortex of the mouse.

Haddara, M. A., and M. A. Nooreddin (1966). *J. Comp. Neurol.* 128:245–254. A quantitative study on the postnatal development of the cerebellar vermis of mouse.

Hadley, R. D., and S. B. Kater (1983). *J. Neurosci.* 3:924–932. Competence to form electrical connections is restricted to growing neurites in the snail, Helisoma.

Hadley, R. D., S. B. Kater, and C. S. Cohan (1983). *Science* 221:466–468. Electrical synapse formation depends on interaction of mutually growing neurites.

Haeckel, E. (1866). *Generelle Morphologie der Organismen*, G. Reimer, Berlin.

Hafen, K., and B. Salzegeber (1977). Les modalités de la régression du mésonephros chez les amniotes. In *Mécanismes de la Rudimentation des Organes chez les Embryons de Vertébrés* (A. Raynaud, ed.), *Colloques Internationaux du CNRS* 266:251–262.

Hagag, N., S. Halegoua, and M. Viola (1986). *Nature* 319: 680–682. Inhibition of growth factor-induced differentiation of PC12 cells by microinjection of antibody to *ras* p21.

Hagan, H. R. (1951). *Embryology of the viviparous Insects.* Ronald Press, New York, 472 pp.

Haggar, R. A. (1957). *J. Comp. Neurol.* 108:269–283. Behavior of the accessory body of Cajal during axon reaction.

Hahn, W. E., and C. D. Laird (1971). *Science* 173:158–161. Transcription of nonrepeated DNA in mouse brain.

Hajós, F., and E. Bascó (1984). *Adv. Anat. Embryol. Cell Biol.* 84:1–81. The surface contact glia.

Halata, Z. (1981). *Bibl. Anat.* 19:210–235. Postnatale Entwicklung sensibler Nervenendigungen in der unbehaarten Nasenhaut der Katze.

Halata, Z., and B. L. Munger (1986). *Brain Res.* 371:205–230. The neuroanatomical basis for the protopathic sensibility of the human glans penis.

Hale, A. J. (1966). Feulgen microspectrophotometry and its correlation with other cytochemical methods, pp. 183–199. In *Introduction to Quantitative Cytochemistry* (G. L. Wied, ed.), Academic Press, New York.

Halfter, W., M. Claviez, and U. Schwarz (1981). *Nature* 292:67–70. Preferential adhesion of tectal membranes to anterior embryonic chick retina neurites.

Halfter, W., W. Reckhaus, and S. Kröger (1987). *J. Neurosci.* 7:3712–3722. Nondirected axonal growth on basal lamina from avian embryonic neural retina.

Halfter, W., R. Chiquet-Ehrismann, and R. P. Tucker (1989). *Dev. Biol.* 132:14–25. The effect of tenascin and embryonic basal lamina on the behavor and morphology of neural crest cells *in vitro*.

Hall, A. K., and U. Rutishauser (1985). *Dev. Biol.* 110:39–46. Phylogeny of a neural cell adhesion molecule.

Hall, B. K., and R. Tremaine (1979). *Anat. Rec.* 194:469–476. Ability of neural crest cells from the embryonic chick to differentiate into cartilage before their migration away from the neural tube.

Hall, D. E., K. M. Neugebauer, and L. F. Reichardt (1987). *J. Cell. Biol.* 104:623–634. Embryonic neural retinal cell response to extracellular matrix proteins: Developmental changes and effects of the cell substratum attachment antibody (CSAT).

Hall, E. K. (1939). *J. Exp. Zool.* 82:173–192. On the duration of the polarization process in the ear primordium of embryos of *Amblystoma punctatum (Linn.)*.

Hall, E. K., and M. A. Schneiderman (1945). *J. Comp. Neurol.* 82:19–34. Spinal ganglion hypoplasia after limb amputation in the fetal rat.

Hall, P. A., and F. M. Watt (1989). *Development* 106:619–633. Stem cells: The generation and maintenance of cellular diversity.

Hall, Z. W. (1973). *J. Neurobiol.* 4:343–361. Multiple forms of acetylcholinesterase and their distribution in endplate and nonendplate regions of rat diaphragm.

Hall, Z. W., and R. B. Kelly (1971). *Nature (New Biol.)* 232:62–63. Enzymatic detachment of endplate acetylcholinesterase from muscle.

Hallermayer, K., C. Harmening, and B. Hamprecht (1981). *J. Neurochem.* 37:43–52. Cellular localization and regulation of glutamine synthetase in primary cultures of brain cells from newborn mice.

Halley, G. (1955). *J. Anat. (London)* 89:133–152. The placodal relations of the neural crest in the domestic cat.

Halliburton, W. D. (1894). *J. Physiol. (London)* 15:90–107. The proteids of nervous tissue.

Hallonet, M. E. R., M.-A. Teillet, and N. M. LeDouarin (1990). *Development* 108:19–31. A new approach to the development of the cerebellum provided by the quail-chick marker system.

Halstead, D. C., and M. G. Larrabee (1972). Early effects of antiserum to the nerve growth factor on metabolism and transmission in superior cervical ganglia of mice, pp. 221–236. In *Immunosympathectomy* (G. Steiner, and E. Schönbaum, eds.), Elsevier, Amsterdam.

Hamberger, A., C. Bloomstrand, and A. L. Lehninger (1970a) *J. Cell Biol.* 45:221–234. Comparative studies on mitochondria isolated from neurons-enriched and glia-enriched fractions of beef brain.

Hamberger, A., H. A. Hansson, and J. Sjöstrand (1970b). *J. Cell Biol.* 47:319–331. Surface structure of isolated neurons: Detachment of nerve terminals during axon regeneration.

Hamburger, V. (1928). *Arch. Entw.-Mech. Organ.* 114:272–363. Die Entwicklung experimentell erzeugter nervloser und schwach innervierter Extremitäten von Anuren.

Hamburger, V. (1934). *J. Exp. Zool.* 68:449–494. The effects of wing bud extirpation on the development of the central nervous system in chick embryos.

Hamburger, V. (1939). *Physiol. Zool.* 12:268–284. Motor and sensory hyperplasia following limb-bud transplantations in chick embryos.

Hamburger, V. (1946). *J. Exp. Zool.* 103:113–142. Isolation of the brachial segments of the spinal cord of the chick embryo by means of tantalum foil blocks.

Hamburger, V. (1948). *J. Comp. Neurol.* 88:221–283. The mitotic patterns in the spinal cord of the chick embryo and their relation to histogenetic processes.

Hamburger, V. (1958). *Am. J. Anat.* 102:365–410. Regression versus peripheral control of differentiation in motor hypoplasia.

Hamburger, V. (1973). Anatomical and physiological basis of embryonic motility in birds and mammals, pp. 51–76. In *Studies on the Development of Behavior and the Nervous System*, Vol. 1, (G. Gottlieb, ed.), Academic Press, New York.

Hamburger, V. (1975). *J. Comp. Neurol.* 160:535–546. Cell death in the development of the lateral motor column of the chick embryo.

Hamburger, V. (1984). *J. Hist. Biol.* 17:1–11. Hilde Mangold, co-discoverer of the organizer.

Hamburger, V. (1988). *The Heritage of Experimental Embryology. Hans Spemann and the Organizer,* Oxford Univ. Press, New York, and Oxford.

Hamburger, V., and H. Hamilton (1951). *J. Morphol.* 88:49–92. A series of normal stages in the development of the chick embryo.

Hamburger, V., and E. L. Keefe (1944). *J. Exp. Zool.* 96:223–242. The effects of peripheral factors on the proliferation and differentiation in the spinal cord of the chick embryo.

Hamburger, V., and R. Levi-Montalcini (1949). *J. Exp. Zool.* 111:457–501. Proliferation differentiation and degeneration in the spinal ganglia of the chick embryo under normal and experimental conditions.

Hamburger, V., and R. W. Oppenheim (1982). *Neurosci. Com.* 1:39–55. Naturally occurring neuronal death in vertebrates.

Hamburger, V., and M. Waugh (1940). *Physiol. Zool.* 13:367–380. The primary development of the skeleton in nerveless and poorly innervated limb transplants in chick embryos.

Hamburger, V., E. Wenger, and R. Oppenheim (1966). *J. Exp. Zool.* 162:133–160. Motility in the chick embryo in the absence of sensory input.

Hamburger, V., J. K. Brunso-Brechtold, and J. W. Yip (1981). *J. Neurosci.* 1:60–71. Neuronal death in the spinal ganglia of the chick embryo and its reduction by nerve growth factor.

Hamburgh, M. (1960). *Experientia* 16:460. Observations on the neuropathology of "Reeler," a neurological mutation in the mouse.

Hamburgh, M. (1963). *Dev. Biol.* 8:165–185. Analysis of the postnatal development of "reeler" a neurological mutation in mice. A study in developmental genetics.

Hamburgh, M. (1968). *Gen. Comp. Endocrinol.* 10:198–213. An analysis of the action of thyroid hormone on development based on *in vivo* and *in vitro* studies.

Hamburgh, M. (1969). *Curr. Top. Dev. Biol.* 4:109–148. The role of thyroid and growth hormones in neurogenesis.

Hamburgh, M., and R. P. Bunge (1964). *Life Sci.* 3:1423–1430. Evidence for a direct effect of thyroid hormone on maturation of nervous tissue grown *in vitro*.

Hamdi, F. A., and D. Whitteridge (1954). *Quart. J. Exp. Physiol.* 39:111–119. The representation of the retina on the optic lobe of the pigeon.

Hamlyn, D. W. (1961). *Sensation and Perception. A History of the Philosophy of Perception,* Routledge, London.

Hammer, R. P., Jr. (1981). *Dev. Brain Res.* 1:191–201. The influence of pre- and postnatal undernutrition on the developing brain stem reticular core: A quantitative Golgi-study.

Hammerschlag, R., G. C. Stone, F. A. Bolen, J. Lindsey, and M. Ellisman (1982). *J. Cell Biol.* 93:568–575. Evidence that all newly synthesized proteins destined for fast axonal transport pass through the Golgi apparatus.

Hammond, W. S. (1949). *J. Comp. Neurol.* 91:67–86. Formation of the sympathetic nervous system in the trunk of the chick embryo following removal of the thoracic neural tube.

Hammond, W. S., and C. L. Yntema (1947). *J. Comp. Neurol.* 86:237–265. Depletions in the thoraco-lumbar sympathetic system following removal of the neural crest in the chick.

Hammond, W. S., and C. L. Yntema (1958). *J. Comp. Neurol.* 110:367–389. Origin of ciliary ganglia in the chick embryo.

Han, V. K. M., J. M. Lauder, and A. J. D'Ercole (1987). *J. Neurosci.* 7:501–511. Characterization of somatomedin/insulin-like growth factor receptors and correlation with biologic action in cultured neonatal rat astroglial cells.

Hanaway, J. (1967). *J. Comp. Neurol.* 131:1–14. Formation and differentiation of the external granular layer of the chick cerebellum.

Hanaway, J., S. I. Lee, and M. G. Netsky (1968). *Neurology* 18:791–799. Pachygyria: Relation of findings to modern embryologic concepts.

Hanaway, J., J. McConnell, and M. G. Netsky (1971). *J. Comp. Neurol.* 142:59–74. Histogenesis of the substantia nigra, ventral tegmental area of Tsai and interpeduncular nucleus: An autoradiographic study of the mesencephalon in the rat.

Handler, L. C., M. B. Stoch, and P. M. Smythe (1981). *Brit. J. Radiol.* 54:953–954. CT brain scans: Part of a 20-year development study following gross undernutrition during infancy.

Haninec, P. (1988). *Anat. Embryol.* 178:553–557. Study of the origin of connective tissue sheaths of peripheral nerves in the limb of avian embryos.

Hankin, M. H., and J. Silver (1988). *J. Comp. Neurol.* 272:177–190. Development of intersecting CNS fiber tracts: The corpus callosum and its perforating fiber pathway.

Hankin, M. H., B. F. Schneider, and J. Silver (1988). *J. Comp. Neurol.* 272:191–202. Death of the subcallosal glial sling is correlated with formation of the cavum septi pellucidi.

Hanna, R. B., A. Hirano, and G. D. Pappas (1976). *J. Cell Biol.* 68:403–410. Membrane specialization of dendrite spines and glia in the weaver mouse cerebellum: A freeze-fracture study.

Hannah, R. S., and E. J. H. Nathaniel (1974). *Anat. Rec.* 178:691–710. The post-natal development of blood vessels in the substantia gelatinosa of rat cervical cord. An ultrastructural study.

Hansson, E., L. Ronnback, and A. Sellstrom (1984). *Neurochem. Res.* 9:679–689. Is there a "Dopaminergic glial cell"?

Hansson, H. A., and J. Sjöstrand (1971). *Brain Res.* 35:379–396. Ultrastructural effects of colchicine on the hypoglossal and dorsal vagal neurons of the rabbit.

Hansson, H. A., and P. Sourander (1964). *Z. Zellforsch* 62:26–47. Studies on cultures of mammalian retina.

Hanström, B (1926). *Z. Mikroskop.-Anat. Forsch.* 7:135–190. Untersuchungen über die relative Grösse der Gehirnzentren verschiedener Arthropoden unter Berücksichtigung der Lebensweise.

Harcombe-Smith, E., and R. J. Wyman (1970). *J. Exp. Biol.* 53:255–263. Diagonal locomotion in deafferented toads.

Hardesty, I. (1904). *Am. J. Anat.* 3:229–268. On the development and nature of the neuroglia.

Hardesty, I. (1905). *Am. J. Anat.* 4:329–354. On the occurrence of sheath cells and the nature of the axone sheaths in the central nervous system.

Harding, K., C. Weeden, W. McGinnis, and M. Levine (1985). *Science* 229:1236–1242. Spatially regulated expression of homeotic genes in *Drosophila.*

Hardman, V. J., and M. C. Brown (1985). *Dev. Brain Res.* 19:1–9. Absence of postnatal death among motoneurons supplying the inferior gluteal nerve of the rat.

Hardman, V. J., and M. C. Brown (1987). *J. Neurosci.* 7:1031–1036. Accuracy of reinnervation of rat internal intercostal muscles by their own segmental nerves.

Hare, W. K., and J. C. Hinsey (1940). *J. Comp. Neurol.* 73:489–502. Reaction of dorsal root ganglion cells to section of peripheral and central processes.

Hargreaves, A., B. Yusta, A. Aranda, J. Avila, and A. Pascual (1988). *Dev. Brain Res.* 38:141–148. Triiodothyronine (T3) induces neurite formation and increased synthesis of a protein related to MAP 1B in cultured cells of neuronal origin.

Harkmark, W. (1954). *J. Comp. Neurol.* 100:115–209. Cell migrations from the rhombic lip to the inferior olive, the nucleus raphe and the pons. A morphological and experimental investigation on chick embryos.

Harkmark, W. (1956). *J. Exp. Zool.* 131:333–371. The influence of the cerebellum on development and maintenance of the inferior olive and the pons. An experimental investigation on chick embryos.

Harman, A. M., and L. D. Beazley (1986). *Anat. Embryol.* 175:181–188. Development of visual projections in the marsupial, *Setonix brachyurus.*

Harman, A. M., L. L. Snell, and L. D. Beazley (1989). *J. Comp. Neurol.* 289:1–10. Cell death in the inner and outer nuclear layers of the developing retina in the wallaby *Setonix brachyurus* (Quokka).

Harman, J. (1947). *Anat. Rec.* 97:342. Quantitative analysis of the brain-isocortex relationship in mammals.

Harms, J. W. (1927). *Zool. Anz.* 74:249–256. Alterscheinungen im Hirn von Affen und Menschen.

Harper, G. P., and H. Thoenen (1980). *J. Neurochem.* 34:5–16. Nerve growth factor: Biological significance, measurement and distribution.

Harris, A. (1972). *Acta Protozool.* 11:145–151. Surface movement in fibroblast locomotion.

Harris, A., and G. Dunn (1972). *Exp. Cell Res.* 73:519–522. Centripetal transport of attached particles on both surfaces of moving fibroblasts.

Harris-Flannagan, A. E. (1969). *J. Morphol.* 129:281–306. Differentiation and degeneration in the motor horn of the foetal mouse.

Harris, A. J. (1974). *Ann. Rev. Physiol.* 36:251–305. Inductive functions of the nervous system.

Harris, A. J. (1981). *Phil. Trans. Roy. Soc. (London) B.* 293:287–314. Embryonic growth and innervation of rat skeletal muscles. III. Neural regulation of junctional and extra-junctional acetylcholine receptor clusters.

Harris, A. J., R. B. Fitzsimons, and J. C. McEwan (1989a). *Development* 107:751–769. Neural control of the sequence of expression of myosin heavy chain isoforms in foetal mammalian muslce.

Harris, A. J., M.. J. Duxson, R. B. Fitzsimons, and F. Rieger (1989b). *Development* 107:771–784. Myonuclear birthdates distinguish the origins of primary and secondary myotubes in embryonic mammalian skeletal muscles.

Harris, G. W. (1964). *Endocrinol.* 75:627–648. Sex hormones, brain development and brain functions.

Harris, G. W., and S. Levine (1962). *J. Physiol. (London)* 163:42–43. Sexual differentiation of the brain and its experimental control.

Harris, G. W., and S. Levine (1965). *J. Physiol. (London)* 181:379–400. Sexual differentiation of the brain and its experimental control.

Harris, H. (1954). *Physiol. Res.* 34:529–562. Role of chemotaxis in inflammation.

Harris, H., J. J. Watkins, C. E. Ford, and G. I. Schoefl (1966). *J. Cell Sci.* 1:1–30. Artificial heterokaryons of animal cells from different species.

Harris, J. B., and S. Thesleff (1972). *Nature (New Biol.)* 236:60–61. Nerve stump length and membrane changes in denervated skeletal muscle.

Harris, K. M., and J. K. Stevens (1988). *J. Neurosci.* 8:4455–4469. Dendritic spines of rat cerebellar Purkinje cells: Serial electron microscopy with reference to their biophysical characteristics.

Harris, K. M., and J. K. Stevens (1989). *J. Neurosci.* 9:2982–2997. Dendritic spines of CA1 pyramidal cells in the rat hippocampus: Serial electron microscopy with reference to their biophysical characteristics.

Harris, L. J. (1978). Sex differences in spatial ability. Possible environmental, genetic and neurological factors. In *Asymmetrical function of the brain* (J. Kinsbourne, ed.), Cambridge University Press, Cambridge, Mass.

Harris, R. M., and T. A. Woolsey (1981). *J. Comp. Neurol.* 196:357–376. Dendritic plasticity in mouse barrel cortex following postnatal vibrissa follicle damage.

Harris, W. A. (1980). *J. Comp. Neurol.* 194:303–317. The effects of eliminating impulse activity on the development of the retinotectal projection in salamanders.

Harris, W. A. (1982). *J. Neurosci.* 2:339–353. The transplantation of eyes to genetically eyeless salamanders: Visual projections and somatosensory interactions.

Harris, W. A. (1984). *J. Neurosci.* 4:1153–1162. Axonal pathfinding in the absence of normal pathways and impulse activity.

Harris, W. A., C. E. Holt, and F. Bonhoeffer (1987). *Development* 101:123–133. Retinal axons with and withouit their somata growing to and arborizing in the tectum of *Xenopus* embryos: A time-lapse video study of single fibres *in vivo*.

Harrison, P. J., H. Hultborn, E. Jankowska, R. Katz, B. Storai, and D. Zytnicki (1984). *Neurosci. Lett.* 45:15–19. Labelling of interneurones by retrograde transsynaptic transport of horseradish peroxidase from motoneurones in rats and cats.

Harrison, R. G. (1901). *Arch. Mikroskop. Anat.* 57:354–444. Ueber die Histogenese des peripheren Nervensystems bei Salmo salar.

Harrison, R. G. (1903). *Arch. Mikroskop. Anat.* 63:35–149. Experimentelle Untersuchungen über die Entwicklung der Sinnesorgane der Seitenlinie bei den Amphibien.

Harrison, R. G. (1904). *Am. J. Anat.* 3:197–220. An experimental study of the relation of the nervous system to the developing musculature in the embryo of the frog.

Harrison, R. G. (1906). *Am. J. Anat.* 5:121–131. Further experiments on the development of peripheral nerves.

Harrison, R. G. (1907a). *J. Exp. Zool.* 4:239–281. Experiments in transplanting limbs and their bearing upon the problem of the development of nerves.

Harrison, R. G. (1907b). *Anat. Rec.* 1:116–118. Observations on the living developing nerve fiber.

Harrison, R. G. (1910). *J. Exp. Zool.* 9:787–846. The outgrowth of the nerve fiber as a mode of protoplasmic movement.

Harrison, R. G. (1911). *Science* 34:279. On the stereotropism of embryonic cells.

Harrison, R. G. (1912). *Anat. Rec.* 6:181–193. The cultivation of tissues in extraneous media as a method of morphogenetic study.

Harrison, R. G. (1914). *J. Exp. Zool.* 17:521–544. The reaction of embryonic cells to solid structures.

Harrison, R. G. (1918). *J. Exp. Zool.* 25:413–461. Experiments on the development of the fore limb of *Amblystoma*, a self-differentiating equipotential system.

Harrison, R. G. (1921). *J. Exp. Zool.* 32:1–136. On relations of symmetry in transplanted limbs.

Harrison, R. G. (1924a). *J. Comp. Neurol.* 37:123–205. Neuroblast versus sheath cell in the development of peripheral nerves.

Harrison, R. G. (1924b). *Proc. Natl. Acad. Sci. U.S.A.* 10:69–74. Some unexpected results of the heteroplastic transplantation of limbs.

Harrison, R. G. (1925). *Arch. Entw.-Mech. Organ.* 106:469–502. The effect of reversing the medio-lateral or transverse axis of the forelimb bud in the salamander embryo (*Amblystoma punctatum Linn*).

Harrison, R. G. (1929). *Arch. Entw.-Mech. Organ.* 120:1–55. Correlation in the development and growth of the eye studied by means of heteroplastic transplantation.

Harrison, R. G. (1935). *Proc. Roy. Soc. (London) Ser. B.* 118:155–196. On the origin and development of the nervous system studied by the methods of experimental embryology.

Harrison, R. G. (1936). *Proc. Natl. Acad. Sci. U.S.A.* 22:238–247. Relations of symmetry in the developing ear of *Amblystoma punctatum*.

Harrison, R. G. (1937–38). *Anat. Anz.* 85:4–30. Die Neuralleiste.

Harrison, R. G. (1945). *Trans. Conn. Acad. Arts Sci.* 36:277–330. Relations of symmetry in the developing embryo.

Harrison, R. G. (1947). *J. Exp. Zool.* 106:27–83. Wound healing and reconstitution of the central nervous system of the amphibian embryo after removal of parts of the neural plate.

Hartenstein, V., and J. A. Campos-Ortega (1984). *Roux Arch. Dev. Biol.* 193:308–325. Early neurogenesis in wild-type *Drosophila melanogaster*.

Hartlieb, E., and C. A. O. Stuermer (1989). *J. Comp. Neurol.* 284:148–168. Pathfinding and target selection of goldfish retinal axons regenerating under TTX-induced impulse blockade.

Hartschuh, W., E. Weihe, M. Büchler, V. Helmstaedter, G. E. Feurle, and W. G. Forssmann (1979). *Cell Tissue Res.* 201:343–348. Met-enkephalin-like immunoreactivity in Merkel cells.

Hartschuh, W., E. Weihe, and M. Büchler (1980). *J. Invest. Dermatol.* 74:453. Met-enkephalin-like immunoreactivity in Merkel cells of various species.

Hartschuh, W., E. Weihe, N. Yanaihara, and M. Reinecke (1983). *J. Invest. Dermatol.* 81:361–364. Immunohistochemical localization of vasoactive intestinal polypeptide (VIP) in Merkel cells of various mammals: Evidence for a neuromodulator function of the Merkel cell.

Hartschuh, W., M. Reinecke, E. Weihe, and N. Yanaihara (1984). *Peptides* 5:239–245. VIP-immunoreactivity in the skin of various mammals: Immunohistochemical, radioimmunological and experimental evidence for a dual localization in cutaneous nerves and Merkel cells.

Hartschuh, W., E. Weihe, and M. Reinecke (1986). The Merkel cell, pp. 605–620. In *Biology of the integument*, Vol. 2 *Vertebrates* (J. Bereiter-Hahn, A. G. Matoltsy, and K. S. Richards, eds.), Springer Verlag, Berlin.

Hartwell, L. H., and T. A. Weinert (1989). *Science* 246:629–634. Checkpoints: Controls that ensure the order of cell cycle events.

Hartzell, H. C., and D. M. Fambrough (1972). *J. Gen. Physiol.* 60:248–262. Acetylcholine receptors. Distribution and extrajunctional density in rat diaphragm after denervation correlated with acetylcholine sensitivity.

Hartzell, H. C., S. W. Kuffler, D. Yoshikami (1976). *Cold Spring Harbor Symp. Quant. Biol.* 40:175–186. The number of acetylcholine molecules in a quantum and the interaction between quanta at the subsynaptic membrane of the skeletal neuromuscular synapse.

Harvey, R. P., C. J. Tabin, and D. A. Melton (1986). *EMBO J.* 5:1237–1244. Embryonic expression and nuclear localization of *Xenopus* homeobox (Xhox) gene products.

Harvey, S. C., and H. S. Burr (1926). *Arch. Neurol. Psychiatry* 15:545. The development of the meninges.

Harvey, S. C., H. S. Burr, and E. VanCampenhout (1933). *Arch. Neurol. Psychiatry* 29:683–690. Development of the meninges. Further experiments.

Hashimoto, K. (1972). *J. Anat. (London)* 111:99–120. The ultrastructure of human embryos. X. Merkel tactile cells in the finger and nail.

Hassan, S., and E. M. Lieberman (1988). *J. Neurosci.* 25:961–969. Studies of axon-glial cell interactions and periaxonal K homeostasis. II. The effect of axonal stimulation, cholinergic agents and transport inhibitors on the resistance in series with the axon membrane.

Hassler, R. (1966). Comparative anatomy of the central visual systems in day- and night-active primates, pp. 419–434. In *Evolution of the Forebrain* (R. Hassler, and H. Stephen, eds.), Stuttgart: Thieme.

Hatai, S. (1901). *J. Comp. Neurol.* 11:25–39. On the presence of the centrosome in certain nerve cells of the white rat.

Hatai, S. (1902). *J. Comp. Neurol.* 12:291–296. On the origin of neuroglia tissue from the mesoblast.

Hatai, S. (1910). *J. Comp. Neurol.* 20:1l9–47. On the length of the internodes in the sciatic nerve of *Rana temporaria* (fusca) and *Rana pipiens:* Being a reexamination by biometric methods of the data studied by Boycott (1904) and Takahashi (1908).

Hatta, K., and M. Takeichi (1986). *Nature* 320:447–449. Expression of N-cadherin adhesion molecules associated with early morphogenetic events in chick development.

Hatta, K., S. Takagi, H. Fujisawa, and M. Takeichi (1987). *Dev. Biol.* 120:215–227. Spatial and temporal expression pattern of N-cadherin cell adhesion molecules correlated with morphogenetic processes of chicken embryos.

Hatta, K., A. Nose, A. Nagafuchi, and M. Takeichi (1988). *J. Cell Biol.* 106:873–881. Cloning and expression of cDNA encoding a neural calcium-dependent cell adhesion molecule: Its identity in the cadherin gene family.

Hatten, M. E. (1985). *J. Cell Biol.* 100:384–396. Neuronal regulation of astroglial morphology and proliferation *in vitro*.

Hatten, M. E., M. B. Furie, and D. B. Rifkin (1982). *J. Neurosci.* 2:1195–1206. Binding of developing mouse cerebellar cells to fibronectin: A possible mechanism for the formation of the external granular layer.

Hatten, M. E., R. K. H. Liem, and C. A. Mason (1984). *J. Neurosci.* 4:1163–1172. Defects in specific associations between astroglia and neurons occur in microcultures of weaver mouse cerebellar cells.

Hatten, M. E., R. K. H. Liem, and C. A. Mason (1986). *J. Neurosci.* 6:2676–2683. Weaver mouse cerebellar granule neurons fail to migrate on wild-type astroglial processes *in vitro*.

Hatten, M. E., M. Lynch, R. E. Rydel, J. Sanchez, J. Joseph-Silverstein, D. Moscatelli, and D. B. Rifkin (1988). *Dev. Biol.* 125:280–289. *In vitro* neurite extension by granule neurons is dependent upon astroglial-derived fibroblast growth factor.

Hatton, G. I. (1985). Reversible synapse formation and modulation of cellular relationships in the adult hypothalamus under physiological conditions, pp. 373–404. In *Synaptic Plasticity* (C. W. Cotman, ed.), Guilford Press, New York.

Hatton, G. I. (1986). *Fed. Proc.* 45:2328–2333. Plasticity in the hypothalamic magnocellular neurosecretory system.

Haug, H. (1956). *J. Comp. Neurol.* 104:473–492. Remarks on the determination and significance of the grey cell coefficient.

Haug, H. (1960). Die Quantitative Zellvolumenverhaltnisse der Hirnrinde. In *Structure and Function of the Cerebral Cortex* (D. B. Tower, and J. P. Schadé, eds.), Elsevier, Amsterdam.

Haug, H. (1967a). *Z. Zellforsch. Mikroskop. Anat. Abt. Histochem.* 83:265–278. Die Länge der Internodien der Markfasern im Bereich der Sehrinde der erwachsenen Katze.

Haug, H. (1967b). Acta Anat. (Basel) 67:53–73. Über die exakte Feststellung der Anzahl Nervenzellen pro Volumeneinheit des Cortex cerebri, zugleich ein Beispiel für die Durchführung genauer Zählungen.

Haug, H. (1970). *Ergebn. Anat. EntwGesch* 43:6–70. Der makroskopische Aufbau des Grosshirns.

Haug, H. (1972). *Z. Zellforsch. Mikrosk. Anat.* 123:544–565. Die post-natale Entwicklung der Gliadeckschicht der sehrinde der Katze. Eine electronenmikroskopische Studie über die Ausbildung von Lamellenstapeln.

Haug, H. (1981). *Nova Acta Leopoldina N. F.* 245:763–777. Die Evolution der Interneurone in der Hirnrinde von Affen und Delphinen sowie ihre Bedeutung für komplexe Funktionen einschließich der Sprache.

Haug, H. (1984). *Gegenbaurs Morphol. Jahrb.* 130:481–500. Der Einfluß der säkularen Akzeleration auf das Hirngewicht des Menschen und dessen Änderung während der Alterung.

Haug, H. (1987). *Am. J. Anat.* 180:126–142. Brain sizes, surfaces and neuronal sizes of the cortex cerebri. A stereological investigation of man and his variability and a comparison with some mammals (primates, whales, marsupialia, insectivores and one elephant).

Hauser, K. F., P. J. McLaughlin, and I. S. Zagon (1989). *J. Comp. Neurol.* 281:13–22. Endogenous opioid systems and the regulation of dendritic growth and spine formation.

Hauser, K. F., P. J. McLaughlin, and I. S. Zagon (1987). *Brain Res.* 416:157–161. Endogenous opioids regulate dendritic growth and spine formation in developing rat brain.

Hausman, R. E., and A. A. Moscona (1975). *Proc. Natl. Acad. Sci. U.S.A.* 72: 916–920. Purification and characterization of the retina-specific cell-aggregating factor.

Hausmann, B., and J. Sievers (1985). *J. Comp. Neurol.* 241:50–62. Cerebellar external granule cells are attached to the basal lamina from the onset of migration up to the End of their proliferative activity.

Hauw, J. J., B. Berger, and R. Escourolle (1975). *Acta Neuropathol.* 31:229–242. Electron microscopic study of the developing capillaries of human brain.

Hawkes, R., and N. Leclerc (1987). *J. Comp. Neurol.* 256:29–41. Antigenic map of the rat cerebellar cortex: The distribution of parasagittal bands as revealed by monoclonal anti-Purkinje cell antibody mabQ113.

Hawkes, R., E. Niday, and J. Gordon (1982). *Anal. Biochem.* 119:142–147. A dot-immunobinding assay for monoclonal and other antibodies.

Hawkes, R., M. Colonnier, and N. Leclerc (1985). *Brain Res.* 333:359–365. Monoclonal antibodies reveal sagittal banding in the rodent cerebellar cortex.

Hawkins, A., and J. Olszewski (1957). *Science* 126:76–77. Glia/nerve cell index for cortex of the whale.

Hawrot, E. (1980). *Dev. Biol.* 74:136–151. Cultured sympathetic neurons: Effects of cell-derived and synthetic substrata on survival and development.

Hay, E. D. (1981). Collagen and embryonic development, pp. 379–409. In *Cell Biology of Extracellular Matrix* (E. D. Hay, ed.), Plenum Press, New York and London.

Hayashi, M. (1924). *Dtsch. Z. Nervenheilk.* 81:74–82. Einige wichtige Tatsachen aus der ontogenetischen Entwicklung des menschlichen Kleinhirns.

Hayashi, M., D. Edgar, and H. Thoenen (1985). *Dev. Biol.* 118:49–55. Nerve growth factor changes the relative levels of neuropeptides in developing sensory and sympathetic ganglia of the chick embryo.

Haydon, P. G., D. P. McCobb, and S. B. Kater (1987). *J. Neurobiol.* 18:197–215. The regulation of neurite outgrowth, growth cone motility, and electrical synaptogenesis by serotonin.

Hayes, B. P. (1976). *Anat. Embryol.* 150:99–111. The distribution of intercellular gap junctions in the developing retina and pigment epithelium of *Xenopus laevis*.

Hayes, B. P., and A. Roberts (1973). *Z. Zellforsch Mikrosk. Anat.* 137:251–269. Synaptic junction development in the spinal cord of an amphibian embryo: An electron microscope study.

Hayes, B. P., and A. Roberts (1974). *Cell Tissue Res.* 153:227–244. The distribution of synapses along the spinal cord of an amphibian embryo: An electron microscope study of junction development.

Hayes, W. P., and R. L. Meyer (1989a). *J. Neurosci.* 9:1400–1413. Normal numbers of retinotectal synapses during the activity-sensitive period of optic regeneration in goldfish: HRP-EM evidence implicating synapse reearrangement and collateral elimination during map refinement.

Hayes, W. P., and R. L. Meyer (1989b). *J. Neurosci.* 9:1414–1423. Impulse blockade by intraocular tetrodotoxin during optic regeneration in goldfish: HRP-EM evidence that the formation of normal numbers of optic synapses and the elimination of exuberant optic fibers is activity independent.

Hayles, J., and P. Nurse (1986). *J. Cell Sci. Suppl.* 4:155–170. Cell cycle regulation in yeast.

Haymaker, W. (1953). *The Founders of Neurology. One Hundred and Thirty-Three Biographical Sketches*, Thomas, Springfield.

Haymaker, W., and F. Schiller (1970). *The Founders of Neurology*, 2nd edn. Thomas, Springfield, Illinois.

Hayman, E. G., M. D. Pierschbacher, Y. Ohgren, and E. Ruoslahti (1983). *Proc. Natl. Acad. Sci. U.S.A.* 80:4003–4007. Serum spreading factor (vitronectin) is present at the cell surface and in tissues.

Hayman, E. G., M. D. Pierschbacher, S. Suzuki, and E. Ruoslahti (1985). *Exp. Cell Res.* 160:245–258. Vitronectin-a major cell attachment-promoting protein in fetal bovine serum.

Hearnshaw, L. S. (1964). *A Short History of British Psychology (1840–1940)*, Methuen, London.

Heathcote, R. D., and P. B. Sargent (1985). *J. Neurosci.* 5:1940–1946. Loss of supernumerary axons during neuronal morphogenesis.

Heaton, M. B. (1977). *Dev. Biol.* 58:421–427. Retrograde axonal transport in lateral motor neurons of chick embryo prior to limb bud innervation.

Heaton, M. B., and S. A. Moody (1980). *J. Comp. Neurol.* 189:61–99. Early development and migration of the trigeminal motor nucleus in the chick embryo.

Heaysman, J. E. M. (1978). *Int. Rev. Cytol.* 55:49–66. Contact inhibition of locomotion: A reappraisal.

Hebb, D. H. (1949). *The organization of Behavior.* John Wiley, New York.

Hebb, D. H. (1966). *A Textbook of Psychology.* 2nd edn. Saunders, Philadelphia.

Hebb, D. O. (1959). A neuropsychological theory, pp. 622–643. In *Psychology: A Study of a Science. Study I*, Vol. 1, McGraw-Hill, New York.

Heckroth, J. A., D. Goldowitz, and L. M. Eisenman (1989). *J. Comp. Neurol.* 279:546–555. Purkinje cell reduction in the Reeler mutant mouse: A quantitative immunohistochemical study.

Hefti, F. (1986). *J. Neurosci.* 6:2155–2162. Nerve growth factor promotes survival of septal cholinergic neurons after fimbrial transections.

Hefti, F., and W. J. Weiner (1986). *Ann. Neurol.* 20:275–281. Nerve growth factor and Alzheimer's disease.

Hefti, F., J. Hartikka, F. Eckenstein, H. Gnahn, R. Heumann, and M. Schwab (1985). *Neuroscience* 14:55–68. Nerve growth factor increases choline acetyltransferase but not survival or fiber outgrowth of cultured fetal septal cholinergic neurons.

Hefti, F., J. Hartikka, A. Salvatierra, W. J. Weinger, and D. C. Mash (1986). *Neurosci. Lett.* 69:37–41. Localization of nerve growth factor receptors in cholinergic neurons of the human basal forebrain.

Heidemann, S. R., and J. R. McIntosh (1980). *Nature* **286**:517–519. Visualization of the structural polarity of microtubules.

Heidemann, S. R., J. M. Landers, and M. A. Hamborg (1981). *J. Cell Biol.* **91**:661–665. Polarity orientation of axonal microtubules.

Heidmann, O., A. Buonanno, B. Goeffroy, B. Robert, J. L. Guénet, J. P. Merlie, and J. P. Changeux (1986). *Science* **234**:866–868. Chromosomal localization of the nicotinic acetylcholine receptor genes in the mouse.

Heilbronn, E., C. Mattsson, L. E. Thornell, M. Sjöström, E. Stålberg, P. Hilton-Brown, and D. Elmqvist (1976). *Ann. N.Y. Acad. Sci.* **274**:337–353. Experimental myasthenia in rabbits: Biochemical, immunological, electrophysiological and morphological aspects.

Heimann, R., M. L. Shelanksi, and R. K. H. Liem (1985). *J. Biol. Chem.* **260**:12160–12166. Microtubule-associated proteins bind specifically to the 70-kDa neurofilament protein.

Heine, U. I., E. F. Munoz, K. C. Flanders, L. R. Ellingsworth, H.-Y. P. Lam, N. L. Thompson, A. B. Roberts, and M. B. Sporn (1987). *J. Cell Biol.* **105**:2861–2876. Role of transforming growth factor-β in the development of the mouse embryo.

Held, H. (1891). *Arch. Anat. Physiol. Lpz.* 270–291. Die centralen Bahnen des Nervous acusticus bei der Katze.

Held, H. (1897a). *Arch. Anat. Physiol. Anat. Abt.* **21**:204–294. Beiträge zur Struktur der Nervenzellen und ihrer Fortsätze (Zweite Abhandlung).

Held, H. (1897b). *Arch. Anat. Physiol. Anat. Abt. Leipzig Suppl.* pp. 273–312. Beiträge zur Struktur der Nervenzellen und ihre Fortsätze. Dritte Abhandlung.

Held, H. (1904). *Abhandl. Math. Physikal. Klasse Kgl. Sachs. Ges. Wiss.* **28**:199–318. Über den Bau der Neuroglia und über die Wand der Lymphgefasse in Haut und Schleimhaut.

Held, H. (1905). *Arch. Anat. Physiol.* Leipzig 55–78. Zur Kenntniss einer neurofibrillären. Continuität im Centralnervensystem der Wirbelthiere.

Held, H. (1909). *Die Entwicklung des Nervengewebes bei den Wirbeltieren.* Barth, Leipzig.

Held, H. (1929). *Forschr. Naturwissen. Forsch. Neue Folge., Heft 8.* Die Lehre von den Neuronen und vom Neurencytium und ihre heutiger Stand.

Heller, I. H., and K. A. C. Elliott (1954). *Con. J. Biochem. Physiol.* **32**:584–592. Desoxyribonucleic acid content and cell density in brain and human brain tumors.

Helmholtz, H. (1847). Ueber die Erhaltung der Kraft. Vortrag in der physikalischen Gesellschaft zu Berlin.

Hempel, C. G. (1966). *Philosophy of Natural Science.* Prentice-Hall, Englewood Cliffs, New Jersey.

Hempstead, B. L., L. S. Schleifer, and M. V. Chao (1989). *Science* **243**:373–375. Expression of functional nerve growth factor receptors after gene transfer.

Hendelman, W. J., and A. S. Aggerwal (1980). *J. Comp. Neurol.* **193**:1063–1079. The Purkinje neuron: I. A Golgi study of its development in the mouse and in culture.

Henderson, C. E. (1988). The role of muscle in the development and differentiation of spinal motoneurons: *In vitro* studies. In *Plasticity of the Neuromuscular System, Ciba Foundation Symposium* **138**:172–191. (D. Evered, and J. Whelan, eds.), Wiley, Chichester.

Henderson, L. P., and N. C. Spitzer (1986). *Dev. Biol.* **113**:381–387. Autonomous early differentiation of neurons and muscle cells in single cell cultures.

Henderson, L. P., M. A. Smith, and N. C. Spitzer (1984). *J. Neurosci.* **4**:3140–3150. The absence of calcium blocks impulse-evoked release of acetylcholine but not de novo formation of functional neuromuscular synaptic contacts in culture.

Hendrickson, A., and R. Boothe (1976). *Vision Res.* **16**:517–521. Morphology of the retina and dorsal lateral geniculate nucleus in dark-reared monkeys (*Macaca nemestrina*).

Hendrickson, A., and C. Kupfer (1976). *Invest. Ophthalmol.* **15**:746–756. The histogenesis of the fovea in the macaque monkey.

Hendrickson, A., and C. Yuodelis (1984). *Ophthalmology* **91**:603–612. The morphological development of the human fovea.

Hendrickson, A. E., and W. M. Cowan (1971). *Exp. Neurol.* **30**:403–422. Changes in the rate of axoplasmic transport during postnatal development of the rabbit's optic nerve and tract.

Hendrickson, A. E., S. P. Hunt, and J.-Y. Wu (1981). *Nature* **292**:605–607. Immunocytochemical localization of glutamic acid decarboxylase in monkey striate cortex.

Hendrikson, C. K., and J. E. Vaughn (1974). *J. Neurocytol.* **3**:659–675. Fine structural relationships between neurites and radial glial processes in developing mouse spinal cord.

Hendry, I. A. (1976). *J. Neurocytol.* **5**:337–349. A method to correct adequately for the change in neuronal size when estimating neuronal numbers after nerve growth factor treatment.

Hendry, I. A., and J. Campbell (1976). *J. Neurocytol.* **5**:351–360. Morphometric analysis of rat superior cervical ganglion after axotomy and nerve growth factor treatment.

Hendry, I. A., and L. L. Iversen (1971). *Brain Res.* **29**:159–162. Effect of nerve growth factor and its antiserum on tyrosine hydroxylase activity in mouse superior cervical sympathetic ganglion.

Hendry, I. A., and L. L. Iversen (1973). *Nature* **243**:500–504. Reduction in the concentration of nerve growth factor in mice after sialectomy and castration.

Hendry, I. A., K. Stockel, H. Thoenen, and L. L. Iversen (1974a). *Brain Res.* **68**:103–121. The retrograde axonal transport of nerve growth factor.

Hendry, I. A., R. Stach, and K. Herrup (1974b). *Brain Res.* **82**:117–128. Characteristics of the retrograde axonal transport system for nerve growth factor in the sympathetic nervous system.

Henkin, R. I., and L. J. Kopin (1964). *Life Sci.* **3**:1319–1325. Abnormalities of taste and smell thresholds in familial dysautonomia: improvement with methacholine.

Henle, J. (1871). *Handbuch der systematischen Anatomie des Menschen, Bd. 3, Nervenlehre.* F. Vieweg, Braunschweig.

Henneman, E., and C. B. Olson (1965). *J. Neurophysiol.* **28**:581–598. Relations between structure and function in the design of skeletal muscles.

Henneman, E., G. Somien, and D. O. Carpenter (1965). *J. Neurophysiol.* **28**:560–580. Functional significance of cell size in spinal motoneurons.

Henrikson, C. K., and J. E. Vaughn (1974). *J. Neurocytol.* **3**:659–675. Fine structural relationships between neurites and radial glial processes in developing mouse spinal cord.

Henry, E. W., and R. L. Sidman (1988). *Science* 241:344–346. Long lives for homozygous trembler mutant mice despite virtual absence of peripheral nerve myelin.

Henry, G. H. (1991). Afferent inputs, receptive field properties and morphological cell types in different laminae of the striate cortex, pp. 223–245. In *The Neural Basis of Visual Function* (A. G. Leventhal, ed.), Macmillan, London.

Herbst, C. (1894). *Biol. Centralbl.* 14. Ueber die Bedeutung der Reizphysiologie für die kausale Auffassung von Vorgängen in die Thierische Ontogenie.

Heringa, G. C. (1918). *Arch. Néerl. Sci. Ex. Nat.* 3:235–315. Le développement des corpuscles de Grandry et de Herbst.

Herlant, M. (1964). *Int. Rev. Cyto.* 17:299–382. The cells of the adenohypophysis and their functional significance.

Herman, C. J., and L. W. Lapham (1968). *Science* 160:537. DNA content of neurons in the cat hippocampus.

Herman, C. J., and L. W. Lapham (1969). *Brain Res.* 15:35–48. Neuronal polyploidy and nuclear volumes in the cat central nervous system.

Herman, L., and S. L. Kauffman (1966). *Dev. Biol.* 13:145–162. The fine structure of the embryonic mouse neural tube with special reference to cytoplasmic microtubules.

Herman, R. K. (1989). *J. Neurogen.* 5:1–24. Mosaic analysis in the nematode *caenorhabditis elegans.*

Hermann, F. (1884). *Arch. f. mikr. Anat.* 24:216–229. Beitrag zur Entwicklungsgeschigte des Geschmacksorgans beim Kaninchen.

Herndon, R. M. (1963). *J. Cell Biol.* 18:167–180. The fine structure of the Purkinje cell.

Herndon, R. M. (1968). *Exp. Brain Res.* 6:49–68. Thiophen induced granule cell necrosis in the rat cerebellum.

Herndon, R. M., and M. L. Oster-Granite (1975a). *Adv. Neurol.* 12:361–371. Effect of granule cell destruction on development and maintenance of Purkinje cell dendrite.

Herndon, R. M., and M. L. Oster-Granite (1975b). Effect of the granule cell destruction on development and maintenance of the Purkinje cell dendrite, pp. 361–371. In *Physiology and Pathology of Dendrites* (G. W. Kreutzberg, ed.), Raven Press, New York.

Herndon, R. M., G. Margolis, and L. Kilham (1971a). *J. Neuropathol. Exp. Neurol.* 30:196–205. The synaptic organization of the malformed cerebellum induced by perinatal infection with the feline panleukopenia virus (PLV). I. Elements forming the cerebellar glomeruli.

Herndon, R. M., G. Margolis, and L. Kilham (1971b). *J. Neuropathol. Exp. Neurol.* 30:557–570. The synaptic organization of the malformed cerebellum induced by perinatal infection with the feline panelukopenia virus (PLV). II. The Purkinje cell and its afferents.

Herre, W. (1936). *Verhandl, Deut. Zool. Ges. Freiburg* 200–211. Untersuchungen an Hirnen von Wild und Hausschweinen.

Herre, W. (1958). *Deut. Med. Wochschr.* 83:1568–1574. Einflüsse der Umwelt auf das Säugetiergehirn.

Herre, W. (1966). Einige Bemerkungen zur Modifikabilität, Vererbung und Evolution von Merkmalen des Vorderhirns bei Säugetieren, pp. 162–174. In *Evolution of the Forebrain* (R. Hassler, and H. Stephan, eds.), Plenum Press, New York.

Herre, W., and M. Röhrs (1971). Domestikation und Stammesgeschichte, pp. 29–174. In *Heberer, Die Evolution der Organismen*, Bd. II/2, Fischer, Stuttgart.

Herre, W., and U. Thiede (1965). *Zool. Jahrb. Abt. Anat. Ontog. Tiere* 82:155–176. Studien an Gehirnen südamerikanischer Tylopoden.

Herrick, C. J. (1908). *J. Comp. Neurol.* 18:373- . The morphological subdivisions of the brain.

Herrick, C. J. (1925). *J. Comp. Neurol.* 39:433–489. The amphibian forebrain. III. The optic tracts and centers of *Amblystoma* and the frog.

Herrick, C. J. (1930). *Proc. Natl. Acad. Sci. U.S.A.* 16:643–650. Localization of function in the nervous system.

Herrick, C. J. (1948). *The Brain of the Tiger Salamander.* Univ. Chicago Press, Chicago.

Herrick, C. J., and C. L. Herrick (1920). Nervous system, *Dictionary of Philosophy and Psychology*, Vol. II, pp. 153–166, In (J. M. Baldwin, ed.), Macmillan, New York.

Herrick, C. L., and C. J. Herrick (1897). *J. Comp. Neurol.* 7:162–168. Inquiries regarding current tendencies in neurological nomenclature.

Herrmann, K., and H.-J. Bischof (1988). *J. Comp. Neurol.* 277:141–154. Development of neurons in the ectostriatum of normal and monocularly deprived zebra finches: A quantitative golgi study.

Herrnstein, R. J., and E. G. Boring (1965). *A Source Book in the History of Psychology*. Harvard Univ. Press, Cambridge, Mass.

Herrup, K., and R. J. Mullen (1979). *Brain Res.* 178:443–457. Staggerer chimeras: Intrinsic nature of Purkinje cell defects and implications for normal cerebellar development.

Herrup, K., and R. J. Mullen (1981). *Dev. Brain Res.* 1:475–485. Role of the staggerer gene in determining Purkinje cell number in the cerebellar cortex of mouse chimeras.

Herrup, K., and E. M. Shooter (1973). *Proc. Natl. Acad. Sci. U.S.A.* 70:3884–3888. Properties of the β nerve growth factor receptor of avian dorsal root ganglia.

Herrup, K., and E. M. Shooter (1975). *J. Cell Biol.* 67:118–125. Properties of the β-nerve growth factor receptor in development.

Herrup, K., and K. Sunter (1987). *J. Neurosci.* 7:829–836. Numerical matching during cerebellar development: Quantitative analysis of granule cell death in staggerer mouse chimeras.

Herrup, K., and E. Trenkner (1987). *Neuroscience* 23:871–885. Regional differences in cytoarchitecture of the weaver cerebellum suggest a new model for weaver gene action.

Herrup, K., R. Stickgold, and E. M. Shooter (1974). *Ann. N.Y. Acad. Sci.* 228:381–392. The role of the nerve growth factor in the development of sensory and sympathetic ganglia.

Hersh, A. H. (1941). *Growth* 5:Suppl. 113–145. Allometric growth: the ontogenic and phylogenetic significance of differential rates of growth.

Hertwig, O. (1893–1898). *Die Zelle und die Gewebe*. 2 vols. Gustav Fischer, Jena.

Hertwig, O. (1906). *Handbuch der vergleichenden und experimentellen Entwickelungslehre der Wirbeltiere*. 3 vols., 5013 pp. Verlag von Gustav Fischer, Jena.

Hertwig, O. (1911–1912). *Arch. mikr. Anat.* 79:113–120. Methoden und Versuche zur Erforschung der Vita propria abgetrennter Gewebs- und Organstückchen von Wierbeltieren.

Hertzig, M. E., H. G. Birch, S. A. Richardson, and J. Tizard

(1972). *Pediatrics* **49**:814–824. Intellectual levels of school children severely malnourished during the first two years of life.

Herzen, A. (1915–1925). *Complete Works and Letters*, K. Lemke, ed. Translated (in part), C. Garnett. Chatto and Windus, London, 1924–27.

Herzig, M. E., H. G. Birch, S. A. Richardson, and J. Tizard (1972). *Pediatrics* **49**:814–824. Intellectual levels of school children severely malnourished during the first two years of life.

Heslop, J. P. (1975). *Adv. Comp. Physiol. Biochem.* **6**:75–161. Axonal flow and fast transport in nerves.

Hess, A., and J. Z. Young (1949). *Nature* **164**:490. Correlation of internodal length and fibre diameter in the central nervous system.

Hesse, M. (1967). Models and analogy in science. In *The Encyclopedia of Philosophy* (P. Edwards, ed.), Macmillan, Free Press, New York.

Hetier, E., J. Ayala, P. Denèfle, A. Bousseau, P. Rouget, M. Mallat, and A. Prochiantz (1988). *J. Neurosci. Res.* **21**:391–397. Brain macrophages synthesize interleukin-1 and interleukin-1 mRNAs *in vitro*.

Heumann, D., and T. Rabinowicz (1980). *Exp. Brain Res.* **38**:75–85. Postnatal development of the dorsal lateral geniculate nucleus in the normal and enucleated albino mouse.

Heumann, D., and G. Leuba (1983). *Neuropathol. Appl. Neurobiol.* **9**:297–311. Neuronal death in the development and aging of the cerebral cortex of the mouse.

Heumann, D., G. Leuba, and T. Rabinowicz (1977). *J. Hirnforsch.* **18**:483–500. Postnatal development of the mouse cerebral cortex. II. Quantitative architectonics of visual and auditory areas.

Heumann, D., G. Leuba, and T. Rabinowicz (1978). *J. Hirnforsch.* **19**:385–393. Postnatal development of the mouse cerebral cortex. IV. Evolution of the total cortical volume of the population of neurons and glia.

Heumann, R., M. Schwab, and H. Thoenen (1981). *Nature* **292**:838–840. A second messenger required for nerve growth factor biological activity?

Heumann, R., S. Korsching, C. Bandtlow, and H. Thoenen (1987a). *J. Cell Biol.* **104**:1623–1631. Changes of nerve growth factor synthesis in nonneuronal cells in response to sciatic nerve transection.

Heumann, R., D. Lindholm, C. Bandtlow, M. Meyer, M. J. Radeke, T. P. Misko, E. Shooter, and H. Thoenen (1987b). *Proc. Natl. Acad. Sci. U.S.A.* **84**:8735–8739. Differential regulation of mRNA encoding nerve growth factor and its receptor in rat sciatic nerve during development, degeneration, and regeneration: Role of macrophages.

Heuser, J., and L. Evans (1980). *J. Cell. Biol.* **84**:560–583. Three-dimensional visualization of coated vesicle formation in fibroblasts.

Heuser, J. E., and T. S. Reese (1973). *J. Cell Biol.* **57**:315–344. Evidence for recycling of synaptic vesicle membrane during transmitter release at the frog neuromuscular junction.

Heuser, J. E., and S. R. Salpeter (1979). *J. Cell Biol.* **82**:150–173. Organization of acetylcholine receptors in quick-frozen, deep-etched, and rotary-replicated *Torpedo* postsynaptic membrane.

Heuser, J. E., T. S. Reese, and D. M. D. Landis (1974). *J.*

Neurocytol. **3**:109–131. Functional changes in frog neuromuscular junctions studied with freeze-fracture.

Hibbard, E. (1959). *J. Exp. Zool.* **141**:323–351. Central integration of developing nerve tracts from supernumerary grafted eyes and brain in the frog.

Hibbard, E. (1964). *Exp. Neurol.* **10**:271–283. Selective innervation and reciprocal functional suppression from grafted extra labyrinths in amphibians.

Hibbard, E. (1965a). *Exp. Neurol.* **13**:289–301. Orientation and directed growth of Mauthner's cell axons from duplicated vestibular nerve roots.

Hibbard, E. (1965b). *Anat. Rec.* **151**:360–361. Innervation of intrinsic limb musculature by cranial nerves in *Pleurodeles waltlii*.

Hibbard, E. (1967). *Exp. Neurol.* **19**:350–356. Visual recovery following regeneration of the optic nerve through oculomotor nerve root in *Xenopus*.

Hickey, T. L. (1975). *J. Comp. Neurol.* **161**:359–382. Translaminar growth of axons in the kitten dorsal lateral geniculate nucleus following removal of one eye.

Hickey, T. L., and R. W. Guillery (1974). *J. Comp. Neurol.* **156**:239–253. An autoradiographic study of retinogeniculate pathways in the cat and the fox.

Hicks, S. P. (1954). *J. Cell. Comp. Physiol.* **43**: Suppl. 1:151–178. The effects of ionizing radiation, certain hormones, and radiomimetic drugs on the developing nervous system.

Hicks, S. P. (1958). *Physiol. Rev.* **38**:337–356. Radiation as an experimental tool in mammalian developmental neurology.

Hicks, S. P., and C. J. D'Amato (1963). Malformation and regeneration of the mammalian retina following experimental radiation, pp. 45–51. In *Les Phakomatoses Cérébrales, Deuxiéme Colloque International, Malformations Congénitales de l'Encéphale* (L. Michaux, and M. Field, eds.), SPEI, Paris.

Hicks, S. P., and C. J. D'Amato (1966). Effects of ionizing radiations on mammalian development, pp. 196–250. In *Advances in Teratology* (D. H. M. Woollam, ed.), Logos Press, London.

Hicks, S. P., and C. J. D'Amato (1968). *Anat. Rec.* **160**:619–634. Cell migrations to the isocortex in the rat.

Hicks, S. P., C. J. D'Amato, and M. J. Lowe (1959). *J. Comp. Neurol.* **113**:435–469. The development of the mammalian nervous system. Malformations of the brain, especially the cerebral cortex, induced in rats by radiation.

Hicks, S. P., C. J. D'Amato, M. A. Coy, E. D. O'Brien, J. M. Thurston, and D. L. Joftes (1961). Migrating cells in the developing central nervous system studied by their radiosensitivity and tritiated thymidine uptake, pp. 246–261. In *Fundamental Aspects of Radiosensitivity*, Brookhaven Symposium in Biology, No. 14, Upton, New York.

Hier, D. B., B. G. W. Arnason, and M. Young (1972). *Proc. Natl. Acad. Sci. U.S.A.* **69**:2268–2272. Studies on the mechanism of action of nerve growth factor.

Hild, W. (1957). *Z. Zellforsch. Mikroskop. Anat.* **46**:71–95. Myelogenesis in cultures of mammalian central nervous system.

Hild, W. (1966). *Z. Zellforsch. Mikroskop. Anat.* **69**:155–188. Cell types and neuronal connections in cultures of mammalian central nervous tissue.

Hildebrand, C. (1971). *Acta Physiol. Scand. (Suppl.)* **364**:109–144. Ultrastructural and light microscopic studies of the developing feline spinal cord white matter. II. Cell death and myelin sheath disintegration in the early postnatal period.

Hildebrand, C. (1989). *J. Neurocytol.* 18:285–294. Myelin sheath remodelling in remyelinated rat sciatic nerve.

Hildebrand, C., and S. Skoglund (1971). *Acta Physiol. Scand. Suppl.* 364:5–41. Caliber spectra of some fiber tracts in the feline central nervous system during postnatal development.

Hildebrand, C., J. D. Kocsis, S. Berglund, and S. G. Waxman (1985). *Brain Res.* 358:163–170. Myelin sheath remodelling in regenerated rat sciatic nerve.

Hildebrand, C., G. Y. Mustafa, and S. G. Waxman (1986). *J. Neurocytol.* 15:681–692. Remodelling of internodes in regenerated rat sciatic nerve: electron microscopic observations.

Hilfer, R. S., and R. L. Searls (1985). Cytoskeletal dynamics in animal morphogenesis, pp. 3–29. In *Developmental Biology a Comprehensive Synthesis*, Vol. 2, (L. W. Browder, ed.), Plenum, New York.

Hilgard, E. R. (1958). *Theories of Learning*, 2nd edn., Methuen, London.

Hill, A. (1896). *Brain* 19:1–42. The chrome-silver method: A study of the conditions under which the reaction occurs and a criticism of its results.

Hill, D. L., and C. R. Almli (1980). *Brain Res.* 197:27–38. Ontogeny of chorda tympani nerve responses to gustatory stimuli in the rat.

Hillman, D. E. (1969). *J. Neurophysiol.* 32:818–846. Morphological organization of frog cerebellar cortex: A light and electron microscopic study.

Hillman, D. E., and S. Chen (1981a). *Neuroscience* 6:1249–1262. Vulnerability of cerebellar development in malnutrition. I. quantitation of layer volume and neuron numbers.

Hillman, D. E., and S. Chen (1981b). *Neuroscience* 6:1263–1275. Vulnerability of cerebellar development in malnutrition. II. Intrinsic determination of total synaptic area on Purkinje cell spines.

Hinds, J. W. (1966). *Anat. Rec.* 154:358–359. Autoradiographic study of histogenesis in the olfactory bulb and accessory olfactory bulb in the mouse.

Hinds, J. W. (1968a). *J. Comp. Neurol.* 134:287–304. Autoradiographic study of histogenesis in the mouse olfactory bulb. I. Time of origin of neurons and neuroglia.

Hinds, J. W. (1968b). *J. Comp. Neurol.* 134:305–322. Autoradiographic study of histogenesis in the mouse olfactory bulb. II. Cell proliferation and migration.

Hinds, J. W., and J. B. Angevine, Jr. (1965). *Anat. Rec.* 151:456–457. Autoradiographic study of histogenesis in the area pyriformis and claustrum in the mouse.

Hinds, J. W., and P. L. Hinds (1972). *J. Neurocytol.* 1:169–187. Reconstruction of dendritic growth cones in neonatal mouse olfactory bulb.

Hinds, J. W., and P. O. Hinds (1974). *Dev. Biol.* 37:381–416. Early ganglion cell differentiation in the mouse retina: An electron microscopic analysis utilizing serial sections.

Hinds, J. W., and P. L. Hinds (1976a). *J. Comp. Neurol.* 169:15–40. Synapse formation in the mouse olfactory bulb. I. Quantitative studies.

Hinds, J. W., and P. L. Hinds (1976b). *J. Comp. Neurol.* 169:41–62. Synapse formation in the mouse olfactory bulb. II. Morphogenesis.

Hinds, J. W., and T. L. Ruffett (1971). *Z. Zellforsch. Mikrosk.*

Anat. 115:226–264. Cell proliferation in the neural tube: An electron microscopic and Golgi analysis in the mouse cerebral vesicle.

Hine, R. J., and G. D. Das (1974). *Z. Anat. Entwickl. Gesch.* 144:173–186. Neuroembryogenesis in the hippocampal formation of the rat. An autoradiographic study.

Hines, M. (1947a). *J. Neurophysiol.* 3:442–466. Movements elicited from precentral gyrus of adult chimpanzee by stimulation with sine wave currents.

Hines, M. (1947b). *Fed. Proc.* 6:441–447. The motor areas.

Hines, M., and R. W. Goy (1985). *Horm. Behav.* 19:331–347. Estrogens before birth and development of sex-related reproductive traits in the female guinea pig.

Hines, H. M., W. H. Wehrmacher, and J. D. Thompson (1945). *Am. J. Physiol.* 145:48–53. Functional changes in nerve and muscle after partial denervation.

Hines, M., F. C. Davis, A. Coquelin, R. W. Goy, and R. A. Gorski (1985). *J. Neurosci.* 5:40–47. Sexually dimorphic regions in the medial preoptic area and bed nucleus of the stria terminalis of the guinea pig: a description and an investigation of their relationship to gonadal steroids in adulthood.

Hinkle, L, C. D. McCaig, and K. R. Robinson (1981). *J. Physiol. (London)* 314:121–135. The direction of growth of differentiating neurones and myoblasts from frog embryos in an applied electric field.

Hinsey, J. C. (1934). *Physiol. Rev.* 14:514–585. Innervation of skeletal muscle.

Hinsey, J. C., M. A. Krupp, and W. T. Lhamon (1937). *J. Comp. Neurol.* 67:205–214. Reaction of spinal ganglion cells to section of dorsal roots.

Hirano, A. (1968). *J. Cell Biol.* 38:637–640. A confirmation of oligodendroglial origin of myelin in the adult rat.

Hirano, A. (1989). *Dev. Neurosci.* 11:112–117. Review of the morphological aspects of remyelination.

Hirano, A., and H. M. Dembitzer (1967). *J. Cell Biol.* 34:555–567. A structural analysis of the myelin sheath in the central nervous system.

Hirano, A., and H. M. Dembitzer (1973). *J. Cell Biol.* 56:478–486. Cerebellar alterations in the weaver mouse.

Hirano, A., and H. M. Dembitzer (1975). *Adv. Neurol.* 12:353–360. Aberrant development of the Purkinje cell dendritic spine.

Hirano, A., H. M. Zimmerman, and S. Levine (1966). *J. Cell Biol.* 31:397–411. Myelin in the central nervous system as observed in experimentally induced edema in the rat.

Hirano, A., H. M. Zimmerman, and S. Levine (1969). *Acta Neuropathol.* 12:348–365. Electron microscopic observations of peripheral myelin in a central nervous system lesion.

Hirano, A., H. M. Dembitzer, and M. Jones (1972). *J. Neuropathol. Exp. Neuronal* 31:113–125. An electron microscope study of cycasin-induced cerebellar alterations.

Hirano, A., H. M. Dembitzer, and C. H. Yoon (1977). *Acta Neuropathol.* 40:85–90. Development of Purkinje cell somatic spines in weaver mouse.

Hirano, H. (1967). *Z. Zellforsch. Mikroskop. Anat.* 79:198–208. Ultrastructural study on the morphogenesis of the neuromuscular junction in the skeletal muscle of the chick.

Hirano, M, and J. E. Goldman (1988). *J. Neurosci. Res.* 21:155–167 Gliogenesis in rat spinal cord: Evidence of origin of astrocytes and oligodendrocytes from radial precursors.

Hirokawa, N. (1982). *J. Cell Biol.* 94:129–142. Cross-linker system between neurofilaments, microtubules, and membranous organelles in frog axons revealed by the quick-freeze, deep-etching method.

Hirokawa, N. (1983). Membrane specialization and cytoskeletal structures in the synapse and axon revealed by the quick-freeze deep-etch method, pp. 113–141. In *Structure and Function in Excitable Cells* (D. Chang, I. Tasaki, W. J. Adelman, and H. R. Leuchtag, eds.), Plenum Press, New York.

Hirokawa, N., and J. E. Heuser (1982). *J. Neurocytol.* 11:487–510. Internal and external differences of the postsynaptic membrane at the neuromuscular junction.

Hirokawa, N., M. A. Glicksman, and M. B. Willard (1984). *J. Cell Biol.* 98:1523–1536. Organization of mammalian neurofilament polypeptides within the neuronal cytoskeleton.

Hirokawa, N., S.-I. Hisanaga, and Y. Shiomura (1988a). *J. Neurosci.* 8:2769–2779. MAP2 is a component of crossbridges between microtubules and neurofilaments in the neuronal cytoskeleton: Quick-freeze, deep-etch immunoelectron microscopy and reconstituition studies.

Hirokawa, N, Y. Shiomura, and S. Okabe (1988b). *J. Cell Biol.* 107:1449–1459. Tau proteins: The molecular structure and mode of binding on microtubules.

Hirokawa, N., K. Sobue, K. Kanda, A. Harada, and H. Yorifuji (1989a). *J. Cell Biol.* 108:111–126. The cytoskeletal architecture of the presynaptic terminal and molecular structure of synapsin.

Hirokawa, N., K. K. Pfister, H. Yorifuji, M. C. Wagner, S. T. Brady, and G. S. Bloom (1989b). *Cell* 56:867–878. Submolecular domains of bovine brain kinesin identified by electron microscopy and monoclonal antibody decoration.

Hirose, G., and M. Jacobson (1979). *Dev. Biol.* 71:191–202. Clonal organization of the central nervous system of the frog. I. Clones stemming from individual blastomeres of the 16-cell and earlier stages.

Hirsch, H. V. B. (1970). Controlled visual stimulation and deprivation. In *Genesis of Neuronal Patterns* (M. V. Edds, Jr., ed.), NRP Work Session, Brookline, Mass.

Hirsch, H. V. B., and M. Jacobson (1973). *Brain Res.* 49:67–74. Development and maintenance of connectivity in the visual system of the frog. II. The effects of eye removal.

Hirsch, H. V. B., and M. Jacobson (1975). The perfectible brain. Principles of neuronal development, pp. 107–137. In *Foundations of Psychobiology* (M. Gazzaniga, and C. Blakemore, eds.), Academic Press, New York.

Hirsch, H. V. B., and A. G. Leventhal (1978). Functional modification of the developing visual system. In *Handbook of Sensory Physiology*, Vol. IX, *Development of Sensory Systems* (M. Jacobson, ed.) Springer-Verlag, New York.

Hirsch, H. V. B., and D. N. Spinelli (1970). *Science* 168:869–871. Visual experience modifies distribution of horizontally and vertically oriented receptive fields in cats.

Hirsch, H. V. B., and D. N. Spinelli (1971). *Exp. Brain Res.* 13:509–527. Modification of the distribution of receptive field orientation in cats by selective visual exposure during development.

His, W. (1856). *Beiträge zur normalen und pathologischen Histologie der Kornea.* Schweighauser, Basel.

His, W. (1868). *Untersuchungen über die erste Anlage des Wirbeltierleibes: Die erste Entwicklung des Hühnchens im Ei.* Vogel, Leipzig.

His, W. (1870). *Arch. mikr. Anat.* 6:229–232. Beschreibung eines Mikrotoms.

His, W. (1873). *Untersuchungen über die erste Anlage des Wirbelthierleibes. Über das ei und die eientwickelung bei Knochenfischen.* Vogel, Leipzig.

His, W. (1874). *Unserer Körperform und das Physiologische Problem ihrer Entstehung.* Engelmann, Leipzig.

His, W. (1878). *Arch. Anat. Physiol. Leipzig, Anat. Abth.* Untersuchungen über die Bildung des Knochenfischembryo.

His, W. (1879). *Arch. Anat. Physiol. Leipzig, Anat. Abth.,* pp. 455–482. Ueber die Anfänge des peripherischen Nervensystemes.

His, W. (1887a). *Abh. kgl. sächs. Ges. Wissensch. math. phys. Kl.* 13:479–513. Zur Geschichte des menschlichen Rückenmarks und der Nervenwurzeln.

His, W. (1887b). *Arch. Anat. Physiol. Leipzig, Anat. Abth.,* 92:368–378. Die Entwickelung der ersten Nervenbahnen beim menschlichen Embryo. Übersichtliche Darstellung.

His, W. (1888a). *Abh. kgl. sächs. Ges. Wissensch. math. phys. Kl.* 24:339–392. Zur Geschichte des Gehirns sowie der centralen und peripherischen Nervenbahnen beim menschlichen Embryo.

His, W. (1888b). *Proc. Roy. Soc. Edin.* 15:287–297. On the principles of animal morphology.

His, W. (1889a). *Abh. kgl. sächs. Ges. Wissensch. math. phys. Kl.* 15:311–372. Die Neuroblasten und deren Entstehung im embryonalen Mark.

His, W. (1889b). *Abh. kgl. sächs. Ges. Wissensch. math. phys. Kl.* 15:673–736. Die Formentwickelung des menschlichen Vorderhirns vom Ende des ersten bis zum Beginn des dritten Monats.

His, W. (1889c). Über die Entwicklung des Riechlappens und des Riechganglions und über diejenige des verlängerten Markes. *Verhandl. der anatom. Ges. auf der 3. Versammlung zu Berlin.*

His, W. (1890a). *Abh. kgl. sächs. Ges. Wissensch. math. phys. Kl.* 29:1–74. Die Entwickelung des menschlichen Rautenhirns vom Ende des ersten bis zum Beginn des dritten Monats. I. Verlängertes Mark.

His, W. (1890b). *Arch. Anat. Physiol. Leipzig, Anat. Abt. Suppl.* 95:95–119. Histogenese und Zusammenhang der Nervenelemente.

His, W. (1891). *Abh. kgl. sächs. Ges. Wissensch. math. phys. Kl.* 17:1–74. Die Entwickelung des menschlichen Rautenhirns vom Ende des ersten bis zum Beginn des dritten Monats.

His, W. (1892). *Arch. Anat. Physiol. Leipzig, Anat. Abth.,* pp. 346–383. Zur allgemeinen Morphologie des Gehirns.

His, W. (1893a). *Arch. Anat. Physiol. Leipzig, Anat. Abth.,* pp. 157–171. Ueber das frontale Ende des Gehirnrohres.

His, W. (1893b). *Arch. Anat. Physiol. Leipzig, Anat. Abth.,* pp. 172–179. Vorschläge zur Eintheilung des Gehirns.

His, W. (1894a). *Arch. Anat. Physiol. Leipzig, Anat. Abth.,* 1:1–80. Ueber mechanische Grundvorgänge thierischer Formenbildung.

His, W. (1894b). *Arch. Anat. Physiol. Leipzig, Anat. Abth.,* pp. 313–336. Ueber die Vorstufen der Gehirn und der Kopfbildung bei Wirbelthieren.

His, W. (1895a). *Arch. Anat. Physiol. Leipzig, Anat. Abth., Suppl.,* pp. 1–180. Die anatomischer Nomenclature. Nomina anatomica.

His, W. (1895b). *Abh. math.-phys. Cl. Königl. Sächs. Gesellsch. Wissench.* 22:379–420. Anatomische Forschungen über Johann Sebastian Bach's Gebeine und Antlitz.

His, W. (1901). *Zeitschr. ges. Neurol. Psychiat.* 87:167. Das Princip der organbildende Keimbezirke und die Verwandschaft der Gewebe.

His, W. (1904a). *Die Entwicklung des menschlichen Gehirns waehrend der ersten Monate.* S. Hirzel, Leipzig.

His, W. (1904b). *Lebenserinnerungen.* Als Manuskript gedruckt, Leipzig.

His, W. Jr. (1897). *Arch. Anat. Physiol. Leipzig Suppl.*, pp. 137–170. Ueber die Entwicklung des Bauchsympathicus beim Hühnchen und Menschen.

Hisanaga, S., and N. Hirokawa (1988). *J. Mol. Biol.* 202:297–305. Structure of the peripheral domains of neurofilaments revealed by low angle rotary shadowing.

Hiscock, J., and C. Straznicky (1986). *J. Embryol. Exp. Morph.* 93:281–290. The formation of axonal projections of the mesencephalic trigeminal neurones in chick embryos.

Hiscoe, H. B. (1947). *Anat. Rec.* 99:447–475. Distribution of nodes and incisures in normal and regenerated nerve fibers.

Hitchock, P. F., and T. L. Hickey (1980). *Brain Res.* 182:176–179. Ocular dominance columns: Evidence for their presence in humans.

Hitzig, E. (1877). *Über den Heutigen Stand der Frage von der Lokalisation im Grosshirn.* Volkmann's Sammlung No. 112. Leipzig.

Hník, P., I. Jirmanová, L. Vyklicky, and J. Zelená (1967). *J. Physiol. (London)* 193:309–325. Fast and slow muscles of the chick after nerve cross-union.

Ho, K.-C., U. Roessmann, J. V. Straumfjord, and G. Monroe (1980a). *Arch. Pathol. Lab. Med.* 104:635–639. Analysis of brain weight. I. Adult brain weight in relation to sex, race, and age.

Ho, K.-C., U. Roessmann, J. V. Straumfjord, and G. Monroe (1980b). *Arch. Pathol. Lab. Med.* 104:640–645. Analysis of brain weight. II. Adult brain weight in relation to body weight, weight and surface area.

Hoch-Ligeti, C. (1963). *J. Am. Geriatr. Soc.* 11:403–408. Effect of aging on the central nervous system.

Hockfield, S. (1987). *Science* 237:67–70. A Mab to a unique cerebellar neuron generated by immunosuppression and rapid immunization.

Hockfield, S. and R. D. G. McKay (1985). *J. Neurosci.* 5:3310–3328. Identification of major cell classes in the developing mammalian nervous system.

Hockfield, S., R. D. McKay, S. H. C. Hendry, and E. G. Jones (1983). *Cold Spring Harbor Symp. Quant. Biol.* 48:877–899. A surface antigen that identifies ocular dominance columns in the visual cortex and laminar features of the lateral geniculate nucleus.

Hoerr, N. L. (1936). *Anat. Record* 66:81–90. Cytological studies by the Altmann-Gersh freezing-drying method. III. The preexistence of neurofibrillae and their disposition in the nerve fiber.

Hoey, T., H. J. Doyle, K. Harding, C. Weeden, and M. Levine (1986). *Proc. Natl. Acad. Sci. U.S.A.* 83:4809–4813. Homeobox gene expression in anterior and posterior regions of the *Drosophila* embryo.

Hofbauer, A., and J. A. Campos-Ortega (1976). *Wilhelm Roux's Arch. Dev. Biol.* 179:275–289. Cell clones and pattern formation: Genetic eye mosaics in *Drosophila melanogaster.*

Hofer, M. M., and Y.-A. Barde (1988). *Nature* 331:261–262. Brain-derived neurotrophic factor prevents neuronal death *in vivo.*

Hoff, E. C. (1932). *Proc. Roy. Soc. (London) Ser. B.* 111:175–188. Central nerve terminals in the mammalian spinal cord and their examination by experimental degeneration.

Hoff, E. C., and W. Riese (1950). *J. Hist. Med.* 5:51–71. A history of the doctrine of cerebral localization. Sources, anticipation and basic reasoning.

Hoff, E. C., and W. Riese (1951). *J. Hist. Med.* 6:439–470. A history of the doctrine of cerebral localization. II. Methods and main results.

Hoff, H. H., and P. Kellaway (1952). *J. Hist. Med.* 7:211–212. The early history of the reflex.

Hoffman, H. (1950). *Aust. J. Exp. Biol. Med. Sci.* 28:383–397. Local re-innervation in partially denervated muscle: A histophysiological study.

Hoffman, H. (1951a). *Austr. J. Exp. Biol. Med. Sci.* 29:211–219. Fate of interrupted nerve fibers regenerating into partially denervated muscles.

Hoffman, H. (1951b). *Austr. J. Exp. Biol. Med. Sci.* 29:289–307. A study of the factors influencing innervation of muscles by implanted nerves.

Hoffman, H. (1952). *Aust. J. Exp. Biol. Med. Sci.* 30:541–566. Acceleration and retardation of the process of axon-sprouting in partially denervated muscles.

Hoffman, H., and P. H. Springell (1951). *Austr. J. Exp. Biol. Med. Sci.* 29:417–424. An attempt at the chemical identification of "neurocletin." (The substance evoking axon-sprouting.)

Hoffman, P. (1922). *Untersuchungen über die Eigenreflexe (Sehnenreflexe) menschlicher Muskeln.* Springer, Berlin.

Hoffman, P. N., and R. J. Lasek (1975). *J. Cell Biol.* 66:351–366. The slow component of axonal transport. Identification of major structural polypeptides of the axon and their generality among mammalian neurons.

Hoffman, S., and G. M. Edelman (1983). *Proc. Natl. Acad. Sci. U.S.A.* 80:5762–5766. Kinetics of homophilic binding by E and A forms of neural cell adhesion molecule.

Hoffman, S., B. C. Sorkin, P. C. White, R. Brackenbury, R. Mailhammer, U. Rutishauser, B. A. Cunningham, and G. M. Edelman (1982). *J. Biol. Chem.* 257:7720–7729. Chemical characterization of a neural cell adhesion molecule (N-CAM) purified from embryonic brain membranes.

Hoffman, W. W., and J. H. Peacock (1973). *Exp. Neurol.* 41:345–356. Postjunctional changes induced by partial interruption of axoplasmic flow in motor nerves.

Hoffmann, K.-P. (1973). *J. Neurophysiol.* 36:409–424. Conduction velocity in pathways from retina to superior colliculus in the cat: A correlation with receptive-field properties.

Hoffmann, K.-P., and M. Cynader (1975). *Brain Res.* 85:179. Recovery in the LGN of the cat after early visual deprivation.

Hoffmann, K.-P., and S. M. Sherman (1974). *J. Neurophysiol.* 37:1276–1286. Effects of early monocular deprivation on visual input to cat superior colliculus.

Hoffmann, K.-P., and S. M. Sherman (1975). *J. Neurophysiol.*

38:1049–1059. Effects of early binocular deprivation on visual input to cat superior colliculus.

Hoffmann, K.-P., and J. Stone (1971). *Brain Res.* 32:460–466. Conduction velocity of afferents to cat visual cortex: A correlation with cortical receptive field properties.

Hofman, M. A. (1982). *Brain Behav. Evol.* 20:84–96. Encephalization in mammals in relation to the size of the cerebral cortex.

Hofman, M. A. (1983). *J. Theor. Biol.* 105:317–332. Evolution of brain size in neonatal and adult placental mammals. A theoretical approach.

Hofman, M. A. (1985a). *Brain Behav. Evol.* 27:28–40. Size and shape of the cerebral cortex in mammals. I. The cortical surface.

Hofman, M. A. (1985b). *J. Theor. Biol.* 112:77–95. Neuronal correlates of corticalization in mammals: A theory.

Hofman, M. A. (1988). *Brain Behav. Evol.* 32:17–26. Size and shape of the cerebral cortex in mammals. II. The cortical volume.

Hofman, M. A. (1989). *Pro. Neurobiol.* 32:137–158. On the evolution and geometry of the brain in mammals.

Hofman, M. A., and D. F. Swaab (1989). *J. Anat. (London)* 164:55–72. The sexually dimorphic nucleus of the preoptic area in the human brain: A comparative morphometric study.

Hogan, B., P. Holland and P. Schofield (1985). *Trends Genet.* 1:67–74. How is the mouse segmented?

Hogan, E. L., and S. Greenfield (1984). Animal models of genetic disorders of myelin, pp. 489–534. In *Myelin,* 2nd edn., (P. Morell, ed.), Plenum, New York.

Hogan, E. L., D. M. Dawson, and F. C. A. Romanul (1965). *Arch. Neurol.* 13:274–282. Enzymic changes in denervated muscle. II. Biochemical studies.

Hoh, J. F. Y. (1971). *Exp. Neurol.* 30:263–276. Selective reinnervation of fast-twitch and slow-graded muscle fibers in the toad.

Hoh, J. F. Y., and S. Hughes (1988a). *J. Musc. Res. Cell Motility* 9:59–72. Myogenic and neurogenic regulation of myosin gene expression in cat jaw-closing muscle regenerating in fast and slow limb muscle beds.

Hoh, J. F. Y., S. Hughes, P. T. Hale, and R. B. Fitzsimons (1988b). *J. Musc. Res. Cell Motil.* 9:30–47. Immunocytochemical and electrophoretic analyses of changes in myosin gene expression in cat limb fast and slow muscles during postnatal development.

Hohmann, A., and O. D. Creutzfeldt (1975). *Nature* 254:613–614. Squint and the development of binocularity in humans.

Hokin, L. E. (1985). *Ann. Rev. Biochem.* 54:205–236. Receptors and phosphoinositide-generated second messengers.

Holder, N., J. Mills, and D. A. Tonge (1982). *J. Physiol. (London)* 326:371–384. Selective reinnervation of skeletal muscle in the newt *Triturus cristatus.*

Holder, N., D. A. Tonge, and M. Jesani (1984). *Proc. Roy. Soc. (London) Ser. B.* 222:477–489. Directed regrowth of axons from a misrouted nerve to their correct target muscles in the limb of the adult newt.

Holland, P. W. H. (1990). *Seminars Dev. Biol.* 1:135–145. Homeobox genes and segmentation: co-option, co-evolution, and convergence.

Holland, P. W. H., and B. L. M. Hogan (1986). *Nature* 321:251–253. Phylogenetic distribution of *Antennapedia*-like homeoboxes.

Holland, P. W. H., and B. L. M. Hogan (1988). *Development* 102:159–174. Spatially restricted patterns of expression of the homeobox-containing gene *Hox-2.1* during mouse embryogenesis.

Holland, R. L., and M. C. Brown (1980). *Science* 207:649–651. Postsynaptic transmission block can cause motor nerve terminal sprouting.

Holley, J. A., C. C. Wimer, and J. E. Vaughn (1982). *J. Comp. Neurol.* 207:333–343. Quantitative analyses of neuronal development in the lateral motor column of mouse spinal cord. III. Generation and settling patterns of large and small neurons.

Hollingworth, T., and M. Berry (1975). *Phil. Trans. Roy. Soc. (London) Ser. B.* 270:227–264. Network analysis of dendritic fields of pyramidal cells in neocortex and Purkinje cells in the cerebellum of the rat.

Holloway, R. L. (1982). *Science* 216:1431–1432. Sexual Dimorphism in the Human Corpus Callosum.

Holloway, R. L., and M. C. de Lacoste (1986). *Human Neurobiol.* 5:87–91. Sexual dimorphism in the human corpus callosum: an extension and replication study.

Holloway, R. L., Jr. (1966). *Brain Res.* 2:393–396. Dendritic branching: Some preliminary results of training and complexity in rat visual cortex.

Hollyday, M. (1980). *Curr. Top Dev. Biol.* 15:181–215. Motoneuron histogenesis and the development of limb innervation.

Hollyday, M. (1981). *J. Comp. Neurol.* 202:439–465. Rules of motor innervation in chick embryos with supernumerary limbs.

Hollyday, M. (1983). Development of motor innervation of chick limb. In *Limb Development and Regeneration,* Pt. A (J. F. Fallon, and A. J. Caplan, eds.), Alan R. Liss, New York.

Hollyday, M., and V. Hamburger (1976a). *J. Comp. Neurol.* 170:311–320. Reduction of the naturally occurring motor neuron loss by enlargement of the periphery.

Hollyday, M., and L. Mendell (1975). *J. Comp. Neurol.* 162:205–220. Area specific reflexes from normal and supernumerary limbs of *Xenopus laevis.*

Hollyday, M., and L. Mendell (1976). *Exp. Neurol.* 51:316–329. Analysis of moving supernumerary limbs of *Xenopus laevis.*

Hollyfield, J. G. (1968). *Dev. Biol.* 18:163–179. Differential addition of cells to the retina in *Rana pipiens* tadpoles.

Hollyfield, J. G. (1971). *Dev. Biol.* 24:264–286. Differential growth of the neural retina in *Xenopus laevis* larvae.

Hollyfield, J. G. (1972). *J. Comp. Neurol.* 144:373–380. Histogenesis of the retina in the killifish.

Hollyfield, J. G., and R. Adler (1970). *Exp. Cell Res.* 59:76–84. Localization of embryonic cells and polystyrene particles within chick embryos after vascular dissemination.

Holmdahl, D. E. (1928). *Z. Mikroskop. Anat. Forsch.* 14:99–298. Die Entstehung und weitere Entwicklung der Neuralleiste (Ganglienleiste) bei Vögeln und Säugetieren.

Holt, C. E. (1980). *Nature* 287:850–852. Cell movements in *Xenopus* eye development.

Holt, C. E. (1984). *J. Neurosci.* 4:1130–1152. Does timing of axon outgrowth influence initial retinotectal topography in *Xenopus?*

Holt, C. E. (1989). *J. Neurosci.* 9:3123–3145. A single-cell analysis of early retinal ganglion cell differentiation in *Xenopus:* From soma to axon tip.

Holt, C. E., and W. A. Harris (1983). *Nature* 301:150–152. Order in the initial retinotectal maps in *Xenopus:* A new technique for labelling growing nerve fibers.

Holt, C. E., T. W. Bertsch, H. M. Ellis and W. A. Harris (1988). *Neuron* 1:15–26. Cellular determination in the *Xenopus* retina is independent of lineage and birth date.

Holt, E. B. (1931). *Animal Drive and the Learning Process.* Holt, New York.

Holtfreter, J. (1929) *Wilhelm Roux Arch. EntwMech. Organ.* 117:421–510. Über die Aufsucht isolierter Teile des Amphibienkeime. I. Methode einer Aufsucht *in vitro.*

Holtfreter, J. (1933). *Arch. Entw.-Mech. Organ.* 137:619–775. Der Einfluss von Wirtsalter und Verschiedenen Organbezirken auf die Differenzierung von angelagertem Gastrulaektoderm.

Holtfreter, J. (1938a). *Arch. Entw.-Mech. Organ.* 138:163–196. Veränderungen der Reaktionsweise im alternden isolierten Gastrulaektoderm.

Holtfreter, J. (1938b). *Arch. Entw.-Mech. Organ.* 138:522–656. Differenzierungspotenzen isolierter Teile der Urodelen gastrula.

Holtfreter, J. (1939). *Arch. Exp. Zellforsch.* 23:169–209. Gewebeaffinität, ein Mittel der embryonalen Formbildung.

Holtfreter, J. (1944). *J. Exp. Zool.* 95:307–343. Neural differentiation of ectoderm through exposure to saline solution.

Holtfreter, J. (1945). *J. Exp. Zool.* 98:161–209. Neurulization and epidermization of gastrula ectoderm.

Holtfreter, J., and V. Hamburger (1955). Amphibians, pp. 230–296. In *Analysis of Development* (B. H. Willier, P. A. Weiss, and V. Hamburger, eds.), Saunders, Philadelphia.

Holton, B., and J. A. Weston (1982a). *Dev. Biol.* 89:64–71. Analysis of glial cell differentiation in peripheral nervous tissue.

Holton, B., and J. A. Weston (1982b). *Dev. Biol.* 89:72–81. Analysis of glial cell differentiation in peripheral nervous tissue. II. Neurons promote S100 synthesis by purified glial precursor cell populations.

Holtzer, H. (1951). *J. Exp. Zool.* 117:523–558. Reconstitution of the urodele spinal cord following unilateral ablation. Part I. Chronology of neuron regulation.

Holtzer, H. (1952). *J. Exp. Zool.* 119:263–302. Reconstitution of the urodele spinal cord following unilateral ablation. Part II. Regeneration of the longitudinal tracts and ectopic synaptic unions of the Mauthner's fibers.

Holtzer, H. (1968). Induction of chondrogenesis: A concept in quest of mechanisms, pp. 152–164. In *Epithelial-Mesenchymal Interactions* (R. Fleischmajer, ed.), Williams & Wilkins, Baltimore.

Holtzman, E. (1971). *Phil. Trans. Roy. Soc. (London) Ser. B.* 261:407–421. Cytochemical studies of protein transport in the nervous system.

Holtzman, E., and E. R. Peterson (1969). *J. Cell Biol.* 40:863–869. Uptake of protein by mammalian neurons.

Holtzman, E., A. B. Novikoff, and H. Villaverde (1967). *J. Cell Biol.* 33:419–435. Lysosomes and GERL in normal and chromatolytic neurons of the rat ganglion nodosum.

Holtzman, E., A. R. Freeman, and L. A. Kashner (1971). *Science* 173:733–736. Stimulation-dependent alterations in peroxidase uptake at lobster neuromuscular junctions.

Hommes, O. R., and C. P. Leblond (1967). *J. Comp. Neurol.* 129:269–278. Mitotic division of neuroglia in the normal adult rat.

Honegger, P., and D. Lenoir (1982). *Dev. Brain Res.* 3:229–238. Nerve growth factor (NGF) stimulation of cholinergic telencephalic neurons in aggregating cell cultures.

Honig, M. G. (1977). *Soc. Neurosci. Abstr.* 3:108. Outgrowth of cutaneous and proprioceptive neurons from chick embryo dorsal root ganglia.

Honig, M. G. (1982). *J. Physiol. (London)* 330:175–202. The development of sensory projection patterns in embryonic chick hind limb.

Honig, M. G., and R. I. Hume (1986). *J. Cell Biol.* 103:171–187. Fluorescent carbocyanine dyes allow living neurons of identified origin to be studied in long-term cultures.

Honig, M. G., and R. I. Hume (1989). *Trends Neurosci.* 12:333–341. DiI and DiO: Versatile fluorescent dyes for neuronal labelling and pathway tracing.

Honig, M. G., C. Lance-Jones, and L. Landmesser (1986). *Dev. Biol.* 118:532–548. The development of sensory projection patterns in embryonic chick hindlimb under experimental conditions.

Hoober, J. K., and S. Cohen (1967). *Biochim. Biophys. Acta* 138:347–356. Epidermal growth factor. I. The stimulation of protein and ribonucleic acid synthesis in chick embryo epidermis.

Hooker, D. (1911). *J. Exp. Zool.* 11:159–186. The development and function of voluntary and cardiac muscle in embryos without nerves.

Hooker, D. (1944). *The Origin of Overt Behavior.* University of Michigan, Ann Arbor.

Hooker, D. (1952). *The Prenatal Origin of Behavior.* Univ. Kansas Press, Lawrence, Kansas.

Hope, R. A., B. J. Hammond, and R. M. Gaze (1976). *Proc. Roy. Soc. (London) Ser. B.* 194:447–466. The arrow model: Retinotectal specificity and map formation in the goldfish visual system.

Höpker, W. (1951). *Z. Alternforsch.* 5:256–279. Das altern des Nucleus Dentatus.

Horch, K. W. (1979). *J. Neurophysiol.* 42:1437–1449. Guidance of regrowing sensory axons after cutaneous nerve lesions in the cat.

Horder, T. J. (1974a). *Brain Res.* 72:41–52. Changes of fibre pathways in the goldfish optic tract following regeneration.

Horder, T. J. (1974b). *J. Physiol. (London)* 241:84–85P. Electron microscopic evidence in goldfish that different optic nerve fibres regenerate selectively through specific routes into the tectum.

Horder, T. J., and P. J. Weindling (1985). Hans Spemann and the organiser, pp. 183–242. In *A History of Embryology* (T. J. Horder, J. A. Witkowski, and C. C. Wylie, eds.), Cambridge Univ. Press, Cambridge.

Hornung, J. P., H. Koppel, and P. G. H. Clarke (1989). *J. Comp. Neurol.* 283:425–437. Endocytosis and autophagy in dying neurons: An ultrastructural study in chick embryos.

Horsburgh, G. M., and A. J. Sefton (1986). *J. Comp. Neurol.* 243:547–560. The early development of the optic nerve and chiasm in embryonic rat.

Horsburgh, G. M., and A. J. Sefton (1987). *J. Comp. Neurol.* 263:553–566 Cellular degeneration and synaptogenesis in the developing retina of the rat.

Horsley, V. A. H. (1909). *Br. Med. J.* 2:125–132. The function of the so-called motor area of the brain.

Hörstadius, S. (1950). *The Neural Crest*, Oxford Univ. Press, London.

Hörstadius, S., and S. Sellman (1946). *Nova Acta Regiae Soc. Sci. Upsal. IV* 13:1–170. Experimenteler Untersuchungen über die Determination des Knorpeligen Kopfskelettes bei Urodelen.

Horstmann, E., and H. Meves (1959). *Z. Zellforsch. Mikroskop. Anat. Abt. Histochem.* 49:569–589. Die Feinstruktur des molekularen Rindengraus und ihre physiologische Bedeutung.

Horton, J. C. (1984). *Phil. Trans. Roy. Soc. (London) B.* 304:199–253. Cytochrome oxidase patches: A new cytoarchitectonic feature of monkey visual cortex.

Horton, J. C., and E. T. Hedley-White (1984). *Phil. Trans. Roy. Soc. (London) B.* 304:255–272. Mapping of cytochrome oxidase patches and ocular dominance columns in human visual cortex.

Horton, J. C., and D. H. Hubel (1981). *Nature* 292:762–764. Regular patchy distribution of cytochrome oxidase staining in primary visual cortex of macaque monkey.

Horton, J. C., M. M. Greenwood, and D. H. Hubel (1980). *Nature* 282:720–722. Non-retinotopic arrangement of fibres in the cat optic nerve.

Horvat, J.-C., M. Pécot-Dechavassine, and J.-C. Mira (1987). *C. R. Hebd. Séanc. Acad. Sci., Paris* 304:143–148. Réinnervation fonctionelle d'un muscle squelettique du Rat adulte au moyen d'un greffon de nerf périphérique introduit dans la moëlle épiniere par voie dorsale.

Horvitz, H. R., H. M. Ellis, and P. W. Sternberg (1982). *Neurosci. Com.* 1:56–65. Programmed cell death in nematode development.

Horwitz, A., K. A. Knudsen, C. H. Damsky, C. Decker, A. Buck and N. T. Neff (1984). Adhesion-related integral membrane glycoproteins identified by monoclonal antibodies, pp. 103–118. In *Monoclonal Antibodies and Functional Cell Lines* (H. Kennett, K. B. Bechtel, and T. J. McKearn, eds.), Plenum, New York.

Hoshino, K., T. Matsuzawa, and U. Murakami (1973). *Exp. Cell Res.* 77:89–94. Characteristics of the cell cycle of matrix cells in the mouse embryo during histogenesis of telencephalon.

Hoskins, S. G. (1986). *J. Neurobiol.* 17:203–229. Control of the development of the ipsilateral retinothalamic projection in *Xenopus leavis* by thyroxine: Results and speculation.

Hoskins, S. G., and P. Grobstein (1984). *Nature* 307:730–733. Induction of the ipsilateral retinothalamic projection in *Xenopus laevis* by thyroxine.

Hoskins, S. G., and P. Grobstein (1985). *J. Neurosci.* 5:930–940. Development of the ipsilateral retinothalamic projection in the frog, *Xenopus laevis*. III. The role of thyroxine.

Hosley, M. A., and B. Oakley (1987). *Anat. Rec.* 218:216–222. Postnatal development of the vallate papilla and taste buds in rats.

Hosley, M. A., S. E. Hughes, and B. Oakley (1987a). *J. Comp. Neurol.* 260:224–232. Neural induction of taste buds.

Hosley, M. A., S. E. Hughes, L. L. Morton, and B. Oakley (1987b). *J. Neurosci.* 7:2075–2080. A sensitive period for the neural induction of taste buds.

Hotta, Y., and S. Benzer (1970). *Proc. Nat. Acad. Sci. U.S.A.* 67:1156–1163. Genetic dissection of the *Drosophila* nervous system by means of mosaics.

Hotta, Y., and S. Benzer (1972). *Nature* 240:527–535. Mapping of behavior in *Drosophila* mosaics.

Hotta, Y., and S. R. Pele (1953). Mapping of behavior of *Drosophila* mosaics, pp. 129–167. In *Genetic Mechanisms of Development* (F. H. Ruddle, ed.), Academic Press, New York.

Howard, A., and S. R. Pele (1953). *Heredity* 6:261–273. Synthesis of deoxyribonucleic acid in normal and irradiated cells and its relation to chromosome breakage.

Howard, E. (1965). *J. Neurochem.* 12:181–191. Effects of corticosterone and food restriction on growth and on DNA, RNA and cholesterol contents of the brain and liver in infant mice.

Howard, E. (1968). *Exp. Neurol.* 22:191–208. Reductions in size and total DNA of cerebrum and cerebellum in adult mice after corticosterone treatment in infancy.

Howard, E. (1973). *Prog. Brain Res.* 40:91–114. DNA content of rodent brains during maturation and aging, and autoradiography of postnatal DNA synthesis in monkey brain.

Howard, E., and J. A. Benjamins (1975). *Brain Res.* 92:73–87. DNA, ganglioside and sulfatide in brains of rats given corticosterone in infancy, with an estimate of cell loss during development.

Howard, E., and D. M. Granoff (1968). *J. Nutr.* 95:111–121. Effect of neonatal food restriction in mice on brain growth, DNA and cholesterol, and on adult delayed response learning.

Howard, E., D. M. Granoff, and P. Bujnovszky (1969). *Brain Res.* 14:697–706. DNA, RNA, and cholesterol increases in cerebrum and cerebellum during development of human fetus.

Hoy, R. R. (1973) The curious nature of degeneration and regeneration in motor neurons and central connectives of the crayfish, pp. 203–232. In *Developmental Neurobiology of Arthropods* (D. Young, ed.), Cambridge Univ. Press, London.

Hoy, R. R., G. D. Bittner, and D. Kennedy (1967). *Science* 156:251–252. Regeneration in crustacean motoneurons: Evidence for axonal fusion.

Hsu, L., D. Natyzak, and J. D. Laskin (1984). *Cancer Res.* 44:4607–4614. Effects of the tumor promoter 12-o-tetradecanoylphorbol-13-acetate on neurite outgrowth from chick embryonic sensory ganglia.

Hsu, T. C., and C. E. Somer (1961). *Proc. Natl. Acad. Sci. U.S.A.* 47:396–403. Effect of 5-bromodeoxyuridine on mammalian chromosomes.

Huang, S., and M. Jacobson (1986a). *Acta Biol. Exp. Sinica* 19:469–479. Differentiation gradients of the nerve fibers in *Xenopus* spinal cord.

Huang, S., and M. Jacobson (1986b). *J. Neurobiol.* 17:593–604. Neurites show pathway specificity but lack directional specificity or predetermined lengths in *Xenopus* embryos.

Hubel, D. H., and M. S. Livingstone (1987). *J. Neurosci.* 7:3378–3415. Segregation of form, color and stereopsis in primate area 18.

Hubel, D. H., and T. N. Wiesel (1962). *J. Physiol. (London)* 160:106–154. Receptive fields, binocular interaction and functional architecture in the cat's visual cortex.

Hubel, D. H., and T. N. Wiesel (1963a). *J. Neurophysiol.* 26:994–1002. Receptive fields of cells in striate cortex of very young, visually inexperienced kittens.

Hubel, D. H., and T. N. Wiesel (1963b). *J. Neurophysiol. (London)* 165:559–568. Shape and arrangement of columns in the cat's striate cortex.

Hubel, D. H., and T. N. Wiesel (1965a). *J. Neurophysiol.* 28:

229–289. Receptive fields and functional architecture in two nonstriate areas (18 and 19) of the cat.

Hubel, D. H., and T. N. Wiesel (1965b). *J. Neurophysiol.* 28:1041–1059. Binocular interaction in striate cortex of kittens reared with artificial squint.

Hubel, D. H., and T. N. Wiesel (1968). *J. Physiol. (London)* 195:215–243. Receptive fields and functional architecture of monkey striate cortex.

Hubel, D. H., and T. N. Wiesel (1969). *Nature* 221:747–750. Anatomical demonstration of columns in the monkey striate cortex.

Hubel, D. H., and T. N. Wiesel (1970). *J. Physiol. (London)* 206:419–436. The period of susceptibility to the physiological effects of unilateral eye closure in kittens.

Hubel, D. H., and T. N. Wiesel (1971). *J. Physiol. (London)* 218:33–62. Aberrant visual projections in the Siamese cat.

Hubel, D. H., and T. N. Wiesel (1972). *J. Comp. Neurol.* 146:421–450. Laminar and columnar distribution of geniculocortical fibers in the macaque monkey.

Hubel, D. H., and T. N. Wiesel (1974a). *J. Comp. Neurol.* 158:267–294. Sequence regularity and geometry of orientation columns in the monkey striate cortex.

Hubel, D. H., and T. N. Wiesel (1974b). *J. Comp. Neurol.* 158:295–306. Uniformity of monkey striate cortex: A parallel relationship between field size, scatter and magnification factor.

Hubel, D. H., and T. N. Wiesel (1974c). *J. Comp. Neurol.* 158:307–318. Ordered arrangement of orientation columns in monkeys lacking visual experience.

Hubel, D. H., T. N. Wiesel, and S. LeVay (1975). *Cold Spring Harbor Symp. Quant. Biol.* 15:581–590. Functional architecture of area 17 in normal and monocularly deprived Macaque monkeys.

Hubel, D. H., T. N. Wiesel, and S. LeVay (1977). *Phil. Trans. Roy. Soc. (London) Ser. B.* 278:377–409. Plasticity of ocular dominance in monkey striate cortex.

Hubel, D. H., T. N. Wiesel, and M. P. Stryker (1978). *J. Comp. Neurol.* 177:361–380. Anatomical demonstration of orientation columns in macaque monkey.

Huber, G., and A. Matus (1984). *J. Cell Biol.* 98:777–781. Immunohistochemical localization of microtubule-associated protein 1 in rat cerebellum using monoclonal antibodies.

Huber, G., D. Alaimo-Beuret, and A. Matus (1985). *J. Cell Biol.* 100:496–507. Characterization of a novel microtubule-associated protein.

Huber, G. C., and E. C. Crosby (1933). *Psychiat. Neurol. Bladen* 4:459–474. The influences of afferent paths on the cytoarchitectonic structure of the submammalian optic tectum.

Huber, H. (1943). *Arch. Entw.-Mech. Organ.* 142:100–120. Experimentelle Studien zum Schicksal des Rumpfganglienleistenmaterials.

Hudson, R. C. L. (1969). *J. Exp. Biol.* 50:47–67. Polyneuronal innervation of the fast muscles of the marine teleost *Cottus scorpius L.*

Hughes, A. F. (1934). *Philos. Trans. Roy. Soc. (London) Ser. B.* 224:75–129. On the development of the blood vessels in the head of the chick.

Hughes, A. F. (1952). *The Mitotic Cycle, The Cytoplasm and Nucleus During Interphase and Mitosis.* Academic Press, New York.

Hughes, A. F. (1953). *J. Anat. (London)* 87:150–162. The growth of embryonic neurites. A study on cultures of chick neural tissue.

Hughes, A. F. (1955). *J. Embryol. Exp. Morph.* 3:305–325. The development of the neural tube of the chick embryo. A study with the ultraviolet microscope.

Hughes, A. F. (1957). *J. Anat. (London)* 91:323–338. The development of the primary sensory system in *Xenopus laevis* (Daudin).

Hughes, A. F. (1959). *A History of Cytology.* Abelard-Schuman, New York.

Hughes, A. F. (1961). *J. Embryol. Exp. Morphol.* 9:269–284. Cell degeneration in the larval ventral horn of *Xenopus laevis* (Daudin).

Hughes, A. F. (1966). *J. Embryol. Exp. Morphol.* 16:401–430. The thyroid and the development of the nervous system in *Eleutherodactylus martinicensis*: An experimental study.

Hughes, A. F. (1968a). *Aspects of Neural Ontogeny*, Logos, London.

Hughes, A. F. (1968b). Development of limb innervation, pp. 110–117. In *Ciba Foundation Symposium on Growth of the Nervous System* (G. E. W. Wolstenholme, and M. O'Connor, eds.), Churchill, London.

Hughes, A. F. (1968c). *Adv. Morphogenesis* 7:79–113. The development of innervation in tetrapod limbs.

Hughes, A. F. (1973). *J. Embryol. Exp. Morphol.* 30:359–376. The development of dorsal root ganglia and ventral horns in the opossum.

Hughes, A. F. (1974). Endocrines, neural development and behavior, pp. 223–243. In *Aspects of Neurogenesis*, Vol. 2, *Studies on the Development of Behavior and the Nervous System* (G. Gottlieb, ed.), Academic Press, New York.

Hughes, A. F., and M. Egar (1972). *J. Embryol. Exp. Morphol.* 27:389–412. The innervation of the hindlimb of *Eleutherodactylus martinicensis*: further comparison of cell and fiber number during development.

Hughes, A. F., and V. McM. Carr (1978). The interaction of periphery and center in the development of dorsal root ganglia. In *Handbook of Sensory Physiology*, Vol. 9, *Development of Sensory Systems* (M. Jacobson, ed.), Springer-Verlag, New York.

Hughes, A. F., and M. C. Prestige (1967). J. Zool. (London) 152:347–359. Development of behaviour in the hindlimb of *Xenopus laevis.*

Hughes, A. F., and P.-A. Tschumi (1958). *J. Anat. (London)* 92:498–527. The factors controlling the development of the dorsal root ganglia and ventral horn in *Xenopus laevis.*

Hughes, S. M., L. Lillien, M. C. Raff, H. Rohrer, and M. Sendtner (1988). *Nature* 335:70–73. Ciliary neurotrophic factor (CNTF) as an inducer of type-2 astrocyte differentiation in rat optic nerve.

Hughes, W. F., and A. LaVelle (1975). *J. Comp. Neurol.* 163:265–284. The effects of early tectal lesions on development in the retinal ganglion cell layer of chick embryos.

Hughes, W. F., and S. C. McLoon (1979). *Exp. Neurol.* 66:587–601. Ganglion cell death during normal retinal development in the chick: Comparisons with cell death induced by early target field destruction.

Hugosson, R., B. Källen, and O. Nilsson (1968). *Acta Neu-*

ropathol. (Berl.) 11:210–220. Neuroglia proliferation studied in tissue culture.

Hui, R. W., and A. A. Smith (1972). Exp. Neurol. 34:331–341. Degeneration of taste buds and lateral line organs in the salamander treated with cholinolytic drugs.

Huizinga, J. (1955). Homo Ludens, Beacon Press, Boston.

Humphreys, T. (1967). The cell surface and specific cell aggregation, pp. 195–210. In The Specificity of Cell Surfaces (B. D. Davis, and L. Warren, eds.), Prentice-Hall, Englewood Cliffs, New Jersey.

Hull, D. (1974). Philosophy of Biological Science. Prentice-Hall, Englewood Cliffs, New Jersey.

Hume, D. A., V. H. Perry, and S. Gordon (1983). J. Cell. Biol. 97:253–257. Immunohistochemical localisation of a macrophage-specific antigen in developing mouse retina: Phagocytosis of dying neurons and differentiation of microglial cells to form a regular array in the plexiform layers.

Hume, R. I., L. W. Role, and G. D. Fischback (1983). Nature 305:632–634. Acetylcholine release from growth cones detected with patches of acetylcholine receptor rich membranes.

Humphrey, A. L., L. C. Skeen, and T. T. Norton (1980). J. Comp. Neurol. 192:549–566. Topographic organization of the orientation columns in the striate cortex of the tree shrew (Tupai glis). II. Deoxyglucose mapping.

Humphrey, A. L., M. Sur, D. J. Uhlrich, and S. M. Sherman (1984). J. Comp. Neurol. 233:159–189. Projection patterns of individual X- and Y-cell axons from the lateral geniculate nucleus to cortical area 17 in the cat.

Humphrey, D. R. (1986). Fed. Proc. 45:2687–2699. Representation of the movements and muscles within the primate precentral motor cortex: Historical and current perspectives.

Humphrey, M. F. (1988). J. Neurocytol. 17:293–304. A morphometric study of the retinal ganglion cell response to optic nerve severance in the frog Rana pipiens.

Humphrey, M. F., and L. D. Beazley (1985). J. Comp. Neurol. 236:382–402. Retinal ganglion cell death during optic nerve regeneration in the frog Hyla moorei.

Humphrey, M. F., J. E. Darby, and L. D. Beazley (1989). J. Comp. Neurol. 279:187–198. Prevention of optic nerve regeneration in the frog Hyla moorei transiently delays the death of some Ganglion cells.

Humphrey, T. (1940). J. Comp. Neurol. 73:431–468. The development of the olfactory and the accessory olfactory formations in human embryos and fetuses.

Huneeus, F. C., and P. F. Davison (1970). J. Mol. Biol. 52:415–428. Fibrillar proteins of the squid axoplasm. I. Neurofilament protein.

Hunt, C. C. (1974). The physiology of muscle receptors, pp. 191–234. In Handbook of Sensory Physiology, Vol. 3, Pt. 2, Muscle Receptors (C. C. Hunt, ed.), Springer-Verlag, Berlin.

Hunt, C. C., and W. K. Riker (1966). J. Neurophysiol. 29:1096–1114. Properties of frog sympathetic neurones in normal ganglia and after axon section.

Hunt, E. A. (1932). J. Exp. Zool. 62:57–91. The differentiation of the chick limb bud in chorio-allantoic grafts, with special reference to the muscle.

Hunt, R. K. (1975). Developmental programming for retinotectal patterns, pp. 131–150. In Cell Patterning, Ciba Foundation Symposium 29, Elsevier, New York.

Hunt, R. K., and E. Frank (1975). Science 189:563–565. Neuronal locus specificity: Trans-repolarization of Xenopus embryonic retina after the time of axial specification.

Hunt, R. K., and M. Jacobson (1970). Science 170:342–344. Brain enhancement in tadpoles: Increased DNA concentration after somatotrophin or prolactin.

Hunt, R. K., and M. Jacobson (1971). Dev. Biol. 26:100–124. Neurogenesis in frogs after early larval treatment with somatotropin or prolactin.

Hunt, R. K., and M. Jacobson (1972a). Proc. Natl. Acad. Sci. U.S.A. 69:780–783. Development and stability of positional information in Xenopus retinal ganglion cells.

Hunt, R. K., and M. Jacobson (1972b). Proc. Natl. Acad. Sci. U.S.A. 69:2860–2864. Specification of positional information in retinal ganglion cells of Xenopus: Stability of the unspecified state.

Hunt, R. K., and M. Jacobson (1973a). Proc. Natl. Acad. Sci. U.S.A. 70:507–511. Specification of positional information in retinal ganglion cells of Xenopus: Assay systems for analysis of the unspecified state.

Hunt, R. K., and M. Jacobson (1973b). Science 180:509–511. Neuronal locus specificity: Altered pattern of spatial deployment in fused fragments of embryonic Xenopus eyes.

Hunt, R. K., and M. Jacobson (1974a). Neuronal specificity revisited, pp. 203–258. In Current Topics in Developmental Biology, Vol. 8, (A. Moscona, and A. Monray, eds.), Academic Press, New York.

Hunt, R. K., and M. Jacobson (1974b). J. Physiol. (London) 241:90–91P. Rapid reversal of retinal axes in embryonic Xenopus eyes.

Hunt, R. K., and M. Jacobson (1974c). Dev. Biol. 40:1–15. Development of neuronal locus specificity in Xenopus retinal ganglion cells after surgical eye transection or after fusion of while eyes.

Hunt, R. K., and M. Jacobson (1974d). Proc. Natl. Acad. Sci. U.S.A., 71:3616–3620. Specification of positional information in retinal ganglion cells of Xenopus laevis: Intraocular control of the time of specification.

Hunt, S. P., and H. Künzle (1976). J. Comp. Neurol. 170:153–172. Observations on the projections and intrinsic organization of the pigeon optic tectum: An autoradiographic study based on anterograde and retrograde, axonal and dendritic flow.

Hunt, S. P., and K. E. Webster (1975). J. Comp. Neurol. 162:433–446. The projection of the retina upon the optic tectum of the pigeon.

Hunter, D. D., V. Shah, J. P. Merlie, and J. R. Sanes (1989). Nature 338:229–233. A laminin-like adhesive protein concentrated in the synaptic cleft of the neuromuscular junction.

Hunter, R., and I. Macalpine (1963). Three Hundred Years of Psychiatry, 1535–1860, Oxford University Press, London.

Huntington, H. W., and R. D. Terry (1966). The origin of reactive cells in cerebral stab wounds.

Hurle, J., and J. R. Hinchliffe (1978). J. Embryol. exp. Morph. 43:123–136. Cell death in the posterior necrotic zone (PNZ) of the chick wing-bud: A stereoscan and ultrastructural survey of autolysis and cell fragmentation.

Hurle, J. M. (1988). Meth. Achiev. exp. Pathol. 13:55–86. Cell death in developing systems.

Hursch, J. B. (1939). Amer. J. Physiol. 127:131–139. Conduction velocity and diameter of nerve fibers.

Hutchins, J. B., and V. A. Casagrande (1988). *Proc. Natl. Acad. Sci. U.S.A.* **85**:8316–8320. Glial cells develop a laminar pattern before neuronal cells in the lateral geniculate nucleus.

Hutchins, J. B., and V. A. Casagrande (1989). *GLIA* **2**:55–66. Vimentin: Changes in distribution during brain development.

Hutchins, J. B., and V. A. Casagrande (1990). *J. Comp. Neurol.* **298**:113–128. Development of lateral geniculate nucleus: Interactions between retinal afferents, cytoarchitectonic, and glial cell process lamination in ferrets and tree shrews.

Huttenlocher, P. R. (1966). *Nature* **211**:91–92. Development of neuronal activity in neocortex of the kitten.

Huttenlocher, P. R. (1967). *Exp. Neurol.* **17**:247–262. Development of cortical neuronal activity in the neonatal cat.

Huttenlocher, P. R. (1970). *Exp. Neurol.* **29**:405–415. Myelination and the development of function in immature pyramidal tract.

Huttenlocher, P. R., and C. de Courten (1987). *Human Neurobiol.* **6**:1–9. The development of synapses in striate cortex of man.

Huttenlocher, P. R., C. de Courten, L. J. Garey, and H. van der Loos (1982). *Neurosci. Lett.* **33**:247–252. Synaptogenesis in human visual cortex—Evidence for synapse elimination during normal development.

Huxley, A. F., and R. Stämpfli (1949). *J. Physiol. (London)* **108**:315–339. Evidence for saltatory conduction in peripheral myelinated nerve fibres.

Huxley, J. S. (1932). Problems of Relative Growth, Methuen, London, p. 276.

Huxley, J. S., and G. R. De Beer (1934). *The Elements of Experimental Embryology.* Cambridge Univ. Press, London, 514 pp.

Huxley, T. H. (1849). *Phil. Trans. Roy. Soc. (London) Ser. B.* ii, 413. On the anatomy and the affinities of the family of the Medusae.

Hyafil, F., D. Morello, C. Babinet, and F. Jacob (1980). *Cell* **21**:927–934. A cell surface glycoprotein involved in the compaction of embryonal carcinoma cells and cleavage stage embryos.

Hyafil, F., C. Babinet, and F. Jacob (1981). *Cell* **26**:447–454. Cell-cell interactions in early embryogenesis: A molecular approach to the role of calcium.

Hydén, H. (1943). *Acta Physiol. Scand. Suppl.* **17** 6:1–136. Protein metabolism in the nerve cell during growth and function.

Hydén, H. (1960). The neuron, pp. 215–323. In *The Cell*, Vol. 4, (J. Brachet, and A. E. Mirsky, eds.), Academic Press, New York.

Hydén, H. (1962). *Endeavour* **21**:144–155. The neuron and its glia—a biochemical and functional unit.

Hynes, R. (1985). *Ann. Rev. Cell Biol.* **1**:67–90. Molecular biology of fibronectin.

Hynes, R. O. (1987). *Cell* **48**:549–554. Integrins: A family of cell surface receptors.

Hynes, R. O. and K. M. Yamada (1982). *J. Cell Biol.* **95**:369–377. Fibronectins: Multifunctional modular glycoproteins.

Hynes, R. O., R. Patel, and R. H. Miller (1986). *J. Neurosci.* **6**:867–876. Migration of neuroblasts along preexisting axonal tracts during prenatal cerebellar development.

Hyyppä, M. (1969). *Z. Anat. Entwicklungsgesch.* **129**:41–52. Differentiation of the hypothalamic nuclei during ontogenetic development in the rat.

Ibrahim, M. Z. M. (1974). *J. Neurol. Sci.* **21**:431–478. The mast cell of the mammalian central nervous system. I. Morphology, distribution and histochemistry.

Ibrahim, M. Z. M., M. Z. Al-Wirr, and N. Bahuth (1979). *Acta Anat.* **104**:134–154. The mast cell of the mammalian central nervous system. III. Ultrastructural characteristics in the adult rat brain.

Ide, C (1982). *Amer. J. Anat.* **163**:73–85. Regeneration of mouse digital corpuscles.

Ide, C., K. Tohyana, R. Yokota, T. Nitatori, and S. Onodera (1983). *Brain Res.* **288**:61–75. Schwann cell basal lamina and nerve regeneration.

Ide, C. F., S. E. Fraser, and R. L. Meyer (1983). *Science* **221**:293–295. Eye dominance columns from an isogenic double-nasal frog eye.

Ifft, J. D. (1972). *J. Comp. Neurol.* **144**:139–204. An autoradiographic study of the time of final division of neurons in rat hypothalamic nuclei.

Iggo, A., and A. R. Muir (1969). *J. Physiol. (London)* **200**:763–796. The structure and function of a slowly adapting touch corpuscle in hairy skin.

Iggo, A., and K. H. Andres (1982). *Ann. Rev. Neurosci.* **5**:1–31. Morphology of cutaneous receptors.

Ikeda, K., and W. D. Kaplan (1970a). *Proc. Natl. Acad. Sci. U.S.A.* **66**:765–772. Patterned activity of a mutant *Drosophila melanogaster.*

Ikeda, K., and W. D. Kaplan (1970b). *Proc. Natl. Acad. Sci. U.S.A.* **67**:1480–1487. Unilaterally patterned neural activity of gynandromorphs, mosaic for a neurological mutant of *Drosophila melanogaster.*

Iles, J. F., and B. Mulloney (1971). *Brain Res.* **30**:397–400. Procion yellow staining of cockroach motor neurons without the use of microelectrodes.

Illing, R. B., and H. Wässle (1981). *J. Comp. Neurol.* **202**:265–285. The retinal projection to the thalamus in the cat: A quantitative investigation and a comparison with the retinotectal pathway.

Ilyinsky, O. B., N. C. Chalisova, and V. F. Kuznetsov (1973). *Experientia* **29**:1129–1131. Development of the new Pacinian corpuscles. Studies on the foreign innervation of mesentery.

Imamoto, K., and C. P. Leblond (1977). *J. Comp. Neurol.* **174**:255–280. Presence of labelled monocytes, macrophages and microglia in a stab wound of the brain following an injection of bone marrow cells labelled with ^{3}H-uridine into rats.

Imamoto, K., and C. P. Leblond (1978). *J. Comp. Neurol.* **180**:139–164. Radioautographic investigation of gliogenesis in the corpus callosum of young rats. II. Origin of microglial cells.

Imamoto, K., T. Nagai, and T. Maeda (1982a). *Arch. Histol. Jpn.* **45**:191–206. Effects of neonatal administrations of 6-OHDA on brain development. II. Changes in the central noradrenaline system.

Imamoto, K., R. Fujiwara, T. Nagai, and T. Maeda (1982b). *Arch. Histol. Jpn.* **45**:505–518. Distribution and fate of macrophogic amoeboid cells in the rat brain.

Inestrosa, I. C., H. L. Fernandez, and J. Garrido (1976). *Neurosci. Lett.* **2**:217–221. Actin-like filaments in synaptosomes detected by heavy meromyosin binding.

Inestrosa, N. C., and J. Alvarez (1988). *Brain Res.* **441**:331–

338. Axons grow in the aging rat but fast transport and acetylcholinesterase content remain unchanged.

Ingebrigtsen, R. (1913a). *J. Exper. Med.* 17:182–191. Studies of the degeneration and regeneration of the axis cylinders *in vitro*.

Ingebrigtsen, R. (1913b). *J. Exper. Med.* 18:412–415. Regeneration of axis cylinders *in vitro*. Second communication.

Ingham, P. W. (1988). *Nature* 335:25–34. The molecular genetics of embryonic pattern formation in *Drosophila*.

Ingham, P. W., D. Ish-Horowicz and K. R. Howard (1986). *EMBO J.* 5:1659–1665. Correlative changes in homoeotic and segmentation gene expression in Krüppel mutant embryos of *Drosophila*.

Ingram, D. K., and T. P. Corfman (1980). *Neurosci. Biobehav. Rev.* 4:421–435. An overview of neurobiological comparison in mouse strains.

Ingram, V. M., M. P. Ogren, C. L. Chatot, J. M. Gossels, and B. Blanchard Owens (1985). *Proc. Natl. Acad. Sci. U.S.A.* 82:7131–7135. Diversity among Purkinje cells in the monkey cerebellum.

Ingvar, D. (1947). *Acta Physiol. Scand.* 13:150–154. Experiments on the influence of electric currents upon growing nerve cell processes *in vitro*.

Ingvar, S. (1920). *Proc. Soc. Exp. Biol. Med. N.Y.* 17:198–199. Reaction of cells to galvanic current in tissue cultures.

Innocenti, G. M. (1981). *Science* 212:824–827. Growth and reshaping of axons in the establishment of visual callosal connections.

Innocenti, G. M., and S. Clarke (1984). *Dev. Brain Res.* 14:143–148. Bilateral transitory projections to visual areas from auditory cortex in kittens.

Innocenti, G. M., L. Fiore, and R. Caminiti (1977). *Neurosci. Lett.* 4:237–242. Exuberant projection into the corpus callosum from the visual cortex of newborn cats.

Innocenti, G. M., S. Clarke, and H. Koppel (1983a). *Dev. Brain Res.* 11:39–54. Transitory macrophage in the white matter of the developing visual cortex. I. Light and electron microscopic characteristics and distribution.

Innocenti, G. M., S. Clarke, and H. Koppel (1983b). *Dev. Brain Res.* 11:55–66. Transitory macrophages in the white matter of the developing visual cortex. II. Development and relations with axonal pathways.

Innocenti, G. M., S. Clarke, and R. Kraftsik (1986). *J. Neurosci.* 6:1384–1409. Interchange of callosal and association projections in the developing visual cortex.

Inouye, E. (1970). *Japan. J. Human Genet.* 15:1–25. Twin studies and human behavioral genetics.

Inouye, M., and U. Murakami (1980). *J. Comp. Neurol.* 194:499–503. Temporal and patial patterns of Purkinje cell formation in the mouse cerebellum.

Insausti, R., C. Blakemore, and W. M. Cowan (1984). *Nature* 308:362–365. Ganglion cell death during development of ipsilateral retino-collicular projection in golden hamster.

Inukai, T. (1928). *J. Comp. Neurol.* 45:1–31. On the loss of Purkinje cells, with advancing age, from the cerebellar cortex of the albino rat.

Irwin, L. N., D. B. Michael, and C. C. Irwin (1980). *J. Neurochem.* 34:1527–1530. Ganglioside patterns of fetal rat and mouse brain.

Irwin, M., R. E. Klein, J. W. Townshend, W. Owens, P. L. Engle, A. Lechtig, R. Martorell, C. Yarbrough, R. E. Lasky, and H. L. Delgado (1979). The effect of food supplementation on cognitive development and behavior among rural Guatemalan Children, pp. 239–254. In Brozek, *Behavioral effects of energy and protein deficits*, US Department of Health, Education and Welfare, NIH Publ. No. (NIH) 79-1906.

Ishii, K. (1967). *Sci. Rep. Tohoku Univ.* Series IV (Biol.) 33:97–104. Morphogenesis of the brain in Medaka, *Oryzias latipes*. I. Observations on morphogenesis.

Itakura, T., T. Kasamatsu, and J. D. Pettigrew (1981). *Neuroscience* 6:159–175. Norepinephrine-containing terminals in kitten visual cortex: Laminar distribution and ultrastructure.

Itaya, S. K., and G. W. Van Hoesen (1982). *Brain Res.* 236:199–204. WGA-HRP as a transneuronal marker in the visual pathways of monkey and rat.

Ito, M. (1984). *The Cerebellum and Neural Control.* Raven, New York.

Itoyama, Y., H. deF. Webster, E. P. Richardson, Jr., and B. D. Trapp. (1983). *Ann. Neurol.* 14:339–346. Schwann cell remyelination of demyelinated axons in spinal cord multiple sclerosis lesions.

Ivanov, A., and D. Purves (1989). *J. Comp. Neurol.* 284:398–404. Ongoing electrical activity of superior cervical ganglion cells in mammals of different size.

Iversen, L. L. (1984). *Proc. Roy. Soc. (London) Ser. B.* 221:245–260. The Ferrier lecture, 1983. Amino acids and peptides: Fast and slow chemical signals in the nervous system?

Iversen, L. L., J. F. Mitchell, and V. Srinivasan (1971). *J. Physiol. (London)* 212:519–534. The release of gamma-amino-butyric acid during inhibition in the cat.

Iversen, O. H. (1976). The history of chalones, p. 37. In *Chalones* (J. C. Houck, ed.). American Elsevier Publishing Company, Inc., New York.

Iversen, O. H. (1981). The Chalones, p. 491. In *Handbook of Experimental Pharmacology*, Vol. 57 (R. Baserga, ed.), Springer-Verlag, New York.

Ivy, G. O., and H. P. Killackey (1978). *Brain Res.* 158:213–218. Transient populations of glial cells in developing rat telencephalon revealed by horseradish peroxidase.

Ivy, G. O., and H. P. Killackey (1981). *J. Comp. Neurol.* 195:367–389. The ontogeny of the distribution of callosal projections in the rat parietal cortex.

Ivy, G. O., and H. P. Killackey (1982). *J. Neurosci.* 2:735–743. Ontogenetic changes in the projections of neocortical neurons.

Jacklet, J. W., and M. J. Cohen (1967a). *Science* 156:1638–1640. Synaptic connections between a transplanted insect ganglion and muscles of the host.

Jacklet, J. W., and M. J. Cohen (1967b). *Science* 156:1640–1643. Nerve regeneration: Correlation of electrical histological and behavioral events.

Jackson, C. A., J. D. Peduzzi, and T. L. Hickey (1989). *J. Neurosci.* 9:1242–1253. Visual cortex development in the ferret. I. Genesis and migration of visual cortical neurons.

Jackson, H., and T. N. Parks (1982). *J. Neurosci.* 2:1736–1743. Functional synapse elimination in the developing avian cochlear nucleus with simultaneous reduction in cochlear nerve axon branching.

Jackson, H., and T. N. Parks (1988). *J. Comp. Neurol.* 271:106–114. Induction of novel functional afferents to the chick cochlear nucleus.

Jackson, J. H. (1898). *Br. Med. J.* 1:65–69. Remarks on the relations of different divisions of the central nervous syustem to one another and to parts of the body.

Jackson, J. H. (1931). *Selected writings of John Hughlings Jackson,* vol. 1. (J. Taylor, ed.), Hodder and Stoughton, London.

Jackson, P. C., and E. Frank (1987). *J. Comp. Neurol.* 255:538–547. Development of synaptic connections between muscle sensory and motor neurons: Anatomical evidence that postsynaptic dendrites grow into a preformed sensory neuropil.

Jacob, F. (1982). *The Possible and The Actual.* Univ. Washington Press, Seattle.

Jacob, M., B. Christ, and H. J. Jacob (1978). *Anat. Embryol.* 153:179–193. On the migration of myogenic stem cell into the prospective wing region of chick embryos.

Jacobs, D. S., V. H. Perry, and M. J. Hawken (1984). *J. Neurosci.* 4:2425–2433. The postnatal reduction of the uncrossed projection from the nasal retina in the cat.

Jacobs, H. L., and K. N. Sharma (1969). *Ann. N.Y. Acad. Sci.* 157:1084–1125. Taste versus calories: sensory and metabolic signals in the control of food intake.

Jacobs, M., Q. L. Choo, and C. Thomas (1982). *J. Neurochem.* 38:969–977. Vimentin and 70 K neurofilament protein co-exist in embryonic neurones from spinal ganglia.

Jacobs-Cohen, R. J., R. F. Payette, M. D. Gershon, and T. P. Rothman (1987). *J. Comp. Neurol.* 255:425–438. Inability of neural crest cells to colonize the presumptive aganglionic bowel of *ls/ls* mutant mice: Requirement for a permissive microenvironment.

Jacobsen, S. (1963). *J. Comp. Neurol.* 121:5–129. Sequence of myelination in the brain of the albino rat. A. Cerebral cortex, thalamus and related structures.

Jacobson, A. G. (1988). *Development* 104:Suppl. 209–220. Somitomeres: Mesodermal segments of vertebrate embryos.

Jacobson, A. G., and S. Meier (1984) *Dev. Biol.* 106:181–193. Morphogenesis of the head of a newt: Mesodermal segments, neuromeres, and distribution of neural crest.

Jacobson, A. G., and P. P. L. Tam (1982). *Anat. Rec.* 203:375–396. Cephalic neurulation in the mouse embryo analyzed by SEM and morphometry.

Jacobson, A. G., G. F. Oster, G. M. Odell, and L. Y. Cheng (1986). *J. Embryol. Exp. Morph.* 96:19–49. Neurulation and the cortical tractor model for epithelial folding.

Jacobson, C.-O. (1959). *J. Embryol. Exp. Morph.* 7:1–21. The localization of the presumptive cerebral regions in the neural plate of the axolotl larva.

Jacobson, C.-O. (1962). *Zool. Bidrag. Uppsala.* 35:433–449. Cell migration in the neural plate and the process of neurulation in the axolotl larva.

Jacobson, C.-O. (1964). *Zool. Bidrag. Uppsala* 36:73–160. Motor nuclei, cranial nerve roots, and fibre pattern in the medulla oblongata after reversal experiments on the neural plate of Axolotl larvae. I. Bilateral operations.

Jacobson, C.-O. (1969). *Zool. Bidrag, Uppsala* 38:241–247. Production of artificial heterokaryons from mammalian neurons and various undifferentiated cells.

Jacobson, C. O., and A. Jacobson (1973). *Zoon* 1:17–21. Studies on morphogenetic movements during neural tube closure in amphibia.

Jacobson, M. (1960a). Studies in the organization of visual mechanisms in Amphibians, Ph.D. Thesis, Edinburgh Univ.

Jacobson, M. (1960b). *J. Physiol. (London)* 154:31–32P. The representation of the visual field on the optic tectum of the frog: Evidence for the presence of an area centralis retinae.

Jacobson, M. (1961a). *J. Physiol. (London)* 157:27–29P. The recovery of an electrical activity in the optic tectum of the frog during early regeneration of the optic nerve.

Jacobson, M. (1961b). *Proc. Roy. Phys. Soc. Edin.* 28:131–137. Recovery of electrical activity in the optic tectum of the frog during early regeneration of the optic nerve.

Jacobson, M. (1962). *Quart. J. Exp. Physiol.* 47:170–178. The representation of the retina on the optic tectum of the frog. Correlation between retinotectal magnification factor and retinal ganglion cell count.

Jacobson, M. (1964). *Quart. J. Exp. Physiol.* 49:384–393. Spectral sensitivity of single units in the optic tectum of the goldfish.

Jacobson, M. (1966). Starting points for research in the ontogeny of behavior, pp. 339–383. In *Major Problems in Developmental Biology* (M. Locke, ed.), Academic Press, New York.

Jacobson, M. (1967). *Science* 155:1106–1108. Retinal ganglion cells: Specification of central connections in larval *Xenopus laevis*.

Jacobson, M. (1968a). *Dev. Biol.* 17:202–218. Development of neuronal specificity in retinal ganglion cells of *Xenopus*.

Jacobson, M. (1968b). *Dev. Biol.* 17:219–232. Cessation of DNA synthesis in retinal ganglion cells correlated with the time of specification of their central connections.

Jacobson, M. (1969). *Science* 163:543–547. Development of specific neuronal connections.

Jacobson, M. (1970a). Development, specification and diversification of neuronal connections. In *The Neurosciences: Second Study Program* (F. O. Schmitt, ed.), The Rockefeller Univ. Press, New York.

Jacobson, M. (1970b). *Developmental Neurobiology,* First edn., Holt Rinehart and Winston, New York.

Jacobson, M. (1971a). Formation of neuronal connections in sensory systems. In *Handbook of Sensory Physiology,* Vol. 1, Chap. 6, (W. Loewenstein, ed.), Springer-Verlag, New York.

Jacobson, M. (1971b). *Proc. Natl. Acad. Sci. U.S.A.* 68:528–532. Absence of adaptive modification in developing retinotectal connections in frogs after visual deprivation or disparate stimulation of the eyes.

Jacobson, M. (1973). Genesis of neuronal specificity, pp. 105–119. In *Development and Ageing in the Nervous System* (M. Rockstein, ed.), Academic Press, New York.

Jacobson, M. (1974a). *Ann. N.Y. Acad. Sci.* 228:63–67, Through the jungle of the brain: Neuronal specificity and typology re-explored.

Jacobson, M. (1974b). A plentitude or neurons, pp. 151–166. In *Studies on the Development of Behavior and the Nervous System,* Vol. 2, (G. Gottlieb, ed.), Academic Press, New York.

Jacobson, M. (1974c). Neuronal plasticity: concepts in pursuit of cellular mechanisms, pp. 31–43, In *Plasticity and Recovery of Function in the Central Nervous System,* Vol. 2, (G. Gottlieb, ed.), Academic Press, New York.

Jacobson, M. (1975a). Development and evolution of Type II neurons: Conjectures a century after Golgi. In *Golgi Centennial Symposium* (M. Santini, ed.), Raven Press, New York.

Jacobson, M. (1975b). Differentiation and Growth of Nerve

Cells. In *Differentiation and Growth of Cells in Vertebrate Tissues*, Chap. 2, (G. Golspink, ed.), Chapman & Hall, London.

Jacobson, M. (1975c). Brain development in relation to language, pp. 105–119. In *Foundations of Language Development*, Vol. 1, (E. H. Lenneberg, and E. Lenneberg, eds.), UNESCO and Academic Press, Paris and New York.

Jacobson, M. (1976a). *Brain Res.* 103:541–545. Histogenesis of retina in the clawed frog with implications for the pattern of development of retinotectal connections.

Jacobson, M. (1976b). *Science* 191:288–290. Premature specification of the retina in embryonic *Xenopus* eyes treated with ionophore X537A.

Jacobson, M. (1976c). Neuronal recognition in the retinotectal system. In *Neuronal Recognition*, (S. Barondes, ed.), Plenum Press, New York.

Jacobson, M. (1977). *Brain Res.* 127:55–67. Mapping the developing retino-tectal projection in frog tadpoles by a double label autoradiographic technique.

Jacobson, M. (1978). *Zoon* 6:149–156. Clonal origins of the central nervous system: Towards a developmental anatomy.

Jacobson, M. (1980). *Trends Neurosci.* 1:3–5. Clones and compartments in the vertebrate central nervous system.

Jacobson, M. (1981a). *J. Neurosci.* 1:918–922. Rohon-Beard neuron origin from blastomeres of the 16-cell frog embryo.

Jacobson, M. (1981b). *J. Neurosci.* 1:923–927. Rohon-Beard neurons arise from a substitute ancestral cell after removal of the cell from which they normally arise in the 16-cell frog embryo.

Jacobson, M. (1982). Origins of the nervous system in amphibians, pp. 45–99. In *Current Topics in Neurobiology* (N. C.Spitzer, ed.), Plenum, New York.

Jacobson, M. (1983). *J. Neurosci.* 3:1019–1038. Clonal organization of the central nervous system of the frog. III. Clones stemming from individual blastomeres of the 128-, 256-, and 512-cell stages.

Jacobson, M. (1984). *Dev. Biol.* 102:122–129. Cell lineage analysis of neural induction: Origins of cells forming the induced nervous system.

Jacobson, M. (1985a). *Ann. Rev. Neurosci.* 8:71–102. Clonal analysis and cell lineages of the vertebrate central nervous system.

Jacobson, M. (1985b). *Trends Neurosci.* 8:151–155. Clonal analysis of the vertebrate central nervous system.

Jacobson, M. (1985c). *Modern masters of Chinese painting from the People's Republic of China*. Utah Museum of Fine Arts, Salt Lake City, Utah.

Jacobson, M. (1988). Neural cell adhesion molecule (NCAM) expression in *Xenopus* embryos during formation of central and peripheral neural maps, pp. 128–148. In *The Making of the Nervous System* (J. G. Parnavelas, C. D Stern, and R. V. Stirling, eds.), Oxford Univ. Press, Oxford.

Jacobson, M. (1990a). Methods for clonal analysis and tracing cell lineages in the vertebrate CNS. In *Methods In Neuroscience* (P. M. Conn, ed.), Academic Press, Orlando, Florida.

Jacobson, M. (1990b). *Semin. Dev. Biol.* 1:101–108. Segmentation and homeosis of vertebrate limbs.

Jacobson, M. (in preparation). *Conceptual Foundations of Neuroscience*, Plenum, New York.

Jacobson, M., and R. E. Baker (1968). *Science* 160:543–545. Neuronal specification of cutaneous nerves through connections with skin grafts in the frog.

Jacobson, M., and R. E. Baker (1969). *J. Comp. Neurol.* 137:121–142. Development of neuronal connections with skin grafts in frogs: Behavioral and electrophysiological studies.

Jacobson, M., and R. M. Gaze (1964). *Quart. J. Exp. Physiol.* 49:199–209. Types of visual response from single units in the optic tectum and optic nerve of the goldfish.

Jacobson, M., and R. M. Gaze (1965). *Exp. Neurol.* 13:418–430. Selection of appropriate tectal connections by regenerating optic nerve fibres in adult goldfish.

Jacobson, M., and G. Hirose (1978). *Science* 202:637–639. Origin of the retina from both sides of the embryonic brain: A contribution to the problem of crossing at the optic chiasma.

Jacobson, M., and G. Hirose (1981). *J. Neurosci.* 1:271–284. Clonal organization of the central nervous system of the frog. II. Clones stemming from individual blastomeres of the 32- and 64-cell stages.

Jacobson, M., and H. V. B. Hirsch (1973a). *Brain Res.* 49:47–65. Development and maintenance of connectivity in the visual system of the frog. I. The effects of eye rotation and visual deprivation.

Jacobson, M., and H. V. B. Hirsch (1973b). *Brain Res.* 49:67–74. Development and maintenance of connectivity in the visual system of the frog. II. The effects of eye removal.

Jacobson, M., and S. Huang (1985). *Dev. Biol.* 110:102–113. Neurite outgrowth traced by means of horseradish peroxidase inherited from neuronal ancestral cells in frog embryos.

Jacobson, M., and R. K. Hunt (1973). *Sci. Amer.* 228:26–35. Origins of nerve-cell specificity.

Jacobson, M., and S. L. Klein (1985). *Phil. Trans. Roy. Soc. (London) B.* 312:57–65. Analysis of clonal restriction of cell mingling in *Xenopus*.

Jacobson, M., and R. L. Levine (1975a). *Brain Res.* 88:339–345. Plasticity in the adult frog brain: Filling the visual scotoma after excision or translocation of parts of the optic tectum.

Jacobson, M., and R. L. Levine (1975b). *Brain Res.* 92:468–471 Stability of implanted duplicate tectal positional markers serving as targets for optic axons in adult frogs.

Jacobson, M., and S. A. Moody (1984). *J. Neurosci.* 4:1361–1369. Quantitative lineage analysis of the frog's nervous system. I. Lineages of Rohon-Beard neurons and primary motoneurons.

Jacobson, M., and U. Rutishauser (1986). *Dev. Biol.* 116:524–531. Induction of neural cell adhesion molecule (NCAM) in *Xenopus* embryos.

Jacobson, M., and W. L. Xu (1989). *Dev. Biol.* 131:119–125. States of determination of single cells transplanted between 512-cell *Xenopus* embryos.

Jacobson, S. (1963). *J. Comp. Neurol.* 121:5–29. Sequence of myelinization in the brain of the albino rat. A. cerebral cortex, thalamus and related structures.

Jacoby, J., and C. B. Kimmel (1982). *J. Comp. Neurol.* 204:364–376. Synaptogenesis and its relation to growth of the postsynaptic cell: A quantitative study of the developing Mauthner neuron of the axolotl.

Jacubowitsch, I. (1857). *Mittheilungen über den feineren Bau von Gehirn und Mark.* Breslau.

Jaenisch, R. (1985). *Nature* 318:181–183. Mammalian neural

crest cells participate in normal embryonic development on microinjection into post-implantation mouse embryos.

Jaffe, L. (1955). *Proc. Nat. Acad. Sci. U.S.A.* 41:267–270. Do *Fucus* eggs interact through a CO_2-pH gradient?

Jaffe, L. (1968). *Adv. Morphogenesis* 7:295–328. Localization in the developing Fucus egg and the general role of localizing currents.

Jaffe, L. F. (1977). *Nature* 265:600–602. Electrophoresis along cell membranes.

Jaffe, L. F., and R. Nuccitelli (1974). *J. Cell Biol.* 63:614–628. An ultrasensitive vibrating probe for measuring steady extracellular currents.

Jaffe, L. F., and R. Nuccitelli (1977). *Ann. Rev. Biophys. Bioeng.* 6:445–476. Electrical controls of development.

Jaffe, L. F., and M.-M. Poo (1979). *J. Exp. Zool.* 209:115–128. Neurites grow faster towards the cathode than the anode in a steady field.

Jaffe, L. F., and C. D. Stern (1979). *Science* 206:569–571. Strong electrical currents leave the primitive streak of chick embryos.

Jahn, T. L., and E. C. Boyee (1969). *Physiol. Rev.* 49:793–862. Protoplasmic movements within cells.

James, D. W., and R. L. Tresman (1969). *Z. Zellforsch. Mikroskop. Anat. Abt. Histochem.* 100:126–140. An electron microscopic study of the de novo formation of neuromuscular junctions in tissue culture.

Jande, S. S., L. Maler, and D. E. M. Lawson (1981). *Nature* 294:765–767. Immunohistochemical mapping of vitamin D-dependent calcium binding protein in brain.

Jankowska, E., Y. Padel, and R. Tanaka (1975). *J. Physiol. (London)* 249:637–669. Projections of pyramidal tract cells to alpha-motoneurons innervating hindlimb muscles in the monkeys.

Janning, W. (1978). Gynandromorph fate maps in *Drosophila*, pp. 1–28. In *Genetics Mosaics and Cell Differentiation* (W. J. Gehring, ed.), Springer Verlag, Berlin/Heidelberg.

Janowsky, J. S., and B. L. Finlay (1983). *Anat. Embryol.* 167:439–447. Cell degeneration in early development of the forebrain and cerebellum.

Jansen, J. K., T. Lomo, K. Nicolaysen, and R. H. Westgaard (1973). *Science* 181:559–561. Hyperinnervation of skeletal muscle fibers: Dependence on muscle activity.

Jansen, J. K., D. C. van Essen, and M. C. Brown (1975). Formation and elimination of synapses in skeletal muscles of rat, pp. 425–434. In *Cold Spring Harbor Symposium on Quantitative Biology, The Synapse*, Vol. 40.

Jansen, J. K. S., and J. G. Nicholls (1972). *Proc. Natl. Acad. Sci. U.S.A.* 69:636–639. Regeneration and changes in synaptic connections between individual nerve cells in the central nervous system of the leech.

Jansen, J. K. S., T. Lomo, K. Nicolaysen, and R. H. Westgaard (1973). *Science* 181:559–561. Hyperinnervation of skeletal muscle fibers: Dependence on muscle activity.

Jansen, J. K. S., W. Thompson, and D. P. Kuffler (1978). *Prog. Brain Res.* 48:3–18. The formation and maintenance of synaptic connections as illustrated by studies of the neuromuscular junction.

Janzer, R. C., and M. C. Raff (1987). *Nature* 325:253–257. Astrocytes induce blood-brain barrier properties in endothelial cells.

Jarlstedt, J. and J.-O. Karlsson (1973). *Exp. Brain Res.* 16:501–506. Evidence for axonal transport of RNA in mammalian neurons.

Jaros, E., W. G. Bradley (1979). *Neuropath. Appl. Neurobiol.* 5:133–147. Atypical axon-Schwann cell relationships in the common peroneal nerve of the dystrophic mouse: An ultrastructural study.

Jarvik, E. (1980). *Basic Structure and Evolution of Vertebrates*, 2 Vols. Academic Press, New York.

Jeffery, G. (1984). *Dev. Brain Res.* 13:81–96. Retinal ganglion cell death and terminal field retraction in the developing rodent visual system.

Jeffery, G., and V. H. Perry (1982). *Dev. Brain Res.* 2:176–180. Evidence for ganglion cell death during development of the ipsilateral retinal projection in the rat.

Jeffery, W. R. (1985). *J. Embryol. Exp. Morphol.* 89:275–287. Identification of proteins and mRNAs in isolated yellow crescents of ascidian eggs.

Jeffrey, P. L., and L. Austin (1973). *Prog. Neurobiol.* 2:207–255. Axoplasmic transport.

Jeffrey, P. L., K. A. C. James, A. D. Kidman, A. M. Richards, and L. Austin (1972). *J. Neurobiol.* 3:199–208. The flow of mitochondria in chicken sciatic nerve.

Jelínek, R. (1959). *Csk. Morfologie,* 7:163–173. Proliferace v centrálním nervovém kurecich zárodku I. Doba trávaní mitosy v germinální zone míchy od 2. do 6. dne zárodeckého vyvoje.

Jelínek, R., and Z. Friebova (1966). *Nature* 209:822–823. Influence of mitotic activity on neurulation movements.

Jelínek, R., and T. Pexieder (1970). *Folia morph.* 18:102–110. Pressure of the CSF and the morphogenesis of the CNS.

Jellies, J. (1990). *Trends Neurosci.* 13:126–131. Muscle assembly in simple systems.

Jellinger, K. (1972). *Z. Anat. Entwicklungsgesch.* 138:145–154. Embryonal cell nests in human cerebellar nuclei.

Jen, L. S., K.-F. So, and H. H. Woo (1984). *Brain Res.* 294:169–173. An anterograde HRP study of the retinocollicular pathways in normal hamsters and hamsters with one eye enucleated at birth.

Jenkins, S., and C. Straznicky (1986). *Anat. Embryol.* 174:59–66. Naturally occurring and induced ganglion cell death. A retinal whole-mount autoradiographic study in *Xenopus*.

Jensen, K. F., and H. P. Killackey (1984). *Proc. Natl. Acad. Sci. U.S.A.* 81:964–968. Subcortical projections from ectopic neocortical neurons.

Jerison, H. J. (1963) *Human Biol.* 35:263–291. Interpreting the evolution of the brain.

Jerison, H. J. (1969). *Amer. Naturalist* 103:575–588. Brain evolution and dinosaur brains.

Jerison, H. J. (1970). *Science* 170:1224–1225. Brain evolution: New light on old principles.

Jerison, H. J. (1974). *Science* 184:677–679. On the meaning of brain size.

Jessell, T. M. (1988). *Neuron* 1:3–13. Adhesion molecules and the hierarchy of neural development.

Jessen, K. R., and R. Mirsky (1983). *J. Neurosci.* 3:2206–2218. Astrocyte-like glia in the peripheral nervous system: An immunohistochemical study of enteric glia.

Jessen, K. R., R. Mirsky, and L. Morgan (1987). *J. Neurosci.* 7:3362–3369. Axonal signals regulate the differentiation of non-myelin forming Schwann cells: An immunohistochemical study of galactocerebroside in transected and regenerating nerves.

Jirmanová, I., and S. Thesleff (1972). *Z. Zellforsch.* 131:77–97. Ultrastructural study of experimental muscle degeneration and regeneration in the adult rat.

Jirmanová, I., and J. Zelená (1970). *Z. Zellforsch. Mikrosk. Anat.* 106:333–347. Effect of denervation and tenotomy on slow and fast muscles of the chicken.

Jirmanová, I., and J. Zelena (1973). *Z. Zellforsch. Mikrosk. Anat.* 146:103–121. Ultrastructural transformation of fast chicken muscle fibres induced by nerve cross-union.

Jirmanová, I., and J. Zelena (1974). *Folia Morphol. (Praha)* XXII:270–272. Ultrastructural transformation of fast chicken muscles reinnervated with slow-type nerves.

Johannsen, O. A., and F. H. Butt (1941). *Embryology of Insects and Myriapods.* McGraw-Hill, New York.

Johanson, C. E. (1989). Ontogeny and phylogeny of the blood-brain barrier, pp. 101–129. In *Implications of The Blood-Brain Barrier and Its Manipulation, Vol. 1, Basic Science Aspects* (E. Neuwelt, ed.), Plenum Press, New York.

Johnen, A. G. (1964). *Arch. Entwmech. Organ.* 155:302–313. Experimentelle Untersuchungen über die Bedeutung des Zeitfaktors beim Vorgang der Neuralen Induktion.

Johns, P. R., A. Rusoff, and M. W. Dubin (1979). *J. Comp. Neurol.* 187:545–556. Postnatal neurogenesis in the kitten retina.

Johns, T. R., and S. Thesleff (1961). *Acta Physiol. Scand.* 51:136–141. Effects of motor inactivation on the chemical sensitivity of skeletal muscle.

Johnson, D., A. Lanahan, C. R. Buck, A. Sehgal, C. Morgan, E. Mercer, M. Bothwell, and M. Chao (1986). *Cell* 47:545–554. Expression and structure of the human NGF receptor.

Johnson, E. M., M. T. Caserta, and L. L. Ross (1977). *Brain Res.* 136:455–464. Effect of destruction of the postganglionic sympathetic neurons in neonatal rats on development of choline acetyltransferase and survival of preganglionic cholinergic neurons.

Johnson, E. M., Jr., and M. Taniuchi (1987). Nerve growth factor (NGF) receptors in the central nervous system.

Johnson, E. M., Jr., P. M. Gorin, L. D. Brandeis, and J. Pearson (1980). *Science* 210:916–918. Dorsal root ganglion neurons are destroyed by exposure *in utero* to maternal antibody to nerve growth factor.

Johnson, E. M., Jr., K. M. Rich, and H. K. Yip (1986). *Trends Neurosci.* 9:33–37. The role of NGF in sensory neurons *in vivo.*

Johnson, E. M., Jr., M. Taniuchi, H. B. Clark, J. E. Springer, S. Koh, M. W. Tayrien, and R. Loy (1987). *J. Neurosci.* 7:923–929. Demonstration of the retrograde transport of nerve growth factor receptor in the peripheral and central nervous system.

Johnson, G. D., and G. M. C. Nogueira Araujo (1981). *J. Immunol. Methods* 43:349–350. A simple method of reducing the fading of immunofluorescence during microscopy.

Johnson, J. E., Y.-A. Barde, M. Schwab, and H. Thoenen (1986). *J. Neurosci.* 6:3031–3038. Brain-derived neurotrophic factor supports the survival of cultured rat retinal ganglion cells.

Johnson, L. R., L. E. Westrum, M. A. Henry, and R. C. Canfield (1985). *Brain Res.* 345:379–383. Toxic ricin demonstrates a dual dental projection.

Johnson, M. H., B. Maro, and M. Takeichi (1986). *J. Embryol. Exp. Morph.* 93:239–255. The role of cell adhesion in the synchronization and orientation of polarization in 8-cell mouse blastomeres.

Johnson, R., and M. Armstrong-James (1970). *Z. Zellforsch.*

Mikrosk. Anat. 110:540–558. Morphology of superficial postnatal cerebral cortex with special reference to synapses.

Johnston, J. B. (1902). *J. Comp. Neurol.* 12:87–106. An attempt to define the primitive functional divisions of the central nervous system.

Johnston, J. B. (1905). *J. Comp. Neurol.* 15:175–275. The morphology of the vertebrate head from the viewpoint oif the functional divisions of the nervous system.

Johnston, J. B. (1906). *The Nervous System of Vertebrates.* P. Blakiston's Son & Co., Philadelphia.

Johnston, J. B. (1909). *J. Comp. Neurol.* 19:593–644. The radix mesencephalica trigemini.

Johnston, J. B. (1914). *Anat. Rec.* 8:185–198. The nervus terminalis in man and mammals.

Johnston, J. G., and D. van der Kooy (1989). *Proc. Natl. Acad. Sci. U.S.A.* 86:1066–1070. Protooncogene expression identifies a transient columnar organization of the forebrain within the late embryonic ventricular zone.

Johnston, M. C. (1966). *Anat. Rec.* 156:143–156. A radioautographic study of the migration and fate of cranial neural crest cells in the chick embryo.

Jolly, W. A. (1911). *Quart. J. exp. Physiol.* 4:67–87. The time relations of the knee-jerk and simple reflexes.

Jones, B., and T. Anuza (1982). *Neuropsychology* 20:347–350. Sex differences in cerebral lateralization in 3- and 4-year-old children.

Jones, D. G. (1973). *Z. Zellforsch. Mikrosk. Anat.* 143:301–312. Some factors affecting the PTA staining of synaptic junctions. A preliminary comparison of PTA stained junctions in various regions of the CNS.

Jones, D. G. (1983). Development, maturation, and aging of synapses, pp. 163–222. In *Advances in Cellular Neurobiology*, Vol. 4, (S. Federoff, and L. Hertz, eds.), Academic Press, New York.

Jones, D. G., and B. J. Smith (1980). *Prog. Neurobiol.* 15:19–69. The hippocampus and its response to differential environments.

Jones, D. G., M. M. Dittmer, and L. C. Reading (1974). *Brain Res.* 70:245–259. Synaptogenesis in guinea-pig cerebral cortex: A glutaraldehyde-PTA study.

Jones, D. S. (1939). *Anat. Rec.* 73:343–357. Studies on the origin of sheaths cells and sympathetic ganglia in the chick.

Jones, E. A. and H. R. Woodland (1987). *Development* 101:557–563. The development of animal cap cells in *Xenopus:* A measure of the start of animal cap competence to form mesoderm.

Jones, E. A., and H. R. Woodland (1989). *Development* 107:785–791. Spatial aspects of neural induction in *Xenopus laevis.*

Jones, E. G. (1970). *J. Anat. (London)* 106:507–520. On the mode of entry of blood vessels into the cerebral cortex.

Jones, E. G. (1972). *J. Hist. Med. Allied Sci.* 27:298–311. The development of the 'muscular sense' concept during the nineteenth century and the work of H. Charlton Bastian.

Jones, E. G. (1984). Cellular Components of the Cerebral Cortex, pp. 521–553. In *Cerebral Cortex*, Vol. 1 (A. Peters, and E. G. Jones, eds.), Plenum, New York.

Jones, E. G., and S. P. Wise (1977). *J. Comp. Neurol.* 175:391–438. Size, laminar and columnar distribution of efferent cells in the cerebral cortex of the monkeys.

Jones, E. G., H. Burton, and R. Porter (1975). *Science*

190:572–574. Commissural and cortico-cortical 'columns' in the somatic sensory cortex of primates.

Jones, F. S., S. Hoffman, B. A. Cunningham, and G. M. Edelman (1989). *Proc. Natl. Acad. Sci. U.S.A.* 86:1905–1909. A detailed structural model of cytotactin: Protein homologies, alternative RNA splicing, and binding regions.

Jones, W. H., and D. B. Thomas (1962). *J. Anat. (London)* 96:375–381. Changes in the dendritic organization of neurons in the cerebral cortex following deafferentation.

Jonson, K. M., J. G. Lyle, M. J. Edwards, and R. H. C. Penny (1976). *Brain Res. Bull.* 1:133–150. Effect of prenatal heat stress on brain growth and serial discrimination reversal learning in the guinea-pig.

Joó, F. (1987). *Int. J. Dev. Neurosci.* 5:369–372. Current aspects of the development of the blood-brain barrier.

Jordan, C., V. Friedrich, Jr., and M. Dubois-Dalcq (1989). *J. Neurosci.* 9:248–257. *In situ* hybridization analysis of myelin gene transcripts in developing mouse spinal cord.

Jordan, C. L., M. S. Letinsky, and A. P. Arnold (1988). *J. Neurobiol.* 19:335–356. Synapse elimination occurs late in the hormone-sensitive levator ani muscle of the rat.

Jordan, C. L., M. S. Letinsky, and A. P. Arnold (1989a). *J. Neurosci.* 9:229–238. The role of gonadal hormones in neuromuscular synapse elimination in rats. I. Androgen delays the loss of multiple innervation in the levator ani muscle.

Jordan, C. L., M. S. Letinsky, and A. P. Arnold (1989b). *J. Neurosci.* 9:239–247. The role of gonadal hormones in neuromuscular synapse elimination in rats. II. Multiple innervation persists in the adult levator ani muscle after juvenile androgen treatment.

Joseph, B., and D. Whitlock (1968). *Anat. Rec.* 160:279–288. Central projections of selected spinal dorsal roots in anuran amphibians.

Joseph, J. (1948). *J. Anat. (London)* 82:146–152. Changes in nuclear population following twenty-one days degeneration in a nerve consisting of small myelinated fibers.

Jouan, P., S. Samperez, M. L. Thieulant, and L. Mercier (1971). *J. Steroid. Biochem.* 2:223–236. Etude du récepteur cytoplasmique de la (1,2-³H) testostérone dans l'hypothalamus du rat.

Jouan, P., S. Samperez, and M. L. Thieulant (1973). *J. Steroid Biochem.* 4:65–74. Testosterone 'receptors' in purified nuclei of rat anterior hypothysis.

Jourdan, A.-J.-L. (1834). *Dictionnaire des Termes usités dans les Sciences Naturelles,* 2 vols. J.-B. Balliére, Paris.

Julien, J. P., and W. E. Mushynski (1982). *J. Biol. Chem.* 258:4019–4025. The distribution of phosphorylation sites among identified proteolytic fragments of mammalian neurofilaments.

Juntunen, J. (1973a). *Z. Anat. Entwicklungsgesch.* 143:1–12. Morphogenesis of the myoneural junctions after immobilization of the muscle in the rat.

Juntunen, J. (1973b). *Z. Zellforsch. Mikrosk. Anat.* 142:193–204. Effects of colchicine and vinblastine on neurotubules of the sciatic nerve and cholinesterases in the developing myoneural junction of the rat.

Juraska, J. M. (1984). *Brain Res.* 295:27–35. Sex differences in dendritic response to differential experience in the rat visual cortex.

Juurlink, B. H., J. A. Schousboe, O. S. Jørgensen, and L. Hertz (1981). *J. Neurochem.* 36:136–142. Induction by hydrocortisone of glutamine synthetase in mouse primary astrocyte cultures.

Kaas, J. H. (1983). *Physiol. Rev.* 63:206–231. What, if anything is S-I?: The organization of the "first somatosensory area" of cortex.

Kaas, J. H., and R. W. Guillery (1973). *Brain Res.* 59:61–95. The transfer of abnormal visual field representations from the dorsal lateral geniculate nucleus to the visual cortex in siamese cats.

Kaas, J. H., M. M. Merzenich, and H. P. Killackey (1983). *Ann. Rev. Neurosci.* 6:325–356. The reorganization of somatosensory cortex following peripheral nerve damage in adult and developing mammals.

Kadanoff, D. (1925). *Arch. Entw.-Mech. Organ.* 106:249–278. Untersuchungen über die Regeneration der sensiblen Nervenendigungen nach Vertauschung verschieden innervierten Hautstücke.

Kageyama, G. H., and M. T. T. Wong-Riley (1982). *Neuroscience* 7:2337–2361. Histochemical localization of cytochrome oxidase in the hippocampus: Correlation with specific neuronal types and afferent pathways.

Kageyama, G. H., and M. Wong-Riley (1986). *J. Comp. Neurol.* 246:212–237. Differential effect of visual deprivation on cytochrome oxidase levels in major cell classes of the cat LGN.

Kahn, A. J. (1973). *Brain Res.* 63:285–290. Ganglion cell formation in the chick neural retina.

Kahn, A. J. (1974). *Dev. Biol.* 38:30–40. An autoradiographic analysis of the time of appearance of neurons in the developing chick neural retina.

Kahn, D., and H. G. Birch (1968). *Percept. Mot. Skills* 27:459–468. Development of auditory-visual integration and reading achievement.

Kahn, M. A., and S. Ochs (1975). *Brain Res.* 96:267–277. Slow axoplasmic transport of mitochondria (MAO) and lactic dehydrogenase in mammalian nerve fibers.

Kalaska, J., and B. Pomeranz (1979). *J. Neurophysiol.* 42:618–633. Chronic paw deafferentation causes an age-dependent appearance of novel responses from forearm in "paw cortex" of kittens and adult cats.

Kalcheim, C., and N. M. DeDouarin (1986). *Dev. Biol.* 116:451–466. Requirement of a neural tube signal for the differentiation of neural crest cells into dorsal root ganglia.

Kalcheim, C., Y.-A. Barde, H. Thoenen, and N. M. LeDourin (1987). *EMBO J.* 6:2871–2873. *In vivo* effect of brain-derived neurotrophic factor on the survival of developing dorsal root ganglion cells.

Kalil, K., and J. H. P. Skene (1986). *J. Neurosci.* 6:2563–2570. Elevated synthesis of an axonally transported protein correlates with axonal outgrowth in normal and injured pyramidal tracts.

Kalil, R. E. (1972). *Anat. Rec.* 172:339–340. Formation of new retino-geniculate connections in kittens after removal of one eye.

Kalil, R. E. (1973) *Anat. Rec.* 175:353. Formation of new retinogeniculate connections in kittens: Effects of age and visual experience.

Kalil, R. E. (1980). *J. Comp. Neurol.* 189:483–524. A quantitative study of the effects of monocular enucleation and deprivation on cell growth in the dorsal lateral geniculate nucleus of the cat.

Kalil, R. E., and G. E. Schneider (1975). *Brain Res.* 100:690–698. Abnormal synaptic connections of the optic tract in the thalamus after midbrain lesions in newborn hamster.

Kalil, R. E., M. W. Dubin, G. Scott, and L. A. Stark (1986).

Nature 323:156–158. Elimination of action potentials blocks the structural development of retinogeniculate synapses.

Källén, B. (1955). *J. Anat. (London)* 89:153–161. Cell degeneration during normal ontogenesis of the rabbit brain.

Källén, B. (1958). *Z. Zellforsch. Mikroskop. Anat. Abt. Histochem.* 47:469–480. Studies on the differentiation capacity of neural epithelium cells in chick embryos.

Källén, B. (1961). *Z. Anat. Entwicklungsgeschichte* 122:388–401. Studies on cell proliferation in the brain of chick embryos with special reference to the mesencephalon.

Källén, B. (1962). *Z. Anat. Entwicklungsgeschichte* 123:309–319. Mitotic patterning in the central nervous system of chick embryos studied by a colchicine method.

Kallen, B. (1965). *Prog. Brain Res.* 14:77–96. Degeneration and regeneration in the vertebrate central nervous system during embryogenesis.

Kallius, E. (1896). *Ergebn. Anat. Entw. Gesch.* 5:55–94. Endigungen sensibler Nerven bei Wirbeltieren.

Kallius, E. (1926). Golgische Methode, pp. 909–944. In *Enzyklopädie der mikroskopischen Technik*, Vol. II, 3rd edn. (R. Krause, ed.), Urban and Schwarzenberg, Berlin.

Kaltenbach, J. C., and A. W. Hobbs (1972). *J. Exp. Zool.* 179:157–165. Local action of thyroxine on amphibian metamorphosis. V. Cell division in the eye of anuran larvae affected by thyroxine—cholesterol implants.

Kalter, H. (1968). *Teratology of the Central Nervous System.* Univ. Chicago Press, Chicago, 483 pp.

Kalugina, M. A. (1956). *Ark. Anat. Gistol. i Embriol.* 33:59–63. On the question of the development of proprioceptors in the striated muscle of mammals. (In Russian.)

Kamrin, R. P., and M. Singer (1953). *Am. J. Physiol.* 174:146–148. Influence of sensory neurons isolated from central nervous system on maintenance of taste buds and regeneration of barbels in the catfish.

Kanai, Y., R. Takemura, T. Oshima, H. Mori, Y. Ihara, M. Yanagisawa, T. Masaki, and N., Hirokawa (1989). *J. Cell Biol.* 109:1173–1184. Expression of multiple Tau isoforms and microtubule bundle formation in fibroblasts transfected with a single Tau cDNA.

Kane, E. C. (1974). *Anat. Rec.* 179:67–92. Patterns of degeneration in the caudal cochlear nucleus of the cat after cochlear ablation.

Kanetmitsu, A., and Y. Kobayashi (1988). *Anat. Anz. Jena* 165:167–175. Time of origin of purkinje cells and neurons of the deep cerebellar nuclei of the chick embryo examined by ^{3}H-thymidine autoradiography.

Kanigel, R. (1986). *Apprentice to a Genius. The Making of Scientific Discovery.* Macmillan, New York.

Kankel, D. R., and J. C. Hall (1976). *Dev. Biol.* 48:1–24. Fate mapping of nervous system and other internal tissues in genetic mosaics of *Drosophila melanogaster.*

Kao, C. C. (1974). *Exp. Neurol.* 44:424–439. Comparison of healing process in transected spinal cords grafted with autogenous brain tissue, sciatic nerve and nodose ganglion.

Kao, C. C., L. W. Chang, and J. M. B. Bloodworth, Jr. (1977). *Exp. Neurol.* 54:591–615. Axonal regeneration across transected mammalian spinal cords: An electron microscopic study of delayed nerve grafting.

Kapfhammer, J. P., B. E. Grunewald, and J. A. Raper (1986). *J. Neurosci.* 6:2527–2534. The selective inhibition of growth cone extension by specific neurites in culture.

Kaplan, B. B., and C. E. Finch (1982). The sequence complexity of brain ribonucleic acids, pp. 71–98. In *Molecular Approaches to Neurobiology* (I. R. Brown, ed.), Academic, New York.

Kaplan, M. S. (1981). *J. Comp. Neurol.* 195:323–338. Neurogenesis in the 3-month-old rat visual cortex.

Kaplan, M. S., and J. W. Hinds (1977). *Science* 197:1092–1094. Neurogenesis in the adult rat: Electron microscopic analysis of light radioautographs.

Kaplan, M. S., and J. W. Hinds (1980). *J. Comp. Neurol.* 193:711–727. Gliogenesis of astrocytes and oligodendrocytes in the neocortical gray and white matter of the adult rat: Electron microscopic analysis of light radioautographs.

Kappers, J. A. (1958). Structural and functional changes in the telencephalic choroid plexus during human ontogenesis, pp. 3–31. In *Ciba Foundation Symposium on Cerebrospinal Fluid* (G. E. W. Wolstenholme, and C. M. O'Connor, eds.), Little Brown & Co., Boston.

Karfunkel, P. (1971). *Dev. Biol.* 25:30–56. The role of microtubules and microfilaments in neurulation in *Xenopus.*

Karfunkel, P. (1972). *J. Exp. Zool.* 181:289–302. The activity of microtubules and microfilaments in neurulation in the chick.

Karfunkel, P. (1974). *Int. Rev. Cytol.* 38:245–271. The mechanisms of neural tube formation.

Karlsson, J.-O., and J. Sjöstrand (1968). *Brain Res.* 11:431–439. Transport of labelled protein in the optic nerve and tract of the rabbit.

Karlsson, J.-O., and J. Sjöstrand (1969). *Brain Res.* 13:617–619. The effect of colchicine on the axonal transport of protein in the optic nerve and tract of the rabbit.

Karlsson, J.-O., and J. Sjostrand (1971a). *J. Neurochem.* 18:749–767. Synthesis, migration and turnover of protein in retinal ganglion cells.

Karlsson, J.-O., and J. Sjöstrand (1971b). *J. Neurochem.* 18:975–982. Transport of microtubular protein in axons of retinal ganglion cells.

Karlsson, J.-O., and J. Sjöstrand (1971c). *J. Neurochem.* 18:2209–2216. Rapid intracellular transport of fucose-containing glycoproteins in retinal ganglion cells.

Karlsson, J.-O., H.-A. Hansson, and J. Sjöstrand (1971). *Z. Zellforsch. Mikrosk. Anat.* 115:265–283. Effect of colchicine on axonal transport and morphology of retinal ganglion cells.

Karlsson, U. (1966b). *J. Ultrastruct. Res.* 16:429–481. Three-dimensional studies of neurons in the lateral geniculate nucleus of the rat. I. Organelle organization in the perikaryon and its proximal branches.

Karlsson, U. (1966c). *J. Ultrastruct. Res.* 16:482–504. Three-dimensional studies of neurons in the lateral geniculate nucleus of the rat. II. Environment of perikarya and proximal parts of their branches.

Karlsson, U. (1967). *J. Ultrastr. Res.* 17:158–175. Observations on the postnatal development of neuronal structures in the lateral geniculate nucleus of the rat by electron microscopy.

Karpati, G., and W. K. Engel (1967). *Nature* 215:1509. Transformation of the histochemical profile of skeletal muscle by "foreign" innervation.

Karssen, A., and B. Sager (1934). *Arch. Exp. Zellforsch.* 16:255–259. Sur l'influence du courant électrique sur la croissance des neuroblastes *in vivo.*

Kasamatsu, T. (1983). *Prog. Psychobiol. Physiol. Psychol.*

10:1–111. Neuronal plasticity maintained by the central norepinephrine system in the cat visual cortex.

Kasamatsu, T., and J. D. Pettigrew (1976). *Science* 194:206–208. Depletion of brain catecholamines: Failure of ocular dominance shift after monocular occlusion in kittens.

Kasamatsu, T., and J. D. Pettigrew (1979). *J. Comp. Neurol.* 185:139–162. Preservation of binocularity after monocular deprivation in the striate cortex of kittens treated with 6-hydroxydopamine.

Kastchenko, N. (1888). *Anat. Anz.* 3:445–467. Zür Entwicklungsgeschichte des Selachierembryos.

Kater, S., and P. C. Letourneau (1985). *J. Neurosci. Res.* 13:1–335. Biology of the nerve growth cone.

Kater, S. B., C. Nicholson, and W. J. Davis (1973). A guide to intracellular staining techniques, pp. 307–325. In *Intracellular Staining in Neurobiology* (S. B. Kater, and C. Nicholson, eds.), Springer-Verlag, New York.

Kater, S. K., M. P. Mattson, C. Cohan, and J. Connor (1988). *Trends Neurosci.* 11:317–323. Calcium regulation of the neuronal growth cone.

Kato, J., and T. Onouchi (1973). *Endocrinol. Jap.* 20:429–432. 5a-Dehydrotestosterone 'receptor' in the rat hypothalamus.

Kato, J., and C. A. Villee (1967). *Endocrinol.* 80:567–575. Preferential uptake of estradiol by the anterior hypothalamus of the rat.

Katz, B., and R. Miledi (1964). *J. Physiol. (London)* 170:389–396. The development of acetylcholine sensitivity in nerve free segments of skeletal muscle.

Katz, L. C., and M. Constantine-Paton (1988). *J. Neurosci.* 8:3160–3180. Relationships between segregated afferents and postsynaptic neurons in the optic tectum of three-eyed frogs.

Katz, L. C., A. Burkhalter, and W. J. Dreyer (1984). *Nature* 310:498–500. Fluorescent latex microspheres as a retrograde neuronal marker for *in vivo* and *in vitro* studies of visual cortex.

Katz, L. C., C. D. Gilbert, and T. N. Wiesel (1989). *J. Neurosci.* 9:1389–1399. Local circuits and ocular dominance columns in monkey striate cortex.

Katz, M. J. (1984). *Dev. Biol.* 104:199–209. Stereotyped and variable growth of redirected mauthner axons.

Kauffman, R. C., J. E. Warnick, and E. X. Albuquerque (1974). *Exp. Neurol.* 44:404–416. Uptake of (^{3}H) colchicine from silastic implants by mammalian nerves and muscles.

Kauffman, S. L. (1968). *Exp. Cell Res.* 49:420–424. Lengthening of the generation cycle during embryonic differentiation of the mouse neural tube.

Kaufman, M. H. (1983). *J. Histochem. Cytochem.* 12:219–221. Occlusion of the neural lumen in early mouse embryos analysed by light and electron microscopy.

Kaufman, T. C., R. Lewis, and B. Wakimoto (1980). *Genetics* 94:115–133. Cytogenetic analysis of chromosome 3 in *Drosophila melanogaster:* The homeotic gene complex in polytene chromosome interval 84A-B.

Kaur, C., E. A. Ling, and W. C. Wong (1984). *J. Anat. (London)* 139:1–7. Cytochemical localisation of 5'-nucleotidase in amoeboid microglial cells in postnatal rats.

Kaur, C., E. A. Ling, and W. C. Wong (1986). *Acta anat.* 125:132–137. Labelling of amoeboid microglial cells in rats of various ages following an intravenous injection of horseradish peroxidase.

Kaur, C., E. A. Ling, and W. C. Wong (1987a). *J. Anat. (London)* 152:13–22. Localization of thiamine pyrophosphatase in the amoeboid microglial cells in the brain of postnatal rats.

Kaur, C., E. A. Ling, and W. C. Wong (1987b). *J. Anat. (London)* 154:215–227. Origin and fate of neural macrophages in a stab wound of the brain of the young rat.

Kawana, E., C. Sandri, and K. Akert (1971). *Z. Zellforsch. Mikrosk. Anat.* 115:284–298. Ultrastructure of growth cones in the cerebellar cortex of the neonatal rat and cat.

Kawana, E., C. San, M. Irwin, P. L. Engle, and C. Yarborough (1977). Malnutrition and mental development in rural Guatemala. An applied cross-cultural research study, pp. 92–121. In Warren *Advances in cross-cultural psychology.* Academic Press, New York.

Keating, M. J. (1968). *J. Physiol. (London)* 198:75P. Functional interaction in the development of specific nerve connexions.

Keating, M. J. (1974). *Br. Med. Bull.* 30:145–151. The role of visual function in the patterning of binocular visual connections.

Keating, M. J. (1975a). *J. Physiol. (London)* 248:36–37P. Plasticity of intertectal connexions in adult *Xenopus.*

Keating, M. J. (1975b). *Proc. Roy. Soc. (London) Ser. B.* 189:603–610. The time course of experience-dependent synaptic switching of visual connections in *Xenopus laevis.*

Keating, M. J., and J. D. Feldman (1975). *Proc. Roy. Soc. (London) Ser. B.* 191:467–474. Visual deprivation and intertectal neuronal connections in *Xenopus laevis.*

Keating, M. J., and R. M. Gaze (1970a). *Brain Behav. Evol.* 3:102–120. Rigidity and plasticity in the amphibian visual system.

Keating, M. J., and R. M. Gaze (1970b). *Am. J. Exp. Physiol.* 55:284–292. The ipsilateral retinotectal pathway in the frog.

Keating, M. J., and C. Kennard (1987). *Neuroscience* 21:519–528. Visual experience and the maturation of the ipsilateral visuotectal projection in *Xenopus laevis.*

Keefer, D. A. (1978). *Brain Res.* 140:15–32. Horseradish peroxidase as a retrogradely-transported, detailed dendritic marker.

Keene, M. F. L., and E. E. Hewer (1931). *J. Anat. (London)* 66:1–13. Some observations on myelination in the human central nervous system.

Keene, M. F. L., and E. E. Hewer (1933). *J. Anat. (London)* 67:522–536. The development and myelination of the posterior longitudinal bundle in the human.

Kelahan, A. M., and G. S. Doetsch (1981). *Soc. Neurosci. Abstr.* 7:540. Short-term changes in the functional organization of somatosensory (SmI) cortex of adult raccoons after digit amputation.

Keller, H. U., and E. Sorkin (1968). *Experientia* 24:641–652. Chemotaxis of leucocytes.

Keller, R. (1978). *J. Morphol.* 157:223–248. Time lapse cinemicrographic analysis of superficial cell behavior during and prior to gastrulation.

Keller, R. E. (1975). *Dev. Biol.* 42:222–241. Vital dye mapping of the gastrula and neurula of *Xenopus laevis.*

Keller, R. E. (1976). *Dev. Biol.* 51:118–137. Vital dye mapping of the gastrula and neurula of *Xenopus laevis.* II. Prospective areas and morphogenetic movements of the deep layer.

Keller, R. E. (1986). The cellular basis of amphibian gastrulation, pp. 241–327. In *Developmental Biology: A Comprehensive Synthesis*, Vol. 2, (L. Browder, ed.), Plenum, New York.

Keller, R. E., and G. C. Schoenwolf (1977). *Wilhelm Roux Arch. Entw. Mech. Org.* 182:165–186. An SEM study of cellular morphology, contact, and arrangement, as related to gastrulation in *Xenopus laevis.*

Keller, R. E., M. Danilchik, R. Gimlich, and J. Shih (1985). *J. Embryol. Exp. Morph.* 89:Suppl. 185–209. The function and mechanism of convergent extension during gastrulation of *Xenopus laevis.*

Kellerth, J.-O., A. Mellstrom, and S. Skoglund (1971). *Acta Physiol. Scand.* 83:31–41. Postnatal excitability changes of kitten motoneurones.

Kelly, A. M. (1983). Emergence of specialization of skeletal muscle, section 10, pp. 507–537. In *Handbook of Physiology* (L. D. Peachey, ed.).

Kelly, A. M. (1987). *J. Cell Biol.* 104:447–459. Slow myosin in developing rat skeletal muscle.

Kelly, A. M., and N. A. Rubinstein (1980). *Nature* 288:266–269. Why are fetal muscles slow?

Kelly, A. M., and S. I. Zacks (1969a). *J. Cell Biol.* 42:135–153. The histogenesis of rat intercostal muscle.

Kelly, A. M., and S. I. Zacks (1969b). *J. Cell Biol.* 42:154–169. The fine structure of motor endplate morphogenesis.

Kelly, J. P., and W. M. Cowan (1972). *Brain Res.* 42:263–288. Studies on the development of the chick optic tectum. III. Effects of early eye removal.

Kelly, J. P., and C. D. Gilbert (1975). *J. Comp. Neurol.* 163:65–80. The projection of different morphological types of ganglion cells in the cat retina.

Kelly, J. P., and D. C. Van Essen (1974). *J. Physiol. (London)* 238:515–547. Cell structure and function in the visual cortex of the cat.

Kelly, S. S., N. Anis, and N. Robbins (1985). *Pfluegers Arch.* 404:97–99. Fluorescent staining of living mouse neuromuscular junctions.

Kemali, M. (1976). *Experientia* 32:747–748. An 'ultra' rapid Golgi method for vertebrate neuroanatomy.

Kemali, M., and V. Braitenberg (1969). *Atlas of the Frog's Brain.* Springer-Verlag, Berlin, 74 pp.

Kemper, T. L., and A. M. Galaburda (1984). Principles of cytoarchitectonics, pp. 35–58. In *Cerebral Cortex*, Vol. 1, *Cellular Components of the Cerebral Cortex* (A. Peters, and E. G. Jones, eds.), Plenum, New York.

Kemplay, S., and C. Stolkin (1980). *Cell Tissue Res.* 212:333–339. Endplate classification and spontaneous sprouting in the sternocostalis muscle of the rat: A new whole mount preparation.

Kennard, C. (1981). *J. Embryol. Exp. Morphol.* 65:199–217. Factors involved in the development of ipsilateral retinothalamic projections in *Xenopus laevis.*

Kennard, C., and M. J. Keating (1985). *Neurosci. Lett.* 58:365–370. A species difference between *Rana* and *Xenopus* in the occurrence of intertectal neuronal plasticity.

Kennard, D. W. (1959). *J. Comp. Neurol.* 111:447–467. The anatomical organization of neurons in the lumbar region of the spinal cord of the frog *(Rana temporaria).*

Kennard, M. A. (1940). *Arch. Neurol. Psychiatr.* 44:377–397. Relation of age to motor impairment in man and in subhuman primates.

Kennard, M. A. (1942). *Arch. Neurol. Psychiatr.* 48:227–240. Cortical reorganization of motor function. Studies on series of monkeys of various ages from infancy to maturity.

Kennedy, H., C. Dehay, and C. Bourdet (1988). Inter- and intra-hemispheric transient pathways in the cat, pp. 142–145. In *Seeing Contour and Colour* (J. J. Kulikowski, C. M. Dickenson, and I. J. Murray, eds.), Pergamon Press, Oxford.

Kennedy, T. C., M. H. Des Rosiers, M. Reivich, F. Sharpe, and L. Sokoloff (1975). *Science* 187:850–853. Mapping of functional neural pathways by autoradiographic survey of local metabolic rate with [14C] deoxyglucose.

Kennedy, T.C., M. H. Des Rosiers, O. Sakurada, M. Shinohara, M. Reivich, J. Jehle, and L. Sokoloff (1976). *Proc. Natl. Acad. Sci. U.S.A.* 73:4230–4234. Metabolic mapping of the primary visual system of the monkey by means of the autoradiographic [14C]deoxyglucose technique.

Kerkut, G. A., A. Shapira, and R. J. Walker (1967). *Comp. Biochem. Physiol.* 23:729–748. The transport of 14C-labelled material from CNS–muscle along a nerve trunk.

Kerns, J. M., and E. J. Hinsman (1973a). *J. Comp. Neurol.* 151:237–254. Neuroglial response to sciatic neurectomy. I. Light microscopy and autoradiography.

Kerns, J. M., and E. J. Hinsman (1973b). *J. Comp. Neurol.* 151:255–280. Neuroglial response to sciatic neurectomy. II. Electron microscopy.

Kerr, F. W. L. (1972). *Brain Res.* 43:547–560. The potential of cervical primary afferents to sprout in the spinal nucleus of V following long term trigeminal denervation.

Kerr, F. W. L. (1975a). *Exp. Neurol.* 48:16–31. Structural and functional evidence of plasticity in the central nervous system.

Kerr, F. W. L. (1975b). *J. Comp. Neurol.* 163:305–328. Neuroplasticity of primary afferents in the neo-natal cat and some results of early deafferentation of the trigeminal spinal nucleus.

Kerr, J. F. R., A. H. Wyllie, and A. R. Currie (1972). *Br. J. Cancer* 26:239–257. Apoptosis: A basic biological phenomenon with wide-ranging implications in tissue kinetics.

Kershman, J. (1938). *Arch. Neurol. Psychiat.* 40:937–967. The medulloblast and the medulloblastoma; a study of human embryos.

Kershman, J. (1939). *Arch. Neurol. Psychiat.* 41:24–50. Genesis of microglia in the human brain.

Kessler, J. A., and I. B. Black (1981). *Proc. Natl. Acad. Sci. U.S.A.* 78:4644–4647. Similarities in development of substance P and somatostatin in peripheral sensory neurons: Effects of capsaicin and nerve growth factor.

Ketelslegers, J.-M., W. D. Hetzel, R. J. Sherins, and K. J. Catt (1978). *Endocrinology* 103:212–222. Developmental changes in testicular gonadotropin receptors: Plasma gonadotropins and plasma testosterone in the rat.

Kett, N. A., and E. D. Pollack (1985). *J. Exp. Zool.* 236:59–66. Retention of lateral motor column neurons during the phase of rapid cell loss after limb amputation in *Rana pipiens* tadpoles.

Key, A., and G. Retzius (1876). *Studien in der Anatomie des Nervensystems und des Bindegewebes*, 2 Vols. Samson and Wallin, Stockholm.

Key, B., and P. P. Giorgi (1987). *Neuroscience* 22:1135–1144. Uptake and axonal transport of horseradish peroxidase isoenzymes by different neuronal types.

Keynes, R. J. (1987). *Trends Neurosci.* 10:137–139. Schwann cells during neural development and regeneration: Leaders or followers?

Keynes, R. J., and C. D. Stern (1984). *Nature* 310:786–789. Segmentation in the vertebrate nervous system.

Keynes, R. J., and C. D. Stern (1985). *Trends Neurosci.* 8:220–223. Segmentation and neural development in vertebrates.

Keynes, R. J., and C. D. Stern (1988). *Development* 103:413–431. Mechanisms of vertebrate segmentation.

Khan, M. A., and S. Ochs (1974). *Brain Res.* 81:413–426. Magnesium or calcium activated ATPase in mammalian nerve.

Kicliter, E., L. J. Misantone, and D. J. Stelzner (1974) *Brain Res.* 82:293–297. Neuronal specificity and plasticity in frog visual system: Anatomical correlates.

Kidokoro, Y., and B. Brass (1985). *J. Physiol. (Paris)* 80:212–220. Redistribution of acetylcholine receptors during neuromuscular junction formation in *Xenopus* cultures.

Kidokoro, Y., B. Brass, and H. Kuromi (1986). *J. Neurosci.* 6:1941–1951. Concanavalin A prevents acetylcholine receptor redistribution in *Xenopus* nerve-muscle cultures.

Kiehlman, B. A. (1966). *The Actions of Chemicals on Dividing Cells*, Prentice Hall, New Jersey.

Kieny, M., A. Mauger, and P. Sengel (1972). *Dev. Biol.* 28:142–161. Early regionalization of the somitic mesoderm as studied by the development of the axial skeleton of the chick embryo.

Kilham, L., and G. Margolis (1964). *Science* 143:1047–1048. Cerebellar ataxia in hamsters inoculated with rat virus.

Kilham, L., and G. Margolis (1965). *Science* 148:244–246. Cerebellar disease in cats induced by inoculation of rat virus.

Kilham, L., and G. Margolis (1966a). *Am. J. Pathol.* 48:991–1011. Viral etiology of spontaneous ataxia of cats.

Kilham, L., and G. Margolis (1966b). *Am. J. Pathol.* 49:457–485. Spontaneous hepatitis and cerebellar "hypoplasia" in suckling rats due to congenital infections with rat virus.

Killackey, H. P. (1980a). *Trends Neurosci.* 3:303–306. Pattern formation in the trigeminal system of the rat.

Killackey, H. P. (1980b). *Am. Soc. Zool. Abstr.* 20:770. Spatial and temporal variables in pattern formation in the rat trigeminal system.

Killackey, H. P., and G. R. Belford (1979). *J. Comp. Neurol.* 183:285–304. The formation of afferent patterns in the somatosensory cortex of the neonatal rat.

Killackey, H. P., and L. M. Chalupa (1986). *J. Comp. Neurol.* 244:331–348. Ontogenetic change in the distribution of callosal projection neurons in the postcentral gyrus of the fetal rhesus monkey.

Killackey, H. P., and D. R. Dawson (1989). *Europ. J. Neurosci.* 1:210–221. Expansion of the central hindpaw respresentation following foetal forelimb removal in the rat.

Killackey, H. P., and R. F. Erzurumlu (1982). *Neuroscience* 7:S116. Interactions between fiber terminals during pattern formation in the rat trigeminal system.

Killackey, H. P., and A. Shinder (1981). *Dev. Brain Res.* 1:121–126. Central correlates of peripheral pattern alterations in the trigeminal system of the rat.

Killackey, H. P., G. Belford, R. Ryugo, and D. K. Ryugo (1976). *Brain Res.* 104:309–315. Anomalous organization of thalamocortical projections consequent to vibrissae removal in the newborn rat and mouse.

Kim, S. U. (1975). *Brain Res.* 88:52–58. Formation of unattached spines of Purkinje cell dendrite in organotypic cultures of mouse cerebellum.

Kimble, J. (1981). *Dev. Biol.* 87:286–300. Alterations in cell lineage following laser ablation of cells in the somatic gonad of *Caenorhabditis elegans*.

Kimelman, D., and M. Kirschner (1987). *Cell* 51:869–877. Synergistic induction of mesoderm by FGF and TGFβ and the identification of mRNA coding for FGF in early *Xenopus* embryos.

Kimmel, C. B., and R. C. Eaton (1976). Development of the Mauthner cell, pp. 186–302. In *Simpler Networks and Behavior* (J. C. Fentress, ed.), Sinauer Assoc., Inc., Sunderland, Mass.

Kimmel, C. B., and R. D. Law (1985). *Dev. Biol.* 108:94–101. Cell lineage of zebrafish blastomeres. III. Clonal analysis of the blastula and gastrula stages.

Kimmel, C. B., and E. Schabtach (1974). *J. Comp. Neurol.* 156:49–80. Patterning in synaptic knobs which connect with Mauthner's cell (*Ambystoma mexicanum*).

Kimmel, C. B., and R. M. Warga (1986). *Science* 231:365–368. Tissue-specific cell lineages originate in the gastrula of the zebrafish.

Kimmel, C. B., and R. M. Warga (1987). *Dev. Biol.* 124:269–280. Indeterminate cell lineages of the zebrafish embryo.

Kimmel, C. B., S. K. Sessions, and R. J. Kimmel (1981). *J. Comp. Neurol.* 198:101–120. Morphogenesis and synaptogenesis of the zebrafish mauthner neuron.

Kimura, D. (1980). *Behav. Brain Sci.* 3:240–241. Sex differences in intrahemispheric organization of speech.

Kimura, D. (1983). *Can. J. Psychol.* 37:19–35. Sex differences in cerebral organization for speech and praxic functions.

Kimura, D., and R. A. Harshman (1984). *Prog. Brain Res.* 61:423–441. Sex differences in brain organization for verbal and non-verbal functions.

Kimura, M., H. Inoko, M. Katsuki, A. Ando, T. Sato, T. Hirose, T. Takashima, S. Inayama, H. Okano, K. Takamatsu, K. Mikoshiba, Y. Tsukada, and I. Watanabe (1985). *J. Neurochem.* 44:692–696. Molecular genetic analysis of myelin-deficient mice: Shiverer mutant mice show deletion in gene(s) coding for myelin basic protein.

Kimura, M., M. Sato, A. Akatsuka, S. Nozawa-Kimura, R. Takahashi, M. Yokoyama, T. Nomura, and M. Katsuki (1989). *Proc. Natl. Acad. Sci. U.S.A.* 86:5661–5665. Restoration of myelin formation by a single type of myelin basic protein in transgenic shiverer mice.

Kinders, R. J., and T. C. Johnson (1982). *Biochem. J.* 206:527–534. Isolation of cell surface glycopeptides from bovine cerebral cortex that inhibit cell growth and protein synthesis in normal but not in transformed cells.

King, A. E., E. Cherubini, and A. Nistri (1987). *Neurosci. Lett.* 76:179–184. A study of amino acid-activated currents recorded from frog motoneurones *in vitro*.

King, T. J., and R. Briggs (1956). *Cold Springs Harbor Symp. Quant. Biol.* 21:271–290. Serial transplantation of embryonic nuclei.

Kingsbury, B. F. (1920). *J. Comp. Neur.* 32:113–135. The extent of the floor-plate of His and its significance.

Kingsbury, B. F. (1922). *J. Comp. Neur.* 34:461–491. The fundamental plan of the vertebrate brain.

Kingsbury, B. F. (1930). *J. Comp. Neur.* 50:117–207. The developmental significance of the floor-plate of the brain and spinal cord.

Kinnman, E., and H. Aldskogius (1986). *Brain Res.* 377:73–82. Collateral sprouting of sensory axons in the glabrous skin of the hindpaw after chronic sciatic nerve lesion in adult and neonatal rats: A morphological study.

Kinnman, E., and H. Aldskogius (1988). *J. Comp. Neurol.* 270:569–574. Collateral reinnervation of taste buds after chronic sensory denervation: A morphological study.

Kintner, C. and D. Melton (1987). *Development* 99:311–325. Expression of *Xenopus* NCAM RNA is an early response of ectoderm to induction.

Kintner, C. R. and J. P. Brockes (1984). *Nature* 308:67–69. Monoclonal antibodies identify blastemal cells derived from differentiating muscle in newt limb regeneration.

Kirby, M. L., and S. A. Gilmore (1976). *Anat. Rec.* 186:437–450. A Correlative histofluorescence and light microscopic study of the formation of the sympathetic trunks in chick embryos.

Kirby, M. L., T. F. Gale, and D. E. Stewart (1983). *Science* 220:1059–1061. Neural crest cells contribute to normal aorticopulmonary septation.

Kirby, M. L., and D. E. Stewart (1983). *Dev. Biol.* 97:433–443. Neural crest origin of cardiac ganglion cells in the chick embryo: Identification and extirpation.

Kirkpatrick, J. B., J. J. Bary, and S. M. Palmer (1972). *Brain Res.* 43:1–10. Visualization of axoplasmic flow *in vitro* by Nomarski microscopy. Comparison to rapid flow of radioactive proteins.

Kirkwood, P. A., and C. J. Shatz (1983). *J. Physiol. (London)* 336:27–28. Development of binocular inputs to dorsal lateral geniculate neurones in the fetal cat.

Kirn, J. R., and T. J. DeVoogd (1989). *J. Neurosci.* 9:3176–3187. Genesis and death of vocal control neurons during sexual differentiation in the zebra finch.

Kirsche, W., and K. Kirsche (1961). *Z. Mikroskop. Anat. Forsch.* 67:140–182. Experimentelle Untersuchungen zur Frage der Regeneration und Funktion des Tectum opticum von Carassius carassius L.

Kirschner, D. A., and A. L. Ganser (1980). *Nature* 283:207–210. Compact myelin exists in the absence of basic protein in the Shiverer mutant mouse.

Kirschner, M. W. (1980). *J. Cell Biol.* 86:330–334. Implications of treadmilling for the stability and polarity of actin and tubulin polymers *in vivo*.

Kirschner, M. W., and T. Mitchison (1986a). *Cell* 45:329–342. Beyond self-assembly: From microtubules to morphogenesis.

Kirschner, M. W., and T. Mitchison (1986b). *Nature* 324:621. Microtubule dynamics.

Kitamura, T., H. Hattori, and S. Fujita (1972). *J. Neuropathol. Exp. Neurol.* 31:502–518. Autoradiographic studies on histogenesis of rat brain macrophages in the mouse.

Kitamura, T., Y. Tsuchirashi, A. Tatebe, and S. Fujita (1977). *Acta Neuropath.* 38:195–201. Electron-microscopic features of the resting microglia in the rabbit hippocampus, identified by silver carbonate staining.

Kitchin, I. C. (1949). *J. Exp. Zool.* 112:393–415. The effects of notochordectomy in *Amblystoma mexicanum*.

Kitraki, E., M. N. Alexis, and F. Stylianopoulou (1984). *J. Steroid Biochem.* 20:263–269. Glucocorticoid receptors in developing rat brain and liver.

Klagsbrun M., and Y. Shing (1985). *Proc. Natl. Acad. Sci. U.S.A.* 82:805–809. Heparin affinity of anionic and cationic capillary endothelial cell growth factors: Analysis of hypothalamus-derived growth factors and fibroblast growth factors.

Klarsfeld, A., and J.-P. Changeux (1985). *Proc. Natl. Acad. Sci. U.S.A.* 82:4558–4562. Activity regulates the level of acetylcholine receptor alpha-subunit mRNA in cultured chick myotubes.

Klarsfeld, A., P. Daubas, B. Bourachot, and J. P. Changeux (1987). *Mol. Cell. Biol.* 7:951–955. A 5' flanking region of the chicken acetylcholine receptor alpha-subunit gene confers tissue-specificity and developmental control of expression in transfected cells.

Klatzko, I., and J. Miquel (1960). *J. Neuropathol. Exp. Neurol.* 19:475–487. Observations on pinocytosis in nervous tissue.

Klauer, G. (1986). *Z. Mikrosk. Anat. Forsch Leipzig* 100:273–289. Die Mechanoreceptoren in der Haut der Wirbeltiere: Morphologie und Klassifizierung.

Kleihues, P., P. L. Lantos, and P. N. Magee (1976). *Int. Rev. Exp. Pathol.* 15:153–232. Chemical carcinogenesis in the nervous system.

Klein, A. H., S. Meltzer, and F. N. Kenney (1972). *J. Pediat.* 81:912–915. Improved prognosis in congenital hypothyroidism treated before age 3 months.

Klein, R. E., M. Irwin, P. L. Engle, and C. Yarborough (1977). Malnutrition and mental development in rural Guatemala, pp. 92–121. An applied cross-cultural research study. In Warren, *Advances in cross-cultural psychology*. Academic Press, New York.

Klein, S. L., and M. Jacobson (1990). *Roux's Arch. Dev. Biol.* 199:237–245. In vitro evidence that interactions between *Xenopus* blastomeres restrict cell migration.

Kleinebeckel, D., and R., Schulte (1988). *Monogr. Dev. Biol.* 21:84–88. Influence of temperature on speed of nerve regeneration and on the quality of reestablished muscle function in frogs.

Kleinfeld, R. G., and J. E. Sisken (1966). *J. Cell Biol.* 31:369–380. Morphological and kinetic aspects of mitotic arrest by and recovery from colcemid.

Kleinman, H. K., R. C. Ogle, F. B. Cannon, C. D. Little, T. M. Sweeney, and L. Luckenbill-Edds (1988). *Proc. Natl. Acad. Sci. U.S.A.* 85:1282–1286. Laminin receptors for neurite formation.

Klingman, G. I., and J. D. Klingman (1967). *Int. J. Neuropharmacol.* 6:501–508. Catecholamines in peripheral tissues of mice and cell counts of sympathetic ganglia after the prenatal and postnatal administration of the nerve growth factor antiserum.

Kliot, M., and C. J. Shatz (1982). *Soc. Neurosci. Abstr.* 8:815. Genesis of different ganglion cell types in the cat.

Knapp, P. E., R. P. Skoff, and D. W. Redstone (1986). *J. Neurosci.* 6:2813–2822. Oligodendroglial cell death in jimpy mice: An explanation for the myelin deficit.

Knobler, R. L., and J. G. Stempak (1973). *Prog. Brain Res.* 40:407–423. Serial section analysis of myelin development in the central nervous system of the albino rat: An electron microscopical study of early axonal ensheathment.

Knouff, R. A. (1927). *J. Comp. Neurol.* 44:259–361. Origin of the cranial ganglia of *Rana*.

Knouff, R. A. (1935). *J. Comp. Neurol.* 62:17–71. The developmental pattern of ectodermal placodes in *Rana pipiens*.

Ko, C.-P. (1987). *J. Neurocytol.* 16:567–576. A lectin, peanut agglutinin, as a probe for the extracellular matrix in living neuromuscular junctions.

Kobayashi, T., O. R. Inman, W. Buno, and H. E. Himwich (1964) *Prog. Brain Res.* 9:87–88. Neurohistological studies of developing mouse brain.

Koch, C., and T. Poggio (1983). *Proc. Roy. Soc. (London) Ser. B.* 218:455–477. A theoretical analysis of electrical properties of spines.

Koch, W. E. (1967). *J. Exp. Zool.* 165:155–170. *In vitro* differentiation of tooth rudiments of embryonic mice. I. Transfilter interaction of embryonic incisor tissues.

Koch, W. E., and C. Grobstein (1963). *Dev. Biol.* 7:303–323. Transmission of radioisotopically labeled materials during embryonic induction *in vitro*.

Koda, L. Y., and L. M. Partlow (1976). *J. Neurobiol.* 7:157–172. Membrane marker movement on sympathetic axons in tissue culture.

Koeke, H. U. (1960). *Arch. Entw.-Mech. Organ.* 151:612–659. Untersuchungen über die regionalen Potenzen der Neuralleiste zur Bildung von Melanoblasten bei der Hausente (*Anas domestica*).

Koelliker, R. A. (1844). *Die Selbständigkeit und Abhängigkeit des sympathischen Nervensystems durch anatomische Beobachtungen beweisen. Ein akad. Programm,* 40 pp. 4°. Meyer and Zeller, Zürich.

Koelliker, R. A. (1852). *Handbuch der Gewebelehre des Menschen.* Engelmann, Leipzig. (The 6th Edition, in 3 volumes, was published in 1896).

Koelliker, R. A. (1887). *Anat. Anz.* 15:480. Die Untersuchungen von Golgi über den feineren Bau des centralen Nervensystems.

Koelliker, R. A. (1890). *Z. wiss. Zool.* 49:663–689. Zur feineren Anatomie des centralen Nervensystems.

Koelliker, R. A. (1892). *Sitzungsber. phys.-med. Gesellsch. Würzburg,* No. 1, pp. 1–5. Ueber den feineren Bau des Bulbus olfactorius.

Koelliker, R. A. (1893). *Handbuch der Gewebelchre des Menschen,* Vol. 2, second edition. Wilhelm Engelmann, Leipzig.

Koelliker, R. A. (1896). *Handbuch der Gewebelehre des Menschen.* Bd. 2, *Nervensystem des Menschen und der Thiere,* 6, Aufl., W. Engelmann, Leipzig.

Koelliker, R. A. (1899). *Erinnerungen aus meinem Leben.* Engelmann, Leipzig.

Koelliker, R. A. (1905). *Z. wiss. Zool.* 82:1–38. Die Entwicklung der Elemente des Nervensystems.

Koenig, E. (1965). *J. Neurochem.* 12:357–361. Synthetic mechanisms in the axon. II. RNA in myelin-free axons of the cat.

Koenig, E. (1967). *J. Neurochem.* 14:437–446. Synthetic mechanisms in the axon. IV. *In vitro* incorporation of [³H] precursors into axonal protein and RN.

Koenig, H. L., L. DiGiamberardino, and G. Bennett (1973). *Brain Res.* 62:413–417. Renewal of proteins and glycoproteins of synaptic constituents by means of axonal transport.

Koenig, J. (1971). *Arch. Anat. Microscop. Morph. Exp.* 60:1–26. Contribution a l'étude de la réaformation expérimentale des plaques motrices de rat.

Koenig, J. (1973). *Brain Res.* 62:361–365. Morphogenesis of motor end-plates 'in vivo' and 'in vitro'.

Köhler, W. (1938). *The Place of Value in a World of Facts.* Liveright, New York.

Koles, Z. J., K. D. McLeod, and R. S. Smith (1982). *J. Physiol. (London)* 328:469–484. A study of the motion of organelles which undergo retrograde and anterograde rapid axonal transport in *Xenopus.*

Kolle, K. (1959). *Grosse Nervenärtzte,* 2 Vols. Georg Thieme Verlag, Stuttgart.

Kollros, J. J. (1942). *Proc. Soc. Exp. Biol. Med.* 49:204–206. Localized maturation of lid-closure reflex mechanism by thyroid implants into tadpole hindbrain.

Kollros, J. J. (1943a). *Physiol. Zool.* 16:269–279. Experimental studies on the development of the corneal reflex in Amphibia. II. Localized maturation of the reflex mechanism effected by thyroxin-agar implants into the hindbrain.

Kollros, J. J. (1943b). *J. Exp. Zool.* 92:121–142. Experimental studies on the development of the corneal reflex in amphibia. III. The influence of the periphery upon the reflex center.

Kollros, J. J. (1953). *J. Exp. Zool.* 123:153–187. The development of the optic lobes in the frog. I. The effects of unilateral enucleation in embryonic stages.

Kollros, J. J. (1958). *Science* 128:1505. Hormonal control of onset of corneal reflex in the frog.

Kollros, J. J. (1982). *J. Comp. Neurol.* 205:171–178. Peripheral control of midbrain mitotic activity in the frog.

Kollros, J. J. (1984). *J. Comp. Neurol.* 224:386–394. Growth and death of cells of the mesencephalic fifth nucleus in *Rana pipiens* larvae.

Kollros, J. J., and V. M. McMurray (1955). *J. Comp. Neurol.* 102:47–64. The mesencephalic V nucleus in anurans. I. Normal development in *Rana pipiens.*

Kollros, J. J., and M. L. Thiesse (1985). *J. Comp. Neurol.* 233:481–489. Growth and death of cells of the mesencephalic fifth nucleus in *Xenopus laevis* larvae.

Kolmer, W. (1910). *Anat. Anz.* 36:281–299. Über Strukturen im Epithel des Sinnesorgane.

Konat, G. , M. Trojanowska, G. Gantt, and E. L. Hogan (1988). *J. Neurosci. Res.* 20:19–22. Expression of myelin protein genes in quaking mouse brain.

König, N., and R. Marty (1981). *Bibl. Anat.* 19:152–162. Early neurogenesis and synaptogenesis in cerebral cortex.

König, N., G. Roch, and R. Marty (1975). *Z. Anat. Entwicklungsgesch.* 148:73–87. The onset of synaptogenesis in rat temporal cortex.

König, N., and M. Schachner (1981). *Neurosci. Lett.* 26:227–231. Neuronal and glial cells in the superficial layers of early postnatal mouse neocortex: Immunofluorescence observations.

König, N., J. P. Nornung, and H. Van der Loos (1981). *Neurosci. Lett.* 27:225–229. Identification of Cajal-Retzius cells in immature rodent cerebral cortex: A combined Golgi-EM study.

König, N., J. Valat, J. Fulcrang, and R. Marty (1977). *Neurosci. Lett.* 4:21–26. The time of origin of Cajal-Retzius cells in the rat temporal Cortex. An autoradiographic study.

Konigsmark, S. W., and R. L. Sidman (1963). *J. Neuropath. Exp. Neurol.* 22:643–676. Origin of brain macrophages in the mouse.

Konishi, M., and E. Akutagawa (1985). *Nature* 315:145–147. Neuronal growth, atrophy and death in a sexually dimorphic song nucleus in the zebra finch brain.

Konkol, R. J., R. B. Mailman, E. G. Bendeich, A. M. Garrison, R. A. Mueller, and G. R. Breese (1978). *Brain Res.*

144:277–285. Evaluation of the effects of nerve growth factor and anti-nerve growth factor on the development of central catecholamine-containing neurons.

Konorski, J. (1958). *J. Ment. Sci.* 104:1100–1110. Trends in the development of physiology of the brain.

Koppel, H., and G. M. Innocenti (1983). *Neurosci. Lett.* 41:33–40. Is there a genuine exuberancy of callosal projections in development? A quantitative electron microscopic study in the cat.

Koppel, H., P. D. Lewis, and J. S. Wigglesworth (1982). *J. Anat. (London)* 134:73–84. A study of the vascular supply to the external granular layer of the postnatal rat cerebellum.

Koppisch, E. (1935). *Z. Hyg. Infektionskrankh.* 117:386–398. Zur Wanderungsgeschwindigkeit neurotroper Virusarten in peripheren Nerven.

Kordower, J. H., R. T. Bartus, M. Bothwell, G. Schatteman, and D. M. Gash (1988). *J. Comp. Neurol.* 277:465–486. Nerve growth factor receptor immunoreactivity in the non-human primate *(Cebus apella)*: Distribution, morphology, and colocalization with cholinergic enzymes.

Korn, E. D., and J. A. Hammer (1988). *Ann. Rev. Biophys. Biophys. Chem.* 17:23–45. Myosins of nonmuscle cells.

Korneliussen, H., and J. K. S. Jansen (1976). *J. Neurocytol.* 5:591–604. Morphological aspects of the elimination of polyneuronal innervation of skeletal muscle fibres in new-born rats.

Korneliussen, H. K. (1967). *J. Hirnforsch.* 9:151–185. Cerebellar corticogenesis in Cetacea, with special reference to regional variations.

Korner, A. (1968). *Prog. Biophys. Molec. Biol.* 17:63–98. Ribonucleic acid and hormonal control of protein synthesis.

Korner, A. (1970). *Proc. Roy. Soc. (London) Ser. B.* 176:287–290. Hormonal control of protein synthesis.

Kornguth, S. E., and G. Scott (1972). *J. Comp. Neurol.* 146:61–82. The role of climbing fibers in the formation of Purkinje cell dendrites.

Kornguth, S. E., J. W. Anderson, and G. Scott (1967). *J. Comp. Neurol.* 130:1–24. Observations on the ultrastructure of the developing cerebellum of the *Macaca mulatta*.

Kornguth, S. E., J. W. Anderson, and G. Scott (1968). *J. Comp. Neurol.* 132:531–546. The development of synaptic contacts in the cerebellum of *Macaca mulatta*.

Korr, H. (1968). *Z. Morphol. Oekol. Tiere* 62:389–422. Das postembryonale Wachstum verschiedener Hirnbereiche bei *Orchesella villosa* L. (Ins. Collembola).

Korr, H. (1978). *Histochemistry* 59:111–116. Combination of metallic impregnation and autoradiography of brain sections. A method for differentiation of proliferating glial cells in the brain of adult rats and mice.

Korr, H. (1980). *Adv. Anat. Embryol. Cell Biol.* 61:1–72. Proliferation of different cell types in the brain.

Korr, H. (1982). *Exp. Brain Res. Suppl.* 5:51–57. Proliferation of different cell types in the brain of senile mice. Autoradiographic studies with ^{3}H- and ^{14}C-Thymidine.

Korr, H., B. Schultze, and W. Maurer (1973). *J. Comp. Neurol.* 150:169–176. Autoradiographic investigations of glial proliferation in the brain of adult mice. I. The DNA synthesis phase of neuroglia and endothelial cells.

Korr, H., B. Schultze, and W. Maurer (1975). *J. Comp. Neurol.* 160:477–490. Autoradiographic investigations of glial

proliferation in the brain of adult mice. II. Cycle time and mode of proliferation of neuroglia and endothelial cells.

Korr, I. M., and G. S. L. Appeltauer (1974). *Exp. Neurol.* 43:452–463. The time-course of axonal transport of neuronal proteins to muscle.

Korr, I. M., P. N. Wilkinson, and F. W. Chornock (1967). *Science* 155:342–346. Axonal delivery of neuroplasmic components to muscle cells.

Korschelt, E., and K. Heider (1902–1909). *Lehrbuch der vergleichenden Entwicklungsgeschichte der Wirbellosen Thiere.* 4 vols., Gustav Fischer, Jena.

Korsching, S. (1986). *Trends Neurosci.* 9:570–573. The role of nerve growth factor in the CNS.

Korsching, S., and H. Thoenen (1977). *Proc. Natl. Acad. Sci. U.S.A.* 74:3513–3516. Nerve growth factor in sympathetic ganglia and corresponding target organs of the rat: Correlation with density of sympathetic innervation.

Korsching, S., and H. Thoenen (1983a). *Proc. Natl. Acad. Sci. U.S.A.* 80:3513–3516. Nerve growth factor in sympathetic ganglia and corresponding target organs of the rat: Correlation with density of sympathetic innervation.

Korsching, S., and H. Thoenen (1983b). *Neurosci. Lett.* 39:1–4. Quantitative demonstration of the retrograde axonal transport of endogenous nerve growth factor.

Korsching, S., G. Auburger, R. Heumann, J. Scott, and H. Thoenen (1985). *EMBO J.* 4:1389–1393. Levels of nerve growth factor and its mRNA in the central nervous system correlate with cholinergic innervation.

Korsching, S., R. Heumann, H. Thoenen, and F. Hefti (1986a). *Neurosci. Lett.* 66:175–180. Cholinergic denervation of the rat hippocampus by fimbrial transection leads to a transient accumulation of nerve growth factor (NGF) without change in mRNA NGF content.

Korsching, S., R. Heumann, A. Davies, and H. Thoenen (1986b). *Soc. Neurosci. Abstr.* 12:1096. Levels of nerve growth factor and its mRNA during development and regeneration of the peripheral nervous system.

Koshtoyantz, C., and A. Ryabinovskaya (1935). *Pfluegers Arch. Ges. Physiol.* 235:416–421. Beitrag zur Physiologie der Skelettmuskeln der Säugetiere in verschiedenen Stadien ihrer individuellen Entwicklung.

Kosik, K.S., and E. A. Finch (1987). *J. Neurosci.* 7:3142–3153. MAP2 and tau segregate into dendritic and axonal domains after the elaboration of morphologically distinct neurites: An immunocytochemical study of cultured rat cerebrum.

Kossut, M. (1988). *Acta Neurobiol. Exp.* 48:83–115. Modifications of the single cortical vibrissal column.

Kostovic, I., and P. Rakic (1980). *J. Neurocytol.* 9:219–242. Cytology and time of origin of interstitial neurons in the white matter in infant and adult human and monkey telencephalon.

Kostrzewa, R. M., and C. T. Harston (1986). *Neuroscience* 18:809–815. Altered histofluorescent pattern of noradrenergic innervation of the cerebellum of the mutant mouse Purkinje cell degeneration.

Kosunen, T. U., and B. H. Waksman (1963). *J. Neuropath. Exp. Neurol.* 22:324–326. Radioautographic studies of experimental allergic encephalomyelitis (EAE) in rats.

Kosunen, T. U., B. H. Waksman, and I. K. Samuelson (1963). *J. Neuropath. Exp. Neurol.* 22:367–380. Radio-autographic study of cellular mechanisms in delayed hypersensitivity. II. Experimental allergic encephalomyelitis in the rat.

Kotani, S., E. Nishida, H. Kumagai, and H. Sakai (1985). *J. Biol. Chem.* 260:10779–10783. Calmodulin inhibits interaction of actin with MAP2 and Tau, two major microtubule-associated proteins.

Koyré, A. (1956). *Bull. Soc. Francaise Philosophie* 50:59–97. L'hypothèse et l'expérience chez Newton.

Krahn, V. (1962). *Anat. Embryol.* 164:257–263. The pia mater at the site of the entry of blood vessels into the central nervous system.

Kratz, K. E., and P. D. Spear (1976). *J. Comp. Neurol.* 170:141–151. Effects of visual deprivation and alterations in binocular competition on responses of striate cortex neurons in the cat.

Kratz, K. E., P. D. Spear, and D. C. Smith (1976). *J. Neurophysiol.* 39:501–511. Postcritical-period reversal of effects of monocular deprivation on striate cortex cells in the cat.

Krause, R. (1926). *Enzyklopädie der mikroskopischen Technik.* Urban & Schwarzenberg, Berlin.

Kraus-Ruppert, R., N. Herschkowitz, and S. Furst (1973). *J. Neuropathol. Exp. Neurol.* 32:197–203. Morphological studies on neuroglia cells in the corpus callosum of the jimpy mutant mouse.

Krawiec, L., C. A. Garcia Argiz, C. J. Gomez, and J. M. Pasquini (1969). *Brain Res.* 15:209–218. Hormonal regulation of brain development. III. Effects of triiodothyronine and growth hormone on the biochemical changes in the cerebral cortex and cerebellum of neonatally thyroidectomized rats.

Krech, D. (1962). Cortical Localization of Function, pp. 31–72. In *Psychology in the Making. Histories of Selected Research Problems* (L. Postman, ed.), Knopf, New York.

Krech, D., M. R. Rosenzweig, and E. L. Bennett (1963). *Arch. Neurol.* 8:403–412. Effects of complex environment and blindness on rat brain.

Kreutzberg, G. W. (1966). *Acta Neuropathol.* 7:149–161. Autoradiographische Untersuchung über die Beteiligung von Gliezellen an der axonalen Reaktion im Facilialiskern der Ratte.

Kreutzberg, G. W., and I. C. D. Barron (1976). *J. Neurocytol.* 7:601–610. 5′ nucleotidase of microglial cells in the facial nucleus during axonal reaction.

Kreutzberg, G. W., and G. W. Gross (1977). *Cell Tiss. Res.* 181:443–457. General morphology and axonal ultrastructure of the olfactory nerve of the Pike, *Esolucius.*

Krey, L. C., I. Lieberburg, N. J. MacLusky, P. G. Davis, and R. Robbins (1982). *Endocrinology* 110:2168–2176. Testosterone increases cell nuclear estrogen receptor levels in the brain of the Stanley-Gumbreck pseudohermaphrodite male rat: Implications for testosterone modulation of neuroendocrine activity.

Krigman, M. R., and E. L. Hogan (1976). *Brain Res.* 107:239–255. Undernutrition in the developing rat: Effect upon myelination.

Krikorian D., M. Manthorpe, and S. Varon (1982). *Dev. Neurosci.* 5:77–91. Purified mouse Schwann cells: Mitogenic effects of fetal calf serum and fibroblast growth factor.

Krishnan, N., and M. Singer (1973). *J. Anat. (London)* 136:1–14. Penetration of peroxidase into peripheral nerve fibers.

Kriss, J. P., and L. Revesz (1961). *Cancer Res.* 22:254–265.

The distribution and fate of bromodeoxyuridine and bromodeoxycytidine in the mouse and rat.

Kristensson, K. (1975). Retrograde axonal transport of protein tracers. In *The Use of Axonal Transport for Studies of Neuronal Connectivity* (W. M. Cowan, and M. Cuenod, eds.), Elsevier, Amsterdam.

Kristensson, K. (1978). *Ann. Rev. Pharmacol. Toxicol.* 18:97–110. Retrograde transport of macromolecules in axons.

Kristensson, K. (1984). Retrograde signaling after nerve injury, pp. 31–43. In *Axonal Transport in Neuronal Growth and Regeneration* (J. S. Elam, and P. Cancalon, eds.), Plenum, New York.

Kristensson, K., and Y. Olsson (1971). *Brain Res.* 29:363–365. Retrograde axonal transport of protein.

Kristensson, K., and Y. Olsson (1973). *Acta Neuropathol.* 23:43–47. Uptake and retrograde axonal transport of protein tracers in hypoglossal neurons.

Kristensson, K., and Y. Olsson (1974). *Brain Res.* 79:101–109. Retrograde transport of horseradish peroxidase in transected axons. I. Time relationships between transport and induction of chromatolysis.

Kristensson, K., and Y. Olsson (1975). *J. Neurocytol.* 4:653–661. Retrograde transport of horseradish peroxidase in transected axons. II. Relations between rate of transfer from the site of injury to the perikaryon and onset of chromatolysis.

Kristensson, K., and Y. Olsson (1976). *Brain Res.* 115:201–213. Retrograde transport of horseradish in transected axons. III. Entry into injured axons and subsequent localization in perikaryon.

Kristensson, K., Y. Olsson, and J. Sjöstrand (1971). *Brain Res.* 32:399–406. Axonal uptake and retrograde transport of exogenous proteins in the hypoglossal nerve.

Kristensson, K., B. Ghetti, and H. M. Wisniewski (1974). *Brain Res.* 79:189–201. Study on the propagation of Herpes simplex virus (type 2) into the brain after intraocular injection.

Kristensson, K., I. Nenmesmo, L. Persson, and E. Lycke (1978). *J. Neurol. Sci.* 35:331–340. Neuron to neuron transmission of herpes simplex virus. Transport of virus from skin to brain stem nuclei.

Kristensson, K., N. K. Zeller, M. E. Dubois-Dalcq, and R. A. Lazzarini (1986). *J. Histochem.* 34:467–473. Expression of myelin basic protein gene in the developing rat brain as revealed by *in situ* hybridization.

Kristt, D. A. (1979). *Brain Res.* 178:69–88. Development of neocortical circuitry: Quantitative ultrastructural analysis of putative monoaminergic synapses.

Kristt, D. A., and M. E. Molliver (1976). *Brain Res.* 108:180–186. Synapses in newborn rat cerebral cortex: A quantitative ultrastructural study.

Kromer, L. F. (1987). *Science* 235:214–216. Nerve growth factor treatment after brain injury prevents neuronal death.

Kromer, L. F., and C. J. Cornbrooks (1986). *Proc. Natl. Acad. Sci. U.S.A.* 82:6330–6334. Transplants of Schwann cell cultures promote axonal regeneration in the adult mammalian brain.

Krotoski, D., C. Domingo, and M. Bronner-Fraser (1986). *J. Cell. Biol.* 103:1061–1071. Distribution of a putative cell surface receptor for fibronectin and laminin in the avian embryo.

Krotoski, D. M., S. E. Fraser, and M. Bronner-Fraser (1988).

Dev. Biol. **127**:119–132. Mapping of neural crest pathways in *Xenopus laevis* using inter- and intra-specific cell markers.

Kruger, L., and D. S. Maxwell (1966). *Am. J. Anat.* **118**:411–435. Electron microscopy of oligodendrocytes in normal rat cerebrum.

Kruger, L., and D. S. Maxwell (1967). *J. Comp. Neur.* **129**:115–142. Comparative fine structure of vertebrate neuroglia teleosts and reptiles.

Krüger, P., and P.G. Günther (1955). *Z. Ges. Anat.* **118**:313–323. Fasern mit "Filbrillenstruktur" und Fasern mit "Felderstruktur" in der quergestreiften skeletmuskulatur der Saüger und des Menschen.

Krum, J. M., and J. M. Rosenstein (1989). *Exp. Neurol.* **103**:203–212 (1989). The fine structure of vascular-astroglial relations in transplanted fetal neocortex.

Krumlauf, R., P. W. H. Holland, J. H. McVey, and B. L. M. Hogan (1987). *Development* **99**:603–617. Developmental and spatial patterns of expression of the mouse homeobox gene, *Hox-2.1*.

Kruska, D. (1970a). *Z. Anat. Entwicklungsgeschichte* **131**:291–324. Vergleichend cytoarchitektonische Untersuchungen an Gehirnen von Wild- und Hausschweinen.

Kruska, D. (1970b). *Z. Säugetierk.* **35**:214–238. Über die Evolution des Gehirns in der Ordnung Artiodactyla Owen, 1848, insbesondere der Teilordnung Suina Gray, 1868.

Kruska, D. (1972). *Z. Anat. Entwicklungsgesch.* **138**:265–282. Volumenvergleich optischer Hirnzentren bei Wild- und Hausschweinen.

Kruska, D. (1987). *J. Hirnforsch.* **28**:59–70. How fast can total brain size change in mammals?

Kruska, D., and M. Rohrs (1974). *Z. Anat. Entwicklungsgesch.* **144**:61–73. Comparative-quantitative investigations on brains of feral pigs from the Galapagos Islands and of European domestic pigs.

Kruska, D., and H. Stephan (1973). *Acta Anat. (Basel)* **84**:387–415. Volumenvergleich allokortikaler Hirnzentren bei Wild- und Hausschweinen.

Krystosek, A., and N. W. Seeds (1981a). *Proc. Natl. Acad. Sci. U.S.A.* **78**:7810–7814. Plasminogen activator secretion by granule neurons in cultures of developing cerebellum.

Krystosek, A., and N. W. Seeds (1981b). *Science* **213**:1523–1534. Plasminogen activator release at the neuronal growth cone.

Krystosek, A., and N. W. Seeds (1984). *J. Cell Biol.* **98**:773–776. Peripheral neurons and Schwann cells secrete plasminogen activator.

Kucera, J. (1980). *Histochemistry* **66**:221–228. Myofibrillar ATPase activity of intrafusal fibers in chronically deafferented rat muscle spindles.

Kucera, J., and J. M. Walro (1987). *Anat. Embryol.* **176**:449–461. Postnatal maturation of spindles in deafferented rat soleus muscles.

Kucera, J., and J. M. Walro (1989). *Anat. Embryol.* **179**:369–376. Postnatal expression of myosin heavy chains in muscle spindles of the rat.

Kucera, J., J. M. Walro, and J. Reichler (1988a). *Anat. Embryol.* **177**:427–436. Motor and sensory innervation of muscle spindles in the neonatal rat.

Kucera, J., J. M. Walro, and J. Reichler (1988b). *Amer. J. Anat.* **183**:344–358. Innervation of developing intrafusal muscle fibers in the rat.

Kucera, P., M. Dolivo, P Coulon, and A. Flamand (1985). *J. Virol.* **55**:158–162. Pathways of the early progression of virulent and avirulent rabies strains from the eye to the brain.

Kuffler, D. P. (1986a). *J. Comp. Neurol.* **250**:228–235. Accurate reinnervation of motor end plates after disruption of sheath cells and muscle fibers.

Kuffler, D. P. (1986b). *J. Comp. Neurol.* **250**:236–244. Thickness of the basal lamina at the frog neuromuscular junction.

Kuffler, D. P., and K. J. Muller (1974). *J. Neurobiol.* **5**:331–348. The properties and connections of supernumerary sensory and motor nerve cells in the central nervous system of an abnormal leech.

Kuffler, D. P., W. Thompson, and J. K. S. Jansen (1980). *Proc. Roy. Soc. (London) Ser. B.* **208**:189–222. The fate of foreign endplates in cross-innervated rat soleus muscle.

Kuffler, S. W. (1967). *Proc. Roy. Soc. (London) Ser. B.* **168**:1–21. Neuroglial cells: Physiological properties and a potasssium mediated effect of neuronal activity on the glial membrane potential.

Kuffler, S. W., and J. G. Nicholls (1966a). *Perspect. Biol. Med.* **9**:69–76. How do materials exchange between blood and nerve cells in the brain?

Kuffler, S. W., and J. G. Nicholls (1966b). *Ergeb. Physiol.* **57**:1–90. The physiology of neuroglial cells.

Kuffler, S. W., and J. G. Nicholls (1976). *From Neuron to Brain*, Sinauer, Mass.

Kuffler, S. W., J. G. Nicholls, and R. K. Orkand (1966). *J. Neurophysiol.* **29**:768–787. Physiological properties of glial cells in the central nervous system of amphibia.

Kuhlenbeck, H. (1938). *J. Comp. Neurol.* **69**:273–301. The ontogenic development and significance of the cortex telencephali in the chick.

Kuhlenbeck, H. (1954). *Confin. Neurol.* **14**:329–342. Some histologic age changes in the rat's brain and their relationship to comparable changes in the human brain.

Kuhlenbeck, H. (1957). *Brain and Consciousness: Some Prolegomena to an Approach of the Problem*, Karger, Basel.

Kuhlenbeck, H. (1967–1978). *The Central Nervous System of Vertebrates*. 5 volumes in 7. Vols. 1 and 2, Academic Press, New York, Vols. 3 to 5, Karger, Basel.

Kuhlenbeck, H. (1973). Neuromery; definitive main subdivisions, pp. 304–350. *The Central Nervous System of Vertebrates*, Vol. 3, Part 2: *Overall Morphologic Pattern*. Karger, Basel.

Kuhlenkampf, H. (1952). *Z. Anat. Entwicklungsgeschichte* **116**:304–312. Das Verhalten der Neuroglia in den Vorderhörnern des Rückenmarkes der weissen Maus unter dem Reiz physiologischer Tätigkeit.

Kuhlman, R. E., and O. H. Lowry (1956). *J. Neurochem.* **1**:173–180. Quantitative histochemical changes during the development of the rat cerebral cortex.

Kuhn, T. (1962). *The Structure of Scientific Revolutions.* Chicago University Press, Chicago.

Kuhn, T. S. (1970). *The Structure of Scientific Revolutions*, 2nd edn. Chicago Univ. Press, Chicago.

Kuhn, T. S. (1974). Second thoughts on paradigms, pp. 459–482. In *The Structure of Scientific Theories* (F. Suppe, ed.), Univ. Illinois Press, Urbana.

Kuhn, T. S. (1977). *The Essential Tension.* Univ. Chicago Press, Chicago.

Kühne, W. (1863). *Virchow's Arch. Path. Anat.* **28**:528–538.

Die Muskelspindeln. Ein Beitrag zur Lehre von der Entwickelung der Muskeln und Nervenfasern.

Kühne, W. (1870). The relation of the ultimate fibres of nerve to muscle, pp. 202–234. In *Manual of Human and Comparative Histology*, Vol. 1, (S. Stricker, ed.), H. Power, transl. The New Sydenham Society, London.

Kühne, W. (1888). *Proc. Roy. Soc. (London) Ser. B.* 44:427–447. On the origin and the causation of vital movement.

Kullberg, R. W., T. L. Lentz, and M. W. Cohen (1977). *Dev. Biol.* 60:101–129. Development of the myotomal neuromuscular junction in *Xenopus laevis:* An electrophysiological and fine-structural study.

Kumar, A., O. P. Ghai, N. Singh, and R. Singh (1977). *J. Pediat.* 90:149–153. Delayed nerve conduction velocities in children with protein-calorie malnutrition.

Kumé, M., and K. Dan (1968). *Invertebrate Embryology*, Nolit, Belgrade, 605 pp.

Kumpulainen T., D. Dahl, L. K. Korhoren, and S. H. M. Nystrom (1983). *J. Histochem. Cytochem.* 31:879–888. Immunolabeling of carbonic anhydrase isoenzyme C and glial fibrillary acidic protein in paraffin-embedded tissue section of human brain and retina.

Kuno, M., and R. Llinás (1970). *J. Physiol. (London)* 210:807–821. Enhancement of synaptic transmission by dendritic potentials in chromatolyzed motoneurones of the cat.

Kuno, M., Y. Miyata, and E. J. Munoz-Martinex (1974a). *J. Physiol. (London)* 240:725–739. Differential reaction of fast and slow α-motoneurons to axotomy.

Kuno, M., Y. Miyata, and E. J. Munoz-Martinez (1974b). *J. Physiol. (London)* 242:273–288. Properties of fast and slow alpha motoneurones following motor reinnervation.

Kupfer, C., and P. Palmer (1964). *Exp. Neurol.* 9:400–409. Lateral geniculate nucleus: Histological and cytochemical changes following afferent denervation and visual deprivation.

Kupffer, C. von (1895). *Studien zür vergleichenden Entwicklungsgeschichte des Kopfes der Cranioten. Heft III: Die Entwicklung der Kopfnerven von Ammocoetes planeri.* Munich.

Kurz, E. M., D. R. Sengelaub, and A. P. Arnold (1986). *Science* 232:395–398. Androgens regulate the dendritic length of mammalian motoneurons in adulthood.

Kurz, E. M., C. A. Bowers, and D. R. Sengelaub (1990). *J. Comp. Neurol.* 292:638–650. Morphology of rat spinal motoneurons with normal and hormonally altered specificity.

Kutsch, W., and D. Bentley (1987). *Dev. Biol.* 123:517–525. Programmed death of peripheral pioneer neurons in the grasshopper embryo.

Kuwano, R., H. Usui, T. Maeda, T. Fukui, N. Yamanari, E. Ohtsuka, M. Ikehara, and Y. Takahashi. (1984). *Nucl. Acids Res.* 12:7455–7465. Molecular cloning and the complete nucleotide sequence of cDNA to mRNA for S-100 protein of rat brain.

Kuwano, R., T. Maeda, H. Usui, K. Araki, T. Yamakuni, et al. (1986). *FEBS Lett.* 202:97–101. Molecular cloning of cDNA of S100 subunit mRNA.

Laatsch, R. H. (1962). *J. Neurochem.* 9:487–492. Glycerol phosphate dehydrogenase activity of developing rat central nervous system.

Lackie, J. M. (1985). *Cell Movement and Cell Behaviour.* Allen and Unwin, London.

Laemmli, U. K. (1970). *Nature* 227:680–685. Cleavage of structural protein during assembly of the head of a bacteriophage T4.

Lahousse, E. (1888). *Arch. Biol. (Liège)* 8:43–110. Recherches sur l'ontogenése du cervelet.

Lai, C., M. A. Brow, K.-A. Naxe, A. B. Noronha, R. H. Quarles, F. E. Bloom, R. J. Milner, and J. G. Sutcliffe (1987). *Proc. Natl. Acad. Sci. U.S.A.* 84:4337–4341. Two forms of 1B236/myelin associated glycoprotein, a cell adhesion molecule for postnatal neural development, are produced by alternative splicing.

Lai, M., and P. D. Lewis (1980). *J. Comp. Neurol.* 193:973–982. Effects of undernutrition on myelination in rat corpus callosum.

Lai, M., P. D. Lewis, and A. J. Patel (1980). *J. Comp. Neurol.* 193:965–972. Effects of undernutrition on gliogenesis and glial maturation in rat corpus callosum.

Laing, N. G. (1982a). *Dev. Brain Res.* 5:181–186. Timing of motoneuron death in brachial and lumbar regions of the chick embryo.

Laing, N. G. (1982b). *J. Embryol. Exp. Morphol.* 72:269–286. Motor projection patterns in the hind limb of normal and paralysed chick embryos.

Laing, N. G., and A. H. Lamb (1983a). *J. Embryol. Exp. Morphol.* 78:67–82. The distribution of muscle fibre types in chick embryo wings transplanted to the pelvic region is normal.

Laing, N. G., and A. H. Lamb (1983b). *J. Embryol. Exp. Morphol.* 78:53–66. Development and motor innervation of a distal pair of fast and slow wing muscles in the chick embryo.

Lakatos, I. (1978). *Philosophical Papers*, 2 Vols., (J. Worrall, and G. Currie, eds.), Cambridge Univ. Press, Cambridge.

Lam, K., A. J. Sefton, and M. R. Bennett (1982). *Dev. Brain Res.* 3:487–491. Loss of axons from the optic nerve of the rat during early postnatal development.

Lamb, A. H. (1974). *Brain Res.* 67:527–530. The timing of the earliest motor innervation in the hind limb bud in the *Xenopus* tadpole.

Lamb, A. H. (1976). *Dev. Biol.* 51:82–99. The projection patterns of the ventral horn to the hindlimb during development.

Lamb, A. H. (1977). *Brain Res.* 134:145–150. Neuronal death in the development of the somatotopic projections of the ventral horn in *Xenopus.*

Lamb, A. H. (1979a). *Dev. Biol.* 71:8–21. Evidence that some developing limb motorneurones die for reasons other than peripheral competition.

Lamb, A. H. (1979b). *J. Embryol. Exp. Morphol.* 49:13–16. Ventral horn cell counts in a *Xenopus* with naturally occurring supernumerary hindlimbs.

Lamb, A. H. (1981a). *Brain Res.* 209:315–324. Axon regeneration by developing limb motoneurones in *Xenopus laevis.*

Lamb, A. H. (1981b). *J. Comp. Neurol.* 203:157–171. Target dependency of developing motoneurons in *Xenopus laevis.*

Lamb, A. H. (1981c). *J. Embryol. Exp. Morphol.* 65:149–163. Selective bilateral motor innervation in *Xenopus* tadpoles with one hind limb.

Lamborghini, J. E. (1980). *J. Comp. Neurol.* 189:323–333. Rohon-Beard cells and other large neurons in *Xenopus* originate during gastrulation.

Lamborghini, J. E. (1987). *J. Comp. Neurol.* 264:47–55. Disappearance of Rohon-Beard neurons from the spinal cord of larval *Xenopus laevis*.

La Mettrie, J. O. de (1747). *Man a Machine*. Including Frederick the Great's "Eulogy" on La Mettrie and extracts from La Mettrie's "The Natural History of the Soul." Open Court, La Salle, Illinois, 1961.

Lance-Jones, C. (1979). *J. Morphol.* 162:275–310. The morphogenesis of the thigh of the mouse with special reference to tetrapod muscle homologies.

Lance-Jones, C. (1982). *Dev. Brain Res.* 4:473–479. Motoneuron cell death in the developing lumbar spinal cord of the mouse.

Lance-Jones, C. (1988a). *Dev. Biol.* 126:394–407. The somitic level of origin of embryonic chick hindlimb muscles.

Lance-Jones, C. (1988b). *Dev. Biol.* 126:408–419. The effect of somite manipulation on the development of motoneuron projection patterns in the embryonic chick hindlimb.

Lance-Jones, C., and L. Landmesser (1980). *J. Physiol. (London)* 302:559–580. Motorneurone projection patterns in embryonic chick limbs following partial deletions of the spinal cord.

Lance-Jones, C., and L. Landmesser (1981a). *Proc. Roy. Soc. (London) Ser. B.* 214:1–18. Pathway selection by chick lumbosacral motoneurons during normal development.

Lance-Jones, C., and L. Landmesser (1981b). *Proc. Roy. Soc. (London) Ser. B.* 214:19–52. Pathway selection by embryonic chick motoneurons in an experimentally altered environment.

Landacre, F. L. (1910). *J. Comp. Neurol.* 20:389–411. The origin of the cranial ganglia in *Ameiurus*.

Landacre, F. L. (1912). *J. Comp. Neurol.* 22:1–69. The epibranchial placodes of *Lepidosteus osseus* and their relation to the cerebral ganglia.

Landacre, F. L. (1914). *Folia Neurobiol.* 8:601–615. Embryonic cerebral ganglia and the doctrine of nerve components.

Landacre, F. L. (1916). *J. Comp. Neurol.* 27:20–55. The cerebral ganglia and early nerves of *Squalus acanthias*.

Landacre, F. L. (1921). *J. Comp. Neurol.* 33:1–43. The fate of the neural crest in the head of the urodeles.

Lander, A. D. (1987). *Molec. Neurobiol.* 1:213–245. Molecules that make axons grow.

Lander, A. D. (1989). *Trends Neurosci.* 12:189–195. Understanding the molecules of neural cell contacts: Emerging patterns of structure and function.

Lander, A. D., D. K. Fujii, D. Gospodarowics, and L. F. Reichardt (1982). *J. Cell Biol.* 94:574–585. Characterization of a factor that promotes neurite outgrowth: Evidence linking activity to a heparan sulfate proteoglycan.

Lander, A. D., D. K. Fujii and L. F. Reichardt (1985a). *J. Cell Biol.* 101:898–913. Purification of a factor that promotes neurite outgrowth: Isolation of laminin and associated molecules.

Lander, A. D., D. K. Fujii and L. F. Reichardt (1985b). *Proc. Natl. Acad. Sci. U.S.A.* 82:2183–2187. Laminin is associated with 'neurite outgrowth promoting factors' found in conditioned media.

Landgren, S., C. G. Phillips, and R. Porter (1962). *J. Physiol. (London)* 161:112–125. Cortical fields of origin of the monosynaptic pyramidal pathways to some alpha motoneurones of the baboon's hand and forearm.

Landis, D. M. D. (1983). *Dev. Brain Res.* 8:231–245. Development of synaptic junctions in cerebellar glomeruli.

Landis, D. M. D. (1987). *J. Comp. Neurol.* 260:513–525. Initial junctions between developing parallel fibers and Purkinje cells are different from mature synaptic junctions.

Landis, D. M. D., and T. S. Reese (1974). *J. Comp. Neurol.* 155:93–126. Differences in membrane structure between excitatory and inhibitory synapses in the cerebellar cortex.

Landis, D. M. D., and T. S. Reese (1977). *J. Comp. Neurol.* 171:247–260. Structure of the Purkinje cell membrane in staggerer and weaver mutant mice.

Landis, D. M. D., and T. S. Reese (1983). *J. Cell Biol.* 97:1169–1178. Cytoplasmic organization in cerebellar dendritic spines.

Landis, D. M. D., and R. L. Sidman (1978). *J. Comp. Neurol.* 179:831–864. Electron microscopic analysis of postnatal histogenesis in the cerebellar cortex of staggerer mutant mice.

Landis, S. C. (1973) *Brain Res.* 61:175–189. Granule cell heterotopia in normal and nervous mutant mice of the BALB/c-strain.

Landis, S. C. (1983). *Ann. Rev. Physiol.* 45:567–580. Neuronal growth cones.

Landis, S. C., and D. Keefe (1983). *Dev. Biol.* 98:349–372. Evidence for neurotransmitter plasticity *in vivo*: Developmental changes in properties of cholinergic sympathetic neurons.

Landis, S. C., and R. J. Mullen (1978). *J. Comp. Neurol.* 177:124–144. The development and degeneration of Purkinje cells in *pcd* mutant mice.

Landis, S. C. and P. H. Patterson (1981). *Trends Neurosci.* 4:172–175. Neural crest cell lineages.

Landis, S. C., W. J. Shoemaker, M. Schlumpf, and F. E. Bloom (1975). *Brain Res.* 93:253–266. Catecholamines in mutant mouse cerebellum: Fluorescence microscopic and chemical studies.

Landmesser, L. (1971). *J. Physiol. (London)* 213:707–725. Contractile and electrical responses of vagus-innervated frog sartorius muscle.

Landmesser, L. (1972). *J. Physiol. (London)* 220:243–256. Pharmacological properties, cholinesterase activity and anatomy of nerve-muscle junctions in vagus-innervated frog sartorius.

Landmesser, L. (1978). *J. Physiol. (London)* 284:391–414. The development of motor projection patterns in the chick hindlimb.

Landmesser, L. (1984). *Trends Neurosci.* 7:336–339. The development of specific motor pathways in the chick embryo.

Landmesser, L. (1987). *J. Anat. (London)* 152:245–247. Growth cone guidance in the chick limb *in vivo* and in cultured slices.

Landmesser, L., and M. G. Honig (1986). *Dev. Biol.* 118:511–531. Altered sensory projections in the chick hind limb following the early removal of motoneurons.

Landmesser, L., and D. G. Morris (1975). *J. Physiol. (London)* 249:301–326. The development of functional innervation in the hind limb of the chick embryo.

Landmesser, L., and M. O'Donovan (1984b). *J. Physiol. (London)* 347:205–224. The activation patterns of embryonic chick motoneurones projecting to inappropriate muscles.

Landmesser, L., and G. Pilar (1970). *J. Physiol. (London)*

211:203–216. Selective reinnervation of two cell populations in the adult pigeon ciliary ganglion.

Landmesser, L., and G. Pilar (1972). *J. Physiol. (London)* 222:691–713. The onset and development of transmission in the chick ciliary ganglion.

Landmesser, L., and G. Pilar (1974a). *J. Physiol. (London)* 241:715–736. Synapse formation during embryogenesis on ganglion cells lacking a periphery.

Landmesser, L., and G. Pilar (1974b). *J. Physiol. (London)* 241:737–749. Synaptic transmission and cell death during normal ganglionic development.

Landmesser, L., and G. Pilar (1976). *J. Cell Biol.* 68:357–374. Fate of ganglionic synapses and ganglion cell axons during normal and induced cell death.

Landmesser, L., and G. Pilar (1978). *Fed. Proc.* 37:2016–2022. Interactions between neurons and their targets during *in vivo* synaptogenesis.

Landmesser, L., and M. Szente (1986). *J. Physiol. (London)* 280:157–174. Activation patterns of embryonic chick hind-limb muscles following blockade of activity and motoneuron cell death.

Landmesser, L. T. (1980). *Ann. Rev. Neurosci.* 3:279–302. The generation of neuromuscular specificity.

Landon, D. N. (1972a). *J. Anat. (London)* 111:512–513. The fine structure of developing muscle spindles in the rat.

Landon, D. N. (1972b). *J. Neurocytol.* 1:189–210. The fine structure of the equatorial regions of developing spindles in the rat.

Landreth, G. E., and E. M. Shooter (1980). *Proc. Natl. Acad. Sci. U.S.A.* 8:4751–4755. Nerve growth factor receptors on PC12 cells: Ligand-induced conversion from low- to high-affinity states.

Landsteiner, K. (1899). *Centr. Bakt. Orig.* 25:546–549. Zur Kenntnis der Specifisch auf Blutkörperchen wirkenden Sera.

Landsteiner, K. (1936). *The Specificity of Serological Reactions*, Thomas, Springfield, Illinois (Reprint, Dover, New York, 1962).

Landstrom, H., T. Caspersson, and G. Wohlfart (1941). *Z. Mikroskop. Anat. Forsch.* 49:534–548. Uber den Nucleontidumsatz der Nervenzelle.

Landstrom, U., and S. Lovtrup (1975). *J. Embryol. Exp. Morphol.* 33:879–895. On the determination of the dorso-ventral polarity in *Xenopus laevis* embryos.

Lange, F. A. (1925). *The History of Materialism and Criticism of its Present Importance*, 3rd edn., 3 vols. in 1 (1875), Routledge, London.

Lange, W. (1982). *Exp. Brain Res.* 6:Suppl. 93–107. Regional differences in the cytoarchitecture of the cerebellar cortex.

Langford, L. A., S. Porter, and R. P. Bunge (1988). *J. Neurocytol.* 17:521–529. Immortalized rat Schwann cells produce tumours *in vivo*.

Langille, R. M. and B. K. Hall (1988). *Anat. Embryol.* 177:297–305. Role of the neural crest in development of the cartilaginous cranial and visceral skeleton of the medaka, *Orysias latipes* (Teleostei).

Langley, J. N. (1895). *J. Physiol. (London)* 18:280–284. Note on regeneration of pre-ganglionic fibres of the sympathetic.

Langley, J. N. (1897). *J. Physiol. (London)* 22:215–230. On the regeneration of pre-ganglionic and post-ganglionic visceral nerve fibres.

Langley, J. N. (1898). *J. Physiol. (London)* 23:240–270. On the union of cranial autonomic (visceral) fibres with the nerve cells of the superior cervical ganglion.

Langley, J. N., and H. K. Anderson (1904a). *J. Physiol. (London)* 30:439–442. On the union of the fifth cervical nerve with the superior cervical ganglion.

Langley, J. N., and H. K. Anderson (1904b). *J. Physiol. (London)* 31:365–391. The union of different kinds of nerve fibres.

Langley, O. K., M. S. Ghaundour, G. Vincendon, and G. Gombos (1980). *Histochem. J.* 12:473–483. Carbonic anhydrase: An ultrastructural study in rat cerebellum.

Langley, O. K., A. Reeber, G. Vincendon, and J. P. Zanetta (1982). *J. Comp. Neurol.* 208:335–344. Fine structural localization of a new Purkinje cell specific glycoprotein subunit: Immunoelectron microscopal study.

Langman, J., and C. Haden (1970). *J. Comp. Neurol.* 138:419–432. Formation and migration of neuroblasts in the spinal cord of the chick embryo.

Langman, J., and M. Shimada (1971). *Am. J. Anat.* 132:355–374. Cerebral cortex of the mouse after prenatal chemical insult.

Langman, J., and G. W. Welch (1967). *J. Comp. Neurol.* 131:15–26. Excess vitamin A and development of the cerebral cortex.

Langman, J., R. Guerrant, and B. Freeman (1966). *J. Comp. Neurol.* 127:399–412. Behavior of neuroepithelial cells.

Langworthy, O. R. (1928a). *J. Comp. Neurol.* 46:201–248. The behavior of pouch-young opossums correlated with the myelinization of tracts in the nervous system.

Langworthy, O. R. (1928b). *Contrib. Embryol. Carnegie Inst.* 20:127–172. A correlated study of the development of reflex activity in fetal and young kittens and the myelinization of tracts in the nervous system.

Langworthy, O. R. (1933). *Contrib. Embryol. Carnegie Inst.* 24:1–58. Development of behavior patterns and myelinization of the nervous system in the human fetus and infant.

Lankester, E. Ray (1911). *Encyclopaedia Brittannica*, Vol. 18, pp. 215–217, 11th edn. Metamerism.

Lankford, K. L., F. G. DeMello, and W. L. Klein (1988). *Proc. Natl. Acad. Sci. U.S.A.* 85:2839–2843. D1-type dopamine receptors inhibit growth cone motility in cultured retina neurons: Evidence that neurotransmitters act as morphogenic growth regulators in the developing central nervous system.

Lanterman, A. J. (1876). *Arch. Mikr. Anat.* 12:1. Ueber den feineren Bau der markhaltigen Nervenfasern.

Lapham, L. W. (1962). *Amer. J. Pathol.* 41:1–21. Cytologic and cytochemical studies of neuroglia. I. A study of the problem of amitosis in reactive protoplasmic astrocytes.

Lapham, L. W. (1968). *Science* 159:310–312. Tetraploid DNA content of Purkinje neurons of human cerebellar cortex.

Lapham, L. W., and M. A. Johnstone (1963). *Arch. Neurol.* 9:194–202. Cytologic and cytochemical studies of neuroglia. II. The occurrence of two DNA classes among glial nuclei in the Purkinje cell layer of normal adult human cerebellar cortex.

Large, T. H., S. C. Bodary, D. O. Clegg, G. Weskamp, U. Otten, and L. F. Reichardt (1986). *Science* 234:352–355. Nerve growth factor gene expression in the developing rat brain.

Lärkfors, L., and T. Ebendal (1987). *J. Immunol. Meth.* 97:41–47. Highly sensitive enzyme immunoassays for β-nerve growth factor.

Larkfors, L., I. Stromberg, T. Ebendahl, and L. Olson (1987). *J. Neurosci. Res.* 18:525–531. Nerve growth factor protein level increases in the adult rat hippocampus after a specific cholinergic lesion.

Laron, Z., A. Pertzelan, S. Mannheimer, J. Goldman, and S. Guttman (1966). *Acta Endocrinol.* 53:687–692. Lack of placental transfer of human growth hormone.

Larrabee, M. G. (1969). *Prog. Brain Res.* 31:95–110. Metabolic effects of nerve impulses and nerve-growth factor in sympathetic ganglion.

Larramendi, L. M. H. (1969). Analysis of synaptogenesis in the cerebellum of the Mouse, pp. 803–843. In *Neurobiology of Cerebellar Evolution and Development* (R. Llinas, ed.), A. M. A. Educ. and Res. Fdn., Chicago.

Larroche, J.-C. (1981). *Anat. Embryol.* 162:301–312. The marginal layer in the neocortex of a 7-week-old human embryo.

Larroche, J.-C., and O. Houcine (1982). *Reprod. Nutr. Dev.* 22:163–170. Le néo-cortex chez l'embryon et le fetus humain: Apport du microscope electronique et du Golgi.

Larsell, O. (1923). *J. Comp. Neurol.* 36:89–112. The cerebellum of the frog.

Larsell, O. (1925). *J. Comp. Neurol.* 39:249–289. The development of the cerebellum in the frog *(Hyla regilla)* in relation to the vestibular and lateral-line systems.

Larsell, O. (1929). *J. Comp. Neurol.* 48:331–353. The effect of experimental excision of one eye on the development of the optic lobe and opticus layer in larvae of the tree frog *(Hyla regilla).*

Larsell, O. (1931). *J. Exp. Zool.* 58:1–20. The effect of experimental excision of one eye on the development of the optic lobe and opticus layer in larvae of the tree frog *(Hyla regilla).* II. The effect on cell size and differentiation of cell processes.

Larsell, O. (1947). *J. Comp. Neurol.* 87:85–129. The development of cerebellum in man in relation to its comparative anatomy.

Larsell, O. (1967). *The Comparative Anatomy and Histology of the Cerebellum from Myxinoids Through Birds.* Minnesota Univ. Press, Minneapolis.

Larsen, W. J., and S. E. Wert (1988). *Tiss. Cell* 20:809–848. Roles of cell junctions in gametogenesis and in early embryonic development.

Lasek, R. J. (1970). *Int. Rev. Neurobiol.* 13:289–324. Protein transport in neurons.

Lasek, R. J. (1975). *Fed. Proc.* 34:1603–1611. Axonal transport and the use of intracellular markers in neuroanatomical investigations.

Lasek, R. J. (1982). *Phil. Trans. Roy. Soc. (London) Ser. B.* 229:313–327. Translocation of the cytoskeleton in neurons and axonal locomotion.

Lasek, R. J., and P. N. Hoffman (1976). *Cold Spring Harbor Conf. Cell Prolif.* 3:1021–1049. The neuronal cytoskeleton, axonal transport and axonal growth.

Lasek, R. J., and B. S. Joseph (1967). *Anat. Rec.* 157:275–276. Radioautography as a neuroanatomical tracing method.

Lasek, R. J., H. Gainer, and R. J. Przybylski (1974). *Proc. Natl. Acad. Sci. U.S.A.* 71: 1188–1192. Transfer of newly synthesized proteins from Schwann cells to the squid giant axon.

Lasek, R. J., H. Gainer, and J. L. Barker (1977). *J. Cell Biol.* 74:501–523. Cell to cell transfer of glial proteins of the squid giant axon.

Lasek, R. J., J. A. Garner., and S. T. Brady (1984). *J. Cell. Biol.* 99:212–221. Axonal transport of the cytoplasmic matrix.

Lasek, R. J., L. Phillips, M. J. Katz, and L. Autilio-Gambetti (1985). *Ann. N.Y. Acad. Sci.* 455:462–478. Function and evolution of neurofilament proteins.

Lash, J., S. Holtzer, and H. Holtzer (1957). *Exp. Cell Res.* 13:292–303. An experimental analysis of the development of the spinal column. VI. Aspects of cartilage induction.

Lasher, R., and R. D. Cahn (1969). *Dev. Biol.* 19:415–435. The effect of 5-bromodeoxyuridine on the differentiation of chondrocytes *in vitro.*

Lashley, K. S. (1929). *Brain Mechanisms and Intelligence. A Quantitative Study of Injuries to the Brain.* Univ. Chicago Press, Chicago.

Lashley, K. S. (1937). *Arch. Neurol. Psychiatry* 38:371–387. Functional determinants of cerebral localization.

Laskey, R. A., and J. B. Gurdon (1970). *Nature* 228:1332–1334. Genetic content of adult somatic cells tested by nuclear transplantation from cultured cells.

Laskowski, M. B., and J. R. Sanes (1988). *J. Neurosci.* 8:3094–3099. Topographically selective reinnervation of adult mammalian skeletal muscles.

Lassek, A. M., and J. H. Perry (1944). *J. Comp. Neurol.* 81:270–284. Retrograde degeneration. Effect of hemisections on the axons of the fasciculus gracilis and cuneatus in the newborn cat.

Lauder, J. M. (1977a). *Brain Res.* 126:31–51. The effects of early hypo- and hyperthyroidism on the development of rat cerebellar cortex. III. Kinetics of cell proliferation in the external granular layer.

Lauder, J. M. (1977b). Effects of thyroid state on development of rat cerebellar cortex, pp. 235–254. In *Thyroid Hormones and Brain Development* (G. D. Grave, ed.), Raven Press, New York.

Lauder, J. M. (1978). *Brain Res.* 142:25–39. Effects of early hypo- and hyperthyroidism on development of rat cerebellar cortex. IV. The parallel fibers.

Lauder, J. M. (1979). *Dev. Biol.* 70:105–115. Granule cell migration in developing rat cerebellum. Influence of neonatal hypo- and hyperthyroidism.

Lauder, J. M. (1983). *Psychoneuroendocrinology* 8:121–155. Hormonal and humoral influences on brain development.

Lauder, J. M., and F. E. Bloom (1974). *J. Comp. Neurol.* 155:469–482. Ontogeny of monoamine neurons in the locus coeruleus, raphe nuclei and substantia nigra of the rat. I. Cell differentiation.

Lauder, J. M., and F. E. Bloom (1975). *J. Comp. Neurol.* 163:251–264. Ontogeny of monoamine neurons in the locus coeruleus, raphe nuclei and substantia nigra of the rat. II. Synaptogenesis.

Lauder, J. M., and E. Mugnaini (1977). *Nature* 268:335–337. Early hyperthyroidism alters the distribution of mossy fibers in the rat hippocampus.

Lauder, J. M., and E. Mugnaini (1980). *Dev. Neurosci.* 3:248–265. Infrapyramidal mossy fibers in the hyperthyroid hippocampus: A light and electron microscopic study in the rat.

Laufer, R., and J. P. Changeux (1987). *EMBO J.* 6:901–906.

Calcitonin gene-related peptide elevates cyclic AMP levels in chick skeletal msucle: Possible neurotrophic role for a coexisting neuronal messenger.

Laufer, R., B. Fontaine, A. Klarsfeld, J. Cartaud, and J.-P. Changeux (1989). *News Physiol. Sci.* 4:5–9. Regulation of acetylcholine receptor biosynthesis during motor endplate morphogenesis.

Laurence, E. B., and A. L. Thornley (1976). Chalone tissue specificity and the embryonic derivation of organs. An appraisal of the problems, p. 273. In *Chalones* (J. C. Houck, ed.), American Elsevier Publishing Company, New York.

LaVail, J. H. (1975). *Fed. Proc.* 34: 1618–1624. The retrograde transport method.

LaVail, J. H., and W. M. Cowan (1971a). *Brain Res.* 28: 391–419. The development of the chick optic tectum. I. Normal morphology and cytoarchitectonic development.

LaVail, J. H., and W. M. Cowan (1971b). *Brain Res.* 28: 421–441. The development of the chick optic tectum. II. Autoradiographic studies.

LaVail, J. H., and M. M. LaVail (1972). *Science* 176: 1416–1417. Retrograde axonal transport in the central nervous system.

LaVail, J. H., and M. M. LaVail (1974). *J. Comp. Neurol.* 157:303–358. The retrograde intraaxonal transport of horseradish peroxidase in the chick visual system: A light and electron microscopic study.

LaVail, J. H., K. R. Winston, and A. Tish (1973). *Brain Res.* 58:470–477. A method based on retrograde intraaxonal transport of protein for identification of cell bodies of origin of axons terminating within the CNS.

LaVail, M. M., J. C. Blanks, and R. J. Mullen (1982). *J. Comp. Neurol.* 212:217–230. Retinal degeneration in the *pcd* cerebellar mutant mouse. I. Light microscopic and autoradiographic analysis.

Lavelle, A. (1951). *J. Comp. Neurol.* 94:453–473. Nucleolar changes and development of Nissl substance in the cerebral cortex of fetal guinea pigs.

Lavelle, A. (1956). *J. Comp. Neur.* 104:175–206. Nucleolar and nissl substance development in nerve cells.

Lavelle, A. (1973). *Prog. Brain Res.* 40:161–166. Levels of maturation and reactions to injury during neuronal development.

Lavelle, A., and F. W. Lavelle (1958). *J. Exp. Zool.* 137:285–316. The nucleolar apparatus and neuronal reactivity to injury during development.

LaVelle, A., and F. W. LaVelle (1984). Neuronal reaction to injury during development, pp. 3–16. In *Early Brain Damage*, Vol. 2 (S. Finger, and C. R. Almli, eds.), Academic Press, New York.

Law, M. I., and M. P. Stryker (1983). *Invest. Opthalmol.* 24:227. The projection of the visual world onto area 17 of the ferret.

Lawson, S. H., K. W. Caddy, and T. J. Biscoe (1974). *Cell Tiss. Res.* 153:399–413. Development of rat dorsal root ganglion neurones. Studies of cell birthdays and changes in mean cell diameter.

Laxson, L. C., and J. S. King (1983). *J. Comp. Neurol.* 214:290–308. The development of the Purkinje cell in the cerebellar cortex of the opossum.

Lazar, G. (1973). *J. Anat. (London)* 116:347–355. The development of the optic tectum in *Xenopus laevis*: A Golgi study.

Lazar, G., and G. Szekely (1967). *J. Hirnforsch.* 9:329–344. Golgi studies on the optic center of the frog.

Lazar, G., and G. Szekely (1969). *Brain Res.* 16:1–14. Distribution of optic terminals in the different optic centers of the frog.

Lazarides, E. (1982). *Ann. Rev. Biochem.* 51:219–250. Intermediate filaments: A chemically heterogeneous, developmentally regulated class of proteins.

Lebert, H. (1845). *Physiologie pathologique ou recherches cliniques, expérimentales et microscopiques sur l'inflammation, la tuberculisation, les tumeurs, la formation dur cal etc.* Baillière, Paris.

LeBeux, Y. J. (1973). *Z. Zellforsch. Mikrosk. Anat.* 143:239–272. An ultrastructural study of the synaptic densities, nematosomes, neurotubules, neurofilaments and of a further three-dimensional filamentous network as disclosed by the E-PTA staining procedure.

LeBlond, C. P., and S. Inoue (1989). *Amer. J. Anat.* 185:367–390. Structure, composition, and assembly of basement membrane.

Lebowitz, P., and M. Singer (1970). *Nature* 225:824–827. Neurotrophic control of protein synthesis in the regenerating limb of the newt, *Triturus*.

Le Douarin, N. M. (1969). *Bull. Biol. Fr. Belg.* 103:435–452. Particularités du noyau interphasique chez la Caille japonaise (*Coturnix coturnix japonica*). Utilisation de ces particularités comme "marquage biologique" dans les recherches sur les interactions tissulaires et les migrations cellulaires au cours de l'ontogenèse.

Le Douarin, N. M.(1973). *Dev. Biol.* 30:217–222. A biological cell labelling technique and its use in experimental embryology.

Le Douarin, N. M. (1982). *The Neural Crest.* Cambridge Univ. Press, Cambridge.

Le Douarin, N. M. (1986a). *Harvey Lect.* 80:137–186. Ontogeny of the peripheral nervous system from the neural crest and the placodes. A developmental model studied on the basis of the quail-chick chimaera system.

Le Douarin, N. M. (1986b). *Science* 231:1515–1522. Cell line segregation during peripheral nervous system ontogeny.

Le Douarin, N. M. (1986c). *Ann. N.Y. Acad. Sci.* 486:66–86. Investigations on the neural crest. Methodological aspects and recent advances.

Le Douarin, N. M., and M.-A. Teillet (1973). *J. Embryol. Exp. Morphol.* 30:31–48. The migration of neural crest cells to the wall of the digestive tract in avian embryos.

Le Douarin, N. M., and M.-A. Teillet (1974). *Dev. Biol.* 41:162–184. Experimental analysis of the migration and differentiation of neuroblasts of the autonomic nervous system and of neurectodermal mesenchymal derivatives, using a biological cell marking technique.

Le Douarin, N. M., M.-A. Teillet, C. Ziller, and J. Smith (1978). *Proc. Natl. Acad. Sci U.S.A.* 75:2030–2034. Adrenergic differentiation of cells of the cholinergic ciliary and Remak ganglia in avian embryo after *in vivo* transplantation.

Lee, C., and L. B. Chen (1988). *Cell* 54:37–46. Dynamic behavior of endoplasmic reticulum in living cells.

Lee, H.-Y., and R. G. Nagele (1979). *Teratology* 20:321–332. Neural tube closure defects caused by papaverine in explanted early chick embryos.

Lee, H.-Y., and R. G. Nagele (1985). *J. Exp. Zool.* 235:205–215. Studies on the mechanisms of neurulation in the chick: Interrelationship of contractile proteins, microfilaments, and the shape of neuroepithelial cells.

Lee, J. H., C. L. Jordan, and A. P. Arnold (1989). *Neurosci. Lett.* 98:79–84. Critical period for androgenic regulation of soma size of sexually dimorphic motoneurons in rat spinal cord.

Lee, K. S., F. Schottler, M. Oliver, and G. Lynch (1980). *J. Neurophysiol.* 44:247–258. Brief bursts of high-frequency stimulation produce two types of structural change in the rat hippocampus.

Lee, M., and P. Nurse (1988). *Trends Genet.* 4:287. Cell cycle control genes in fission yeast and mammalian cells.

Lee, M. T., and P. B. Farel (1988). *J. Neurosci.* 8:2430–2437. Guidance of regenerating motor axons in larval and juvenile bullfrogs.

Lee, V. M.-Y., M. J. Carden, and W. W. Schlaepfer (1986). *J. Neurosci.* 6:2179–2186. Structural similarities and differences between neurofilament proteins from five different species as revealed using monoclonal antibodies.

Lee, V. M.-Y., M. J. Carden, W. W. Schlaepfer, and J. Q. Trojanowski (1987). *J. Neurosci.* 7:3474–3488. Monoclonal antibodies distinguish several differentially phosphorylated states of the two largest rat neurofilament subunits (NF-H and NF-M) and demonstrate their existence in the normal nervous system of adult rats).

Leech, R. W., and P. Kohnen (1974). *Am. J. Path.* 77:465–474. Subependymal and intraventricular hemorrhages in the newborn.

Lees, M. B., and S. W. Brostoff (1984). Proteins of myelin, pp. 197–224. In *Myelin* (P. Morell, ed.), Plenum Press, New York.

Lees, M. B., and V. S. Sapirstein (1983). Myelin-associated enzymes, pp. 435–460. In *Handbook of Neurochemistry*, Vol. 4, 2nd edn., (A. Lajtha, ed.), Plenum, New York.

Legendre, R. (1912). *Nature* 40:359–363. La survie des organes et la "culture" des tissus vivants.

Leghissa, S. (1951). *Bol. Zool.* 18:355–365. A proposito dello svilupo del tetto ottico nei Teleostei *(Salmo fario).*

Leghissa, S. (1955). *Z. Anat. Entwicklungsgeschichte* 118:427–463. La struttura microscopica e la citoarchitettonica del tetto ottico dei pesci teleostei.

Leghissa, S. (1957). *Arch. Sci. Biol.* 12:601–628. Il differenziamento ontogenetico ed istogenetico del tetto ottico nell'embrione di pollo.

Leghissa, S. (1959). *Atti Accad. Sci. Bologna* 6:56–75. Studio sperimentale sul differenziamento dei neuroni del tetto ottico di gallus. I. Esperienze de asportazione della vesicola ottica.

Leghissa, S. (1962). *Arch. Ital. Anat. Embriol.* 67:343–413. L'evoluzione del tetto ottico nei bassi vertebrati.

Legrand, C., J. Clos, J. Legrand, O. K. Langley, M. S. Ghandour, G. Labourdette, G. Gombos, and G. Vincendon (1981). *Neurobiol.* 7:299–306. Localization of S100 protein in the rat cerebellum: An electron microscope study coupled to immunoperoxidase technique.

Legrand, J. (1963). *Arch. Anat. Microscop. Morphol. Exp.* 52:205–214. Maturation du cervelet et deficience thyroidienne données chronologiques.

Legrand, J. (1965). *C. R. Acad. Sci. (Paris)* 261:544–547. Influence de l'hypothyroïdisme sur la maturation du cortex cérébelleux.

Legrand, J. (1967a). *Arch. Anat. Microsc. Morph. Exp.* 56:205–244. Analyse de l'action morphogénétique des hormones thyroïdiennes sur le cervelet du jeune rat.

Legrand, J. (1967b). *Arch. Anat. Microsc. Morphol. Exp.* 56:291–307. Variations, en fonction de l'âge, de la response du cervelet á l'action morphogénétique de la thyroide chez le Rat.

Legrand, T., A. Kriegel, and A. Jost (1961). *Arch. Anat. Microscop. Morphol. Exp.* 50:507–519. Deficience thyroidienne et maturation du cervelet chez le rat blanc.

Le Gros Clark, W. E. (1945). *Essays on Growth and Form*, pp. 1–22. (W. E. Le Gros Clark, and P. B. Medawar, eds.), Oxford Univ. Press, London.

Lehman, F. E. (1927). *J. Exp. Zool.* 49:93–132. Further studies on the morphogenetic role of the somite in the development of the nervous system of amphibians.

Lehman, O. (1918). *Ergeb. Physiol.* 16:255–509. Die Lehre von den flüssigen Kristallen und ihre Beziehung zu den Problemen der Biologie.

Lehmann, H. (1959). Die Nervenfaser, pp. 515–701. In *Handbuch der Mikroskopischen Anatomie des Menschen.* Vol. 4, part 3, (W. Bargmann, ed.), Springer-Verlag, Berlin.

Leibovich, S. J., P. J. Polverini, H. M. Shepard, D. M. Wiseman, V. Shively, and N. Nuseir (1987). *Nature* 329:630–635. Macrophage-induced angiogenesis is mediated by tumor necrosis factor-alpha.

Leibrock, J., F. Lottspeich, A. Hohn, M. Hofer, B. Hengerer, P. Masiakowski, H. Thoenen, and Y.-A. Barde (1989). *Nature* 341:149–152. Molecular cloning and expression of brain-derived neurotrophic factor.

Leifer, D., S. A. Lipton, C. J. Barnstable, and R. H. Masland (1984). *Science* 224:303–306. Monoclonal antibody of *Thy-1* enhances regeneration of processes by rat retinal ganglion cells in culture.

Lemay, M. (1976). *Ann. N.Y. Acad. Sci.* 280:349–366. Morphological cerebral asymmetries of modern man, fossil man, and nonhuman primate.

Lemay, M., and N. Geschwind (1975). *Brain Beh. Evol.* 11:48–52. Hemispheric differences in the brains of great apes.

Lemke, G. (1988). *Neuron* 1:535–543. Unwrapping the myelin genes.

Lemke, G., and R. Axel (1985). *Cell* 40:501–508. Isolation and sequence of a cDNA encoding the major structural protein of peripheral nerve.

Lemmon, V., and D. I. Gottlieb (1982). *J. Neurosci.* 2:531–535. Monoclonal antibodies selective for the inner portion of the chick retina.

Lemons, J. A., R. L. Schreiner, and E. L. Gresham (1981). *Human Biol.* 53:351–354. Relationship of brain weight to head circumference in early infancy.

LeMouellic, H., H. Condamine, and P. Brûlet (1988). *Genes Dev.* 2:125–135. Pattern of transcription of the homeo gene *Hox-3.1* in the mouse embryo.

Lenhossék, M. von (1890). *Verhandl. des X internat. med. Congresses, Berlin* 2:115. Zur Kenntniss der ersten Entstehung der Nervenzellen und Nervenfasern beim Vogelembryo.

Lenhossék, M. von (1891). *Verh. Anat. Ges.* 5:193–221. Zur Kenntnis der Neuroglia des menschlichen Rückenmarkes.

Lenhossék, M. von (1892–93). *Anat. Anz.* 8:121–127. Der feinere Bau und die Nervenendigungen der Geschmacksknospen.

Lenhossék, M. von (1893). *Der feinere Bau des Nervensystems im Lichte neuester Forschungen.* Fischer's Medicinische Buchhandlung, H. Kornfeld, Berlin.

Lenhossék, M. von (1895). *Arch. Mikr. Anat.* **46:**345–369. Centrosom und sphäre in den Spinalganglienzellen des Frosches.

Lenhossék, M. von (1896–1897). *Arch. f. Psychiat. u. Nervenkr. Berlin* **29:**346–380. Ueber den Bau der Spinalganglienzellen des Menschen.

Lenneberg, E. H. (1967). *Biological Foundations of Language.* Wiley, New York, 489 pp.

Lenneberg, E. H. (1975). The concept of language differentiation, pp. 17–33. In *Foundations of Language Development*, Vol. 1, (E. H. Lenneberg, and E. Lenneberg, eds.), UNESCO and Academic Press, Paris and New York.

Lentz, R. D., and L. W. Lapham (1969). *J. Neurochem.* **16:**379–384. A quantitative cytochemical study of the DNA content of neurons of rat cerebellar cortex.

Lentz, R. D., and L. W. Lapham (1970). *J. Neuropath. Exp. Neurol.* **29:**43–56. Postnatal development of tetraploid DNA content in rat Purkinje cells: A quantitative cytochemical study.

Leonard, J. L., and P. R. Larsen (1985). *Brain Res.* **327:**1–13. Thyroid hormone metabolism in primary cultures of fetal rat brain cells.

Leong, S. K., and C. K. Tan (1987). *J. Anat. (London)* **154:**15–26. Central projection of rat sciatic nerve fibres as revealed by Ricinus communis agglutinin and horseradish peroxidase tracers.

Leong, S. K., J. Y. Shieh, E. A. Ling, and W. C. Wong (1983). *J. Anat. (London)* **136:**367–377. Labelling of amoeboid microglial cells in the supraventricular corpus callosum following the application of horseradish peroxidase to the cerebrum and spinal cord in rats.

Lester, B. M., R. E. Klein, and S. J. Martínez (1975). *Dev. Psychobiol.* **8:**541. The use of habituation in the study of the effects of infantile malnutrition.

Letinsky, M. S. (1974). *Dev. Biol.* **40:**129–153. The development of nerve-muscle junctions in *Rana catesbeiana* tadpoles.

Letinsky, M. S., and K. Morrison-Graham (1980). *J. Neurocytol.* **9:**321–342. Structure of developing frog neuromuscular junctions.

Letinsky, M. S., K. H. Fischbeck, and U. J. McMahan (1976). *J. Neurocytol.* **5:**691–718. Precision of reinnervation of original postsynaptic sites in frog muscle after a nerve crush.

Letourneau, P. C. (1975a). *Dev. Biol.* **44:**77–91. Possible roles for cell-to-substratum adhesion in neuronal morphogenesis.

Letourneau, P. C. (1975b). *Dev. Biol.* **44:**92–101. Cell-to-substratum adhesion and guidance of axonal elongation.

Letourneau, P. C. (1979). *Exp. Cell Res.* **124:**127–138. Cell-substratum adhesion and guidance of axonal elongation.

Letourneau, P. C. (1982). Nerve fiber growth and its regulation by extrinsic factors, pp. 213–254. In *Neuronal Development* (N. C. Spitzer, ed.), Plenum Press, New York.

Letourneau, P. C. (1983). *J. Cell Biol.* **97:**963–973. Differences in the organization of actin in the growth cones compared with the neurites of cultured neurons from chick embryos.

Letourneau, P. C., and A. H. Ressler (1984). *J. Cell Biol.* **98:**1355–1362. Inhibition of neurite initiation and growth by taxol.

Letourneau, P. C., T. A. Shattuck, and A. H. Ressler (1986). *J. Neurosci.* **6:**1912–1917. Branching of sensory and sympathetic neurites *in vitro* is inhibited by treatment with taxol.

Letourneau, P. C., T. A. Shattuck, and A. H. Ressler (1987). *Cell Motility Cytoskel.* **8:**193–209. "Pull" and "push" in neurite elongation: Observations on the effects of different concentrations of cytochalasin B and taxol.

Letourneau, P. C., I. V. Pech, S. L. Rogers, S. L. Palm, J. B. McCarthy, and L. T. Furcht (1988a). *J. Neurosci. Res.* **21:**286–297. Growth cone migration across extracellular matrix components depends on integrin, but migration across glioma cells does not.

Letourneau, P. C., A. M. Madsen, S. L. Palm, and L. T. Furcht (1988b). *Dev. Biol.* **125:**135–144. Immunoreactivity for laminin in the developing ventral longitudinal pathway of the brain.

Letterier, J. F., R. Lime, and M. Shelanski (1982). *J. Cell Biol.* **95:**982–986. Interactions between neurofilaments and microtubule-associated proteins: A possible mechanism for intra-organellar bridging.

Lettvin, J. Y., H. R. Maturana, W. S. McCulloch, and W. H. Pitts (1959). *Proc. Inst. Radio Engr. N.Y.* **47:**1940–1951. What the frog's eye tells the frog's brain.

Lettvin, J. Y., H. R. Maturana, W. H. Pitts, and W. S. McCulloch (1961). Two remarks on the visual system of the frog, pp. 757–776. In *Sensory Communication* (W. A. Rosenblith, ed.), The M.I.T. Press, Cambridge.

Leussink, J. A. (1970). *Neth. J. Zool.* **20:**1–79. The spatial distribution of inductive capacities in the neural plate and archenteron roof of urodeles.

LeVay, S., and S. B. Nelson (1990). Columnar organization of the visual cortex, pp. 266–314. In *The Neural Bases of Visual Function* (A. G. Leventhal, ed.), MacMillan, London.

LeVay, S., and M. P. Stryker (1979). The development of ocular dominance columns in the cat, pp. 83–98. In *Aspects of Developmental Neurobiology (Soc. Neurosci. Symp.)* (J. A. Ferrendelli, ed.), Society for Neuroscience, Bethesda.

LeVay, S., D. H. Hubel, and T. N. Wiesel (1975). *J. Comp. Neurol.* **159:**559–576. The pattern of ocular dominance columns in macaque visual cortex revealed by a reduced silver stain.

LeVay, S., M. P. Stryker, and C. J. Shatz (1978). *J. Comp. Neurol.* **179:**223–244. Ocular dominance columns and their development in layer IV of the cat's visual cortex: A quantitative study.

LeVay, S., T. N. Wiesel, and D. H. Hubel (1980). *J. Comp. Neurol.* **191:**1–51. The development of ocular dominance columns in normal and visually deprived monkeys.

Leveille, P. J., J. F. McGinnis, D. S. Maxwell, and J. De Vellis (1980). *Brain Res.* **196:**287–305. Immunocytochemical localization of glycerol-3-phosphate dehydrogenase in rat oligodendrocytes.

Leventhal, A. G. (1982). *J. Neurosci.* **2:**1024–1042. Morphology and distribution of retinal ganglion cells projecting to different layers of the lateral geniculate nucleus in normal and Siamese cats.

Leventhal, A. G., and D. J. Creel (1985). *J. Neurosci.* **5:**795–807. Retinal projections and functional architecture of cortical areas 17 and 18 in the tyrosinase-negative albino cat.

Leventhal, A. G., and H. V. B. Hirsch (1975). *Science* 190:902–904. Cortical effect of early selective exposure to diagonal lines.

Leventhal, A. G., and H. V. B. Hirsch (1980). *J. Neurophysiol.* 43:1111–1132. Receptive-field properties of different classes of neurons in visual cortex of normal and dark-reared cats.

Leventhal, A. G., R. W. Rodieck, and B. Dreher (1985a). *J. Comp. Neurol.* 237:216–226. Central projections of cat retinal ganglion cells.

Leventhal, A. G., D. J. Vitek, and D. J. Creel (1985b). *Science* 229:1395–1397. Abnormal visual pathways in normally pigmented cats that are heterozygous for albinism.

Leventhal, A. G., J. D. Schall, S. J. Ault, J. M. Provis, and D. J. Vitek (1988a). *J. Neurosci.* 8:2011–2027. Class-specific cell death shapes the distribution and pattern of central projection of cat retinal ganglion cells.

Leventhal, A. G., J. D. Schall, and S. J. Ault (1988b). *J. Neurosci.* 8:2028–2038. Extrinsic determinants of retinal ganglion cell structure in the cat.

Leventhal, A. G., S. J. Ault, D. J. Vitek, and T. Shou (1989). *J. Comp. Neurol.* 286:170–189. extrinsic determinants of retinal ganglion cell development in primates.

Levi, G., and H. Meyer (1945). *J. Exp. Zool.* 99:141–181. Reactive, regressive and regenerative processes of neurons, cultivated *in vitro* and injured with a micromanipulator.

Levi, G., K. L. Crossin, and G. M. Edelman (1987). *J. Cell Biol.* 105:2359–2372. Expression sequences and distribution of two primary cell adhesion molecules during embryonic development of *Xenopus laevis*.

Levi-Montalcini, R. (1949). *J. Comp. Neurol.* 91:209–242. The development of the acoustico-vestibular centers in the chick embryo in the absence of the afferent root fibers and of descending fiber tracts.

Levi-Monatalcini, R. (1950). *J. Morphol.* 86:253–283. The origin and development of the visceral system in the spinal cord of the chick embryo.

Levi-Montalcini, R. (1952). *Ann. N.Y. Acad. Sci.* 55:330–343. Effects of mouse tumor transplantation on the nervous system.

Levi-Montalcini, R. (1964a). *Prog. Brain Res.* 4:1–29. Events in the developing nervous system.

Levi-Montalcini, R. (1964b). Growth and differentiation in the nervous system, pp. 261–295. In *The Nature of Biological Diversity* (J. M. Allen, ed.), McGraw-Hill, New York.

Levi-Montalcini, R. (1964c). *Ann N.Y. Acad. Sci.* 118:149–168. The nerve growth factor.

Levi-Montalcini, R. (1965). *Arch. Biol. (Liége)* 76:387–414. Morphological and metabolic effects of the nerve growth factor.

Levi-Montalcini, R. (1966). *Harvey Lectures* 60:217–259. The nerve growth factor: Its mode of action on sensory and sympathetic nerve cells.

Levi-Montalcini, R. (1972). The morphological effects of immunosympathectomy, pp. 55–77. In *Immunosympathectomy* (G. Steiner, and E. Schonbaum, eds.), Elsevier, New York.

Levi-Montalcini, R. (1987). *Science* 237:1154–1162. The nerve growth factor 35 years later.

Levi-Montalcini, R., and R. Amprino (1947). *Arch. de Biol.* 58:265–288. Recherches experimentals sur l'origine du ganglion ciliaire dans l'embryon de Poulet.

Levi-Montalcini, R., and P. U. Angeletti (1963). *Dev. Biol.* 7:653–659. Essential role of the nerve growth factor in the survival and maintenance of dissociated sensory and sympathetic nerve cells *in vitro*.

Levi-Montalcini, R., and P. U. Angeletti (1966). *Pharmacol. Rev.* 18:619–628. Immunosympathectomy.

Levi-Montalcini, R., and P. U. Angeletti (1968). *Physiol. Rev.* 48:534–569. Nerve growth factor.

Levi-Montalcini, R., and B. Booker (1960a). *Proc. Natl. Acad. Sci. U.S.A.* 42:373–384. Excessive growth of the sympathetic ganglia evoked by a protein isolated from mouse salivary glands.

Levi-Montalcini, R., and B. Booker (1960b). *Proc. Natl. Acad. Sci. U.S.A.* 42:384–391. Destruction of the sympathetic ganglia in mammals by an antiserum to the nerve-growth promoting factor.

Levi-Montalcini, R., and S. Cohen (1956). *Proc. Natl. Acad. Sci. U.S.A.* 42:695–699. *In vitro* and *in vivo* effects of a nerve growth stimulating agent isolated from snake venom.

Levi-Montalcini, R., and S. Cohen (1960). *Ann. N.Y. Acad. Sci.* 85:324–341. Effects of the extract of the mouse salivary glands on the sympathetic system of mammals.

Levi-Montalcini, R., and V. Hamburger (1951). *J. Exp. Zool.* 116:321–362. Selective growth stimulating effects of mouse sarcoma on the sensory and sympathetic nervous system of the chick embryo.

Levi-Montalcini, R., and V. Hamburger (1953). *J. Exp. Zool.* 123:233–288. A diffusible agent of mouse sarcoma producing hyperplasia of sympathetic ganglia and hyperneurotization of the chick embryo.

Levi-Montalcini, R., and G. Levi (1943). *Arch. Biol. (Liége)* 54:183–206. Recherches quantitatives sur la marche du processus de differenciation des neurones dans les ganglions spinaux de l'embryon de poulet.

Levi-Montalcini, R., H. Meyer, and V. Hamburger (1954). *Cancer Res.* 14:49–57. *In vitro* experiments on the effects of mouse Sarcoma 180 and 37 on the spinal and sympathetic ganglia of the chick embryo.

Levi-Montalcini, R., F. Caramia, S. A. Luse, and P. U. Angeletti (1968). *Brain Res.* 8:347–362. *In vitro* effects of the nerve growth factor on the fine structure of the sensory nerve cells.

Levi-Montalcini, R., F. Caramia, and P. U. Angeletti (1969). *Brain Res.* 12:54–73. Alterations in the fine structure of nucleoli in sympathetic neurons following NGF antiserum treatment.

Levi, V., V. Gallo, M. T. Ciotti (1986). *Proc. Natl. Acad. Sci. U.S.A.* 83:1504–1508. Bipotential precursors of putative fibrous astrocytes and oligodendrocytes in rat cerebellar cultures express distinct surface features and "neuronlike" gamma-aminobutyric acid transport.

Levick, W. R., and L. N. Thibos (1983). *Prog. Retinal Res.* 2:267–319. Receptive fields of cat ganglion cells: Classification and construction.

Levin, M. (1953). *J. Nerv. Ment. Dis.* 118:481–493. Reflex action in the highest cerebral centers: A tribute to Hughlings Jackson.

Levin, M. (1960). *Am. J. Psychiat.* 116:718–722. The mind-brain problem and Hughlings Jackson's doctrine of concomitance.

Levine, J., and M. Willard (1981). *J. Cell Biol.* 90:631–643. Fodrin; axonally transported polypeptides associated with the internal periphery of many cells.

Levine, J. M., and W. B. Stallcup (1987). *J. Neurosci.* 7:2721–2731. Plasticity of developing cerebellar cells *in vitro* studied with antibodies against the NG2 antigen.

Levine, R. (1975). *J. Exp. Zool.* 192:363–380. Regeneration of the retina in the adult newt, *Triturus cristatus*, following surgical division of the eye by a limbal incision.

Levine, R., and J. R. Cronly-Dillon (1974). *Brain Res.* 68:319–329. Specification of regenerating retinal ganglion cells in the adult newt, *Triturus cristatus*.

Levine, R., and M. Jacobson (1974). *Exp. Neurol.* 43:527–538. Deployment of optic nerve fibers is determined by positional markers in the frog's tectum.

Levine, R., and M. Jacobson (1975). *Brain Res.* 98:172–176. Discontinuous mapping of retina onto tectum innervated by both eyes.

Levine, S., and R. F. Mullins (1966). *Science* 152:1585–1592. Hormonal influence on brain organization in infant rats.

LeVine, S. M., and J. E. Goldman (1988a). *J. Comp. Neurol.* 277:456–464. Ultrastructural characteristics of GD_3 ganglioside-positive immature glia in rat forebrain white matter.

LeVine, S. M., and J. E. Goldman (1988b). *J. Neurosci.* 8:3992–4006. Embryonic divergence of oligodendrocyte and astrocyte lineages in developing rat cerebrum.

LeVine, S. M., and J. E. Goldman (1988d). *J. Comp. Neurol.* 277:441–455 Spatial and temporal patterns of oligodendrocyte differentiation in rat cerebrum and cerebellum.

Levinthal, C., and R. Ware (1972). *Nature* 236:207–210. Three dimensional reconstruction from serial sections.

Levitsky, D. A., and R. H. Barnes (1970). *Nature* 225:468–469. Effect of early malnutrition on the reaction of adult rats to aversive stimuli.

Levitt, P., and R. Y. Moore (1978). *Brain Res.* 139:219–231. Noradrenaline neuron innervation of the neocortex in the rat.

Levitt, P., and R. Y. Moore (1979). *Brain Res.* 162:243–259. Development of the noradrenergic innervation of neocortex.

Levitt, P. and P. Rakic (1980). *J. Comp. Neurol.* 193:815–840. Immunoperoxidase localization of glial fibrillary acidic protein in radial glial cells and astrocytes of the developing rhesus monkey brain.

Levitt, P., M. C. Cooper, and P. Rakic (1981). *J. Neurosci.* 1:27–39. Coexistence of neural and glial precursor cells in the cerebral ventricular zone of the fetal monkey: An ultrastructural immunoperoxidase study.

Lewes, G. H. (1864). *The Life of Goethe.* Smith, Elder and Co., London.

Lewis, A. (1958). J. C. Reil's concepts of brain function, pp. 154–166. In *The Brain and its Functions* (F. N. L. Poynter, ed.), Blackwell, Oxford.

Lewis, B. (1876). *M. Micr. J.* 16:105–110. A new process for preparing and staining fresh brain for microscopic examination.

Lewis, E. B. (1963). *Am. Zool.* 3:33–56. Genes and developmental pathways.

Lewis, E. B. (1978). *Nature* 276:565–570. A gene complex controlling segmentation in *Drosophila*.

Lewis, J. (1978). *Zoon* 6:Suppl. 175–179. Pathways of axons in the developing chick wing: Evidence against chemospecific guidance.

Lewis, J., L. Al-Ghaith, G. Swanson, and A. Khan (1983). The control of axon outgrowth in the developing chick wing, pp. 195–205. In *Limb Development and Regeneration, Part A* (J. F. Fallon, and A. I. Caplan, eds.), Alan R. Liss Inc., New York.

Lewis, J. H. (1975). *J. Embryol. Exp. Morphol.* 33:419–434. Fate maps and the pattern of cell division: A calculation for the chick wing-bud.

Lewis, J. H., and L. Wolpert (1976). *J. Theor. Biol.* 62:479–490. The principle of non-equivalence in development.

Lewis, J. H., D. Summerbell, and L. Wolpert (1972). *Nature* 239:276–279. Chimaeras and cell lineage in development.

Lewis, M. R., and W. H. Lewis (1911). *Anat. Rec.* 5:277–293. The cultivation of tissues from chick embryos in solutions of NaCl, $CaCl_2$, KCl and $NaHCO_3$.

Lewis, M. R., and W. H. Lewis (1912). *Anat. Rec.* 6:207–211. The cultivation of chick tissues in media of known chemical constitution.

Lewis, P. D. (1968a). *Exp. Neurol.* 20:203–207. A quantitative study of cell proliferation in the subependymal layer of the adult rat brain.

Lewis, P. D. (1968b). *Nature* 217:974–975. Mitotic activity in the primate subependymal layer and the genesis of gliomas.

Lewis, P. D. (1968c). *Brain* 91:721–736. The fate of subependymal cell in the adult brain, with a note on the origin of microglia.

Lewis, P. D. (1968d). *Exp. Neurol.* 20:208–214. Radiosensitivity of the subependymal cell layer of the adult rat brain.

Lewis, P. D. (1975). *Neuropathol. Appl. Neurobiol.* 1:21–29. Cell death in the germinal layers of the postnatal rat brain.

Lewis, P. D. (1978). *Neuropathol. Appl. Neurobiol.* 4:191–195. Kinetics of cell proliferation in the postnatal rat dentate gyrus.

Lewis, P. D., and M. Lai (1974). *Brain Res.* 77:520–525. Cell generation in the subependymal layer of the rat brain during the early postnatal period.

Lewis, P. D., R. Balázs, A. J. Patel, and A. L. Johnson (1975). *Brain Res.* 83:235–247. The effect of undernutrition in early life on cell generation in the rat brain.

Lewis, P. D., A. J. Patel, A. L. Johnson, and R. Balazs (1976). *Brain Res.* 104:49–62. Effect of thyroid deficiency on cell acquisition in the postnatal rat brain: A quantitative histological study.

Lewis, S., and C. Straznicky (1979). *J. Comp. Neurol.* 183:633–646. The time of origin of the mesencephalic trigeminal neurons in *Xenopus*.

Lewis, S. A., and N. J. Cowan (1985a). *J. Neurosci.* 45:913–919. Temporal expression of mouse glial fibrillary acidic protein mRNA studied by a rapid *in situ* hybridization procedure.

Lewis, S. A., and N. J. Cowan (1985b). *J. Cell Biol.* 100:843–850. Genetics, evolution, and expression of the 68,000 mol. wt. neurofilament protein: Isolation of a cloned cDNA probe.

Lewis, S. A., and N. J. Cowan (1986). *Mol. Cell. Biol.* 6:1529–

1534. Anomalous placement of introns in a member of the intermediate filament multigene family: An evolutionary conundrum.

Lewis, V. G., J. Money, and R. Epstein (1968). *Johns Hopkins Med. J.* 122:192–195. Concordance of verbal and nonverbal ability in the adrenogenital syndrome.

Lewis, W. B. (1878). *Brain* 1:79–96. On the comparative structure of the cortex cerebri.

Lewis, W. B. (1880). *Phil. Trans. Roy. Soc. (London) Ser. B.* 171:33–64. Researches on the comparative structure of the cortex cerebri.

Lewis, W. B., and H. Clarke (1878). *Proc. Roy. Soc. (London) Ser. B.* 27:38–49. The cortical lamination of the motor area of the brain.

Lewis, W. H. (1910a). *Anat. Rec.* 4:191–200. Localization and regeneration in the neural plate of amphibian embryos.

Lewis, W. H. (1910b). *J. Anat. (London)* 4:191–198. Localization and regeneration in the neural plate of amphibian embryos.

Lewis, W. H. (1931). *Bull. Johns Hopkins Hosp.* 49:17–26. Pinocytosis.

Lewis, W. H., and M. R. Lewis (1912). *Anat. Rec.* 6:7–31. The cultivation of sympathetic nerves from the intestine of chick embryos in saline solutions.

Leyton, A. S. F., and C. S. Sherrington (1917). *Quarterly J. Exp. Physiol.* 11:135–222. Observations on the excitable cortex of the chimpanzee, orang-utan and gorilla.

Lia, B., R. W. Williams, and L. M. Chalupa (1986). *Dev. Brain Res.* 25:296–301. Does axonal branching contribute to the overproduction of optic nerve fibres during early development of the cat's visual system?

Liang, P. H., T. T. Hie, O. H. Jan, and L. T. Giok (1967). *Am. J. Clin. Nutr.* 20:1290–1294. Evaluation of mental development in relation to early malnutrition.

Liao, S. (1975). *Int. Rev. Cytol.* 41:87–172. Cellular receptors and mechanisms of action of steroid hormones.

Libby, P., S. Bursztajn, and A. J. Goldberg (1980). *Cell* 9:481–491. Degradation of the acetylcholine receptor in cultured muscle cells: Selective inhibitors and the fate of undegraded receptors.

Lichtman, J. (1977). *J. Physiol. (London)* 273:155–177. The reorganization of synaptic connexions in the rat submandibular ganglion during post-natal development.

Lichtman, J. W., and E. Frank (1984). *J. Neurosci.* 4:1745–1753. Physiological evidence for specificity of synaptic connections between individual sensory and motor neurons in the brachial cord of the bullfrog.

Lichtman, J. W., D. Purves, and J. W. Yip (1979). *J. Physiol. (London)* 292:69–84. On the purpose of selective innervation of guinea-pig superior cervical ganglion cells.

Lichtman, J. W., D. Purves, and J. W. Yip (1980). *J. Physiol. (London)* 298:285–299. Innervation of sympathetic neurones in the guinea-pig thoracic chain.

Lichtman, J. W., S. Jhaveri, and E. Frank (1984). *J. Neurosci.* 4:1754–1763. Anatomical basis of specific connections between sensory axons and motor neurons in the brachial spinal cord of the bullfrog.

Lichtman, J. W., L. Magrassi, and D. Purves (1987). *J. Neurosci.* 7:1215–1222. Visualization of neuromuscular junctions over periods of several months in living mice.

Lichtman, J. W., R. S. Wilkinson, and M M. Rich (1985). *Nature* 314:357–359. Multiple innervation of tonic end-plates revealed by activity-dependent uptake of fluorescent probes.

Liddell, E. G. T. (1960). *The Discovery of Reflexes.* Clarendon Press, Oxford.

Liddell, E. G. T., and C. S. Sherrington (1925). *Proc. Roy. Soc. (London) Ser. B.* 97:488–518. Recruitment and some other features of reflex inhibition.

Lidov, H. G. W., M. E. Molliver, and N. R. Zecevic (1978). *J. Comp. Neurol.* 181:663–680. Characterization of the monoaminergic innervation of immature rat neocortex: A histofluorescence analysis.

Lieberburg, I., and B. S. McEwen (1975). *Brain Res.* 85:165–170. Estradiol-17B: A metabolite of testosterone recovered in cell nuclei from limbic areas of neonatal rat brains.

Lieberman, A. R. (1968). *J. Anat. (London)* 104:49–54. Absence of ultrastructural changes in ganglionic neurons after supranodose vagotomy.

Lieberman, A. R. (1969). *J. Anat. (London)* 104:309–325. Light and electron microscope observations on the Golgi apparatus of normal and axotomised primary sensory neurons.

Lieberman, A. R. (1971). The axon reaction: A review of the principle features of perikaryal response to axon injury, pp. 49–124. In *Int. Rev. Neurobiology*, Vol. 14, (C. C. Pfeiffer, and J. R. Smythies, eds.), Academic Press, New York.

Lieberman, A. R. (1974). "Some factors affecting retrograde neuronal responses to axonal lesions", pp. 71–105. In *Essays on the Nervous System* (R. Bellairs, and E. G. Gray, eds.), Clarendon Press, Oxford.

Liebig, J. (1842). *Die Thier-Chemie, oder die organische Chemie in ihrer Anwendung auf Physiologie und Pathologie.* 2 Bd. Braunschweig.

Liem, R. K. H., S.-H. Yen, G. E. Solomon, and M. L. Shelanski (1978). *J. Cell Biol.* 79:637–645. Intermediate filaments in nervous tissues.

Liesi, P. (1985a). *EMBO J.* 4:1163–1170. Do neurons in the vertebrate CNS migrate on laminin?

Liesi, P. (1985b). *EMBO J.* 4:2505–2511. Laminin-immunoreactive glia distinguish regenerative adult CNS systems from nonregenerative ones.

Lilien, J. (1968). *Dev. Biol.* 17:657–678. Specific enhancement of cell aggregation *in vitro*.

Lillien, L. E., M. Sendtner, H. Rohrer, S. M. Hughes, and M. C. Raff (1988). *Neuron* 1:485–494. Type-2 astrocyte development in rat brain cultures is initiated by a CNTF-like protein produced by type-1 astrocytes.

Lim, R. (1985). Glia maturation factor and other factors acting on glia, pp. 119–147. In *Growth and Maturation Factors*, Vol. 3, (G. Guroff, ed.). Wiley, New York.

Lim, R., and J. F. Miller (1988). *J. Cell Biol.* 107:270a. Isolation and sequence analysis of GMF-beta: A neural growth factor.

Lim, R., J. F. Miller, D. J. Hicklin, and A. A. Andresen (1985). *Biochemistry* 24:8070–8074. Purification of bovine glia maturation factor and characterization with monoclonal antibody.

Lim, R., D. J. Hicklin, J. F. Miller, T. H. Williams, and J. B. Crabtree (1987). *Dev. Brain Res.* 33:93–100. Distribution of immunoreactive glia maturation factor-like molecule in organs and tissues.

Lim, R., J. F. Miller, and A. Zaheer (1989). *Proc. Natl. Acad. Sci. U.S.A.* 86:3901–3905. Purification and characterization of glia maturation factor-beta: A growth regulator for neurons and glia.

Lim, R., A. Zahar, and W. S. Lane (1990). *Proc. Natl. Acad. Sci. USA* 87:5233–5237. Complete amino acid sequence of bovine glia maturation factor β.

Lim, S.-S., P. J. Sammak, and G. G. Borisy (1989). *J. Cell Biol.* 109:253–263. Progressive and spatially differentiated stability of microtubules in developing neuronal cells.

Lin, J. J. C., J. R. Feramisco, S. H. Blose, and F. Matsumura (1984). Monoclonal antibodies to cytoskeletal proteins. In *Monoclonal Antibodies and Functional Cell Lines* (R. H. Kennett, K. B. Bechtol, and T. J. McKearn, eds.), Plenum, 1984.

Lin, J.-W., D. S. Faber, and M. R. Wood (1983). *Brain Res.* 274:319–324. Organized projection of the goldfish saccular nerve onto the Mauthner cell lateral dendrite.

Lin, L.-F. H., D. Mismer, J. D. Lile, L. G. Armes, E. T. Butler III, J. L. Vannice, and F. Collins (1989). *Science* 246:1023–1025. Purification, cloning, and expression of ciliary neurotrophic factor (CNTF).

Lin, L.-F. H., L. G. Armes, A. Sommer, D. J. Smith, and F. Collins (1990). *J. Biol. Chem.* 265:8942–8947. Isolation and characterization of ciliary neurotrophic factor from rabbit sciatic nerves.

Linden, D. C., R. W. Guillery, and J. Cucchiaro (1981). *J. Comp. Neurol.* 203:189–211. The dorsal lateral geniculate nucleus of the normal and visually deprived monkeys.

Linden, R., and V. H. Perry (1982). *Neuroscience* 7:2813–2827. Ganglion cell death within the developing retina: A regulatory role for retinal dendrites.

Linden, R., and C. A. Serfaty (1985). *Neuroscience* 15:853–868. Evidence for differential effects of terminal and dendritic competition upon developmental neuronal death in the retina.

Lindholm, D. R. Heumann, M. Meyer, and H. Thoenen (1987). *Nature* 330:658–659. Interleukin-1 regulates synthesis of nerve growth factor in non-neuronal cells of the rat sciatic nerve.

Lindner, J., F. G. Rathjen, and M. Schachner (1983). *Nature* 305:427–430. L1 mono- and polyclonal antibodies modify cell migration in early postnatal mouse cerebellum.

Lindner, J., J. Guenther, H. Nick, G. Zinser, H. Antonicek, M. Schachner, and D. Monard (1986). *Proc. Natl. Acad. Sci. U.S.A.* 83:4568–4571. Modulation of granule cell migration by a glia-derived protein.

Lindsay, H. A., and M. L. Barr (1955). *J. Anat. (London)* 89:47–63. Further observations on the behaviour of nuclear structures during depletion and restoration of Nissl substance.

Lindsay, R. M. (1979). *Nature* 282:80–82. Adult rat brain astrocytes support survival of both NGF-dependent and NGF-insensitive neurons.

Lindsay, R. M. (1985). *Dev. Biol.* 112:319–328. Placode and neural crest-derived sensory neurons are responsive at early developmental stages to brain-derived neurotrophic factor.

Lindsay, R. M., Y.-A. Barde, A. M. Davies, and H. Rohrer (1985a). *J. Cell Sci.* 3:Suppl. 115–129. Differences and similarities in the neurotrophic growth factor require-ments of sensory neurons derived from neural crest and neural placode.

Lindsay, R. M., H. Thoenen, and Y.-A. Barde (1985b). *Dev. Biol.* 112:319–328. Placode and neural crest-derived sensory neurons are responsive at early developmental stages to brain-derived neurotrophic factor.

Lindvall, O., A. Björklund, R. Y. Moore, and U. Stenevi (1974). *Brain Res.* 81:325–331. Mesencephalic dopamine neurons projecting to neocortex.

Linell, E. A., and M. I. Tom (1931). *Anat. Rec. Suppl.* 48:27. The postnatal development of the oligodendroglia cell in the brain of the white rat and the possible role of this cell in myelogenesis.

Ling, E. A. (1976a). *J. Anat. (London)* 121:29–45. Some aspects of amoeboid microglia in the corpus callosum and neighbouring regions of neonatal rats.

Ling, E. A. (1976b). *Acta anat.* 96:600–609. Electron microscopy identification of amoeboid microglia in the spinal cord of newborn rats.

Ling, E. A. (1977). *J. Anat. (London)* 123:637–648. Light and electron microscopic demonstration of some lysosomal enzymes in the amoeboid microglia in neonatal rat brain.

Ling, E. A. (1978). *J. Anat. (London)* 126:111–121. Electron microscopic studies of macrophages in Wallerian degeneration of rat optic nerve after intravenous injection of colloidal carbon.

Ling, E. A. (1979). *Arch. Histol. Jap.* 42:41–50. Electron microscopic study of macrophages appearing in a stab wound of the brain of rats following intravenous injection of carbon particles.

Ling, E. A. (1981). The origin and nature of microglia, pp. 33–82. In *Advances in Cellular Neurobiology*, Vol. 2, (S. Fedoroff, and L. Hertz, eds.), Academic, New York.

Ling, E. A., and S. K. Leong (1987). *J. Neurocytol.* 16:373–387. Effects of intraneural injection of Ricinus communis agglutinin-60 into the rat vagus nerve.

Ling, E. A., and S. K. Leong (1988). *J. Anat. (London)* 159:207–218. Infiltration of carbon-labelled monocytes into the dorsal motor nucleus following an intraneural injection of ricinus communis agglutinin-60 into the vagus nerve in rats.

Ling, E. A., J. A. Paterson, A. Privat, S. Mori, and C. P. Leblond (1973). *J. Comp. Neurol.* 149:43–72. Investigation of glial cells in simithin sections I. Identification of glial cells in the brain of young rats.

Ling, E. A., D. Penney, and C. P. Leblond (1980). *J. Comp. Neurol.* 193:631–657. The use of carbon labeling to demonstrate the role of blood monocytes as precursors of the ameboid cells' present in the corpus callosum of postnatal rats.

Ling, E. A., C. Kaur, and W. C. Wong (1982). *J. Anat. (London)* 135:385–394. Light and electron microscopic demonstration of non-specific esterase in amoeboid microglial cells in the corpus callosum in postnatal rats: A cytochemical link to monocytes.

Ling, E. A., W. C. Wong, T. Y. Yick, and S. K. Leong (1986). *J. Neurocytol.* 15:1–15. Ultrastructural changes in the dorsal motor nucleus of monkey following bilateral cervical vagotomy.

Ling, E. A., C. Y. Wen, J. Y. Shieh, T. Y. Yick, and S. K. Leong (1989). *J. Anat. (London)* 164:201–213. Neuroglial response to neuron injuiry. A study using intraneural injection of ricinus communis agglutinin-60.

Ling, T., J. Mitrofanis, and J. Stone (1989). *J. Comp. Neurol.* 286:345–352. Origin of retinal astrocytes in the rat: Evidence of migration from the optic nerve.

Linnemann, D., D. Edvardsen, and E. Bock (1988). *Dev. Neurosci.* 10:34–42. Developmental study of the cell adhesion molecule L1.

Linser, P., and A. A. Moscona (1979). *Proc. Natl. Acad. Sci. U.S.A.* 76:6476–6480. Induction of glutamine synthetase in embryonic neural retina: localization in Müller fibers and dependence on cell interactions.

Linville, G. P., and T. H. Shepard (1972). *Nature (New Biol.)* 236:246–247. Neural tube closure defects caused by cytochalasin B.

Lippe, W. R., O. Steward, and E. W. Rubel (1980). *Brain Res.* 196:43–58. The effect of unilateral basilar papilla removal upon nuclei laminaris and magnocellularis of the chick examined with [³H]2-deoxy-D-glucose autoradiography.

Lipton, S. A., J. A. Wagner, R. D. Madison, and P. A. D'Amore (1988). *Proc. Natl. Acad. Sci. U.S.A.* 85:2388–2392. Acidic fibroblast growth factor enhances regeneration of processes by postnatal mammalian retinal ganglion cells in culture.

Lisanti, M. P., L. S. Shapiro, N. Moskowits, E. L. Hua, S. Puszkin, and W. Schook (1982). *Eur. J. Biochem.* 125:463–470. Isolation and preliminary characterization of clathrin-associated proteins.

Liu, C. N., and W. W. Chambers (1958). *Arch. Neurol. Psychiatry* 79:46–61. Intraspinal sprouting of dorsal root axons.

Liu, C. N., and C. Y. Liu (1971). *Anat. Rec.* 169:369. Role of afferents in maintenance of dendritic morphology.

Liu, L., P. G. Layer, and A. Gierer (1983). *Dev. Brain Res.* 8:223–229. Binding of FITC-coupled peanut-agglutinin (FITC-PNA) to embryonic chicken retina reveals developmental spatio-temporal patterns.

Liuzzi, F. J., and R. J. Lasek (1985). *J. Comp. Neurol.* 232:456–465. Regeneration of lumbar dorsal root axons into the spinal cord of adult frogs *(Rana pipiens),* an HRP study.

Liuzzi, F. J., and R. H. Miller (1987). *Brain Res.* 403:385–388. Radially oriented astrocytes in the normal adult spinal cord.

Livingston, M. S., and D. H. Hubel (1984). *J. Neurosci.* 4:309–356. Anatomy and physiology of a color system in primate visual cortex.

Livingston, W. K. (1947). *J. Neurosurg.* 4:140–145. Evidence of active invasion of denervated areas by sensory fibers from neighboring nerves in man.

Llinas, R., D. E. Hillman, and W. Precht (1973). *J. Neurobiol.* 4:69–94. Neuronal circuit reorganization in mammalian agranular cerebellar cortex.

Lnenicka, G. A., H. L. Atwood, and L. Marin (1986). *J. Neurosci.* 6:2252–2258. Morphological transformation of synaptic terminals of a phasic motoneuron by longterm tonic stimulation.

Lo, R. Y. S., and R. L. Levine (1980). *J. Comp. Neurol.* 191:295–314. Time course and pattern of optic fiber regeneration following tectal lobe removal in the goldfish.

Lockerbie, R. O. (1987). *Neuroscience* 20:719–729. The neuronal growth cone: A review of its locomotory, navigational and target recognition capabilities.

Lockshin, R. A. (1981). Cell death in metamorphosis, pp. 79–121. In *Cell death in biology and pathology* (I. D. Bowen, and R. A. Lockshin, eds.), Chapman & Hall, London.

Lockshin, R. A., and J. Beaulaton (1974a). *Life Sci.* 15:1549–1566. Programmed cell death.

Lockshin, R. A., and J. Beaulaton (1974b). *J. Ultrastruct. Res.* 46:43–62. Programmed cell death. Cytochemical evidence for lysosomes during the normal breakdown of the intersegmental muscles.

Lockwood, M. (1989). *Mind, Brain and the Quantum: The Compound "I".* Blackwell, Oxford.

Loeb, J. (1916). *The Organism as a Whole from a Physicochemical Viewpoint.* Putnam's, New York.

Loeb, L. (1893). *J. Morphol.* 8. A contribution to the physiology of coloration in animals.

Loeb, L. (1902). *Arch. Entw.Mech. Organ.* 13:487–506. Ueber das Wachstum des Epithels.

Loeb, L. (1912). *Anat. Rec.* 6:109–120. Growth of tissue in culture media and its significance for the analysis of growth phenomena,

Loeb, L., and M. S. Fleisher (1917). *J. Med. Res.* 37:75–99. On the factors which determine the movements of tissues in culture media.

Loeser, J. D., R. J. Lemire, and E. C. Alvord, Jr. (1972). *Anat. Rec.* 173:109–114. The development of the folia in the human cerebellar vermis.

Loewenstein, W. R. (1968a). *Perspect. Biol. Med.* 11:260–272. Some reflections on growth and differentiation.

Loewenstein, W. R. (1968b). *Dev. Biol. Suppl.* 2:151–183. Communication through cell junctions. Implications in growth control and differentiation.

Loewenstein, W. R. (1970). *Sci. Am.* 222:78–86. Intercellular communication.

Loewenstein, W. R. (1973). *Fed. Proc.* 32:60–64. Membrane junctions in growth and differentiation.

Loewenstein, W. R. (1975). Permeable junctions: Permeability, formation, and genetic aspects, pp. 419–436. In *The Nervous System,* Vol. 1, (D. B. Tower, ed.), Raven Press, New York.

Loewenstein, W. R. (1987). *Cell* 48:725–726. The cell-to-cell channel of gap junctions.

Loewi, O. (1921). *Pflüg. Arch. ges. Physiol.* 189:239–242. Uber humorale Ubertragbarkeit der Herznervenwirkung.

Loewi, O. (1933). *Proc. Roy. Soc. (London) Ser. B.* 118:299–316. The Ferrier lecture on problems connected with the principle of humoral transmission of nervous impulses.

Löfberg, J., K. Ahlfors, and C. Fällström (1980). *Dev. Biol.* 75:148–167. Neural crest cell migration in relation to extracellular matrix organization in the embryonic axolotl trunk.

Löfberg, J., A. Nynäs-McCoy, C. Olsson, L. Jönsson, and R. Perris (1985). *Dev. Biol.* 107:442–459. Stimulation of initial neural crest cell migration in the axolotl embryo by tissue grafts and extracellular matrix transplanted on microcarriers.

Löfberg, J., R. Perris, and H. H. Epperlein (1989). *Dev. Biol.* 131:168–181. Timing in the regulation of neural crest cell migration: Retarded "maturation" of regional extracellular matrix inhibits pigment cell migration in embryos of the white axolotl mutant.

Lohka, M. J. (1989). *J. Cell Sci.* 92:131–135. Mitotic control by metaphase-promoting factor and *cdc* proteins.

Lømo, T., and J. Rosenthal (1972). *J. Physiol. (London)* 221:493–513. Control of ACh sensitivity by muscle activity in the rat.

Lømo, T., and C. R. Slater (1980a). *J. Physiol. (London)*

303:173–189. Acetylcholine sensitivity of developing ectopic nerve-muscle junctions in adult rat soleus muscles.

Lømo, T., and C. R. Slater (1980b). *J. Physiol. (London)* 303:191–202. Control of junctional acetylcholinesterase by neural and muscular influences in the rat.

Lømo, T., R. H. Westgaard, and H. A. Dahl (1974). *Proc. Roy. Soc. (London) Ser. B.* 187:99–103. Contractile properties of muscle: Control by pattern of muscle activity in the rat.

London, C., R. Akers, and C. R. Phillips (1988). *Dev. Biol.* 129:380–389. Expression of Epi 1, an epidermal specific marker, in *Xenopus laevis* embryos is specified prior to gastrulation.

Long, W. L. (1983). *J. Exp. Zool.* 228:91–97. The role of the yolk syncytial layer in determination of the plane of bilateral symmetry in the rainbow trout, *Salmo gairdneri* Richardson.

Longet, F. A. (1842). *Anatomie et physiologie du système nerveux de l'homme et des animaux vertébrés*, 2 vols. Fortin, Masson & Cie, Paris.

Longo, A. M., and E. E. Penhoet (1974). *Proc. Natl. Acad. Sci. U.S.A.* 71:2347–2349. Nerve growth factor in rat glioma cells.

Lopresti, V., E. R. Macagno, and C. Levinthal (1973) *Proc. Natl. Acad. Sci. U.S.A.* 70:433–437. Structure and development of neuronal connections in isogenic organisms: Cellular interactions in the development of the optic lamina of *Daphnia*.

Lopresti, V., E. R. Macagno, and C. Levinthal (1974). *Proc. Natl. Acad. Sci. U.S.A.* 71:1098–1102. Structure and development of neuronal connections in isogenic organisms: Transient gap junctions between growing optic axons and lamina neuroblasts.

Lord, K., and I. D. Duncan (1987). *J. Comp. Neurol.* 265:34–46. Early postnatal development of glial cells in the canine cervical spinal cord.

Lorente de Nó, R. (1922). *Trab. Lab. Invest. Biol. Univ. Madr.* 29:41–78. La corteza cerebral del raton.

Lorente de Nó, R. (1933a). *Laryngoscope* 43:327–350. Anatomy of the eighth nerve. III. General plan of structure of the primary cochlear nuclei.

Lorente de Nó, R. (1933b). *J. Psychol. Neurol. (Leipzig)* 45:381–438. Studies on the structure of the cerebral cortex.

Lorente de Nó, R. (1935). *Amer. J. Physiol.* 111:272–281. The synaptic delay of motoneurons.

Lorente de Nó, R. (1938a). *J. Neurophysiol.* 1:187–194. Limits of variation of the synaptic delay of motoneurons.

Lorente de Nó, R. (1938b). The cerebral cortex: Architecture, intracortical connections and motor projections, pp. 291–325. In *Physiology of the Nervous System* (J. F. Fulton, ed.), Oxford Univ. Press, London.

Lorente de Nó, R. (1943). Cerebral cortex: Architecture, intracortical connections, motor projections. Chap. 15, pp. 274–301. In *Physiology of the Nervous System*, 2nd edn., (J. F. Fulton, ed.), Oxford Univ. Press, London.

Loring, J., B. Glimelius, C. Erickson, and J. A. Weston (1981). *Dev. Biol.* 82:86–94. Analysis of developmentally homogeneous neural crest cell populations *in vitro*.

Loring, J., B. Glimelius, and J. A. Weston (1982). *Dev. Biol.* 90:165–174. Extracellular matrix materials influence quail neural crest cell differentiation *in vitro*.

Loring, J. F., D. L. Barker, and C. A. Erickson (1988). *J. Neurosci.* 8:1001–1015. Migration and differentiation of

neural crest and ventral neural crest and ventral neural tube cells *in vitro*: Implications for *in vitro* and *in vivo* of the neural crest.

Lossinsky, A. S., A. W. Vorbrodt, and H. M. Wisniewski (1986). *Dev. Neurosci.* 8:61–75. Characterization of endothelial cell transport in the developing mouse blood-brain barrier.

Lovell, K. L., M. G. Goetting, and M. Z. Jones (1980). *Dev. Neurosci.* 3:128–139. Regeneration in the cerebellum following methylazoxymethanol-induced destruction of the external germinal layer.

Lovinger, D. M., K. L. Wong, K. Murakami, and A. Routtenberg (1987). *Brain Res.* 436:177–183. Protein kinase C inhibitors eliminate hippocampal long-term potentiation.

Löwit, M. (1875). *Wien. Akad. Sitzber.* 71:355–376. Die Nerven der glatten Musculatur.

Lu, B., C. R. Buck, C. F. Dreyfus, and I. B. Black (1989). *Exp. Neurol.* 104:191–199. Expression of NGF and NGF receptor mRNAs in the developing brain: Evidence for local delivery and action of NGF.

Lubinska, L. (1958). *Nature* 181:957–958. "Intercalated" internodes in nerve fibers.

Lubinska, L. (1961). *Exp. Cell Res. Suppl.* 8:74–90. Sedentary and migratory states of Schwann cells.

Lubinska, L. (1964). *Prog. Brain Res.* 13:1–66. Axoplasmic streaming in regenerating and in normal nerve fibers.

Lubinska, L., and S. Niemierko (1971). *Brain Res.* 27:329–342. Velocity and intensity of bidirectional migration of acetylcholinesterase in transected nerves.

Lubinska, L, and M. Olekiewicz (1950). *Acta Biol. Exp.* 15:125–145. The rate of regeneration of amphibian peripheral nerves at different temperatures.

Lucas, K. (1909). *J. Physiol. (London)* 38:113–133, 39:207–227. The "all or none" contraction of the amphibian skeletal muscle fibre.

Luciani, L. (1884). *Brain* 7:145–160. On the sensorial localisations in the cortex cerebri.

Luco, C. F., and J. V. Luco (1971). *J. Neurophysiol.* 34:1066–1071. Sympathetic effects on fibrillary activity of denervated striated muscles.

Luco, J. V., and C. Eyzaguirre (1955). *J. Neurophysiol.* 18:65–73. Fibrillation and hypersensitivity to Ach in denervated muscle: Effect of length of degenerating nerve fibers.

Ludena, R. F., and D. O. Woodward (1975). *Ann. N.Y. Acad. Sci.* 253:272–283. A and B -tubulin: Separation and partial sequence analysis.

Luduena, M. A., and N. K. Wessells (1973). *Dev. Biol.* 30:427–440. Cell locomotion, nerve elongation, and microfilaments.

Ludwig, W. (1932). *Das Rechte-Links-Problem im Tierreich und beim Menschen. Mit einem Anhang: Rechts-Links-Merkmale der Pflanzen.* Julius Springer, Berlin. (Reprinted, 1970, Springer-Verlag, Berlin).

Ludwin, S. K. (1984). *Nature* 308:274–275. Proliferation of mature oligodendrocytes after trauma to the central nervous system.

Lugaro, E. (1907). *Riv. Pat. Nerv. Ment.* 12:225–233. Sulle funzioni della nevroglia.

Luizzi, A., F. H. Foppen, J. M. Saavedra, D. Jacobowitz, and I. J. Kopin (1977). *J. Neurochem.* 28:1215–1220. Effect of NGF and dexamethasone on phenylethanolamine-N-methyltransferase (PNMT) activity in neonatal rat superior cervical ganglia.

Lullman-Rauch, R. (1971). *Z. Zellforsch. Mikrosk. Anat.* 121:593. The regeneration of neuromuscular junctions during spontaneous reinnervation of the rat diaphragm.

Lumsden, A. (1990). *Trends Neurosci.* 13:329–335. The cellular basis of segmentation in the developing hindbrain.

Lumsden, A., and R. Keynes (1989). *Nature* 337:424–428. Segmental patterns of neuronal development in the chick hindbrain.

Lumsden, A. G. S., and A. M. Davies (1983). *Nature* 306:786–788. Earliest sensory nerve fibres are guided to peripheral targets by attractants other than nerve growth factor.

Lumsden, A. G. S., and A. M. Davies (1986). *Nature* 323:538–539. Chemotropic effect of specific target epithelium in the developing mammalian nervous system.

Lumsden, C. E. (1968). Nervous tissue in culture, pp. 67–142. In *The Structure and Function of Nervous Tissue* Vol. 1, (G. Bourne, ed.), Academic Press, New York.

Lumsden, C. E., and C. M. Pomerat (1951). *Exp. Cell Res.* 2:103–114. Normal oligodendrocytes in tissue culture.

Lunau, H. (1956). *Anat. Anz.* 62:673–698. Vergleichend-metrische Untersuchungen am Allocortex von Wild- und Hausschweinen.

Lund, E. J. (1923). *Botan. Gaz.* 76:288–301. Electrical control of organic polarity in the egg of *Fucus.*

Lund, E. J. (1947). *Bioelectric Fields and Growth,* Univ. Tex. Press, Austin.

Lund, J. S. (1988). *Ann. Rev. Neurosci.* 11:253–288. Anatomical organization of macaque monkey striate visual cortex.

Lund, R. D. (1965). *Science* 149:1506–1507. Uncrossed visual pathways of hooded albino rats.

Lund, R. D. (1978). *Development and Plasticity of the Brain.* Oxford University Press, New York.

Lund, R. D., and J. S. Lund (1972). *Brain Res.* 42:1–20. Development of synaptic patterns in the superior colliculus of the rat.

Lund, R. D., and J. S. Lund (1973). *Exp. Neurol.* 40:377–390. Reorganization of the retinotectal pathway in rats after neonatal retinal lesions.

Lund, R. D., T. J. Cunningham, and J. S. Lund (1973). *Brain Behav. Evol.* 8:51–72. Modified optic projections after unilateral eye removal in young rats.

Lund, R. D., R.-L. F. Chang, and P. W. Land (1984). *Dev. Brain Res.* 14:139–142. The development of callosal projections in normal and one eyed rats.

Lund, R. K. (1975). *Exp. Eye Res.* 21:193–203. Variations in the laterality of the central projections of retinal ganglion cells.

Lunn, E. R., J. Scourfield, R. J. Keynes, and C. D. Stern (1987). *Development* 101:247–254. The neural tube origin of ventral root sheath cells in the chick embryo.

Lunn, E. R., V. H. Perry, M. C. Brown, H. Rosen, and S. Gordon (1989). *Europ. J. Neurosci.* 1:27–33. Absence of Wallerian degeneration does not hinder regeneration in peripheral nerve.

Luo, M., R. Faure, and J. H. Dussault (1986). *Brain Res.* 381:275–280. Ontogenesis of nuclear T_3 receptor in primary cultured astrocytes and neurons.

Luse, S. A. (1956). *J. Biophys. Biochim. Cytol.* 2:777–784. Formation of myelin in the central nervous system of mice and rats, as studied with the electron microscope.

Luse, S. A. (1958). *Lab. Invest.* 7:401–417. Ultrastructure of reactive and neoplastic astrocytes.

Luse, S. A. (1960). *Anat. Rec.* 138:461–492. The ultrastructure of normal and abnormal oligodendroglia.

Luskin, M. B., and C. J. Shatz (1985a). *J. Comp. Neurol.* 242:611–631. Neurogenesis of the cat's primary visual cortex.

Luskin, M. B., and C. J. Shatz (1985a). *J. Neurosci.* 5:1062–1075. Cogeneration of subplate and marginal zone cells in the cat's primary visual cortex.

Luskin, M. B., A. L. Pearlman, and J. R. Sanes (1988). *Neuron* 1:635–647. Cell lineage in the cerebral cortex of the mouse studied *in vivo* and *in vitro* with a recombinant retrovirus.

Luzzatto, A. C., G. Mangano, and N. Vonesch (1988). *Int. J. Dev. Neurosci.* 6:211–216. Prenatal development of the hippocampus in two strains of inbred mice.

Lycke, E., and H. Tsiang (1987). *J. Virol.* 61:2733–2741. Rabies virus infection of cultured rat sensory neurons.

Lycke, E., K. Kristensson, B. Svennerholm, A. Vahlne, and R. Ziegler (1984). *J. Gen. Virol.* 65:55–64. Uptake and transport of Herpes Simplex virus in neurites of rat dorsal root ganglia cels in culture.

Lynch, G., S. Deadwyler, and C. Cotman (1973a). *Science* 180:1364–1366. Postlesion axonal growth produces permanent functional connections.

Lynch, G., B. Stanfield, and C. W. Cotman (1973b). *Brain Res.* 59:155–168. Developmental differences in post-lesion axonal growth in the hippocampus.

Lynch, G., S. Mosko, T. Parks, and C. Cotman (1973c). *Brain Res.* 50:174–178. Relocation and hyperdevelopment of the dentate gyrus commissural system after entorhinal lesions in immature rats.

Lynch, G., B. Stanfield, T. Parks, and C. W. Cotman (1974). *Brain Res.* 69:1–11. Evidence for selective postlesion axonal growth in the dentate gyrus of the rat.

Lyon, M. F., S. G. (1970). *Nature* 227:1217–1219. X-linked gene for testicular feminization in the mouse.

Lyser, K. M. (1964). *Dev. Biol.* 10:433–466. Early differentiation of motor neuroblast in the chick embryo as studied by electron microscopy.

Lyser, K. M. (1966). *J. Embryol. Exp. Morphol.* 16:497–517. The development of the chick embryo diencephalon and mesencephalon during the initial phases of neuroblast differentiation.

Lyser, K. M. (1968a). *Dev. Biol.* 17:117–142. Early differentiation of motor neuroblasts in the chick embryo as studied by electron microscopy. II. Microtubules and neurofilaments.

Lyser, K. M. (1968b). *J. Embryol. Exp. Morphol.* 20:343–354. An electron-microscope study of centrioles in differentiating motor neuroblasts.

Lyser, K. M. (1971). *Tissue Cell* 3:395–404. Microtubules and filaments in developing axons and optic stalk cells.

Macagno, E. R., V. Lopresti, and C. Levinthal (1973). *Proc. Natl. Acad. Sci. U.S.A.* 70:57–61. Structure and development of neuronal connections in isogenic organisms: Variations and similarities in the optic system of *Daphnia magna.*

MacArthur, C. G., and E. A. Doisy (1919). *J. Comp. Neurol.* 30:445–486. Quantitative chemical changes in the human brain during growth.

MacInnis, A. J., W. M. Bethel, and E. M. Cornford (1974).

Nature 248:361–363. Identification of chemicals of snail origin that attract *Schistosoma mansoni* miracidia.

Macintyre, L., and J. Diamond (1981). *Proc. Roy. Soc. (London) Ser. B.* 211:471–499. Domains and mechanosensory nerve fields in salamander skin.

Mackie, E. J., R. P. Tucker, W. Halfter, R. Chiquet-Ehrismann, and H. H. Epperlein (1988). *Development* 102:237–250. The distribution of tenascin coincides with neural crest cell migration.

Mackie, K., M. DePasquale, and H. F. Cserr (1986). *Ann. J. Physiol.* 251:1186–1192. Increased permeability of a glial blood-brain barrier during acute hyperosmolar stress.

MacLean, P. D. (1970). The triune brain, emotion, and scientific bias, pp. 336–349. In *The Neurosciences, 2nd study program* (F. O. Schmitt, ed.), Rockefeller University Press, New York.

MacLean, P. D. (1972). *Ann. N.Y. Acad. Sci.* 193:137–149. Cerebral evolution and emotional processes: New findings on the striatal complex.

Macphail, E. M. (1985). *Phil. Trans. Roy. Soc. (London) Ser. B.* 308:37–51. Vertebrate intelligence: The null hypothesis.

Maden, M., D. E. Ong, D. Summerbell, F. Chytil, and E. A. Hirst (1989). *Dev. Biol.* 135:124–132. Cellular retinoic acid-binding protein and the role of retinoic acid in the development of the chick embryo.

Maderdrut, J. L., I. Merchenthaler, and R. W. Oppenheim (1984). *Neurosci. Soc. Abst.* 10:639. Reduction and enhancement of naturally-occurring cell death in the ciliary ganglion of the chick embryo following blockade of ganglionic and neuromuscular transmission.

Maderdrut, J. L., R. W. Oppenheim, and D. Prevette (1988). *Brain Res.* 444:189–194. Enhancement of naturally occurring cell death in the sympathetic and parasympathetic ganglia of the chicken embryo following blockade of ganglionic transmission.

Madrid, R. E., E. Jaros, M. J. Cullen, and W. G. Bradley (1975). *Nature* 257:319–321. Genetically determined defect of Schwann cell basement membrane in dystrophic mouse.

Madsen, A., S. Palm, L. Furcht, and P. Letourneau (1986). *Soc. Neurosci. Abstr.* 12:1210. Distribution of laminin and collagen type IV during early axonal growth in the mouse CNS.

Maekawa, T., and J. Tsuchiya (1968). *Exp. Cell Res.* 53:55–64. A method for the direct estimation of the length of G1, S and G2 phase.

Magendie, F. (1822). *J. Physiol. exp. Paris* 2:276–279. Expériences sur les fonctions des racines des nerfs rachidiens. *J. Physiol. Exp. Paris* 2:366–371. Expériences sur les fonctions des racines des nerfs qui naissent de la moelle épinière. Reprinted in Cranefield (1974).

Magini, G. (1888). *Arch. Ital. Biol.* 9:59–60. Sur la neuroglie et les cellules nerveuses cérébrales chez les foetus.

Magnani, J. L., W. A. Thomas, and M. S. Steinberg (1981). *Dev. Biol.* 81:96–105. Two distinct adhesion mechanisms in embryonic neural retina cells.

Magrassi, L., D. Purves, and J. W. Lichtman (1987). *J. Neurosci.* 7:1207–1214. Fluorescent probes that stain living nerve terminals.

Maheras, H. M., and E. D. Pollack (1985). *Dev. Brain Res.* 19:150–154. Quantitative compensation by lateral motor column neurons in response to four functional hindlimbs in a frog tadpole.

Maienschein, J. (1978). *J. Hist. Biol.* 11:129–158. Cell lineage, ancestral reminiscence, and the biogenetic law.

Maier, A., B. Gambke, and D. Pette (1986). *Cell Tiss. Res.* 244:635–643. Degeneration-regeneration as a mechanism contributing to the fast to slow conversion of chronically stimulated fast-twitch rabbit muscle.

Maier, A., B. Gambke, and D. Pette (1988). *Histochemistry* 88:267–271. Immunohistochemical demonstration of embryonic myosin in adult mammalian intrafusal fibers.

Maier, C. E., and M. Singer (1984). *J. Comp. Neurol.* 230:459–464. Gangliosides stimulate protein synthesis, growth, and axon number of regenerating limb buds.

Maier, C. E., J. Geraudie, and M. Singer (1982). *Dev. Brain Res.* 3:155–159. The effect of electrical stimulation of brachiospinal nerves on protein synthesis in the forelimb regenerate of the newt.

Maier, C. E., R. A. Grimm, and M. Singer (1984a). *Brain Res.* 301:363–369. Neurotrophic and neuronotrophic effects in the regenerating newt limb bud after electrical stimulation of brachiospinal nerves.

Maier, C. E., I. G. McQuarrie, and M. Singer (1984b). *J. Exp. Zool.* 232:181–186. A nerve conditioning lesion accelarates limb regeneration in the newt.

Maier, C. E., I. G. McQuarrie, and M. Singer (1984c). *Exp. Neurol.* 83:443–447. Parent and daughter axon density in the limb stump and regenerating limb bud of the newt.

Mair, R. G., R. L. Gellman, and R. C. Gesteland (1982). *Neuroscience* 7:3105–3116. Postnatal proliferation and maturation of olfactory bulb neurons in the rat.

Maisonpierre, P. C., L. Belluscio, S. Squinto, N. Y. Ip, M. E. Furth, R. M. Lindsay, and G. D. Yancopoulos (1990). *Science* 247:1446–1451. Neurotrophin-3: A neurotrophic factor related to NGF and BDNF.

Majno, G., and M. L. Karnofsky (1958). *J. Exp. Med.* 107:475–496. A biochemical and morphologic study of myelination and demyelination. I. Lipid biosynthesis *in vitro* by normal nervous tissue.

Major, R. H. (1939). *Classic Descriptions of Disease*, 2nd edition. Thomas, Springfield, Illinois.

Malacinski, G. M., and B. W. Youn (1981). *Dev. Biol.* 88:352–357. Neural plate morphogenesis and axial stretching in "notochord-defective" *Xenopus laevis* embryos.

Malhotra, S. K. (1960). *Quart. J. Microscop. Sci.* 101:75–93. The cytoplasmic inclusions of the neurones of crustacea.

Malhotra, S. K., and A. van Harreveld (1966). *J. Anat. (London)* 100:99–110. Distribution of extracellular material in central white matter.

Mall, F. (1893). *J. Morphol.* 8:415–432. Histogenesis of the retina in amblystoma and necturus.

Mall, F. P. (1909). *Am. J. Anat.* 9:1–32. On several anatomical characters of the human brain, said to vary according to race and sex, with special reference to the weight of the frontal lobe.

Mallatt, M., and B. Chamak (1989). *Neurosci. Lett.* 99:12–17. Lineage relationship between oligodendrocytes and brain macrophages?

Mallat, M., R. Houlgatte, P. Brachet, and A. Prochiantz (1989). *Dev. Biol.* 133:309–311. Lipopolysaccharide-stimulated rat brain macrophages release NGF *in vitro*.

Maller, J. (1985). *Cell. Diff.* 16:211–221. Regulation of amphibian oocyte maturation.

Mallory, F. B. (1900). *J. Exp. Med.* 5:15–20. A contribution to staining methods.

Malmgren L., Y. Olsson, T. Olsson, and K. Kristensson

(1978). *Brain Res.* 153:477–493. Uptake and retrograde axonal transport of various exogenous macromolecules in normal and crushed hypoglossal nerves.

Malzacher, P. (1968). *Z. Morphol. Oekol. Tiere* 62:103–161. Die Embryogenese des Gehirns paurometaboler Insekten. Untersuchungen an *Carausius morosus* und *Periplaneta americana*.

Manchot, E. (1929). *Arch. Entw.-Mech. Organ.* 116:689–708. Abgrenzung des Augenmaterials und andere Teilbezirke in der Medullarplatte: die Teilbewegungen Während der Auffaltung.

Mandelbrot, B. B. (1982). *The Fractal Geometry of Nature.* Freeman, New York.

Mangelsdorf, D. J., E. S. Ong, J. A. Dyck, and R. M. Evans (1990). *Nature* 345:224–229. Nuclear receptor that identifies a novel retinoic acid response pathway.

Mangold-Wirz, K. (1966). *Acta Anat.* 63:449–508. Cerebralisation und Ontogenese-Modus bei Eutherien.

Mangold, O. (1931). *Ergeb. Biol.* 7:193–403. Das Determinationsprobleme. III. Das Wirbeltierauge in der Entwicklung und Regeneration.

Mangold, O. (1933). *Naturwissen* 21:394–397. Isolationsversuche zur Analyse der Entwicklung bestimmter Kopforgane.

Mangold, O. and Spemann, H. (1927). *Roux Arch. EntusMech. Organ.* 3:341–422. Über Induktion von Medullarplatte durch Medullarplatte im jüngeren Keim, ein Beispiel homoeögenetischer oder assimilatorische Induktion.

Mani, R. B., J. B. Lohr, and D. V. Jeste (1986). *Exp. Neurol.* 94:29–40. Hippocampal pyramidal cells and aging in the human: a quantitative study of neuronal loss in sectors CA1 to CA4.

Mann, D. M. A., and P. O. Yates (1973a). *J. Neurol. Sci.* 18:183–196. Polyploidy in the human nervous system. I. The DNA content of neurones and glia of the cerebellum.

Mann, D. M. A., and P. O. Yates (1973b). *J. Neurol. Sci.* 18:197–205. Polyploidy in the human nervous system. II. Studies of the glial cell populations of the Purkinje cell layer of the human cerebellum.

Mann, W. S., and B. Salafsky (1970). *J. Physiol. (London)* 208:33–47. Enzymic and physiological studies on normal and disused developing fast and slow cat muscle.

Mannen, H. (1965). *Arch. Ital. Biol.* 103:197–219. Arborizations dendritiques. Étude topographique et quantitative dans le noyau vestibulaire du chat.

Mannen, H. (1966). *J. Comp. Neurol.* 126:75–90. Contributions to the quantitative study of the nervous tissue. A new method for measurement of the volume and surface area of neurons.

Manocha, S. L. (1972). *Malnutrition and Retarded Human Development.* Charles Thomas, Springfield, Illinois.

Manthorpe, M., E. Engvall, E. Ruoslahti, F. M. Longo, G. E. Davis, and S. Varon (1983). *J. Cell Biol.* 97:1882–1890. Laminin promotes neuritic regeneration from cultured peripheral and central neurons.

Manthorpe, M., S. Skaper, L. R. Williams, and S. Varon (1986). *Brain Res.* 367:282–286. Purification of adult rat sciatic nerve ciliary neuronotrophic factor.

Manuelidis, L., and M. Bornstein (1970). *Z. Zellforsch. Mikrosk. Anat.* 106:189–199. I-125 labelled thyroid hormones in cultured mammalian nerve tissue.

Manuelidis, L., and E. E. Manuelidis (1974). *Exp. Neurol.* 43:192–206. On the DNA content of cerebellar Purkinje cells *in vivo* and *in vitro*.

Marani, E., and J. Voogd (1973). *Acta Morphol. Neerl. Scand.* 11:353–354. Some aspects of the localization of the enzyme 5′-nucleotidase in the molecular layer of the cerebellum of the mouse.

Marani, E., and J. Voogd (1977). *J. Anat. (London)* 124:335–345. An acetylcholinesterase band pattern in the molecular layer of the cerebellum of the cat.

Marano, N., B. Dietzschold, J. J. Early, Jr., G. Schatteman, S. Thompson, P. Gorb, A. H. Ross, M. Bothwell, B. F. Atkinson, and H. Koprowski (1987). *J. Neurochem.* 48:225–232. Purification and amino acid sequencing of human melanoma nerve growth factor receptor.

March, B. (1935). *Some Technical Terms of Chinese Painting.* American council of learned societies, studies in Chinese and related civilizations, no. 2, Baltimore.

Marchase, R. B. (1976). Biochemical investigations of retinotectal adhesive specificity, Ph.D. Thesis, Johns Hopkins Univ.

Marchase, R. B., A. J. Barbera, and S. Roth (1975). A molecular approach to retinotectal specificity, pp. 315–327. In *Cell Patterning*, Ciba Foundation Symposium 29, Elsevier, New York.

Marchesi, V. T. (1985). *Ann. Rev. Cell. Biol.* 1:531–561. Stabilizing infrastructure of cell membranes.

Marchi, V., and G. Algeri (1885–1886). *Riv. Sper. Freniatria Med. Legal.* 11:492–494, 12:208–252. Sulla degenerazioni discendenti consecutive a lesioni sperimentali in diverse zone della corteccia cerebrale.

Marchisio, P. C. (1969). *J. Neurochem.* 16:665–671. Choline acetyltransferase (ChAc) activity in developing chick optic centres and the effects of monolateral removal of retina at an early embryonic stage and at hatching.

Marchisio, P. C., and J. Sjöstrand (1972). *J. Neurocytol.* 1:101–108. Radioautographic evidence for protein transport along the optic pathway of early chick embryos.

Marchisio, P. C., J. Sjöstrand, M. Aglietta, and J.-O. Karlesson (1973). *Brain Res.* 63:273–284. The development of axonal transport of proteins and glycoproteins in the optic pathway of chick embryos.

Mareck, A., A. Fellous, A. Francon, and J. Nunez (1980). *Nature* 284:353–355. Changes in composition and activity of microtubule-associated proteins during brain development.

Mares, V., and Z. Lodin (1970). *Brain Res.* 23:343–352. The cellular kinetics of the developing mouse cerebellum. II. The function of the external granular layer in the process of gyrification.

Mares, V., Z. Lodin, and J. Srajer (1970). *Brain Res.* 23:323–342. The cellular kinetics of the developing mouse cerebellum. I. The generation cycle, growth fraction and rate of proliferation of the external granular layer.

Mares, V., Z. Lodin, and J. Sacha (1973). *Brain Res.* 53:273–289. A cytochemical and autoradiographic study of nuclear DNA in mouse Purkinje cells.

Mares, V., B. Schultze, and W. Maurer (1974). *J. Cell Biol.* 63:665–674. Stability of DNA in Purkinje cell nuclei of the mouse.

Margolis, F. L. (1969). *J. Neurochem.* 16:447–456. DNA and DNA polymerase activity in chicken brain regions during ontogeny.

Mariani, J. (1982). *J. Neurobiol.* 13:119–126. Extent of multiple innervation of Purkinje cells by climbing fibers in the olivocerebellar system of weaver, reeler, and staggerer mutant mice.

Mariani, J., and J.-P. Changeux (1980). *J. Neurobiol.* 11:41–50. Multiple innervation of Purkinje cells by climbing fibers in the cerebellum of the adult staggerer mutant mouse.

Mariani, J., and J.-P. Changeux (1981a). *J. Neurosci.* 1:696–702. Ontogenesis of olivocerebellar relationships. I. Studies by intracellular recordings of the multiple innervation of Purkinje cells by climbing fibers in the developing rat cerebellum.

Mariani, J., and J.-P. Changeux (1981b). *J. Neurosci.* 1:703–709. Ontogenesis of olivocerebellar relationships. II. Spontaneous activity of inferior olivary neurons and climbing fiber-mediated activity of cerebellar Purkinje cells in developing rats.

Mariani, J., F. Crepel, K. Mikoshiba, J. P. Changeux, and C. Sotelo (1977). *Phil. Trans. Roy. Soc. (London) Ser. B.* 281:1–28. Anatomical, physiological and biochemical studies of the cerebellum from reeler mutant mouse.

Marin-Padilla, M. (1970a). *Brain Res.* 23:167–183. Prenatal and early postnatal ontogenesis of the human motor cortex: A Golgi study. I. The sequential development of the cortical layer.

Marin-Padilla, M. (1970b). *Brain Res.* 23: 185–191. Prenatal and early postnatal ontogenesis of the human motor cortex: A Golgi Study. II. The basket-pyramidal system.

Marin-Padilla, M. (1971). *Z. Anat. Entwicklungsgesch.* 134: 117–145. Early prenatal ontogenesis of the cerebral cortex (neocortex) of the cat *(Felis domestica).* A Golgi study.

Marin-Padilla, M. (1972). *Z. Anat. Entwicklungsgesch.* 136:125–142. Prenatal ontogenetic history of the principal neurons of the neocortex of the cat *(Felis domestica).* A Golgi study. II. Developmental differences and their significances.

Marin-Padilla, M. (1983). *Anat. Embryol.* 168:21–40. Structural organization of the human cerebral cortex prior to the appearance of the cortical plate.

Marin-Padilla, M. (1984). Neurons of layer I, pp. 447–477. In *Cerebral Cortex,* Vol. l, (A. Peters, and E. G. Jones, eds.), Plenum, New York.

Marin-Padilla, M. (1985). *J. Comp. Neurol.* 241:237–249. Early vascularization of the embryonic cerebral cortex: Golgi and electron microscopic studies.

Marin-Padilla, M. (1988a). Early ontogenesis of the human cerebral cortex, pp. 1–34. In *Cerebral Cortex,* Vol. 7, (A. Peters, and E. G. Jones, eds.), Plenum, New York.

Marin-Padilla, M. (1988b). Embryonic vascularization of the mammalian cerebral cortex, pp. 479–509. In *Cerebral Cortex,* Vol. 7, Plenum, New York.

Marín-Padilla, M. (1990). *J. Comp. Neurol.* 299:89–105. Three-dimensional structural organization of layer I of the human cerebral cortex: A Golgi study.

Marin-Padilla, M., and T. M. Marin-Padilla (1982). *Anat. Embryol.* 164:161–206. Origin, prenatal development and structural organization of layer I of the human cerebral (motor) cortex.

Marinesco, G. (1892). *Neurol. Centralbl.* 11:463, 505, 564. Ueber Veränderungen der Nerven und des Rückenmarks nach Amputationen; ein Beitrag zur Nerventrophik.

Marinesco, G. (1896). *C. R. Soc. Biol. (Paris)* 48:989–991. Lésions des centres nerveux produites par la toxine du Bacillus Botulinus.

Marinesco, G. (1907). *Rev. Neurologique* No 21, 15 Nov. 17pp; Plasticité et amiboisme des cellules des ganglions sensitifs.

Marinesco, G. (1909). *La cellule nerveuse.* O. Doin, Paris.

Marinesco, G. (1919). *Phil. Trans. Roy. Soc. (London) B* 209:229. Nouvelles contributions à l'étude de la régénération nerveuse et du neurotropisme.

Marinesco, G., and J. Minea (1912a). *Soc. Biol. Compt. Rend.* 73:668–670. Croissance des fibres nerveuses dans le milieu de culture, *in vitro,* des ganglions spinaux.

Marinesco, G., and J. Minea (1912b). *Acad. nat. méd. Paris. Bull.* ser. 3, 68:37–40. Culture des ganglions spinaux des mamifères *(in vitro).* Suivant le procédé de M. Carrel.

Marinesco, G., and J. Minea (1912c). *Soc. Biol. Compt. Rend.* 73:346–348. Culture des ganglions spinaux des mamifères *'in vitro'* suivant la méthode de Harrison et Montrose T. Burrows.

Marinesco, G., and J. Minea (1912d). *Rev. Neurol.* 24:469–482. La culture des ganglions spinaux de mammifères *in vitro.* Contribution à l'étude de la neurogenèse.

Mark, H. von der, K. von der Mark, and S. Gay (1976). *Dev. Biol.* 48:237–249. Study of differential collagen synthesis during development of the chick embryo by immunofluorescence.

Mark, R. F. (1965). *Exp. Neurol.* 12:292–302. Fin movements after regeneration of neuromuscular connections: And investigation of myotypic specificity.

Mark, R. F. (1969). *Brain Res.* 14:245–254. Matching muscles and motoneurones. A review of some experiments on motor nerve regeneration.

Mark, R. F. (1974a). *Britt. Med. Bull.* 30:122–126. Selective innervation of muscle.

Mark, R. F. (1974b). *Memory and Nerve Cell Connections,* Clarendon Press, Oxford.

Mark, R. F. (1975). Topography and topology in functional recovery of regenerated sensory and motor systems, pp. 289–307. In *Cell Patterning,* Ciba Foundation Symposium 29, Elsevier, New York.

Mark, R. F., G. von Campenhausen, and D. J. Lischinsky (1966). *Exp. Neurol.* 16:438–499. Nerve-muscle relations in salamander: Possible relevance to nerve regeneration and muscle specificity.

Mark, R. F., L. R. Marotte, and J. R. Johnstone (1970). *Science* 170:193–194. Reinnervated eye muscles do not respond to impulses in foreign nerves.

Mark, R. J., and J. Feldman (1972). *Invest. Ophthalmol.* 11:402–410. Binocular interaction in the development of optokinetic reflexes in tadpoles of *Xenopus laevis.*

Markham, J. A., and E. Fifková (1986). *Dev. Brain Res.* 27:263–269. Actin filament organization within dendrites and dendritic spines during development.

Marko, P., and M. Cuenod (1973). *Brain Res.* 62:419–423. Contribution of the nerve cell body to renewal of axonal and synaptic glycoproteins in the pigeon visual system.

Markus, E. J., and T. L. Petit (1989). *Synapse* 3:1–11. Synaptic structural plasticity: Role of synaptic shape.

Marler, P. (1971). *Amer. Sci.* 58:669–673. Birdsong and speech development: Could there be parallels?

Marler, P. (1981). *Trends Neurosci.* 4:88–94. Birdsong: The acquisition of a learned motor skill.

Marotte, L. R., and R. F. Mark (1970a). *Brain Res.* 19:41–51. The mechanism of selective reinnervation of fish eye muscle. I. Evidence from muscle function during recovery.

Marotte, L. R., and R. F. Mark (1970b). *Brain Res.* 19:53–62. The mechanism of selective reinnervation of fish eye muscle. II. Electron microscopy of nerve endings.

Marsh, G., and H. W. Beams (1946a). *Anat. Rec.* 94:370. Orientation of chick nerve fibers by direct electric currents.

Marsh, G., and H. W. Beams (1946b). *J. Cell Comp. Physiol.* 27:139–157. *In vitro* control of growing chick nerve fibers by applied electric currents.

Marsh, L., and P. C. Letouneau (1984). *J. Cell Biol.* 99:2041–2047. Growth of neurites without filopodial or lamellipodial activity in the presence of cytochalasin B.

Martin, A. H. (1967). *Nature* 216:1133–1134. Significance of mitotic spindle fibre orientation in the neural tube.

Martin, A. H., and J. Langman (1965). *J. Embryol. Exp. Morphol.* 14:23–35. The development of the spinal cord examined by autoradiography.

Martin, D. P., R. E. Schmidt, P. S. DiStefano, O. H. Lowry, J. G. Carter, and E. M. Johnson, Jr. (1988). *J. Cell Biol.* 106:829–844. Inhibitors of protein synthesis and RNA synthesis prevent neuronal death caused by nerve growth factor deprivation.

Martin, D. P., T. L. Wallace, and E. M. Johnson, Jr. (1990). *J. Neurosci.* 10:184–193. Cytosine arabinoside kills postmitotic neurons in a fashion resembling trophic factor deprivation : Evidencce that a deoxycytidine-dependent proces may be required for nerve growth factor signal transduction.

Martin, G. R., and R. Timpl (1987b). *Cell Biol.* 3:57–85. Laminin and other basement membrane components.

Martin, G. R., R. Timpl, P. K. Müller, and K. Kühn (1985). *Trends Biochem. Sci.* 10:285–287. The genetically distinct collagens.

Martin, H. P. (1970). *Am. J. Dis. Child.* 119:128–131. Microcephaly and mental retardation.

Martin, J. R., and H. deF. Webster (1973). *Dev. Biol.* 32:417–431. Mitotic Schwann cells in developing nerve: Their changes in shape, fine structure, and axon relationships.

Martin, M. R. (1981). *J. Comp. Neurol.* 197:141–152. Morphology of the cochlear nucleus of the normal and reeler mutant mouse.

Martin, M. R., and C. Rickets (1981). *J. Comp. Neurol.* 197:169–184. Histogenesis of the cochlear nucleus of the mouse.

Martin, P. R., A. J. Sefton, and B. Dreher (1983). *Neurosci. Lett.* 41:219–226. The retinal location and fate of ganglion cells which project to the ipsilateral superior colliculus in neonatal albino and hooded rats.

Martin, R. D. (1983). *Human Brain Evolution in an Ecological Context.* James Arthur Lecture on the evolution of the human brain, No. 52. Am. Mus. Nat. Hist., New York.

Martinez-Arias, A., and P. A. Lawrence (1985). *Nature* 313:639–642. Parasegments and compartments in the *Drosophila* embryo.

Martinez-Palomo, A. (1970). *Int. Rev. Cytol.* 29:29–76. The surface coats of animal cells.

Martini, R., and M. Schachner (1986). *J. Cell Biol.* 103:2439–2448. Immunoelectron microscopic localisation of neural cell adhesion molecules (L1, N-CAM and MAG) and their shared carbohydrate epitope and myelin basic protein in developing sciatic nerve.

Martini, R., E. Bollensen, and M. Schachner (1988). *Dev. Biol.* 129:330–338. Immunocytological localization of the major peripheral nervous system glycoprotein P$_0$ and the L2/HNK-1 and L3 carbohydrate structures in developing and adult mouse sciatic nerve.

Martins-Green, M. (1988). *Development* 103:687–706. Origin of the dorsal surface of the neural tube by progressive delamination of epidermal ectoderm and neuroepithelium: Implications for neurulation and neural tube defects.

Martuza, R. L., B. R. Seizinger, L. B. Jacoby, G. A. Rouleau, and J. F. Gusella (1988). *Trend Neurosci.* 11:22–27. The molecular biology of human glial tumors.

Marty, R., and J. Scherrer (1964). *Prog. Brain Res.* 4:222–234. Criteres de maturation des systemes afferents corticaux.

Martz, D., R. J. Lasek, S. T. Brady, and R. D. Allen (1984). *Cell Motil.* 4:89–101. Mitochondrial movement in axons: Membranous organelles may interact with the force generating system through multiple surface binding sites.

Marusich, M. F., K. Pourmehr, and J. A. Weston (1986a). *Dev. Biol.* 118:494–504. A monoclonal antibody (SN1) identifies a subpopulation of avian sensory neurons whose distribution is correlated with axial level.

Marusich, M. F., K. Pourmehr, and J. A. Weston (1986b). *Dev. Biol.* 118:505–510. The development of an identified subpopulation of avian sensory neurons is regulated by interaction with the periphery.

Maruyama, S., and A. N. D'Agostino (1967). *Neurol.* 17:550–558. Cell necrosis in the central nervous system of normal rat fetuses. An electron microscope study.

Maruyama, S., M. Chiga, and A. N. D'Agostino (1968). *J. Neuropathol. Exp. Neurol.* 27: 96–107. Selective necrosis in the fetal rat central nervous system produced by 5-fluoro–2′-deoxyuridine. A morphologic study.

Marx, M. H., and W. A. Hillix (1963). *Systems and Theories in Psychology,* McGraw-Hill, New York.

Mason, C. A. (1982). *Neuroscience* 7:541–559. Development of terminal arbors of retino-geniculate axons in the kitten. I..Light microscopical observations.

Mason, C. A. (1985). *J. Neurosci. Res.* 13:55–73. Growing tips of embryonic cerebellar axons *in vivo*.

Mastronarde, D. N. (1983a). *J. Neurophysiol.* 49:303–324. Correlated firing of cat retinal ganglion cells. I. Spontaneously active inputs to X- and Y-cells.

Mastronarde, D. N. (1983b). *J. Neurophysiol.* 49:325–349. Correlated firing of cat retinal ganglion cells. II. Responses of X- and Y-cells to single quantal events.

Mathers, L. H., K. L. Chow, P. D. Spear, and P. Grobstein (1974). *Exp. Brain Res.* 19: 20–35. Ontogenesis of receptive fields in the rabbit striate cortex.

Matiegka, H. (1902). Über das hirngewicht die Schadelkapacitat und die Kopfform, sowie deren Beziehungen zur psychischen Thatigkeit des Menschen: I. Über das Hirngewicht des Menschen, F. Rivnac, Prague.

Matlin, K. S. (1986). *J. Cell Biol.* 103:2565–2568. The sorting of proteins to the plasma membrane in epithelial cells.

Mato, M., and S. Ookawara (1982). *Experientia* 38:499–500. Ultrastructural observation on the tips of growing vascular cords in the rat cerebral cortex.

Mato, M., S. Ookawara, M. Sugamata, and E. Aikawa (1984). *Experientia* 40:399–402. Evidences for the possible function of the fluorescent granular perithelial cells in brain as scavengers of high molecular-weight waste products.

Mato, M., S. Ookawara, T. K. Mato, and T. Namiki (1985). *Amer. J. Anat.* 172:125–140. An attempt to differentiate further between microglia and fluorescent granular perithelial (FGP) cells by their capacity to incorporate exogenous protein.

Matsumoto, A., and Y. Arai (1981). *Neuroendocrinology* 33:166–169. Effect of androgen on sexual differentiation of synaptic organization in the hypothalamic arcuate nucleus: An ontogenetic study.

Matsumoto, S. G., and R. K. Murphey (1977). *J. Physiol. (London)* 268:533–548. Sensory deprivation during development decreases the responsiveness of cricket giant interneurones.

Matsumoto, T. (1920). *Bull. Johns Hopkins Hosp.* 30:91–93. The granules, vacuoles and mitochondria in the sympathetic nerve fibers cultivated *in vitro*.

Matsunaga, M., K. Hatta, and M. Takeichi (1988). *Neuron* 1:289–295. Role of N-cadherin cell adhesion molecules in the histogenesis of neural retina.

Mattanza, G. G. (1973). *Acta Anat. (Basel)* 85:206–215. Significance of embryonic cell necrosis in the forebrain. II. Histochemical studies in the mouse.

Matthews-Bellinger, J., and M. M. Salpeter (1978). *J. Physiol. (London)* 279:197–213. Distribution of acetylcholine receptors at frog neuromuscular junctions with a discussion of some physiological implications.

Matthews-Bellingers, J. A., and M. M. Salpeter (1983). *J. Neurosci.* 3:644–657. Fine structural distribution of acetylcholine receptors at developing mouse neuromuscular junctions.

Matthews, M. A. (1968). *Anat. Rec.* 161:337–352. An electron microscopic study of the relationship between axon diameter and the initiation of myelin production in the peripheral nervous system.

Matthews, M. A. (1974). *Cell Tiss. Res.* 148:477–491. Microglia and reactive "M" cells of degenerating central nervous system: Does similar morphology and function imply a common origin?

Matthews, M. R., and V. H. Nelson (1975). *J. Physiol. (London)* 245:91–135. Detachment of structurally intact nerve endings from chromatolytic neurones of rat superior cervical ganglion during the depression of synaptic transmission induced by postganglionic axotomy.

Matthews, M. R., and G. Raisman (1972). *Proc. Roy. Soc. (London) Ser. B.* 181:43–79. A light and electron microscopic study of the cellular response to axonal injury in the superior cervical ganglion of the rat.

Matthews, M. R., W. M. Cowan, and T. P. S. Powell (1960). *J. Anat. (London)* 94:145–169. Transneuronal cell degeneration in the lateral geniculate nucleus of the macaque monkey.

Matthews, P. B. C. (1972). *Mammalian Muscle Receptors and their Central Actions.* Edward Arnold, London.

Matthews, S. A., and S. R. Detwiler (1926). *J. Exp. Zool.* 45:279–292. The reactions of Amblystoma embryos following prolonged treatment with chloretone.

Mattson, M. P. (1988). *Brain Res. Rev.* 13:179–212. Neurotransmitters in the regulation of neuronal cytoarchitecture.

Mattson, M. P. (1990). Second messengers in neuronal growth and degeneration, pp. 1–48. In *Current Aspects of the Neurosciences.* Vol 2. (N. N. Osborne, ed.), Macmillan Press.

Mattson, M. P., and S. B. Kater (1987). *J. Neurosci.* 7:4034–4043. Calcium regulation of neurite elongation and growth cone motility.

Mattson, M. P., P. Dou, and S. B. Kater (1988a). *J. Neurosci.* 8:2087–2100. Outgrowth-regulating actions of glutamate in isolated hippocampal pyramidal neurons.

Mattson, M. P., P. B. Guthrie, and S. B. Kater (1988b). *J. Neurosci. Res.* 20:331–345. Components of neurite outgrowth which determine neuroarchitecture: Influence of calcium and the growth substrate.

Mattson, M. P., R. E. Lee, M. E. Adams, P. B. Guthrie, and S. B. Kater (1988c). *Neuron* 1:865–876. Interactions between entorhinal axons and target hippocampal neurons: A role for glutamate in the development of hippocampal circuitry.

Mattson, M. P., A. Taylor-Hunter, and S. B. Kater (1988d). *J. Neurosci.* 8:1704–1711. Neurite outgrowth in individual neurons of a neuronal population is differentially regulated by calcium and cyclic. AMP.

Mattson, M. P., M. Murrain, P. B. Guthrie, and S. B. Kater (1989a). *J. Neurosci.* 9:3728–3740. Fibroblast growth factor and glutamate: Opposing roles in the generation and degeneration of hippocampal neuroarchitecture.

Mattson, M. P., P. B. Guthrie, B. C. Hayes, and S. B. Kater (1989b). *J. Neurosci.* 9:1223–1232. Roles of mitotic history in the generation and degeneration of hippocampal neuroarchitecture.

Maturana, H. R. (1959). *Nature* 183:1406. Number of fibers in the optic nerve and the number of ganglion cells in the retina of anurans.

Maturana, H. R. (1960). *J. Biophys. Biochem. Cytol.* 7:107–120. The fine anatomy of the optic nerve of anurans: An electron microscope study.

Maturana, H. R., J. Y. Lettvin, W. S. McCulloch, and W. H. Pitts (1959). *Science* 130:1709–1710. Evidence that cut optic nerve fibers in a frog regenerate to their proper places in the tectum.

Maturana, H. R., J. Y. Lettvin, W. S. McCulloch, and W. H. Pitts (1960). *J. Gen. Physiol. Suppl.* 43:129–175. Anatomy and physiology of vision in the frog (*Rana pipiens*).

Matus, A. (1988). *Ann. Rev. Neurosci.* 11:29–44. Microtubule-associated proteins: Their potential role in determining neuronal morphology.

Matus, A., and S. Mughal (1975). *Nature* 258:746–748. Immunohistochemical localization of S100 protein in brain.

Matus, A., M. Ackermann, G. Pehling, H. R. Byers, and K. Fujiwara (1982). *Proc. Natl. Acad. Sci. U.S.A.* 79:7590–7594. High actin concentrations in brain dendritic spines and postsynaptic densities.

Maunsell, J. H. R., and W. T. Newsome (1987). *Ann. Rev. Neurosci.* 10:363–401. Visual processing in monkey extrastriate cortex.

Mauro, A. (1961). *J. Biophys. Biochem. Cytol.* 9:493–495. Satellite cells of skeletal muscle fibers.

Mauthner, L. (1860). *Sitzungsber. Akad. Wien. Math-naturw. Kl.* 39:1. Beiträge zur näheren Kenntniss der morphologischen Elemente des Nervensystems.

Mauthner, L. (1863). *Denkschr. Akad. Wiss. Wien.* 21:1–56. Beiträge zur näheren Kenntniss der morphologischen Elemente des Nervensystems.

Mauthner, L. (1895). *Sitzber. Akad. Wiss. Wien.* 34:31–36. Untersuchungen über den Bau des Rückenmarks der Fische.

Max, S. R., and E. X. Albuquerque (1975). *Exp. Neurol.* 49:852–857. Neurotrophic regulation of acetylcholinesterase in regenerating skeletal muscle.

Maxwell, D. S., and L. Kruger (1965). *Exp. Neurol.* 12:33–54.

Small blood vessels and the origin of phagocytes in the rat cerebral cortex following heavy particle irradiation.

Maxwell, D. S., and L. Kruger (1966). *Am. J. Anat.* 118:437–460. The reactive oligodendrocyte. An electron microscopic study of cerebral cortex following alpha particle irradiation.

Maxwell, G. D., M. E. Forbes, and D. S. Christie (1988). *Neuron* 1:557–568. Analysis of the development of cellular subsets present in the neural crest using cell sorting and cell culture.

May, M. K., and T. J. Biscoe (1973). *Brain Res.* 53:181–186. Preliminary observations on synaptic development in the foetal rat spinal cord.

May, R. M. (1925). *J. Exp. Zool.* 42:371–410. The relation of nerves to degenerating and regenerating taste buds.

May, R. M. (1927a). *Proc. Natl. Acad. Sci. U.S.A.* 13:372–374. Modification of nerve centers due to the transplantation of the eye and olfactory organ in anuran embryos.

May, R. M. (1927b). *Arch. Biol. (Liége)* 37:336–396. Modifications des centres nerveux dues a la transplantation de l'oeil et de l'organe olfactif chez les embryos d'Anoures.

May, R. M. (1930). *Bull. Biol. Liége* 64:355–387. Répercussions de la greffe de moelle sur le systéme nerveux chez l'embryon de l'anoure, *Discoglossus pictus* Otth.

May, R. M. (1933). *Bull. Biol. Liége* 67:327–349. Réactions neurogéniques de la moelle á la greffe en surnombre, ou á l'ablation d'une ébauche de patte postérieure chez l'embryon de l'anoure, *Discoglossus pictus* Otth.

May, R. M., and S. R. Detwiler (1925). *J. Exp. Zool.* 43:83–103. The relation of transplanted eyes to developing nerve centers.

Mayer, B. W., Jr., E. D. Hay, and R. O. Hynes (1981). *Dev. Biol.* 82:267–286. Immunocytochemical localization of fibronectin in embryonic chick trunk area vasculosa.

Maynard, D. M. (1965). *J. Exp. Biol.* 43:79–106. The occurrence and functional characteristics of heteromorph antennules in an experimental population of spiny lobsters, *Panulirus argus.*

Maynard, D. M., and M. J. Cohen (1965). *J. Exp. Biol.* 43:55–78. The function of a heteromorph antennule in a spiny lobster, *Panulirus argus.*

Mayr, E. (1965). Cause and effect in biology, pp. 33–50. In *Cause and Effect* (D. Lerner, ed.), Free Press, New York.

Mayr, E. (1970). *Populations, Species and Evolution*, Belknap. Harvard Univ. Press, Cambridge, Mass.

Mayr, E. (1974). Teleological and teleonomic, a new analysis, pp. 91–117. In *Boston Studies in the Philosophy of Science, XIV* (R. S. Cohen, and W. W. Wartofsky, eds.), Reidel, Boston.

Mayr, E. (1982). *The Growth of Biological Thought. Diversity, Evolution and Inheritance.* Belknap, Harvard Univ. Press, Cambridge, Mass.

Mayr, E., and W. Provine (eds.) (1980). *The Evolutionary Synthesis.* Harvard Univ. Press, Cambridge, Mass.

McBride, W. G. (1974). *Teratology* 10:283–292. Fetal nerve cell degeneration produced by the thalidomide in rabbits.

McCaig, C. D. (1986). *J. Embryol. Exp. Morph.* 94:245–255. Electric fields, contact guidance and the direction of nerve growth.

McCaig, C. D., and K. R. Robinson (1982). *Dev. Biol.* 90:335–339. The ontogeny of trans-epidermal potential difference in frog embryos.

McCarthy, K. D., and J. de Vellis (1980). *J. Cell Biol.* 85:890–902. Preparation of separate astroglial and oligodendroglial cell cultures from rat cerebral tissues.

McCarthy, K. D., and L. M. Partlow (1976a). *Brain Res.* 114:391–414. Preparation of pure neuronal and non-neuronal cultures from embryonic chick sympathetic ganglia: A new method based on both differential cell adhesiveness and the formation of homotypic neuronal aggregates.

McCarthy, K. D., and L. M. Partlow (1976b). *Brain Res.* 114:415–426. Neuronal stimulation of [³H] thymidine incorporation by primary cultures of highly purified non-neuronal cells.

McCarthy, M. P., J. P. Earnest, E. F. Young, S. Choe, and R. M. Stroud (1986). *Ann. Rev. Neurosci.* 9:383–413. The molecular neurobiology of the acetylcholine receptor.

McCasland, J. S., and T. A. Woolsey (1988). *J. Comp. Neurol.* 278:555–569. High-resolution 2-deoxyglucose mapping of functional cortical columns in mouse barrel cortex.

McClain, D. A., and G. M. Edelman (1982). *Proc. Natl. Acad. Sci. U.S.A.* 79:6380–6384. A neural cell adhesion molecule from human brain.

McClay, D. R., et al. (1977). *J. Cell Biol.* 75:56–66. A requirement for trypsin-sensitive cell-surface components for cell-cell interactions of embryonic neural retina cells.

McClellan, A. D., and P. B. Farel (1985). *Brain Res.* 332:119–130. Pharmacological activation of locomotor patterns in larval and adult frog spinal cords.

McConnel, P., and M. Berry (1978). *J. Comp. Neurol.* 177:159–172. The effects of undernutrition on Purkinje cell dendritic growth in the rat.

McConnell, C. H. (1933). *Quart. J. Microscop. Sci.* 75:495–509. Development of the ectodermal nerve net in the buds of hydra.

McConnell, J. A. (1981). *J. Comp. Neurol.* 200:273–288. Identification of early neurons in the brainstem and spinal cord. II. An autoradiographic study in the mouse.

McConnell, J., and J. B. Angevine, Jr. (1983). *Brain Res.* 272:150–156. Time of neuron origin in the amygdaloid complex of the mouse.

McConnell, P., and M. Berry (1978a). *J. Comp. Neurol.* 177:159–172. Effects of under-nutrition on Purkinje cell dendritic growth in the rat.

McConnell, P., and M. Berry (1978b). *J. Comp. Neurol.* 178:759–772. The effect of refeeding after neonatal starvation on Purkinje cell dendritic growth in the rat.

McConnell, P., and M. Berry (1981). *J. Comp. Neurol.* 200:463–479. The Effects of refeeding after varying periods of neonatal undernutrition on the morphology of Purkinje cells in the cerebellum of the rat.

McConnell, P., and M. Berry (1982). *Brain Res.* 241:362–365. Regeneration of ganglion cell axons in the adult mouse retina.

McConnell, S, K. (1985). *J. Neurosci.* 8:945–974. Fates of visual cortical neurons in the ferret after isochronic and heterochronic transplantation.

McConnell, S. K. (1988a). *Brain Res. Rev.* 13:1–23. Development and decision-making in the mamallian cerebral cortex.

McConnell, S. K. (1988b). *J. Neurosci.* 8:945–974. Fates of visual cortical neurons in the ferret after isochronic and heterochronic transplantation.

McConnell, S. K. (1989). *Trends Neurosci.* 12:342–349. The determination of neuronal fate in the cerebral cortex.

McCouch, G. P., G. M. Austin, C.-N. Liu, and C. Y. Liu (1958).

J. Neurophysiol. 21:205–216. Sprouting as a cause of spasticity.

McCutcheon, M. (1946). *Physiol. Rev.* 26:319–336. Chemotaxis in leukocytes.

McDonald, J. K., J. G. Parnavelas, A. N. Karamanlidis, N. Brecha, and J. I. Koenig (1982a). *J. Neurocytol.* 11:809–824. The morphology and distribution of peptide-containing neurons in the adult and developing visual cortex of the rat. I. Somatostatin.

McDonald, J. K., J. G. Parnavelas, A. N. Karamanlidis, and N. Brecha (1982b). *J. Neurocytol.* 11:825–837. The morphology and distribution of peptide-containing neurons in the adult and developing visual cortex of the rat. II. Vasoactive intestinal polypeptide.

McDonald, J. K., J. G. Parnavelas, A. N. Karamanlidis, G. Rosenquist, and N. Brecha (1982c). *J. Neurocytol.* 11:881–895. The morphology and distribution of peptide-containing neurons in the adult and developing visual cortex of the rat. III. Cholecystokinin.

McDonald, J. K., J. G. Parnavelas, A. N. Karamanlidis, and N. Brecha (1982d). *J. Neurocytol.* 11:985–995. The morphology and distribution of peptide-containing neurons in the adult and developing visual cortex of the rat. IV. Avian pancreatic polypeptide.

McDonald, W. I. (1974) *Br. Med. Bull.* 30: 186–189. Remyelination in relation to clinical lesions of the central nervous system.

McEwen, B. S., and B. Parsons (1982). *Ann. Rev. Pharmacol. Toxicol.* 22:565–598. Gonadal steroid action on the brain. Neurochemistry and neuropharmacology.

McEwen, B. S., and D. W. Pfaff (1970). *Brain Res.* 21:1–16. Factors influencing sex hormone uptake by rat brain regions. I. Effects of neonatal treatment, hypophysectomy, and competing steroids on estradiol uptake.

McEwen, B. S., J. M. Weiss, and L. S. Schwartz (1969). *Brain Res.* 16:227–241. Uptake of corticosterone by rat brain and its concentration by certain limbic structures.

McEwen, B. S., G. Wallach, and C. Magnus (1974). *Brain Res.* 70:321–334. Corticosterone binding to hippocampus: Immediate and delayed influences of the absence of adrenal secretion.

McEwen, B. S., L. Plapinger, C. Chaptal, J. Gerlach, and G. Wallach (1975). *Brain Res.* 96:400–406. Role of feto-neonatal estrogen binding proteins in the association of estrogen with neonatal brain cell nuclear receptors.

McEwen, B. S., I. Lieberburg, N. Maclusky, and L. Plapinger (1976). *Ann Biol. Anim. Biochem. Biophys.* 16:471–478. Interactions of testosterone and estradiol with the neonatal rat brain: Protective mechanism and possible relationship to sexual differentiation.

McGinnis, W. (1985). *Cold Spring Harbor Symp. Quant. Biol.* 50:263–270. Homeobox sequences of the *Antennapedia* class are conserved only in higher animals.

McGinnis, W., R. L. Garber, J. Wirz, A. Kuroiwa, and W. J. Gehring (1984). *Cell* 37:403–408. A homologous protein-coding sequence in *Drosophila* homoeotic genes and its conservation in other metazoans.

McGlone, J. (1980). *Behav. Brain Sci.* 3:215–263. Sex differences in human brain asymmetry: A critical survey.

McGrath, P. A., and M. R. Bennett (1979). *Dev. Biol.* 69:133–145. Development of the synaptic connections between different segmental motoneurons and striated muscles in an axolotl limb.

McGraw, C. F., B. J. McLaughlin, and L. G. Boykins (1980). *J. Neurocytol.* 9:95–106. A freeze-fracture study of synaptic junction development in the superficial layers of the chick optic tectum.

McHenry, L. C. (1969). *Garrison's History of Neurology.* Thomas, Springfield, Illinois.

McIlwain, H. (1959). *Biochemistry and the Central Nervous System,* 2nd edn., Little, Brown and Co., Boston.

McIntosh, J. R. (1987). Progress in Research on Mitosis. *Biomechanics of Cell Division* (N. Akkas, ed.), Plenum, New York.

McIntyre, A. K., and G. Robinson (1958). *Proc. Otago. Univ. Med. School* 36:25. Stability of spinal reflex patterns.

McIntyre, A. R. (1947). *Curare, Its History, Nature, and Clinical Use.* Chicago Univ. Press, Chicago.

McKanna, J. A., and S. Cohen (1989). *Science* 243:1477–1479. The EGF receptor kinase substrate p35 in the floor plate of the embryonic rat CNS.

McKay, D. D. G., and S. V. Hockfield (1982). *Proc. Natl. Acad. Sci. U.S.A.* 79:6747–6751. Monoclonal antibodies distinguish antigenically discrete neuronal types in the vertebrate central nervous system.

McKay, H., A. McKay, and L. Sinisterra (1972). Behavioral intervention studies with malnourished children. A review of experiences, pp. 121–145. In Kallen, *Nutrition, Development and Social Behavior.* DHEW Publ. No. (NIH) 73–242. U.S. Government Printing Office, Washington.

McKay, S., and R. W. Oppenheim (1988). *Soc. Neurosci. Abst.* 14:116. An apparent absence of cell death among spinal cord interneurons in the chick embryo.

McKeehan, M. S. (1966). *Anat. Rec.* 154:705–712. The mitotic pattern in the neural tube of *Amblystoma maculatum.*

McKeever, P. E. (1978). *Am. J. Pathol.* 93:155–164. Macrophage migration through the brain parenchyma to the perivascular space following particle ingestion.

McKenna, O. C. (1979). *J. Comp. Neurol.* 187:169–190. Endocytic activity of subependymal microglial cells in the toad brain: A cytochemical study of peroxidase uptake.

McKeown, T., and R. G. Record (1952). *J. Endocrinol.* 8:386–401. Observations on foetal growth in multiple pregnancy in man.

McKinney, R. V., and B. J. Panner (1972). *Lab. Invest.* 26:100–113. Regenerating capillary basement membrane in skeletal muscle wounds.

McLachlan, E. M. (1974). *J. Physiol. (London)* 237:217–242. The formation of synapses in mammalian sympathetic ganglia reinnervated with preganglionic or somatic nerves.

McLaughlin, B. J., J. G. Wood, K. Saito, E. Roberts, and J.-Y. Wu (1975). *Brain Res.* 85:355–371. The fine structural localization of glutamate decarboxylase in developing axonal processes and presynaptic terminals of rodent cerebellum.

McLennan, I. S. (1982). *Dev. Biol.* 92:263–265. Size of motoneuron pool may be related to number of myotubes in developing muscle.

McLennan, I. S. (1983). *Dev. Biol.* 98:287–294. Neural dependence and independence of myotube production in chicken hindlimb muscles.

McLoon, L. K., and A. LaVelle (1981). *Exp. Neurol.* 73:762–774. Long-term effects of regeneration and prevention of regeneration on nucleolar morphology after facial nerve injury during development.

McLoon, S. C., and W. F. Hughes (1978). *Brain Res.* 150:398–

402. Ganglion cell death during retinal development in chick eyes explanted to the chorioallantoic membrane.

McLoon, S. C., and R. D. Lund (1982). *Exp. Brain Res.* 45:277–284. Transient retinofugal pathways in the developing chick.

McLoon S. C., L. K. McLoon, S. L. Palm,and L. T. Furcht (1986). *Soc. Neurosci. Abstr.* 12:1211. Laminin is transiently expressed in the developing rat optic nerve during the time retinal axons are growing.

McLoughlin, C. B. (1968). Interaction of epidermis with various types of foreign mesenchyme, pp. 244–251. In *Epithelial-Mesenchymal Interactions* (R. Fleischmajer, and R. Billingham, eds.), Williams and Wilkins Co., Baltimore.

McMahon, D. (1973). *Proc. Natl. Acad. Sci. U.S.A.* 70:2396–2400. A cell-contact model for cellular position determination in development.

McMahon, D. (1974). *Science* 185:1012–1021. Chemical messengers in development: A hypothesis.

McMahon, T. (1973). *Science* 179:1201–1204. Size and shape in biology.

McMorris, F. A., and F. H. Ruddle (1974). *Dev. Biol.* 39:226–246. Expression of neuronal phenotypes in neuroblastoma cell hybrids.

McMorris, F. A., A. R. Kolber, B. W. Moore, and A. S. Perumal (1974). *J. Cell. Physiol.* 84:473–480. Expression of the neuron-specific protein, 14-3-2, and steroid sulfatase in neuroblastoma cell hybrids.

McMorris, F. A., T. M. Smith, S. DeSalvo, and R. W. Furlanetto (1986). *Proc. Natl. Acad. Sci. U.S.A.* 83:822–826. Insulin-like growth factor I/somatomedin C: A potent inducer of oligodendrocyte development.

McMurray, V. (1954). *J. Exp. Zool.* 125:247–263. The development of the optic lobes in *Xenopus laevis*. The effect of repeated crushing of the optic nerve.

McNaughton, B. L., R. M. Douglas, and G. V. Goddard (1978). *Brain Res.* 157:277–293. Synaptic enhancement in fascia dentata: Cooperativity among coactive afferents.

McPherson, A., and J. Tokunaga (1967). *J. Physiol. (London)* 188:121–129. The effects of cross-innervation on the myoglobin concentration of tonic and phasic muscles.

Meakin, P. A. (1986). *J. Theor. Biol.* 118:101–113. A new model for biological pattern formation.

Mearow, K. M., and J. Diamond (1988). *Neuroscience* 26:695–708. Merkel cells and the mechanosensitivity of normal and regenerating nerves in *Xenopus* skin.

Medvedev, Z. A. (1969). *The Rise and Fall of T. D. Lysenko.* Transl. by I. M. Lerner, Columbia Univ. Press, New York.

Meek, E. S., and J. F. A. Harbison (1967). *J. Anat. (London)* 101:487–489. Nuclear area and deoxyribonucleic acid content in human liver cell nuclei.

Meier, C. (1976). *Brain Res.* 104:21–32. Some observations on early myelination in the human spinal cord, light and electron microscope study.

Meier, C., and A. Bischoff (1975). *J. Neurol. Sci.* 26:5517–5528. Oligodendroglial cell development in jimpy mice and controls, and electron-microscopic study in optic nerve.

Meier, G., and W. G. Hoag (1962). *J. Neuropath. Exp. Neurol.* 21:649–654. The neuropathology of "reeler," a neuromuscular mutation in mice.

Meier, R., M. Becker-André, R. Götz, R. Heumann, A. Shaw, and H. Thoenen (1986). *EMBO J.* 5:1489–1493. Molecular cloning of bovine and chick nerve growth factor (NGF): Delineation of conserved and unconserved domains and that relationship to the biological activity and antigenicity of NGF.

Meier, S. (1979). *Dev. Biol.* 73:25–45. Development of the chick mesoblast. Formation of the embryonic axis and establishment of the metameric pattern.

Meier, S. (1981). *Dev. Biol.* 83:49–61. Development of the chick embryo mesoblast: Morphogenesis of the prechordal plate and cranial segments.

Meier, S. (1984). *Cell Differ.* 14:235–243. Somite formation and its relationship to metameric patterning of the mesoderm.

Meier, S., and P. P. L. Tam (1982). *Differentiation* 21:95–108. Metameric pattern development in the embryonic axis of the mouse. I. Differentiation of the cranial segments.

Meinecke, F. (1928). Values and causalities in history, pp. 267–288, transl. J. H. Franklin. In *The Varieties of History*, 2nd edn. (1970), (F. Stern, ed.), Macmillan, London.

Meinertzhagen, I. A. (1972). *Brain Res.* 41:39–49. Erroneous projection of retinula axons beneath a dislocation in the retinal equator of *Calliphora*.

Meinertzhagen, I. A. (1975). The development of neuronal connection patterns in the visual system of insects, pp. 265–283. In *Cell Patterning*, Ciba Foundation Symposium 29, Elsevier, New York.

Meinhardt, H. (1982). *Models of Biological Pattern Formation*, Academic Press, London.

Meinhardt, H., and A. Gierer (1974). *J. Cell Sci.* 15:321–346. Applications of a theory of biological pattern formation based on lateral inhibition.

Meiri, K. F., and P. R. Gordon-Weeks (1990). *J. Neurosci.* 10:256–266. GAP-43 in growth cones is associated with areas of membrane that are tightly bound to substrate and is a component of a membrane skeleton subcellular fraction.

Meiri, K. F., K. H. Pfenninger, and M. B. Willard (1986). *Proc. Natl. Acad. Sci. U.S.A.* 83:3537–3541. Growth-associated protein, GAP-43, a polypeptide that is induced when neurons extend axons, is a component of growth cones and corresponds to pp46, a major polypeptide of a subcellular fraction enriched in growth cones.

Meisami, E. (1976). *Brain Res.* 107:437–444. Effects of olfactory deprivation on postnatal growth of the rat olfactory bulb utilizing a new method for production of neonatal unilateral anosmia.

Meisami, E., and E. Noushinfar (1986). *Int. J. Dev. Neurosci.* 4:431–444. Early olfactory deprivation and the mitral cells of the olfactory bulb: A golgi study.

Meisami, E., and L. Safari (1981). *Brain Res.* 221:81–107. A quantitative study of the effects of early unilateral olfactory deprivation on the number and distribution of mitral and tufted cells and of glomeruli in the rat olfactory bulb.

Meller, K., and R. Haupt (1967). *Z. Zellforsch. Mikroskop. Anat. Abt. Histochem.* 76:260–277. Die Feinstruktur der Neuro-, Glio- und Ependymoblasten von Hühnerembryonen in der Gewebekultur.

Meller, K., W. Breipohl, and P. Glees (1968a). *Z. Zellforsch. Mikroskop. Anat. Abt. Histochem.* 86:171–183. The cytology of the developing molecular layer of mouse motor cortex. An electron microscopical and Golgi impregnation study.

Meller, K., W. Breipohl, and P. Glees (1968b). *Z. Zellforsch.*

Mikroskop. Anat. Abt. Histochem. 92:217–231. Synaptic organization of the molecular and outer granular layer in the motor cortex in the white mouse during post-natal development. A Golgi and electron-microscopical study.

Melton, D. A. (1987). *Nature* 328:80–82. Translocation of a localized maternal mRNA to the vegetal pole of *Xenopus* oocytes.

Mendell, L. M. (1984). *Physiol. Rev.* 64:260–324. Modifiability of spinal synapses.

Mendell, L. M., and E. Henneman (1968). *Science* 160:96–98. Terminals of single Ia fibers: Distribution within a pool of 300 homonymous motor neurons.

Mendell, L. M., and E. Henneman (1971). *J. Neurophysiol.* 24:171–187. Terminals of single Ia fibers: Location, density, and distribution within a pool of 300 homonymous motoneurons.

Mendell, L. M., and J. G. Scott (1975). *Exp. Brain Res.* 22:221–234. The effect of peripheral nerve cross-union on connections of single Ia fibers to motoneurons.

Mendell, L. M., J. B. Munson, and J. G. Scott (1974). *Brain Res.* 73:338–342. Connectivity changes of Ia efferents on axotomized motoneurons.

Mendelsohn, E. (1963). *Arch. Intern. Hist. Sci.* 6:419–429. Cell theory and the development of general physiology.

Mendoza, A. S., W. Breipohl, and F. Miragall (1982). *J. Embryol. Exp. Morph.* 69:47–59. Cell migration from the chick olfactory placode: A light and electron microscopic study.

Menesini-Chen, M. G., J. S. Chen, and R. Levi-Montalcini (1978). *Arch. Ital. Biol.* 116:53–84. Sympathetic nerve fiber ingrowth in the central nervous system of neonatal rodents upon intracerebral NGF injections.

Menezes-Ferreira, M. M., P. A. Petrick, and B. D. Weintraub (1986). *Endocrinology* 118:2125–2130. Regulation of thyrotropin (TSH) bioactivity by TSH-releasing hormone and thyroid hormone.

Mercola, M., D. A. Melton, and C. D. Stiles (1988). *Science* 241:1223–1225. Platelet-derived growth factor A chain is maternally encoded in *Xenopus* embryos.

Meredith, H. V. (1971). *Growth* 35:233–251. Human head circumference from birth to early adulthood: Racial, regional and sex comparisons.

Merkel, F. (1875). *Arch. mikr. Anat. Bonn.* 11:636–652. Tastzellen und Tastkörperchen bei den Hausthieren und beim Menschen.

Merkel, F. (1880). *Ueber die Endigungen der sensiblen Nerven in der Haut der Wirbeltiere.* Schmidt, Rostock.

Merlie, J. P., and J. R. Sanes (1985). *Nature* 317:66–68. Concentration of acetylcholine receptor mRNA in synaptic regions of adult muscle fibers.

Merlie, J. P., and M. M. Smith (1986). *J. Membr. Biol.* 91:1–10. Synthesis and assembly of acetylcholine receptor, a multisubunit membrane glycoprotein.

Merrell, R., and L. Glaser (1973). *Proc. Natl. Acad. Sci. U.S.A.* 70:2794–2798. Specific recognition of plasma membranes by embryonic cells.

Merrill, E. G., and P. D. Wall (1972). *J. Physiol. (London)* 226:825–846. Factors forming the edge of a receptive field: The presence of relatively ineffective afferent terminals.

Merrill, J. E., S. Kutsunai, C. Mohlstrom, F. Hofman, J. Groopman, and D. W. Golde (1984). *Science* 224:1428–1430. Proliferation of astroglia and oligodendroglia in response to human T cell-derived factors.

Merton, R. K. (1961). *Proc. Amer. Phil. Soc.* 105:470–486. Singletons and multiples in Scientific discovery: A chapter in the sociology of science.

Merz, J. T. (1904–1912). *A History of European Thought in the Nineteenth Century.* 4 Vols. William Blackwood & Son, London.

Merzenich, M. M., R. J. Nelson, M. Sur, J. T. Wall, D. H. Felleman, and J. H. Kaas (1983). *Neuroscience* 10:639–666. Progression of change following median nerve section in the cortical representation of the hand in areas 3b and 1 in adult owl and squirrel monkeys.

Mescher, A. L. (1982). *J. Embryol. Exp. Morph.* 69:183–192. Neurotrophic control of events in injured forelimbs of larval urodeles.

Messer, A., G. L. Snodgrass, and P. Maskin (1984). *Cell. Molec. Neurosci.* 4:285–290. Enhanced survival of cultured cerebellar Purkinje cells by plating on antibody of *Thy-1.*

Messier, B., C. P. Leblond, and I. Smart (1958). *Exp. Cell Res.* 14:224–226. Presence of DNA synthesis and mitosis in the brain of young adult mice.

Messier, P. E., and C. Auclair (1973). *J. Embryol. Exp. Morphol.* 30:661–671. Inhibition of nuclear migration in the absence of microtubules in the chick embryo.

Messier, P. E., and C. Auclair (1974). *Dev. Biol.* 36:218–223. Effect of cytochalasin B on interkinetic nuclear migration in the chick embryo.

Messier, P. E., and C. Auclair (1975). *J. Embryol. Exp. Morphol.* 34:339–354. Neurulation et migration nucleaire intercinetique chez des embryons de poulet.

Mesulam, M. M. (1982). Principles of horseradish peroxidase neurohistochemistry and their applications for tracing neural pathways axonal transport, enzyme histochemistry and light microscopic analysis, pp. 1–151. In *Tracing Neural Connections with Horseradish Peroxidase* (M M. Mesulam, ed.), John Wiley, Chichester.

Metcalf, D. (1985). *Science* 229:16–22. The granulocyte-macrophage colony-stimulating factors.

Metin, C., and D. O. Frost (1989). *Proc. Natl. Acad. Sci. U.S.A* 86:357–361. Visual responses of neurons in somatosensory cortex of hamsters with experimentally induced retinal projections to somatosensory thalamus.

Metuzals, J. (1969). *J. Cell Biol.* 43:480–505. Configuration of a filamentous network in the axoplasm of the squid.

Metuzals, J., and I. Tasaki (1978). *J. Cell Biol.* 78:597–621. Subaxolemmal filamentous network in the giant nerve fiber of the squid *(Loligo pealei L.)* and its possible role in excitability.

Metuzals, J., V. Montepetit, and D. F. Clapin (1981). *Cell Tissue Res.* 214:455–482. Organization of the neurofilamentous network.

Meyer, A. (1971). *Historical Aspects of Cerebral Anatomy.* Oxford Univ. Press, London.

Meyer, A. (1978). *Brain* 101:673–685. The concept of a sensorimotor cortex. Its early history, with especial emphasis on two early experimental contributions by W. Bechterew.

Meyer, A. W. (1939). *The Rise of Embryology,* Stanford Univ. Press, Stanford.

Meyer, J. S. (1983). *Exp. Neurol.* 82:432–446. Early adrenalectomy stimulates subsequent growth and development of the rat brain.

Meyer, J. S. (1985). *Physiol. Rev.* 65:946–1020. Biochemical effects of corticosteroids on neural tissues.

Meyer, J. S., and K. R. Fairman (1985). *Dev. Brain Res.* 17:1–9. Early adrenalectomy increases myelin content of the rat brain.

Meyer, J. S., P. J. Leveille, J. De Vellis, J. L. Gerlach, and B. S. McEwen (1982). *J. Neurochem.* 39:423–434. Evidence for glucocorticoid target cells in the rat optic nerve. Hormone binding and glycerolphosphate dehydrogenase induction.

Meyer, M. R., and J. S. Edwards (1982). *J. Neurosci.* 2:1651–1659. Metabolic changes in deafferented central neurons of an insect, *Acheta domesticus*. I. Effects upon amino acid uptake and incorporation.

Meyer, R. L. (1982). *Science* 218:589–591. Tetrodotoxin blocks the formation of ocular dominance columns in goldfish.

Meyer, R. L. (1983a). *Dev. Brain Res.* 6:279–291. The growth and formation of ocular dominance columns by deflected optic fibers in goldfish.

Meyer, R. L. (1983b). *Dev. Brain Res.* 6:293–298. Tetrodotoxin inhibits the formation of refined retinotopography in goldfish.

Meyer, R. L. (1987). *Dev. Brain Res.* 37:115–124. Intratectal targeting by optic fibers in goldfish under impulse blockade.

Meyer, R. L., and R. W. Sperry (1973). *Exp. Neurol.* 40:525–539. Tests for neuroplasticity in the anural retinotectal system.

Meyer, R. L., and L. L. Wolcott (1984). *Soc. Neurosci. Abstr.* 10:467. Retinotopic expansion and compression in the retinotectal system of goldfish in the absence of impulse activity.

Meyer, R. L., K. Sakurai, and E. Schauwecker (1985). *J. Comp. Neurol.* 239:27–43. Topography of regenerating optic fibers in goldfish traced with local wheat germ injections into retina: Evidence for discontinuous microtopography in the retinotectal projection.

Meynert, T. (1867). *Der Bau der Grosshirnrinde und seine örtlichen Verschiedenheiten, nebst einem pathologisch-anatomischen Corollarium*. Engelmann, Leipzig.

Meynert, T. (1868–1869). *Vschr. Psychiat. Vienna* 1:77–93, and 2:88–113. Der Bau der Gross-Hirnrinde und seine örtlichen Verschiedenheiten, nebst einem pathologisch-anatomischen Corollarium.

Meynert, T. (1872). Vom Gehirne der Saugethiere, pp. 694–808. In *Handbuch der Lehre von den Geweben des Menschen und die Thiere*, Vol. 2, (S. Stricker, ed.), Engelmann, Leipzig.

Miale, I. L., and R. L. Sidman (1961). *Exp. Neurol.* 4:277–296. An autoradiographic analysis of histogenesis in the mouse cerebellum.

Miani, N., A. Di Girolamo, and M. Girolamo (1966). *J. Neurochem.* 13:755–759. Sedimentation characteristics of axonal RNA in rabbit.

Michelson, A. M., E. S. Russel, and P. J. Harman (1955). *Proc. Natl. Acad. Sci. U.S.A.* 61:1079–1084. Dystrophia muscularis: A hereditary primary myopathy in the house mouse.

Michetti, F., N. Miami, G. De Renzis, A. Caniglia, and S. Correr (1974). *J. Neurochem.* 22:239–244. Nuclear localization of S-100 protein.

Miescher, F. J. (1871). *Med. Chem. Untersuch.* 1:441–460. Ueber die chemische Zusammensetzung der Eiterzellen.

Mikoshiba, K., K. Nagaike, S. Kohsaka, K. Takamatsu, E. Aoki, and Y. Tsukada (1980). *Dev. Biol.* 79:64–80. Developmental studies on the cerebellum from reeler mutant mouse *in vivo* and *in vitro*.

Milburn, A. (1973a). *J. Cell Sci.* 12:175–195. The early development of muscle spindles in the rat.

Milburn, A. (1973b). The development of the muscle spindle in the rat. Ph.D. Thesis, Durham University.

Milburn, A. (1984). *J. Embryol. Exp. Morphol.* 82:177–216. Stages in the development of cat muscle spindles.

Milburn, N. S., and D. R. Bentley (1971). *J. Insect Physiol.* 17:607–623. On the dendritic topology and activation of cockroach giant interneurons.

Miledi, R. (1960a). *J. Physiol. (London)* 151:1–23. The acetylcholine sensitivity of frog muscle fibres after complete or partial denervation.

Miledi, R. (1960b). *J. Physiol. (London)* 151:24–30. Junctional and extra- junctional acetylcholine receptors in skeletal muscle fibres.

Miledi, R. (1962). *Nature* 193:281–282. Induced innervation of end plate free muscle segments.

Miledi, R. (1963). *Nature* 199:1191–1192. Formation of extra nerve-muscle junctions in innervated muscle.

Miledi, R., and P. Orkand (1966). *Nature* 209:717–718. Effect of a "fast" nerve on "slow" muscle fibres in the frog.

Miledi, R., and C. R. Slater (1970). *J. Physiol. (London)* 207:507–528. On the degeneration of rat neuromuscular junctions after nerve section.

Miledi, R., and E. Stefani (1969). *Nature* 222:569–571. Nonselective re-innervation of slow and fast muscle fibres in the rat.

Miledi, R., and J. Zelena (1966). *Nature* 210:855–856. Sensitivity to acetylcholine in rat slow muscle.

Millar, J., A. I. Basbaum, and P. D. Wall (1976). *Exp. Neurol.* 50:658–672. Restructuring of the somatotopic map and appearance of abnormal neuronal activity in the gracile nucleus after partial deafferentation.

Miller, J. B., and F. E. Stockdale (1987). *J. Cell Biol.* 103:2197–2208. Developmental regulation of the multiple myogenic cell lineages of the avian embryo.

Miller, K. D., J. B. Keller, and M. P. Stryker (1989). *Science* 245:605–615. Ocular dominance column development: Analysis and simulation.

Miller, R. H. (1989). *Ann. Rev. Neurosci.* 12:517–34. The macroglial cells of the rat optic nerve.

Miller, R. H., and M. C. Raff (1984). *J. Neurosci.* 4:585–592. Fibrous and protoplasmic astrocytes are biochemically and developmentally distinct.

Miller, R. H., S. David, R Patel, E. R. Abney, and M. C. Raff (1985). *Dev. Biol.* 111:35–41. A quantitative immunocytochemcial study of macroglia cell development in the rat optic nerve: *In vivo* evidence for two distinct astrocyte lineages.

Miller, R. H., E. R. Abney, S. David, C. ffrench-Constant, R. Lindsay, R. Patel, J. Stone, and M. C. Raff (1986). *J. Neurosci.* 6:22–29. Is reactive gliosis a property of a distinct subpopulation of astrocytes?

Miller, R. L. (1966). *J. Exp. Zool.* 161:23–44. Chemotaxis during fertilization in the hydroid *Campanularia*.

Miller, R. L., and C. J. Brokaw (1970). *J. Exp. Biol.* 52:699–

706. Chemotactic turning behavior of *Tubularia* spermatozoa.

Millhouse, O. E. (1981). The Golgi methods, pp. 311–344. In *Neuroanatomical Tract-Tracing Methods* (L. Heimer, and M. J. RoBards, eds.), Plenum, New York.

Mills, L., C. A. Nurse, and J. Diamond (1984). *Soc. Neurosci. Abstr.* 10:1088. Regional differences in the sensory nerve dependence of Merkel cell development in at skin.

Mills, L. R., C. A. Nurse, and J. Diamond (1989). *Dev. Biol.* 136:61–74. The neural dependency of merkel cell development in the rat: The touch domes and foot pads contrasted.

Milne-Edwards, H. (1857–1881). *Leçons sur la physiologie et l'anatomie comparée de l'homme et des animaux.* 14 vols. and Index vol. Victor Masson, Paris.

Miner, N. (1956). *J. Comp. Neurol.* 105:161–170. Integumental specification of sensory fibers in the development of cutaneous local sign.

Minkowski, M. (1920). *Schweiz. Arch. Neurol. Psychiat.* 6:201–252; 7:268–303. Über den Verlauf, die Endigung und die zentrale Repräsentation von gekreuzten und ungekreuzien sehnervenfasern bei einigen Säugetieren und beim Menschen.

Mintz, B. (1971). *Symp. Soc. Exp. Biol.* 25:345–370. Clonal basis of mammalian differentiation.

Mintz, B., and S. Sanyal (1970). *Genetics* 64:Suppl. 43–44. Clonal origin of the mouse visual retina mapped from genetically mosaic eyes.

Mintz, B., and L. S. Stone (1934). *Proc. Soc. Exp. Biol. Med.* 31:1080–1082. Transplantation of taste organs in adult *Triturus viridescens.*

Mirsky, R., J. Winter, E. R. Abney, R. M. Pruss, J. Gavrilovic, and M. C. Raff (1980). *J. Cell Biol.* 84:483–494. Myelin-specific proteins and glycolipids in rat Schwann cells and oligodendrocytes in culture.

Misantone, L. J., and D. J. Stelzner (1974). *Exp. Neurol.* 45:364–376. Behavioral manifestations of competition of retinal endings for sites in doubly innervated frog optic tectum.

Misson, J.-P., M. A. Edwards, M. Yamamoto, and V. S. Caviness, Jr. (1988a). *Dev. Brain Res.* 44:95–108. Identification of radial glial cells within the developing murine central nervous system: Studies based upon a new immunohistochemical marker.

Misson, J.-P., M. A. Edwards, M. Yamamoto, and V. S. Caviness, Jr. (1988b). *Dev. Brain Res.* 38:183–190. Mitotic cycling of radial glial cells of the fetal murine cerebral wall: A combined autoradiographic and immunohistochemical study.

Mistretta, C. M. (1972). Topographical and histological study of the developing rat tongue, palate and taste buds, pp. 163–187. In *Third Symposium on Oral Sensation and Perception: The Mouth of the Infant* (J. F. Bosma, ed.), Thomas, Springfield, Ill.

Mistretta, C. M., and R. M. Bradley (1978). *Science* 202:535–537. Taste responses in sheep medulla: Changes during development.

Mitra, N. L. (1955). *J. Anat. (London)* 89:467–483. Quantitative analysis of cell types in mammalian neo-cortex.

Miyata, Y., and K. Yoshioka (1980). *J. Physiol. (London)* 309:631–646. Selective elimination of motor nerve terminals in the rat soleus muscle during development.

Miyata, Y., Y. Kashihara, S. Homma, and M. Kuno (1986). *J. Neurosci.* 6:2012–2018. Effects of nerve growth factor on the survival and synaptic function of Ia sensory neurons axotomized in neonatal rats.

Miyayama, Y., and T. Fujimoto (1977). *Okajimas Fol. Anat. Jap.* 54:97–120. Fine morphological study of neural tube formation in the teleost, *Oryzias latipes.*

Mize, R. R., and E. H. Murphy (1973). *Science* 180:320–323. Selective visual experience fails to modify receptive field properties of rabbit striate cortex neurons.

Mizel, S. B. (1989). *FASEB J.* 3:2379–2388. The interleukins.

Mizel, S. B., and J. R. Bamburg (1976). *Dev. Biol.* 49:20–28. Studies on the action of nerve growth factor.

Mizel, S. B., and L. Wilson (1972). *Biochemistry* 11:2573–2578. Nucleoside transport in mammalian cells. Inhibition by colchicine.

Mizell, M. (1968). *J. Exp. Zool.* 229:247–258. Cell cycle and histological effects of reinnervation in denervated forelimb stumps of larval Ambystoma.

Mizuno, N., M. Uemura-Sumi, K. Matsuda, Y. Takeuchi, M. Kume, and R. Matsushima (1980). *Neurosci. Lett.* 19:33–37. Non-selective distribution of hypoglossal nerve fibers after section and resuture: A horseradish peroxidase study in the cat.

Mjaatvedt, A. E., and M. T. T. Wong-Riley (1988). *J. Comp. Neurol.* 277:155–182. Relationship between synaptogenesis and cytochrome oxidase activity in Purkinje cells of the developing rat cerebellum.

Mobley, W. C., J. L. Rutkowski, G. I. Tennekoon, K. Buchanan, and M. V. Johnson (1985). *Science* 229:284–287. Choline acetyltransferase activity in striatum of neonatal rats increased by nerve growth factor.

Model, P. G., M. B. Bornstein, S. M. Crain, and G. D. Pappas (1971). *J. Cell Biol.* 49:362–371. An electron microscopic study of the development of synapses in cultured fetal mouse cerebrum continuously exposed to xylocaine.

Moffatt, D. B. (1962). *Ann. R. Coll. Surg. Engl.* 30:368–382. The embryology of the arteries of the brain.

Moll, R., I. Moll, and W. W. Franke (1984). *Differentiation* 28:136–154. Identification of Merkel cells in human skin by specific cytokeratin antibodies: Changes of cell density and distribution in fetal and adult plantar epidermis.

Möller, A. (1950). *Zool. Jahrb., Abt. Allgem. Zool. Physiol. Tiere* 62:138–182. Die Struktur des Auges bei Urodelen verschiedener Körpergrösse.

Møllgård, K., and N. R. Saunders (1975). *J. Neurocytol.* 4:453–468. Complex tight junctions of epithelial and of endothelial cells in early foetal brain.

Møllgård, K., and N. R. Saunders (1986). *Neuropathol. Appl. Neurobiol.* 12:337–358. The development of the human blood-brain and blood-CSF barriers.

Molliver, M. E., and H. Van der Loos (1970). *Ergebn. Anat. Ent. Gesch.* 42:7–53. The ontogenesis of cortical circuitry: The spatial distribution of synapses in somesthetic cortex of newborn dog.

Molliver, M. E., I. Kostovic, and H. Van der Loos (1973). *Brain Res.* 50:403–407. The development of synapses in the cerebral cortex of the human fetus.

Monagle, R. D., and H. Brody (1974). *J. Comp. Neurol.* 155:61–66. The affects of age upon the main nucleus of the inferior olive in the human.

Monard, D. (1988). *Trends Neurosci.* 11:541–544. Cell-derived proteases and protease inhibitors as regulators of neurite outgrowth.

Monard, D., F. Solomon, M. Rentsch, and R. Gysin (1973). *Proc. Natl. Acad. Sci. U.S.A.* 70:1894–1897. Glia-induced morphological differentiation in neuroblastoma cells.

Monard, D., K. Stockel, R. Goodman, and H. Thoenen (1975). *Nature* 258:444–445. Distinction between nerve growth factor and glial factor.

Monard, D., E. Niday, A. Limat, and F. Solomon (1983). *Prog. Brain Res.* 58:359–364. Inhibition of protease activity can lead to neurite extension in neuroblastoma cells.

Mönckeberg, F. (1968). Effect of early marasmic malnutrition on subsequent physical and psychological development, pp. 269–278. In Scrimshaw, Gordon, *Malnutrition, learning and behavior*, Vol. 10. MIT Press, Cambridge.

Mönckeberg, F. (1979). Recovery of severely malnourished infants: effects of early sensory-affective stimulation, pp. 120–130. In Brozek, *Behavioral Effects of Energy and Protein Deficits*. U.S. Department of Health, Education, and Welfare. NIH Publ. No. (NIH) 79-1906.

Money, J. (1971). *Impact Sci. Soc.* 22:285–290. Prenatal hormones and intelligence: A possible relationship.

Money, J., and A. A. Ehrhardt (1972). *Man and Woman, Boy and Girl*, Johns Hopkins Univ. Press, Baltimore, Maryland.

Money, J., and V. Lewis (1966). *Bull. Johns Hopkins Hosp.* 118:365–373. IQ, genetics and accelerated growth: Adrenogenital syndrome.

Monro, A. (Primus) (1732). *The Anatomy of the Human Bones, to Which are Added an Anatomical Treatise of the Nerves*, W. Monro, Edinburgh.

Montero, C. N., and E. Hefti (1988). *J. Neurosci.* 8:2986–2999. Rescue of lesioned septal cholinergic neurons by nerve growth factor: Specificity and requirements for chromic treatment.

Montgomery, A. (1972). A study of the effects of disuse upon the isometric characteristics of fast twitch and slow twitch mammalian skeletal muscle. Ph.D. Thesis, Univ. of Bristol.

Montz, H. P. M., G. E. Davis, S. D. Skaper, M. Manthorpe, and S. Varon (1985). *Dev. Brain Res.* 23:150–154. Tumor promoting phorbol diester mimics two distinct neuronotrophic factors.

Moody, S. A. (1987a). *Dev. Biol.* 119:560–578. Fates of the blastomeres of the 16-cell stage *Xenopus* embryo.

Moody S. A. (1987b). *Dev. Biol.* 122:300–319. Fates of the blastomeres of the 32-cell stage *Xenopus* embryo.

Moody, S. A. (1989). *J. Neurosci.* 9:2919–2930. Quantitative lineage analysis of the origin of frog primary motor and sensory neurons from cleavage stage blastomeres.

Moody, S. A., and M. B. Heaton (1983a). *J. Comp. Neurol.* 213:327–343. Developmental relationships between trigeminal ganglia and trigeminal motoneurons in chick embryos. I. Ganglion development is necessary for motoneuron migration.

Moody, S. A., and M. B. Heaton (1983b). *J. Comp. Neurol.* 213:344–349. Developmental relationships between trigeminal ganglia and trigeminal motoneurons in chick embryos. II. Ganglion axon ingrowth guides motoneuron migration.

Moody, S. A., and M. B. Heaton (1983c). *J. Comp. Neurol.* 216:20–35. Ultrastructural observations of the migration and early development of trigeminal motoneurons in chick embryos.

Moody, S. A. and M. Jacobson (1983). *J. Neurosci.* 3:1670–1682. Compartmental relationships between anuran primary spinal motoneurons and somitic muscle fibers that they first innervate.

Moody, S. A., M. S. Quigg, and A. Frankfurter (1989). *J. Comp. Neurol.* 279:567–580. Development of the peripheral trigeminal system in the chick revealed by an isotype-specific anti-beta-tubulin monoclonal antibody.

Moor, H., K. Pfenninger, and K. Akert (1969). *Science* 164:1405–1407. Synaptic vesicles in electron micrographs of freeze etched nerve terminals.

Moore, B. W. (1972). *Int. Rev. Neurobiol.* 15:215–225. Chemistry and biology of two proteins, S-100 and 14-3-2, specific to the nervous system.

Moore, B. W., and V. J. Perez (1968). Specific acidic proteins of the nervous system, pp. 343–360. In *Physiological and Biochemical Aspects of Nervous Integration* (F. D. Carlson, ed.), Prentice-Hall, Englewood Cliffs, New Jersey.

Moore, K. E., and O. T. Phillipson (1975). *J. Neurochem.* 25:289–294. Effects of dexamethasone on phenylethanolamine *N*-methyltransferase and adrenaline in the brains and superior cervical ganglia of adult and neonatal rats.

Moore, R. Y., and M. E. Bernstein (1989). *J. Neurosci.* 9:2151–2162. Synaptogenesis in the rat suprachiasmatic nucleus demonstrated by electron microscopy and synapsin I immunoreactivity.

Moore, R. Y., A. Bjorklund, and U. Stenevi (1971). *Brain Res.* 33:13–35. Plastic changes in the adrenergic innervation of the rat septal area in response to denervation.

Moore, R. Y., A. Bjorklund, and U. Stenevi (1973). Growth and plasticity of adrenergic neurons, pp. 961–977. In *The Neurosciences, Third Study Program* (F. O. Schmitt, ed.), MIT Press, Cambridge.

Moorman, S. J., and R. I. Hume (1990). *J. Neurosci.* 10:3158–3163. Growth cones of chick sympathetic preganglionic neurons *in vitro* with other neurons in a cell-specific manner.

Moos, M., R. Tacke, H. Scherer, D. Teplow, K. Früh and M. Schachner (1988). *Nature* 334:701–703. Neural adhesion molecule L1 as a member of the immunoglobulin superfamily with binding domains similar to fibronectin.

Mora, J. O., J. Clement, N. Christiansen, N. Ortiz, L. Vuori, M. Wagner, and M. G. Herrera (1978). The effects of nutritional supplementation and early home stimulation on child development, pp. 132–153. In *The Jonxis Lectures: Growth and development of the full-term and premature infant*, Vol. 1. Excerpta medica, Amsterdam.

Mora, J. O., J. Clement, N. Christiansen, N. Ortiz, L. Vuori, and M. Wagner (1979). Nutritional supplementation, early stimulation and child development, pp. 255–269. In Brozek, *Proc. Int. Nutr. Conf. Behavioral Effects of Energy and Protein Deficits*, NIH Publ. No. 79-106.

Morales, M., and E. Fifková (1989). *J. Comp. Neurol.* 279:666–674. *In situ* localization of myosin and actin in dendritic spines with the immunogold technique.

Moran, D. J. (1976). *J. Exp. Zool* 198:409–416. A scanning electron microscopic and flame spectrometry study on the role of Ca^{2+} in amphibian neurulation using papaverine inhibition and ionophore induction of morphogenetic movement.

Moran, D. J., and R. W. Rice (1976). *Nature* 261:497–499. Action of papaverine and ionophore A 23187 on neurulation.

Moran, D. T., and J. C. Rowley III (1974). *Brain Res.* 74:373–377. Cytoplasmic order in an invertebrate neuron.

Morest, D. K. (1968). *Z. Anat. Entwicklungsgesch.* 127:201–220. The growth of synaptic endings in the mammalian brain: A study of the calyces of the trapezoid body.

Morest, D. K. (1969a). *Z. Anat. Entwicklungsgesch.* 128:271–289. The differentiation of cerebral dendrites: A study of the post-migratory neuroblast in the medial trapezoid body.

Morest, D. K. (1969b). *Z. Anat. Entwicklungsgesch.* 128:290–317. The growth of dendrites in the mammalian brain.

Morest, D. K. (1970a). *Z. Anat. Entwicklungsgesch.* 130:265–305. A study of neurogenesis in the forebrain of opossum pouch young.

Morest, D. K. (1970b). *Z. Anat. Entwicklungsgesch.* 131:45–67. The pattern of neurogenesis in the retina of the cat.

Morest, D. K. (1971). *Z. Anat. Entwicklungsgesch.* 133:216–246. Dendrodendritic synapses of cells that have axons: The fine structure of the Golgi type II cell in the medial geniculate body of the cat.

Morest, D. K. (1981). The Golgi methods, pp. 124–138. In *Techniques in Neuroanatomical Research* (C. Heym, and W. G. Forssmann, eds.), Springer, Berlin.

Morest, D. K., and R. R. Morest (1966). *Am. J. Anat.* 118:811–832. Perfusion-fixation of the brain with chrome-osmium solutions for the rapid Golgi method.

Morgan, M. J., J. M. O'Donnell, and R. F. Oliver (1973). *J. Comp. Neurol.* 149:203–214. Development of left-right asymmetry in the habenular nuclei of *Rana temporaria*.

Morgan, T. H. (1905). *J. Exp. Zool.* 2:495–506. Polarity considered as a phenomenon of gradation of materials.

Morgane, P. J., M. S. Jacobs, and W. L. McFarland (1980). *Brain Res. Bull.* 5:Suppl. 3. The anatomy of the brain of the bottlenose dolphin (*Tursiops truncatus*). Surface configurations of the telencephalon of the bottlenose dolphin with comparative anatomical observations in four other Cetacean species.

Morgane, P. J., M. S. Jacobs, and A. Galaburda (1985). *Brain Behav. Evol.* 26:176–184. Conservative features of neocortical evolution in dolphin brain.

Mori, H., Y. Komiya, and M. Kurokawa (1979). *J. Cell Biol.* 82:174–184. Slowly migrating axonal polypeptides. Inequalities in their rate and amount of transport between two branches of bifurcating axons.

Mori, K., S. C. Fujita, Y. Watanabe, and K. Obata (1987). *Proc. Natl. Acad. Sci. U.S.A.* 84:3921–3925. Telencephalic-specific antigen identified by monoclonal antibody.

Mori, S., and C. P. Leblond (1969). *J. Comp. Neurol.* 135:57–80. Identification of microglia in light and electron microscopy.

Morrell, J. I., D. B. Kelley, and D. W. Pfaff (1975). Sex steroid binding in the brains of vertebrates, pp. 230–256. In *Brain-Endocrine Interaction II. The Ventricular System* (K. M. Knigge, and D. E. Scott, eds.), S. Karger AG, Basel.

Morris, D. G. (1978). *J. Neurophysiol.* 41:1450–1465. Development of functional motor innervation in supernumerary hindlimbs of the chick embryo.

Morris, G. M., and M. Solursh (1978a). *J. Embryol. Exp. Morphol.* 46:37–52. Regional differences in mesenchymal cell morphology and glycosaminoglycans in early neural-fold stage rat embryos.

Morris, G. M., and M. Solursh (1978b). *Zoon* 6:33–38. The role of primary mesenchyme in normal and abnormal morphogenesis of mammalian neural folds.

Morris-Kay, G. M, F. Tuckett, and M. Solursh (1986). *J. Embryol. Exp. Morphol.* 98:59–70. The effects of *Streptomyces* hyaluronidase on tissue organization and cell cycle time in rat embryos.

Morris, J. E. (1979). *Exp. Cell Res.* 120:141–153. Steric exclusion of cells. A mechanism of glycosaminoglycan induced cell aggregation.

Morris, J. M. (1953). *Amer. J. Obstet. Gynecol.* 65:1192. The syndrome of testicular feminization in male pseudo-hermaphroditism.

Morris, J. R., and R. J. Lasek (1984). *J. Cell Biol.* 92:192–198. Stable polymers of the axonal cytoskeleton: the axoplasmic ghost.

Morris, R. (1985). *J. Neurocytol.* 7:133–160. *Thy-1* in developing nervous tissue.

Morris, V. B. (1973). *J. Comp. Neurol.* 151:323–330. Time differences in the formation of the receptor types in the developing chick retina.

Morris, V. B. (1975). *J. Comp. Neurol.* 164:95–104. Non-randomness in the sequential formation of principal cones in small areas of the developing chick retina.

Morrison, J. H., and S. L. Foote (1986). *J. Comp. Neurol.* 243:117–138. Noradrenergic and serotoninergic innervation of cortical, thalamic, and tectal visual structures in old and new world monkeys.

Morrison, J. H., R. Grzanna, M. E. Molliver, and J. T. Coyle (1978). *J. Comp. Neurol.* 181:17–40. The distribution and orientation of noradrenergic fibers in neocortex of the rat: An immunofluorescence study.

Morrison, J. H., S. L. Foote, M. E. Molliver, F. E. Bloom, and H. G. W. Lidov (1982). *Proc. Natl. Acad. Sci. U.S.A.* 79:2401–2405. Noradrenergic and serotonergic fibers innervate complementary layers in monkey primary visual cortex: An immunohistochemical study.

Morrison-Graham, K. (1983). *Dev. Biol.* 99:298–311. An anatomical and electrophysiological study of synapse elimination at the developing frog neuromuscular junction.

Morrison, L. R. (1932). *Arch. Neurol. Psychiat.* 28:204–205. Role of oligodendroglia in myelogenesis.

Morrison, R. S. (1987). *J. Neurosci. Res.* 17:99–101. Fibroblast growth factors: Potential neurotrophic agents in the central nervous system.

Morrison, R. S., A. Sharma, J. DeVellis, and R. A. Bradshaw (1986). *Proc. Natl. Acad. Sci. U.S.A.* 83:7537–7541. Basic fibroblast growth factor supports the survival of cerebral cortical neurons in primary cultures.

Morriss, G. M., and M. Solursh (1978a). *J. Embryol. Exp. Morphol.* 46:37–52. Regional differences in mesenchymal cell morphology and glycosaminoglycans in early neural-fold stage rat embryos.

Morriss, G. M., and M. Solursh (1978b). *Zoon* 6:33–38. The role of primary mesenchyme in normal and abnormal morphogenesis of mammalian neural folds.

Morriss-Kay, G. M., F. Tuckett, and M. Solursh (1986). *J. Embryol. Exp. Morph.* 98:59–70. The effects of *Streptomyces* hyaluronidase on tissue organization and cell cycle time in rat embryos.

Morriss-Kay, G. M. (1983). *J. Physiol. (London)* 345:52P. The effect of cytochalasin-D on structure and function of microfilament bundles during cranial neural tube formation in cultured rat embryos.

Moscona, A., and H. Moscona (1952). *J. Anat.* 86:287–301.

Dissociation and aggregation of cells from organ rudiments of the early chick embryos.

Moscona, A. A. (1956). *Proc. Soc. Exp. Biol. Med.* **92**:410–416. Development of heterotypic combinations of dissociated embryonic chick cells.

Moscona, A. A. (1957). *Proc. Natl. Acad. Sci. U.S.A.* **43**:184–194. The development *in vitro* of chimeric aggregates of dissociated embryonic chick and mouse cells.

Moscona, A. A. (1962). *J. Cell Comp. Physiol.* **60**:Suppl. 65–80. Analysis of cell recombinations in experimental synthesis of tissues *in vitro*.

Moscona, A. A. (1968). *Dev. Biol.* **18**:250–277. Cell aggregation properties of specific cell ligands and their role in the formation of multicellular systems.

Moscona, A. A. (1974). Surface specification of embryonic cells: Lectin receptors, cell recognition and specific ligands, pp. 69–99. In *The Cell Surface in Development* (A. A. Moscona, ed.), Wiley, New York.

Moscona A. A., and R. Piddington (1966). *Biochim. Biophys. Acta* **121**:409–411. Stimulation by hydrocortisone of premature changes in the developmental pattern of glutamine synthetase in embryonic retina.

Moscona, A. A., and R. Piddington (1967). *Science* **158**:496–497. Enzyme induction by corticosteroids in embryonic cells: Steroid structure and inductive effect.

Moscona, M., N. Frenkel, and A. A. Moscona (1972). *Dev. Biol.* **28**:229–241. Regulatory mechanisms in the induction of glutamine synthetase in the embryonic retina: Immunochemical studies.

Moshkov, D. A., L. L. Petrovskaia, and A. G. Bragin (1977). *Dokl. Akad. Nauk. SSSR* **237**:1525–1528. Post-tetanic changes in the ultrastructure of the giant spinal synapses in hippocampal field CA3.

Moshkov, D. A., L. L. Petrovskaia, and A. G. Bragin (1980). *Tsitologiya.* **22**:20–26. Ultrastructural study of the bases of postsynaptic potentiation in hippocampal sections by the freeze-substitution method.

Moss, F. P., and C. P. Leblond (1971). *Anat. Rec.* **170**:421–436. Satellite cells as the source of nuclei in muscles of growing rats.

Mott, F. W. (1894). *J. Physiol., (London)* **15**:464–487. The sensory motor functions of the central convolutions of the cerebral cortex.

Mott, F. W., and C. S. Sherrington (1895). *Proc. Roy. Soc. (London) Ser. B.* **57**:481–488. Experiments upon the influence of sensory nerves upon movement and nutrition of the limbs. Preliminary communication.

Mottet, K. (1952). *J. Comp. Neurol.* **96**:519–553. The effect of removal of somatopleur on the development of motor and sensory neurons in the spinal cord and ganglia.

Mottet, K., and D. H. Barron (1954). *Yale J. Biol. Med.* **26**:275–284. Some effects of the peripheral field on the cytochemical differentiation of neurons.

Moulton, J. M., A. Jurand, and H. Fox (1968). *J. Embryol. Exp. Morphol.* **19**:415–431. A cytological study of Mauthner's cells in *Xenopus laevis* and *Rana temporaria* during metamorphosis.

Mountcastle, V. B. (1957). *J. Neurophysiol.* **20**:408–432. Modality and topographic properties of single neurons of cat's somatic sensory cortex.

Mountcastle, V. B. (1974). Neural mechanisms in somesthesia, pp. 307–347. In *Medical Physiology*, Vol. 1, (V. B. Mountcastle, ed.), Mosby, St. Louis.

Mountcastle, V. B. (1979). An organising principle for cerebral function: The unit module and the distributed system, pp. 21–42. In *Neuroscience: Fourth Study Program* (F. O. Schmidt, and F. G. Worden, eds.), MIT Press, Cambridge.

Moussa, T. A. (1955–1956). *Cellule* **57**: 321–334. An experimental study of the effect of axon sectioning on the cytoplasmic components of the corresponding neurones.

Movshon, J. A., and R. C. Van Sluyters (1981). *Ann. Rev. Psychol.* **32**:477–522. Visual neural development.

Mower, G. D., D. Berry, J. L. Burchfiel, and F. H. Duffy (1981). *Brain Res.* **220**:255–267. Comparison of the effects of dark rearing and binocular suture on development and plasticity of cat visual cortex.

Mower, G. D., C. J. Caplan, W. G. Christen, and F. Duffy (1985). *J. Comp. Neurol.* **235**:448–466. Dark rearing prolongs physiological but not anatomical plasticity of the cat visual cortex.

Mugnaini, E. (1969). Maturation of nerve cell populations and establishment of synaptic connections in the cerebellar cortex of the chick, pp. 749–782. In *Neurobiology of Cerebellar Evolution and Development* (R. Llinas, ed.), American Medical Association, Chicago.

Mugnaini, E. (1983). *J. Comp. Neurol.* **220**:7–15. The length of cerebellar parallel fibers in chicken and rhesus monkey.

Mugnaini, E., and J. I. Morgan (1987). *Proc. Natl. Acad. Sci. U.S.A.* **84**:8692–8696. The neuropeptide cerebellin is a marker for two similar neuronal circuits in rat brain.

Mugnaini, E., A. S. Berrebi, A.-L. Dahl, and J. I. Morgan (1987). *Arch. Ital. Biol.* **126**:41–67. The polypeptide PEP-19 is a marker for Purkinje neurons in cerebellar cortex and cartwheel neurons in the dorsal cochlear nucleus.

Mullen, R. J. (1975). *Nature* **258**:528–530. Two new types of retinal degeneration in cerebellar mutant mice.

Mullen, R. J. (1977). *Nature* **270**:245–247. Site of *pcd* gene action and Purkinje cell mosaicism in cerebella of chimaeric mice.

Mullen, R. J. (1978a). Genetic dissection of the CNS with mutant-normal mouse and rat chimeras, pp. 47–65. In *Society for Neuroscience, Symposium 2.* (W. M. Cowan, and J. A. Ferrendelli, eds.) Bethesda: Society for Neuroscience.

Mullen, R. J. (1978b). Mosaicism in the central nervous system of mouse chimeras, pp. 83–101. In *The Clonal Basis of Development* (S. Subtelny, and I. M. Sussex, eds.), Academic Press, New York.

Mullen, R. J. (1982). Analysis of CNS development with mutant mice and chimeras, pp. 183–193. In *Genetic Approaches to Developmental Neurobiology*, (Y. Tsukada, ed.), Springer-Verlag, Berlin, Heidelberg, New York.

Mullen, R. J., and K. Herrup (1979). Chimeric analysis of mouse cerebellar mutants, pp. 173–196. In *Neurogenetics: Genetic Approaches to the Nervous System* (X. O. Breakefield, ed.), Elsevier, New York.

Mullen, R. J., and M. M. LaVail (1975). *Nature* **258**:528–530. Two new types of retinal degeneration in cerebellar mutant mice.

Mullen, R. J., E. M. Eicher, and R. L. Sidman (1976). *Proc. Natl. Acad. Sci. U.S.A* **73**:208–212. Purkinje cell degeneration, a new neurological mutation in the mouse.

Muller, K., and G. Gerisch (1978). *Nature* **274**:445–449. A specific glycoprotein as the target site of adhesion blocking Fab in aggregating *Dictyostelium* cells.

Munchnick, N., and E. Hibbard (1980). *Exp. Neurol.* 68:205–216. Avian retinal ganglion cells resistant to degeneration after optic nerve lesion.

Munger, B. L. (1965). *J. Cell Biol.* 26:79–97. The intraepidermal innervation of the snout skin of the opossum: A light and electronmicroscope study, with observations on the nature of Merkel's Tastzellen.

Munk, H. (1890). *Über die Functionen der Grosshirnrinde: Gesammelte Mitteilungen mit Anmerkungen*, 2nd edn. Berlin, Hirschwald.

Munoz-Garcia, D., and S. K. Ludwin (1985). *J. Neuroimmunol.* 8:237–254. Intermediate glial cells and reactive astrocytes revisited.

Munoz-Garcia, D., and S. K. Ludwin (1986a). *J. Neurocytol.* 15:273–290. Gliogenesis in organotypic tissue culture of the spinal cord of the embryonic mouse. I. Immunocytochemical and ultrastructural studies.

Munoz-Garcia, D., and S. K. Ludwin (1986b). *J. Neurocytol.* 15:291–302. Gliogenesis in organotypic tissue culture of the spinal cord of the embryonic mouse. II. Autoradiographic studies.

Muñoz-Martínez, E. J., R. Núñez, and A. Sanderson (1981). *J. Neurobiol.* 12:15–26. Axonal transport: A quantitative study of retained and transported protein fraction in the cat.

Munro, M., and F. H. C. Crick (1971). *Symp. Soc. Exp. Biol.* 25:439–453. The time needed to set up a gradient: Detailed calculations.

Munson, R. (1971). *Phil. Sci.* 38:200–215. Biological adaptation.

Munson, R. (1972). *Phil. Sci.* 39:529–532. Biological adaptation: A reply.

Muntz, W. R. A. (1962a). *J. Neurophysiol.* 25:699–711. Microelectrode recordings from the diencephalon of the frog, *(Rana pipiens)* and a blue sensitive system.

Muntz, W. R. A. (1962b). *J. Neurophysiol.* 25:712–720. Effectiveness of different colors of light in releasing the positive phototactic behavior of frogs, and a possible function of the retinal projection to the diencephalon.

Murabe, Y., and Y. Sano (1982a). *Cell Tiss. Res.* 223:493–506. Morphological studies on neuroglia. V. microglial cells in the cerebral cortex of the rat with special reference to their possible involvement in synaptic function.

Murabe, Y., and Y. Sano (1982b). *Cell Tissue Res.* 225:464–485. Morphological studies on neuroglia. VI. Postnatal development of microglial cells.

Murphey, R. K., B. Mendenhall, J. Palka, and J. S. Edwards (1975). *J. Comp. Neurol.* 159:407–418. Deafferentation slows the growth of specific dendrites of identified giant interneurons.

Murphy, C., and C. Tokunaga (1970). *J. Exp. Zool.* 175:197–220. Cell lineage in the dorsal mesothoracic disc of *Drosophila*.

Murphy, R. A., N. J. Pantazis, B. G. W. Arnason, and M. Young (1975). *Proc. Natl. Acad. Sci. U.S.A.* 72:1895–1898. Secretion of a nerve growth factor by mouse neuroblastoma cells in culture.

...hy, S., and J. Rudge (1985). *Dev. Brain Res.* 21:73–81. ...lycoprotein composition and turnover in subcellular ...ctions from the cerebral cortex of normal and reeler ...tant mice.

..., T. H., R. L. Schnaar, and J. T. Coyle (1990). *FASEB J.* ...624–1633. Immature cortical neurons are uniquely sensitive to glutamate toxicity by inhibition of cystine uptake.

Murray, B. A., J. J. Hemperly, W. J. Gallin, J. S. MacGregor, and G. M. Edelman (1984). *Proc. Natl. Acad. Sci. U.S.A.* 81:5584–5588. Isolation of cDNA clones for the chicken neural cell adhesion molecule (N-CAM).

Murray, C. D. (1926a). *J. Gen. Physiol.* 9:835–841. The physiological principle of minimum work applied to the angle of branching of arteries.

Murray, C. D. (1926b). *Proc. Natl. Acad. Sci. U.S.A.* 12:207–214. The physiological principle of minimum work. I. The vascular system and the cost of blood volume.

Murray, G. R. (1920). *Br. Med. J.* 1:359–360. The life history of the first case of myxoedema treated by thyroid extract.

Murray, H. M., and B. E. Walker (1973). *Exp. Neurol.* 41:290–302. Comparative study of astrocytes and mononuclear leukocytes reacting to brain trauma in mice.

Murray, J. G., and J. W. Thompson (1957). *J. Physiol. (London)* 135:133–162. The occurrence and function of collateral sprouting in the sympathetic nervous system of the cat.

Murray, M. (1968). *Exp. Neurol.* 20:460–468. Effects of dehydration on the rate of proliferation of hypothalamic neuroglia cells.

Murray, M. (1982). *J. Comp. Neurol.* 209:352–362. A quantitative study of regenerative sprouting by optic axons in goldfish.

Murray, M., and M. E. Goldberger (1974). *J. Comp. Neurol.* 158:19–36. Restitution of function and collateral sprouting in the cat spinal cord: The partially hemisected animal.

Murray, M. A., and N. Robbins (1982). *Neuroscience* 7:1823–1833. Cell proliferation in denervated muscle: Identity and origin of dividing cells.

Murray, M. R. (1959). *Prog. Neurobiol.* 4:201–221. Factors bearing on myelin formation *in vitro*. The biology of myelin.

Murray, M. R. (1965). Nervous tissue *in vitro*. In *Cells and Tissues in Culture* (E. D. Wilmer, ed.), Academic Press, New York.

Murray, M. R., and H. H. Benitez (1967). *Science* 155:1021–1024. Deuterium oxide: Direct action on sympathetic ganglia isolated in culture.

Murray, M. R., and H. H. Benitez (1968). Action of heavy water (D_2O) on growth and development of isolated nervous tissues, pp. 148–178. In *Ciba Foundation Symposium on Growth of the Nervous System* (G. E. W. Wolstenholme, and M. O'Connor, eds.), Little, Brown and Company, Boston.

Murray, R. G. (1973). The ultrastructure of taste buds, pp. 1–81. In *The Ultrastructure of Sensory Organs* (I. Friedmann, ed.), Elsevier, New York.

Murray, R. G. (1986). *J. Ultrastruct. Mol. Struct. Res.* 95:175–188. The mammalian taste bud type III cell: A critical analysis.

Murthy, A. S., and M. Flavin (1983). *Eur. J. Biochem.* 137:37–46. Microtubule assembly using microtubule-associated protein MAP-2 prepared in defined states of phosphorylation with protein kinase and phosphatase.

Muthukkaruppan, V. (1966). *J. Exp. Zool.* 159:269–288. Inductive tissue interaction in the development of the mouse lens *in vitro*.

Myers, M. W., R. A. Lazzarini, V. M.-Y. Lee, W. W.

Schlaepfer, and D. L. Nelson (1987). *EMBO J.* 6:1617–1626. The human mid-size neurofilament subunit: A repeated protein sequence and the relationship of its gene to the intermediate filament gene family.

Myslivecek, J. (1968). *Brain Res.* 10:418–430. The development of the response to light flash in the visual cortex of the dog.

Nabeshima, S., R. S. Reese, and M. D. Landis (1975). *J. Comp. Neurol.* 164:127–170. Junction of meninges and marginal glia.

Naegele, J. R., and C. J. Barnstable (1989). *Trends Neurosci.* 12:28–34. Molecular determinants of GABAergic local-circuit neurons in visual cortex.

Naess, O., E. Haug, A. Attramadel, A. Aakvaag, V. Hansson, and F. French (1976). *Endocrinology* 99:1295–1303. Androgen receptors in the anterior pituitary and central nervous system of the androgen "insensitive" (Tfm) rat: Correlation between receptor binding and effects of androgens on gonadotropin secretion.

Nafstad, P. H. J. (1986). *J. Anat. (London)* 145:25–33. On the avian Merkel cells.

Nafstad, P. H. J., and R. E. Baker (1973). *Z. Zellforsch* 139:451–462. Comparative ultrastructural study of normal and grafted skin in the frog, *Rana pipiens*, with special reference to neuroepithelial connections.

Naftolin, F., K. J. Ryan, and Z. Petro (1971a). *J. Clin. Endocrinol.* 33:368–370. Aromatization of androstenedione by the diencephalon.

Naftolin, F., K. J. Ryan, and Z. Petro (1971b). *J. Endocrinol.* 51:797–796. Aromatization of androstenedione by the limbic system tissue from human foetuses.

Naftolin, F., K. J. Ryan, and Z. Petro (1972). *Endocrinol.* 90:295–298. Aromatization of androstenedione by the anterior hypothalamus of adult male and female rats.

Naftolin, F., K. J. Ryan, I. J. Davies, V. V. Reddy, F. Flores, Z. Petro, and M. Kuhn (1975). *Rec. Prog. Horm. Res.* 31:295–319. The formation of estrogens by central neuroendocrine tissues.

Nagafuchi, A., Y. Shirayoshi, K. Okazaki, K. Yasuda, and M. Takeichi (1987). *Nature* 329:341–343. Transformation of cell adhesion properties by exogenously introduced E-cadherin cDNA.

Nagajski, D. J., S. C. Guthrie, C. C. Ford, and A. E. Warner (1989). *Development* 105:747–752. The correlation between patterns of dye transfer through gap junctions and future developmental fate in *Xenopus*: The consequences of u.v. irradiation and lithium treatment.

Nagel, E. (1961). *The Structure of Science*. Routledge and Kegan Paul, London.

Nagel, E. (1965). Types of causal explanation in science, pp. 11–26. In *Cause and Effect* (D. Lerner, ed.), Free Press, New York.

Nagele, R. G., and H.-Y. Lee (1987). *J. Exp. Zool.* 241:197–205. Studies on the mechanisms of neurulation in the chick: Morphometric analysis of the relationship between regional variations in cell shape and sites of motive force generation.

Nageotte, J. (1907). Cited in Ramón y Cajal (1928) *Degeneration and Regeneration in the Nervous System*, p. 429.

Nageotte, J. (1910). *C. R. Soc. Biol. (Paris)* 68:1068–1069. Phénomènes de sécrétion dans le protoplasma des cellules névrogliques de la substance grise.

Nageotte, J. (1918). See Ramon y Cajal, S., 1933, p. 310.

Nagy, A. R., and P. Witkovsky (1981). *J. Neurocytol.* 10:897–919. A freeze-fracture study of synaptogenesis in the distal retina of larval *Xenopus*.

Naidoo, S., T. Valcana, and P. S. Timiras (1978). *Amer. Zool.* 18:545–552. Thyroid hormone receptors in the developing rat brain.

Nairn, J. G., K. S. Bedi, T. M. Mayhew, and L. F. Campbell (1989). *J. Comp. Neurol.* 290:527–532. On the number of Purkinje cells in the human cerebellum: Unbiased estimates obtained by using the "fractionator."

Naismith, A. L., E. Hoffman-Chudzik, L.-C. Tsui, and J. R. Riordan (1985). *Nucleic Acids Res.* 13:7413–7425. Study of the expression of myelin proteolipid protein (lipophilin) using a cloned complementary DNA.

Naito, J. (1989). *J. Comp. Neurol.* 284:174–186. Retinogeniculate projection fibers in the monkey optic nerve: A demonstration of the fiber pathways by retrograde axonal transport of WGA-HRP.

Naka, K.-I. (1964). *J. Gen. Physiol.* 47:1003–1022. Electrophysiology of the fetal spinal cord. I. Action potentials of the motoneuron.

Nakai, J. (1956). *Am. J. Anat.* 99:81–130. Dissociated dorsal root ganglia in tissue culture.

Nakai, J. (1960). *Z. Zellforsch. Mikrosk. Anat.* 52:427–449. Studies on the mechanism determining the course of nerve fibres in tissue culture. II. The mechanism of fasciculation.

Nakai, J. (1965). *Texas Rep. Biol. Med.* 23:Suppl. 371–375. Tridimensional nerve formation *in vitro*.

Nakai, J. (1969). *J. Exp. Zool.* 170:85–106. The development of neuromuscular junctions in cultures of chick embryo tissue.

Nakai, J., and Y. Kawasaki (1959). *Z. Zellforsch. Mikroskop. Anat.* 51:108–122. Studies on the mechanism determining the course of nerve fibers in tissue culture. I. The reaction of the growth cone to various obstructions.

Nakajima, S. (1965). *J. Comp. Neurol.* 125:193–205. Selectivity in fasciculation of nerve fibres *in vitro*.

Nakamura, H., and D. D. M. O'Leary (1989). *J. Neurosci.* 9:3776–3795. Inaccuracies in initial growth and arborization of chick retinotectal axons followed by course corrections and axon remodeling to develop topographic order.

Nakamura, O., and S. Toivonen (1978). *Organizer—a Milestone of Half-Century from Spemann*, Elsevier/North-Holland, Amsterdam.

Nakao, T., and A. Ishizawa (1984). *Am. J. Anat.* 170:55–71. Light and electron neuroscopic observations of the tail bud of the larval lamprey (*Lampetra japonica*), with special reference to neural tube formation.

Nakatsuji, N., and K. E. Johnson (1982). *Cell Motil.* 2:149–161. Cell locomotion *in vitro* by *Xenopus laevis* gastrula mesodermal cells.

Nakazawa, S. (1959). *Naturwissen* 46:333–334. General mechanism of the polarity determination in some fucoid eggs.

Nansen, F. (1887). *The Structure and Combination of the Histological Elements in the Central Nervous System*. Bergen.

Narayanan, C. H., and Y. Narayanan (1978a). *J. Embryol. Exp. Morphol.* 43:85–105. Determination of the embryonic origin of the mesencephalic nucleus of the trigeminal nerve in birds.

Narayanan, C. H., and Y. Narayanan (1978b). *J. Embryol. Exp. Morphol.* 44:53–70. Neuronal adjustments in developing nuclear centers of the chick embryo following transplantation of an additional optic primordium.

Narayanan, C. H., and Y. Narayanan (1978c). *J. Embryol. Exp. Morphol.* 47:137–148. On the origin of the ciliary ganglion in birds studied by the method of interspecific transplantation of embryonic brain regions.

Narayanan, C. H., and Y. Narayanan (1980). *Anat. Rec.* 196:71–82. Neural crest and placodal contributions in the development of the glossopharyngeal-vagal complex in the chick.

Nass, M. M. K. (1969). *Science* 165:25–35. Mitochondrial DNA: Advances, problems and goals.

Nastuk, W. L., W. D. Niemi, J. T. Alexander, H. W. Change, and M. A. Nastuk (1979). *Ann. J. Physiol.* 236:C53–57. Myasthenia in frogs immunized against cholinergic-receptor protein.

Nathanson, N., G. A. Cole, and H. Van der Loos (1969). *Brain Res.* 15:532–536. Heterotopic cerebellar granule cells following administration of cyclophosphamide to suckling rats.

Natyzak, L. H. D., and J. D. Laskin (1984). *Cancer Res.* 44:4607–4614. Effects of the tumor promoter 12-o-tetradecanoylphorbol-13-acetate on neurite outgrowth from chick embryo sensory ganglia.

Nauta, W. J. H. (1950). *Arch. Neurol. Psychiat.* 66:353–376. Über die sogenannte terminale Degeneration im Zentralnervensystem und ihre Darstellung durch silberimprägnation.

Nauta, W. J. H. (1957). Silver impregnation of degenerating axons. In *New Research Techniques of Neuroanatomy* (W. F. Windle, ed.), Thomas, Springfield, Illinois.

Navascués, J., L. Rodriguez-Gallardo, G. Martin-Partido, and I. S. Alvarez (1985). *Anat. Embryol.* 172:19–31. Proliferation of glial precursors during the early development of the chick optic nerve.

Navascués, J., G. Martín-Partido, I. S. Alvarez, and L. Rodríguez-Gallardo (1988). *J. Comp. Neurol.* 278:34–46. Cell death in suboptic necrotic centers of chick embryo diencephalon and their topographic relationship with the earliest optic fiber fascicles.

Nave, K.-A., C. Lai, F. E. Bloom, and R. J. Milner (1986). *Proc. Natl. Acad. Sci. U.S.A.* 83:9264–9268. Jimpy mutant mouse: A 74 base deletion in the mRNA for myelin proteolipid protein and evidence for a primary defect in RNA splicing.

Navone, F., R. Jahn, G. DiGioia, H. Stukenbrok, P. Greengard, and P. DeCamilli (1986). *J. Cell Biol.* 103:2511–2527. Protein-p38: An integral membrane protein specific for small vesicles of neurons and neuroendocrine cells.

Nawar, G. (1956). *Am. J. Anat.* 99:473–506. Experimental analsis of the origin of the autonomic ganglia in the chick embryo.

Neal, H. V. (1918). *J. Morphol.* 10:293–315. Neuromeres and metameres.

Neder, R. (1959). *Zool. Jahrb. Abt. Anat. Ontog. Tiere* 77:411–464. Allometrisches Wachstum von Hirnteilen bei drei verschieden grossen Schabenarten.

Needham, J. (1931). *Chemical Embryology*, 3 Vols. Macmillan, New York; Cambridge Univ. Press, Cambridge.

Needham, J. (1942). *Biochemistry and Morphogenesis.* Cambridge Univ. Press, London, 758 pp.

Needham, J. (1954–1956). *Science and Civilization In China.* Vol. 1. *Introductory orientations.* Vol. 2. *History of Scientific Thought.* Cambridge Univ. Press, Cambridge.

Needham, J. (1970). The roles of Europe and China in the evolution of oecumenical science, pp. 396–418. In *Clerks and Craftsmen in China and the West.* Cambridge Univ. Press, Cambridge.

Nellhaus, G. (1968). *Pediatrics* 41:106–114. Head circumference from birth to eighteen years.

Nelson, E., K. Blinzinger, and H. Hager (1961). *Neurol.* 11:285–295. Electron microscopic observations on subarachnoid and perivascular spaces of the Syrian hamster brain.

Nelson, R. B., D. J. Linden, C. Hyman, K. H. Pfenninger, and A. Routtenberg (1989). *J. Neurosci.* 9:381–389. The two major phosphoproteins in growth cones are probably identical to two protein kinase C substrates correlated with persistence of long-term potentiation.

Nes, N. (1966). *Nord Vet. Med.* 18:19. Testikulaer feminiseniz has storfe.

Neubuerger, K. T. (1970). Carl Weigert, pp. 388–391. In *The Founders of Neurology*, 2nd edn., (W. Haymaker, and F. Schiller, eds.), Thomas, Springfield, Illinois.

Neuburger, M. (1897). *Die historische Entwickelung der experimentellen Gehirn und Rückenmarksphysiologie vor Flourens.* Enke, Stuttgart.

Neufeld, G., D. Gospodarowicz, L. Dodge, and D. K. Fuji (1987). *J. Cell Physiol.* 131:131–140. Heparin modulation of the neurotrophic effects of acidic and basic fibroblast growth factors and nerve growth factors on PC12 cells.

Neugebauer, K. M., K. J. Tomaselli, J. Lilien, and L. F. Reichardt (1988). *J. Cell Biol.* 107:1177–1187. N-cadherin, NCAM and integrins promote retinal neurite outgrowth on astrocytes *in vitro*.

Neumayer, L. (1906). *Histogenese und Morphogenese des peripheren Nervensystems, der Spinalganglien und des Nervus sympathicus*, Vol. 2, Part 3, pp. 513–626. In Handbuch der vergleichenden und experimentellen Entwickelungslehre der Wirbeltiere. Oskar Hertwig, editor, Gustav Fischer Verlag, Jena.

Neurath, O. (1932). *Erkenntnis* 3:206. Protokollsätze.

New, H. V., and A. W. Mudge (1986a). *Dev. Biol.* 116:337–346. Distribution and ontogeny of SP, CGRP, SOM, and VIP chick sensory and sympathetic ganglia.

New, H. V., and A. W. Mudge (1986b). *Nature* 323:809–811. Calcitonin gene-related peptide regulates muscle acetylcholine receptor synthesis.

Newgreen, D. (1984). *Cell Tiss. Res.* 236:265–277. Spreading of explants of embryonic chick mesenchymes and epithelia on fibronectin and laminin.

Newgreen, D., and J. P. Thiery (1980). *Cell Tissue Res.* 221:269–291. Fibronectin in early avian embryos: Synthesis and distribution along migration pathways of neural crest cells.

Newgreen, D. F. (1989). *Dev. Biol.* 131:136–148. Physical influence on neural crest cell migration in avian embryos: Contact guidance and spatial restriction.

Newgreen, D. F., and C. A. Erickson (1986). *Int. Rev. Cytol.* 103:89–145. The migration of neural crest cells.

Newgreen, D. F. and D. Gooday (1985). *Cell Tiss. Res.* 239:329–336. Control of the onset of migration of neural crest cells in avian embryos: Role of Ca^{++}-dependent cell adhesions.

Newgreen, D. F., I. L. Gibbins, J. Sauter, B. Wallenfels and R. Wütz (1982). *Cell Tiss. Res.* 221:521–549. Ultrastructural and tissue-culture studies on the role of fibronectin, collagen and glycosaminoglycans in the migration of neural crest cells in the fowl embryo.

Newman, E. A. (1986). *Science* 233:453–454. High potassium conductance in astrocyte endfeet.

Newman, S., K. Kitamura, and A. T. Campognoni (1987). *Proc. Natl. Acad. Sci. U.S.A.* 84:886–890. Identification of a cDNA coding for a fifth form of myelin basic protein in mouse.

Ng, A. Y. K., and J. Stone (1982). *Dev. Brain Res.* 5:263–271. The optic nerve of the cat: Appearance and loss of axons during normal development.

Nicholas, J. S. (1924). *J. Exp. Zool.* 39:27–41. Ventral and dorsal implantations of the limb bud in *Amblystoma punctatum*.

Nicholas, J. S. (1930a). *Anat. Rec.* 45:234. Movements in transplanted limbs innervated by eye muscle nerves.

Nicholas, J. S. (1933). *J. Comp. Neurol.* 57:253–283. The correlation of movement and nerve supply in transplanted limbs of *Amblystoma*.

Nicholas, J. S. (1957). *Proc. Natl. Acad. Sci. U.S.A.* 43:542–545. Results of inversion of neural plate material.

Nicholls, J. G., and D. A. Baylor (1968). *J. Neurophysiol.* 31:740–756. Specific modalities and receptive fields of sensory neurons in CNS of the leech.

Nichols, D. H. (1981). *J. Embryol. Exp. Morph.* 64:105–120. Neural crest formation in the head of the mouse embryo as observed using a new histological technique.

Nichols, D. H. (1986). *Am. J. Anat.* 176:19–31. Mesenchyme formation from the trigeminal placodes of the mouse embryo.

Nicholson, J. L., and J. Altman (1972a). *Brain Res.* 44:13–23. The effects of early hypo- and hyperthyroidism on the development of rat cerebellar cortex. I. Cell proliferation and differentiation.

Nicholson, J. L., and J. Altman (1972b). *Brain Res.* 44:25–36. The effects of early hypo- and hyperthyroidism on the development of rat cerebellar cortex. II. Synaptogenesis in the molecular layer.

Nicholson, J. L., and J. Altman (1972c). *Science N.Y.* 176:530–532. Synaptogenesis in rat cerebellum: Effects of early hypo- and hyperthyroidism.

Nicklas, R. B. (1987). Chromosomes and kinetochores do more in mitosis than previously thought. In *Chromosome Structure and Function: The Impact of New Concepts (18th Stadler Genetics Symposium)*, J. P. Gustafson, R. Appels, and R. J. Kaufman, eds.), Plenum, New York.

Nicklas, R. B. (1988). *A. Rev. Biophys. Biophys. Chem.* 17:431–449. The forces that move chromosomes in mitosis.

Nicoll, R. A. (1988). *Science* 241:545–551. The coupling of neurotransmitters to ion channels in the brain.

Nieuwenhuys, R. (1964). *Prog. Brain Res.* 25:1–93. Comparative anatomy of the cerebellum.

Nieuwenhuys, R. (1974). *J. Comp. Neurol.* 156:255–276. Topological analysis of the brain stem: A general introduction.

Nieuwenhuys, R., J. G. Veening, and P. Van Domburg (1988/89). *Acta Morphol. Neerl.-Scand.* 26:131–163. Core and paracores: Some new chemoarchitectural entities in the mammalian neuraxis.

Nieuwkoop, P. D. (1952). *J. Exp. Zool.* 120:1–130. Activation and organization of the amphibian central nervous system.

Nieuwkoop, P. D. (1955). *Proc. Koninkl. Ned. Adak. Wetenschap.* 58:219–239; 356–370. Origin and establishment of organization patterns in embryonic fields during early development in amphibians and birds especially in the nervous system and its substrate.

Nieuwkoop, P. D. (1962). *Acta Biotheoret.* 16:57–68. The "organization centre." I. Induction and determination.

Nieuwkoop, P. D. (1967a). *Acta Biotheoret.* 17:151–177. The "organization centre." II. Field phenomena, their origin and significance.

Nieuwkoop, P. D. (1967b). *Acta Biotheoret.* 17:178–194. The "organization centre." III. Segregation and pattern formation in morphogenetic fields.

Nieuwkoop, P. D. (1969). *Wilhelm Roux Arch.* 162:341–373. The formation of mesoderm in urodelan amphibians. I. Induction by the endoderm.

Nieuwkoop, P. D. (1973). *Adv. Morphog.* 10:1–39. The "organization center" of the amphibian embryo: Its origin, spatial organization, and morphogenetic action.

Nieuwkoop, P. D. (1977). *Curr. Top. Dev. Biol.* 11: 115–132. Origin and establishment of embryonic polar axes in amphibian development.

Nieuwkoop, P. D. (1985). *J. Embryol. Exp. Morphol.* 89:Suppl. 333–347. Inductive interactions in early amphibian development and their general nature.

Nieuwkoop, P. D., and J. Faber (1967). *Normal Table of Xenopus Laevis (Daudin)*, 2nd edn., Elsevier/North-Holland, Amsterdam.

Nieuwkoop, P. D., A. G. Johnen, and B. Albers (1985). *The Epigenetic Nature of Early Chordate Development.* Cambridge University Press.

Niklowitz, W., and I. J. Bak (1965) *Z. Zellforsch. Mikroskop. Anat.* 66:529–547. Elektronenmikroskopische Untersuchungen am Ammonshorn.

Nilaver, G., R. Defendini, E. A. Zimmerman, M. C. Beinfeld, and T. L. O'Donohue (1982). *Nature* 295:597–598. Motilin in the Purkinje cell of the cerebellum.

Nilsson, I., and C.-H. Berthold (1988). *J. Anat. (London)* 156:71–96. Axon classes and internodal growth in the ventral spinal root L7 of adult and developing cats.

Nishida, H., and N. Satoh (1983). *Dev. Biol.* 99:382–394. Cell lineage analysis in ascidian embryos by intracellular injection of a tracer enzyme. I. Up to the eight cell stage.

Nishida, H., T. Kuwaki, and H. Sakai (1981). *J. Biochem. Tokyo* 90:575–578. Phosphorylation of microtubule associated proteins (MAPs) and pH of the medium control interaction between MAPs and actin filaments.

Nishizuka, M., and Y. Arai (1981). *Brain Res.* 212:31–38. Sexual dimorphism in synaptic organization in the amygdala and its dependence on neonatal hormone environment.

Nishizuka, Y. (1988). *Nature* 334:661–665. The molecular heterogeneity of protein kinase C and its implications for cellular regulation.

Nissl, F. (1892). *Allgem. Z. Psychiat.* 48:197–198. Über die Veränderungen der Ganglienzellen am Facialiskern des Kaninchens nach Ausreissung der Nerven.

Nissl, F. (1894). *Neurol. Centralbl.* 13:676–685, 781–789, 810–814. Ueber die sogenannten Granula der Nervenzellen.

Nissl, F. (1894). *Neurol. Centralbl.* 13:507–508. Ueber eine neue Untersuchungsmethode des Centralorgans speciell zur Feststellung der Localisation der Nervenzellen.

Nissl, F. (1903). *Die Neuronlehre und ihre Anhänger.* Fischer, Jena.

Nissley, S. P., and M. M. Rechler (1984). Insulin-like growth factors: Biosynthesis, receptors and carrier proteins, pp. 128–203. In *Hormonal Proteins and Peptides,* Vol. 12, (C. H. Li, ed.), Academic, New York.

Nixdorf, B., and H.-J. Bischof (1987). *Brain Res.* 405:326–336. Ultrastructural effects of monocular deprivation in the neuropil of nucleus rotundus in the zebra finch: A quantitative electron microscopic study.

Nixon, R. A., B. A Brown, and C. A. Marotta (1982). *J. Cell Biol.* 94:150–158. Posttranslational modification of a neurofilament protein during axoplasmic transport: Implications for regional specialization of CNS axons.

Nja, A., and D. Purves (1977). *J. Physiol. (London)* 264:565–583. Specific innervation of guinea pig superior cervical ganglion cells by preganglionic fibres arising from different levels of the spinal cord.

Njolstad, P. R., A. Molven, I. Hordvik, J. Apold, and A. Fjose (1988). *Nucl. Acids Res.* 16:9097–9111. Primary structure, developmentally regulated expression and potential duplication of the zebrafish homeobox gene ZF-21.

Noakes, P. G., and M. R. Bennett (1987). *J. Comp. Neurol.* 259:330–347. Growth of axons into developing muscles of the chick forelimb is preceded by cells that stain with Schwann cell antibodies.

Noakes, P. G., A. W. Everett, and M. R. Bennett (1986). *J. Comp. Neurol.* 246:245–256. The growth of muscle nerves in relation to the formation of primary myotubes in the developing chick forelimb.

Noback, C. R., and M. L. Moss (1956). *J. Comp. Neurol.* 117:291–308. Postnatal ontogenesis of neurons in cat neocortex.

Noble, M., and K. Murray (1984). *EMBO J.* 3:2243–2247. Purified astrocytes promote the *in vitro* division of a bipotential progenitor cell.

Noble, M., K. Murray, P. Stroobant, M. D. Waterfield, and P. Riddle (1988). *Nature* 333:560–562. Platelet derived growth factor promotes division and motility and inhibits premature differentiation of the oligodendrocyte/type 2 astrocyte progenitor cell.

Noble, R.G. (1973). *Horm. Behav.* 4:45–52. The effects of castration at different intervals after birth on the copulatory behavior of male hamsters *(Mesocricetus auratus).*

Noden, D. M. (1978a). *Dev. Biol.* 67:296–312. The control of avian cephalic neural crest cyto-differentiation. I. Skeletal and connective tissue.

Noden, D. M. (1978b). *Dev. Biol.* 67:313–329. The control of avian cephalic neural crest cytodifferentiation. II. Neural tissues.

Noden, D. M. (1983). *Dev. Biol.* 96:144–165. The role of the neural crest in patterning of avian cranial skeletal, connective and muscle tissues.

Noden, D. M. (1986). *J. Craniofacial Genetics Dev. Biol. Supp.* 2:15–31. Origins and patterning of craniofacial mesenchymal tissues.

Noden, D. M. (1988). *Development* 103 suppl:121–140. Interactions and fates of avian craniofacial mesenchyme.

Noell, W. K., and R. Albrecht (1971). *Science* 172:76–80. Irreversible effects of visible light on the retina: Role of vitamin A.

Noell, W. K., V. S. Walker, B. S. Kang, and S. Berman (1966). *Invest. Ophthal.* 5:450–473. Retinal damage by light in rats.

Noetzel, H., and J. Rox (1964) *Acta Neuropathol.* 3:326–342. Autoradiographische Untersuchungen über Zellteilung und Zellentwicklung im Gehirn der erwachsenen Maus und der erwachsenen Rhesus-affen nach Injektion von radioaktiven Thymidin.

Noguchi, T. (1988). *Prog. Neurobiol.* 31:149–170. Brain development in dwarf mice.

Nolte, A. (1953). *Zool. Jahrb. Abt. Allgem. Zool. Physiol. Tiere* 64:538–594. Die Abhängigkeit des Proportionierung und Cytoarchitektonik des Gehirns von der Körpergrösse bei Urodelen.

Nomura, K., M. Uchida, H. Kageura, K. Shiokawa, and K. Yamana (1986). *Dev. Growth and Differ.* 28:311–319. Cell to cell adhesion systems in *Xenopus laevis,* the South African clawed frog. I. Detection of Ca^{2+}-dependent and independent adhesions systems in adult and embryonic cells.

Nomura, S., K. Itoh, T. Sugimoto, Y. Yasui, H. Kamiya, and N. Mizuno (1986). *J. Comp. Neurol.* 253:121–133. Mystacial vibrissae representation within the trigeminal sensory nuclei of the cat.

Nonidez, J. F. (1944). *Biol. Rev.* 19:30–40. The present status of the neurone theory.

Nordeen, E. J., and K. W. Nordeen (1988). *J. Neurosci.* 8:2869–2874. Sex and regional differences in the incorporation of neurons born during song learning in zebra finches.

Nordeen, E. J., K. W. Nordeen, D. R. Sengelaub, and A. P. Arnold (1985). *Science* 229:671–673. Androgens prevent normally occurring cell death in a sexually dimorphic spinal nucleus.

Nordeen, E. J., K. W. Nordeen, and A. P. Arnold (1987). *J. Comp. Neurol.* 259:393–399. Sexual differentiation of androgen accumulation within the zebra finch brain through selective cell loss and addition.

Nordenskiöld, E. (1928). *The History of Biology.* Knopf, New York.

Nordling, S., H. Mietinen, J. Wartiovaara, and L. Saxén (1971). *J. Embryol. Exp. Morphol.* 26:231–252. Transmission and spread of embryonic induction. I. Temporal relationships in transfilter induction of kidney tubules *in vitro.*

Nordquist, D. T., C. A. Kozak, and H. T. Orr (1988). *J. Neurosci.* 8:4780–4789. cDNA cloning and characterization of three genes uniquely expressed in cerebellum by Purkinje neurons.

Norenberg, M. D. (1979). *J. Histochem. Cytochem.* 27:756–762. The distribution of glutamine synthetase in the rat central nervous system.

Norenberg, M. D., K. Dutt, and L. Reif-Lehrer (1980). *J. Cell Biol.* 84:803–807. Glutamine synthetase localization in cortisol induced chick embryo retinas.

Norman, M. G. (1986). *J. Neuropathol. Exp. Neurol.* 45:222–232. The growth and development of microvasculature in human cerebral cortex.

Norman, R. M. (1966). *Dev. Med. Child Neurol.* 8:170–177. Neuropathological findings in trisomies 13–15 and 17–18 with special reference to the cerebellum.

Normand, G., J. Clos, F. Vitiello, and G. Gombos (1989). *Int. J. Dev. Neurosci.* 7:323–328. Developing rat cerebellum. I. Effects of abnormal thyroid states and undernutrition on sulfated glycosaminoglycans.

Nornes, H. O., and M. Carry (1978). *Brain Res.* **159**:1–16. Neurogenesis in spinal cord of mouse: An autoradiographic analysis.

Nornes, H. O., and G. D. Das (1974). *Brain Res.* **73**:121–138. Temporal pattern of neurogenesis in spinal cord of rat. I. An autoradiographic study—time and sites of origin and migration and settling patterns of neuroblasts.

Nornes, H. O., and M. Morita (1979). *Dev. Neurosci.* **2**:101–114. Time of origin of the neurons in the caudal brain stem of rat.

Norr, S. C. (1973). *Dev. Biol.* **34**:16–38. *In vitro* analysis of sympathetic neuron differentiation from chick neural crest cells.

Norr, S. C., and S. Varon (1975). *Neurobiol.* **5**:101–118. Dynamic, temperature-sensitive association of 125I-nerve growth factor *in vitro* wih ganglionic and non-ganglionic cells from embryonic chick.

Nörstrom, A., H. A. Hansson, and J. Sjöstrand (1971). *Z. Zellforsch. Mikrosk. Anat.* **113**:271–293. Effects of colchicine on axonal transport and ultrastructure of the hypothalamoneurohypophyseal system of the rat.

Northcutt, R. G. (1981). *Ann. Rev. Neurosci.* **4**:301–350. Evolution of the telencephalon in nonmammals.

Norton, W. T. (1976). Formation, structure, and biochemistry of myelin, pp. 74–99. In *Basic Neurochemistry*, 2nd edn., (G. J. Siegel, R. W. Albers, R. Katzman, and B. W. Agranoff, eds.), Little, Brown and Company, Boston.

Norton, W. T., and W. Cammer (1984). Isolation and characterization of myelin, pp. 147–180. In *Myelin* (P. Morell, ed.), Plenum, New York.

Norton, W. T., and M. Farooq (1989). *J. Neurosci.* **9**:769–775. Astrocytes cultured from mature brain derive from glial precursor cells.

Norton, W. T., and S. E. Poduslo (1970). *Science* **167**:1144–1146. Neuronal soma and whole neuroglia of rat brain: A new isolation technique.

Norton, W. T., and S. E. Poduslo (1973). *J. Neurochem.* **21**:759–773. Myelination in rat brain: Changes in myelin composition during brain maturation.

Nottebohm, F. (1969). *Ibis* **111**:386–387. The "critical period" for song learning.

Nottebohm, F. (1970). *Science* **167**:950–956. Ontogeny of bird song.

Nottebohm, F. (1977). Asymmetries in neural control of vocalization in the canary, pp. 23–45. In *Lateralization in the Nervous System* (S. Harnard, R. W. Doty, L. Goldstein, J. Jaynes, and G. Krauthamer, eds.), Academic Press, New York.

Nottebohm, F. (1981). *Trends Neurosci.* **4**:104–106. Laterality, seasons and space govern the learning of a motor skill.

Nottebohm, F., T. M. Stokes, and C. M. Leonard (1976). *J. Comp. Neurol.* **165**:457–486. Central control of song in the canary (*Serinus canarius*).

Nousek-Goebl, N. A., and M. F. Press (1986). *Dev. Brain Res.* **30**:67–73. Golgi-electron microscopic study of sprouting endothelial cells in the neonatal rat cerebellar cortex.

Novéková, V., J. Pilny, W. Sandritter, and G. Kiefer (1968). Changes in nucleic acids of the central nervous system neuron in the postnatal ontogenesis of the rat, pp. 285–289. In *Ontogenesis of the Brain*, (L. Jílek, and S. Trojan, eds.), Charles Univ. Press, Prague.

Novelli, A., J. A. Reilly, P. G. Lysko, and R. C. Henneberry (1988). *Brain Res.* **451**:205–212. Glutamate becomes neurotoxic via the N-methyl-d-aspartate receptor when intracellular energy levels are reduced.

Nowakowski, R. S. (1984). *J. Neurogenet.* **1**:249–258. The mode of inheritance of a defect in lamination in the hippocampus of BALB/c mice.

Nowakowski, R. S., and P. Rakic (1974). *Cell Tiss. Kinet.* **7**:189–194. Clearance rate of exogenous 3H-thymidine from the plasma of rhesus monkey.

Nowakowski, R. S., and P. Rakic (1981). *J. Comp. Neurol.* **196**:129–154. The site of origin and route and rate of migration of neurons to the hippocampal region of the rhesus monkey.

Nuccitelli, R. (1983). *Mod. Cell Biol.* **2**:451–481. Transcellular ion currents: Signals and effectors of cell polarity.

Nunez, J. (1984). *Mol. Cell. Endocrinol.* **37**:125–132. Effects of thyroid hormones during brain differentiation.

Nunez, J. (1985). *Neurochem. Int.* **7**:959–968. Microtubules and brain development: The effects of thyroid hormone.

Nunez, J. (1986). *Dev. Neurosci.* **8**:125–141. Differential expression of microtubule components during brain development.

Nurcombe, V., P. A. McGrath, and M. R. Bennett (1981). *Neurosci. Lett.* **27**:249–254. Postnatal death of motor neurons during the development of brachial spinal cord of the rat.

Nurnberger, J. I., and M. W. Gordon (1957). The cell density of neural tissues: Direct counting method and possible applications as a biologic referent, pp. 100–128. In *Progress in Neurobiology* (H. Waelsch, ed.), Hoeber, New York.

Nurse, C. A., L. Macintyre, and J. Diamond (1984a). *Neuroscience* **11**:521–533. A quantitative study of the time course of the reduction in Merkel cell number within denervated rat touch domes.

Nurse, C. A., L. Macintyre, and J. Diamond (1984b). *Neuroscience* **13**:563–571. Reinnervation of the rat touch dome restores the Merkel cell population reduced after denervation.

Nurse, P. (1985). *Trends Genet.* **1**:51–55. Cell cycle control genes in yeast.

Nussbaum, J. L., N. Neskovic, and P. Mandel (1971). *J. Neurochem.* **18**:1529–1543. The fatty acid composition of phospholipids and glycolipids in Jimpy mouse brain.

Nüsslein-Volhard, C. and E. Wieschaus (1980). *Nature* **287**:795–801. Mutations affecting segment number and polarity in *Drosophila*.

Nüsslein-Volhard, C., C. Frohnhöfer, and R. Lehmann (1987). *Science* **238**:1675–1681. Determination of anteroposterior polarity in *Drosophila*.

Nuttall, R. P., and P. P. Zinsmeister (1983). *Cell Motil.* **3**:307–320. Differential response to contact during embryonic nerve-nonnerve cell interactions.

Nyholm, M., S. Saxen, S. Toivonen, and T. Vainio (1962) *Exp. Cell Res.* **28**:209–212. Electron microscopy of trans-filter neural induction.

Oakley, B. (1967). *J. Physiol. (Lond.)* **188**:353–371. Altered temperature and taste responses from cross-regenerated sensory nerves in the rat's tongue.

Oakley, B. (1970). *Acta Physiol. Scand.* **79**:88–94. Reformation of taste buds by crossed sensory nerves in the rat's tongue.

Oakley, B. (1974a). *Brain Res.* **75**:85–96. On the specification of taste neurons in the rat tongue.

Oakley, B. (1974b). Problems in the development of taste

receptor properties and synaptic connections, pp. 319–329. In *Transduction Mechanisms in Taste* (T. M. Pointer, ed.), Retrieval, Ltd., London.

Oakley, B., L. B. Jones, and M. A. Hosley (1980). *Brain Res.* **194**:213–218. The effect of nerve stump length upon mammalian taste responses.

Oakley, B., J. S. Chu, and L. B. Jones (1981). *Brain Res.* **221**:289–298. Axonal transport maintains taste responses.

Obar, R. A., C. A. Colins, J. A. Hammarback, H. S. Shpetner, and R. B. Vallee (1990). *Nature* **347**:256–261. Molecular cloning of the microtubule-associated mechanochemical enzyme dynamin reveals homology with a new family of GTP-binding proteins.

Obersteiner, H. (1883). *Biol. Zentralbl.* **3**:145–155. Der feinere Bau der Kleinhirnrinde beim Menschen und bei Tieren.

O'Brien, R. A. D. (1981). *J. Physiol. (London)* **371**:89–90. A difference in transmitter release between surviving and non-surviving nerve terminals in developing rat skeletal muscles.

O'Brien, R. A. D., A. J. Ostberg, and G. Vrbova (1978). *J. Physiol.* **282**:571–582. Observations on the elimination of polyneuronal innervation in developing mammalian skeletal muscle.

O'Brien, R. A. D., A. J. Ostberg, and G. Vrbová (1980). *Neuroscience* **5**:1367–1379. The effect of acetylcholine on the function and structure of the developing mammalian neuromuscular junction.

O'Brien, R. A. D., A. J. C. Ostberg, and G. Vrbova (1984). *Neuroscience* **12**:637–646. Protease inhibitors reduce the loss of nerve terminals induced by activity and calcium in developing rat soleus muscles *in vitro*.

Ochs, S. (1971a). *J. Neurobiol.* **2**:331–345. Characteristics and a model for fast axoplasmic transport in nerve.

Ochs, S. (1971b). *Proc. Natl. Acad. Sci. U.S.A.* **68**:1279–1282. Local supply of energy to the fast axoplasmic transport mechanism.

Ochs, S. (1972a). *Science* **176**:252–260. Fast transport of materials in mammalian nerve fibers.

Ochs, S. (1972b). *J. Physiol. (Lond.)* **227**:627–645. Rate of fast axoplasmic transport in mammalian nerve fibres.

Ochs, S. (1973). *Prog. Brain Res.* **40**:349–362. Effect of maturation and aging on the rate of fast axoplasmic transport in mammalian nerve.

Ochs, S. (1975). *J. Physiol.* **253**:459–475. Retention and redistribution of proteins in mammalian nerve fibres by axoplasmic transport.

Ochs, S. (1977). *Med. Hist.* **21**:261–274. The early history of nerve regeneration beginning with Cruikshanks observations in 1776.

Ochs, S. (1981). Axoplasmic transport, pp. 425–444. In *Basic Neurochemistry* (G. J. Siegel, R. W. Albers, B. W. Agranoff, and R. Katzman, eds.), Little, Brown and Co., Boston.

Ochs, S., and D. Hollingsworth (1971). *J. Neurochem.* **18**:107–114. Dependence of fast axoplasmic transport in nerve on oxidative metabolism.

Ochs, S., and C. Smith (1971). *Fed. Proc.* **30**:665. Effect of temperature and rate of stimulation on fast axoplasmic transport in mammalian nerve fibers.

Ochs, S., and C. Smith (1975). *J. Neurobiol.* **6**:85–102. Low temperature slowing and cold-block of fast axoplasmic transport in mammalian nerves *in vitro*.

O'Connor, T. M., and C. R. Wyttenbach (1974). *J. Cell Biol.* **60**:448–459. Cell death in the embryonic chick spinal cord.

Oda, M. A. S., and P. R. Huttenlocher (1974). *Yale J. Biol. Med.* **3**:155–165. The effect of corticosteroids on dendritic development in the rat brain.

O'Dell, D. S., R. Tencer, A. Monroy, and J. Brachet (1974). *Cell Differ.* **3**:193–198. The pattern of concanavalin A-binding sites during the early development of *Xenopus laevis*.

Odenwald, W. F., C. F. Taylor, F. J. Palmer-Hill, V. Friederich, Jr., M. Tani, and R. A. Lazzarini (1987). *Genes Dev.* **1**:482–496. Expression of a homeo domain protein in non-contact-inhibited cultured cells and postmitotic neurons.

Oehmichen, M. (1983). *Prog. Neuropathol.* **5**:277–325. Inflammatory cells in the central nervous system.

O'Farrell, P. H., B. A. Edgar, D. Lakich, and C. F. Lehner (1989). *Science* **246**:635–640. Directing cell division during development.

Ogawa, F. (1934). *Sci. Rep. Tohoku Univ., Fourth Ser.* **8**:345–368. The number of ganglion cells and nerve fibers in the nervous system of the earthworm.

Ogawa, F. (1939). *Sci. Rep. Tohoku Univ., Fourth Ser.* **13**:395–488. The nervous system of earthworm (*Pheretima communissima*) in different ages.

Ogawa, M., T. Ishikawa, and A. Irimajiri (1984). *Nature* **307**:66–68. Adrenal chromaffin cells form functional cholinergic synapses in culture.

Oger, J., B. G. W. Arnason, N. Pantazis, J. Lehrich, and M. Young (1974). *Proc. Natl. Acad. Sci. U.S.A.* **71**:1554–1558. Synthesis of nerve growth factor by L and 3T3 cells in culture.

Oja, S. S. (1966). *Ann. Acad. Sci. Fennicae, Ser. A. V.* **125**:1–67. Postnatal changes in the concentration of nucleic acids, nucleotides and amino acids in the rat brain.

Okabe, S., and N. Hirokawa (1990). *Nature* **343**:479–482. Turnover of fluorescently labelled tubulin and actin in the axon.

Okada, A., S. Furber, N. Okado, S. Homma, and R. W. Oppenheim (1989). *J. Neurobiol.* **20**:219–233. Cell death of motoneurons in the chick embryo spinal cord. X. synapse formation on motoneurons following the reduction of cell death by neuromuscular blockade.

Okada, E., V. Mizuhira, H. Nakamura (1976). *J. Neurol. Sci.* **28**:505–520. Dysmyelination in the sciatic nerves of dystrophic mice.

Okado, N., and R. W. Oppenheim (1985). *J. Neurosci.* **4**:1639–1652. Cell death of motoneurons in the chick embryo spinal cord. IX. The loss of motoneurons following removal of afferent inputs.

Olavarria, J., and R. C. Van Sluyters (1985). *J. Comp. Neurol.* **239**:1–26. Organization and postnatal development of callosal connections in the visual cortex of the rat.

Olavarria, J., R. C. Van Sluyters, and H. P. Killackey (1984). *Brain Res.* **391**:362–368. Evidence for complementary organization of callosal and thalamic connections within rat somatosensory cortex.

Olby, R. C. (1966). *Origins of Mendelism.* Schocken, New York.

Oldfield, R. C., and K. Oldfield, (1951). *Annals of Science* **7**:371–381. Hartley's "Observations on Man".

O'Leary, D. D. M. (1987). Remodelling of early axonal projections through the selective elimination of neurons and long axon collaterals, pp. 113–142. In *Selective Neuronal Death* (G. Bock, and M. O'Connor, eds.), Ciba Foundation Symposium 126, Wiley, Chichester.

O'Leary, D. D. M. (1989). *Trends Neurosci.* **12**:400–406. Do cortical areas emerge from a protocortex?

O'Leary, D. D. M., and W. M. Cowan (1982). *J. Comp. Neurol.* **212**:399–416. Further studies on the development of the isthmo-optic nucleus with special reference to the occurrence and fate of ectopic and ipsilaterally projecting neurons.

O'Leary, D. D. M., and W. M. Cowan (1983). *Proc. Natl. Acad. Sci. U.S.A.* **80**:6131–6135. Topographic organization of certain tectal afferent and efferent connections can develop normally in the absence of retinal input.

O'Leary, D. D. M., and W. M. Cowan (1984). *Dev. Brain Res.* **12**:293–310. Survival of isthmo-optic neurons after early removal of one eye.

O'Leary, D. D. M., and B. B. Stanfield (1985). *Brain Res.* **336**:326–333. Occipital cortical neurons with transient pyramidal tract axons extend and maintain collaterals to subcortical but not intracortical targets.

O'Leary, D. D. M., and B. B. Stanfield (1986). *Dev. Brain Res.* **27**:87–99. A transient pyramidal tract projection from the visual cortex in the hamster and its removal by selective collateral elimination.

O'Leary, D. D. M., and B. B. Stanfield (1989). *J. Neurosci.* **9**:2230–2246. Selective elimination of axons extended by developing cortical neurons is dependent on regional locale: Experiments utilizing fetal cortical transplants.

O'Leary, D. D. M., B. B. Stanfield, and W. M. Cowan (1981). *Dev. Brain Res.* **1**:607–617. Evidence that the early postnatal restriction of the cells of origin of the callosal projection is due to the elimination of axonal collaterals rather than to the death of neurons.

O'Leary, D. D. M., C. R. Gerffen, and W. M. Cowan (1983). *Dev. Brain Res.* **10**:93–109. The development and restriction of the ipsilateral retinofugal projection in the chick.

O'Leary, D. D. M., J. W. Fawcett, and M. Cowan (1986). *J. Neurosci.* **6**:3692–3705. Topographic targeting errors in the retinocollicular projection and their elimination by selective ganglion cell death.

O'Leary, J. L. (1941). *J. Comp. Neurol.* **75**:131–161. A structure of area striata of the cat.

O'Leary, J. L., J. Imukai, and J. M. Smith (1971). *J. Comp. Neurol.* **142**:377–391. Histogenesis of the cerebellar climbing fiber in the rat.

Olek, A. J., P. A. Pudimat, and M. P. Daniels (1983). *Cell* **34**:255–264. Direct observation of the rapid aggregation of acetylcholine receptors on identified cultured myotubes after exposure to embryonic brain extract.

Olmsted, J. B. (1986). *Ann. Rev. Cell Biol.* **2**:421–457. Microtubule-associated proteins.

Olmsted, J. B., G. B. Witman, K. Carlson, and J. L. Rosenbaum (1974). *Proc. Natl. Acad. Sci. U.S.A.* **68**:2273–2277. Comparison of the microtubule proteins of neuroblastoma cells, brain, and *Chlamydomonas* flagella.

Olmsted, J. B., C. F. Asnes, L. M. Parysek, H. D. Lyon, and G. M. Kidder (1986). *Ann. N.Y. Acad. Sci.* **466**:292–305. Distribution of MAP-4 in cells and in adult and developing mouse tissues.

Olmsted, J. M. D. (1920a). *J. Comp. Neurol.* **31**:465–468. The nerve as a formative influence in the development of taste-buds.

Olmsted, J. M. D. (1920b). *J. Exp. Zool.* **31**:369–401. The results of cutting the seventh cranial nerve in *Ameiurus nebulosus* (Lesueur).

Olmsted, J. M. D. (1925). *J. Comp. Neurol.* **33**:149–154. Effects of cutting the lingual nerve of the dog.

Olmsted, J. M. D. (1944). *François Magendie*. Schuman's, New York.

Olmsted, J. M. D. (1946). *Charles-Édouard Brown-Séquard. A Nineteenth Century Neurologist and Endocrinologist.* Johns Hopkins, Baltimore.

Olney, J. W. (1968). *Invest. Ophthal.* **7**:250–268. An electron microscopic study of synapse formation, receptor outer segment development, and other aspects of developing mouse retina.

Olpe, H.-R., and B. S. McEwen (1976). *Brain Res.* **105**:121–128. Glucocorticoid binding to receptor-like proteins in rat brain and pituitary: Ontogenetic and experimentally induced changes.

Olson, C. B., and C. P. Swett, Jr. (1966). *J. Comp. Neurol.* **128**:475–497. A functional and histochemical characterization of motor units in a heterogeneous muscle (flexor digitorum longus) of the cat.

Olson, C. B., and C. P. Swett, Jr. (1969). *Arch. Neurol.* **20**:263–270. Speed of contraction of skeletal muscle. The effect of hypoactivity and hyperactivity.

Olson, C. R., and R. D. Freeman (1975). *J. Neurophysiol.* **38**:26–32. Progressive changes in kitten striate cortex during monocular vision.

Olson, L., and T. Malmfors (1970). *Acta Physiol. Scand.* **348**:Suppl. 1–112. Growth characteristics of adrenergic nerves in the adult rat. Fluorescence, histochemical and ^{3}H-noradrenaline uptake studies using tissue transplantation to the anterior chamber of the eye.

Olsson, Y., and J. Sjöstrand (1969). *Exp. Neurol.* **23**:102–112. Origin of macrophages in Wallerian degeneration of peripheral nerves demonstrated autoradiographically.

O'Malley, B. W. (1969). *Trans. N.Y. Acad. Sci.* **31**:478–503. Hormonal regulation of nucleic acid and protein synthesis.

O'Malley, B. W., and A. R. Means (1974). *Science* **183**:610–620. Female steroid hormones and target cell nuclei.

Omlin, F. X., H. deF. Webster, C. G. Paklovitz, and S. R. Cohen (1982). *J. Cell Biol.* **95**:242–248. Immunocytochemical localization of basic protein in major dense line regions of central and peripheral myelin.

Onteniente, B., N. Konig, J. Sievers, S. Jenner, H. P. Klemm, and R. Marty (1980). *Anat. Embryol.* **159**:245–256. Structural and biochemical changes in rat cerebral cortex after neonatal 6-hydroxydopamine administration.

Opalski, A. (1933). *Z. Ges. Neurol. Psychiat.* **149**:221–254. Ueber lokale Unterschiede im Bau der Ventrikelwände beim Menschen.

Oppel, A. (1913). *Zentr. Zool. allgem. exp. Biol.* **3**:209–232. Explantation (Deckglaskultur, *in vitro*-Kultur).

Oppenheim, R. W. (1981a). *J. Neurosci.* **1**:141–151. Cell death of motoneurons in the chick embryo spinal cord. V. Evidence on the role of cell death and neuromuscular function in the formation of specific peripheral connections.

Oppenheim, R. W. (1981b). Neuronal cell death and some related regressive phenomena during neurogenesis: A selective historical review and progress report, pp. 74–133. In *Studies in Developmental Neurobiology: Essays in Honor of Viktor Hamburger* (W. M. Cowan, ed.), Oxford Univ. Press, Oxford.

Oppenheim, R. W. (1984). *Dev. Biol.* **101**:35–39. Cell death of motoneurons in the chick embryo spinal cord. VIII. Motoneurons prevented from dying in the embryo persist after hatching.

Oppenheim, R. W. (1986). *J. Comp. Neurol.* **246**:281–286. The absence of significant postnatal motoneuron death in the brachial and lumbar spinal cord of the rat.

Oppenheim, R. W. (1989). *Trends Neurosci.* **12**:252–255. The neurotrophic theory and naturally occurring motoneuron death.

Oppenheim, R. W., and M. B. Heaton (1975). *Brain Res.* **98**:291–302. The retrograde transport of horseradish peroxidase from the developing limb of the chick embryo.

Oppenheim, R. W., and L. J. Haverkamp (1988). Neurotrophic interactions in the development of spinal cord motoneurons, pp. 152–171. In *Plasticity of the Neuromuscular System* Vol. 138, (D. Evered, and J. Whelan, eds.), Wiley, Chichester.

Oppenheim, R. W., and J. L. Maderdrut (1981). *Neurosci. Soc. Abst.* **7**:291. Pharmacological modulation of neuromuscular transmission and cell death in the lateral motor column of the chick embryo.

Oppenheim, R. W., and R. Nunez (1982). *Nature* **295**:57–59. Electrical stimulation of hindlimb increases neuronal cell death in chick embryo.

Oppenheim, R. W., I.-W. Chu-Wang, and R. F. Foelix (1975). *J. Comp. Neurol.* **161**:383–418. Some aspects of synaptogenesis in the spinal cord of the chick embryo: A quantitative electron microscopic study.

Oppenheim, R. W., I.-W. Chu-Wang, and J. L. Maderdrut (1978). *J. Comp. Neurol.* **177**:87–112. Cell death of motoneurons in the chick embryo spinal cord. III. The differentiation of motoneurons prior to their induced degeneration following limb removal.

Oppenheim, R. W., J. L. Maderdrut, and D. J. Wells (1982a). *J. Comp. Neurol.* **210**:174–189. Cell death of motoneurons in the chick embryo spinal cord. VI. Reduction of naturally occurring cell death in the thoracolumbar column of Terni by nerve growth factor.

Oppenheim, R. W., J. L. Maderdrut, and D. Wells (1982b). *Dev. Brain Res.* **3**:134–139. Reduction of naturally occurring growth factor and hemicholimium-3.

Oppenheim, R. W., L. Houenou, M. Pincon-Raymond, J. A. Powell, F. Rieger, and L. J. Standish (1986). *Dev. Biol.* **114**:426–436. The development of motoneurons in the embryonic spinal cord of the mouse mutant, muscular dysgenesis (*mdg/mdg*): Survival, morphology and biochemical differentiation.

Oppenheim, R. W., L. Haverkamp, D. Prevette, J. McManaman, and S. Appel (1988). *Science* **240**:919–922. Reduction of naturally occurring motoneuron death *in vivo* by a target-derived neurotrophic factor.

Oppenheim, R. W., T. Cole, and D. Prevette (1989a). *Dev. Biol.* **133**:468–474. Early regional variations in motoneuron numbers arise by differential proliferation in the chick embryo spinal cord.

Oppenheim, R. W., S. Bursztajn, and D. Prevette (1989b). *Development* **107**:331–341. Cell death of motoneurons in the chick embryo spinal cord. XI. Acetylcholine receptors and synaptogenesis in skeletal muscle following the reduction of motoneuron death by neuromuscular blockade.

Oppenheimer, J. M. (1936). *J. Exp. Zool.* **72**:409–437. Trans-

plantation experiments on developing teleosts (*Fundulus and Perca*).

Oppenheimer, J. M. (1941). *J. Comp. Neurol.* **74**:131–167. The anatomical relationships of abnormally located Mauthner's cells in *Fundulus* embryos.

Oppenheimer, J. M. (1942). *J. Comp. Neurol.* **77**:577–587. The decussation of Mauthner's fibers in *Fundulus* embryos.

Oppenheimer, J. M. (1966). *Bull. Hist. Med.* **40**:525–543. Ross Harrison's contributions to experimental embryology.

Oppenheimer, J. M. (1970a). *Bull. Hist. Med.* **44**:241–250. Some diverse backgrounds for Curt Herbst's ideas about embryonic induction.

Oppenheimer, J. M. (1970b). *Bull. Hist. Med.* **44**:378–382. Hans Driesch and the theory and practice of embryonic transplantation.

Oppenheimer, J. M. (1971). *Trans. Stud. Coll. Physic. Philadel., Ser. 4,* **39**:26–33. Historical relationships between tissue culture and transplantation experiments.

O'Rahilly, R., and E.Gardner (1971). *Z. Anat. Entwicklungsgesch.* **134**:1–12. The timing and sequence of events in the development of the human nervous system during the embryonic period proper.

Orbach, H. S., L. B. Cohen, and A. Grinvald (1985). *J. Neurosci.* **5**:1886–1895. Optical mapping of electrical activity in rat somatosensory and visual cortex.

O'Reilly, P. M. R., and M. J. T. Fitzgerald (1985). *J. Anat. (London)* **140**:645–650. Internodal segments in human laryngeal nerves.

O'Rourke, N. A., and S. E. Fraser (1986a). *Dev. Biol.* **114**:265–276. Dynamic aspect of retinotectal map formation revealed by a vital-dye fiber-tracting technique.

O'Rourke, N. A., and S. E. Fraser (1986b). *Dev. Biol.* **114**:277–288. Pattern regulation in the eyebud of *Xenopus* studied with a vital-dye fiber-tracing technique.

Ortiz-Caro, J., B. Yusta, F. Montiel, A. Villa, A. Aranda, and A. Pascual (1986). *Endocrinology* **119**:2163–2167. Identification and characterization of L-triiodothyronine (T3) receptors in cells of glial and neuronal origin.

Ortmann, R. (1943). *Anat. Entwicklungsgesch.* **112**:537–587. Ueber Placoden und Neuralleiste beim Entenembryo, ein Beitrag zum Kopfproblem.

Osborn, H. F. (1929). *From the Greeks to Darwin,* 2nd edn. Charles Scribner's Sons, New York.

O'Shea, K. S. (1981). *Prog. Anat.* **1**:35–60. The cytoskeleton in neurulation: Role of cations.

O'Shea, K. S. (1982). *Birth Defects* **18**:95–106. Calcium and neural tube closure defects: An *in vitro* study.

Osowski, H. E. (1914). *Roux Arch. EntwMech. Organ.* **38**:547–583. Über aktive Zellbewegungen im Explantat von Wirbeltierembryonen.

Ostberg, A. J. C., G. Raisman, P. M. Field, L. L. Iverson, and R. E. Zigmond (1976). *Brain Res.* **107**:445–470. A quantitative comparison of the formation of synapses in the rat superior cervical sympathetic ganglion by its own and foreign nerve fibers.

Ostberg, B. (1956). Missbildungen, Grundzüge der Entwicklung und Fehlentwicklung: Die Formbestimmenden Faktoren, p. 283. In *Handbuch der speziellen pathologischen Anatomie und Histologie,* Vol. 12, Part 4: *Nervensystem* (O. Lubarsch, F. Henke, and R. Rössle, eds.), Springer-Verlag, Berlin.

O'Steen, W. K., and K. V. Andreson (1972). *Z. Zellforsch.*

127:306–313. Photoreceptor degeneration after exposure of rats to incandescent illumination.

Oster-Granite, M. L., and R. M. Hendon (1976). *J. Comp. Neurol.* 169:443–480. The development of the cerebellar cortex of the Syrian hamster *Mesocricetus auratus*. Foliation, cytoarchitectonic, Golgi and electronmicroscopic studies.

Ostrach, L. H., and L. H. Mathers (1979). *J. Comp. Neurol.* 183:415–428. Evidence for a critical period of neuronal tropism late in the development of the chick visual system.

Otsuka, N. (1962). *Z. Zellforsch. Mikrosk. Anat. Abt. Histochem.* 58:33–50. Histologisch-entwicklungsgeschichtliche Untersuchungen an Mauthnerschen Zellen von Fischen.

Otsuka, N. (1964). *Z. Zellforsch. Mikrosk. Anat. Abt. Histochem.* 62:61–71. Weitere vergleichend-anatomische Untersuchungen an Mauthnerschen Zellen von Fischen.

Otte, A. P., C. H. Koster, G. T. Snoek, and A. J. Durston (1988). *Nature* 334:618–620. Protein kinase C mediates neural induction in *Xenopus laevis*.

Otten, U., and H. Thoenen (1976). *Mol. Pharmacol.* 12:353–361. Selective induction of tyrosine hydroxylase and dopamine β-hydroxylase in sympathetic ganglia in organ culture: Role of glucocorticoids as modulators.

Otten, U., and H. Thoenen (1976). *Brain Res.* 111:438–441. Modulatory role of glucocorticoids on NGF-mediated enzyme induction in organ cultures of sympathetic ganglia.

Otten, U., and H. Thoenen (1977). *J. Neurochem.* 29:69–75. Effect of glucocorticoids on nerve growth factor-mediated enzyme induction in organ cultures of rat sympathetic ganglia: Enhanced response and reduced time requirement to initiate enzyme induction.

Otten, U., and M. Towbin (1980). *Brain Res.* 193:304–308. Permissive action of glucocorticoids in induction of tyrosine hydroxylase by nerve growth factor in a pheochromocytoma cell line.

Otten, U. H., and H. P. Lorez (1983). *Neurosci. Lett.* 34:153–158. NGF increases substance P, cholecystokinin and vasoactive intestinal polypeptide immunoreactivities in primary sensory neurons of newborn rats.

Otten, U., M. Goedert, N. Mayer, and F. Lembeck (1980). *Nature* 301:158–159. Requirements of nerve growth factor for development of substances P-containing sensory neurones.

Otto, K. B., and W. Lierse (1970). *Acta Anat.* 77:25–36. Die Kapillarisierung verschiedener Teile des menschlichen Gehirns in der Fetalperiode und in den ersten Lebensjahren.

Ovalle, W. K., and R. S. Smith (1972). *Can. J. Physiol. Pharmacol.* 50:195–202. Histochemical identification of three types of intrafusal muscle fibers in the cat and monkey based on the myosin ATPase reaction.

Owens, G. C., and R. P. Bunge (1989). *Glia* 2:119–128. Evidence for an early role for myelin-associated glycoprotein in the process of myelination.

Owsjannikow, P. (1860). *Müller's Arch. f. Anat. Physiol. und wissensch. Med. Leipzig* pp. 469–477. Ueber die feinere Struktur der Lobi olfactorii der Säugethiere.

Pác. (1984). *Z. Mikrosk. Anat. Forsch Leipzig* 98:36–48. Contribution to ontogenesis of Merkel cells.

Pachter, J. S., and R. K. H. Liem (1984). *Dev. Biol.* 103:200–210. The differential appearance of neurofilament triplet polypeptides in the developing rat optic nerve.

Packard, A., and V. Albergoni (1970). *J. Exp. Biol.* 52:539–552. Relative growth, nucleic acid content and cell numbers of the brain in *Octopus vulgaris* (Lamarck).

Padget, D. H. (1948). *Contrib. Embryol. Carnegie Inst.* 32:207–261. The development of the cranial arteries in the human embryo.

Padget, D. H. (1957). *Contrib. Embryol. Carnegie Inst.* 34:79–140. The development of the cranial venous system in man: From the view point of comparative anatomy.

Pagel, W. (1945). *Bull. Hist. Med.* 18:1–43. The speculative basis of modern pathology.

Paillard, J. (1960). The patterning of skilled movements, pp. 1679–1708. In *Handbook of Physiology, Neurophysiology*, Vol. III (J. Field, H. W. Magoun, and V. E. Hall, eds.), American Physiology Society, Washington, D.C.

Päivärinta, H., and O. Eränkö (1982). *J. Auton. Nerv. Syst.* 5:219–236. Number of neurons and dexamethasone-induced SIF cells in developing sympathetic ganglia and in intraocular ganglion transplants.

Päivärinta, H., S. Soinila, and O. Eränkö (1984). *Int. J. Dev. Neurosci.* 2:557–566. Effect of hydrocortisone on the number of small intensely fluorescent cells in the rat superior cervical ganglion during pre- and postnatal development.

Pakkenberg, H. (1967). *J. Comp. Neurol.* 128:17–20. The number of nerve cells in the cerebral cortex of man.

Pakkenberg, H., and H. J. G. Gundersen (1988). *J. Microsc.* 150:1–20. Total number of neurons and glial cells in human brain nuclei estimated by the disector and the fractionator.

Pakkenberg, H., and J. Voigt (1979). *Acta Anat.* 59:297–307. Brain weight of the Danes.

Palacios-Prü, L. Palacios, and R. V. Mendoza (1981). *J. Submicrosc. Cytol.* 13:145–167. Synaptogenetic mechanisms during chick cerebellar cortex development.

Palade, G. E., and S. L. Palay (1954). *Anat. Record* 118:335–336. Electron microscope observations of interneuronal and neuromuscular synapses.

Palay, S. L. (1956). *J. Biophys. Biochem. Cytol.* 2:193–202. Synapses in the central nervous system.

Palay, S. L. (1958a). An electron microscopical study of neuroglia, pp. 24–49. In *Biology of Neuroglia* (W. F. Windle, ed.), Thomas, Springfield, Ill.

Palay, S. L. (1958b). *Exp. Cell Res.* 5:275–293. The morphology of synapses in the central nervous system.

Palay, S. L. (1961). *Anat. Rec.* 139:262. Structural peculiarities of the neurosecretory cells in the preoptic nucleus of the goldfish, *Carassius auratus*.

Palay, S. L. (1989). *Nature* 341:493–494. The neuroanatomist.

Palay, S. L., and V. Chan-Palay (1974). *Cerebellar cortex. Cytology and organization.* Springer, Berlin.

Palay, S. L., and G. E. Palade (1955). *J. Biophys. Biochem. Cytol.* 1:69–88. The fine structure of neurons.

Palay, S. L., C. Sotelo, A. Peters, and P. M. Orkand (1968). *J. Cell Biol.* 38:193–201. The axon hillock and the initial segment.

Palka, J., and J. S. Edwards (1974). *Proc. Roy. Soc. (London) Ser. B.* 185:105–121. The cerci and abdominal giant fibres of the house cricket, *Acheta domesticus*. II. Regeneration and effects of chronic deprivation.

Palkovits, M., P. Magyar, and J. Szentágothai (1971). *Brain Res.* 32:1–13. Quantitative histological analysis of the cerebellar cortex in the cat. I. Number and arrangement in space of the Purkinje cells.

Pallas, S. L., S. M. Gilmour, and B. L. Finlay (1988). *Dev. Brain Res.* 43:1–11. Control of cell number in the developing neocortex. I. Effects of early tectal ablation.

Palm, S. L., and L. T. Furcht (1983). *J. Cell. Biol.* 96:1218–1226. Production of laminin and fibronectin by Schwannoma cells: Cell-protein interactions *in vitro* and protein localization in peripheral nerve *in vivo*.

Palmatier, M. A., B. K. Hartman, and E. M. Johnson, Jr. (1984). *J. Neurosci.* 4:751–756. Demonstration of retrogradely transported endogenous nerve growth factor in axons of sympathetic neurons.

Palmiter, R. D. (1986). *Ann. Rev. Genet.* 20:465–499. Germline transformation of mice.

Pandazis, G. (1930). *Z. Morphol. Oekol. Tiere* 18:114–169. Über die relative verschiedene Ausbildung der Gehirnzentren bei biologisch verschiedenen Ameisenarten.

Pander, H. C. (1817). *Beiträge zur Entwickelungsgeschichte des Hühnchens im Eye.* Würzburg.

Panem, S. (1989). *Science* 246:1329–1330. The discovery track.

Pannese, E. (1963a). *Z. Zellforsch. Mikroskop. Anat.* 60:711–740. Investigations on the ultrastructural changes of the spinal ganglion neurons in the course of axon regeneration and cell hypertrophy. I. Changes during axon regeneration.

Pannese, E. (1963b). *Z. Zellforsch. Mikroskop. Anat.* 61:561–586. Investigations on the ultrastructural changes of the spinal ganglion neurons in the course of axon regeneration and cell hypertrophy. II. Changes during cell hypertrophy and comparison between the ultrastructure of nerve cells of the same type under different functional conditions.

Pannese, E. (1968). *J. Comp. Neurol.* 132:331–364. Developmental changes of the endoplasmic reticulum and ribosomes in nerve cells of the spinal ganglia of the domestic fowl.

Pannese, E. (1969). *J. Comp. Neurol.* 135:381–422. Electron microscopical study on the development of the satellite cell sheath in spinal ganglia.

Pannese, E. (1974). *Adv. Anat. Embryol. Cell Biol.* 47:6–97. The histogenesis of the spinal ganglia.

Pannese, E. (1976). *Neuropathol. Appl. Neurobiol.* 2:247–267. An electron microscopic study of cell degeneration in chick embryo spinal ganglia.

Pannese, E., L. Luciano, S. Iurato, and E. Reale (1971). *J. Ultrastruct. Res.* 36:46–67. Cholinesterase activity in spinal ganglia neuroblasts: A histochemical study at the electron microscope.

Panov, A. A. (1960). *Dokl. Akad. Nauk SSR* 132:689–692. Origin of neuroblasts, neurilemma cells and neuroglia in the brain of the larva of Antheraea pernid. Guer. (In Russian).

Panov, A. A. (1962). *Dokl. Akad. Nauk SSR Biol. Sci. Sect. (Transl.)* 145:904–907. The nature of cell reproduction in the central nervous system of the house cricket (*G. domesticus.* orthoptera, Insecta).

Papadopoulos, G. C., J. G. Parnavelas, and R. M. Buijs (1989a). *J. Neurocytol.* 18:1–10. Light and electron microscopic immunocytochemical analysis of the noradrenaline innervation of the rat visual cortex.

Papadopoulos, G. C., J. G. Parnavelas, and R. M. Buijs (1989b). *J. Neurocytol.* 18:303–310. Light and electron microscopic immunocytochemical analysis of the dopamine innervation of the rat visual cortex.

Papasozomenos, S. C., and L. I. Binder (1986). *J. Neurosci.* 6:1748–1756. Microtubule-associated protein 2 (MAP2) is present in astrocytes of the optic nerve but absent from astrocytes of the optic tract.

Papasozomenos, S. C., and L. I. Binder (1987). *Cell Moltil. Cytoskel.* 8:210–226. Phosphorylation determines two distinct species of tau in the central nervous system.

Papasozomenos, S. C., L. Autilio-Gambetti, and P. Gambetti (1981). *J. Cell Biol.* 91:866–871. Reorganization of axoplasmic organelles following iminodipropionitrile administration.

Papasozomenos, S. C., L. I. Binder, P. Bender, and M. R. Payne (1985). *J. Cell Biol.* 100:74–85. Microtubule-associated protein 2 within axons of spinal motor neurons: Associations with microtubules and neurofilaments in normal and b,b'-iminoproprionitrile (IDPN)-treated axons.

Pappas, G. D., and M. V. L. Bennett (1966). *Ann. N. Y. Acad. Sci.* 137:495–508. Specialized junctions involved in electrical transmission between neurons.

Pappas, G. D., and D. P. Purpura (1961). *Exp. Neurol.* 4:507–530. Fine structure of dendrites in the superficial neocortical neuropil.

Pappas, G. D., G. Q. Fox, E. B. Masurovsky, E. R. Peterson, and S. M. Crain (1975). Neuronal growth cone relationships and their role in synaptogenesis in the mammalian central nervous system, pp. 163–180. In *Advances in Neurology: Physiology and Pathology of Dendrites* (G. W. Kreutzberg, ed.), Raven Press, New York.

Paradiso, M. A., M. F. Bear, and J. D. Daniels (1983). *Exp. Brain Res.* 51:413–422. Effects of intracortical infusion of 6-hydroxydopamine on the response of kitten visual cortex to monocular deprivation.

Paravicini, U., K. Stoeckel, and H. Thoenen (1975). *Brain Res.* 84:279–291. Biological importance of retrograde axonal transport of nerve growth factor in adrenergic neurons.

Pardanaud, L., C. Altman, P. Kitos, F. Dieterlen-Liévre, and C. A. Buck (1987). *Development* 100:339–349. Vasculogenesis in the early quail blastodisc as studied with a monoclonal antibody recognizing endothelial cells.

Pardee, A. B. (1989). *Science* 246:603–608. G_1 events and regulation of cell proliferation.

Pardee, A. B., R. Dubrow, J. L. Hamlin, and R. F. Kletzien (1978). *Ann. Rev. Biochem.* 47:715–750. Animal cell cycle.

Pardridge, W. M. (1983). *Physiol. Rev.* 63:1481–1535. Brain metabolism: A perspective from the blood-brain barrier.

Pardridge, W. M., and L. J. Mietus (1979a). *J. Clin. Invest.* 64:145–154. Transport of steroid hormones through the rat blood-brain barrier. Primary role of albumin-bound hormone.

Pardridge, W. M., and L. J. Mietus (1979b). *J. Neurochem.* 33:579–581. Regional blood-brain transport of the steroid hormones.

Pardridge, W. M., T. L. Moeller, L. J. Mietus, and W. H. Oldendorf (1980). *Am. J. Physiol.* 239:96–102. Blood-brain barrier transport and brain sequestration of steroid hormones.

Park, C. M., and M. J. Hollenberg (1989). *Dev. Biol.* 134:201–

205. Basic fibroblast growth factor induces retinal regeneration *in vivo*.

Parker, G. H. (1922). *Smell, Taste and Allied Senses in the Vertebrates,* Chap. 6, pp. 110–131. Lippincott Co., Philadelphia.

Parker, G. H. (1929). *Quart. Rev. Biol.* **4**:251–264. The neurofibril hypothesis.

Parker, G. H. (1932). *Am. Naturalist* **66**:147–158. On the trophic impulse so-called, its rate and nature.

Parker, G. H., and V. L. Paine (1934). *Am. J. Anat.* **54**:1–25. Progressive nerve degeneration and its rate in the lateral-line nerve of the catfish.

Parks, T. N. (1979). *J. Comp. Neurol.* **183**:665–678. Afferent influences on the development of the brainstem auditory nuclei of the chicken: Otocyst ablation.

Parks, T. N. (1981). *J. Comp. Neurol.* **202**:47–57. Changes in the length and organization of nucleus laminaris dendrites after unilateral otocyst ablation in chick embryos.

Parks, T. N., and E. W. Rubel (1975). *J. Comp. Neurol.* **164**:435–448. Organization and development of the brain stem auditory nuclei of the chicken: Organization of projections from n. magnocellularis to n. laminaris.

Parks, T. N., D. A. Taylor, and H. Jackson (1990). *J. Neurosci.* **10**:975–984. Adaptations of synaptic form in an aberrant projection to the avian cochlear nucleus.

Parnavelas, J. G. (1978). *Prog. Brain Res.* **48**:247–259. Influence of stimulation on cortical development.

Parnavelas, J. G., and M. E. Blue (1982). *Dev. Brain Res.* **3**:140–144. The role of the noradrenergic system on the formation of synapses in the visual cortex of the rat.

Parnavelas, J. G., and M. E. Cavanagh (1988). *Trends Neurosci.* **11**:92–93. Transient expression of neurotransmitters in the developing neocortex.

Parnavelas, J. G., and S. M. Edmunds (1983). *J. Neurocytol.* **12**:863–871. Further evidence that Retzius-Cajal cells transform to nonpyramidal neurons in the developing rat visual cortex.

Parnavelas, J. G., and G. C. Papadopoulos (1989). *Trends Neurosci.* **12**:315–319. The monoaminergic innervation of the cerebral cortex is not diffuse and nonspecific.

Parnavelas, J. G., A. Globus, and P. Kaups (1973). *Exp. Neurol.* **40**:742–747. Continuous illumination from birth affects spine density of neurons in the visual cortex of the rat.

Parnavelas, J. G., G. Lynch, N. Brecha, C. W. Cotman, and A. Globus (1974). *Nature* **248**:71–73. Spine loss and regrowth in hippocampus following deafferentation.

Parnavelas, J. G., R. Luder, S. G. Pollard, K. Sullivan, and A. R. Lieberman (1983). *Phil. Trans. Roy. Soc. (London) Ser. B.* **301**:55–84. A qualitative and quantitative ultrastructural study of glial cells in the developing visual cortex of the rat.

Partington, J. R. (1937). *A Short History of Chemistry.* Macmillan, London.

Partlow, L. M., and M. G. Larrabee (1969). *Fed. Proc.* **28**:886. Metabolic effects of nerve growth factor on chick sympathetic ganglia *in vitro*. Inhibitory effects of actinomycin-D and cycloheximide.

Partlow, L. M., and N. G. Larrabee (1971). *J. Neurochem.* **18**:2101–2118. Effects of a nerve-growth factor, embryo age and metabolic inhibitors on growth of fibres and on synthesis of ribonucleic acid and protein in embryonic sympathetic ganglia.

Partlow, L. M., C. D. Ross, R. Motwani, and D. V. McDougal, Jr. (1972). *J. Gen. Physiol.* **60**:388–405. Transport of axonal enzymes in surviving segments of frog sciatic nerve.

Parysek, L. M., J J. Wolosewick, and J. Olmsted (1984). *J. Cell Biol.* **99**:2287–2296. A novel microtubule-associated protein specific for a subset of tissue microtubules.

Paschal, B. M., H. S. Shpetner, and R. B. Vallee (1987). *J. Cell Biol.* **105**:1273–1282. MAP 1C is a microtubule-activated ATPase which translocates microtubules *in vitro* and has dynein-like properties.

Pasquini, J. M., B. Kaplun, C. A. Garcia Argiz, and C. J. Gomez (1967). *Brain Res.* **6**:621–634. Hormonal regulation of brain development. I. The effect of neonatal thyroidectomy upon nucleic acids, protein and two enzymes in developing cerebral cortex and cerebellum of the rat.

Pasquini, P. (1927). *Boll. Ist. Zool. Univ. Roma,* **5**:1–83. Ricerche di Embriologia sperimentale sui trapianti omeoplastici della vescicola ottica primaria in *Pleurodeles waltli.*

Passingham, R. E. (1975). *Brain Behav. Evol.* **11**:1–15. The brain and intelligence.

Passingham, R. E. (1979). *Brain Behav. Evol.* **16**:253–270. Brain size and intelligence in man.

Passingham, R. E. (1981). *Symp. Zool. Soc. Lond.* **46**:361–388. Primate specialization in brain and intelligence.

Pasternak, J. F., and T. A. Woolsey (1975a). *J. Comp. Neurol.* **160**:291–306. The number, size and spatial distribution of neurons in lamina IV of the mouse Sml neocortex.

Pastore, N. (1971). *Selective History of Theories of Visual Perception 1650–1950.* Oxford Univ. Press, New York.

Patel, A. J., A. Rabie, P.D. Lewis and R. Balazs (1976). *Brain Res.* **104**:33–48. Effect of thyroid deficiency on postnatal cell formation in the rat brain. A biochemical investigation.

Patel, A. J., P. D. Lewis, R. Balázs, P. Bailey, and M. Lai (1979). *Brain Res.* **172**:57–72. Effects of thyroxine on postnatal cell acquisition in the rat brain.

Patel, A. J., A. Hunt, and C. S. M. Tahourdin (1983). *Dev. Brain Res.* **10**:83–91. Regulation of *in vivo* glutamine synthetase activity by glucocorticoids in the developing rat brain.

Patel, N., and M.-M. Poo (1982). *J. Neurosci.* **2**:483–496. Orientation of neurite growth by extracellular electric fields.

Patel, N. B., and M.-M. Poo (1984). *J. Neurosci.* **4**:2939–2947. Perturbation of the direction of neurite growth by pulsed and focal electric fields.

Patel, N. B., Z.-P. Xie, S. H. Young, and M.-M. Poo (1985). *J. Neurosci. Res.* **13**:245–256. Response of nerve growth cone to focal electric currents.

Patel, S. N., and M. G. Stewart (1988). *Brain Res.* **449**:34–46. Changes in the number and structure of dendritic spines 25 hours after passive avoidance training in the domestic chick, *Gallus domesticus.*

Patel-Vaidya, U. (1985). *J. Neurosci. Res.* **14**:357–371. Ultrastructural organization of posterior and anterior barrels in the somatosensory cortex of the rat.

Paterson, J. A., A. Privat, E. A. Ling, and C. P. Leblond (1973). *J. Comp. Neurol.* **149**:83–102. Investigation of glial cells in semithin sections. III. Transformation of subependymal cells into glial cells, as shown by radioautography after ³H-thymidine injection into the lateral ventricle of the brain of young rats.

Pattee, H. H., ed. (1973). *Hierarchy Theory, The Challenge of Complex Systems.* George Braziller, New York.

Patterson, C. (1988). *Mol. Biol. Evol.* 5:603–625. Homology in classical and molecular biology.

Patterson, P. H. (1978). *Ann. Rev. Neurosci.* 1:1–17. Environmental determination of autonomic neurotransmitter functions.

Paulson, O. B., and E. A. Newman (1987). *Science* 237:896–898. Does the release of potassium from astrocyte endfeet regulate cerebral blood flow?

Pauly, P. J. (1987). *Controlling Life: Jacques Loeb and the Engineering Ideal in Biology.* Oxford Univ. Press, London.

Pavlík, A., and M. Buresová (1984). *Dev. Brain Res.* 12:13–20. The neonatal cerebellum: The highest level of glucocorticoid receptors in the brain.

Paweletz, N., and M. Little (1980). *Interdisciplinary Sci. Rev.* 5:138–148. Cell division problems and solutions.

Payer, A. F. (1979). *J. Comp. Neurol.* 183:365–384. An ultrastructural study of Schwann cell response to axonal degeneration.

Payette, R. F., G. S. Bennett, and M. D. Gershon (1984). *Dev. Biol.* 105:273–287. Neurofilament expresson in vagal neural crest-derived precursors of enteric neurons.

Payette, R. F., V. M. Tennyson, H. D. Pomeranz, T. D. Pham, T. P. Rothman, and M. D. Gershon (1988). *Dev. Biol.* 125:341–360. Accumulation of components of basal laminae: Association with the failure of neural crest cells to colonize the presumptive aganglionic bowel of *Is/Is* mutant mice.

Pearl, R. (1905). *Biometrika* 4:13–104. Variation and correlation in brain weight.

Pearlman, A. L., H. G. Kim, and G. Schmitt (1986). *Soc. Neurosci. Abstr.* 12:502. Early cortical afferents arrive after fibronectinlike immunoreactivity appears in their migratory pathway.

Pearse, B. M. F. (1976). *Proc. Natl. Acad. Sci. U.S.A.* 73:1255–1259. Clathrin: A unique protein associated with intracellular transfer of membrane by coated vesicles.

Pearse, B. M. F., and R. A. Crowther (1982). *Cold Spring Harbor Symp. Quant. Biol.* 46:703–706. Packing of clathrin into coats.

Pearson, J., E. M. Johnson, Jr., and L. Brandeis (1983). *Dev. Biol.* 96:32–36. Effects of antibodies to nerve growth factor on intrauterine development of derivatives of cranial neural crest and placode in the guinea pig.

Pearson, K. G., and A. B. Bradley (1972). *Brain Res.* 47:492–496. Specific regeneration of excitatory motor neurons to leg muscles in the cockroach.

Pearson, R. (1972). *The Avian Brain.* Acad. Press, New York.

Pearson, R. C. A., K. C. Gatter, and T. P. S. Powell (1983). *Brain Res.* 261:321–326. Retrograde cell degeneration in the basal nucleus in monkey and man.

Pease, D. C. (1964). *Histological Techniques for Electron Microscopy.* Academic Press, New York.

Pease, D. C., and T. A. Quilliam (1957). *J. Biophys. Biochem. Cytol.* 3:331–342. Electron microscopy of the Pacinian corpuscle.

Peck, C. K., and C. Blakemore (1975). *Exp. Brain Res.* 22:57–68. Modification of single neurons in the kitten's visual cortex after brief periods of monocular visual experience.

Peduzzi, J. D., and W. J. Crossland (1983). *J. Comp. Neurol.* 213:287–300. Anterograde transneuronal degeneration in the ectomamillary nucleus and ventral lateral geniculate nucleus of the chick.

Pei, Y. F., and J. A. G. Rhodin (1970). *Anat. Rec.* 168:105–126. The prenatal development of the mouse eye.

Pelton, E. W., R. E. Grindeland, E. Young, and N. H. Bass (1977). *Neurology* 27:282–288. Effects of immunologically induced growth hormone deficiency on myelinogenesis in developing rat cerebrum.

Penfield, W. (1920). *Brain* 43:290–305. Alterations of the Golgi apparatus in nerve cells.

Penfield, W. (1924). *Brain* 47:430–452. Oligodendroglia and its relation to classical neuroglia.

Penfield, W. (1928). Neuroglia and microglia. The interstitial tissue of the central nervous system, pp. 1032–1067. In *Special Cytology*, Vol. 2, (E. V. Cowdry, ed.), Hoeber, New York.

Penfield, W. (1932). Neuroglia: Normal and pathological, pp. 423–479. In *Cytology and Cellular Pathology of the Nervous System*, Vol. 2, (W. Penfield, ed.), Hoeber, New York.

Penfield, W. (1954). Ramón y Cajal, an appreciation. In *Neuron Theory or Reticular Theory?* Translated by M. U. Purkiss and C. A. Fox. C.S.I.C. Instituto "Ramón y Cajal," Madrid.

Penfield, W. (1958). *The excitable cortex in conscious man.* Liverpool University Press, Liverpool.

Penfield, W. (1977). *No Man Alone. A Neurosurgeon's Life.* Little Brown, Boston.

Penfield, W., and W. Cone (1929). Neuroglia and microglia (the metallic methods). In *Handbook of Microscopical Technique* (C. E. McClung, ed.), Hoeber, New York.

Penfield, W., and T. Rasmussen (1950). *The Cerebral Cortex of Man: A Clinical Study of Localization of Function.* Macmillan, London.

Penfield, W., and K. Welch (1949). *Trans. Amer. Neurol. Assoc.* 74:179–184. The supplementary motor area in the cerebral cortex of man.

Penfield, W., and K. Welch (1951). *A.M.A. Arch. Neurol. Psychiat.* 66:289–317. The supplementary motor area of the cerebral cortex: A clinical and experimental study.

Peng, H. B., (1983). *J. Cell Biol.* 97:489–498. Cytoskeletal organization of the presynaptic nerve terminal and the acetylcholine receptor cluster in cell cultures.

Peng, H. B., and L. F. Jaffe (1976). *Dev. Biol.* 53:277–284. Polarization of fucoid eggs by steady electrical fields.

Peng, H. B., D. R. Markey, W. L. Muhlach, and E. D. Pollack (1987). *Synapse* 1:10–19. Development of presynaptic specializations induced by basic polypeptide-coated latex beads in spinal cord cultures.

Peng, H. B., Q. Chen, M. W. Rochlin, D. Zhu, and B. Kay (1988). Mechanisms of neuromuscular junction development studied in tissue culture, pp. 103–119. In *Developmental Neurobiology of the Frog.* Alan R. Liss, Inc.

Peng, I., L. I. Binder, and M. M. Black (1986). *J. Cell Biol.* 102:252–262. Biochemical and immunological analyses of cytoskeletal domains of neurons.

Peng, Y.-Y., and E. Frank (1988). *J. Neurobiol.* 19:727–742. Anatomical specificity of regenerated muscle sensory afferents in the spinal cord of the bullfrog.

Penrose, R. (1989). *The Emperor's New Mind: Concerning Computers, Minds and the Laws of Physics.* Oxford Univ. Press.

Peper, K., and U. McMahan (1972). *Proc. Roy. Soc. (London)*

Ser. B. 181:431–440. Distribution of acetylcholine receptors in the vicinity of nerve terminals on skeletal muscle of the frog.

Percheron, G. (1979a). *Neurosci. Lett.* 14:287–293. Quantitative analysis of dendritic branching. I. Simple formulae for the quantitative analysis of dendritic branching.

Percheron, G. (1979b). *Neurosci. Lett.* 14:295–302. Quantitative Analysis of dendritic branching. II. Fundamental dendritic numbers as a tool for the study of neuronal groups.

Perdrau, J. R. (1937). *Brain* 6:204–210. The axis cylinder as a pathway for dyes and salts in solution with observations on the node of Ranvier in the rabbit.

Perkel, D. H., and D. J. Perkel (1985). *Brain Res.* 325:331–335. Dendritic spines: Role of active membrane in modulating synaptic efficacy.

Perri, T. (1956). *Arch. Zool. Ital.* 41:369–410. Ricerche sulla correlazioni tra midollo spinale, gangli spinali ed arti negli Anfibi anuri. Esperienze d'asportazione di un abbozzo d'arto in *Bufo Vulgaris*.

Perris, R., Y. von Boxberg, and J. Löfberg (1988). *Science* 241:86–89. Local embryonic matrices determine region-specific phenotypes in neural crest cells.

Perris, R., M. Paulsson, and M. Bronner-Fraser (1989). *Dev. Biol.* 136:222–238. Molecular mechanisms of avian neural crest cell migration on fibronectin and laminin.

Perry, R. P. (1966). *Nat. Cancer Inst. Monogr.* 23:527–545. On ribosome biogenesis.

Perry, V. H., and R. Linden (1982). *Nature* 297:683–685. Evidence for dendritic competition in the developing retina.

Perry, V. H., and S. Gordon (1988). *Trends Neurosci.* 11:273–277. Macrophages and microglia in the nervous system.

Perry, V. H., and L. Maffei (1988). *Dev. Brain Res.* 41:195–208. Dendritic competition: Competition for what?

Perry, V. H., D. A. Hume, and S. Gordon (1985). *Neuroscience* 15:313–326. Immunohistochemical localisation of macrophages and microglia in the adult and developing mouse brain.

Persson, L., and A. Sima (1975). *Neurobiology* 5:151–166. The effect of pre- and postnatal undernutrition on the development of the cerebellar cortex in the rat. II. Histochemical observations.

Pesetsky, I. (1960). *Anat. Rec.* 136:257. Maintenance and regression of Mauthner's neuron in larval *Rana pipiens*.

Pesetsky, I. (1962). *Gen. Comp. Endocrinol.* 2:229–235. The thyroxine-stimulated enlargement of Mauthner's neuron in anurans.

Pesetsky, I. (1966). *Z. Zellforsch. Mikroskop. Anat.* 75:138–145. The role of the thyroid in the development of Mauthner's neuron. A karyometric study in thyroidectomized anuran larvae.

Pesetsky, I., and J. J. Kollros (1956). *Exp. Cell Res.* 11:477–482. A comparison of the influence of locally applied thyroxine upon Mauthner's cell and adjacent neurons.

Pessacq, T. P., and N. J. Reissenweber (1972). *Acta Anat. (Basel)* 8:1–12. Structural aspects of vasculogenesis in the central nervous system. I. Postnatal development of the capillary blood vessels.

Pestronk, A. (1985). *J. Neurosci.* 5:1111–1117. Intracellular acetylcholine receptors in skeletal muscles of the adult rat.

Pestronk, A., D. B. Drachman, and J. W. Griffin (1976a).

Nature 260:352–353. Effect of muscle disuse on acetylcholine receptors.

Pestronk, A., D. B. Drachman, and J. W. Griffin (1976b). *Nature* 264:787–789. Effect of botulinum toxin on trophic regulation of acetylcholine receptors.

Peterfi, T., and St. C. Williams (1933). *Arch. Exp. Zellforsch.* 14:210–254. Elektrische Reizversuche an gezüchten Gewebezellen. I. Versuche an Nervenzellen.

Peters, A. (1959). *Am. J. Anat.* 93:177–195. Experimental studies on the staining of nervous tissue with silver proteinates.

Peters, A. (1960). *J. Biophys. Biochem. Cytol.* 8:431–446. The formation and structure of myelin sheaths in the central nervous system.

Peters, A. (1964a). *J. Anat. (London)* 98:125–134. Observations on the connections between myelin sheaths and glial cells in the optic nerve of young rats.

Peters, A. (1964b). *J. Cell Biol.* 20:281–296. Further observations on the structure of myelin sheaths in the central nervous system.

Peters, A. (1966). *Quart. J. Exp. Physiol.* 51:229–236. The node of Ranvier in the central nervous system.

Peters, A., and A. R. Muir (1959). *Quart. J. Exp. Physiol.* 44:117–130. The relationship between axons and Schwann cells during development of peripheral nerves in the rat.

Peters, A., and J. E. Vaughn (1967). *J. Cell Biol.* 32:113–119. Microtubules and filaments in the axons and astrocytes of early postnatal rat optic nerve.

Peters, A., S. L. Palay, and H. DeF. Webster (1970). *The Fine Structure of the Nervous System*, Harper and Row, New York.

Peters, A., S. L. Palay, and H. Webster de F. (1976). *The Fine Structure of the Nervous System: The Neurons and Supporting Cells*. Saunders, Philadelphia.

Peters, H. G., and H. Bademan (1963). *J. Anat. (London)* 97:111–117. The form and growth of stellate cells in the cortex of the guinea-pig.

Peters, V. B., and L. B. Flexner (1950). *Amer. J. Anat.* 86:133–161. Biochemical and physiological differentiation during morphogenesis. VII. Quantitative morphologic studies on the developing cerebral cortex of the fetal guinea pig.

Petersen, H. (1923). *Ergeb. Anat. Entw.-Gesch.* 24:327–347. Berichte über Entwicklungsmechanik. I. Entwicklungsmechanik des Auges.

Peterson, A. C., and G. M. Bray (1984). *J. Cell Biol.* 99:1831–1837. Normal basal laminas are realized on dystrophic Schwann cells in dystrophic ↔ shiverer chimera nerves.

Peterson, E. R., and S. M. Crain (1968). *Anat. Rec.* 160:408–409. Reinnervation of denervated mammalian skeletal muscle *in vitro*.

Peterson, E. R., and M. R. Murray (1955). *Am. J. Anat.* 96:319–355. Myelin sheath formation in cultures of avian spinal ganglia.

Peterson, E. R., and M. R. Murray (1965). *Ann. N.Y. Acad. Sci.* 122:39–49. Patterns of peripheral demyelination *in vitro*. Research in demyelinating disease.

Peterson, E. R., S. M. Crain, and M. R. Murray (1958). *Anat. Rec.* 130:357. Activities of Schwann cells during myelin formation *in vitro*.

Peterson, J. A., J. J. Bray, and L. Austin (1968). *J. Neurochem.* 15:741–745. An autoradiographic study of the flow of protein and RNA along peripheral nerve.

Peterson, R. P., R. M. Hurwitz, and R. Lindsay (1967). *Exp. Brain Res.* 4:138–145. Migration of axonal protein: Absence of a protein concentration gradient and effect of inhibition of protein synthesis.

Petit, T. L. (1988). Synaptic plasticity and the structural basis of learning and memory, pp. 201–234. In *Neural Plasticity: A Lifespan Approach* (T. L. Petit, and G. O. Ivy, eds.), Alan R. Liss, New York.

Petkovich, M., N. J. Brand, A. Krust, and P. Chambon (1987). *Nature* 330:444–450. A human retinoic acid receptor which belongs to the family of nuclear receptors.

Pettigrew, A. G., R. Lindeman, and M. R. Bennett (1979). *J. Embryol. Exp. Morphol.* 49:115–137. Development of the segmental innervation of the chick forelimb.

Pettigrew, J. D. (1974a). *Ann. N.Y. Acad. Sci.* 228:393–405. The effects of selective visual experience on stimulus trigger features of kitten cortical neurons.

Pettigrew, J. D. (1974b). *J. Physiol. (London)* 237:49–74. The effects of visual experience on the development of stimulus specificity by kitten cortical neurones.

Pettigrew, J. D., and M. Konishi (1976b). *Nature* 264:753–754. Effects of monocular deprivation on binocular neurones in the owl's visual wulst.

Pettmann, B., M. Weibel, M. Sensenbrenner, and G. Labourdette (1985). *FEBS* 189:102–108. Purification of two astroglial growth factors from bovine brain.

Petukhov, V. V., and V. I. Popov (1986). *Neuroscience* 18:823–835. Quantitative analysis of ultrastructural changes in synapses of the rat hippocampal field CA3 *in vitro* in different functional states.

Peusner, K. D., and D. K. Morest (1977). *Neuroscience* 2:253–270. Neurogenesis in the nucleus vestibularis tangentialis of the chick embryo in the absence of the primary afferent fibers.

Peyrieras, N., F. Hyafil, D. Louvard, H. L. Ploegh, and F. Jacob (1983). *Proc. Natl. Acad. Sci. U.S.A.* 80:6274–6277. Uvomorulin: A nonintegral membrane protein of early mouse embryo.

Peyronnard, J. M., L. C. Terry, and A. Aguayo (1975). *Arch. Neurol.* 32:36–38. Schwann cell internuclear distances in developing rat unmyelinated nerve fibers.

Pfaff, D. W. (1968a). *Experientia* 24:958–959. Autoradiographic localization of testosterone-³H in the female rat brain and estradiol-³H in the male rat brain.

Pfaff, D. W. (1968b). *Science* 161:1355–1356. Autoradiographic localization of radioactivity in rat brain after injection of tritiated sex hormones.

Pfaff, D. W. (1968c). *Endocrinol.* 82:1149–1155. Uptake of ³H-estradiol by the female rat brain. An autoradiographic study.

Pfaff, D. W., and M. Keiner (1973). *J. Comp. Neurol.* 151:121–158. Atlas of estradiol-concentrating cells in the central nervous system of the female rat.

Pfaff, D. W., and B. S. McEwen (1983). *Science* 219:808–814. Actions of estrogens and progestins on nerve cells.

Pfaff, D. W., J. L. Gerlach, B. S. McEwen, M. Ferin, P. Carmel, and E. A. Zimmerman (1976). *J. Comp. Neurol.* 170:279–294. Autoradiographic localization of hormone-concentrating cells in the brain of the female rhesus monkey.

Pfeffer, W. (1884). *Untersuch. Bot. Inst. Tübingen.* 1:397–500. Locomotorische Richtungsbewegungen durch chemische Reize.

Pfenninger, K. H. (1984). *Adv. Exp. Med. Biol.* 181:1–14. Molecular biology of the nerve growth cone: A perspective.

Pfenninger, K. H., and J.-F. Maylié-Pfenninger (1981a). *J. Cell Biol.* 89:536–546. Lectin labeling of sprouting neurons. I. Regional distribution of surface glycoconjugates.

Pfenninger, K. H., and M.-F. Maylié-Pfenninger (1981b). *J. Cell Biol.* 89:547–559. Lectin labeling of sprouting neurons. II. Relative movement and appearance of glycoconjugates during plasmalemmal expansion.

Pfenninger, K. H., M.-F. Maylié-Pfenninger, L. B. Friedman, and P. Simkowitz (1984). *Dev. Biol.* 106:97–108. Lectin labeling of sprouting neurons. III. Type-specific glycoconjugates on growth cones of different origin.

Pflugfelder, O (1952). *Roux Arch. Entw.-Mech.* 145:549–560. Weitere volumetrische Untersuchungen über die Wirkung der Augenextirpation und der Dunkelhaltung auf das Mesencephalon und die Pseudobranchien von Fischer.

Pflugfelder, O. (1958). *Entwicklungsphysiologie der Insekten*, 2nd edn. Geest and Portig, Leipzig, 490 pp.

Phelps, C. H. (1972). *Z. Zellforsch. Mikrosk. Anat.* 128:555–563. The development of glio-vascular relationships in the rat spinal cord.

Phemister, R. D., and S. Young (1968). *J. Comp. Neurol.* 134:243–254. The postnatal development of the canine cerebellar cortex.

Phemister, R. D., J. N. Shively, and S. Young (1969). *J. Neuropathol. Exp. Neurol.* 28:128–138. The effects of gamma irradiation on the postnatally developing canine cerebellar cortex. II. Sequential histogenesis of radiation-induced changes.

Phillips, C. G. (1967). *Arch. Neurol.* 17:188–195. Corticomotoneuronal organization. Projection from the arm area of the baboon's motor cortex.

Phillips, C. G. (1969). *Proc. Roy. Soc. (London) Ser. B.* 173:141–174. Motor apparatus of the baboon's hand.

Phillips, C. G. (1975). *Can. J. Neurol. Sci.* 2:209–218. Laying the ghost of 'muscles versus movements'.

Phillips, C. G., and R. Porter (1964). *Prog. Brain Res.* 12:222–242. The pyramidal projection to motoneurones of some muscle groups of the baboon's forelimb.

Phillips, C. G., and R. Porter (1977). *Corticospinal neurones.* Academic, New York.

Phillips, D. E. (1973). *Z. Zellforsch. Mikrosk. Anat.* 140:145–167. An electron microscopic study of macroglia and microglia in the lateral funiculus of the developing spinal cord in the fetal monkey.

Phillips, L. L., L. Autilio-Gambetti, and R. J. Lasek (1983). *Brain Res.* 278:219–223. Bodian's silver method reveals molecular variation in the evolution of neurofilament proteins.

Phillips, R. J. P. (1954). *Z. Vererbungsl.* 86:322–326. Jimpy, a totally new sex-linked gene in the house mouse.

Phillips, R. J. S. (1960). *J. Genet.* 57:35–42. "Lurcher," a new gene in linkage group XI of the house mouse.

Piatt, J. (1939). *J. Morphol.* 65:155–185. A study of nerve-muscle specificity in the forelimb of *Triturus pyrrogaster*.

Piatt, J. (1940). *J. Exp. Zool.* 85:211–241. Nerve-muscle specificity in *Amblystoma*, studied by means of heterotopic cord grafts.

Piatt, J. (1941). *J. Exp. Zool.* 86:77–85. Grafting of limbs in place of the eye in *Amblystoma*.

Piatt, J. (1942). *J. Exp. Zool.* 91:79–101. Transplantation of aneurogenic forelimbs in *Amblystoma punctatum*.

Piatt, J. (1943). *J. Comp. Neurol.* 79:165–183. The course and decussation of ectopic Mauthner's fibers in *Amblystoma punctatum*.

Piatt, J. (1944). *J. Comp. Neurol.* 80:335–353. Experiments on the decussation and course of Mauthner's fibers in *Amblystoma punctatum*.

Piatt, J. (1945). *J. Comp. Neurol.* 82:35–54. Origin of the mesencephalic V cells in *Amblystoma*.

Piatt, J. (1946). *J. Exp. Zool.* 102:109. The influence of the peripheral field on the development of the mesencephalic V nucleus in *Amblystoma*.

Piatt, J. (1947). *J. Comp. Neurol.* 86:199–236. A study of the factors controlling the differentiation of Mauthner's cell in *Amblystoma*.

Piatt, J. (1948). *Biol. Rev.* 23:1–45. Form and causality in neurogenesis.

Piatt, J. (1949). *J. Comp. Neurol.* 90:47–93. A study of the development of fiber tracts in the brain of *Amblystoma* after excision or inversion of the embryonic dimesencephalic region.

Piatt, J. (1951). *J. Comp. Neurol.* 94:105–121. An experimental approach to the problem of pallial differentiation.

Piatt, J. (1952). *J. Exp. Zool.* 120:247–285. Transplantation of aneurogenic forelimbs in place of the hindlimb in *Amblystoma*.

Piatt, J. (1955). *J. Exp. Zool.* 129:177–207. Regeneration of the spinal cord in the salamander.

Piatt, J. (1957a). *J. Exp. Zool.* 134:103–125. Studies on the problem of nerve pattern. II. Innervation of the intact forelimb by different parts of the central nervous system in *Amblystoma*.

Piatt, J. (1957b). *J. Exp. Zool.* 136:229–247. Studies on the problem of nerve pattern. III. Innervation of the regenerated forelimb in *Amblystoma*.

Piatt, J. (1958). *J. Exp. Zool.* 120:247–286. Transplantation of aneurogenic forelimbs in place of the hindlimb in *Amblystoma*.

Piatt, J. (1969). *Dev. Biol.* 19:608–616. The influence of VIIth and VIIIth cranial nerve roots upon the differentiation of Mauthner's cell in *Amblystoma*.

Picard, A., J.-C. Cavadore, P. Lory, J.-C. Bernengo, C. Ojeda, and M. Dorée (1990). *Science* 247:327–329. Microinjection of a conserved peptide sequence of p34^cdc2 induces a Ca^{2+} transient in oocytes.

Piccolino, M. (1988). *Trends Neurosci.* 11:521–525. Cajal and the retina: A 100-year retrospective.

Pickel, V. M., J. Chan, and D. Ganten (1986). *J. Neurosci.* 6:2457–2469. Dual peroxidase and colloidal gold-labeling study of angiotensin-like immunoreactivity in the rat subfornical organ.

Picken, L. (1956). *Nature* 178:1162–1165. The fate of Wilhelm His.

Piddington, R. (1967). *Dev. Biol.* 16:168–188. Hormonal effects on the development of glutamine synthetase in the embryonic chick retina.

Piddington, R., and A. A. Moscona (1967). *Biochim. Biophys. Acta* 141:429–432. Precocious induction of retinal glutamine synthetase by hydrocortisone in the embryo and in culture. Age-dependent differences in tissue response.

Pierce, E. T. (1973). *Prog. Brain Res.* 40:53–65. Time of origin of neurons in the brain stem of the mouse.

Pilar, G., and L. Landmesser (1972). *Science* 177:1116–1118. Axotomy mimicked by localized colchicine application.

Pilar, G., L. Landmesser, and L. Burstein (1980). *J. Neurophysiol.* 43:233–254. Competition for survival among developing ciliary ganglion cells.

Pilbeam, D., and S. J. Gould (1974). *Science* 186:892–901. Size and scaling in human evolution.

Pilleri, G. (1959). Camillo Golgi. In *Grosse Nervenärzte*, Vol. 2. Georg Thieme Verlag, Stuttgart.

Pillsbury, W. B. (1929). *The History of Psychology*, Norton, New York.

Pinot, M. (1969). *J. Embryol. Exp. Morph.* 21:149–164. Etude experimentale de la morphogenèse de la cage thoracique chez l'embryon de poulet.

Pintar, J. E. (1978). *Dev. Biol.* 67:444–464. Distribution and synthesis of glycosaminoglycans during quail neural crest morphogenesis.

Pinto-Lord, M. C., P. Evrard, and V. S. Caviness, Jr. (1982). *Dev. Brain Res.* 4:379–393. Obstructed neuronal migration along radial glial fibers in the neocortex of the reeler mouse: A Golgi-EM analysis.

Pishak, M. R., and A. T. Phillips (1980). *J. Neurochem.* 34:866–872. Glucocorticoid stimulation of glutamine synthetase production in cultured rat glioma cells.

Pitman, R. M., C. D. Tweedle, and M. J. Cohen (1972). *Science* 176:412–414. Branching of central neurons: Intracellular cobalt injection for light and electron microscopy.

Pitot, H. C., and M. D. Yatvin (1973). *Physiol. Rev.* 53:228–325. Interrelationships of mammalian hormones and enzyme levels *in vivo*.

Pittendrigh, C. S. (1958). Adaptation, natural selection and behavior, pp. 390–416. In *Behavior and Evolution* (A. Roe, and G. G. Simpson, eds.), Yale Univ. Press, New Haven, Conn.

Pittman, R. H., and R. W. Oppenheim (1978). *Nature* 271:364–365. Neuromuscular blockade increases motoneurone survival during normal cell death in the chick embryo.

Pittman, R. H., and R. W. Oppenheim (1979). *J. Comp. Neurol.* 187:425–446. Cell death of motorneurons in the chick embryo spinal cord. IV. Evidence that a functional neuromuscular interaction is involved in the regulation of naturally occurring cell death and the stabilization of synapses.

Pittman, R. N. (1985). *Dev. Biol.* 110:91–101. Release of plaminogen activator and a calcium-dependent metalloprotease from cultured sympathetic and sensory neurons.

Pittman, R. N., and H. M. Buettner (1989). *Dev. Neurosci.* 11:361–375. Degradation of extracellular matrix by neuronal proteases.

Pituello, F., P. Deruntz, L. Pradayrol, and A.-M. Duprat (1989). *Development* 105:529–540. Peptidergic properties expressed *in vitro* by embryonic neuroblasts after neural induction.

Pixley, S. K. R., and J. DeVellis (1984). *Dev. Brain Res.* 15:201–209. Transition between immature radial glia and mature astrocytes sudied with a monoclonal antibody to vimentin.

Plapinger, L., and B. S. McEwen (1973). *Endocrinol.* 93:1119–1128. Ontogeny of estradiol-binding sites in rat brain. I. Appearance of presumptive adult receptors in cytosol and nuclei.

Plapinger, L., B. S. McEwen, and L. E. Clemens (1973). *Endocrinol.* 93:1129–1139. Ontogeny of estradiol-binding sites in rat brain. II. Characteristics of a neonatal binding macromolecule.

Platel, R., and C. Delfini (1986). *J. Hirnforsch.* 27:279–293. L'Encéphalisation chez la Lamproie marine, *Petromyzon marinus* (L.). Analyse quantifiée des principales subdivisions encéphaliques.

Platel, R., R. Bauchot, and C. Delfini (1972). *Z. wiss. Zool.* 185:88–104. Les relations pondérales encéphalo-somatiques chez *Gallus domesticus* L. (Galliformes, Phasianidae). Analyse au cours de l'incubation et de la période post natale.

Platt, J. B. (1891). *J. Morphpol.* 5:79–106. A contribution to the morphology of the vertebrate head, based on a study of *Acanthias vulgaris*.

Platt, J. B. (1893). *Anat. Anz.* 8:506–509. Ectodermic origin of the cartilages of the head.

Pleasure, D., B. Kreider, S. Shuman, and G. Sobue (1985). *Dev. Neurosci.* 7:364–373. Tissue culture studies of Schwann cell proliferation and differentiation.

Pleet, H., J. M. Graham, and D. W. Smith (1981). *Pediatrics* 67:785–789. Central nervous system and facial defects associated with hyperthermia at four to 14 weeks' gestation.

Poduslo, J. F., C. T. Berg, and P. J. Dyck (1984). *Proc. Natl. Acad. Sci. U.S.A* 81:1864–1866. Schwann cell expression of a major myelin glycoprotein in the absence of myelin assembly.

Poduslo, J. F., P. J. Dyck, and C. T. Berg (1985). *J. Neurochem.* 44:388–400. Regulation of myelination: Schwann cell transition from a myelin-maintaining state to a quiescent state after permanent nerve transection.

Poenie, M., J. Alderton, R. Steinhardt, and R. Tsien (1986). *Science* 233:886–889. Calcium rises abruptly and briefly throughout the cell at the onset of anaphase.

Polacek, P. (1966). *Acta Fac. Med. Univ. Brun.* 23:1–107. Receptors of the joints.

Poliak, S. (1932). *Univ. Calif. Publ. Anat.* 2:1–370. The main afferent fiber systems of the cerebral cortex of primates.

Poliakov, G. I. (1953) *Arkh. Anat. Gistol. Embriol.* 30: 48–63. Fine structural characteristics of man's cortex and functional interrelations among neurons. (In Russian).

Poliakov, G. I. (1956). *Zhurn. Vyss. Nerv. Vyssh. Nerv. Deiat. imeni I.P. Pavlova* 6:461–478. The ratio of main types of neurons in man's cerebral cortex. (In Russian).

Poliakov, G. I. (1959). Progressive neuron differentiation of the human cerebral cortex in ontogenesis, pp. 37–38. In *Razvitic Tsentral'noi Nervnoi Systemy* (Development of the Central Nervous System), (S. A. Sarkisov, and N. S. Preobrazhenskaya, eds.), Medgiz, Moscow.

Poliakov, G. I. (1961). *J. Comp. Neurol.* 117:197–212. Some results of research into the development of the neuronal structure of the cortical ends of the analyzers in man.

Poliakov, G. I. (1965). Development of the cerebral neocortex during the first half of intrauterine life, pp. 22–52. In *Development of the Child's Brain* (S. A. Sarkisov, ed.), Meditsina, Leningrad (In Russian).

Politis, M. J., N. Sternberger, K. Ederle, and P. S. Spencer (1982). *J. Neurosci.* 2:1252–1266. Studies on the control of myelinogenesis. IV. Neuronal induction of Schwann cell myelin-specific protein synthesis during nerve fiber regeneration.

Pollack, E. D. (1969). *Anat. Rec.* 163:111–120. Normal development of the lateral motor column in the brachial cord in *Rana pipiens*.

Pollack, E. D., and W. L. Muhlach (1982). *J. Neurosci. Res.* 8:343–355. Target control of neuronal development during formation of the spinal reflex arc: An operant model.

Pollak, R. D., and J. F. Fallon (1974). *Exp. Cell Res.* 86:9–14. Autoradiographic analysis of macromolecular synthesis in prospectively necrotic cells of the chick limb bud. I. Protein synthesis.

Pollak, R. D., and J. F. Fallon (1976). *Exp. Cell Res.* 100:15–22. Autoradiographic analysis of macromolecular synthesis in prospectively necrotic cells of the chick limb bud. II. Nucleic acids.

Pollard, T. D., and J. A. Cooper (1986). *Ann. Rev. Biochem.* 55:987–1035. Actin and actin-binding proteins. A critical evaluation of mechanisms and functions.

Polley, E. H., R. P. Zimmerman, and R. L. Fortney (1989). Neurogenesis and maturation of cell morphology in the development of the mammalian retina, pp. 3–30. In *Development of the Vertebrate Retina* (D. R. Sengelaub, and B. L. Finlay, eds.), Plenum Press, New York.

Pollit, E., and G. Granoff (1967). *Revista. Interamer. Psicol.* I:93–102. Mental and motor development of Peruvian children treated for severe malnutrition.

Poltorak, M., R. Sadoul, G. Keilhauer, C. Landa, T. Fahrig, and M. Schachner (1987). *J. Cell Biol.* 105:1893–1899. Myelin associated glycoprotein, a member of the L2/HNK-1 family of neural cell adhesion molecules, is involved in neuron–oligodendrocyte and oligodendrocyte–oligodendrocyte interaction.

Polyak, S. L. (1941). *The Retina.* University of Chicago Press, Chicago.

Polyak, S. L. (1957). *The Vertebrate Visual System.* Univ. Chicago Press, Chicago.

Pomerat, C. M. (1961). *Int. Rev. Cytol.* 11:307–339. Cinematology, indispensible tool for cytology.

Pomeranz, B. (1972). *Exp. Neurol.* 34:187–199. Metamorphosis of frog vision: Changes in ganglion cell physiology and anatomy.

Pomeranz, B., and S. H. Chung (1970). *Science,* 170:983–984. Dendritic-tree anatomy codes form-vision physiology in tadpole retina.

Pomerat, C. M., W. J. Hendelman, C. W. Raiborn, and J. F. Massey (1967). Dynamic activities of nervous tissue *in vitro*, pp. 120–178. In *The Neuron* (H. Hyden, ed.), Elsevier Science Publishing Co., Inc., New York.

Poo, M. M., and K. R. Robinson (1977). *Nature* 265:602–605. Electrophoresis of concanavalin A receptors along embryonic muscle cell membrane.

Popper, K. R. (1959). *The Logic of Scientific Discovery.* Hutchinson, London.

Popper, K. R. (1961). *The Poverty of Historicism,* 3rd edn. Routledge and Kegan Paul, London.

Popper, K. R. (1962). *Conjectures and Refutations: The Growth of Scientific Knowledge,* Basic Books, New York.

Popper, K. R. (1972). *Objective Knowledge.* Clarendon Press, Oxford.

Popper, K. R., and J. C. Eccles (1977). *The Self and its Brain.* Springer International, Berlin.

Poritsky, R. L., and M. Singer (1963). *J. Exp. Zool.* 153:211–218. The fate of taste buds in tongue transplants in the orbit in the urodele *triturus*.

Porter, K. R. (1966). Cytoplasmic microtubules and their functions, pp. 308–345. In *Ciba Foundation Symposium: Principles of Biomolecular Organization* (G. E. W. Wolstenholme, and M. O'Connor, eds.), Little, Brown, Boston.

Porter, K. R., and M. B. Bowers (1963). *J. Cell Biol.* 19:56A–57A. A study of chromatolysis in motor neurons of the frog *Rana pipiens*.

Porter, S., M. B. Clark, L. Glaser, and R. P. Bunge (1986). *J. Neurosci.* 6:3070–3078. Schwann Cells stimulated to proliferate in the absence of neurons retain full functional capability.

Porter, S., L. Glaser, and R. P. Bunge (1987). *Proc. Natl. Acad. Sci. U.S.A.* 84:7768–7772. Release of autocrine growth factor by primary and immortalized Schwann cells.

Potter, D. D., E. J. Furshpan, and E. S. Lennox (1966). *Proc. Natl. Acad. Sci. U.S.A.* 55:328–336. Connections between cells of the developing squid as revealed by electrophysiological methods.

Potter, H. D. (1969). *J. Comp. Neurol.* 136:203–232. Structural characteristics of cell and fiber populations in the optic tectum of the frog *(Rana catesbiana).*

Potter, V. R., W. C. Schneider, and G. J. Leibl (1945). *Cancer Res.* 5:21–24. Enzyme changes during growth and differentiation in the tissues of the newborn rat.

Potts, R. A., B. Dreher, and M. R. Bennett (1982). *Dev. Brain Res.* 3:481–486. The loss of ganglion cell in the developing retina of the rat.

Poulson, D. F. (1950). Histogenesis, organogenesis, and differentiation in the embryo of *Drosophila melanogaster* Meigen, pp. 168–274. In *Biology of Drosophila* (M. Demerec, ed.), Wiley, New York.

Povlishock, J. T., A. J. Martinez, and J. Moossy (1977). *Am. J. Anat.* 149:439–452. The fine structure of blood vessels of the telencephalic germinal matrix in the human fetus.

Powell, J. A., F. Rieger, B. Blondet, P. Dreyfus, and M. Pincon-Raymond (1984). *Dev. Biol.* 101:168–180. Distribution and quantification of ACh receptors and innervation in diaphragm muscle of normal and *mdg* mouse embryos.

Powell, T. P. S., and W. M. Cowan (1964). *J. Anat. (London)* 98:579–585. A note on retrograde fiber degeneration.

Powell, T. P. S., and S. D. Erulkar (1962). *J. Anat. (London)* 91:249–268. Transneuronal cell degeneration in the auditory relay nuclei of the cat.

Powell, T. P. S., and V. B. Mountcastle (1959). *Bull. Johns Hopkins Hosp.* 105:133–162. Some aspects of the functional organization of the cortex of the postcentral gyrus of the monkey: A correlation of findings obtained in single unit analysis with cytoarchitecture.

Power, M. E. (1952). *J. Morphol.* 91:389–411. A quantitative study of the growth of the central nervous system of a holometalbolous insect, *Drosophila melanogaster*.

Prasad, K. N., and A. W. Hsie (1971). *Nature (New Biol.)* 233:141–142. Morphologic differentiation of mouse neuroblastoma cells induced *in vitro* by dibutyryl adenosine 3':5'-cyclic monophosphate.

Pratt, F. H. (1917a). *Am. J. Physiol.* 43:159–168. The excitation of microscopic areas: A non-polarizable capillary electrode.

Pratt, F. H. (1917b). *Am. J. Physiol.* 44:517–542. The all-or-none principle in graded response of skeletal muscle.

Pratt, R. M., M. A. Larsen, and M. C. Johnston. *Dev. Biol.* 44:298–305. Migration of cranial neural crest cells in a cell-free hyaluronate-rich matrix.

Prensky, A. L., S. Carr, and H. W. Moser (1968). *Arch. Neurol. (Chicago)* 19:522–558. Development of myelin in inherited disorders of amino acid metabolism.

Prescott, D. M. (1964). *Natl. Cancer Inst. Monograph.* 14:57–72. Comments on the cell life cycle.

Prestige, M. C. (1965). *J. Embryol. Exp. Morphol.* 13:63–72. Cell turnover in the spinal ganglia of *Xenopus laevis* tadpoles.

Prestige, M. C. (1967a). *J. Embryol. Exp. Morphol.* 17:453–471. The control of cell number in the lumbar spinal ganglia during the development of *Xenopus laevis* tadpoles.

Prestige, M. C. (1967b). *J. Embryol. Exp. Morphol.* 18:359–387. The control of cell number in the lumbar ventral horns during the development of *Xenopus laevis* tadpoles.

Prestige, M. C. (1970). Differentiation, degeneration and the role of the periphery: quantitative considerations, pp. 73–82. In *The Neurosciences: Second Study Program* (F. O. Schmitt, ed.), Rockefeller Univ. Press, New York.

Prestige, M. C. (1973). *Brain Res.* 59:400–404. Gradients in time of origin of tadpole motoneurons.

Prestige, M. C. (1974). *Br. Med. Bull.* 30:107–111. Axon and cell numbers in the developing nervous system.

Prestige, M. C., and D. J. Willshaw (1975). *Proc. Roy. Soc. (London) Ser. B.* 190:77–98. On a role for competition in the formation of patterned neural connexions.

Prestige, M. C., and M. A. Wilson (1972). *Brain Res.* 41:467–470. Loss of axons from ventral roots during development.

Prestige, M. C., and M. A. Wilson (1974). *J. Embryol. Exp. Morphol.* 32:819–833. A quantitative study of the growth and development of *Xenopus laevis* tadpoles.

Prévost, J. L., and J. B. A. Dumas (1824). *Ann. Sci. Nat. Paris* 3:113–138. De la génération dans les mammifères, et des premiers indices du développement de l'embryon.

Preyer, W. (1885). *Specielle Physiologie des Embryo. Untersuchungen ueber die Lebenserscheinungen vor der Geburt.* Th. Grieben's Verlag (L. Fernau), Leipzig.

Price, D. J., and C. Blakemore (1985). *Nature* 316:721–724. Regressive events in the postnatal development of association projections in the visual cortex.

Price, D. L. (1972). *J. Neuropathol. Exp. Neurol.* 31:267–277. The response to amphibian glial cells to axonal transection.

Price, J., and L. Thurlow (1989). *Development* 104:473–482. Cell lineage in the rat cerebral cortextex: A study using retroviral-mediated gene transfer.

Price, M. T. (1974). *Brain Res.* 77:497–501. The effects of colchicine and lumichochicine on the rapid phase of axonal transport in the rabbit visual system.

Privat, A. (1975). *Int. Rev. Cytol.* 40:281–323. Postnatal gliogenesis in the mammalian brain.

Privat, A., and M. J. Drian (1976). *J. Comp. Neurol.* 166:201–244. Postnatal maturation of rat Purkinje cells cultivated in the absence of two afferent systems: An ultrastructural study.

Privat, A., and J. Fulcrand (1977). In *Cell, Tissue, and Organ Culture in Neurobiology*, pp. 11–37. (S. Fedoroff, and L. Hertz, eds.), Academic, New York.

Privat, A., and C. P. Leblond (1972). *J. Comp. Neurol.* 146:277–302. The subependymal layer and neighboring region in the brain of the young rat.

Privat, A., J. Valat, and J. Fulcrand (1981). *J. Neuropath. Exp. Neurol.* 40:46–60. Proliferation of neuroglial cell lines in the degenerating optic nerve of young rats. A radioautographic study.

Privat, A. C., J. M. Jacque, P. Bourre, P. Dupouey, and N. Baumann (1979). *Neurosci. Lett.* 12:107–112. Absence of the major dense line in myelin of the mutant mouse "shiverer."

Prochaska, G. (1851). *A Dissertation on the Functions of the Nervous System* (1874), Sydenham Society, London.

Prothero, J. W., and J. W. Sundsten (1984). *Brain Behav. Evol.* 24:152–167. Folding of the cerebral cortex in mammals. A scaling model.

Provis, J. M. (1987). *J. Comp. Neurol.* 259:237–246. Patterns of cell death in the ganglion cell layer of the human fetal retina.

Provis, J. M., D. van Driel, F. A. Billson, and P. Russell (1985a). *J. Comp. Neurol.* 233:429–451. Development of the human retina: Patterns of cell distribution and redistribution in the ganglion cell layer.

Provis, J. M., D. van Driel, F. A. Billson, and P. Russell (1985b). *J. Comp. Neurol.* 238:92–100. Human fetal optic nerve: Overproduction and elimination of retinal axons during development.

Pruss, R. M., P. F. Bartlett, J. Gavrilovic, R. P. Lisak, and S. Rattray (1981). *Dev. Brain Res.* 2:19–35. Mitogens for glial cells: Comparison of the response of cultured astrocytes, oligodendrocytes, and Schwann cells.

Pubols, L. M., and G. L. Brenowitz (1982). *J. Neurophysiol.* 47:103–112. Maintenance of dorsal horn somatotopic organization and increased high-threshold response after single-root or spared-root deafferentation in cats.

Pubols, L. M., and M. E. Goldberger (1980). *J. Neurophysiol.* 43:102–117. Recovery of function in dorsal horn following partial deafferentation.

Puck, T. T., and J. Steffen (1963). *Biophys. J.* 3:379–397. Life cycle analysis of mammalian cells. A method for localizing metabolic events within the life cycle, and its application to the action of colcemide and sublethal doses of X-irradiation.

Purkinje, J. E. (1838). Über die gangliöse Natur bestimmter Hirntheile, *Ber. Vers. dtsch. Naturf. Ärzte (Prag.)*, 1837, **15**, 174 ff., in *Opera omnia* (1939), Vol. 3, Prague, pp. 45–49.

Purkyne, J. E. (1837a) Neueste Beobachtungen über die Struktur des Gehirns. *Opera omnia.* 2:88. (12 vols., Prague: Purkynova Spolecnost. 1918–1973).

Purkyne, J. E. (1837b). Neueste Untersuchungen aus der Nerven-und Hirnanatomie. *Opera Omnia* 3:45–49a. (12 vols., Prague: Purkynova. Spolecnost. 1918–1973).

Puro, D. G., and D. J. Woodward (1977). *Brain Res.* 129:141–146. The climbing fiber system in the weaver mutant.

Puro, D. G., and D. J. Woodward (1978). *J. Neurobiol.* 9:195–215. Physiological properties of afferents and synaptic reorganization in the rat cerebellum degranulated by postnatal X-irradiation.

Purpura, D. P., R. J. Shofer, E. M. Housepian, and C. Noback (1964). *Prog. Brain Res.* 4:187–221. Comparative ontogenesis of structure-function relations in cerebral and cerebellar cortex.

Purves, D. (1975). *J. Physiol. (London)* 252:429–463. Functional and structural changes in mammalian sympathetic neurones following interruption of their axons.

Purves, D. (1976). *J. Physiol. (London)* 261:453–475. Competitive and non- competitive re-innervation of mammalian sympathetic neurones by native and foreign fibers.

Purves, D. (1988). *Body and Brain. A Trophic Theory of Neural Connections.* Harvard Univ. Press, Cambridge, Mass.

Purves, D., and J. W. Lichtman (1980). *Science* 210:153–157. Elimination of synapses in the developing nervous system.

Purves, D., and J. W. Lichtman (1983). *Ann. Rev. Physiol.* 45:553–565. Specific connections between nerve cells.

Purves, D., and J. W. Lichtman (1985a). *Principles of Neural Development.* Sinauer, Sunderland, MA.

Purves, D., and J. W. Lichtman (1985b). *Science* 228:298–302. Geometrical differences among homologous neurons in mammals.

Purves, D., and J. T. Voyvodic (1987). *Trends Neurosci.* 10:398–404. Imaging mammalian nerve cells and their connections over time in living animals.

Purves, D., E. Rubin, W. D. Snider, and J. Lichtman (1986a). *J. Neurosci.* 6:158–163. Relation of animal size to convergence, divergence, and neuronal number in peripheral sympathetic pathways.

Purves, D., R. D. Hadley, and J. T. Voyvodic (1986b). *J. Neurosci.* 6:1051–1060. Dynamic changes in the dendritic geometry of individual neurons visualized over periods of up to three months in the superior cervical ganglion of living mice.

Purves, D., J. T. Voyvodic, L. Magrassi, and H. Yawo (1987). *Science* 238:1122–1126. Nerve terminal remodeling visualized in living mice by repeated examination of the same neuron.

Puszkin, S., S. Berl, E. Puszkin, and D. D. Clarke (1968). *Science* 161:170–171. Actomyosin-like protein isolated from mammalian brain.

Puszkin, S., W. J. Nicklas, and S. Berl (1972). *J. Neurochem.* 19:1319–1333. Actomyosin-like protein in brain: Subcellular distribution.

Pysh, J. J. (1969). *Am. J. Anat.* 124:411–430. The development of the extracellular space in neonatal rat inferior colliculus: An electron microscopic study.

Pysh, J. J. (1970). *Brain Res.* 18:325–342. Mitochondrial changes in rat inferior colliculus during postnatal development: An electron microscopic study.

Pysh, J. J. (1978). *Brain Res.* 154:219–230. Evidence for loss of Purkinje cell dendrites during late development: A morphometric Golgi analysis in the mouse.

Pytela, R., M. D. Pierschbacher, and E. Ruoslahti (1985). *Proc. Natl. Acad. Sci. U.S.A.* 82:5766–5770. A 125/115-kDa cell surface receptor specific for vitronectin interacts with the arginine-glycine-aspartic acid adhesion sequence derived from fibronectin.

Quarles, R. H. (1985). *Dev. Neurosci.* 6:285–303. Myelin-associated glycoprotein in development and disease.

Quastler, H. (1959). *Exp. Cell Res.* 17:420–438. Cell population kinetics in the intestinal epithelium of the mouse.

Querido, A., N. Bleichrodt, and R. Djokomoeljanto (1978). Thyroid hormones and human mental development, pp. 337–346. In *Maturation of the Nervous System, Progress in Brain Research*, Vol. 48, (M. A. Corner, N. E. van de

Poll, D. F. Swaab, and H. B. M. Uylings, eds.), Elsevier, Amsterdam.

Quilliam, T. A. (1962). *Anat. Rec.* 142:322. Growth, degrowth and regrowth in the Herbst corpuscle.

Quine, W. V. O. (1960). *Word and Object.* Harvard Univ. Press, Cambridge, Mass.

Quine, W. V. O. (1969). *Ontological Relativity.* Harvard Univ. Press, Cambridge, Mass.

Raaf, J., and J. W. Kernohan (1944). *Am. J. Anat.* 75:151–172. A study of the external granular layer in the cerebellum.

Rabié, A., and J. Legrand (1973). *Brain Res.* 61:267–278. Effects of thyroid hormone and undernourishment on the amount of synaptosomal fraction in the cerebellum of the young cat.

Rabie, A., A. J. Patel, M. C. Clavel, and J. Legrand (1979). *Dev. Neurosci.* 2:183–194. Effect of thyroid deficiency on the growth of the hippocampus in the rat. A combined biochemcial and morphological study.

Rabl-Rückhard, H. (1890). *Neurol. Centralbl. Leipzig* 9:199. Sind die Ganglianzellen amöboid? Eine Hypothese zur Mechanik psychischer Vorgänge.

Race, J., Jr. (1961). *Gen. Comp. Endocrinol.* 1:322–331. Thyroid hormone control of development of lateral motor column cells in the lumbo-sacral cord in hypophysectomized *Rana pipiens.*

Race, J., Jr., and R. J. Terry (1965). *Anat. Rec.* 152:99–106. Further studies on the development of the lateral motor column in Anuran larvae. I. Normal development in *Rana temporaria.*

Radeke, M. J., T. P. Misko, C. Hsu, L. A. Herzenberg, and E. M. Shooter (1987). *Nature* 298:593–597. Gene transfer and molecular cloning of the rat nerve growth factor receptor.

Radinsky, L. (1967). *Science* 155:836–838. Relative brain size: A new measure.

Radinsky, L. (1975). *Am. Scient.* 63:656–663. Primate brain evolution.

Rádl, E. (1930). *The History of Biological Theories.* Oxford University Press, London.

Raedler, A., and J. Sievers (1976). *Anat. Embryol.* 149:173–181. Light and electron microscopical studies on specific cells of the marginal zone in the developing rat cerebral cortex.

Raedler, E., A. Raedler, and S. Feldhaus (1980). *Anat. Embryol.* 158:253–269. Dynamic aspects of neocortical ontogenesis in the rat.

Raff, M. C. (1989). *Science* 243:1450–1455. Glial cell diversification in the rat optic nerve.

Raff, M. C., R. Mirsky, K. L. Fields, R. P. Lisak, S. H. Dorfman, D. H. Silberberg, N. A. Gregson, S. Liebowitz, and M. C. Kennedy (1978). *Nature* 274:813–816. Galactocerebroside is a specific cell surface antigenic marker for oligodendrocytes in culture.

Raff, M. C., K. L. Fields, S.-I. Hakomori, R. Mirsky, R. M. Pruss, and J. Winter (1979). *Brain Res.* 174:283–308. Cell type specific markers for distinguishing and studying neurons and the major classes of glial cells in culture.

Raff, M. C., R. H. Miller, and M. Noble (1983). *Nature* 303:390–396. A glial progenitor cell that develops *in vitro* into an astroctye or an oligodendrocyte depending on the culture medium.

Raff, M. C., E. A. Abney, and A. Miller (1984a). *Dev. Biol.* 106:53–60. Two glial cell lineages diverge prenatally in rat optic nerve.

Raff, M. C., B. P. Williams, and R. H. Miller (1984b). *EMBO J.* 3:1857–1864. The *in vitro* differentiation of a bipotential glial progenitor cell.

Rager, G. (1976a). *Proc. Roy. Soc. (London) Ser. B.* 192:331–352. Morphogenesis and physiogenesis of the retinotectal connection in the chicken. I. The retinal ganglion cells and their axons.

Rager, G. (1976b). *Proc. Roy. Soc. (London) Ser. B* 192:353–370. Morphogenesis and physiogenesis of the retinotectal connection in the chicken. II. The retino-tectal synapse.

Rager, G. (1980). *Adv. Anat. Embryol. Cell Biol.* 63:1–90. Development of the retinotectal projection in the chicken.

Rager, G., and U. Rager (1976). *Exp. Brain Res.* 25:551–553. Generation and degeneration of retinal ganglion cells in the chicken.

Rager, G., and U. Rager (1978). *Exp. Brain Res.* 33:65–78. Systems matching by degeneration. I. A quantitative electron microscopic study of the generation and degeneration of ganglion cells in the chicken.

Raine, C. S. (1984). Morphology of myelin and myelination, pp. 1–50 In *Myelin,* 2nd edn. (P. Morell, ed.), Plenum, New York.

Raine, C. S., S. E. Poduslo, and W. T. Norton (1971). *Brain Res.* 27:11–24. The ultrastructure of purified preparations of neurons and glial cells.

Raisman, G. (1969). *Brain Res.* 14:25–48. Neuronal plasticity in the septal nuclei of the adult rat.

Raisman, G., and P. M. Field (1971). *Science* 173:731–733. Sexual dimorphism in the preoptic area of the rat.

Raisman, G., and P. M. Field (1973a). *Brain Res.* 54:1–29. Sexual dimorphism in the neuropil of the preoptic area of the rat and its dependence on neonatal androgen.

Raisman, G., and P. M. Field (1973b). *Brain Res.* 50:241–264. A quantitative investigation of the development of collateral reinnervation after partial deafferentation of the septal nuclei.

Raivich, G., and G. W. Kreutzberg (1987). *Neuroscience* 20:23–36. The localization and distribution of high affinity βNGF binding sites in the central nervous system in the adult rat. A light microscopic autoradiographic study using [^{125}-I] β-NGF.

Raivich, G., A. Zimmermann, and A. Sutter (1985). *EMBO J.* 4:637–644. The spatial and temporal pattern of βNGF receptor expression in the developing chick embryo.

Raivich, G., A. Zimmermann, and A. Sutter (1987). *J. Comp. Neurol.* 256:229–245. Nerve growth factor (NGF) receptor expression in chicken cranial development.

Raju, T., A. Bignami, and K. Dahl (1981). *Dev. Biol.* 85:344–357. *In vivo* and *in vitro* differentiation of neurons and astrocytes in the rat embryo. Immunofluorescence study with neurofilament and glial filament antisera.

Rakic, P. (1971a). *Brain Res.* 33:471–476. Guidance of neurons migrating to the fetal monkey neocortex.

Rakic, P. (1971b). *J. Comp. Neurol.* 141:283–312. Neuron-glia relationship during granule cell migration in developing cerebellar cortex. A Golgi and electronmicroscopic study in *Macacus rhesus.*

Rakic, P. (1972a). *J. Comp. Neurol.* 145:61–84. Mode of cell migration to the superficial layers of fetal monkey neocortex.

Rakic, P. (1972b). *J. Comp. Neurol.* **146**:335–354. Extrinsic cytological determinants of basket and stellate cell dendritic pattern in the cerebellar molecular layer.

Rakic, P. (1973). *J. Comp. Neurol.* **147**:523–546. Kinetics of proliferation and latency between final cell division and onset of differentiation of cerebellar stellate and basket neurons.

Rakic, P. (1974). *Science* **183**:425–427. Neurons in rhesus monkey visual cortex: Systematic relation between time of origin and eventual disposition.

Rakic, P. (1975a). *Birth Defects* **11**:95–129. Cell migration and neuronal ectopias in the brain.

Rakic, P. (1975b). *Cold Spring Harbor Symp. Quant. Biol.* **40**:333–346. Synaptic specificity in the cerebellar cortex: Study of anomalous circuits induced by single gene mutations in mice.

Rakic, P. (1976a). *Phil. Trans. Roy. Soc. (London) Ser. B.* Prenatal development of the visual system in rhesus monkey.

Rakic, P. (1976b). *Nature* **261**:467–471. Prenatal genesis of connections subserving ocular dominance in the rhesus monkey.

Rakic, P. (1977a). *J. Comp. Neurol.* **176**:23–52. Genesis of the dLGN in the rhesus monkey: Site of origin, kinetics of proliferation, routes of migration and pattern of distribution of neurons.

Rakic, P. (1977b). *Phil. Trans. Roy. Soc. (London) Ser. B.* **278**:245–260. Prenatal development of the visual system in rhesus monkey.

Rakic, P. (1978). *Postgrad. Med. J.* **54**:25–40. Neuronal migration and contact guidance in primate telencephalon.

Rakic, P. (1981a). *Science* **214**:928–931. Development of visual centres in the primate brain depends on binocular competition before birth.

Rakic, P. (1981b). *Trends Neurosci.* **4**:184–187. Neuronal-glial interaction during brain development.

Rakic, P. (1986). *Trends Neurosci.* **9**:11–15. Mechanism of ocular dominance segregation in the lateral geniculate nucleus: Competitive elimination hypothesis.

Rakic, P. (1987). Principles of neuronal migration. In *Handbook of Physiology* (W. M. Cowan, ed.), Am. Physiol. Soc., Bethesda.

Rakic, P. (1988). *Science* **241**:170–176. Specification of cerebral cortical areas.

Rakic, P., and R. S. Nowakowski (1981). *J. Comp. Neurol.* **196**:99–128. The time of origin of neurons in the hippocampal region of the rhesus monkey.

Rakic, P., and R. P. Riley (1983). *Nature* **305**:135–137. Regulation of axon number in primate optic nerve by prenatal binocular competition.

Rakic, P., and R. L. Sidman (1968). *J. Neuropathol. Exp. Neurol.* **27**:246–276. Supravital DNA synthesis in the developing human and mouse brain.

Rakic, P., and R. L. Sidman (1969). *Z. Anat. Entwicklungsgesch.* **129**:53–82. Telencephalic origin of pulvinar neurons in the fetal human brain.

Rakic, P., and R. L. Sidman (1970). *J. Comp. Neurol.* **139**:473–500. Histogenesis of cortical layers in human cerebellum, particularly the lamina dissecans.

Rakic, P., and R. L. Sidman (1972). *J. Neuropathol. Exp. Neurol.* **31**:192. Synaptic organization of displaced and disoriented cerebellar cortical neurons in reeler mice.

Rakic, P., and R. L. Sidman (1973a). *J. Comp. Neurol.* **152**:103–132. Sequence and developmental abnormalities leading to granule cell deficit in cerebellar cortex of weaver mutant mice.

Rakic, P., and R. L. Sidman (1973b). *J. Comp. Neurol.* **152**:133–162. Organization of cerebellar cortex secondary to deficit of granule cells in weaver mutant mice.

Rakic, P., and R. L. Sidman (1973c). *Proc. Natl. Acad. Sci. U.S.A.* **70**:240–244. Weaver mutant mouse cerebellum: Defective neuronal migration secondary to abnormality of Bergmann glia.

Rakic, P., L. J. Stensaas, E. P. Sayre, and R. L. Sidman (1974). *Nature* **250**:31–34. Computer-aided three-dimensional reconstruction and quantitative analysis of cells from serial electron microscopic montages of foetal monkey brain.

Rakic, P., J.-P. Bourgeois, M. F. Eckenhoff, N. Zecevic, and P. S. Goldman-Rakic (1986). *Science* **232**:232–235. Concurrent overproduction of synapses in diverse regions of the primate cerebral cortex.

Rall, W. (1970). Cable properties of dendrites and effects of synaptic location, pp. 175–187. In *Excitatory Synaptic Mechanisms. Proceedings of the 5th International Meeting of Neurobiologists*, Universitets Forlaget, Oslo.

Rall, W. (1974). Dendritic spines, synaptic potency and neuronal plasticity. In *Cellular Mechanisms Subserving Changes in Neuronal Activity* (C. Woody, K. Brown, T. Crow, and J. Knispel, eds.), Brain Information Service, UCLA, Los Angeles.

Rall, W. (1978). Dendritic spines and synaptic potency. In *Studies in Neurophysiology* (A. K. McIntyre, and K. Porter, eds.), Cambridge Univ. Press, Cambridge.

Rall, W., and I. Segev (1988). *Neurol. Neurobiol.* **37**:263–282. Synaptic integration and excitable dendritic spine clusters: Structure/function.

Ralston, H. J., and K. L. Chow (1973). *J. Comp. Neurol.* **147**:321–350. Synaptic reorganization in the degenerating lateral geniculate nucleus of the rabbit.

Rambourg, A., and B. Droz (1980). *J. Neurochem.* **35**:16–25. Smooth endoplasmic reticulum and axonal transport.

Rami, A., A. Rabie, and A. J. Patel (1986a). *Neuroscience* **19**:1207–1216. Thyroid hormone and development of the rat hippocampus: Cell acquisition in the dentate gyrus.

Rami, A., A. Rabie, and A. J. Patel (1986b). *Neuroscience* **19**:1217–1226. Thyroid hormone and development of the rat hippocampus: Morphological alterations in granule and pyramidal cells.

Ramoa, A. S., G. Campbell, and C. J. Shatz (1988). *J. Neurosci.* **8**:4239–4261. Dendritic growth and remodeling of cat retinal ganglion cells during fetal and postnatal development.

Ramón y Cajal, S. (1888a). *Rev. trim. Histol. normal y Pathol.* Estructura de los centros nerviosos de las aves.

Ramón y Cajal, S. (1888b). *Rev. trim. Histol. normal y Pathol.* May 1888. Terminaciones nerviosas los husos musculares de la rana.

Ramón y Cajal, S. (1889a). *Man. de Histol. Normal y Técnica Micrográfica.* Libreria de Pascuel Aguilar, Valencia.

Ramón y Cajal, S. (1889b). *La medicina práctica, Madrid,* 2 Oct. 1889. Connexión general de los elementos nerviosos.

Ramón y Cajal, S. (1890a). *Int. Mschr. Anat. Physiol.* **7**:12–31. A propos de certains éléments bipolaires du cervelet avec quelques détails nouveaux sur l'évolution des fibres cérébelleuses.

Ramón y Cajal, S. (1890b). *Int. Mschr. Anat. Physiol.* **7**:12–31.

Sur les fibres nerveuses de la conche granuleuse du cervelet et sur l'évolution des éléments cérébelleux.

Ramón y Cajal, S. (1890c). *Anat. Anz.* 5:85–95; 111–119; 609–613; 631–639. Sur l'origine et les ramifications des fibres nerveuses de la moelle embryonnaire.

Ramón y Cajal, S. (1890d). *Anat. Anz.* 5:579–587. Réponse à Mr. Golgi à propos des fibrilles collaterales de la moelle épinière, et de la structure générale de la substance grise.

Ramón y Cajal, S. (1890e). *Gac. san Barcelona,* 11 October. Origen y terminación de las fibras nerviosas olfatorias.

Ramón y Cajal, S. (1890f). *Gac. san Barcelona, II(12):* 414–419. Sobre la aparición de las expansiones celulares la médula embrionaria.

Ramón y Cajal, S. (1891a). *Cellule* 7:125–176. Sur la structure de l'écorce cérébrale de quelques mammifères.

Ramón y Cajal, S. (1891b). *Rev. Cien. méd. Barcelona* 17:673. Significación fisiológica de las expansiones protoplasmáticas y nervosias de las células de la substancia gris.

Ramón y Cajal, S. (1892). *Rev. Cien. méd. Barcelona* 18:361–376. Nuevo concepto de la histologia de los centros nerviosos.

Ramón y Cajal, S. (1893). *La Cellule* 9:17–257. La rétine des vertébrés. Translation in Rodiek, R. W. (1973).

Ramón y Cajal, S. (1894a). *Die Retina der Wirbelthiere.* Bergmann-Verlag, Wiesbaden.

Ramón y Cajal, S. (1894b). *Les nouvelles idées sur la structure du système nerveux chez l'homme et chez les vertébrés. Reinwald, Paris.*

Ramón y Cajal, S. (1895a). *Rev. med. cirurg. práct. Madrid* 36:497–508. Algunas conjeturas sobre el mecanismo anatómico de la ideación, asociación y atención. Translated into German in *Arch. Anat. Physiol. Anat. Abt. Leipzig* 4/6:367–378 (1895).

Ramón y Cajal, S. (1895b). *Manual de Histologia Normal y de Técnica Micrográfica.* 1ª edición, N. Moya, Madrid. (2ª ed., 1897; 3ª ed., 1901; 4ª ed., 1905).

Ramón y Cajal, S. (1896a). *Revista trimestral micrográfica* 1:123–136. Las espinas colaterales de las células del cerebro teñidas con el azul de metileno.

Ramón y Cajal, S. (1896b). *Beitrag zur Studium der Medulla oblongata, des Kleinhirns und des Ursprung der Gehirnnerven.* Ambrosius Barth, Leipzig.

Ramón y Cajal, S. (1897). *Rev. Trim. Micrografica* 2:105–127. Las células de cilindro-eje corto de la capa molecular del cerebro.

Ramón y Cajal, S. (1897, 1899–1904). *Textura del sistema nervioso del hombre y de los vertebrados.* 2 vols. in 3. N. Moya, Madrid.

Ramón y Cajal, S. (1900). *Rev. Trim. Micrografica* 5:1–11. Estudios sobre la corteza cerebral humana. III. Corteza motriz.

Ramón y Cajal, S. (1901–1917). *Recuerdos de mi vida,* primera parte *Mi infancia y juventud;* segunda parte: *Historia de mi labor científica.* Third edition 1923 with *"Post scriptum."* English translation (incomplete) of the third edition by E. H. Craigie and J. Cano, *Recollections of My Life,* American Philosophical Society, Philadelphia (1937).

Ramón y Cajal, S. (1903). *Trab. Lab. Invest. Biol. Univ. Madrid.* 2:129–221. Un sencillo método de coloración selectiva del retículo protoplásmatico y sus efectos en los diversos organos nerviosos.

Ramón y Cajal, S. (1905a). *Trab. Lab. Invest. Biol. Univ. Madrid* 4:119–210. Mecanismo de la regeneración de los nervios.

Ramón y Cajal, S. (1905b). *Trab. Lab. Invest. Biol. Univ. Madrid* 4:227–294. Génesis de las fibras nerviosas del embrión.

Ramón y Cajal, S. (1906). *Studien über die Hirnrinde des Menschen. H.5, Vergleichende Strukturbeschreibung und Histogenesis der Hirnrinde.* J. A. Barth, Leipzig.

Ramón y Cajal, S. (1907). *Anat. Anz.* 5:113–144. Die histogenetische Beweise der Neuronentheorie von His und Forel.

Ramón y Cajal, S. (1908). *Anat. Anz.* 23:1–25; 65–87. Nouvelles observationes sur l'évolution des neuroblasts avec quelques remarques sur l'hypothése neurogénétique de Hensen-Held, p. 71. In *Studies in Vertebrate Neurogenesis,* L. Guth (trans.). Thomas, Springfield, Ill.

Ramón y Cajal, S. (1909–1911). *Histologie du Systeme Nerveux de l'Homme et des Vertébrés,* 2 vols. L. Azoulay (trans.). Reprinted by Instituto Ramón y Cajal del C.S.I.C., Madrid, 1952–1955.

Ramón y Cajal, S. (1910). *Trab. Lab. Invest. Biol. Univ. Madrid* 8:63–134. Algunas observaciones favorables á la hipótesis neurotrópica.

Ramón y Cajal, S. (1913a). *Trab. Lab. Invest. biol. Univ. Madrid* 11:219–237. Sobre un nuevo proceder de impregnacion de la neuroglia y sus resultados en los centros nerviosos del hombre y animales.

Ramón y Cajal, S. (1913b). *Trab. Lab. Invest. Biol. Univ. Madrid* 11:255–315. Contribución al conocimiento de la neuroglia del cerebro humano.

Ramón y Cajal, S. (1913–1914). *Estudios sobre la Degeneración y Regeneración del Sistema Nervioso.* N. Moya, Madrid.

Ramón y Cajal, S. (1916). *Trab. Lab. Invest. Biol. Univ. Madrid* 14:155–162. El proceder del oro-sublimado para la coloracion de la neuroglia.

Ramón y Cajal, S. (1919). *Trab. Lab. Invest. Biol. Univ. Madrid* 17:181–228. Acción neurotrópica de los epitelios (Algunas detalles sobre el mecanismo genético de las ramificaciones nerviosas intraepiteliales, sensitivas y sensoriales), pp. 149–200. In *Studies On Vertebrate Neurogenesis,* L. Guth (trans.). Thomas, Springfield, Ill., 1960.

Ramón y Cajal, S. (1920). *Trab. Lab. Invest. Biol. Univ. Madrid* 18:109–127. Algunas consideraciones sobre la mesoglia de Robertson y Río-Hortega.

Ramón y Cajal, S. (1922). Studies on the fine structure of the regional cortex of rodents. I: Subcortical cortex (retrosplenial cortex of Brodmann). *Trab. Lab. Invest. Biol. Univ. Madrid* 20:1–30. Translated by J. De Felipe and E. G. Jones in *Cajal on the Cerebral Cortex.* Oxford Univ. Press, New York, 1988.

Ramón y Cajal, S. (1923). *Recuerdos de mi vida: Historia de mi labor científica.* 3rd edn. Juan Pueyo, Madrid.

Ramón y Cajal, S. (1925). *Trab. Lab. Invest. Biol. Univ. Madrid* 23:245–254. Quelques remarques sur les plaques motrices de la langue des mammiféres.

Ramón y Cajal, S. (1928). *Degeneration and Regeneration of the Nervous System,* R. M. May, (trans.), Hafner, New York, 1959.

Ramón y Cajal, S. (1929a). Étude sur la neurogenése de quelques vertébrés, L. Guth (trans.). In *Studies on Vertebrate Neurogenesis.* Thomas, Springfield, Ill., 1960.

Ramón y Cajal, S. (1929b). *Trab. Lab. Invest. Biol. Univ.*

Madrid 26:107–130. Considérations critiques sur le rôle trophiques des dendrites et leurs prétendues relations vasculaires.

Ramón y Cajal, S. (1933). *Histology.* Translated by M. Fernán-Núñez from the 10th Spanish edition). Wood, Baltimore.

Ramón y Cajal, S. (1933). ¿Neuronismo o reticularismo? Las pruebas objectivas de la unidad anatómica, de las cellulas nerviosas. *Arch. Neurobiol. Psicol. Madr.* 13:217–291; 579–646; French transl. *Trab. Lab. Invest. Biol. Univ. Madrid* 29:1–137 (1934); German transl. Die Neuronenlehre, *Bumke u. Foersters Handb. Neurol.* 1:887–994 (1935); English transl. by M. Ubeda Purkiss and C. A. Fox, *Neuron theory or reticular theory? Objective evidence of the anatomical unity of the nerve cells.* Consejo Superior de Investigaciones Cientificas, Madrid, 1954.

Ramón y Cajal, S. (1937). *Recollections of My Life.* English translation by E. H. Craigie and J. Cano from the third (1923) Spanish edition. Amer. Philos. Soc. Philadelphia.

Ramón y Cajal, S. (1952). *Trab. Inst. Cajal. Invest. Biol.* 44:1–8, originally published in *Trab. Lab. Invest. Biol. Univ. Madrid* 1:1–8. (1901) Significación probable de las células nerviosas de cilindro-eje corto.

Ramón y Cajal, S., and D. Sanchez (1915). *Trab. Lab. Invest. Biol. Univ. Madrid* 13:1–64. Contribución al conocimiento de los centros nerviosos de los insectos.

Ramón-Moliner, E. (1957). *Stain Technol.* 32:105–116. A chlorate-formaldehyde modification of the Golgi method.

Ramón-Moliner, E. (1958). *J. Comp. Neurol.* 110:157–171. A study of neuroglia. The problem of transitional forms.

Ramón-Moliner, E. (1962). *J. Comp. Neurol.* 119:211–227. An attempt at classifying nerve cells on the basis of their dendritic patterns.

Ramón-Moliner, E. (1968). The morphology of dendrites, pp. 205–267. In *The Structure and Function of Nervous Tissue,* Vol. 1, (G. H. Bourne, ed.), Academic Press, New York.

Ramón-Moliner, E. (1970a). The Golgi-Cox technique, pp. 32–55. In *Contemporary Research Methods in Neuroanatomy,* (W. J. H. Nauta, and S. O. E. Ebbeson, eds.), Springer, New York.

Ramón-Moliner, E. (1970b). The Golgi-Cox technique, pp186–216. In *Contemporary Research Methods in Neuroanatomy,* (W. J. H. Nauta, and S. O. E. Ebbeson, eds.), Springer, Berlin, Heidelberg, New York.

Ranish, N. A., W. D. Dettbarn, and L. Wecker (1980). *Brain Res.* 191:379–386. Nerve stump length-dependent loss of acetylcholinesterase activity in endplate regions of rat diaphragm.

Ranke, O. (1910). *Beitr. Pathol. Anat. Allg. Pathol.* 47:51–125. Beiträge zur Kenntnis der normalen und pathologischen Hirnrindenbildung.

Rankin, E. C. C., and J. E. Cook (1986). *Exp. Brain. Res.* 63:409–420. Topographic refinement of the regenerating retinotectal projection of the goldfish in standard laboratory conditions. A quantitative WGS-HRP study.

Ranscht, B., P. A. Clapshaw, J. Price, M. Noble, and W. Seifert (1982). *Proc. Natl. Acad. Sci. U.S.A.* 79:2709–2713. Development of oligodendrocytes and Schwann cells studied with a monoclonal antibody against galactocerebroside.

Ranson, S. W. (1906). *J. Comp. Neurol.* 16:265–293. Retrograde degeneration in the spinal nerves.

Ranson, S. W. (1911). *Am. J. Anat.* 12:67–87. Non-medullated nerve fibers in the spinal nerves.

Ranson, S. W. (1912a). *J. Comp. Neurol.* 22:159–175. The structure of the spinal ganglia and of the spinal nerves.

Ranson, S. W. (1912b). *J. Comp. Neurol.* 22:487–537. Degeneration and regeneration of nerve fibers.

Ranson, S. W. (1913). *J. Comp. Neurol.* 23:259–281. The course within the spinal cord of the non-medullated fibers of the dorsal roots: A study of Lissauer's tract in the cat.

Ranson, S. W. (1914). *J. Comp. Neurol.* 24:531–545. An experimental study of Lissauer's tract and the dorsal roots.

Ranson, S. W. (1915). *Brain* 38:381–389. Unmyelinated nerve-fibers as conductors of protopathic sensation.

Ranson, S. W., W. H. Droegemueller, H. K. Davenport, and C. Fisher (1935). *Assoc. Res. Nerv. Ment. Dis.* 15:3–34. Number, size and myelination of the sensory fibers in the cerebrospinal nerves. Research Publications.

Ranvier, L. (1889). *Traité Technique d'Histologie.* Savy, Paris.

Ranvier, L.-A. (1871). *Compt. rend. hebd. Acad. Sci. Paris* 73:1168–1171. Contributions à l'histologie et à la physiologie des nerfs periphériques.

Ranvier, L.-A. (1872). *Arch. Physiol. norm. path.* 4:129–149. Recherches sur l'histologie et la physiologie des nerfs.

Ranvier, L. A. (1880). *Quart. J. Micr. Sci.* 20:456–458. On the termination of the nerves in the epidermis.

Ranvier, M. L. (1878). *Leçons sur l'histologie du système nerveux,* 2 vols. Savy, Paris.

Rapaport, D. H., and J. Stone (1982). *Dev. Brain Res.* 5:273–279. The site of commencement of maturation in mammalian retina: Observations in the cat.

Rapoport, A., and J. Stempak (1968). *Anat. Rec.* 161:361–376. Ultrastructure of the ventral horn cell in the albino rat.

Rapoport, S. I. (1970). *Am. J. Physiol.* 219:270–274. Effects of concentrated solutions on blood-brain barrier.

Rapoport, S. I., M. Ohata, and E. D. London (1981). *Fed. Proc.* 40:2322–2325. Cerebral blood flow and glucose utilization following opening of the blood-brain barrier and during maturation of the rat brain.

Rash, J. E., and M. H. Ellisman (1974). *J. Cell Biol.* 63:567–586. Studies of excitable membranes. I. Macromolecular specializations of the neuromuscular junction and the nonjunctional sarcolemma.

Rather, L. J. (1958). *Disease, Life and Man, Selected Essays by Rudolph Virchow.* Stanford Univ. Press, Stanford.

Rathjen, F. G., and M. Schachner (1984). *EMBO J.* 3:1–10. Immunocytological and biochemical characterization of a new neuronal cell surface component (L1 antigen) which is involved in cell adhesion.

Rathjen, F. G., J. M. Wolff, R. Frank, F. Bonhoeffer, and U. Rutishauser (1987). *J. Cell Biol.* 104:343–353. Membrane glycoproteins involved in neurite fasciculation.

Ratner, A., and N. J. Adamo (1971). *Neuroendocrinol.* 8:26–35. Arcuate nucleus region in androgen-sterilized female rats: Ultrastructural observations.

Ratner, N., L. Glaser, and R. P. Bunge (1984). *J. Cell Biol.* 98:1150–1155. PC12 cells as a source of neurite-derived cell surface mitogen, which stimulates Schwann cell division.

Ratner, N., C. Eldridge, R. P. Bunge, and L. Glaser (1987). Effects of an inhibitor of proteoglycan biosynthesis on neuron-induced Schwann cell proliferation and basal lamina formation by Schwann cells, pp. 127–139. In *Mesenchymal/Epithelial Interactions in Neural Development* (J. R. Wolff, and J. Sievers, eds.), Springer-Verlag, Berlin.

Rauber, A. (1886a). *Arch. Mikroskop. Anat.* 26:622–644. Die Kerntheilungsfiguren im Medullarrohr der Wirbeltiere.

Rauber, A. (1886b). *Zool. Anz.* 9:159–164. Über die Mitosen des Medullarrohres.

Rausch, G., and H. Scheich (1982). *Neurosci. Lett.* 29:129–133. Dendritic spine loss and enlargement during maturation of the speech-control-system in the mynah bird (*Gracula religiosa*).

Rauschecker, J. P., and S. Hahn (1987). *Nature* 326:183–185. Ketamine-xylazine anaesthesia blocks consolidation of ocular dominance changes in kitten visual cortex.

Raven, C. P. (1931–1933). *Arch. Entw. Mech. Organ* 125:210–292; 129:179–198; 130:517–561. Zur Entwicklung der Ganglienleiste.

Raven, C. P. (1936). *Arch. Entw.-Mech. Organ.* 134:122–146. Zur Entwicklung der Ganglienleiste. V. Differenzierung des Rumpfganglienleistenmaterials.

Raven, C. P. (1937). *J. Comp. Neurol.* 67:221–240. Experiments on the origin of the sheath cells and sympathetic neuroblasts in amphibia.

Ray, K., B. Bhattacharyya, and B. B. Biswas (1980). *Eur. J. Cell Biol.* 2:288. Colcemid and colchicine binding to tubulin: Similarity and dissimilarity.

Raymond, P. A., and S. S. Easter Jr. (1983). *J. Neurosci.* 3:1077–1091. Post-embryonic growth of the optic tectum in goldfish. I. Location of germinal cells and numbers of neurons produced.

Raynaud, J. P., C. Mercier-Bodard, and C. Baulieu (1971). *Steroids* 18:767–788. Rat estradiol binding plasma protein.

Raza, A., H. Preisler, G. Mayers, and R. Bankert (1984). *N. Engl. J. Med.* 310:991. Rapid enumeration of S-phase cells by means of monclonal antibodies.

Ready, D. F., T.E. Hanson, and S. Benzer (1976). *Dev. Biol.* 53:217–240. Development of the *Drosophila* retina, a neurocrystalline lattice.

Rebagliati, M. R., D. L. Weeks, R. P. Harvey and D. A. Melton (1985). *Cell* 42:769–777. Identification and cloning of localized maternal RNAs from *Xenopus* eggs.

Rebière, A., and J. Dainat (1976). *Acta Neuropath.* 35:117–129. Répercussions de l'hypothyroïdie sur la synaptogenèse dans le cortex cérébelleux du rat.

Rebière, A., and J. Legrand (1970a). *Brain Res.* 22:299–312. Absence d'effets marqués de l'hormone hypophysaire de croissance sur la maturation histologique du cortex cérébelleux chez le jeune rat normal ou hypothyroïdien.

Rebière, A., and J. Legrand (1970b). *C. R. Acad. Sci. (Paris)* 274:3581–3584. Données quantitatives sur la synaptogenèse dans le cervelet du rat normal et rendu hypothyroïdien par le propyl-thiouracyle.

Rebière, A., and J. Legrand (1972). *Arch. Anat. Microsc. Morphol. Exp.* 61:105–126. Effets comparés de las sous-alimentation, de l'hypothyroïdisme et de l'hyperthyroïdisme sur la maturation de la zone moléculaire du cortex cérébelleux chez le jeune rat.

Rebiere, A., J. Dainat, and J. C. Bisconte (1983). *Dev. Brain Res.* 6:113–122. Autoradiographic study of neurogenesis in the duck olfactory bulb.

Reddy, D. R., W. J. Davis, R. B. Ohlander, and D. J. Bihary (1973). Computer analysis of neuronal structure, pp. 227–253. In *Intracellular Staining in Neurobiology* (S. B. Kater, and C. Nicholson, eds.), Springer-Verlag, New York.

Reddy, V. V. R., F. Naftolin, and K. J. Ryan (1974). *Endocrinology* 94:117–121. Conversion of androstenedione to estrone by neural tissues from fetal and neonatal rats.

Redfern, P. A. (1970). *J. Physiol. (London)* 209:701–709. Neuromuscular transmission in new-born rats.

Redies, C., M. Diksic, and H. Rimi (1990). *J. Neurosci.* 10:2791–2803. Functional organization in the ferret visual cortex: A double-label 2-deoxyglucose study.

Reeber, A., G. Vincendon, and J. P. Zanetta (1981). *Brain Res.* 229:53–65. Isolation and immunohistochemical localization of a 'Purkinje cell specific glycoprotein subunit' from rat cerebellum.

Rees, R. P., and T. S. Rees (1981). *Neuroscience* 6:247–254. New structural features of feeze-substituted neuritic growth cones.

Rees, R. P., M. P. Bunge, and R. P. Bunge (1976). *J. Cell Biol.* 68:240–263. Morphological changes in the neuritic growth cone and target neuron during synaptic junction development in culture.

Rees, S., and R. Harding (1988). *Int. J. Dev. Neurosci.* 6:461–469. The effects of intrauterine growth retardation on the development of the Purkinje cell dendritic tree in the cerebellar cortex of fetal sheep: A note on the ontogeny of the Purkinje cell.

Reese, T. S., and M. J. Karnovsky (1967). *J. Cell Biol.* 34:204–217. Fine structural localization of a blood-brain barrier to exogenous peroxidase.

Regan, L. J., J. Dodd, S. H. Barondes, and T. M. Jessell (1986). *Proc. Natl. Acad. Sci. U.S.A.* 830:2248–2252. Selective expression of endogenous lactose-binding lectins and lactoseries glycoconjugates in subsets of rat sensory neurons.

Reh, T. A., and M. Constantine-Paton (1984). *J. Neurosci.* 4:442–457. Retinal ganglion cell terminals change their projection sites during larval develpment of *Rana pipiens*.

Reh, T. A., and M. Constantine-Paton (1985). *J. Neurosci.* 5:1132–1143. Eye specific segregation requires neural activity in 3 eyed *Rana pipiens*.

Rehkämper, G., E. Haase, and H. D. Frahm (1988). *Brain Behav. Evol.* 31:141–149. Allometric comparison of brain weight and brain structure volumes in different breeds of the domestic pigeon, *Columba livia f. d.* (Fantails, Homing Pigeons, Strassers).

Reichenbach, H. (1951). *The Rise of Scientific Philosophy*, Univ. of Calif. Press, Berkeley.

Reichert, F., and S. Rotshenker (1979). *Brain Res.* 170:187–189. Motor axon terminal sprouting in intact muscles.

Reinis, S. (1972). *Physiol. Chem. Phys.* 4:391–397. Autoradiographic study of ^{3}H-thymidine incorporation into brain DNA during learning.

Reinisch, J. M., N. G. Simon, W. G. Karow, and R. Gandelman (1978). *Science* 202:436–438. Prenatal exposure to prednisone in humans and animals retards intrauterine growth.

Reisert, I., G. Wildemann, D. Grab, and C. Pilgrim (1984). *J. Comp. Neurol.* 229:121–128. The glial reaction in the course of axon regeneration: A stereological study of the rat hypoglossal nucleus.

Remak, R. (1837). *Froriep's Neue Notizen* 3:35–40. Weitere Beobachtungen über die Primitivfasern des Nervensystem der Wirbelthiere.

Remak, R. (1838a). *Observationes anatomicae et microscopicae de systematis nervosi structura.* G. Reimer, Berlin.

Remak, R. (1838b). *Froriep's Notizen* 7:65–70. Ueber die Verrichtungen des organischen Nervensystems.

Remak, R. (1844). Neurologische Erläuterungen, pp. 463–472. *Virchow's Arch. f. Anat. Physiol. u. wissensch. Med. Berlin.*

Remak, R. (1852). *Müller's Arch. f. Anat. Physiol. wissensch. Medicin,* pp. 47–57. Über extracellulare Entstehung thierische Zellen und über Vermehrung derselben durch Theilung.

Remak, R. (1853). *Ber. Verh. k. preuss. Akad. wiss. Berl.* 293–298. Über gangliöse Nervenfasern beim Menschen und bei den Wirbeltieren.

Remak, R. (1854). *Verhandlungen der König. Preuss. Akad. der Wissenschaften, Berlin* 19:26–32. Ueber multipolare Ganglienzellen. English translation in *Monthly J. Medical Sciences, Edinburgh* 18:362–365. Professor Remak on multipolar ganglion cells.

Remak, R. (1855a). *Untersuchungen über die Entwickelung der Wirbelthiere.* Berlin.

Remak, R., (1855b). *Dtsch. Klinik* 7:295. Über den Bau der grauen Säulen im Rückenmark der Säugethiere.

Renehan, W. E., and B. L. Munger (1986). *J. Comp. Neurol.* 246:129–146. Degeneration and reorganization of peripheral nerve in the rat trigeminal system. I. Identification and characterization of the multiple afferent innervation of the mystacial vibrissae.

Rennels, M. L., and E. Nelson (1975). *Am. J. Anat.* 144:233–241. Capillary innervation in the mammalian central nervous system: An electron microscopic demonstration.

Rennert, P. D., and G. Heinrich (1986). *Biochem. Biophys. Res. Comm.* 138:813–818. Nerve growth factor messenger RNA in brain: Localization by in situ hibridization.

Rensch, B. (1958). *Naturwissenschaften* 45:145–154, 175–180. Die Abhängigkeit der Struktur und der Leistungen tierischer Gehirne von ihrer Grösse.

Rensch, B., and A. Nolte (1949a). *Z. Vergleich. Physiol.* 31:696–710. Über die Funktion auf den Rücken transplantierter Augen.

Rensch, B., and A. Nolte (1949b). *Verhandl. Deutsch. Zool. (Mainz)* 34:208–215. Über die Funktion auf den Rucken transplantierter Augen, 2 Mitteilung.

Resko, J. A., R. W. Goy, and C. H. Phoenix (1967). *Endocrinology* 80:490–498. Uptake and distribution of exogenous testosterone-1-2-^{3}H in neural and genital tissues of the castrate guinea pig.

Resko, J. A., H. H. Feder, and R. W. Goy (1968). *J. Endocrinol.* 40:485–491. Androgen concentrations in plasma and testis of developing rat.

Retzius, G. (1890). *Biol. Untersuch. Neue Folge* 1:1–50. Zur Kenntniss des Nervensystems der Crustaceen.

Retzius, G. (1891a). *Biol. Untersuch. Neue Folge.* 2:1–28. Zur Kentniss des centralen Nervensystems der Würmer.

Retzius, G. (1891b). *Biol. Untersuch. Neue Folge* 2:29–46. Zur Kentniss des centralen Nervensystems von Amphioxus lanceolatus.

Retzius, G. (1892a). *Biol. Untersuch. neue Folge* 3:1–16. Das Nervensystem der Lumbricinen.

Retzius, G. (1892b). *Biol. Untersuch. Neue Folge* 3:17–24. Die nervösen Elemente der Kleinhirnrinde.

Retzius, G. (1892c). *Biol. Untersuch. Neue Folge* 3:25–28. Die endingungsweise des Riechnerven.

Retzius, G. (1892d). *Biol. Untersuch. Neue Folge* 3:41–52. Zur Kenntniss der motorischen Nervenendigungen.

Retzius, G. (1892e). *Biol. Untersuch. Neue Folge* 4:19–32. Die Nervenendigungen in dem Geschmacksorgan der Säugetiere und Amphibien.

Retzius, G. (1892f). *Biol. Untersuch. Neue Folge* 4:45–48. Ueber die Nervenendigungen an den Haaren.

Retzius, G. (1893a). *Biol. Untersuch. Neue Folge* 5:1–8. Die Cajal'schen Zellen des Grosshirnrinde beim Menschen und bei Säugetieren.

Retzius, G. (1893b). *Biol. Untersuch. Neue Folge* 5:48–54. Zur Kenntniss der ersten Entwicklung der nervösen Elemente im Rückenmarke des Hühnchens.

Retzius, G. (1894a). *Biol. Untersuch. Neue Folge* 6:1–28. Die Neuroglia des Gehirns beim Menschen und bei Säugethieren.

Retzius, G. (1894b). *Biol. Untersuch. Neue Folge* 6:29–36. Weitere Beiträge zur Kenntniss der Cajal'schen Zellen der Grosshirnrinde des Menschen.

Retzius, G. (1894c). *Biol. Untersuch. Neue Folge* 6:61–62. Ueber die Endigungsweise der Nerven an den Haaren des Menschen.

Retzius, G. (1896). *Das Menschenhirn.* Königliche Buchdruckerei, P. A. Norstedt & Söner, Stockholm.

Retzius, G. (1898a). *Biol. Untersuch. Neue Folge* 8:23–48. Zur äusseren Morphologie des Riechhirns der Säugethiere und des Menschen.

Retzius, G. M. (1898b). *Biol. Untersuch. Neue Folge* 8:114–117. Zur Frage von der Endigungsweise peripherischer sensibler Nerven.

Retzius, G. (1900). *Biol. Untersuch. Neue Folge* 9:51–68. Über das Hirngewicht der Schweden.

Retzius, G. (1906a). *Biol. Untersuch. Neue Folge* 13:107–112. Zur Kenntniss des Nervensystems der Daphniden.

Retzius, G. (1906b). *Cerebra Simiarum Illustrata. Das Affenhirn in bildlicher Darstellung.* Gustav Fischer, Stockholm, Jena.

Reul, J. M. H. M., and E. R. De Kloet (1985). *Endocrinology* 117:2505–2511. Two receptor systems for corticosteroids in the brain: Microdistribution and differential occupation.

Revel, J. P., and S. Ito (1967). The surface components of cells, pp. 211–234. In *The Specificity of Cell Surfaces* (B. D. Davis, and L. Warren, eds.), Prentice-Hall, Englewood Cliffs, N.J.

Rexed, B. (1944). *Acta Psychiat. Neurol. Scand.* 33:1–206. Contributions to the knowledge of postnatal development of the peripheral nervous system in man.

Rexed, B., and U. Rexed (1951). *Br. J. Ophthalmol.* 35:38–49. Degeneration and regeneration of corneal nerve fibers.

Reyer, R. W. (1983). *J. Exp. Zool.* 226:101–121. Availability time of tritium-labeled DNA precursors in newt eyes following intraperitoneal Injection of ^{3}H-thymidine.

Reynolds, R., and N. Herschkowitz (1986). *Brain Res.* 371:253–266. Selective uptake of neuroactive amino acids by both oligodendrocytes and astrocytes in primary dissociated culture: A possible role for oligodendrocytes in neurotransmitter metabolism.

Reynolds, R., and G. P. Wilkin (1988). *Development* 102:409–0425. Development of macroglial cells in rat cerebellum. II. An *in situ* histochemical study of oligodendroglial lineage from precursor to mature myelinating cell.

Reynolds, W. A. (1963). *J. Exp. Zool.* 153:237–250. The effects of thyroxine upon the initial formation of the lateral motor column and differentiation of motor neurons in *Rana pipiens.*

Reynolds, W. A. (1966). *Gen. Comp. Endocrinol.* 6:453–465. Mitotic activity in the lumbosacral spinal cord of *Rana pipiens* larvae after throxine or thiourea treatment.

Rezai, Z., and C. H. Yoon (1972). *Dev. Biol.* 29:17–26. Abnormal rate of granule cell migration in the cerebellum of "weaver" mutant mice.

Reznikov, K. Y., Z. Fülöp, and F. Hajós (1984). *Anat. Embryol.* 170:99–105. Mosaicism of the ventricular layer as the developmental basis of neocortical columnar organization.

Rhees, R. W., B. I. Grosser, and W. Stevens (1975). *Brain Res.* 83:293–300. Effect of steroid competition and time on the uptake of [³H]-corticosterone in the rat brain: An autoradiographic study.

Rhoades, R. W., and D. D. Dellacroce (1980). *Brain Res.* 202:189–195. Neonatal enucleation induces an asymmetric pattern of visual callosal connections in hamsters.

Rhodin, J. A. (1963). *An Atlas of Ultrastructure*, Saunders, Philadelphia.

Ribot, T. (1873). *English Psychology*, King, London.

Ricciuti, A. J., and E. R. Gruberg (1985). *Brain Res.* 341:399–402. Nucleus isthmi provides most tectal choline acetyltransferase in the frog *R. pipiens*.

Rice, R. L., and H. Van der Loos (1977). *J. Comp. Neurol.* 171:545–560. Development of the barrels and barrel field in the somatosensory cortex of the mouse.

Rich, M. M., and J. W. Lichtman (1989). *J. Neurosci.* 9:1781–1805. *In Vivo* visualization of pre- and postsynaptic changes during synapse elimination in reinnervated mouse muscle.

Richa, J., C. H. Damsky, C. A. Buck, B. B. Knowles, and D. Solter (1985). *Dev. Biol.* 108:513–521. Cell surface glycoproteins mediate compaction, trophoblast attachment, and endoderm formation during early mouse development.

Richards, F. F., W. H. Konigsberg, R. W. Rosenstein, and J. M. Varga (1975). *Science* 187:130–136. On the specificity of antibodies.

Richardson, P. M., U. M. McGuiness, and A. J. Aguayo (1980). *Nature* 284:264–265. Axons from CNS neurones regenerate into PNS grafts.

Richardson, P. M., U. M. McGuiness, and A. J. Aguayo (1982). *Brain Res.* 237:147–162. Peripheral nerve autografts to the rat spinal cord: Studies with axonal tracing methods.

Richardson, P. M., V. M. K. Issa, and A. J. Aguayo (1984). *J. Neurocytol.* 13:165–182. Regeneration of long spinal axons in the rat.

Richardson, P. M., V. M. K. Verge Issa, and R. J. Riopelle (1986). *J. Neurosci.* 6:2312–2321. Distribution of neuronal receptors for nerve growth factor in the rat.

Richardson, S. A., H. G. Birch, E. Grabie, and K. Yoder (1972). *J. Hlth Soc. Behav.* 13:276–284. The behavior of children in school age who were severely malnourished in the first years of life.

Richman, D. P., R. M. Stewart, and V. S. Caviness, Jr. (1973). *Neurolology* 23:413. Microgyria, lissencephaly and neuron migration to the cerebral cortex: An architectonic approach.

Richman, D. P., R. M. Stewart, H. W. Hutchinson, and V. S. Caviness, Jr. (1975). *Science* 189:18–21. Mechanical model of brain convolutional development.

Rickmann, M., and J. R. Wolff (1981). *Biblthca. Anat.* 19:142–146. Differentiation of 'preplate' neurons in the pallium of the rat.

Rickmann, M., B. M. Chronwall, and J. R. Wolff (1977). *Anat. Embryol.* 151:285–307. On the development of nonpyramidal neurons and axons outside the cortical plate: The early marginal zone as a pallial anlage.

Rickmann, M., J. W. Fawcett and R. J. Keynes (1985). *J. Embryol. Exp. Morph.* 90:437–455. The migration of neural crest cells and the growth of motor axons through the rostral half of the chick somite.

Ridge, R. M. A. P. (1967) *Quart. J. Exp. Physiol.* 52:293–304. The differentiation of conduction velocities of slow twitch and fast twitch muscle motor innervation in kittens and cats.

Rieder, R. (1906). *Carl Weigert und seine Bedeutung für die medizinische Wissenschaft unserer Zeit.* Springer, Berlin.

Riederer, B., and A Matus (1985). *Proc. Natl. Acad. Sci. U.S.A.* 82:6006–6009. Differential expression of distinct microtubule-associated proteins during brain development.

Rieger, F., and M. Pincon-Raymond (1981). *Dev. Biol.* 87:85–101. Muscle and nerve in muscular dysgenesis in the mouse at birth: Sprouting and multiple innervation.

Rieger, F., M. Grumet, and G. M. Edelman (1985). *J. Cell Biol.* 101:285–293. N-CAM at the vertebrate neuromuscular junction.

Riese, W. (1949). *Bull. Hist. Med.* 23:111–136. An outline of a history of ideas in neurology.

Riese, W. (1956). *J. Nerv. Ment. Dis.* 124:125–134. The sources of Jacksonian neurology.

Riese, W. (1959). *A History of Neurology*, MD, New York.

Riese, W., and G. E. Arrington (1963). *Bull. Hist. Med.* 37:179–183. The history of Johannes Müller's doctrine of specific nerve energies of the senses: Original and later versions.

Riese, W., and E. C. Hoff (1950a). *J. Hist. Med.* 5:51–71. A history of the doctrine of cerebral localization. I. Sources, anticipations and basic reasoning.

Riese, W., and E. C. Hoff (1950b). *J. Hist. Med.* 6:439–470. A history of the doctrine of cerebral localization. II. Methods and main results.

Rieske, E. (1969). *Z. Zellforsch. Mikrosk. Anat. Abt. Histochem.* 95:546–567. Einfluss eines spezifischen Nervenwachstumsfaktors (NGF) auf Zellkulturen des Ganglion trigeminale.

Rifkin, D. B., and D. Moscatelli (1989). *J. Cell Biol.* 109:1–6. Recent developments in the cell biology of basic fibroblast growth factor.

Riggott, M. J., and S. A. Moody (1987). *J. Comp. Neurol.* 258:580–596. Distribution of laminin and fibronectin along peripheral trigeminal axon pathways in the developing chick.

Riley, D. A. (1977). *Exp. Neurol.* 5:400–409. Multiple innervation of fiber types in the soleus muscles of postnatal rats.

Riley, D. A. (1978). *Soc. Neurosci. Abstr.* 4:534. An investigation of selective reinnervation of rat skeletal muscles.

Riley, D.A., and E.F. Allin (1973). *Exp. Neurol.* 40:391–413. The effects of inactivity, programmed stimulation, and denervation on the histochemistry of skeletal muscle fiber types.

Rinard, R. G. (1988). *J. Hist. Biol.* 21:95–118. Neo-Lamarckism and technique: Hans Spemann and the development of experimental embryology.

Ringwald, M., R. Schuh, D. Vestweber, H. Eistetter, F. Lottspeich, J. Engel, R. Dolz, F. Jahnig, J. Epplen, S. Mayer,

C. Muller, and R. Kemler (1987). *EMBO J.* 6:3647–3653. The structure of cell adhesion molecule uvomorulin. Insights into the molecular mechanism of Ca²⁺-dependent cell adhesion.

Rio-Hortega, P. del (1916a). *Trab. Lab. Inv. Biol. Univ. Madrid* 14:269. Estructura fibrilar del protoplasma neuróglico y origine de las gliofibrillas.

Rio-Hortega, P. del (1916b). *Trab. Lab. Inv. Biol. Univ. Madrid* 14:1. Contribution à l'étude de l'histopathologie de la neuroglie. Les variations dans le ramollissement cerebral.

Rio-Hortega, P. del (1916c). *Trab. Lab Inv. Biol. Univ. Madrid* 14:117–153. Estudios sobre el centrosoma de las células nerviosas y neuróglias de los vertebrados, en sus formas normal y anormales.

Rio-Hortega, P. del (1919). *Bol. Soc. Esp. Biol.* 9:69–129. El tercer elemento de los centros nerviosos. I. La microglia normal. II. Intervención de la microglia en los procesos patológicos. (Celulas en bastoncito y cuerpos granuloadiposos). III. Naturaleza probable de la microglia.

Rio-Hortega, P. del (1920). *Trab. Lab. Inv. Biol. Univ. Madrid* 18:37–82. La microglía y su transformación en células en basoncito y cuerpos gránulo-adiposos.

Rio-Hortega, P. del (1921a). *Mem. de la Real. Soc. Esp. Hist. Nat.* 11:213–268. Histogenesis y evolución normal exodo y distribución regional de la microglia.

Rio-Hortega, P. del (1921b). *Bol. Soc. Esp. Biol.* 21:64–92. Estudios sobre la neuroglia. La glia de escasas radiaciones (oligodendroglia).

Rio-Hortega, P. del (1922). *Bol. Soc. Esp. Biol.* 10. Son homologables la glia de escasas radiacion es y la celula de Schwann?

Rio-Hortega, P. del (1924). *Compt. Rend. Soc. Biol.* 91:818–820. La glie á radiations peu nombreuses et la cellule de Schwann sont elles homologables?

Rio-Hortega, P. del (1928). *Mem. Real. Soc. esp. Hist. Nat.* 14:5–122. Tercera aportacion conocimiento morfologico e interpretacion functional de la oligodendroglia.

Rio-Hortega, P. del (1932). Microglia, pp. 483–534. In *Cytology and Cellular Pathology of the Nervous System*, Vol. 2, (W. Penfield, ed.), Hoeber, New York.

Rio-Hortega, P. del (1933). *Residencia: Rev. Resid. Estudiantes Madrid* 4:191–206. Arte y artificio de la ciencia histologica. Translated by E. W. Wolfe and G. M. Butler (1949). *Texas Rep. Biol. Med.* 7:363–390.

Rio-Hortega, P. del (1939). *Lancet* 1:1023–1026. The microglia.

Rio-Hortega, P. del (1942). *Arch. Histol. Normal Pathol. B. Aires* 1:5–71. La neuroglia normal.

Rio-Hortega, P. del, and F. Jimenez de Asua (1921). *Archiv. de Cardiol. y Hematol.* 2:161. Sobre la fagocitosis en los tumores y en otros procesos patológicos.

Riopelle, R. J., P. M. Richardson, and V. M. K. Verge (1987a). *Neurochem. Res.* 12:923–928. Distribution and characteristics of nerve growth factor binding on cholinergic neurons of rat and monkey forebrain.

Riopelle, R. J., V. M. K. Verge, and P. M. Richardson (1987b). *Mol. Brain Res.* 3:45–53. Properties of receptors for nerve growth factor in the mature rat nervous system.

Risau, W. (1986). *Proc. Natl. Acad. Sci. U.S.A.* 83:3855–3859. Developing brain produces an angiogenic factor.

Risau, W., R. Hallmann, U. Albrecht, and S. Henke-Fahle (1986). *EMBO J.* 5:3179–3183. Brain induces the expression of an early cell surface marker for blood-brain barrier-specific endothelium.

Risau, W., P. Gautschi-Sova, and P. Bühlen (1988). *EMBO J.* 7:959–962. Endothelial cell growth factors in embryonic and adult chick brain are related to human acidic fibroblast growth factor.

Rizzino, A. (1988). *Dev. Biol.* 130:411–422. Transforming growth factor-β: Multiple effects on cell differentiation and extracellular matrices.

Roach, F.C. (1945). *J. Exp. Zool.* 99:53–77. Differentiation of the central nervous system after axial reversals of the medullary plate of *Amblystoma*.

Roback, A. A. (1961). *History of Psychology and Psychiatry*. Philosophical Library, New York.

Roback, H. N., and H. J. Scherrer (1935). *Virchows Arch. Pathol. Anat. Physiol. Klin. Med.* 294:365–413. Über die feinere Morphologie des frühkindlichen Hirnes unter besonderer Berücksichtigung der Gliaentwicklung.

Robain, J., and G. Ponsot (1978). *Brain Res.* 149:379–397. Effects of undernutrition on glial maturation.

Robain, O. (1970). *J. Neurol. Sci.* 11:445–461. Gliogenèse post-natale chez le lapin.

Robbins, E., and N. K. Gonatas (1964a). *J. Cell Biol.* 21:429–463. Ultrastructure of a mammalian cell during the mitotic cycle.

Robbins, E., and N. K. Gonatas (1964b). *J. Histochem. Cytochem.* 12:704. Histochemical and ultrastructural studies on HeLa cell cultures exposed to spindle inhibitors with special reference to the interphase cell.

Robbins, N. (1967a). *Exp. Neurol.* 17:364–380. The role of the nerve in maintenance of frog taste buds.

Robbins, N. (1967b). *J. Physiol. (London)* 192:493–504. Peripheral modification of sensory nerve responses after cross-regeneration.

Robbins, N., and J. Polak (1987). *Soc. Neurosci. Abstr.* 13:1007. Forms of growth and retraction at mouse neuromuscular junctions revealed by a new nerve terminal stain and correlative electron microscopy.

Robbins, N., and T. Yonezawa (1971). *Science* 172:395–398. Developing neuromuscular junctions: First signs of chemical transmission during formation in tissue culture.

Roberts, A., and J. S. H. Taylor (1982). *J. Embryol. Exp. Morphol.* 69:237–250. A scanning electron microscope study of the development of a peripheral sensory neurite network.

Roberts, A. B. and M. B. Sporn (1987). *Adv. Cancer Res.* Transforming growth factor-beta.

Roberts, P. J., and R. A. Yates (1976). *Neuroscience* 1:371–374. Tectal deafferentation in the frog: Selective loss of L-glutamate and lambda-aminobutyrate.

Robertson, J. D. (1953). *Proc. Soc. Exptl. Biol. Med.* 82:219–223. Ultrastructure of two invertebrate synapses.

Robertson, J. D. (1955). *J. Biophys. Biochem. Cytol.* 1:271–278. The ultrastructure of adult vertebrate peripheral myelinated fibers in relation to myelinogenesis.

Robertson, J. D. (1956). *J. Biophys. Biochem. Cytol.* 2:381–394. The ultrastructure of a reptilian myoneural junction.

Robertson, J. D. (1963). *J. Cell Biol.* 19:201–221. The occurrence of a subunit pattern in the unit membranes of club endings in Mauthner cell synapses in goldfish brains.

Robertson, J. D. (1965). *Neurosci. Res. Prog. Bull.* 3:1–79. The synapse: Morphological and chemical correlates of function: A report of an NRP work session.

Robertson, J. D. (1987). *Int. Rev. Cytol.* **100**:129–201. The early days of electron microscopy of nerve tissue and membranes.

Robertson, M. (1987). *Nature* **330**:420–421. Towards a biochemistry of morphogenesis.

Robertson, W. (1897). *J. Ment. Sci.* **43**:733–752. The normal histology and pathology of neuroglia.

Robertson, W. (1899). *Scottish Med. Surg. J.* **4**:23. On a new method of obtaining a black reaction in certain tissue-elements of the central nervous system (platinum method).

Robertson, W. F. (1900). *J. Ment. Sci.* **46**:733–752. A microscopic demonstration of the normal and pathological histology of mesoglia cells.

Robinson, K. R. (1985). *J. Cell Biol.* **101**:2023–2027. The responses of cells to electrical fields: A review.

Robinson, S. M., T. O. Fox, P. Dikkes, and R. A. Pearlstein (1986). *Brain Res.* **371**:380–384. Sex differences in the shape of the sexually dimorphic nucleus of the preoptic area and suprachiasmatic nucleus of the rat: 3D computer reconstructions and morphometrics.

Robinson, S. R. (1988). *J. Comp. Neurol.* **267**:507–515. Cell death in the inner and outer nuclear layers of the developing cat retina.

Rockel, A. J., R. W. Hiorns, and T. P. S. Powell. (1980). *Brain* **103**:221–244. The basic uniformity in structure of the neocortex.

Rodieck, R. W. (1973). *The Vertebrate Retina. Principles of Structure and Function.* Freeman, San Francisco.

Rodieck, R. W. (1979). *Ann. Rev. Neurosci.* **2**:193–225. Visual pathways.

Rodieck, R. W. (1988). The primate retina, pp. 203–278. In *Comparative Primate Biology,* Vol. 4 (H. D. Steklis, and J. Erwin, eds.), Alan R. Liss, New York.

Rodieck, R. W., and R. K. Brening (1983). *Brain Behav. Evol.* **23**:121–164. Retinal ganglion cells: Properties, types, genera, pathways and trans-species comparisons.

Rodriguez-Tébar, A., and Y.-A. Barde (1988). *J. Neurosci.* **8**:3337–3342. Binding characteristics of brain-derived neurotrophic factor to its receptors on neurons in the chick embryo.

Rodriguez-Tébar, A., P. L. Jeffrey, H. Thoenen, and Y.-A. Barde (1989). *Dev. Biol.* **136**:296–303. The survival of chick retinal ganglion cells in response to brain-derived neurotrophic factor depends on their embryonic age.

Roffler-Tarlov, S., and A. M. Grabiel (1984). *Nature* **307**:62–66. Weaver mutation has differential effect on the dopamine-containing innervation of the limbic and non-limbic striatum.

Roffler-Tarlov, S., P. M. Beart, S. O'Gorman, and R. L. Sidman (1979). *Brain Res.* **168**:75–95. Neurochemical and morphological consequences of axon terminal degeneration in cerebellar deep nuclei of mice with inherited Purkinje cell degeneration.

Roffler-Tarlov, S., D. Pugatch, and A. M. Graybiel (1990). *J. Neurosci.* **10**:734–740. Patterns of cell and fiber vulnerability in the mesostriatal system of the mutant mouse weaver. II. High affinity uptake sites for dopamine.

Roger, J. (1963). *Les Sciences de la vie dans la penseé francaise du XVIII siècle. La génération des animaux de Descartes à l'Encyclopédie.* Paris.

Rogers, K. T. (1957). *Anat. Rec.* **127**:97–107. Early development of the optic nerve in the chick.

Rogers, L. A., and W. M. Cowan (1973). *J. Comp. Neurol.* **147**:291–319. The development of the mesencephalic nucleus of the trigeminal nerve in the chick.

Rogers, S. L. (1981). *Dev. Biol.* **94**:265–283. Muscle spindle formation and differentiation in regenerating rat muscle grafts.

Rogers, S. L., and B. M. Carlson (1981). *Neurosci.* **6**:87–94. A quantitative assessment of muscle spindle formation in reinnervated and non-reinnervated grafts of the rat extensor digitorum longus muscle.

Rogers, S. L., P. C. Letourneau, S. L. Palm, J. McCarthy, and L. T. Furcht (1983). *Dev. Biol.* **98**:212–220. Neurite extension by peripheral and central nervous system neurons in response to substratum-bound fibronectin and laminin.

Rogers, S. L., K. J. Edson, P. C. Letourneau, and S. C. McLoon (1986). *Dev. Biol.* **113**:429–435. Distribution of laminin in the developing peripheral nervous system of the chick.

Rogers, W. M. (1934). *Proc. Natl. Acad. Sci. U.S.A.* **20**:247–249. Heterotopic spinal cord grafts in salamander embryos.

Rohde, E. (1923). *Zeitschr. für wissensch. Zool.* **120**:325–535. Der plasmodiale Aufbau des Tier- und Pflanzenkörpers.

Rohon, V. (1884). *Sitzungsberichte Akad. Wien,* pp. 39–57. Zur histogenese des Rückenmarks der Forelle.

Rohrer, H. (1985). *Dev. Biol.* **111**:95–107. Nonneuronal cells from chick sympathetic and dorsal root sensory ganglia express catecholamine uptake and receptors for nerve growth factor during development.

Rohrer, H., R. Heumann, and H. Thoenen (1988a). *Dev. Biol.* **128**:240–244. The synthesis of nerve growth factor (NGF) in developing skin is independent of innervation.

Rohrer, H., M. Hofer, R. Hellweg, S. Korsching, A. D. Stehle, S. Saadat, and H. Thoenen (1988b). *Development* **103**:545–552. Antibodies against mouse nerve growth factor interfere *in vivo* with the development of avian sensory and sympathetic neurones.

Röhrs, M. (1955). *Zool. Anz.* **155**:53–69. Vergleichende Untersuchungen an Wild- und Hauskatzen.

Röhrs, M., and P. Ebinger (1978). *Z. zool. Syst. Evolut.-forsch* **16**:1–14. Die Beurteilung von Hirngrößenunterschieden zwischen Wild- und Haustieren.

Roisen, F. J., R. A. Murphy, and W. G. Braden (1972a). *J. Neurobiol.* **4**:347–368. Neurite development *in vitro.* I. The effects of adenosine 3'5'-clyclic monophosphate (cyclic AMP).

Roisen, F. J., R. A. Murphy, M. E. Pichichero, and W. G. Braden (1972b). *Science* **175**:73–74. Cyclic adenosine monophosphate stimulation of axonal elongation.

Roisen, F. J., W. G. Braden, and J. Friedman (1975). *Ann. N.Y. Acad. Sci.* **253**:545–561. Neurite development *in vitro:* III. The effects of several derivatives of cyclic AMP, colchicine, and colcemid.

Rolando, L. (1809). *Saggio sopra la vera struttura del cervello dell'uomo e degl'animali, e spora le funzioni del sistema nervosa.* Stampa Privileg, Sassari. French translation by P. Flourens (1823), *J. Physiol. Expér. Path.* **3**:95–113. Expériences sur les fonctions du systeme nerveux.

Romanes, G. J. (1941). *J. Anat. (London)* **76**:112–130. The development and significance of the cell columns in the ventral horn of the cervical and upper thoracic spinal cord of the rabbit.

Romanes, G. J. (1946). *J. Anat. (London)* 80:117–131. Motor localization and the effects of nerve injury on the ventral horn cells of the spinal cord.

Romanes, G. J. (1947). *J. Anat. (London)* 81:64–81. The prenatal medullation of the sheep's nervous system.

Romanes, G. J. (1951). *J. Comp. Neurol.* 94:313–364. The motor cell columns of the lumbosacral spinal cord of the cat.

Romanes, G. J. (1964). *Prog. Brain Res.* 11:93–119. The motor pools of the spinal cord.

Romanul, F. C. A., and E. L. Hogan (1965). *Arch. Neurol.* 13:263–273. Enzymatic changes in denervated muscle. I. Histochemical studies.

Romanual, F. C. A., and J. P. van der Meulen (1967). *Arch. Neurol.* 17:387–402. Slow and fast muscle after cross innervation.

Romer, A. S. (1942). *J. Morphol.* 71:251–298. The development of tetrapod limb musculature—the thigh of Lacerta.

Roncali, L. (1970). *Monitore Zool. Ital. N.S.* 4:81–98. The brachial plexus and the wing nerve pattern during early developmental phases in chicken embryo.

Ronnevi, L.-O., and S. Conradi (1974). *Brain Res.* 80:335–359. Ultrastructural evidence for spontaneous elimination of synaptic terminals on spinal motoneurons in the kitten.

Roofe, P. G. (1947). *Science* 105:180–181. Role of the axis cylinder in transport of tetanus toxin.

Rootman, D. S., W. G. Tatton, and M. Hay (1981). *J. Comp. Neurol.* 199:17–27. Postnatal histogenetic death of rat forelimb motoneurons.

Roots, B. (1983). *Science* 221:971–972. Neurofilament accumulation induced in synapses by leupeptin.

Roper, S. D. (1989). *Ann. Rev. Neurosci.* 12:329–353. The cell biology of vertebrate taste receptors.

Rosa, F., A. B. Roberts, D. Danielpour, L. L. Dart, M. B. Sporn, and I. B. Dawid (1988). *Science* 239:783–785. Mesoderm induction in amphibians: The role of TGF-β2-like factors.

Rose, G. H., and D. B. Lindsley (1968). *J. Neurophysiol.* 31:607–623. Development of visually evoked potentials in kittens: Specific and nonspecific responses.

Rose, M. (1926). *J. f. Psychol. u. Neurol.* 32:97–158. Über das histogenetische Prinzip der Einteilung der Grosshirnrinde.

Rose, P. K. (1982). *J. Neurosci.* 2:1596–1607. Branching structure of motoneuron stem dendrites: A study of neck muscle motoneurons intracellularly stained with horseradish peroxidase in the cat.

Rosen, J., D. Stein, and N. Butters (1971). *Science* 173:353–356. Recovery of function after serial ablation of prefrontal cortex in rhesus monkey.

Rosenbluth, J. (1963). *Z. Zellforsch. Mikrosk. Anat.* 60:213–236. The visceral ganglion of *Aplysia californica*.

Rosenfeld, P., J. A. M. Van Eekelen, S. Levine, and E. R. De Kloet (1988). *Dev. Brain Res.* 42:119–127. Ontogeny of the Type 2 glucocorticoid receptor in discrete rat brain regions: An immunocytochemical study.

Rosenheim, O., and M. C. Tebb (1910). *Biochem. Zeit.* 25:151. Die Nicht-Existenz des sogenannten 'Protagons' im Gehirn.

Rosenstein, J. M. (1987). *Science* 235:772–774. Neocortical transplants in the mammalian brain lack a blood-brain barrier to macromolecules.

Rosenzweig, M. R., E. L. Bennett, and M. C. Diamond (1971). Chemical and anatomical plasticity of brain: Replications and extensions, pp. 205–278. In *Macromolecules and Behaviour* (J. Gaito, ed.), Appleton Century Crofts, New York.

Rosner, H., M. Al-Agtum, and S. Henke-Fahle (1984). *Dev. Brain Res.* 18:85–95. Developmental expression of GD_3 and polysialogangliosides in embryonic chicken nervous tissue reacting with monoclonal antiganglioside antibodies.

Roth, H. (1950). *Rev. Suisse Zool.* 57:621–686. Die entwicklung xenoplastischer Neuralchimaeren.

Roth, H. J., M. J. Hunkeler, and A. T. Campagnoni (1985). *J. Neurochem.* 45:572–580. Expression of myelin basic protein genes in serveral dysmyelinating mouse mutants during early postnatal brain development.

Roth, J., D. Baetens, A. W. Norman, and L.-M. Garcia-Segura (1981). *Brain Res.* 222:452–457. Specific neurons in chick central nervous system stain with an antibody against chick intestinal vitamin D-dependent calcium-binding protein.

Rothbard, J. B., R. Brackenbury, B. A. Cunningham, and G. M. Edelman (1982). *J. Biol. Chem.* 257:11064–11069. Differences in the carbohydrate structures of neural cell adhesion molecules from adult and embryonic brains.

Rothman, S. M., and J .W. Olney (1987). *Trends Neurosci.* 10:299–302. Excitotoxicity and the NMDA receptor.

Rothman, T. P., and M. D. Gershon (1982). *J. Neurosci.* 2:381–393. Phenotypic expression in the developing murine enteric nervous system.

Rothman, T. P., and M. D. Gershon (1984). *Neuroscience* 12:1293–1311. Regionally defective colonization of the terminal bowel by the precursors of enteric neurons in lethal spotted mutant mice.

Rothman, T. P., G. Nilaver, and M. D. Gershon (1984). *J. Comp. Neurol.* 225:13–23. Colonization of the developing murine enteric nervous system and subsequent phenotypic expression by the precursors of peptidergic neurons.

Rothman, T. P., V. M. Tennyson, and M. D. Gershon (1986). *J. Comp. Neurol.* 252:493–506. Colonization of the bowel by the precursors of enteric glia: Studies of normal and congenitally aganglionic mutant mice.

Rotshenker, S. (1979). *J. Physiol. (London)* 292:535–547. Synapse formation in intact innervated cutaneous-pectoris muscle of the frog following denervation of the opposite muscle.

Rotshenker, S.and and F. Reichert (1980). *J. Comp. Neurol.* 193:413–422. Motor axon sprouting and site of synapse formation in intact innervated skeletal muscle of the frog.

Roufa, D., M. B. Bunge, M. I. Johnson, and C. J. Cornbrooks (1986). *J. Neurosci.* 6:790–802. Variation in content and function of non-neuronal cells in the outgrowth of sympathetic ganglia from embryos of differing age.

Roussel, G., and J. L. Nussbaum (1981). *Histochem. J.* 13:1029–1047. Comparative localization of Wolfgram W1 and myelin basic protein in the rat brain during ontogenesis.

Rousselet, A., A. Autillo-Touati, D. Araud, and A. Prochiantz (1990). *Dev. Biol.* 137:33–45. *In vitro* regulation of neuronal morphogenesis and polarity by astrocyte-derived factors.

Routtenberg, A. (1985). *Behav. Neural Biol.* 44:186–200. Protein kinase C activation leading to protein F1 phosphorylation may regulate synaptic plasticity by presynaptic terminal growth.

Routtenberg, A. (1986). *Prog. Brain Res.* 69:211–234. Synaptic plasticity and protein kinase C.

Roux, W. (1883). *Arch. Anat. Physiol. Anat. Abtlg.* pp. 76–160. Beiträge zur Morphologie der funktionellen Anpassung: Nr 1. Über die Struktur eines hochdifferenzierten bindegewebigen Organ (der Schwanzflosse des Delphins).

Roux, W. (1885a). *Z. Biol.* 31:429–528. Zur Orientierung ueber einige Probleme der embryonalen Entwicklung.

Roux, W. (1885b). *Z. Biol.* 21:411–524. Beiträge zur Entwickelungsmechanik des Embryo. Nr. 1. Einleitung und Orientierung über einige Probleme der embryonalen Entwickelung.

Roux, W. (1888). *Arch. f. path. Anat. u. Physiol. u. Klin. Med. (Virchow's)* 114:113–153. Beiträge zur Entwickelungsmechanik des Embryo. Über die künstliche Hervorbringung halber Embryonen durch Zerstörung einer der beiden ersten Furchungskugeln, sowie über die Nachentwickelung (Postgeneration) der fehlenden Körperhälfte.

Roux, W. (1895). *Gesammelte Abhandlungen über Entwickelungsmechanik der Organismen.* Vol. 1: Abhandlung I-XII vorwiegend über funktionelle Anpassung pp. 1–816; Vol. 2: Abhandlungen XIII-XXXIII über Entwickelungsmechanik des Embryo, pp. 1–105. W. Engelmann, Leipzig.

Roux, W. (1923). Autobiographie, pp. 141–206. In *Die Medizin der Gegenwart in Selbstdarstellungen* (L. R. Grote, ed.), Verlag von Felix Meiner, Leipzig.

Rovainen, C. M. (1967). *J. Neurophysiol.* 30:1000–1023. Physiological and anatomical studies on large neurons of central nervous system of the sea lamprey *(Petromyzon marinus).*

Rovasio, R. A., A. Delouvée, K. M. Yamada, R. Timpl and J. P. Thiery (1983). *J. Cell. Biol.* 96:462–473. Neural crest cell migration: Requirements for exogenous fibronectin and high cell density.

Rozengurt, E. (1986). *Science* 234:161–166. Early signals in the mitogenic response.

Rubel, E. W. (1978). Ontogeny of structure and function in the vertebrate auditory system, pp. 135–237. In *Handbook of Sensory Physiology, Development of Sensory Systems,* Vol. 9, (M. Jacobson, ed.), Springer-Verlag, New York.

Rubel, E. W., D. J. Smith, and L. C. Miller (1976). *J. Comp. Neurol.* 166:469–490. Organization and development of brain stem auditory nuclei of the chicken: Ontogeny of n. magnocellularis and n. laminaris.

Rubin, E. (1985). *J. Neurosci.* 5:697–704. Development of the rat superior cervical ganglion: Initial stages of synapse formation.

Rubin, G. M. (1988). *Science* 240:1453–1459. *Drosophila melanogaster* as an experimental organism.

Rubin, L. L., S. M. Schuetze, and G. D. Fischbach (1979). *Dev. Biol.* 69:46–58. Accumulation of acetylcholinesterase at newly formed nerve-muscle synapses.

Rubin, L. L., S. M. Schuetze, C. L. Weill, and G. D. Fischbach (1980). *Nature* 283:264–267. Regulation of acetylcholinesterase appearance at neuromuscular junctions *in vitro.*

Rubinstein, H. S. (1936). *J. Comp. Neurol.* 64:469–496. The effect of the growth hormone upon the brain and brain weight-body weight relations.

Ruckmich, C. A. (1913). *Am. J. Psychol.* 24:99–123. The use of the term *function* in English textbooks of psychology.

Ruddle, F. H., C. P. Hart, A. Awgulewitsch, A. Fainsod, M. Utset, D. Dalton, N. Kerk, M. Rabin, A. Ferguson-Smith, A. Fienberg, and W. McGinnis (1985). *Cold Spring Harbor Symp. Quant. Biol.* 50:277–284. Mammalian homeo box genes.

Ruel, J., R. Faure, and J. H. Dussault (1985). *J. Endocrinol. Invest.* 8:343–348. Regional distribution of nuclear T_3 receptors in rat brain and evidence for preferential localization in neurons.

Ruffini, A. (1892). *R. C. Accad. Lincei sér.* 5, 2nd sem. 31–38. Sulla terminazione nervosa nei fusi muscolari e sul loro significato fisiologico.

Ruffini, A. (1898). *J. Physiol. (London)* 23:190–208. On the minute anatomy of the neuromuscular spindles of the cat, and on their physiological significance.

Rugh, R., and J. Wolff (1955a). *Proc. Soc. Exp. Biol. Med.* 89:248–253. Resilience of the fetal eye following radiation insult.

Rugh, R., and J. Wolff (1955b). *Arch. Opthalmol.* 54:351–359. Reparation of the fetal eye following radiation insult.

Ruiz-Marcos, A., and F. Valverde (1969). *Exp. Brain Res.* 8:284–294. The temporal evolution of the distribution of dendritic spines on the visual cortex of normal and dark raised mice.

Ruiz-Marcos, A., and F. Valverde (1970). *Brain Res.* 19:25–39. Dynamic architecture of the visual cortex.

Ruiz-Marcos, A., F. Sanchez-Toscano, F. Escobar del Rey, and G. Morreale de Escobar (1979). *Brain Res.* 162:315–329. Severe hypothyroidism and the maturation of the rat cerebral cortex.

Ruiz-Marcos, A., J. Salas, F. Sanchez-Toscano, F. Morreale de Escobar, and G. Morreale de Escobar (1983). *Dev. Brain Res.* 9:205–213. Effect of neonatal and adult-onset hypothyroidism on pyramidal cells of the rat auditory cortex.

Ruoslahti, E. (1988). *Ann. Rev. Biochem.* 57:375–413. Fibronectin and its receptor.

Ruoslahti, E., and M. D. Pierschbacher (1986). *Cell* 44:517–518. Arg-gly-asp: A versatile cell recognition signal.

Ruoslahti, E., and M. D. Pierschbacher (1987). *Science* 238:491–497. New perspectives in cell adhesion: RGD and integrins.

Ruse, M. (1972). *Phil. Sci.* 39:525–528. Biological adaptation.

Rush, R. A. (1984). *Nature* 312:364–367. Immunohistochemical localization of endogenous nerve growth factor.

Rushton, W. A. H. (1951). *J. Physiol. (London)* 115:101–122. A theory of the effects of fibre size in medullated nerve.

Rusoff, A. C. (1984). *J. Neurosci.* 4:1414–1428. Patterns of axons in the visual system of perciform fish and implications of these paths for rules governing axonal growth.

Rusoff, A. C., and S. S. Easter (1980). *Science* 208:311–312. Order in the optic nerve of goldfish.

Russel, D. A., and J. O. W. Bland (1933). *J. Pathol. Bact.* 36:273–283. A study of gliomas by the method of tissue culture.

Russell, D. S., and L. J. Rubinstein (1977). *Pathology of Tumours of the Nervous System,* pp. 372–401. Williams and Wilkins, Baltimore.

Russell, E. S. (1916). *Form and Function: A Contribution to the History of Animal Morphology.* John Murray, London.

Russell, E. S. (1930). *The Interpretation of Development and Heredity. A Study in Biological Method.* Clarendon Press, Oxford.

Russell, E. S. (1946). *The Directiveness of Organic Activities.* Cambridge Univ. Press, Cambridge.

Rustioni, A., and I. Molenaar (1975). *Exp. Brain Res.* 23:1–13. Dorsal column nuclei afferents in the lateral funiculus of the cat: Distribution pattern and absence of sprouting after chronic deafferentation.

Rustioni, A., and C. Sotelo (1974). *Brain Res.* 73:527–533. Some effects of chronic deafferentation on the ultrastructure of the nucleus gracilis of the cat.

Rutishauser, U. (1984). *Nature* 310:549–554. Developmental biology of a neural cell adhesion molecule.

Rutishauser, U. (1989). *Trends Neurosci.* 12:275–276. N-Cadherin: A cell adhesion molecule in neural development.

Rutishauser, U., and T. M. Jessell (1988). *Physiol. rev.* 68:819–857. Cell adhesion molecules in vertebrate neural development.

Rutishauser, U., W. E. Gall, and G. M. Edelman (1978a). *J. Cell Biol.* 79:386–393. Adhesion among neural cells of the chick embryos. IV. Role of the cell surface molecule N-CAM in the formation of neurite bundles in cultures of spinal ganglia.

Rutishauser, U., S. Hofman, and G. M. Edelman (1982). *Proc. Natl. Acad. Sci. U.S.A* 79:685–689. Binding properties of a cell adhesion molecules from neural tissue.

Rutishauser, U., M. Grumet, and G. M. Edelman (1983). *J. Cell Biol.* 97:145–152. Neural cell adhesion molecule mediates initial interactions between spinal cord neurons and muscle cells in culture.

Rutishauser, U., A. Acheson, A. K. Hall, D. M. Mann, and J. Sunshine (1988). *Science* 240:53–57. The neural cell adhesion molecule (NCAM) as a regulator of cell-cell interactions.

Rutledge, L. T., C. Wright, and J. Duncan (1974). *Exp. Neurol.* 44:209–228. Morphological changes in pyramidal cells of mammalian neocortex associated with increased use.

Ryall, R. W., and M. F. Piercy (1970). *Brain Res.* 23:57–65. Visceral afferent and efferent fibers in sacral ventral roots in cats.

Rydel, R. E., and L. A. Greene (1987). *J. Neurosci.* 7:3639–3653. Acidic and basic fibroblast growth factors promote stable neurite outgrowth and neuronal differentiation in cultures of PC12 cells.

Ryder, R. E., and L. A. Greene (1988). *Proc. Natl. Acad. Sci. U.S.A.* 85:1257–1261. cAMP analogs promote survival and neurite outgrowth in cultures of rat sympathetic and sensory neurons independently of nerve growth factor

Ryser, H. J. P. (1968). *Science* 159:390–396. Uptake of protein by mammalian cells: An underdeveloped area.

Ryugo, D. K., R. Ryugo, and H. P. Killackey (1975). *Brain Res.* 96:82–87. Changes in pyramidal cell spine density consequent to vibrissae removal in the newborn rat.

Rzehak, K., and M. Singer (1966). *Anat. Rec.* 155:537–540. The number of nerve fibers in the limb of the mouse and its relation to regenerative capacity.

Sabatini, D. D., K. Bensch, and R. J. Barnett (1963). *J. Cell Biol.* 17:19–58. Cytochemistry and electron microscopy: The preservation of cellular ustrastructure and enzymatic activity by aldehyde fixation.

Sabatini, M. T., A. P. de Iraldi, and E. de Robertis (1965). *Exp. Neurol.* 12:370–383. Early effects of antiserum against the nerve growth factor on fine structure of sympathetic neurons.

Sabel, B. A., and G. E. Schneider (1988). *Exp. Brain Res.* 73:505–518. The principle of "conservation of total axonal arborizations": Massive compensatory sprouting in the hamster subcortical visual system after early tectal lesions.

Sacher, G. A. (1959). Relation of life span to brain weight in mammals, pp. 115–133. In *The Lifespan of Animals,* CIBA Foundation Colloquia on Aging, Vol. 5. (G. E. W. Wolstonholme, and M. O'Connor, eds.), Churchill, London.

Sacher, G. A., and E. F. Staffeldt (1974). *Am. Nat.* 108:593–615. Relation of gestation time to brain weight for placental mammals: Implications for the theory of vertebrate growth.

Sadaghiani, B., and C. H. Thiébaud (1987). *Dev. Biol.* 124:91–110. Neural crest development in the *Xenopus laevis* embryo, studied by interspecific transplantation and scanning electron microscopy.

Sadoul, K., R. Sadoul, A. Faissner, and M. Schachner (1988). *J. Neurochem.* 50:510–521. Biochemical characterization of different molecular forms of the neural cell adhesion molecule L1.

Sadoul, R., M. Hirn, H. Deagostini-Bazin, G. Rougon, and C. Goridis (1983). *Nature* 304:347–349. Adult and embryonic mouse neural cell adhesion molecules have different binding properties.

Saetersdal, T. A. S. (1956). *Univ. Bergen Arbok. Naturvitenskap. Rekke* 3:1–53. On the ontogenesis of the avian cerebellum. II. Measurements of the cortical layers.

Saetersdal, T. A. S. (1958). *Univ. Bergen Arbok. Naturvitenskap. Rekke* 10:1–20. A critical review of quantitative mitotic recordings in animal tissues with special reference to the central nervous system.

Saetersdal, T. A. S. (1959). *Univ. Bergen Arbok. Naturvitenskap. Rekke* 4:1–39. On the ontogenesis of the avian cerebellum. IV. Mitotic activity in the external granular layer with a summary of certain aspects of cortical development.

Sah, D. W.. Y., and E. Frank (1984). *J. Neurosci.* 4:2784–2791. Regeneration of sensory-motor synapses in the spinal cord of the bullfrog.

Sahota, T. S., and J. S. Edwards (1969). *J. Insect Physiol.* 15:1367–1373. Development of grafted supernumerary legs in the house cricket, *Acheta domesticus.*

Saint-Jeannet, J.-P., F. Foulquier, C. Goridis, and A.-M. Duprat (1989). *Development* 106:675–683. Expression of N-CAM precedes neural induction in *Pleurodeles waltl* (Urodele, amphibian).

Saito, A., and S. I. Zacks (1969). *Exp. Mol. Pathol.* 10:256. Fine structure of neuromuscular junctions after nerve section and implantation of nerve in denervated muscle.

Saito, H.-A. (1983). *J. Comp. Neurol.* 221:279–288. Morphology of physiologically identified X-, Y- and W-type retinal ganglion cells of the rat.

Saitua, F., and J. Alvarez (1988). *J. Comp. Neurol.* 269:203–209. Do axons grow during adulthood? A study of caliber and microtubules of sural nerve axons in young, mature, and aging rats.

Sakaguchi, D. S., and R. K. Murphey (1985). *J. Neurosci.* 5:3228–3245. Map formation in the developing *Xenopus* retinotectal system: An examination of ganglion cell terminal arborizations.

Sakai, Y. (1989). *Anat. Rec.* 223:194–203. Neurulation in the mouse: Manner and timing of neural tube closure.

Sakia, F. B. (1965). *J. Comp. Neurol.* 124:189–202. Post-natal growth of neuroglia cells and blood vessels of the cervical spinal cord of the albino mouse.

Salisbury, J. L., J. S. Condeelis, and P. Satir (1983). *Int. Rev. Exp. Pathol.* 24:1–62. Receptor-mediated endocytosis: Machinery and regulation of the clathrin-coated vesicle pathway.

Salmons, S., and F. A. Sretér (1976). *Nature* 263:30–34. Significance of impulse activity in the transformation of skeletal muscle type.

Salmons, S., and G. Vrbová (1969). *J. Physiol.* 201:535–549. The influence of activity on some contractile characteristics of mammalian fast and slow muscles.

Salpeter, M., and R. H. Loring (1985). *Prog. Neurobiol.* 25:297–325. Nicotinic acetylcholine receptors in vertebrate muscle: Properties, distribution and neural control.

Salpeter, M. M. (1966). General area of autoradiography at the electron microscope level, pp. 229–253. In *Methods in Cell Physiology* (D. M. Prescott, ed.), Academic Press, New York.

Salpeter, M. M., and R. H. Loring (1986). *Prog. Neurobiol.* 25:297–325. Nicotinic acetylcholine receptor in vertebrate muscle: Properties, distribution and neural control.

Salpeter, M. M., L. Bachmann, and E. E. Salpeter (1969). *J. Cell Biol.* 41:1–32. Resolution in electron microscope radioautography.

Salpeter, M. M., G. C. Budd, and S. Mattimoe (1974) *J. Histochem. Biochem.* 22:217–222. Resolution in autoradiography using semithin sections.

Salzer, J. L., and R. P. Bunge (1980). *J. Cell Biol.* 84:739–752. Studies of Schwann cell proliferation. I. An analysis in tissue culture of proliferation during development, Wallerian degeneration and direct injury.

Salzer, J. L., A. K. Williams, L. Glaser, and R. P. Bunge (1980a). *J. Cell Biol.* 84:753–766. Studies of Schwann cell proliferation: II. Characterization of the stimulation and specificity of the response to a neurite membrane fraction.

Salzer, J. L., R. P. Bunge, and L. Glaser (1980b). *J. Cell Biol.* 84:767–778. Studies of Schwann cell proliferation. III. Evidence for the surface localization of the neurite mitogen.

Salzer, J. L., W. P. Holmes, and D. R. Colman (1987). *J. Cell Biol.* 104:957–965. The amino acid sequences of the myelin-associated glycoproteins: Homology to the immunoglobulin gene super-family.

Salzgeber, B., and R. Weber (1966). *J. Embryol. Exp. Morph.* 15:397–419. La régression du mésonéphros chez l'embryon de poulet.

Samaha, F. J., L. Guth, and R. W. Albers (1970). *Exp. Neurol.* 26:120–125. Phenotypic differences between actomyosin ATPase of the three fiber types of mammalian skeletal muscle.

Samorajski, T., R. L. Friede, and P. R. Reimer (1970). *J. Neuropathol. Exp. Neurol.* 29:507–523. Hypomyelination in the quaking mouse. A model for the analysis of disturbed myelin formation.

Samson, F., J. A. Donoso, I. Heller-Bettinger, D. Watson, and R. H. Himes (1979). *J. Pharmacol. Exp. Ther.* 208:411–417. Nocodazole action on tubulin assembly, axonal ultrastructure and fast axoplasmic transport.

Samson, F. E., Jr., W. M. Balfour, and R. J. Jacobs (1960). *Am. J. Physiol.* 199:693–696. Mitochondrial changes in developing rat brain.

Samsonova, V. G. (1965). *Pavlov. J. Higher Nerv. Activ.* (English Trans.) 15:491–499. Functional organization of neurons of different types in the visual center of frogs.

Samuels, L. D., and W. E. Kisielski (1963). *Radiation Res.* 18:620–632. Toxicological studies of tritiated thymidine.

Sánchez y Sánchez, D. (1923). *Trab. Lab. Invest. biol. Univ. Madrid* 23:29–52. L'histogenese dans les centres nerveux des insectes pendent les métamorphoses.

Sánchez-Herrero, E., I. Vernós, R. Marco, and G. Morata (1985). *Nature* 313:108–113. Genetic organization of *Drosophila* bithorax complex.

Sanders, F. K. (1948). *Proc. Roy. Soc. (London) Ser. B.* 135:323–357. The thickness of the myelin sheaths of normal and regenerating peripheral nerve fibers.

Sanders, F. K., and D. Whitteridge (1946). *J. Physiol. (London)* 105:152–174. Conduction velocity and myelin thickness in regenerating nerve fibers.

Sanders, F. K., and J. Z. Young (1946). *J. Exp. Biol.* 22:203–212. The influence of peripheral connexion on the diameter of regenerating nerve fibers.

Sanderson, K. J., R. W. Guillery, and R. M. Shackelford (1974). *J. Comp. Neurol.* 154:225–248. Congenitally abnormal visual pathways in mink (Mustela vison) with reduced retinal pigment.

Sanderson, K. J., L. J. Pearson, and P. G. Dixon (1978). *J. Comp. Neurol.* 180:841–868. Altered retinal projections in brushtailed possum, *Trichosurus vulpecula,* following removal of one eye.

Sanderson, K. J., P. G. Dixon, and L. J. Pearson (1982). *Dev. Brain Res.* 5. Postnatal development of retinal projections in the brushtailed possum, *Trichosurus vulpecula.*

Sandritter, W., V. Nováková, J. Pilny, and G. Kiefer (1967). *Z. Zellforsch. Mikroskop. Anat.* 80:145–152. Cytophotometrische Messungen des Nukleinsäure- und Proteingehaltes von Ganglienzellen der Ratte während der postnatalen Entwicklung und im Alter.

Sanes, J. (1982). *J. Cell Biol.* 93:442–451. Laminin, fibronectin, and collagen in synaptic and extrasynaptic portions of muscle fiber basement membrane.

Sanes, J. R. (1989) *Trends Neurosci.* 12:21–28. Analysing cell lineage with a recombinant retrovirus.

Sanes, J. R., and J. M. Cheney (1982). *Nature* 300:646–647. Lectin binding reveals a synapse-specific carbohydrate in skeletal muscle.

Sanes, J. R., and A. Y. Chiu (1983). *Cold Spring Harbor Symp. Quant. Biol.* 48:667–678. The basal lamina of the neuromuscular junction.

Sanes, J. R., and Z. W. Hall (1979). *J. Cell Biol.* 83:357–370. Antibodies that bind specifically to synaptic sites on muscle fiber basal lamina.

Sanes, J. R., L. M. Marshall, and U. J. McMahan (1978). *J. Cell Biol.* 78:176–198. Reinnervation of muscle fiber basal lamina after removal of myofibers. Differentiation of regenerating axons at original synaptic sites.

Sanes, J. R., M. Schachner, and J. Covault (1986). *J. Cell Biol.* 102:420–431. Expression of several adhesive macromolecules (NCAM, L1, J1, NILE, uvomorulin, laminin, fibronectin, and a heparan sulfate proteoglycan) in embryonic, adult, and denervated adult skeletal muscle.

Sangameswaran, L., J. Hempstead, and J. I. Morgan (1989). *Proc. Natl. Acad. Sci. U.S.A.* 86:5651–5655. Molecular cloning of a neuron-specific transcript and its regulation during normal and aberrant cerebellar development.

Sanides, F. (1964). *J. für Hirnforschung* 6:269–282. The cytomyeloarchitecture of the human frontal lobe and its relations to phylogenetic differentiation of the cerebral cortex.

Sanides, F. (1969). *Ann. N.Y. Acad. Sci.* 167:404–423. Comparative architectonics of the neocortex of mammals and their evolutionary interpretation.

Sanides, F. (1970). Functional architecture of motor and sensory cortices in primates in the light of a new concept of neocortex evolution. In *The Primate Brain: Advances In Primatology*, Vol. 2, (Noback, C., and W. Montagna, eds.), Appleton, New York.

Sanides, F. (1972). Representation in the cerebral cortex and its areal lamination patterns. In *The Structure and Function of Nervous Tissue*, Vol. 5, (Bourne, G. H., ed.), Academic Press, New York.

Santen, R. J., and B. W. Agranoff (1963). *Biochim. Biophys. Acta* 72:251–262. Studies on the estimation of deoxyribonucleic acid and ribonucleic acid in rat brain.

Santos, E., and A. R. Nebreda (1989). *Faseb. J.* 3:2151–2163. Structural and functional properties of *ras* proteins.

Sapolsky, R. M. (1986). *J. Neurosci.* 6:2240–2244. Glucocorticoid toxicity in the hippocampus: Reversal by supplementation with brain fuels.

Sapolsky, R. M., B. S. McEwen, and T. C. Rainbow (1983). *Brain Res.* 271:331–334. Quantitative autoradiography of [³H] corticosterone receptors in rat brain.

Sara, V. R., and L. Lazarus (1974). *Nature* 250:257–258. Prenatal action of growth hormone on brain and behaviour.

Sara, V. R., L. Lazarus, M. C. Stuart, and T. King (1974). *Science* 186:446–447. Fetal brain growth: Selective action by growth hormone.

Sargent, T. D., M. Jamrich, and I. B. Dawid (1986). *Dev. Biol.* 114:238–246. Cell interactions and the control of gene activity during early development of *Xenopus laevis*.

Sariola, H, E. Aufderheide, H. Bernhard, S. Henke-Fahle, W. Dippold, and P. Ekblom (1988). *Cell* 54:235–245. Antibodies to cell surface ganglioside GD3 perturb inductive epithelial-mesenchymal interactions.

Sarkisov, S. A., and N. S. Preobrazhenskaya (eds.) (1959). *Razvitic Tsentral'noi Nervnoi Systemy* (Development of the Central Nervous System). Medgiz, Moscow.

Sarton, G. (1952–1959). *A History of Science. I. Ancient Science Through the Golden Age of Greece; II. Hellenistic Science and Culture in the Last Three Centuries B.C.* Harvard Univ. Press, Cambridge, Mass.

Sasaki, S., J. K. Stevens, and N. Bodick (1983). *Brain Res.* 259:193–206. Serial reconstruction of microtubular arrays within dendrites of the cat retinal ganglion cell: The cytoskeleton of a vertebrate dendrite.

Sato, M. (1968). *Brain Nerve* 20:1239–1250. ³H-Thymidine autoradiographic studies on the origin of reactive cells in the brain of mice infected with Japanese encephalitis virus.

Sato-Yoshitake, R., Y. Shiomura, H. Miyasaka, and N. Hirokawa (1989). *Neuron* 3:229–238. Microtubule-associated protein 1B: Molecular structure, localization, and phosphorylation-dependent expression in developing neurons.

Sato, S. M., and T. D. Sargent (1989). *Dev. Biol.* 134:263–266. Development of neural inducing capacity in dissociated *Xenopus* embryos.

Sauer, F. C. (1935a). *J. Comp. Neurol.* 62:377–405. Mitosis in the neural tube.

Sauer, F. C. (1935b). *J. Comp. Neurol.* 63:13–23. The cellular structure of the neural tube.

Sauer, F. C. (1936). *J. Morphol.* 60:1–11. The interkinetic migration of embryonic epithelial nuclei.

Sauer, F. C. (1937). *J. Morphol.* 61:563–579. Some factors in the morphogenesis of vertebrate embryonic epithelium.

Sauer, M. E., and A. C. Chittenden (1959). *Exp. Cell Res.* 16:1–6. Deoxyribonucleic acid content of cell nuclei in the neural tube of the chick embryo: Evidence for intermitotic migration of nuclei.

Sauer, M. E., and B. E. Walker (1959). *Proc. Soc. Exp. Biol. Med.* 101:557–560. Radiographic study of interkinetic nuclear migration in the neural tube.

Saunders, J. W., and M. T. Gasseling (1968). Ectodermal-Mesenchymal interactions, pp. 78. In *Epithelial-Mesenchymal Interactions* (R. Fleischmajer, and R. E. Billingham, eds.), Williams and Wilkins, Baltimore.

Saunders, J. W., Jr. (1966). *Science* 154:604–612. Death in embryonic systems.

Saunders, J. W., Jr., and J. F. Fallon (1966). Cell death in morphogenesis, pp. 289–314. In *Major Problems in Developmental Biology* (M. Locke, ed.), Academic Press, New York.

Saunders, N. R. (1977). *Exp. Eye Res.* 25:Suppl. 523–550. Ontogeny of the blood-brain barrier.

Saunders, N. R., and K. Møllgård (1984). *J. Dev. Physiol.* 6:45–57. Development of the blood-brain barrier.

Savage, R., and C. R. Phillips (1989). *Dev. Biol.* 133:157–168. Signals from the dorsal blastopore lip region during gastrulation bias the ectoderm toward a nonepidermal pathway of differentiation in *Xenopus laevis*.

Savio, T., and M. E. Schwab (1989). *J. Neurosci.* 9:1126–1133. Rat CNS white matter, but not gray matter, is nonpermissive for neuronal cell adhesion and fiber outgrowth.

Sawaguchi, T., and K. Kubota (1986). *Int. J. Neurosci.* 30:57–64. A hypothesis on the primate neocortex evolution: Column-multiplication hypothesis.

Saxén, L. (1954). *Ann. Acad. Sci. Fennicae Series A. IV.* 23:1–93. The development of the visual cells. Embryological and physiological investigations of *Amphibia*.

Saxén, L. (1961). *Dev. Biol.* 3:140–152. Transfilter neural induction of amphibian ectoderm.

Saxén, L. (1980). *Curr. Topics Dev. Biol.* 15:409–417. Neural induction: Past, present and future.

Saxén. L., and S. Toivonen (1961). *J. Embryol Exp. Morphol.* 9:514–533. The two-gradient hypothesis in primary induction. The combined effect of two types of inductors mixed in different ratios.

Saxén, L., and S. Toivonen (1962). *Primary Embryonic Induction*, Logos Press, London.

Saxén, L., E. Lehtonen, M. Karkinen-Jääskelainen, S. Nordling, and J. Wartiovaara (1976). *Nature* 259:662–663. Are morphogenetic tissue interactions mediated by transmissible signal substances or through cell contacts?

Saxén, L., P. Ekblom, and I. Thesleff (1982). Cell-matrix interaction in organogenesis, pp. 257–264. In *New Trends in Basement Membrane Research* (K. Kuehn, H. Schoene, and R. Timpl, eds), Raven Press, New York.

Saxod, R. (1967). *Arch. Anat. Microscop. Morphol. Exp.* 56:153–166. Histogenése des corpuscules sensoriels cutanés chez le poulet et le canard.

Saxod, R. (1970a). *J. Ultrastruct. Res.* 32:477–496. Etude au microscope electronique de l'histogenese du corpuscule sensoriel cutane de Grandry chez le canard.

Saxod, R. (1970b). *J. Ultrastruct. Res.* 33:463–492. Etude au microscope électronique de l'histogenése du corpuscule sensoriel cutané de Herbst chez le canard.

Saxod, R. (1971). *C. R. Acad. Sci. (D) Paris* 273:89–91. Embryologie expérimentale.—Sur l'origine des differentes catégories cellulaires du corpuscle de Herbst.

Saxod, R. (1972a). *J. Embryol. Exp. Morphol.* 27:277–300. Rôle du nerf et du territoire cutané dans le développement des corpuscules de Herbst et de Grandry.

Saxod, R. (1972b). *J. Embryol. Exp. Morphol.* 27:585–601. Interactions morphogènes au course de l'histogenèse du corpuscule de Herbst, étudiées á l'aide de transplantations hètérochrones.

Saxod, R. (1973a). *Dev. Biol.* 32:167–178. Developmental origin of the Herbst cutaneous sensory corpuscle. Experimental analysis using cellular markers.

Saxod, R. (1973b). *Tiss. Cell* 5:269–280. Les organites périnucléaires du corpuscle sensoriel cutané de Grandry. Organisation ultrastructurale et formation.

Saxod, R. (1978). Development of cutaneous sensory receptors in birds. In *Handbook of Sensory Physiology*, Vol. 9, *Development of Sensory System* (M. Jacobson, ed.), Springer-Verlag, New York.

Saxod, R., and P. Sengel (1968). *Compt. Rend. Acad. Sci. (Paris)* 267:1149–1152. Sur les conditions de la differenciation des corpuscules sensoriels cutanes le Poulet et le Canard.

Scadding, S. R. (1983). *J. Exp. Zool.* 226:75–80. Can differences in limb regeneration ability between individuals within certain amphibian species be explained by differences in the quantity of innervation?

Scadding, S. R. (1984). *J. Exp. Zool.* 229:155–161. Forelimbs of the newt *Notophthalmus viridescens* continuously denervated for up to six weeks prior to amputation do not regenerate.

Scalia, F., and K. Fite (1974). *J. Comp. Neurol.* 158:455–478. A retinotopic analysis of the central connections of the optic nerve in the frog.

Scalia, F., and D. E. Matsumoto (1985). *J. Comp. Neurol.* 231:323–338. The morphology of growth cones of regenerating optic nerve axons.

Scalia, F., H. Knapp, M. Halpern, and W. Riss (1968). *Brain Behav. Evol.* 1:324–353. New observations on the retinal projection in the frog.

Scalia, F., V. Arango, and E. L. Singman (1985). *Brain Res.* 344:267–280. Loss and displacement of ganglion cells after optic nerve regeneration in adult *Rana pipiens*.

Scaravilli, F., and L. W. Duchen (1980). *J. Neurocytol.* 9:373–380. Electron microscopic and quantitative studies of cell necrosis in developing sensory ganglia in normal and Sprawling mutant mice.

Scarr, S. (1969). *Soc. Biol.* 16:249–256. Effects of birth weight on later intelligence.

Sceats, D J., Jr., W. A. Friedman, G. W. Sypert, and W. E.

Ballinger, Jr. (1986). *Brain Res.* 362:149–156. Regeneration in peripheral nerve grafts to the cat spinal cord.

Schachner, M. (1982). *J. Neurochem.* 39:1–8. Cell type-specific surface antigens in the mammalian nervous system.

Schadé, J. P. (1959). *Growth* 23:159–168. Differential growth of nerve cells in cerebral cortex.

Schadé, J. P., and C. F. Baxter (1960). *Exp. Neurol.* 2:158–178. Changes during growth in the volume and surface area of cortical neurons in the rabbit.

Schadé, J. P., and W. B. van Groeningen (1961). *Acta Anat. (Basel)* 47:79–111. Structural organization of the human cerebral cortex.

Schadé, J. P., K. Meeter, and W. B. van Groeningen (1962). *Acta Morphol. Neerl. Scand.* 5:37–48. Maturational aspects of the dendrites in the human cerebral cortex.

Schadewald, M. (1941). *J. Comp. Neurol.* 74:239–246. Effects of cutting the trochlear and abducens nerves on the endbulbs about the cells of the corresponding nuclei.

Schadewald, M. (1942). *J. Comp. Neurol.* 77:739–746. Transynaptic effect of neonatal axon section on bouton appearance about somatic motor cells.

Schäfer, E. A. (1900). *Textbook of Physiology* 2:697–782. Edinburgh and London: Pentland.

Schäfer, K. (1923). *Z. Anat. EntwGesch.* 95:467–482. Histogenese der Hirnfurchung.

Schäfer, K., and R. L. Friede (1988). *J. Anat. (London)* 159:181–195. The onset and rate of myelination in six peripheral and autonomic nerves of the rat.

Schäfer, T., M. E. Schwab, and H. Thoenen (1983). *J. Neurosci.* 3:1501–1510. Increased formation of preganglionic synapses and axons due to a retrograde transsynaptic action of nerve growth factor in the rat sympathetic nervous system.

Schaffer, K. (1893). *Neurol. Centralbl. Leipzig* 12:849–851. Kurze Anmerkung über die morphologische Differenz des Axencylinders im Verhaltnisse zu den protoplasmatischen Fortsätzen bei Nissl's Färbung.

Schaffer, K. (1926). *Z. Anat. Entw. Gesch.* 81:715–719. Über die Hortegasche Mikroglia.

Schaffner, K. (1969). *Br. J. Phil. Sci.* 20:325–348. The Watson-Crick model and reductionism.

Schall, J. D., S. J. Ault, D. J. Vitek, and A. G. Leventhal (1988). *J. Neurosci.* 8:2039–2048. Experimental induction of an abnormal ipsilateral visual field representation in the geniculocortical pathway of normally pigmented cats.

Schaper, A. (1894a). *Anat. Anz.* 9:489–501. Die morphologische und histologische Entwicklung des Kleinhirns der Teleostier.

Schaper, A. (1894b). *Morphol. Jahrb.* 21:625–708. Die morphologische und histologische Entwickung des Kleinhirns der Teleostier.

Schaper, A. (1895). *Anat. Anz.* 10:422–426. Einige kritische Bemerkungen zu Lugaro's Aufsatz: Ueber die Histogenese der Körner der Kleinhirnrinde.

Schaper, A. (1897a). *Arch. Entw.-Mech. Organ.* 5:81–132. Die frühesten Differenzierungsvorgänge im Centralnervensystem.

Schaper, A. (1897b). *Science* 5:430–431. The earliest differentiation in the central nervous system of vertebrates.

Schapiro, S., K. Vukovich, and A. Globus (1973). *Exp. Neurol.* 40:286–296. Effects of neonatal thyroxine and hydrocortisone administration on the development of dendritic spines in the visual cortex of rats.

Scharf, J.-H. (1951). *Morphol. Jahrb.* 91:187–252. Die markhaltigen Ganglienzellen und ihre Beziehung zu den myelogenetischen Theorien.

Scharf, J.-H., and R. Blume (1964). *Z. Zellforsch. Mikroskop. Anat.* 62:454–467. Quantitativ morphologische Befunde zur Hypothese des Mitochondrientransportes im Neuron.

Schatteman, G. C., L. Gibbs, A. A. Lanahan, P. Claude, and M. Bothwell (1988). *J. Neurosci.* 8:860–873. Expression of NGF receptor in the developing and adult primate central nervous system.

Schecter, A. L., and M. A. Bothwell (1981). *Cell* 24:867–874. Nerve growth factor receptors on PC12 cells: Evidence for two receptor classes with differing cytoskeletal association.

Scheff, S. W. (1987). *Neurobiol. Aging* 8:571–573. Methodological considerations when assessing age related changes.

Scheibel, M. E., and A. B. Scheibel (1970). The rapid Golgi method. Indian Summer or renaissance?, pp. 1–11. In *Contemporary Research Methods in Neuroanatomy* (W. J. H. Nauta, and S. O. E. Ebbesson, eds.), Springer, Berlin, Heidelberg, New York.

Scheibel, M. E., and A. B. Scheibel (1978). The methods of Golgi, pp. 89–114. In *Neuroanatomical Research Techniques* (R. T. Robertson, ed.), Academic Press, New York.

Scheibel, M. E., T. L. Davies, and A. B. Scheibel (1973). *Exp. Neurol.* 38:301–310. Maturation of reticular dendrites: Loss of spines and development of bundles.

Schelper, R. L., and E. J. Adrian Jr. (1986). *J. Neuropathol. Exp. Neurol.* 45:1–19. Monoctyes become macrophages: They do not become microglia: A light and electronic microscopic autoradiographic study using 125-Iododeoxyuridine.

Scherer, W. J., and S. B. Udin (1989). *J. Neurosci.* 9:3837–3843. N-methyl-D-aspartate antagonists prevent interaction of binocular maps in *Xenopus* tectum.

Scherrer, J., R. Verley, and L. Garner (1968). Time, flow and velocity in early life, pp. 303–309. In *Ontogenesis of the Brain* (L. Tilek, and S. Trojan, eds.), Charles University, Prague.

Schiaffino, S., and S. Pierobon (1976). *J. Neurocyt.* 5:319–336. Morphogenesis of rat muscle spindles after nerve lesion during early postnatal development.

Schierenberg, E. (1989). *BioEsays* 10:99–104. Cytoplasmic determination and distribution of developmental potential in the embryo of *Caenorhabditis elegans*.

Schierhorn, H., and J. Nagel (1977). *J. Hirnforsch* 18:345–356. Qualitativer Vergleich der Imprägnationsresultate verschiedener Golgi-Techniken. Untersuchungen am Neocortex adulter Albinoratten.

Schiff, J., and W. R. Loewenstein (1972). *Science* 177:712–715. Development of a receptor on a foreign nerve fiber in a Pacinian corpuscle.

Schittny, J. C., R. Timpl, and J. Engel (1988). *J. Cell. Biol.* 107:1599–1610. High resolution immunoelectron microscopic localization of functional domains of laminin, nidogen, and heparan sulfate proteoglycan in epithelial basement membrane of mouse cornea reveals different topological orientations.

Schjeide, O. A., R. I. S. Lin, and J. de Vallis (1968). *Radiation*

Res. 33:107–128. Molecular composition of myelin synthesized subsequent to irradiation.

Schlaepfer, W. W. (1974). *Brain Res.* 69:203–215. Calciuminduced degeneration of axoplasm in isolated segments of rats peripheral nerve.

Schlaepfer, W. W., and L. A. Freeman (1978). *J. Cell Biol.* 78:653–662. Neurofilament proteins of rat peripheral nerve and spinal cord.

Schleiden, M. J. (1838). *Müller's Arch. f. Anat., Physiol. u. wissensch. Medicin,* pp. 137–176. Beiträge zur Phytogenesis.

Schleifenbaum, C. (1973). *Z. Anat. Enticklungsgesch.* 141:179–205. Untersuchungen zur postnatalen Ontogenese des Gehirns von Grosspudeln und Wölfen.

Schlenska, G. (1974). *J. Hirnforsch* 15:401–408. Volumenund Oberflächenmessungen an Gehirnen verschiedener Säugetiere im Vergleich zu einem errechneten Modell.

Schlessinger, A. R., W. M. Cowan, and E. I. Gottlieb (1975). *J. Comp. Neurol.* 159:149–176. An autoradiographic study of the time of origin and the pattern or granule cell migration in the dentate gyrus of the rat.

Schlessinger, A. R., W. M. Cowan, and L. W. Swanson (1978). *Anat. Embryol.* 154:153–173. The time of origin of neurons in Ammon's horn and the associated retrohippocampal fields.

Schliwa, M. (1986). *The Cytoskeleton.* Springer Verlag, New York.

Schlumpf, M., W. J. Shoemaker, and F. E. Bloom (1980). *J. Comp. Neurol.* 192:361–377. Innervation of embryonic rat cerebral cortex by catecholamine-containing fibers.

Schmalbruch, H. (1982). *Dev. Biol.* 91:485–490. Skeletal muscle fibers of newborn rats are coupled by gap junctions.

Schmatolla, E. (1972). *J. Embryol. Exp. Morphol.* 27:555–576. Dependence of tectal neuron differentiation on optic innervation in teleost fish.

Schmechel, D. E., and P. Rakic (1973). *Anat. Rec.* 175:436. Evolution of fetal radial glial cells in the rhesus monkey telencephalon: A Golgi study.

Schmechel, D. E., and P. Rakic (1979). *Anat. Embryol.* 156:115–152. A Golgi study of radial glial cells in developing monkey telencephalon: Morphogenesis and transformation into astrocytes.

Schmidt, H. D. (1874). *Monthly Microscopical J.* 1 March. On the construction of the dark or double-bordered nervefibre.

Schmidt, J. T. (1985a). *Fed. Proc.* 44:2767–2772. Selective stabilization of retinotectal synapses by an activitydependent mechanism.

Schmidt, J. T. (1985b). *Cell Mol. Neurobiol.* 5:65–84. Formation of retinotopic connections: Selective stabilization by an activity-dependent mechanism.

Schmidt, J. T., and D. L. Edwards (1983). *Brain Res.* 269:29–39. Activity sharpens the map during the regeneration of the retinotectal projection in goldfish.

Schmidt, J. T., and L. E. Eisele (1985). *Neuroscience* 14:535–546. Stroboscopic illumination and dark rearing block the sharpening of the regenerated retinotectal map in goldfish.

Schmidt, J. T., J. C. Turcotte, M. Buzzard, and D. G. Tieman (1988). *J. Comp. Neurol.* 269:565–591. Staining of regenerated optic arbors in goldfish tectum: Progressive changes in immature arbors and a comparison of mature regenerated arbors with normal arbors.

Schmidt-Nielson, K. (1970). *Fed. Proc.* 29:1524–1532. Energy metabolism, body size and problems of scaling.

Schmidt-Nielsen, K. (1975). *J. Exp. Zool.* 194:287–308. Scaling in biology: The consequences of size.

Schmidt-Nielsen, K. (1984). *Scaling. Why Is Animal Size So Important.* Cambridge Univ. Press, Cambridge.

Schmidt, M. J., B. D. Sawyer, K. W. Perry, R. W. Fuller, M. M. Foreman, and B. Ghetti (1982). *J. Neurosci.* 2:376–380. Dopamine deficiency in the weaver mutant mouse.

Schmidt, T. J., and G. Litwack (1982). *Physiol. Rev.* 62:1131–1192. Activation of the glucorticoid-receptor complex.

Schmidt, W. J. (1936). *Z. Zellforsch. Mikrosk. Anat.* 23:657–676. Doppelbrechung und Feinbau der Markscheide der Nervenfasern.

Schmidtke, J., M. T. Zenzes, H. Dittes, and W. Engel (1975). *Nature* 254:426–427. Regulation of cell size in fish of tetraploid origin.

Schmitt, C. A., and A. A. Donough (1986). *J. Biol. Chem.* 261:10439–10444. Development and thyroid hormone regulation of two molecular forms of Na^+-K^+-ATPase in brain.

Schmitt, F. O. (1936). *Cold Spring Harbor Symp. Quant. Biol.* 4:7–12. Nerve ultrastructure as revealed by X-ray diffraction and polarized light studies.

Schmitt, F. O. (1950). *Assoc. Res. Nerv. Ment. Dis.* 28:247–254. The ultrastructure of the nerve myelin sheath.

Schmitt, F. O. (1968). *Proc. Natl. Acad. Sci. U.S.A.* 60:1092–1101. Fibrous proteins—Neuronal organelles.

Schmitt, F. O., and R. S. Bear (1939). *Biol. Rev.* 14:27–50. The ultrastructure of the nerve axon sheath.

Schmitt, F. O., R. S. Bear, and G. L. Clark (1935). *Radiology* 25:131–151. X-ray diffraction studies on nerve.

Schmitt, F. O., P. Dev, and B. H. Smith (1976). *Science* 193:114–120. Electrotonic processing of information by brain cells.

Schnapp, B. J., and T. S. Reese (1982). *J. Cell Biol.* 94:667–679. Cytoplasmic structure in rapid-frozen axons.

Schnapp, B. J., R. D. Vale, M. P. Sheetz, and T. S. Reese (1985). *Cell* 40:455–462. Single microtubules from squid axoplasm support bidirectional movement of organelles.

Schneider, G. E. (1970). *Brain Behav. Evol.* 3:295–323. Mechanisms of functional recovery following lesions of visual cortex or superior colliculus in neonatal and adult hamsters.

Schneider, G. E. (1973). *Brain Behav. Evol.* 8:73–109. Early lesions of superior colliculus: Factors affecting the formation of abnormal retinal projections.

Schneider, G. E. (1981). *Trends Neurosci.* 4:187–192. Early lesions and abnormal neuronal connections.

Schneider, H. R. (1968). *J. Comp. Neurol.* 133:411–428. Some findings concerning the relationship between ontogenesis and cytoarchitecture of the primate brain.

Schnepp, G., P. Schnepp, and G. Spaan (1971). *Z. Zellforsch. Mikrosk. Anat.* 119:77–98. Faseranalytische Untersuchungen an peripheren Nerven bei Tieren verschiedener Grösse. I. Fasergesamtzahl Faserkaliber und Nervenleitungsgeschwindigkeit.

Schnepp, P. and G. Schnepp (1971). *Z. Zellforsch. Mikrosk. Anat.* 119:99–114. Faseranalytische Untersuchungen an peripheran Nerven bei Tieren verschiedener Grösse. II. Verhältnis Axondurchmesser, Gesamtdurchmesser und Internodallänge.

Schnitzer, J., W. W. Franke, and M. Schachner (1981). *J. Cell Biol.* 90:435–447. Immunocytochemical demonstration of vimentin in astrocytes and ependymal cells of developing and adult mouse nervous system.

Schoefl, G. I. (1964). *Ann. N.Y. Acad. Sci.* 116:789–802. Electron microscopic observations of the regeneration of blood vessels after injury.

Schoenfeld, T. A., L. McKerracher, R. Obar, and R. B. Vallee (1989). *J. Neurosci.* 9:1712–1730. MAP 1A and MAP 1B are structurally related microtubule associated proteins with distinct developmental patterns in the CNS.

Schoenwolf, G. C. (1982). *Scan. Elec. Microscopy* 1:289–308. On the morphogenesis of the early rudiments of the developing central nervous system.

Schoenwolf, G. C. (1985). *Dev. Biol.* 109:127–139. Shaping and bending of the avian neuroepithelium: Morphometric analysis.

Schoenwolf, G. C. (1988). *J. Comp. Neurol.* 276:498–507. Microsurgical analyses of avian neurulation: Separation of medial and lateral tissues.

Schoenwolf, G. C., and I. S. Alvarez (1989). *Development* 106:427–439. Roles of neuroepithelial cell rearrangement and division in shaping of the avian neural plate.

Schoenwolf, G. C., and J. Delongo (1980). *Am. J. Anat.* 158:43–63. Ultrastructure of secondary neurulation in the chick embryo.

Schoenwolf, G. C., and M. Fisher (1983). *J. Embryol. Exp. Morph.* 73:1–15. Analysis of the effects of *Streptomyces* hyaluronidase on formation of the neural tube.

Schoenwolf, G. C., and M. V. Franks (1984). *Dev. Biol.* 105:257–272. Quantitative analysis of changes in cell shapes during bending of the avian neural plate.

Schoenwolf, G. C., and P. Sheard (1989). *Development* 105:17–25. Shaping and bending of the avian neural plate as analysed with a fluorescent-histochemical marker.

Schoenwolf, G. C., D. Folsom, and A. Moe (1988). *Anat. Rec.* 220:87–102. A reexamination of the role of microfilaments in neurulation in the chick embryo.

Schoenwolf, G. C., H. Bortier, and L. Vakaet (1989). *J. Exp. Zool.* 249:271–278. Fate mapping the avian neural plate with quail/chick chimeras: Origin of prospective median wedge cells.

Scholes, J. H. (1979). *Nature* 278:620–624. Nerve fibre topography in the retinal projection to the tectum.

Scholte, W., and J. W. Boellaard (1983). Role of lipopigment during aging of nerve and glial cells in the human central nervous system, pp. 27–74. In *Brain Aging. Neuropathology and Neuropharmacology* (Aging, Vol. 21), (J. Cervos-Navarro, and H.-I. Sarkander, eds.), Raven Press, New York.

Schonbach, J., K. H. Hu, and R. L. Friede (1968). *J. Comp. Neurol.* 134:21–38. Cellular and chemical changes during myelination: Histologic, autoradiographic, histochemical and biochemical data on myelination in the pyramidal tract and corpus callosum of rat.

Schönheit, B. (1982). *J. Hirnforsch.* 23:681–692. Über den Einfluß einer frühen postnatalen mangelernährung auf die Reifung kortikaler Neurone bei der Ratte.

Schook, P. (1980). *Acta Morphol. Neerl-Scand.* 18:1–30. Morphogenetic movements during early development of the chick eye. A light microscopic and reconstructive study.

Schook, W., S. Puszkin, W. Bloom, C. Ores, and S. Kochwa (1979). *Biochemistry* 76:116–120. Mechanochemical properties of brain clathrin: Interactions with actin and alpha-actinin and polymerization into basketlike structures or filaments.

Schooley, R. A., S. Friedkin, and E. S. Evans (1966). *Endocrinology* 79:1053–1057. Reexamination of the discrepancy between acidophil numbers and growth hormone concentration in the anterior pituitary following thyroidectomy.

Schoppmann, A., R. J. Nelson, M. P. Stryker, M. Cynader, J. Zook, and M. M. Merzenich (1981). *Neurosci. Abstr.* 7;842. Reorganization of hand representation within area 3b following digit amputation in owl monkey.

Schouls, P. A. (1989). *Descartes and the Enlightenment*. Edinburgh Univ. Press, Edinburgh.

Schousboe, A., and I. Divac (1979). *Brain Res.* 177:407–409. Differences in glutamate uptake in astrocytes cultured from different brain regions.

Schrödinger, E. (1944). *What Is Life?* Cambridge Univ. Press, Cambridge.

Schroeder, T. E. (1969). *Biol. Bull.* 137:413–414. The role of "contractile ring" filaments in dividing *Arbacia* egg.

Schroeder, T. E. (1970). *J. Embryol. Exp. Morphol.* 23:427–462. Neurulation in *Xenopus laevis*. An analysis and model based upon light and electron microscopy.

Schroeder, T. E. (1972). *Proc. Natl. Acad. Sci. U.S.A.* 70:1688–1692. Actin in dividing cells: Contractile ring filaments bind heavy meromysin.

Schubert, D., and M. LaCorbiere (1985a). *J. Cell Biol.* 100:56–63. Isolation of a cell-surface receptor for chick neural retina adherons.

Schubert, D., and M. LaCorbiere (1985b). *J. Cell Biol.* 101:1071–1077. Isolation of an adhesion-mediating protein from chick neural retina adherons.

Schubert, D., M. LaCorbiere, and F. Esch (1986). *J. Cell Biol.* 102:2295–2301. A chick neural retina adhesion and survival molecule is a retinol-binding protein.

Schubert, P., and G. W. Kreutzberg (1974). *Brain Res.* 76:526–530. Axonal transport of adenosine and uridine derivatives and transfer to postsynaptic neurons.

Schubert, P., H. D. Lux, and G. W. Kreutzberg (1971). *Acta Neuropathol. (Berl.)* 5:179–186. Single cell isotope injection technique, a tool for studying axonal and dendritic transport.

Schucker, F. (1972). *Exp. Neurol.* 36:59–78. Effects of NGF-antiserum in sympathetic neurons during early postnatal development.

Schuetze, E., and L. Role (1987). *Ann. Rev. Neurosci.* 10:403–457. Developmental regulation of nicotinic acetylcholine receptors.

Schughart, K., M. F. Utset, A. Awgulewitsch, and F. H. Ruddle (1988). *Proc. Natl. Acad. Sci. U.S.A.* 85:5582–5586. Structure and expression of Hox-2.2, a murine homeo box-containing gene.

Schultz, D. M., D. A. Giordano, and D. H. Schulz (1962). *Arch. Pathol.* 74:80–86. Weights of organs of fetuses and infants.

Schultz, M. G. (1962). *J. Amer. Vet. Med. Asso.* 140:241. Male pseudohermaphroditism diagnosed with aid of sex chromatin technique.

Schultz, R. L. (1964). *J. Comp. Neurol.* 122:281–296. Macroglial identification in electron microscopy.

Schultz, R. L., E. A. Maynard, and D. C. Pease (1957). *Am. J. Anat.* 100:369–407. Electron microscopy of neurons and neuroglia of cerebral cortex and corpus callosum.

Schultz, W. (1969). *Zool. Anz.* 183:47–72. Zur Kenntnis des Hallstromhundes (*Canis hallstromi* Throughton, 1957).

Schultze, B., B. Nowak, and W. Maurer (1974). *J. Comp. Neurol.* 158:207–218. Cycle times of the neural epithelial cells of various types of neuron in the rat. An autoradiographic study.

Schultze, B., W. Maurer, and H. Hagenbusch (1976). *Cell Tiss. Kinet.* 9:245–255. A two emulsion autoradiographic technique and the discrimination of the three different types of labelling after double labelling with ^{3}H- and ^{14}C-thymidine.

Schultze, M. J. S. (1858a). *Abh. Naturforsch. Gesellsch. Halle* 4:30–33. Zur Kenntniss der elektrischen Organe der Fische.

Schultze, M. J. S. (1858b). *Müller's Archiv* 1858:343–381. Ueber die Endigungweise des Hörnerven im Labyrinth.

Schultze, M. J. S. (1860). *Centralbl. f. d. med. Wissensch. Berlin* 2:385–390. Das Epithelium der Riechschleimhaut des Menschen.

Schultze, M. J. S. (1862). *Abh. naturforsch. Ges. Halle* 7:1–100. Untersuchungen über der Bau der Nasenschleimhaut, namentlich die Struktur und Endigungsweise der Geruchsnerven bei dem Menschen und den Wirbelthieren.

Schultze, M. J. S. (1866). *Arch. mikr. Anat.* 2:165–286. Zur Anatomie und Physiologie der Retina.

Schultze, M. J. S. (1870). In *Manual of Human and Comparative Histology*, Vol. 1, trans. H. Power, (S. Stricker, ed.), New Sydenham Society, London.

Schulz, C. (1951). *Zool. Jahrb., Abt. Allgem. Zool. Physiol.* 63:64–106. Die relative Grösse cytoarchitektonischer Einheiten im Grosshirn der weissen Ratte, weissen Maus und Zwergmaus.

Schulze, E., and M. Kirschner (1986). *J. Cell Biol.* 102:1020–1031. Microtubule dynamics in interphase cells.

Schulze, E., and M. Kirschner (1987). *J. Cell Biol.* 97:1249–1254. Dynamic and stable populations of microtubules in cells.

Schumacher, U. (1963). *J. Hirnforsch.* 6:137–163. Quantitative Untersuchungen an Gehirnen mitteleuropäischer Musteliden.

Schüz, A. (1981). *J. Hirnforsch.* 22:93–127. Pränatale Reifung und postnatale Veränderung im Cortex des Meerschweinchens: Mikroskopische Auswertung eines natürlichen Deprivationsexperiments. I: Pränatale Reifung, II: postnatale Veränderungen.

Schüz, A. (1986). *J. Comp. Neurol.* 244:277–285. Comparison between the dimensions of dendritic spines in the cerebral cortex of newborn and adult guinea pigs.

Schwab, M., and H. Thoenen (1977). *Brain Res.* 122:459–474. Selective trans-synaptic migration of tetanus toxin after retrograde axonal transport in peripheral sympathetic nerves: A comparison with nerve growth factor.

Schwab, M., and H. Thoenen (1983). Retrograde axonal transport, pp. 381–404. In *Handbook of Neurochemistry* (A. Lajtha, ed.), Plenum, New York.

Schwab, M. E. (1977). *Brain Res.* 130:190–196. Ultrastructural localization of a nerve growth factor-horseradish peroxidase (NGF-HRP) coupling product after retrograde axonal transport in adrenergic neurons.

Schwab, M. E., and P. Caroni (1988). *J. Neurosci.* 8:2381–2393. Oligodendrocytes and CNS myelin are nonpermissive substrates for neurite growth and fibroblast spreading *in vitro*.

Schwab, M. E., and H. Thoenen (1985). *J. Neurosci.* 5:2415–2423. Dissociated neurons regenerate into sciatic but not optic nerve explants in culture irrespective of neurotrophic factors.

Schwann, T. (1839). *Mikroskopische Untersuchungen über die Übereinstimmung in der Struktur und dem Wachstum der Thiere und Pflanzen.* Berlin. Republished in *Ostwald's Klassiker*, Leipzig, 1910. English transl. H. Smith, Microscopical Researches, London, 1847.

Schwann, T. (1847). *Microscopical Researches into the Accordance in the Structure and Growth of Animals and Plants.* (Translated by H. Smith), pp. 129–140. The Sydenham Society, London.

Schwarting, G. A., and M. Yamamoto (1988). *BioEssays* 9:19–23. Expression of glycoconjugates during development of the vertebrate nervous system.

Schwartz, H. L., and J. H. Oppenheimer (1978a). *Endocrinology* 103:267–273. Nuclear triiodothyronine receptor sites in the brain: Probable identity with hepatic receptors and regional distribution.

Schwartz, H. L., and J. H. Oppenheimer (1978b). *Endocrinology* 103:943–948. Ontogenesis of 3,5,3'-triiodothyronine receptors in neonatal rat brain: Dissociation between receptor concentration and stimulation of oxygen consumption by 3,5,3'-triiodothyronine.

Schwartz, M. L., and P. S. Goldman-Rakic (1982). *Nature* 299:154–155. Single cortical neurones have axon collaterals to ipsilateral and contralateral cortex in fetal and adult primates.

Schweichel, J.-U., and H.-J. Merker (1973). *Teratology* 7:253–266. The morphology of various types of cell death in prenatal tissues.

Schweigerer, L., G. Neufeld, J. Friedman, J. A. Abraham, J. C. Fiddes, and D. Gospodarowicz (1987). *Nature* 325:257–259. Capillary endothelial cells express basic fibroblast growth factor, a mitogen that promotes their own growth.

Schweizer, G., C. Ayer-Le Lièvre, and N. M. Le Douarin (1983). *Cell Differ.* 13:191–200. Restrictions of developmental capacities in the dorsal root ganglia during the course of development.

Schwind, J. L. (1931). *J. Exp. Zool.* 59:265–295. Heteroplastic experiments on the limb and shoulder girdle of Amblystoma.

Scott, J. P., J. M. Stewart, and V. J. DeGhett (1974). *Dev. Psychobiol.* 7:489–513. Critical periods in the organization of systems.

Scott, L. J. C., F. Bacou, and J. R. Sanes (1988). *J. Neurosci.* 8:932–944. A synapse-specific carbohydrate at the neuromuscular junction: Association with both acetylcholinesterase and a glycolipid.

Scott, M., and P. H. O'Farrell (1986). *Ann. Rev. Cell Biol.* 2:49–80. Spatial programming of gene expression in early *Drosophila* embryogenesis.

Scott, M. P., and S. B. Carroll (1987). *Cell* 51:689–698. The segmentation and homeotic gene network in early drosophila development.

Scott, M. Y. (1977). *Exp. Neurol.* 54:579–590. Behavioral tests of compression of retinotectal projection after partial tectal ablation in goldfish.

Scott, S. A. (1975). *Science* 189:644–646. Persistence of foreign innervation on reinnervated goldfish extraocular muscles.

Scott, S. A. (1982). *J. Physiol.* 330:203–220. The development of the segmental pattern of skin sensory innervation in embryonic chick hindlimb.

Scott, S. A. (1987). *Trends Neurosci.* 10:468–473. The development of skin sensory innervation patterns.

Scott, S. A. (1988). *Dev. Biol.* 126:362–374. Skin sensory innervation patterns in embryonic chick hindlimbs deprived of motoneurons.

Scott, S. A., E. Cooper, and J. Diamond (1981). *Proc. Roy. Soc. (London) Ser. B.* 211:455–470. Merkel cells as targets of the mechanosensory nerves in salamander skin.

Scott, S. A., L. Macintyre, and J. Diamond (1981b). *Proc. Roy. Soc. (London) Ser. B.* 211:505–511. Competitive reinnervation of salamander skin by regenerating and intact mechanosensory nerves.

Scott, T. G. (1964). *J. Comp. Neurol.* 22:1–7. A unique pattern of localization within the cerebellum of the mouse.

Scott, T. M. (1974). *J. Embryol. Exp. Morphol.* 31:409–414. The development of the retino-tectal projection in *Xenopus laevis:* An autoradiographic and degeneration study.

Scott, T. M., and S. M. Bunt (1986). *J. Embryol. Exp. Morphol.* 91:181–195. An examination of the evidence for the existence of preformed pathways in the neural tube of *Xenopus laevis.*

Scott, T. M., and G. Lazar (1976). *J. Anat.* 121:485–496. An investigation into the hypothesis of shifting neuronal relationships during development.

Scrimshaw, N. S., and J. E. Gordon (eds.), (1968). *Malnutrition, Learning and Behavior.* M. I. T. Press, Cambridge, Mass.

Scriven, M. (1961). The key property of physical laws—Inaccuracy, pp. 91–101. In *Current Issues in the Philosophy of Science* (H. Feigl, and G. Maxwell, eds.), Holt, Reinhart and Winston, New York.

Sechenov, I. M. (1863). *Physiologische Studien über die Hemmungsmechanismen für Reflexthätigkeit des Frosches.* Hirschwald, Berlin. Reprinted in *Selected Works,* pp. 153–176, State Publishing House, Moscow.

Sechrist, J. W. (1969). *Am. J. Anat.* 124:117–134. Neurocytogenesis. I. Neurofibrils, neurofilaments, and the terminal mitotic cycle.

Sechrist, J. W., and A. Lavelle (1966). *Am. Zool.* 6:530–531. Neurofilaments and initial neuroblast differentiation.

Sedgwick, A. (1895). *Quart. J. Microsc. Sci.* 37:87–101. On the inadequacy of the cellular theory of development, and on the early development of nerves etc.

Sedlacek, J. (1967). *Physiol. Bohemoslav.* 16:531–537. Development of optic evoked potentials in chick embryos.

Seeley, P. J., and L. A. Greene (1983). *Proc. Natl. Acad. Sci. U.S.A.* 80:2789–2793. Short-latency local actions of nerve growth factor at the growth cone.

Seeley, P. J., C. H. Keith, M. L. Shelanski, and L. A. Greene (1983). *J. Neurosci.* 3:1488–1494. Pressure microinjection of nerve growth factor and antinerve growth factor into the nucleus and cytoplasm: Lack of effects on neurite outgrowth from pheochromocytoma cells.

Sefton, A. J., and K. Lam (1984). *Exp. Brain Res.* 57:107–117. Quantitative and morphological studies on developing optic axons in normal and enucleated albino rats.

Segal, S. J., and D. C. Johnson (1959). *Arch. Anat. Microscop.* 48:261–265. Inductive influence of steroid hormones on neural growth.

Seiger, Å., and L. Olson (1973). *Z. Anat. Entwicklungsgesch.* 140:281–318. Late prenatal ontogeny of central monoamine neurons in the rat: Fluorescence histochemical observations.

Seil, F. J., and R. M. Herndon (1970). *J. Cell Biol.* **45**:212–220. Cerebellar granule cells *in vitro:* A light and electron microscope study.

Seiler, M., and M. E. Schwab (1984). *Brain Res.* **300**:33–39. Specific retrograde transport of nerve growth factor (NGF) from neocortex to nucleus basalis in the rat.

Seldon, S. C., and T. D. Pollard (1983). *J. Biol. Chem.* **258**:7064–7071. Phosphorylation of microtubule-associated proteins regulates their interaction with actin filaments.

Sellinger, O. Z., and J. M. Azcurra (1970). *Trans. Am. Neurochem.* **1**:22. Separation of neuronal and glial cell fractions.

Sellinger, O. Z., and P. D. Petiet (1973). *Exp. Neurol.* **38**:370–385. Horseradish peroxidase uptake *in vivo* by neuronal and glial lysosomes.

Seltzer, Z., and M. Devor (1984). *Brain Res.* **306**:31–37. Effect of nerve section on the spinal distribution of neighboring nerves.

Sendtner, M., G. W. Kreutzberg, and H. Thoenen (1990). *Nature* **345**:440–441. Ciliary neurotrophic factor prevents the degeneration of motor neurons after axotomy.

Sengel, P. (1976). *Morphogenesis of Skin.* Cambridge University Press, Cambridge.

Sengel, P. (1983). Epidermal-dermal interactions during formation of skin and cutaneous appendages, pp. 102–131. In *Biochemistry and Physiology of the Skin*, Vol. 1 (L. A. Goldsmith, ed.), Oxford University Press, Yew York.

Sengelaub, D. R., and A. P. Arnold (1986). *J. Neurosci.* **6**:1613–1620. Development and loss of early projections in a sexually dimorphic rat spinal nucleus.

Sengelaub, D. R., and B. L. Finlay (1981). *Science* **213**:573–574. Early removal of one eye reduces normally occurring cell death in the remaining eye.

Sengelaub, D. R., and B. L. Finlay (1982). *J. Comp. Neurol.* **204**:311–317. Cell death in the mammalian visual system during normal development: I. Retinal ganglion cells.

Sengelaub, D. R., M. S. Windrem, and B. L. Finlay (1983). *Exp. Brain Res.* **52**:269–276. Increased cell number in the adult hamster retinal ganglion cell layer after early removal of one eye.

Sengelaub, D. R., R. P. Dolan, and B. L. Finlay (1986). *J. Comp. Neurol.* **246**:527–543. Cell generation, death and retinal growth in the development of the hamster retinal ganglion cell layer.

Senglaub, K. (1959). *Morphol Jahrb.* **100**:11–62. Vergleichende metrische und morphologische Untersuchungen an Organen und am Kleinhirn von Wild-, Gefangenschafts- und Hausenten.

Senjo, M., T. Ishibashi, T. Terashima, and Y. Inoue (1986). *Neurosci. Lett.* **66**:39–42. Correlation between astrogliogenesis and blood-brain barrier formation: Immunocytochemical demonstration by using astroglia-specific enzyme glutathione-S-transferase.

Sephel, G. C., B. A. Burrous, and H. K. Kleinman (1989). *Dev. Neurosci.* **11**:313–331. Laminin neural activity and binding proteins.

Serbedzija, G. N., M. Bronner-Fraser, and S. E. Fraser (1989). *Development* **106**:809–816. A vital dye analysis of the timing and pathways of avian trunk neural crest cell migration.

Server, A. C., and E. M. Shooter (1977). *Adv. Protein Chem.* **31**:339–409. Nerve growth factor.

Severinghaus, A. E. (1930). *J. Comp. Neurol.* **51**:237–270. Cellular proliferation in heterotopic spinal cord grafts.

Seymour, R. M., and M. Berry (1975). *J. Comp. Neurol.* **160**:105–125. Scanning and transmission electron microscope studies of interkinetic nuclear migration in the cerebral vesicles of the rat.

Shackney, S., and P. S. Ritch (1986). Percent labeled mitosis curve analysis. In *Techniques in Cell Cycle Analysis* (J. Gray, and Z. Darzynkiewicz, eds.), Humana, New Jersey.

Shackney, S. E. (1974). *J. Theor. Biol.* **44**:49–90. A cytokinetic model for heterogeneous mammalian cell populations. II. Tritiated thymidine studies: The percent labeled mitosis (PLM) curve.

Shafiq, S. A. (1970). Satellite cells and fiber nuclei in muscle regeneration, pp. 122–132. In *Regeneration of Striated Muscle and Myogenesis* (A. Mauro, S. A. Shafiq, and A. T. Milhorat, eds.), Excerpta Medica, Amsterdam.

Shahbazian, F. M., M. S. Jacobs, and A. Lajtha (1989). *J. neurosci. Meth.* **27**:91–101. Rates of protein synthesis: A review.

Shantha, T. R., and G. H. Bourne (1968). The perineural epithelium—A new concept, pp. 379–459. In *The Structure and Function of Nervous Tissue*, Vol. 1, (G. Bourne, ed.), Academic Press, New York.

Shapin, S. (1975). *Ann. Sci.* **32**:219–243. Phrenological knowledge and the social structure of early nineteenth-century Edinburgh.

Shapiro, B. H., D. C. Levine, and N. T. Adler (1980). *Science* **209**:418. The testicular feminized rat: A naturally occurring model of androgen independent brain masculinization.

Shapiro, S., and K. R. Vukovich (1970). *Science* **167**:292–294. Early experience effects upon cortical dendrites: A proposed model for development.

Shariff, G. A. (1953). *J. Comp. Neurol.* **98**:381–400. Cell counts in the primate cerebral cortex.

Sharma, S. C. (1972a). *Exp. Neurol.* **34**:171–182. Reformation of retinotectal projections after various tectal ablations in adult goldfish.

Sharma, S. C. (1972b). *Exp. Neurol.* **35**:358–365. Restoration of the visual projection following tectal lesions in goldfish.

Sharma, S. C. (1972c). *Brain Res.* **39**:213–223. The retinal projections in the goldfish: An experimental study.

Sharma, S. C. (1972d). *Proc. Natl. Acad. Sci. U.S.A.* **69**:2637–2639. Redistribution of visual projections in altered optic tecta of adult goldfish.

Sharma, S. C. (1972e). *Nat. New Biol.* **238**:286–287. Retinotectal connexions of a heterotopic eye.

Sharma, S. C. (1975). *Brain Res.* **93**:497–501. Visual projection in surgically created 'compound' tectum in adult goldfish.

Sharma, S. C., and R. M. Gaze (1971). *Arch. Ital. Biol.* **109**:357–366. The retinotopic organization of visual responses from tectal reimplants in adult goldfish.

Sharma, S. C., and J. C. Hollyfield (1974). *J. Comp. Neurol.* **155**:395–408. Specification of retinal central connections in *Rana pipiens* before the appearance of the first postmitotic ganglion cells.

Sharp, G. A., G. Shaw, and K. Weber (1982). *Exp. Cell Res.* **137**:403–413. Immunoelectron microscopical localization of the three neurofilament triplet proteins along neurofilaments of cultured dorsal root ganglion neurons.

Sharpe, C. R., A. Fritz, E. M. DeRobertis, and J. B. Gurdon (1987). *Cell* **49**:749–758. A homeobox-containing marker of posterior neural differentiation shows the importance of predetermination in neural induction.

Sharpe, P. T., J. R. Miller, E. P. Evans, M. D. Burtenshaw, and S. J. Gaunt (1988). *Development* 102:397–407. *Hox-6:* A new homeobox gene locus.

Shatz, C. J. (1977). *J. Comp. Neurol.* 171:205–228. A comparison of visual pathways in Boston and Midwestern Siamese cats.

Shatz, C. J. (1983). *J. Neurosci.* 3:482–499. The prenatal development of the cat's retinogeniculative pathway.

Shatz, C. J., and P. A. Kirkwood (1984). *J. Neurosci.* 4:1378–1397. Prenatal development of functional connections in the cat's retinogeniculate pathway.

Shatz, C. J., and D. W. Sretavan (1986). *Ann. Rev. Neurosci.* 9:171–207. Interactions between retinal ganglion cells during the development of the mammalian visual system.

Shatz, C. J., and M. P. Stryker (1978). *J. Physiol. (London)* 281:267–283. Ocular dominance in layer IV of the cat's visual cortex and the effects of monocular deprivation.

Shatz, C. J., and M. P. Stryker (1986). *Soc. Neurosci. Abstr.* 12:589. Tetrodotoxin infusion prevents the formation of eye-specific layers during the prenatal development of the cat's retinogeniculate pathway.

Shatz, C. J., S. Lindström, and T. N. Wiesel (1977). *Brain Res.* 131:103–116. The distribution of afferents representing the right and left eyes in the cat's visual cortex.

Shatz, C. J., P. A. Kirkwood, and M. W. Siegel (1982). *Soc. Neurosci. Abstr.* 8:815. Functional retinogeniculate synapses in fetal cats.

Shatz, C. J., J. J. M. Chun, and M. B. Luskin (1988). The role of the subplate in the development of the mammalian telencephalon, pp 35–58. In *The Cerebral Cortex*, Vol. 7, (E. G. Jones, ed.), Plenum Press, New York.

Shaw, C., U. Yinon, and E. Auerbach (1974). *Exp. Neurol.* 45:42–49. Diminution of evoked neuronal activity in the visual cortex of pattern deprived rats.

Shaw, G., and K. Weber (1982). *Nature* 298:277–279. Differential expression of neurofilament triplet proteins in brain development.

Shaw, G., E. Debus, and K. Weber (1984). *Eur. J. Cell Biol.* 34:130–136. The immunological relatedness of neurofilament proteins of higher vertebrates.

Shaw, G., M. Osborn, and K. Weber (1986). *Eur. J. Cell Biol.* 42:1–9. Reactivity of a panel of neurofilament antibodies on phosphorylated and dephosphorylated neurofilaments.

Shaw, M. D., and K. E. Alley (1982). *J. Comp. Neurol.* 207:203–207. Generation of motoneurons in the rabbit brainstem.

Shear, C.R., and G. Goldspink (1971). *J. Morphol.* 135:351–360. Structural and physiological changes associated with the growth of avian fast and slow muscle.

Sheard, P., and M. Jacobson (1987). *Science* 236:851–854. Clonal restriction boundaries in *Xenopus* embryos shown with two intracellular lineage tracers.

Sheard, P., and M. Jacobson (1990). *Ann. N.Y. Acad. Sci.* 599:141–157. Analysis of frequency of intermingling between labeled clones in *Xenopus* embryos.

Sheard, P. W., and L. D. Beazley (1988). *Vision Res.* 28:461–470. Retinal ganglion cell death is not prevented by application of tetrodotoxin during optic nerve regeneration in the frog *Hyla moorei*.

Sheetz, M. P. (1987). *BioEssays* 7:165–168. What are the functions of kinesin?

Shelanski, M., J.-F. LeTerrier, and R. K. Liem (1981). *Neurosci. Res. Program Bull.* 19:32–43. Evidence for interactions between neurofilaments and microtubules.

Shellswell, G. B. (1977). *J. Embryol. Exp. Morphol.* 41:269–277. The formation of discrete muscles from the chick wing dorsal and ventral muscle masses in the absence of nerves.

Shelton, D. L., and L. F. Reichardt (1986). *Proc. Natl. Acad. Sci. U.S.A.* 83:2714–2718. Studies on the expression of the β nerve growth factor (NGF) gene in the central nervous system: Levels and regional distribution of NGF mRNA suggest that NGF functions as a trophic factor for several different populations of neurons.

Shepherd, G. M. (1972). *Yale J. Biol. Med.* 45:584–599. The neuron doctrine: A revision of functional concepts.

Shepherd, G. M., editor (1990). *The Synaptic Organization of the Brain*. Third Edn. Oxford Univ. Press, New York, Oxford.

Sheridan, J. D. (1966). *J. Cell Biol.* 31:C1–5. Electrophysiological study of special connections between cells in the early chick embryo.

Sheridan, J. D. (1968). *J. Cell Biol.* 37:650–659. Electrophysiological evidence for low-resistance intercellular junctions in the early chick embryo.

Sheridan, J. D. (1973). *Am. Zool.* 13:1119–1128. Functional evaluation of low resistance junctions: Influence of cell shape and size.

Sherk, H., and M. P. Stryker (1976). *J. Neurophysiol.* 39:63–70. Quantitative study of cortical orientation selectivity in visually inexperienced kittens.

Sherman, G. F., A. M. Galaburda, and N. Geschwind (1982). *Trends Neurosci.* 5:429–431. Neuroanatomical asymmetries in non-human species.

Sherman, S. M. (1985a). Functional organization of the W-, X-, and Y-cell pathways in the cat: A review and hypothesis, pp. 233–314. In *Progress in Psychobiology and Physiological Psychology*, Vol. 11. (J. M. Sprague, and A. N. Epstein, eds.), Academic Press, New York.

Sherman, S. M. (1985b). *Trend Neurosci.* 8:350–355. Development of retinal projections to the cat's lateral geniculate nucleus.

Sherman, S. M., and K. J. Sanderson (1972). *Brain Res.* 37:126–131. Binocular interaction on cells of the dorsal lateral geniculate nucleus of visually-deprived cats.

Sherman, S. M., and P. D. Spear (1982). *Physiol. Rev.* 62:738–855. Organization of visual pathways in normal and visually deprived cats.

Sherman, S. M., and J. Stone (1973). *Brain Res.* 60:224–230. Physiological normality of the retina in visually deprived cats.

Sherman, S. M., and J. R. Wilson (1975). *J. Comp. Neurol.* 161:183–196. Behavioral and morphological evidence for binocular competition in the postnatal development of the dog's visual system.

Sherman, S. M., K.-P. Hoffmann, and J. Stone (1972). *J. Neurophysiol.* 35:532–541. Loss of a specific cell type from dorsal lateral geniculate nucleus in visually deprived cats.

Sherman, S. M., R. W. Guillery, J. H. Kaas, and R. J. Sanderson (1974). *J. Comp. Neurol.* 158:1–18. Behavioral, electrophysiological and morphological studies of binocular competition in the development of the geniculo-cortical pathways of cats.

Sherman, S. M., J. R. Wilson, and R. W. Guillery (1975). *Brain Res.* 100:441–444. Evidence that binocular competition affects the postnatal development of Y-cells in the cat's lateral geniculate nucleus.

Sherrington, C. S. (1894). *J. Physiol. (London)* 17:211–258. On the anatomical constituion of nerves of skeletal muscles; with remarks on recurrent fibres in the ventral spinal nerve roots.

Sherrington, C. S. (1897a). The central nervous system. In M. Foster, *A Text Book of Physiology*, 7th Edn. Macmillan, London.

Sherrington, C. S. (1897b). *Proc. Roy. Soc. (London) Ser. B.* 60:414–417. On the reciprocal innervation of antagonistic muscles. Third note.

Sherrington, C. S. (1897c). *Proc. Roy. Soc. (London) Ser. B.* 61:247–249. Further note on sensory nerves of muscles.

Sherrington, C. S. (1900). The spinal cord. In *Text book of physiology*, Schäfer, 2:782–883. Pentland, Edinburgh.

Sherrington, C. S. (1904). Correlation of reflexes and the principle of the final common path. *Rep. Br. Assoc. Adv. Sci. 74th meeting, transact.*, Sec. 1, Physiology, pp. 728–741.

Sherrington, C. S. (1906). *The Integrative Action of the Nervous System*. Yale Univ. Press, New Haven.

Sherrington, C. S. (1925). *Proc. Roy. Soc. (London) Ser. B.* 97:519–545. Remarks on some aspects of reflex inhibition.

Sherrington, C. S. (1933a). *Inhibition as a co-ordinative factor. Nobel Lecture*. Norstedt, Stockholm.

Sherrington, C. S. (1933b). *The Brain and Its Mechnaism*. Cambridge Univ. Press, Cambridge.

Sherrington, C. S. (1949). Preface, In Cannon, D. F., *Explorer of the Human Brain: The Life of Santiago Ramón y Cajal*. Schuman, New York.

Shibata, S., and R. Y. Moore (1987). *Dev. Brain Res.* 34:311–315. Development of neuronal activity in the rat suprachiasmatic nucleus.

Shieh, B. H., M. Ballivet, and J. Schmidt (1987). *J. Cell Biol.* 104:1337–1341. Quantitation of an alpha subunit splicing intermediate: Evidence for transcriptional activation in the control of acetylcholine receptor expression in denervated chick skeletal muscle.

Shieh, P. (1951). *J. Exp. Zool.* 117:359–395. The neoformation of cells of preganglionic type in the cervical spinal cord of the chick embryo following its transplantation to the thoracic level.

Shimada, M., and J. Langman (1970). *Am. J. Anat.* 129:247–260. Repair of the external granular layer after postnatal treatment with 5-fluorodeoxyuridine.

Shimada, M., and T. Nakamura (1973). *Exp. Neurol.* 41:163–173. Time of neuron origin in mouse hypothalamic nuclei.

Shinoda, H., A. M. Marini, C. Cosi, and J. P. Schwartz (1989). *Science* 245:415–417. Brain region and gene specificity of neuropeptide gene expression in cultured astrocytes.

Shiomura, Y., and N. Hirokawa (1987a). *J. Neurosci.* 7:1461–1469. The molecular structure of microtubule-associated protein 1A (MAP1A) *in vivo* and *in vitro*. An immunoelectron microscopy and quick-freeze, deep-etch study.

Shiomura, Y., and N. Hirokawa (1987b). *J. Cell Biol.* 103:1911–1919. Colocalization of MAP1 and MAP2 on the neuronal microtubule *in situ* revealed by double-labeling immunoelectron microscopy.

Shiota, K. (1982). *Am. J. Med. Genet.* 12:281–288. Neural tube defects and maternal hyperthermia in early pregnancy: Epidemiology in a human embryo population.

Shirayoshi, Y., T. S. Okada, and M. Takeichi (1983). *Cell* 35:631–638. The calcium-dependent cell-cell adhesion system regulates inner cell mass formation and cell surface polarization in early mouse development.

Shirayoshi, Y., K. Hatta, M. Hosoda, S. Tsunasawa, F. Sakiyama, and M. Takeichi (1986). *EMBO J.* 5:2485–2488. Cadherin cell adhesion molecules with distinct specificities share a common structure.

Shlaer, R. (1971). *Science* 173:638–641. Shifts in binocular disparity causes compensating changes in the cortical structure of kittens.

Shojaeian, H., N. Delhaye-Bouchaud, and J. Mariani (1985a). *J. Comp. Neurol.* 232:309–318. Neuronal death and synapse elimination in the olivocerebellar system. II. Cell counts in the inferior olive of adult X-irradiated rats and *Weaver* and *Reeler* mutant mice.

Shojaeian, H., N. Delhaye-Bouchaud, and J. Mariani (1985b). *Dev. Brain Res.* 21:141–146. Decreased number of cells in the inferior olivary nucleus of the developing staggerer mouse.

Sholl, D. A. (1953). *J. Anat. (London)* 87:387–406. Dendritic organization in the neurons of the visual and motor cortices of the cat.

Sholl, D. A. (1955). *J. Anat. (London)* 89:571–572. The surface area of cortical neurons.

Sholl, D. A. (1956a). *The Organization of the Cerebral Cortex*. Methuen, London.

Sholl, D. A. (1956b) *Prog. Neurobiol.* 2: 324–333. The measurable parameters of the cerebral cortex and their significance in its organization.

Shorey, M. L. (1909). *J. Exp. Zool.* 7:25–64. The effect of the destruction of peripheral areas on the differentiation of the neuroblasts.

Shumway, W. (1940). *Anat. Rec.* 78:139–147. Stages in the normal development of *Rana pipiens*. I. External forms.

Shumway, W. (1942). *Anat. Rec.* 83:309–315. Stages in the normal development of *Rana pipiens*. II. Identification of the stages from sectioned material.

Shupnik, M. A., W. W. Chin, J. F. Habener, and C. Ringway (1985). *J. Biol. Chem.* 260:2900–2903. Transcriptional regulation of the thyrotropin subunit genes by thyroid hormones.

Sidman, R. L. (1961). Histogenesis of the mouse retina studied with tritiated thymidine, pp. 487–505. In *The Structure of the Eye* (G. K. Smelser, ed.), Academic Press, New York.

Sidman, R. L. (1968). Development of interneuronal connections in brains of mutant mice, pp. 163–193. In *Physiological and Biochemical Aspects of Nervous Integration* (F. D. Carlson, ed.), Prentice-Hall, Englewood Cliffs, N.J.

Sidman, R. L. (1970). Autoradiographic methods and principles for study of the nervous system with thymidine-H^3. In *Contemporary Research Techniques of Neuroanatomy* (S. O. E. Ebbesson, and W. J. Nauta, eds.), Springer-Verlag, New York.

Sidman, R. L. (1972). Cell interactions in developing mammalian central nervous system, pp. 1–13. In *Cell Interactions, Proceedings of the Third Lepetit Colloquium* (L. G. Silvestri, ed.), North-Holland, Amsterdam.

Sidman, R. L. (1974). Cell-cell recognition in the central nervous system, pp. 743–758. In *The Neurosciences: Third Study Program* (F. O. Scmitt, and F. G. Worden, eds.), M.I.T. Press, Cambridge, Mass.

Sidman, R. L. (1983). Experimental neurogenetics, pp. 19–

46. In *Genetics of Neurological and Psychiatric Disorders* (S. S. Kety, L. P. Rowland, R. L. Sidman, and S. W. Matthysse, eds.).

Sidman, R. L., and M. C. Green (1970). "Nervous," a new mutant mouse with cerebellar disease. *Symposium of the Centre National de la Recherche Scientifique*, Orleans-la-Source, France.

Sidman, R. L., and P. Rakic (1973). *Brain Res.* 62:1–35. Neuronal migration, with special reference to developing human brain: A review.

Sidman, R. L., I. L. Miale, and N. Feder (1959). *Exp. Neurol.* 1:322–333. Cell proliferation and migration in the primitive ependymal zone: An autoradiographic study of histogenesis in the nervous system.

Sidman, R. L., P. W. Lane, and M. M. Dickie (1962). *Science* 137:610–611. Staggerer, a new mutation in the mouse affecting the cerebellum.

Sidman, R. L., M. N. Dickie, and S. H. Appel (1964). *Science* 144:309–311. Mutant mice (quaking and jimpy) with deficient myelination in the central nervous system.

Sidman, R. L., M. C. Green, and S. H. Appel (1965). *Catalog of the Neurological Mutants of the Mouse.* Harvard Univ. Press, Cambridge, Mass. 82 pp.

Sieber-Blum, M. (1989). *Dev. Biol.* 134:362–375. SSEA-1 is a specific marker for the spinal sensory neuron lineage in the quail embryo and in neural crest cell cultures.

Sieber-Blum, M. (1989). *Science* 243:1608–1611. Commitment of neural crest cells to the sensory neuron lineage.

Sieber-Blum, M., and A. M. Cohen (1980). *Dev. Biol.* 80:96–106. Clonal analysis of quail neural crest cells. They are pluripotent and differentiate *in vitro* in the absence of non-crest cells.

Sieber-Blum, M., and F. Sieber (1984). *Dev. Brain Res.* 14:241–246. Heterogeneity among early quail neural crest cells.

Sieber-Blum, M., and F. Sieber (1985). *In vitro* analysis of quail neural crest cell differentiation, pp. 193–222. In *Cell Culture in the Neurosciences* (J. E. Bottenstein, and G. Sato, eds.), Plenum Press, New York.

Siegers, M. P., J. C. Schaer, H. Hirsiger, and R. Schindler (1974). *J. Cell Biol.* 62:305–315. Determination of rates of DNA synthesis in cultured mammalian cell populations.

Sievers, J., F.-W. Pehlemann, and M. Berry (1986). *Naturwissenschaften* 73:188–194. Influences of meningeal cells on brain development.

Sievers, J., B. Hausmann, K. Unsicker, and M. Berry (1987). *Neurosci. Lett.* 76:157–162. Fibroblast growth factors promote the survival of adult rat retinal ganglion cells after transection of the optic nerve.

Siggins, G. R., S. J. Henriksen, and S. C. Landis (1976). *Brain Res.* 114:53–69. Electrophysiology of Purkinje neurons in the weaver mouse: Iontophoresis of neurotransmitters and cyclic nucleotides, and stimulation of the nucleus locus coeruleus.

Sillito, A. M. (1975a). *J. Physiol. (London)* 250:287–304. The effectiveness of bicuculline as an antagonist of GABA and visually evoked inhibition in the cat's striate cortex.

Sillito, A. M. (1975b). *J. Physiol. (London)* 250:305–329. The contribution of inhibitory mechanisms to the receptive field properties of neurones in the striate cortex of the cat.

Sillito, A. M., J. A. Kemp, J. A. Wilson, and N. Berardi (1980). *Brain Res.* 194:517–520. A re-evaluation of the mechanisms underlying simple cell orientation selectivity.

Silver, J. (1978). Cell death during development of the nervous system. In *Handbook of Sensory Physiology*, Vol. 9, *Development of Sensory Systems* (M. Jacobson, ed.), Springer-Verlag, New York.

Silver, J. (1984). *J. Comp. Neurol.* 223:238–251. Studies on factors that govern directionality of axonal growth in the embryonic optic nerve and at the chiasm of mice.

Silver, J., and A. F. Hughes (1973). *J. Morphol.* 140:159–170. The role of cell death during morphogenesis of the mammalian eye.

Silver, J., and R. M. Robb (1979). *Dev. Biol.* 68:175–190. Studies on the development of the eye cup and optic nerve in normal mice and in mutants with congenital nerve aplasia.

Silver, J., and U. Rutishauser (1984). *Dev. Biol.* 106:485–499. Guidance of optic axons *in vivo* by a preformed adhesive pathway on neuroepithelial endfeet.

Silver, J., and J. Sapiro (1981). *J. Comp. Neurol.* 202:521–538. Axonal guidance during development of the optic nerve: The role of the pigmented epithelia and other extrinsic factors.

Silver, J., and R. L. Sidman (1980). *J. Comp. Neurol.* 189:101–111. A mechanism for the guidance and topographic patterning of retinal ganglion cell axons.

Silver, J., S. E. Lorenz, D. Wahlsten, and J. Coughlin (1982). *J. Comp. Neurol.* 210:10–29. Axonal guidance during development of the great cerebral commissures: Descriptive and experimental studies, *in vivo*, on the role of preformed glial pathways.

Silver, M. L. (1942). *J. Comp. Neurol.* 77:1–39. The motoneurons of the spinal cord of the frog.

Simmler, G. M. (1949). *J. Exp. Zool.* 110:247–257. The effects of wing bud extirpation on the brachial sympathetic ganglia of the chick embryo.

Simmons, P. A., V. Lemmon, and A. L. Pearlman (1982). *J. Comp. Neurol.* 211:295–308. Afferent and efferent connections of the striate and extrastriate visual cortex of the normal and reeler mouse.

Simons, D. J. (1978). *J. Neurophysiol.* 54:615–635. Response properties of vibrissa units in the rat SI somatosensory neocortex.

Simons, D. J., and T. A. Woolsey (1979). *Brain Res.* 163:327–332. Functional organization in mouse barrel cortex.

Simons, D. J., and T. A. Woolsey (1984). *J. Comp. Neurol.* 230:119–132. Morphology of Golgi—Cox impregnated barrel neurons in rat SmI cortex.

Simons, D. J., D. Durham, and T. A. Woolsey (1984). *Somatosen. Res.* 1:207–245. Functional organization of mouse anf rat SmI barrel cortex following vibrissal damage on different postnatal days.

Simons, K., and S. D. Fuller (1985). *Ann. Rev. Cell Biol.* 1:243–288. Cell surface polarity in epithelia.

Simpson, I., B. Rose, and W. R. Loewenstein (1977). *Science* 195:294–296. Size limit of molecules permeating the junctional membrane channels.

Simpson, S. A., and J. Z. Young (1945). *J. Anat. (London)* 79:48–65. Regeneration of fibre diameter after cross-unions of visceral and somatic nerves.

Sims, R. T. (1961). *J. Embryol. Exp. Morphol.* 9:32–41. The blood vessels of the developing spinal cord of *Xenopus laevis*.

Sims, T. J., and J. E. Vaughn (1979). *J. Comp. Neurol.* 183:707–720. The generation of neurones involved in an early reflex pathway of embryonic mouse spinal cord.

Singer, I. I., S. Scott, D. W. Kawka, D. M. Kazazis, J. Gailit, and E. Ruoslahti (1988). J. Cell Biol. 106:2171–2182. Cell surface distribution of fibronectin and vitronectin receptors depends on substrate composition and extracellular matrix accumulation.

Singer, M. (1952). Quart. Rev. Biol. 27:169–200. The influence of the nerve in regeneration of the amphibian extremity.

Singer, M. (1965). A theory of the trophic nervous control of amphibian limb regeneration, including a re-valuation of quantitative nerve requirement, pp. 20–32. In Regeneration in Animals and Related Problems (V. Kiortsis, and H. A. L. Trampusch, eds.), North Holland Publishing Co., Amsterdam.

Singer, M. (1968). Penetration of labelled amino acids into the peripheral nerve fibre from surrounding body fluids, pp. 200–215. In Ciba Foundation Symposium on Growth of the Nervous System (G. E. W. Wolstenholme, and M. O'Connor, eds.), Churchill, London.

Singer, M. (1978). Am. Zool. 18:829–841. On the nature of the neurotrophic phenomenon in urodele limb regeneration.

Singer, M., and M. R. Green (1968). J. Morphol. 124:321–344. Autoradiographic studies of uridine incorporation in peripheral nerve of the newt, Triturus.

Singer, M., and M. M. Salpeter (1966). Nature 210:1225–1227. Transport of tritium-labelled l-histidine through the Schwann and myelin sheaths into the axon of peripheral nerves.

Singer, M., C. E. Maier, and W. S. McNutt (1976). J. Exp. Zool. 196:131–150. Neurotrophic activity of brain extracts in forelimb regeneration of the urodele, Triturus.

Singer, S. J., and A. Kupfer (1986). Ann. Rev. Cell Biol. 2:337–365. The directed migration of eukaryotic cells.

Singer, W., F. Tretter, and M. Cynader (1975). J. Neurophysiol. 38:1080–1098. Organization of cat striate cortex: A correlation of receptive-field properties with afferent and efferent connections.

Sinha, A. K., and S. P. R. Rose (1971). Brain Res. 33:205–217. Bulk separation of neurones and glia: A comparison of techniques.

Sisken, B. F., and S. D. Smith (1975). J. Embryol. Exp. Morphol. 33:29–41. The effects of minute directed electrical currents on cultured chick embryo trigeminal ganglia.

Sisken, B. F., I. Fowler, E. J. Barr, and R. J. Kryscio (1984). J. Neurosci. Res. 12:623–632. The threshold quantity of nerve required to induce limb regeneration in the chick embryo.

Sisto-Daneo, L., and G. Filogamo (1974). J. Submicr. Cytol. 6:219–228. Ultrastructure of developing myo-neural junctions. Evidence for two patterns of synaptic area differentiation.

Sisto-Daneo, L., and G. Filogamo (1975). J. Submicro. Cytol. 7:121–132. Differentiation of synaptic area in slow and fast muscle fibers.

Sjöstrand, J. (1965). Z. Zellforsch. Mikroskop. Anat. Abt. Histochem. 68:481–493. Proliferative changes in glial cells during nerve regeneration.

Sjöstrand, J. (1966a). Acta Physiol. Scand. Suppl. 270 67:1–17. Glial cells in the hypoglossal nucleus of the rabbit during nerve regeneration.

Sjöstrand, J. (1966b). Acta Physiol. Scand. Suppl. 270 67:19–43. Morphological changes in glial cells during nerve regeneration.

Sjöstrand, J. (1971). Exp. Neurol. 30:178–189. Neuroglial proliferation in the hypoglossal nucleus after nerve injury.

Sjöstrand, J., and M. Frizell (1975). Brain Res. 85:325–330. Retrograde axonal transport of rapidly migrating proteins in peripheral nerves.

Sjöstrand, J., and J.-O. Karlsson (1969). J. Neurochem. 16:833–844. Axoplasmic transport in the optic nerve and tract of the rabbit: A biochemical and radioautographic study.

Sjöstrand, J., M. Frizell, and P.-O. Hasselgren (1970). J. Neurochem. 17:1563–1570. Effects of colchicine on axonal transport in peripheral nerves.

Skaper, S., H. P. M. Montz, and S. Varon (1986). Brain Res. 386:130–135. Control of Na^+, K^+-pump activity in dorsal root ganglionic neurons by different neuronotrophic agents.

Skarf, B. (1973). Brain Res. 51:352–357. Development of binocular single units in the optic tectum of frogs raised with disparate stimulation to the eyes.

Skarf, B., and M. Jacobson (1974). Exp. Neurol. 42:669–686. Development of binocularly-driven single units in frogs raised with asymmetrical visual stimulation.

Skeels, H. M. (1966). Monogr. Soc. Res. Child Dev. 31: Serial No. 105. Adult status of children with contrasting early life experiences: A follow-up study.

Skeen, L. C., B. R. Due, and F. E. Douglas (1985). Neurosci. Lett. 54:301–306. Effects of early anosmia on two classes of granule cells in developing mouse olfactory bulbs.

Skeen, L. C., B. R. Due, and F. E. Douglas (1986). Neurosci. Lett. 63:5–10. Neonatal sensory deprivation reduces tufted cell number in mouse olfactory bulb.

Skene, J. H. P., and M. Willard (1981a). J. Cell. Biol. 89:96–103. Axonally transported proteins associated with growth in rabbit central and peripheral nervous system.

Skene, J. H. P., and M. Willard (1981b). J. Neurochem. 37:79–87. Electrophoretic analysis of axonally transported proteins in toad retinal ganglion cells.

Skene, J. H. P., R. D. Jacobson, G. J. Snipes, C. B. MacGuire, J. Norden, and J. A. Freeman (1986). Science 233:783–785. A protein induced during nerve growth, GAP-43, is a major component of growth cone membranes.

Sklar, J. H., and R. K. Hunt (1973). Proc. Natl. Acad. Sci. U.S.A.. 70:3684–3688. The acquisition of specificity in cutaneous sensory neurons: A reconsideration of the integumental specification hypothesis.

Skoff, R. P., and V. Hamburger (1974). J. Comp. Neurol. 153:107–148. Fine structure of dendritic and axonal growth cones in embryonic chick spinal cord.

Skoff, R. P., D. L. Price, and A. Stocks (1976a). J. Comp. Neurol. 169:291–311. Electron microscopic autoradiographic studies of gliogenesis in rat optic nerve. I. Cell proliferation.

Skoff, R. P., D. L. Price, and A. Stocks (1976b). J. Comp. Neurol. 169:313–333. Electron microscopic autoradiographic studies of gliogenesis in rat optic nerve. II. Time of origin.

Skoff, R. P., P. E. Knapp, and W. P. Bartlett (1986). Astrocyte diversity in the optic nerve: A cytoarchitectural study, pp. 269–291. In Astrocytes, Vol. 1, (S. Fedoroff, and A. Vernadakis, eds.), New York, Academic

Slack, J. M. W. (1984). J. Embryol. Exp. Morph. 80:289–319. Regional biosynthetic markers in the early amphibian embryo.

Slack, J. M. W. (1985). *Cell* 41:237–247. Peanut lectin receptors in the early amphibian embryo: Regional markers for the study of embryonic induction.

Slack, J. M. W., and H. V. Isaacs (1989). *Development* 105:147–153. Presence of basic fibroblast growth factor in the early *Xenopus* embryo.

Slack. J. M. W., L. Dale, and J. C. Smith (1984). *Phil. Trans. Roy. Soc. (London) Ser. B.* 307:331–336. Analysis of embryonic induction by using cell lineage markers.

Slack, J. M. W., B. G. Darlington, J. K. Heath, and S. F. Godsave (1987). *Nature* 326:197–200. Mesoderm induction in early *Xenopus* embryos by heparin-binding growth factors.

Slack, J. R. (1978). *Brain Res.* 146:172–176. Interactions between foreign and regenerating axons in axolotl muscles.

Sládecek, F. (1952). *Acta. Soc. Zool. Bohemoslav.* 16:322–333. Regulative tendencies of the central nervous system during embryogenesis of the Axolotl (*Amblystoma mexicanum cope*). I. Regulation after inversion of the mediolateral axes of the medullary plate.

Sládecek, F. (1955). *Acta Soc. Zool. Bohemoslav.* 19:138–149. Regulative tendencies of the central nervous system during embryogenesis of the Axoltl (*Amblystoma mexicanum cope*). II. Regulation after simultaneous inversion of anteroposterior and medio-lateral axes of medullary plate.

Slavkin, H. C. (1972). Intercellular communication during odontogenesis, pp. 165–199. In *Developmental Aspects of Oral Biology* (H. C. Slavkin, and L. A. Bavetta, eds.), Academic Press, New York.

Slemmon, J. R., R. Blacher, W. Danho, J. L. Hempstead, and J. I. Morgan (1984). *Proc. Natl. Acad. Sci U.S.A.* 81:6866–6870. Isolation and sequencing of two cerebellum specific peptides.

Slemmon, J. R., W. Danho, J. L. Hempstead, and J. I. Morgan (1985). *Proc. Natl. Acad. Sci. U.S.A.* 82:7145–7148. Cerebellin: A quantifiable marker for Purkinje cell maturation.

Sloan, H. E., S. E. Hughes, and B. Oakley (1983). *J. Neurosci.* 3:117–123. Chronic impairment of axonal transport eliminates taste responses and taste buds.

Sloviter, R. S., G. Valiquette, G. M. Abrams, E. C. Ronk, A. L. Sollas, L. A. Paul, and S. Neubort (1989). *Science* 243:535–538. Selective loss of hippocampal granule cells in the mature rat brain after adrenalectomy.

Small, R. K., and K. H. Pfenninger (1984). *J. Cell Biol.* 98:1422–1433. Components of the plasma membrane of growing axons. I. Size and distribution of intramembrane particles.

Small, R. K., P. Riddle, M. Noble (1987). *Nature* 328:155–157. Evidence for migration of oligodendrocyte-type-2 astrocyte progenitor cells into the developing rat optic nerve.

Smart, I. (1961). *J. Comp. Neurol.* 116:325–347. The subependymal layer of the mouse brain and its cell production as shown by radioautography after thymidine-H3 injection.

Smart, I., and C. P. Leblond (1961). *J. Comp. Neurol.* 116:349–367. Evidence for division and transformation of neuroglia cells in the mouse brain as derived form radioautography after injection of thymidine-H3.

Smart, I. H. M. (1973). *J. Anat. (London)* 116:67–91. Proliferative characteristics of the ependymal layer during the early development of the mouse neocortex: A pilot study based on recording the number, location and plane of cleavage of mitotic figures.

Smart, I. H. M. (1976). *J. Anat. (London)* 121:71–84. A pilot study of cell production by the ganglionic eminences of the developing mouse brain.

Smart, I. H. M. (1983). *J. Anat. (London)* 137:683–694. Three dimensional growth of the mouse isocortex.

Smart, I. H. M. (1986a). *J. Anat. (London)* 146:141–152. Gyrus formation in the cerebral cortex in the ferret. I. Description of the external changes.

Smart, I. H. M. (1986b). *J. Anat. (London)* 147:27–43. Gyrus formation in the cerebral cortex of the ferret. II. Description of the internal histological changes.

Smart, I. H. M., and M. Smart (1977). *J. Anat. (London)* 123:515–525. The location of nuclei of different labelling intensities in autoradiographs of the anterior forebrain of postnatal mice injected with [^{3}H]thymidine on the eleventh and twelfth days post-conception.

Smart, I. H. M., and M. Smart (1982). *J. Anat.* 134:273–298. Growth patterns in the lateral wall of the mouse telencephalon: I. Autoradiographic studies of the histogenesis of the isocortex and adjacent areas.

Smart, J. L. (1977). Early life malnutrition and later learning ability. A critical analysis, pp. 215–235. In Oliverio, *Genetics, environment and intelligence.* Elsevier/North-Holland, Amsterdam.

Smart, J. L., T. S. Whatson, and J. Dobbing (1975). *Br. J. Nutr.* 34:511–516. Thresholds of response to electric shock in previously undernourished rats.

Smart, N. (1967). Indian philosophy, pp. 155–169. In *The Encyclopedia of Philosophy,* Vol. 3, (P. Edwards, ed.), Macmillan, New York and London.

Smedley, M. J., and M. Stanisstreet (1985). *J. Embryol. Exp. Morphol.* 89:1–14. Calcium and neurulation in mammalian embryos.

Smeyne, R. J., and D. Goldowitz (1989). *J. Neurosci.* 9:1608–1620. Development and death of external granular layer cells in the Weaver mouse cerebellum: A quantitative study.

Smit, G. J., and E. J. Colon (1969). *Brain Res.* 13:485–510. Quantitative analysis of the cerebral cortex. I. Aselectivity of the Golgi-Cox staining technique.

Smith, A. A., and F. W. Hui (1971). *Pharmacologist* 13:235. Familial dysautonomia: A neurotransmitter disease.

Smith, A. A., A. Farbman, and J. Dancis (1965a). *Science* 147:1040–1041. Absence of taste bud papillae in familial dysantonomia.

Smith, A. A., J. I. Hirsch, and J. Dancis (1965b). *Pediatrics* 36:225–230. Responses to infused methacholine in familial dysautonomia.

Smith, C. L., and E. Frank (1987). *J. Neurosci.* 7:1537–1549. Peripheral specification of sensory neurons transplanated to novel locations along the neuraxis.

Smith, D. C., P. D. Spear, and K. E. Kratz (1978). *J. Comp. Neurol.* 178:313–328. Role of visual experience in postcritical-period reversal of effects of monocular deprivation in cat striate cortex.

Smith, D. E. (1974). *Brain Res.* 74:119–130. The effect of deafferentiation on the postnatal development of Clarke's nucleus in the kitten—A Golgi study.

Smith, D. E. (1977). *Prog. Neurobiol.* 8:349–367. The effect of deafferentation on the development of brain and spinal nuclei.

Smith, D. S. (1970). *J. Cell Biol.* 47:195–196. Bridges between vesicles and axoplasmic microtubules.

Smith, D. S. (1971). *Phil. Trans. Roy. Soc. (London) Ser. B.* 261:395–405. On the significance of cross-bridges between microtubules and synaptic vesicles.

Smith, D. S., U. Jarlfors, and M. L. Cayer (1977). *J. Cell Sci.* 27:235–272. Structural cross-bridges between microtubules and mitochondria in central axons of an insect (*Periplaneta americana*).

Smith, D. W., R. M. Blizzard, and L. Wilkins (1957). *Pediatrics* 19:1011–1022. The mental prognosis in hypothyroidism of infancy and childhood. A review of 128 cases.

Smith, D. W., S. K. Clarren, and M. A. S. Harvey (1978). *J. Pediatr.* 92:878–883. Hyperthermia as a possible teratogenic agent.

Smith, G. M., R. H. Miller, and J. Silver (1986). *J. Comp. Neurol.* 251:23–43. Changing role of forebrain astrocytes during development, regenerative failure, and induced regeneration upon transplantation.

Smith, J. C. (1987). *Development* 99:3–14. A mesoderm inducing factor is produced by a *Xenopus* cell line.

Smith, J. C. (1989). *Development* 105:665–677. Mesoderm induction and mesoderm-inducing factors in early amphibian development.

Smith, J. C., and J. M. W. Slack (1983). *J. Embryol. Exp. Morphol.* 78:299–317. Dorsalization and neural induction: Properties of the organizer in *Xenopus laevis*.

Smith, J. C., M. Yaqoob, and K. Symes (1988). *Development* 103:591–600. Purification, partial characterization and biological effects of the XTC mesoderm-inducing factor.

Smith, J. C., B. M. J. Price, K. Van Nimmen, and D. Huylebroeck (1990). *Nature* 345:729–731. Identification of a potent *Xenopus* mesoderm-inducing factor as a homologue of activin A.

Smith, J. L., and G. C. Schoenwolf (1988). *Cell Tiss. Res.* 252:491–500. Role of cell-cycle in regulating neuroepithelial cell shape during bending of the chick neural plate.

Smith, K. A. (1988). *Science* 240:1169–1176. Interleukin-2: Inception, impact, and implications.

Smith, K. J., W. F. Blakemore, J. A. Murray, and R. C. Patterson (1982). *J. Neurolog. Sci.* 55:231–246. Internodal myelin volume and axon surface area. A relationship determining myelin thickness.

Smith-Thomas, L. C., and J. W. Fawcett (1989). *Development* 105:251–262. Expression of Schwann cell markers by mammalian neural crest cells *in vitro*.

Smith-Thomas, L. C., J. P. Davis, and M. L. Epstein (1986). *Dev. Biol.* 115:293–300. The gut supports neurogenic differentiation of periocular mesenchyme, a chondrogenic neural crest-derived cell population.

Smith, L. J. (1985). *J. Embryol. Exp. Morphol.* 89:15–35. Embryonic axis orientation in the mouse and its correlation with blastocyst relationships to the uterus.

Smith, R. S. (1980). *J. Neurocytol.* 9:39–65. The short term accumulation of axonally transported organelles in the region of localized lesions of single myelinated axons.

Smith, R. S., and P. D. Cooper (1980). *Can. J. Physiol. Pharmacol.* 59:857–863. Variability and temperature dependence of the velocity of retrograde particle transport in myelinated axons.

Smith, R. S., and W. K. Ovalle (1972). Structure and function of intrafusal muscle fibres, pp. 147–227. In *Muscle Biology*, Vol. 1, (R. G. Cassens, ed.), Marcel Dekker, Inc, New York.

Smith, U. (1971). *Phil. Trans. Roy. Soc. (London) Ser. B.* 261:391–394. Uptake of ferritin into neurosecretory terminals.

Smits-Van Prooije, A. E., R. E. Poelmann, J. A. Dubbeldam, M. M. T. Mentink, and C. H. R. Vermeij-Keers (1986a). *Stain Tech.* 61:97–106. Wheat germ agglutinin as a novel marker for mesectoderm formation in mouse embryos cultured *in vitro*.

Smits-Van Prooije, A. E., R. E. Poelmann, A. F. Gesnick, M. J. Van Groeningen, and C. Vermeji-Keers (1986b). *Anat. Embryol.* 175:111–117. The cell surface coat in neurulating mouse and rat embryos, studied with lectins.

Snell, O. (1892). *Arch. Psychiat. Nervenkr.* 23:436–446. Die Abhängigkeit des Hirngewichtes von dem Körpergewicht und den geistigen Fähigkeiten.

Snider, R. S., and M. Perez del Cerro (1967). *Exp. Neurol.* 17:466–480. Drug-induced dendritic sprouts on Purkinje cells in the adult cerebellum.

Snider, W. D. (1988). *J. Neurosci.* 8:2628–2634. Nerve growth factor enhances dendritic arborization of sympathetic ganglion cells in developing mammals.

Snider, W. D. (1989). *Ann. Neurol.* 26:489–506. Neurotrophic molecules.

Snow, M. H. L. (1975). *J. Embryol. Exp. Morphol.* 34:707–721. Embryonic development of tetraploid mice during the second half of gestation.

Snow, P. J., P. K. Rose, and A. G. Brown (1976). *Science* 191:312–313. Tracing axons and axon collaterals of spinal neurons using intracellular injection of horseradish peroxidase.

Snyder, R. E. (1986). *J. Neurobiol.* 17:637–647. The kinematics of turnaround and retrograde axonal transport.

Snyder, R. E. (1989). *J. Neurobiol.* 20:81–94. Loss of material from the retrograde axonal transport system in frog sciatic nerve.

Snyder, S. H. (1989). *Brainstorming. The Science and Politics of Opiate Research.* Harvard Univ. Press, Cambridge, Mass.

Snyder, W. D. (1988). *J. Neurosci.* 8:2628–2634. Nerve growth factor enhances dendritic arborization of sympathetic ganglion cells in developing mammals.

So, K.-F., and A. J. Aguayo (1985). *Brain Res.* 328:349–354. Lengthy regrowth of cut axons from ganglion cells after peripheral nerve transplantation into the retina of adult rats.

So, K.-F., G. E. Schneider, and D. O. Frost (1978). *Brain Res.* 142:343–352. Postnatal development of retinal projections to the lateral geniculate body in Syrian hamsters.

So, K.-F, H. H. Wook, and L. S. Jen (1984). *Dev. Brain. Res.* 12:191–205. The normal and abnormal development of retinogeniculate projections in golden hamsters: An anterograde horseradish peroxidase tracing study.

Söderholm, U. (1965). *Acta Physiol. Scand. Suppl.* 65:256. Histochemical localization of esterases, phosphatases and tetrazolium reductases in the motor neurons of the spinal cord of the rat and the effect of nerve division.

Sodersten, P. (1973). *Horm. Behav.* 4:1–17. Increased mounting behavior in the female rat following a single neonatal injection of testosterone propionate.

Sofroniew, M. V., R. C. A. Pearson, F. Eckenstein, A. C. Cuello, and T. P. S. Powell (1983). *Brain Res.* 289:370–374. Retrograde changes in cholinergic neurons in the basal forebrain of the rat following cortical damage.

Sofroniew, M. V., N. P. Galletly, O. Isacson, and C. N. Svendsen (1990). *Science* 247:338–342. Survival of adult basal forebrain cholinergic neurons after loss of target neurons.

Soga, K., and Y. Takahashi (1975). *Nature* 256:233–234. Differences in transcription of unique DNA sequences between neuronal and glial cells.

Soga, K., and Y. Takahashi (1976). *J. Neurochem.* 26:89–94. Transcription of repeated and unique DNA sequences in brain nuclei.

Soha, J. M., C. Yo, and D. C. Van Essen (1987). *Dev. Biol.* 123:136–144. Synapse elimination by fiber type and maturational state in rabbit soleus muscle.

Sohal, G. S. (1976). *Exp. Neurol.* 51:684–698. An experimental study of cell death in the developing trochlear nucleus.

Sohal, G. S. (1977). *Brain Res.* 138:217–228. Development of the oculomotor nucleus, with special reference to the time of cell origin and cell death.

Sohal, G. S., and R. K. Holt (1977). *Exp. Neurol.* 56:227–236. Autoradiographic studies on the time of origin of neurons of the eye muscle nuclei.

Sohal, G. S., and C. H. Narayanan (1974). *Brain Res.* 77:243–255. The development of the isthmo-optic nucleus in the duck (*Anas platyrhynchos*). I. Changes in cell number and cell size during normal development.

Sohal, G. S., and C. H. Narayanan (1975). *Exp. Neurol.* 46:521–533. Effects of optic primordium removal on the development of the isthmo-optic nucleus in the duck (*Anas platyrhynchos*).

Sohal, G. S., and T. A. Weidman (1978). *Brain Res.* 142:455–465. Development of the trochlear nerve: Loss of axons during normal ontogeny.

Sohal, G. S., T. A. Weidman, and S. D. Stoney (1978). *Exp. Neurol.* 59:331–341. Development of the trochlear nerve: Effects of early removal of periphery.

Sohal, G. S., R. T. Leshner, and T. R Swift (1983). *Muscle Nerve* 6:122–127. Myasthenia gravis immunoglobulin augments motor neuron survival without producing muscle paralysis.

Sokol, S., G. G. Wong, and D. A. Melton (1990). *Science* 249:561–564. A mouse macrophage factor induces head structures and organizes a body axis in *Xenopus*.

Solandt, D. Y., C. Partridge, and J. Hunter (1943). *J. Neurophysiol.* 6:17–22. The effects of skeletal fixation on skeletal muscle.

Solomon, F. (1979). *Cell* 16:165–169. Detailed neurite morphologies of sister neuroblastoma cells are related.

Solomon, F. (1980). *Cell* 21:333–338. Neuroblastoma cells recapitulate their detailed neurite morphologies after reversible microtubule disassembly.

Solomon, F. (1981). *J. Cell Biol.* 90:547–533. Specification of cell morphology by endogenous determinants.

Somjen, G. G. (1988). *Glia* 1:2–9. Nervenkitt: Notes on the history of the concept of neuroglia.

Sommer, I., and M. Schachner (1981). *Dev. Biol.* 83:311–327. Monoclonal antibodies (01–04) for oligodendrocyte cell surfaces: An immunological study in the central nervous system.

Sonmez, E., and K. Herrup (1984). *Dev. Brain Res.* 12:271–283. Role of staggerer gene in determining cell number in cerebellar cortex. II. granule cell death and persistence of the external granule cell layer in young mouse chimeras.

Sonnenfield, K. H., and D. N. Ishii (1982). *J. Neurosci. Res.* 8:375–391. Nerve growth factor effects and receptors in cultured human neuroblastoma lines.

Sosula, L., and P. H. Glow (1970). *J. Comp. Neurol.* 141:427–452. Increase in number of synapses in the inner plexiform layer of light deprived rat retinae: Quantitative electron microscopy.

Sotelo, C. (1973). *Brain Res.* 62:345–351. Permanance and fate of paramembranous synaptic specializations in "mutant" and experimental animals.

Sotelo, C. (1975a). *Adv. Neurol.* 12:353–360. Dendritic abnormalities of Purkinje cells of neurologic mutant mice (weaver and staggerer).

Sotelo, C. (1975b). *Brain Res.* 94:19–44. Anatomical physiological and biochemical studies of the cerebellum from mutant mice. II. Morphological study of cerebellar cortical neurons and circuits in the weaver mouse.

Sotelo, C. (1982). *Exp. Brain Res.* 6:50–68. Synaptic remodeling in a-granular cerebellum.

Sotelo, C., and M. C. Arsenio-Nunes (1976). *Brain Res.* 111:389–395. Development of Purkinje cells in absence of climbing fibers.

Sotelo, C., and J.-P. Changeux (1974a). *Brain Res.* 67:519–526. Transsynaptic degeneration 'en cascade' in the cerebellar cortex of staggerer mutant mice.

Sotelo, C., and J.-P. Changeux (1974b). *Brain Res.* 77:484–491. Bergmann fibers and granular cell migration in the cerebellum of homozygous weaver mutant mouse.

Sotelo, C., and S. L. Palay (1971). *Lab. Invest.* 25:653–671. Altered axons and axon terminals in the lateral vestibular nucleus of the rat. Possible example of axonal remodeling.

Sotelo, C., and D. Riche (1974). *Anat. Embryol.* 146:209–218. The smooth endoplasmic reticulum and the retrograde and fast orthograde transport of horseradish peroxidase in the nigro-neostriato-nigral loop.

Sotelo, C., F. Bourrat, and A. Triller (1984). *J. Comp. Neurol.* 222:177–199. Postnatal development of the inferior olivary complex in the rat. II. Topographic organization of the immature olivocerebellar projection.

Sotelo, C., R. M. Alvarado-Mallart, R. Gardette, and F. Crepel (1990). *J. Comp. Neurol.* 295:165–187. Fate of grafted embryonic Purkinje cells in the cerebellum of the adult "Purkinje cell degeneration" mutant mouse. I. Development of reciprocal graft-host interactions.

Souccar, C., A. J. Lapa, and J. R. DoValle (1982). *Exper. Neurol.* 75:576–588. Influence of castration on the electrical excitability and contraction properties of the rat levator ani muscle.

Soury, J. (1899). *Le Système Nerveux Central. Structure et Fonctions. Histoire Critique des Théories et des Doctrines,* 2 Vols. Carré et Naud, Paris.

Spacek, J. (1985). *Anat. Embryol.* 171:235–243. Three-dimensional analysis of dendritic spines. II. Spine apparatus and other cytoplasmic components.

Spacek, J. (1989). *J. Neurocytol.* 18:27–38. Dynamics of the Golgi method: A time-lapse study of the early stages of impregnation in single sections.

Spacek, J., and M. Hartmann (1983). *Anat. Embryol.* 167:289–

310. Three-dimensional analysis of dendritic spines. I. Quantitative observations related to dendritic and synaptic morphology in cerebral and cerebellar cortices.

Spacek, J., J. Parizek, and A. R. Lieberman (1973). *J. Neurocytol.* 2:407–428. Golgi cells, granule cells and synaptic glomeruli in the molecular layer of the rabbit cerebellar cortex.

Speidel, C. C. (1932). *J. Exp. Zool.* 61:279–331. Studies of living nerves. I. The movements of individual sheath cells and nerve sprouts correlated with the process of myelin sheath formation in amphibian larvae.

Speidel, C. C. (1933). *Am. J. Anat.* 52:1–79. Studies of living nerves. II. Activities of ameboid growth cones, sheath cells, and myelin segments, as revealed by prolonged observation of individual nerve fibers in frog tadpoles.

Speidel, C. C. (1935a). *J. Comp. Neurol.* 61:1–82. Studies on living nerves. III. Phenomena of nerve irritation recovery, degeneration and repair.

Speidel, C. C. (1935b). *Biol. Bull.* 68:140–161. Studies of living nerves. IV. Growth, regeneration, and myelination of the peripheral nerves in salamanders.

Speidel, C. C. (1941). *Harvey Lectures* 36:126–158. Adjustments of nerve endings.

Speidel, C. C. (1942). *J. Comp. Neurol.* 76:57–69. Studies of living nerves. VII. Growth adjustments of cutaneous terminal arborizations.

Speidel, C. C. (1948). *Am. J. Anat.* 82:277–320. Correlated studies of sense organs and nerves of the lateral line in living frog tadpoles. II. The trophic influence of specific nerve supply as revealed by prolonged observations of denervated and reinnervated organs.

Speidel, C. C. (1964). *Int. Rev. Cytol.* 16:173–231. *In vivo* studies of myelinated nerve fibers.

Spemann, H. (1905). *Zool. Anz.* 28:419–432. Über Linsenbildung nach experimenteller Entfernung der primären Linsenbildungszellen.

Spemann, H. (1906). *Verhandl. Deut. Ges. Zool.* 16:195–202. Über eine neue Methode der embryonalen Transplantation.

Spemann, H. (1912). *Zool. Jahrb. Suppl.* 15 3:1–48. Über die Entwicklung umgedrehter Hirnteile bei Amphibienembryonen.

Spemann, H. (1918). *Roux' Arch. EntwMech* 43:448–555. Über die Determination der ersten Organanlagen des Amphibienembryo, I-VI.

Spemann, H. (1921). *Arch. Entw. Mech. Organ.* 48:533–570. Die erzeugung tierischer Chimären durch heteroplastische embryonale Transplantation zwischen Triton cristatus und taeniatus.

Spemann, H. (1924a). *Naturwissensch.* 12:1092–1094. Über Organisatoren in der tierischen Entwicklung.

Spemann, H. (1938). *Embryonic Development and Induction,* Yale Univ. Press, New Haven. English Transl. of Spemann (1936) Experimentelle Beiträge zu einer Theorie der Entwicklung. Springer Verlag, Berlin.

Spemann, H. (1941). *Roux' Arch. EntwMech.* 141:1–14. Walther Vogt zum Gedächtnis.

Spemann, H. (1943). *Forschung und Leben.* F. W. Spemann, editor, J. Engelhorn, Stuttgart.

Spemann, H., and H. Mangold (1924). *Arch. Mikr. Anat. Entw. Mech* 100:599–638. Über Induktion von Embryonalanlagen durch Implantation artfremder Organisatoren.

Spencer, H. (1866). *The Principles of Biology,* 2 Vols. Appleton, New York.

Sperry, D. G. (1988a). *J. Comp. Neurol.* 278:446–452. Lumbar lateral motor column development in triploid *Xenopus laevis.*

Sperry, D. G. (1988b). *J. Comp. Neurol.* 278:499–508. Effects of increasing ploidy on the lumbar lateral motor column and hindlimb of newly metamorphosed *Xenopus laevis:* A comparison of diploid and triploid sibling.

Sperry, D. G., and P. Grobstein (1985). *J. Comp. Neurol.* 232:287–298. Regulation of neuron numbers in *Xenopus laevis:* Effects of hormonal manipulation altering size at metamorphosis.

Sperry, R. W. (1940). *J. Comp. Neurol.* 73:379–404. The functional results of muscle transposition in the hindlimbs of the rat.

Sperry, R. W. (1941). *J. Comp. Neurol.* 75:1–19. The effect of crossing nerves to antagonistic muscles in the hindlimb of the rat.

Sperry, R. W. (1942). *J. Comp. Neurol.* 76:283–321. Transplantation of motor nerves and muscles in the forelimb of the rat.

Sperry, R. W. (1943). *J. Comp. Neurol.* 79:33–55. Visuomotor coordination in the newt *(Triturus viridescens)* after regeneration of the optic nerves.

Sperry, R. W. (1944). *J. Neurophysiol.* 7:57–69. Optic nerve regeneration with return of vision in anurans.

Sperry, R. W. (1945a). *Quart. Rev. Biol.* 20:311–369. The problem of central nervous reorganization after nerve regeneration and muscle transposition.

Sperry, R. W. (1945b). *J. Neurophysiol.* 8:15–28. Restoration of vision after uncrossing of optic nerves and after contralateral transposition of the eye.

Sperry, R. W. (1947). *Arch. Neurol. Psychiat.* 58:452–473. Effect of crossing nerves to antagonistic limb muscles in the monkey.

Sperry, R. W. (1948). *Anat. Rec.* 102:63–75. Orderly patterning of synaptic associations in regeneration of intracentral fiber tracts mediating visuomotor coordination.

Sperry, R. W. (1950a). Neuronal specificity, pp. 232–239. In *Genetic Neurology* (P. Weiss, ed.), Univ. Chicago Press, Chicago.

Sperry, R. W. (1950b). *J. Comp. Neurol.* 93:277–287. Myotypic specificity in teleost motoneurons.

Sperry, R. W. (1951a). Mechanisms of neural maturation, pp. 236–280. In *Handbook of Experimental Psychology* (S. S. Stevens, ed.), Wiley, New York.

Sperry, R. W. (1951b). *Growth Symp.* 10:63–87. Regulative factors in the orderly growth of neural circuits.

Sperry, R. W. (1963). *Proc. Natl. Acad. Sci. U.S.A.* 50:703–710. Chemoaffinity in the orderly growth of nerve fiber patterns and connections.

Sperry, R. W. (1965). Embryogenesis of behavioral nerve nets, pp. 161–186. In *Organogenesis* (R. L. DeHaan, and H. Ursprung, eds.), Holt, Rinehart and Winston, New York.

Sperry, R. W. (1966). Selective communication in nerve nets: Impulse specificity vs. connection specificity, pp. 213–219. In *Neuroscience Research Symposium Summaries,* Vol. 1, (F. O. Schmitt, and T. Melnechuk, eds.), M.I.T. Press, Cambridge, Mass.

Sperry, R. W. (1968). *Dev. Biol. Suppl.* 2:306–327. Plasticity of neural maturation.

Sperry, R. W., and H. L. Arora (1965). *J. Embryol. Exp. Morphol.* 14:307–317. Selectivity in regeneration of the oculomotor nerve in the cichlid fish Astronotus ocellatus.

Sperry, R. W., and N. Deupree (1956). *J. Comp. Neurol.* 106:143–158. Functional recovery following alterations in nerve-muscle connections of fishes.

Sperry, R. W., and N. Miner (1949). *J. Comp. Neurol.* 90:403–423. Formation within sensory nucleus V of synaptic associations mediating cutaneous localization.

Spinelli, D. N., and F. E. Jensen (1979). *Science* 203:75–78. Plasticity: The mirror of experience.

Spira, A., S. Hudy, and R. Hannah (1984). *Anat. Embryol.* 169:293–301. Ectopic photoreceptor cells and cell death in the developing rat retina.

Spitz, R., and A. M. Wolf (1946). *Psychoanal. Study Child* 1:53. Hospitalization: An inquiry into the psychiatric conditions in early childhool.

Spitzer, E. A. (1907). *Trans. Amer. Philos. Soc. N.S.* 21:175–308. A study of the brains of six eminent scientists and scholars belonging to the American Anthropometric Society, together with a description of the skull of Professor E. D. Cope.

Spitzer, N. C. (1984). *J. Physiol. (London)* 357:51–65. On the basis of delayed depolarization and its role in repetitive firing of Rohon-Beard neurones in *Xenopus* tadpoles.

Spitzer, N. C. (1984). The differentiation of membrane properties of spinal neuron, pp. 95–106. In *Cellular and Molecular Biology of Neuronal Development* (I. B. Black, ed.), Plenum, 1984.

Spraggett, K., R. A. Wanner, and F. C. Fraser (1982). *Teratology* 25:78A. Teratogenicity of maternal fever in (wo)man-a retrospective study.

Springer, A. D., and B. R. Wilson (1989). *J. Comp. Neurol.* 282:119–132. Light microscopic study of degenerating cobalt-filled optic axons in goldfish: Role of microglia and radial glia in debris removal.

Springer, J. E. (1988). *Exp. Neurol.* 102:354–365. Nerve growth factor receptors in the central nervous system.

Springer, J. E., and R. Loy (1985). *Brain Res. Bull.* 15:629–634. Intrahippocampal injections of antiserum to nerve growth factor inhibit sympathohippocampal sprouting.

Springer, J. E., S. Koh, M. W. Tayrien, and R Loy (1987). *J. Neurosci. Res.* 17:111–118. Basal forebrain magnocellular neurons stain for nerve growth factor receptor: Correlation with cholinergic cell bodies and effects of axotomy.

Springer, J. E., T. J. Collier, J. R. Sladek, Jr., and R. Loy (1988a). *J. Neurosci. Res.* 19:291–296. Transplantation of male mouse submaxillary gland increases survival of axotomized basal forebrain neurons.

Springer, J. E., T. J. Collier, M. F. D. Notter, R. Loy, and J. R. Sladek, Jr. (1988b). *Prog. Brain Res.* 78:401–407 CNS grafts of NGF-rich tissue as an alternative source of trophic support for axotomized cholinergic neurons.

Sretavan, D. W., and C. J. Shatz (1986a). *J. Neurosci.* 6:234–251. Prenatal development of retinal ganglion cell axons: Segregation into eye specific layers within the cat's lateral geniculate nucleus.

Sretavan, D. W., and C. J. Shatz (1986b). *J. Neurosci.* 6:990–1003. Prenatal development of cat retino-geniculate axon arbors in the absence of binocular interactions.

Srihari, T., and G. Vrbová (1978). *J. Neurocytol.* 7:529–540. The role of muscle activity in the differentiation of neuromuscular junctions in slow and fast chick muscles.

Stach, R. W., and J. R. Perez-Polo (1987). *J. Neurosci. Res.* 17:1–10. Binding of nerve growth factor to its receptor.

Stach, R. W., and B. J. Wagner (1982). *J. Neurosci. Res.* 7:103–110. Decrease in the number of lower affinity (type II) nerve growth factor receptors on embryonic sensory neurons does not affect fiber outgrowth.

Stahl, W. R. (1962). *Science* 137:205–212. Similarity and dimensional methods in biology.

Stahl, W. R. (1970). *Physiological similarity and modeling: The application of dimensional analysis and physical similarity theory to mammalian physiology.* Appleton-Century-Crofts, New York.

Stanfield, B. B., and W. M. Cowan (1976). *Brain Res.* 104:129–136. Evidence for a change in the retino-hypothalamic projection in the rat following early removal of one eye.

Stanfield, B. B., and W. M. Cowan (1979a). *J. Comp. Neurol.* 185:393–422. The morphology of the hippocampus and dentate gyrus in normal and reeler mice.

Stanfield, B. B., and W. M. Cowan (1979b). *J. Comp. Neurol.* 185:423–460. The development of the hippocampus and dentate gyrus in normal and reeler mice.

Stanfield, B. B., V. S. Caviness, Jr., and W. M. Cowan (1979). *J. Comp. Neurol.* 185:461–484. The organization of certain afferents to the hippocampus and dentate gyrus in normal and reeler mice.

Stanfield, B. B., D. D. O'Leary, and C. Fricks (1982). *Nature* 298:371–373. Selective collateral elimination in early postnatal development restricts cortical distribution of rat pyramidal tract neurons.

Stanley, A. J., L. G. Gumbreck, J. E. Allison, and R. B. Easley (1973). *Recent Prog. Horm. Res.* 29:43–64. Male pseudohermaphroditism in the laboratory Norway rat.

Stannius, H. (1847). *Arch. Anat. Physiol. Wissensch. Med. Berlin,* pp. 443–462. Untersuchungen über Muskelreizbarkeit.

Stannius, H. (1849). *Das peripherische Nervensystem der Fische anatomisch und physiologisch untersucht.* Druck von Adler's Erben, Rostock.

Stanton, P. K., and J. M. Sarvey (1983). *J. Neurosci.* 4:3080–3088. Blockade of long-term potentiation in rat hippocampal CA1 region by inhibitors of protein synthesis.

Starck, D. (1937). *Morphol. Jahrb.* 79:358–435. Ueber einige Entwicklungsvorgänge am Kopf der Urodelen.

Starre-van der Molen, L. G. (1974). *Cell Tissue Res.* 151:219–230. Embryogenesis of calliphora erythrocephala Meigen. IV. Cell death in the central nervous system during late embryogenesis.

Stasny, F., J. Fröhlich, and J. Svoboda (1968). Development of some essential components in different parts of the chick embryo brain, pp. 37–50. In *Ontogenesis of the Brain* (I. Jilek, and S. Trojan, eds.), Charles Univ. Press, Prague.

State, F. A., and H. I. Dessouky (1977). *Acta Anat.* 98:353–360. Effect of the distal stump of transected nerve upon the rate of degeneration of taste buds.

Stebbins, C. A., and E. D. Pollack (1986). *J. Exp. Zool.* 237:79–85. Neuron number and asynchronous hindlimb development during the period of profound cell loss in the lateral motor column of *Rana pipiens* larvae.

Stebbins, G. L. (1973). *Brookhaven Symp. Biol.* 25:227–243. Evolution of morphogenetic pattterns.

Steck, P. A., J. Blenis, P. G. Voss, and J. L. Wang (1982). *J. Cell Biol.* 92:523–530. Growth control in cultured 3T3 fibroblasts. II. Molecular properties of a fraction enriched in growth inhibitory activity.

Stefanelli, A. (1950). Studies on the development of

Mauthner's cell, pp. 161–165. In *Genetic Neurology* (P. Weiss, ed.), Univ. of Chicago Press, Chicago.

Stefanelli, A. (1951). *Quart. Rev. Biol.* **26**:17–34. The Mauthnerian apparatus in the Ichthyopsida; its nature and function and correlated problems of neurohistogenesis.

Stefanowska, M. (1898). *Trav. Lab. Physiol. Inst. Solvay* **2**:1–44. Évolution des cellules nerveuses corticales chez le souris aprés le naissance.

Steffen, H., and H. Van der Loos (1980). *Exp. Brain Res.* **40**:419–431. Early lesions of mouse vibrissal follicles: Their influence on dendrite orientation in the cortical barrel field.

Stein, D. G., J. J. Rosen, J. Graziadei, D. Mishkin, and J. J. Brink (1969). *Science* **166**:528–529. Central nervous system: Recovery of function.

Stein, J. M., and H. A. Padykula (1962). *Am. J. Anat.* **110**:103–124. Hostochemical classification of individual skeletal muscle fibers of the rat.

Stein, P. S. G. (1984). Central pattern generators in the spinal cord, pp. 647–672. In *Handbook of the Spinal Cord,* Vol 2 and 3: *Anatomy and Physiology* (R. A. Davidoff, ed.), Marcel Dekker, New York.

Stein, Z., M. Susser, G. Saenger, and F. Marolla (1972). *Science* **178**:708–713. Nutrition and mental performance.

Stein, Z., M. Susser, G. Saenger, and F. Marolla (1975). *Famine and human development. The Dutch hunger winter of 1944–45.* Oxford University Press, New York.

Steinbach, J. H. (1981). *Dev. Biol.* **84**:267–276. Developmental changes in acetylcholine receptor aggregates at rat neuromuscular junctions.

Steinbach, J. H., A. J. Harris, J. Patrick, D. Schubert, and S. Heinemann (1973). *J. Gen. Physiol.* **62**:255–270. Nerve-muscle interaction in vitro.

Steinberg, M. S. (1962a). *Proc. Natl. Acad. Sci. U.S.A.* **48**:1577–1582. On the mechanism of tissue reconstruction by dissociated cells. I. Population kinetics, differential adhesiveness and the absence of directed migration.

Steinberg, M. S. (1962b). *Proc. Natl. Acad. Sci. U.S.A.* **48**:1769–1776. On the mechanism of tissue reconstruction by dissociated cells. III. Free energy relations and the reorganization of fused, heteronomic tissue fragments.

Steinberg, M. S. (1963). *Science* **141**:401–408. Reconstruction of tissues by dissociated cells.

Steinberg, M. S. (1964). The problem of adhesive selectivity in cellular interactions, pp. 321–366. In *Cellular Membranes in Development* (M. Locke, ed.), Academic Press, New York.

Steinberg, M. S. (1970). *J. Exp. Zool.* **173**:395–434. Does differential adhesion govern self-assembly processes in histogenesis? Equilibrium configurations and the emergence of a hierarchy among populations of embryonic cells.

Steinberger, W. W., and E. M. Smith (1968). *Arch. Phys. Med. Rehabil.* **49**:573–577. Maintenance of denervated rabbit muscle with direct electrostimulation.

Steindler, A. (1916). *Am. J. Orthopedic Surg.* **14**:707–719. Direct neurotization of paralyzed muscles, further study of the question of direct nerve implantation.

Steindler, D. A., T. F. O'Brien, and N. G. F. Cooper (1988). *J. Comp. Neurol.* **267**:357–369. Glycoconjugate boundaries during early postnatal development of the neostriatal mosaic.

Steindler, D. A., N. G. F. Cooper, A. Faissner, and M. Schachner (1989). *Dev. Biol.* **131**:243–260. Boundaries defined by adhesion molecules during development of the cerebral cortex: The J1/tenascin glycoprotein in the mouse somatosensory cortical barrel field.

Steinert, P. M., and D. R. Roop (1988). *Ann. Rev. Biochem.* **57**:593–625. Molecular and cellular biology of intermediate filaments.

Steinert, P. M., J. C. R. Jones, and R. D. Goldman (1984). *J. Cell Biol.* **99**:22–27. Intermediate filaments.

Steinert, P. M., A. C. Steven, and D. R. Roop (1985). *Cell* **42**:411–419. The molecular biology of intermediate filaments.

Steinman, R. M., J. M. Silver, and Z. A. Cohn (1973). *J. Cell Biol.* **63**:949–969. Pinocytosis in fibroblasts.

Stelzner, D. J. (1982). *Trends Neurosci.* **5**:167–169. Regenerating frog optic and mammalian PNS axons. Are they really so different?

Stelzner, D. J., and J. A. Strauss (1986). *J. Comp. Neurol.* **245**:83–106. A quantitative analysis of frog optic nerve regeneration: Is retrograde ganglion cell death or collateral axonal loss related to selective reinnervation?

Stenevi, U., and A. Björklund (1978). *Neurosci. Lett.* **7**:219–224. Growth of vascular sympathetic axons into the hippocampus after lesions of the septo-hippocampal pathway: A pitfall in brain lesion studies.

Stenevi, U., A. Bjorklund, and R. Y. Moore (1973). *Brain Behav. Evol.* **8**:110–134. Morphological plasticity of central adrenergic neurons.

Stenevi, U., B. Bjerre, A Björklund, and W. Mobley (1974). *Brain Res.* **69**:217–234. Effects of localized intracerebral injections of nerve growth factor on the regenerative growth of lesioned central noradrenergic neurones.

Stensaas, L. J. (1967a). *J. Comp. Neurol.* **129**:59–70. The development of hippocampal and dorsolateral pallial regions of the cerebral hemisphere in fetal rabbits. I. Fifteen millimeter stage, spongioblast morphology.

Stensaas, L. J. (1967b). *J. Comp. Neurol.* **129**:71–84. The development of hippocampal and dorsolateral pallial regions of the cerebral hemisphere in fetal rabbits. II. Twenty millimeter stage, neuroblast morphology.

Stensaas, L. J., and W. H. Reichert (1971). *Z. Zellforsch. Mikrosk. Anat.* **119**:147–163. Round and ameboid microglial cells in the neonatal rabbit brain.

Stensaas, L. J., and S. S. Stensaas (1971). *Brain Res.* **31**:67–84. Light and electron microscopy of motoneurons and neuropile in the amphibian spinal cord.

Stenwig, A. E. (1972). *J. Exp. Neuropathol. Exp. Neurol.* **31**:696–704. The origin of brain macrophages in traumatic lesions, Wallerian degeneration and retrograde degeneration.

Stephan, H. (1951). *Zool. Jahrb. Abt. Anat. Ontog. Tiere* **71**:487–586. Vergleichende Untersuchungen über den Feinbau des Hirnes von Wild- und haustieren. I. Studien am Schwein und Schaf.

Stephan, H. (1960). *Z. wiss. Zool.* **164**:143–172. Methodische Studien über den quantitativen Vergleich architektonischer Struktureinheiten des Gehirns.

Stephens, L. B. (1965). *Am. Zool.* **5**:222–223. The influence of thyroxin upon Rohon-Beard cells of *Rana pipiens* larvae.

Stephens, N., and N. Holder (1987). *Development* **99**:221–

230. Reformation of the pattern of neuromuscular connections in the regenerated axolotl hindlimb.

Stern, C. (1956a). *Cold Spring Harbor Symp. Quant. Biol.* **21**:375–382. Genetic mechanisms on the localized initiation of differentiation.

Stern, C. (1956b). *Arch. Entw. Mech. Organ.* **149**:1–25. The genetic control of developmental competence and morphogenetic tissue interactions in genetic mosaics.

Stern, C. (1968). *Genetic Mosaics and Other Essays.* Harvard Univ. Press, Boston.

Stern, C. D. (1990). *Seminars Dev. Biol.* **1**:109–116. Two distinct mechanisms for segmentation?

Stern, L., and R. Peyrot (1927). *C. R. séance Soc. Biol.* **96**:1124–1126. Le fonctionnement de la barrière hématoencéphalique aux divers stades de développement chez diverses espèces animales.

Sternberg, J. and S. J. Kimber (1986). *J. Embryol. Exp. Morph.* **91**:267–282. Distribution of fibronectin, laminin and entactin in the environment of migrating neural crest cells in early mouse embryos.

Sternberger, L. A., and N. H. Sternberger (1983). *Proc. Natl. Acad. Sci. U.S.A.* **80**:6126–6130. Monoclonal antibodies distinguish phosphorylated and nonphosphorylated forms of neurofilaments *in situ*.

Sternberger, L. A., and L. A. Sternberger (1984). *Ann. N.Y. Acad. Sci.* **420**:90–99. Neurotypy: The heterogeneity of brain proteins.

Sternberger, N. H., R. H. Quarles, Y. Itoyama, and H. deF. Webster (1979). *Proc. Natl. Acad. Sci. U.S.A.* **76**:1510–1514. Myelin-associated glycoprotein demonstrated immunocytochemically in myelin and myelin-forming cells of developing rat.

Sterzi, G. (1914–15). *Anatomia del Sistema Nervoso Centrale dell'Uomo.* 2 vols. Angelo Draghi, Editore, Padova.

Stevens, A. R. (1968). High resolution autoradiography, pp. 255–310. In *Methods in Cell Physiology* (D. M. Prescott, ed.), Academic Press, New York.

Steward, O. (1983a). *J. Neurosci.* **3**:177–188. Alterations in polyribosomes associated with dendritic spines during the reinnervation of the dentate gyrus of the adult rat.

Steward, O. (1983b). *Cold Spring Harbor Symp. Quant. Biol.* **48**:745–759. Polyribosomes at the base of dendritic spines of central nervous system neurons: Their possible role in synapse construction and modification.

Steward, O., and P. M. Falk (1986). *J. Neurosci.* **6**:412–423. Protein-synthetic machinery at postsynaptic sites during synaptogenesis: A quantitative study of the association between polyribosomes and developing synapse.

Steward, O., and B. Fass (1983). *Prog. Brain Res.* **58**:131–136. Polyribosomes associated with dendritic spines in the denervated dentate gyrus: Evidence for local regulation of protein synthesis during reinnervation.

Steward, O., and W. B. Levy (1982). *J. Neurosci.* **2**:284–291. Preferential localization of polyribosomes under the base of dendritic spines in granule cells of the dentate gyrus.

Steward, O., and C. E. Ribak (1986). *J. Neurosci.* **6**:3079–3085. Polyribosomes associated with synaptic specializations on axon initial segments: Localization of protein-synthetic machinery at inhibitory synapses.

Steward, O., and E. W. Rubel (1985). *J. Comp. Neurol.* **231**:385–395. Afferent influences on brain stem auditory nuclei of the chicken: Cessation of amino acid incorporation as an antecedent to age-dependent transneuronal degeneration.

Steward, O., C. W. Cotman, and G. S. Lynch (1974). *Exp. Brain Res.* **20**:45–66. Growth of a new fiber projection in the brain of adult rats: Re-innervation of the dentate gyrus by the contralateral entorhinal cortex following ipsilateral entorhinal lesions.

Steward, O., W. F. White, C. W. Cotman, and G. Lynch (1976). *Exp. Brain Res.* **26**:423–441. Potentiation of excitatory synaptic transmission in the normal and in the reinnervated dentate gyrus of the rat.

Steward, O., L. Davis, C. Dotti, L. L. Phillips, A. Rao, and G. Banker (1988). *Mol. Neurobiol.* **2**:227–261. Protein synthesis and processing in cytoplasmic microdomains beneath postsynaptic sites on CNS neurons.

Stewart, J. A. (1975). *Dev. Biol.* **44**:178–186. Contribution of a change in mRNA half-life to the accumulation of the tissue-specific S-100 protein during postnatal development of the mouse brain.

Stewart, J. A., and M. I. Urban (1972). *Dev. Biol.* **29**:372–384. The postnatal accumulation of S-100 protein in mouse central nervous system. Modulation of protein synthesis and degradation.

Stewart, P. A., and M. J. Wiley (1981). *Dev. Biol.* **84**:183–192. Developing nervous tissue induces formation of blood-brain barrier characteristics in invading endothelial cells: A study using quail-chick transplantation chimeras.

Stewart, R. M., D. P. Richman, and V. S. Caviness, Jr. (1975). *Acta Neuropathol. (Berl.)* **31**:1–12. Lissencephaly and pachygyria. An architectonic and topographical analysis.

Stieda, L. (1899). *Geschichte der Entwickelung der Lehre von den Nervenzellen und Nervenfasern Während des XIX. Jahrhunderts. I. Teil: Von Sömmering bis Deiters.* Verlag von Gustav Fischer, Jena.

Stilling, B. (1859). *Neue Untersuchungen über den Bau des Rückenmarks.* Hotop, Cassel.

Stirewalt, W. S., L. G. Wool, and P. Cavicehi (1967). *Proc. Natl. Acad. Sci. U.S.A.* **57**:1885–1892. The relation of RNA and protein synthesis to the sedimentation of muscle ribosomes: Effect of diabetes and insulin.

Stirling, R. V., and D. Summerbell (1979). *Nature* **278**:640–642. The segmentation of axons from the segmental nerve roots to the chick wing.

Stirling, R. V., and D. Summerbell (1981). *J. Embryol. Exp. Morphol.* **61**:233–247. The innervation of dorsoventrally reversed chick wings: Evidence that motor axons do not actively seek out their appropriate targets.

Stirling, R. V., and D. Summerbell (1985). *J. Embryol. Exp. Morphol.* **85**:251–269. The behavior of growing axons invading developing chick wing buds with dorsoventral or anteroposterior axis reversed.

Stoch, M. B., and P. M. Smythe (1963). *Arch. Dis. Child.* **38**:546–552. Does undernutrition during infancy inhibit brain growth and subsequent intellectual development?

Stoch, M. B., and P. M. Smythe (1967). *S. Afr. Med. J.* **41**:1027–1030. The effect of undernutrition during infancy on subsequent brain growth and intellectual development.

Stoch, M. B., and P. M Smythe (1976). *Arch. Dis. Child.* **51**:327–336. 15-year developmental study on effects of severe undernutrition during infancy on subsequent physical growth and intellectual functioning.

Stoch, M. B., P. M. Smythe, A. D. Moodie, and D. Bradshaw

(1982). *Dev. Med. Child Neurol.* 24:419–436. Psychosocial outcome and CT findings after gross undernourishment during infancy: A 20-year developmental study.

Stockdale, F. E., and H. Holtzer (1961). *Exp. Cell Res.* 24:508–520. DNA synthesis and myogenesis.

Stockdale, F. E., and J. B. Miller (1987). *Dev. Biol.* 123:1–9. The cellular basis of myosin heavy chain isoform expression during development of avian skeletal muscles.

Stöckel, K., M. Schwab, and H. Thoenen (1975). *Brain Res.* 99:1–16. Comparison between the retrograde axonal transport of nerve growth factor and tetanus toxin in motor, sensory and adrenergic neurons.

Stoeckel, K., and H. Thoenen (1975). *Brain Res.* 85:337–341. Retrograde axonal transport of nerve growth factor: Specificity and biological importance.

Stoeckel, K., U. Paravicini, and H. Thoenen (1974). *Brain Res.* 76:413–421. Specificity of the retrograde axonal transport of nerve growth factor.

Stoeckel, K., M. Schwab, and H. Thoenen (1975). *Brain Res.* 89:1–14. Specificity of retrograde transport of nerve growth factor (NGF) in sensory neurons: A biochemical and morphological study.

Stoeckel, K., G. Guroff, M. Schwab, and H. Thoenen (1976). *Brain Res.* 109:271–284. The significance of retrograde axonal transport for the accumulation of systemically administered nerve growth factor (NGF) in the rat superior cervical ganglion.

Stöhre, P. (1935). *Z. Anat. Entw Gesch.* 104:133–158. Beobachtungen und Bemerkungen über die Endausbreitung des vegetativen Nervensystems.

Stoll, G., B. D. Trapp, and J. W. Griffin (1989). *J. Neurosci.* 9:2327–2335. Macrophage function during wallerian degeneration of rat optic nerve: Clearance of degenerating myelin and Ia expression.

Stone, J. (1983). *Parallel Processing in the Visual System: The Classification of Retinal Ganglion Cells and Its Impact on the Neurobiology of Vision.* Plenum Press, New York.

Stone, J., and B. Dreher (1973). *J. Neurophysiol.* 36:551–567. Projection of X- and Y-cells of the cat's lateral geniculate nucleus to areas 17 and 18 of visual cortex.

Stone, J., and Y. Fukuda (1974a). *J. Neurophysiol.* 37:722–748. Properties of cat retinal ganglion cells: A comparison of W-cells with X- and Y-cells.

Stone, J., and Y. Fukuda (1974b). *J. Comp. Neurol.* 155:377–394. The naso-temporal division of the cat's retina reexamined in terms of Y-, X-, and W-cells.

Stone, J., and D. H. Rapaport (1986). The role of cell death in shaping the ganglion cell layer population of the adult cat retina, pp. 157–169. In *Visual Neuroscience* (J. D. Pettigrew, K. J. Sanderson, and W. R. Levick, eds.), Cambridge University Press, Cambridge.

Stone, J., D. H. Rapaport, R. W. Williams, and L. M. Chalupa (1982). *Dev. Brain Res.* 2:231–242. Uniformity of cell distribution in the ganglion cell layer of prenatal cat retina: Implications for mechanisms of retinal development.

Stone, J., J. Maslim, and D. Rapaport (1984). The development of the topographical organisation of the cat's retina, pp. 3–21. In *Development of Visual Pathways in Mammals* (J. Stone, B. Dreher, and D. Rapaport, eds.), Alan R. Liss, New York.

Stone, L. C. (1922). *J. Exptl. Zool.* 35:421–496. Experiments on the development of the cranial ganglia and the lateral line sense organs in *Amblystoma punctatum*.

Stone, L. C. (1929). *Arch. Entwicklungsmech.* 118:40–77. Experiments showing the role of migrating neural crest (mesectoderm) in the formation of head skeleton and loose connective tissue in *Rana palustris*.

Stone, L. S. (1930). *J. Exp. Zool.* 55:193–261. Heteroplastic transplantation of eyes between the larvae of two species of Amblystoma.

Stone, L. S. (1933). *Proc. Soc. Exp. Biol. Med.* 30:1256–1257. Independence of taste organs with respect to their nerve fibers demonstrated in living salamanders.

Stone, L. S. (1940). *J. Exp. Zool.* 83:481–506. The origin and development of taste organs in salamanders observed in the living condition.

Stone, L. S. (1941). *Trans. N.Y. Acad. Sci.* 3:208–212. Transplantation of the vertebrate eye and return of vision.

Stone, L. S. (1944). *Proc. Soc. Exp. Biol. Med.* 57:13–14. Functional polarization in retinal development and its reestablishment in regenerated retinae of rotated eyes.

Stone, L. S. (1948). *Ann. N.Y. Acad. Sci.* 49:856–865. Functional polarization in developing and regenerating retinae of transplanted eyes.

Stone, L. S. (1953). *Arch. Ophthalmol.* 49:28–35. Normal and reversed vision in transplanted eyes.

Stone, L. S. (1960). *J. Exp. Zool.* 145:85–93. Polarization of the retina and development of vision.

Stone, L. S. (1963). *J. Exp. Zool.* 153:57–67. Vision in eyes of several species of adult newts transplanted to adult Triturus viridescens.

Stone, L. S. (1964). *Invest. Ophthalmol.* 3:555–565. Return of vision in eyes exchanged between Amblystoma punctatum and the cave salamander, Typhlotriton spelaeus.

Stone, L. S., and C. H. Cole (1943). *Yale J. Biol. Med.* 15:735–754. Grafted eyes of young and old salamanders (*Amblystoma punctatum*) showing return of vision.

Stone, L. S., and F. S. Ellison (1940). *Proc. Soc. Exp. Biol. Med.* 45:181–182. Exchange of eyes between adult hosts of *Amblystoma punctatum* and Triturus viridescens.

Stone, L. S., and L. S. Farthing (1942). *J. Exp. Zool.* 91:265–285. Return of vision four times in the same adult salamander eye (*Triturus viridescens*) repeatedly transplanted.

Stone, L. S., and J. S. Zaur (1940). *J. Exp. Zool.* 85:243–270. Reimplantation and transplantation of adult eyes in the salamander (Triturus viridescens) with return of vision.

Stossel, T. P., J. H. Hartwig, H. L. Yin, K. S. Zaner, and O. I. Stendahl (1981). *Cold Spring Harbor Symp. Quant. Biol.* 46:569–578. Actin gelation and the structure of cortical cytoplasm.

Stott, D. H. (1960). *Brit. J. Educ. Psychol.* 30:95–102. Interaction of heredity and environment in regard to "measured intelligence."

Stough, H. B. (1930). *J. Comp. Neurol.* 50:217–229. Polarization of the giant nerve fibers of the earthworm.

Straus, W. L. (1939). *Anat. Rec.* Suppl. 273:50–55. Changes in the structure of skeletal muscle at the time of its first visible contraction in living rat embryos.

Straus, W. L. (1946). *Biol. Rev.* 21:75–91. The concept of nerve-muscle specificity.

Straus, W. L., and G. Weddell (1940). *J. Neurophysiol.* 3:358–369. Nature of the first visible contractions of the forelimb musculature in rat foetuses.

Straznicky, C., and M. Chehade (1987). *Development*

100:411–420. The formation of the area centralis of the retinal ganglion cell layer in the chick.

Straznicky, C., and R. A. Rush (1985). *Anat. Embryol.* 171:91–95. The effect of nerve growth factor on developing primary sensory neurons of the trigeminal nerve in chick embryos.

Straznicky, C., D. Tay, and J. Hiscock (1980). *Neurosci. Let.* 19:131–136. Segregation of optic fibre projections into eye-specific bands in dually innervated tecta in *Xenopus*.

Straznicky, C., R. M. Gaze, and M. J. Keating (1981). *J. Embryol. Exp. Morph.* 62:13–35. The development of the retinotectal projections from compound eyes in *Xenopus*.

Straznicky, K. (1963). *Acta Biol. Acad. Sci. Hung.* 14:143–155. Function of heterotopic spinal cord segments investigated in the chick.

Straznicky, K. (1967). *Acta Biol. Acad. Sci. Hung.* 18:437–448. The development of innervation and the musculature of wings innervated by thoracic nerves.

Straznicky, K. (1973). *J. Embryol. Exp. Morphol.* 29:397–409. The formation of the optic fibre projection after partial tectal removal in Xenopus.

Straznicky, K. (1983). *Anat. Embryol.* 167:247–262. The patterns of innervation and movements of ectopic hindlimb supplied by brachial spinal cord segments in the chick.

Straznicky, K., and R. M. Gaze (1971). *J. Embryol. Exp. Morphol.* 26:67–79. The growth of the retina in *Xenopus laevis*: An autoradiographic study.

Straznicky, K., and R. M. Gaze (1972). *J. Embryol. Exp. Morphol.* 28:87–115. The development of the tectum in *Xenopus laevis*: An autoradiographic study.

Straznicky, K., and R. A. Rush (1985). *Anat. Embryol.* 171:91–95. The effect of nerve growth factor on developing primary sensory neurons of the trigeminal nerve in chick embryos.

Straznicky, K., and G. Székely (1967). *Acta Biol. Acad. Sci. Hung.* 18:449–456. Functional adaptation of thoracic spinal cord segments in the newt.

Straznicky, K., and D. Tay (1977). *J. Embryol. Exp. Morphol.* 40:175–185. Retinal growth in double dorsal and double ventral eyes in *Xenopus*.

Straznicky, K., R. M. Gaze, and M. J. Keating (1971). *J. Embryol. Exp. Morphol.* 26:523–542. The retinotectal projections after uncrossing the optic chiasma in *Xenopus* with one compound eye.

Straznicky, K., R. M. Gaze, and M. J. Keating (1974). *J. Embryol. Exp. Morphol.* 31:123–137. The retinotectal projection from a double-ventral compound eye in *Xenopus laevis*.

Streeter, G. L. (1912). The development of the nervous system, pp. 1–156. In *Manual of Human Embryology*, Vol. 2, (F. Keibel, and F. P. Mall, eds.), Lippincott, Philadelphia.

Streeter, G. L. (1918). *Contrib. Embryol. Carnegie Inst.* 8:5–38. The developmental alterations in the vascular system of the brain in the human embryo.

Streeter, G. L. (1919). *Am. J. Anat.* 25:1–11. Factors involved in the formation of the filum terminale.

Streit, W. J., M. B. Graeber, and G. W. Kreutzberg (1988). *GLIA* 1:301–307. Functional plasticity of microglia: A review.

Stretton, A. O. W., and E. A. Kravitz (1968). *Science* 162:132–134. Neuronal geometry: Determination of a technique of intracellular dye injection.

Stroebe, H. (1895). *Centralbl. Path. path. Anat. Jena* 6:849–960. Die allgemeine Histologie der degenerativen und regenerativen Processe im centralen und peripheren Nervensystem nach dem neuesten Forschungen. Zusammend fassendes Referat.

Strome, S. (1989). *Int. Rev. Cytol.* 114:81–123. Generation of cell diversity during early embryogenesis in the nematode *caenorhabditis elegans*.

Strong, L. H. (1961). *Acta Anat.* 44:80–108. The first appearance of vessels within the spinal cord of the mammal: Their developing patterns as far as partial formation of the dorsal septum.

Strong, O. S. (1895). *J. Morphol.* 10:101–230. The cranial nerves of Amphibia; a contribution to the morphology of the vertebrate nervous system.

Strong, O. S. (1896). *J. Comp. Neurol.* 6:101–127. Review of the Golgi method.

Struhl, G., K. Struhl, and P. M. MacDonald (1989). *Cell* 57:1259–1273. The gradient morphogen bicoid is a concentration-dependent transcriptional activator.

Stryker, M. P., and H. Sherk (1975). *Science* 190:904–905. Modification of cortical orientation selectivity in the cat by restricted visual experience: A reexamination.

Stryker, M. P., and W. A. Harris (1986). *J. Neurosci.* 6:2117–2133. Binocular impulse blockade prevents the formation of ocular dominance columns in cat visual cortex.

Stryker, M. P., and S. L. Strickland (1984). *Invest. Opthamol. Suppl.* 25:278. Physiological segregation of ocular dominance columns depends on the pattern of afferent electrical activity.

Stryker, M. P., H. V. B. Hirsch, H. Sherk, and A. G. Leventhal (1976). Orientation selectivity in cat visual cortex following selective orientation deprivation using goggles. Paper presented at ARVO, Sarasota, Florida.

Stubbe, H. (1972). *History of Genetics From Prehistoric Times to the Rediscovery of Mendel's Laws*. T. R. W., transl. M.I.T. Press, Cambridge, Massachusetts.

Stuermer, C. A. O., and S. S. Easter (1984a). *J. Comp. Neurol.* 223:57–76. A comparison of the normal and regenerated retinotectal pathways of goldfish.

Stuermer, C. A. O., and S. S. Easter (1984b). *J. Neurosci.* 4:1045–1051. Rules of order in the retinotectal fascicles of goldfish.

Stuermer, C. A. O. (1988a). *J. Comp. Neurol.* 267:55–68. The trajectories of regenerating retinal axons in the goldfish. I. A comparison of normal and regenerated axons at late regeneration stages.

Stuermer, C. A. O. (1988b). *J. Comp. Neurol.* 267:69–91. The trajectories of regenerating retinal axons in the goldfish tectum. II. Exploratory branches and growth cones on axons at early regeneration stages.

Stuermer, C. A. O. (1988c). *J. Neurosci.* 8:4513–4530. Retinotopic organization of the developing retinotectal projection in the zebrafish embryo.

Stuermer, C. A. O. (1988d). *Soc. Neurosci. Abstr.* 14. Development of the retinotectal projection in zebrafish embryos under TTX-induced blockade of neural activity.

Stultz, W. A. (1942). *Anat. Rec.* 82:450. Alterations in the spinal cord of Amblystoma following changes in the peripheral field.

Stump, R. F., and K. R. Robinson (1983). *J. Cell Biol.* 97:1226–1233. *Xenopus* neural crest cell migration in an applied electrical field.

Stumpf, H. F. (1966a). *Nature* 212:430–431. Mechanism by which cells estimate their location within the body.

Stumpf, H. F. (1966b). *J. Insect Physiol.* 12:601–617. Über Gefälleabhangige Bildungen des Insektensegmentes.

Stumpf, H. F. (1968). *J. Exp. Biol.* 49:49–60. Further studies on gradient-dependent diversification in the pupal cuticle of Galleria mellonella.

Stumpf, W. E. (1971a). *Am. Zool.* 11:725–739. Autoradiographic techniques and the localization of estrogen, androgen, and glucocorticoid in the pituitary and brain.

Stumpf, W. E. (1971b). *J. Neuro-Visceral Relations* 10:51–64. Probable sites for estrogen receptors in brain and pituitary.

Stumpf, W. E., and M. Sar (1975). Anatomical distribution of corticosterone-concentrating neurons in rat brain, pp. 254–261. In *Anatomical Neuroendocrinology* (W. E. Stumpf, and L. E. Grant, eds.), Karger, Basel, 1975.

Sturrock, R. R. (1974a). *J. Anat. (London)* 117:17–25. Histogenesis of the anterior limb of the anterior commissure of the mouse brain. I. A quantitative study of changes in the glial population with age.

Sturrock, R. R. (1974b). *J. Anat. (London)* 117:27–35. Histogenesis of the anterior limb of the anterior commissure of the mouse brain. II. A quantitative study of pre- and postnatal mitosis.

Sturrock, R. R. (1978). *J. Anat. (London)* 129:777–793. A morphological study of the development of the mouse choroid plexus.

Sturrock, R. R. (1979a). *Neuropathol. Appl. Neurobiol.* 5:433–456. A quantitative lifespan study of changes in cell number, cell division and cell death in various regions of the mouse forebrain.

Sturrock, R. R. (1979b). *J. Anat. (London)* 129:31–44. A semithin light microscopic, transmission electron microscopic and scanning electron microscopic study of macrophages in the lateral ventricle of mice from embryonic to adult life.

Sturrock, R. R. (1981a). *J. Anat. (London)* 132:203–221. A quantitative and morphological study of vascularization of the developing mouse spinal cord.

Sturrock, R. R. (1981b). *J. Anat. (London)* 132:429–432. Electron microscopic evidence for mitotic division of oligodendrocytes.

Sturrock, R. R. (1981c). *J. Anat. (London)* 133:499–512. Microglia in the prenatal mouse neostriatum and spinal cord.

Sturrock, R. R. (1982a). *J. Anat. (London)* 134:771–793. Gliogenesis in the prenatal rabbit spinal cord.

Sturrock, R. R. (1982b). *J. Anat. (London)* 135:89–96. A quantitative study of vascularisation of the prenatal rabbit spinal cord.

Sturrock, R. R. (1982c). *Adv. Cell. Neurobiol.* 3:3–33. Cell division in the normal central nervous system.

Sturrock, R. R. (1983). *Applied Neurobiol.* 6:211–219. A morphological lifespan study of neurolipomastocytes in various regions of the mouse forebrain.

Sturrock, R. R. (1983). *J. Anat. (London)* 371:47–55. Identification of mitotic oligodendrocytes in semithin sections of the developing mouse corpus callosum and hippocampal commissure.

Sturrock, R. R., and I. H. M. Smart (1980). *J. Anat. (London)* 130:391–415. A morphological study of the mouse subependymal layer from embryonic life to old age.

Sturrock, R. R., J. L. Smart, and M. D. Tricklebank (1983). *J. Anat. (London)* 136:129–144. A quantitative neurohistological study of the long term effects in the rat brain of stimulation in infancy.

Sturtevant, A. H. (1929). *Z. Wiss. Zool.* 135:325–356. The claret mutant type of *Drosophila simulans:* A study of chromosome elimination and cell lineage.

Stussi, T. (1960). *Arch. Sci. Physiol. (Paris)* 14:261–277. Etudes des localisations motrices du renflement lombaire chez la grenouille.

Suburo, A., N. Carri, and R. Adler (1979). *J. Comp. Neurol.* 184:519–536. The environment of axonal migration in the developing chick retina: a scanning electron microscopic (SEM) study.

Sudarwati, S. and P. D. Nieuwkoop (1971). *Wilhelm Roux Arch. Entw. Mech. Org.* 166:189–204. Mesoderm formation in the Anuran Xenopus laevis (Daudin).

Sudol, M. (1988). *Brain Res. Rev.* 13:391–403. Expression of proto-oncogenes in neural tissues.

Sugiyama, H., P. Benda, J.-C. Meunier, and J.-P. Changeux (1973). *FEBS Lett.* 35:124–128. Immunological characterization of the cholinergic receptor protein from electrophorus electricus.

Sulston, J. E. (1976). *Phil. Trans. Roy. Soc. (London) B.* 275:287–297. Post-embryonic development in the ventral cord of Caenorhabditis elegans.

Sulston, J. E., and H. R. Horwitz (1977). *Dev. Biol.* 56:110–156. Postembryonic cell lineages of the nematode *Caenorhabditis elegans.*

Sulston, J. E., and H. R. Horwitz (1981). *Dev. Biol.* 82:41–55. Abnormal cell lineages in mutants of the nematode *Caenorhabditis elegans.*

Sulston, J. E., and J. G. White (1980). *Dev. Biol.* 78:577–597. Regulation of cell autonomy during postembryonic development of *Caenorhabditis elegans.*

Sulston, J. E., E. Schierenberg, J. G. White, and J. N. Thomson (1983). *Dev. Biol.* 100:64–119. The embryonic cell lineage of the nematode *Caenorhabditis elegans.*

Sumi, S. M. (1970). *Brain* 93:821–830. Brain malformation in the trisomy 18 syndrome.

Sumida, H., N. Akimoto, and H. Nakamura (1989). *Anat. Embryol.* 180:29–35. Distribution of neural crest cells in the heart of birds: A three dimensional analysis.

Summerbell, D., and J. H. Lewis (1975). *J. Embryol. Exp. Morphol.* 33:621–643. Time, place and positional value in the chick limb-bud.

Sumner, B. E. H. (1975). *Exp. Neurol.* 46:605–615. A quantitative analysis of the response of presynaptic boutons to postsynaptic motor neuron axotomy.

Sumner, B. E. H. (1976). *Exp. Brain Res.* 26:141–150. Quantitative ultrastructural observations on the inhibited recovery of the hypoglossal nucleus from the axotomy response when regeneration of the hypoglossal nerve is prevented.

Sumner, B. E. H., and F. I. Sutherland (1973). *J. Neurocytol.* 2:315–328. Quantitative electron microscopy on the injured hypoglossal nucleus in the rat.

Sumner, B. E. H., and W. E. Watson (1971). *Nature* 233:273–275. Retraction and expansion of the dendritic tree of motor neurons of adult rats induced *in vivo.*

Sunderland, S. (1947). *Arch. Neurol. Psychiat.* 58:251–295. Rate of regeneration in human peripheral nerves. Analysis of interval between injury and onset of recovery.

Sunshine, J., K. Balak, U Rutishauser, and M. Jacobson (1987). *Proc. Natl. Acad. Sci U.S.A.* 84:5986–5990. Changes in neural cell adhesion molecule (NCAM) structure during vertebrate neural development.

Sur, M., and S. M. Sherman (1982). *Science* 218:389–391. Retinogeniculate terminations in cats: Morphological differences between X and Y cell axons.

Sur, M., A. L. Humphrey, and S. M. Sherman (1982). *Nature* 300:183–185. Monocular deprivation affects X- and Y-cell retinogeniculate terminations in cats.

Sur, M., R. E. Weller, and S. M. Sherman (1984). *Nature* 310:246–249. Development of X- and Y-cell retinogeniculate terminations in kittens.

Sur, M., P. E. Garraghty, and M. P. Stryker (1985). *Soc. Neurosci. Abstr.* 11:805 (Abstr.). Morphology of physiologically identified retinogeniculate axons in cats following blockade of retinal impulse activity.

Sur, M., M. Esguerra, P. E. Garraghty, M. F. Kritzer, and S. M. Sherman (1987). *J. Neurophysiol.* 58:1–32. Morphology of physiologically identified retinogeniculate X and Y axons in the cat.

Sur, M., P. E. Garraghty, and A. W. Roe (1988a). *Science* 242:1437–1441. Experimentally induced visual projections into auditory thalamus and cortex.

Sur, M., D. O. Frost, and S. Hockfield (1988b). *J. Neurosci.* 8:874–882. Expression of a surface-associated antigen on Y-cells in the cat lateral geniculate nucleus is regulated by visual experience.

Sur, M., S. L. Pallas, and A. W. Roe (1990). *Trends Neurosci.* 13:227–233. Cross-modal plasticity in cortical development: Differentiation and specification of sensory neocortex.

Sutcliffe, J. G. (1988). *Ann. Rev. Neurosci.* 11:157–198. mRNA in the mammalian central nervous system.

Sutherland, E. W. (1972). *Science* 177:401–408. Studies on the mechanism of hormone action.

Sutter, A., R. J. Riopelle, R. M. Harris-Warrick, and E. M. Shooter (1979). *J. Biol. Chem.* 254:5972–5982. Nerve growth factor receptors: Characterization of two distinct classes of binding sites on chick embryo sensory ganglia cells.

Sutton, A. C. (1915). *Am. J. Anat.* 18:117–144. On the development of the neuro-muscular spindle in the extrinsic eye muscles of the pig.

Suzuki, A., and K. Kuwabara (1974). *Dev. Growth Diff.* 16:29–40. Mitotic activity and cell proliferation in primary induction of newt embryo.

Suzuki, A., K. Kuwabara, and Y. Kuwabara (1975). *Dev. Growth Diff.* 17:343–353. Temporal relations between extension of archenteron roof and realization of neural induction during gastrulation of newt embryo.

Suzuki, D. T., T. Grigliatti, and R. Williamson (1971). *Proc. Natl. Acad. Sci. U.S.A.* 68: 890–893. Temperature-sensitive mutations in Drosophila melanogaster. VII. A mutation (parats) causing reversible adult paralys.

Suzuki, S., A. Oldberg, E. G. Hayman, M. D. Pierschbacher, and E. Ruoslahti (1985). *EMBO J.* 4:2519–2524. Complete amino acid sequence of human vitronectin deduced from cDNA. Similarity of cell attachment sites in vitronectin and fibronectin.

Suzuki, S., W. S. Argraves, R. Pytela, H. Artai, T. Krusius, M. D. Pierschbacher and E. Ruoslahti (1986). *Proc. Natl. Acad. Sci. U.S.A.* 83:8614–8618. cDNA and amino acid sequences of the cell adhesion protein receptor recogniz-

ing vitronectin reveal a transmembrane domain and homologies with other adhesion protein receptors.

Swaab, D. F., and E. Fliers (1985). *Science* 228:1112–1115. A Sexually Dimorphic Nucleus in the Human Brain.

Swaab, D. F., and M. A. Hofman (1988). *Dev. Brain Res.* In press. Sexual differentiation of the human hypothalamus: Ontogeny of the sexually dimorphic nucleus of the preoptic area.

Swaab, D. F., and D. F. Swaab (1984). *Prog. Brain Res.* 61:361–374. Sexual differentiation of the human brain. A historic perspective.

Swaab, D. F., E. Fliers, and T. S. Partiman (1985). *Brain Res.* 342:37–44. The suprachiasmatic nucleus of the human brain in relation to sex, age and senile dementia.

Swanson, G. J., and J. Lewis (1982). *J. Embryol. Exp. Morphol.* 71:121–137. The timetable of innervation and its control in the chick wing bud.

Swanson, G. J., and J. Lewis (1986). *J. Embryol. Exp. Morphol.* 95:37–52. Sensory nerve routes in chick wing buds deprived of motor innervation.

Swanson, L. W. (1983). The use of retrogradely transported fluorescent markers in neuroanatomy, pp. 219–240. In *Current Methods in Cellular Neurobiology*, Vol. 1. *Anatomical Techniques* (J. L. Barker, and J. F. McKelvy, eds.), Wiley, New York.

Swash, M., and K. P. Fox (1974). *J. Neurol. Sci.* 22:1–24. The pathology of the human muscle spindle: Effect of denervation.

Swazey, J. P. (1969). *Reflexes and Motor Integration: Sherrington's Concept of Integrative Action.* Harvard Univ. Press, Cambridge, Mass.

Sweet, J. E., E. Eldred, and J. S. Buchwald (1970). *Am. J. Phsyiol.* 219:762–766. Somatotopic cord-to-muscle relations in efferent innervation of cat gastrocnemius.

Swett, F. H. (1927). *J. Exp. Zool.* 47:385–439. Differentiation of the amphibian limb.

Swett, F. H. (1937). *Quart. Rev. Biol.* 12:322–339. Determination of limb-axes.

Swett, F. H. (1938). *J. Exp. Zool.* 78:47–79. Experiments designed to hasten polarization of the dorsoventral limb axis in Amblystoma punctatum.

Swift, H. (1950). *Physiol. Zool.* 23:169–198. The desoxyribose nucleic acid content of animal nuclei.

Swindale, N. V. (1981a). *Nature* 290:332–333. Absence of ocular dominance patches in dark-reared cats.

Swindale, N. V. (1981b). *Trends Neurosci.* 4:240–241. Dendritic spines only connect.

Swindale, N. V. (1988). *J. Comp. Neurol.* 267:472–488. Role of visual experience in promoting segregation of eye dominance patches in the visual cortex of the cat.

Swisher, D. A., and D. B. Wilson (1977). *J. Comp. Neurol.* 173:205–218. Cerebellar histogenesis in the lurcher (*Lc*) mutant mouse.

Szaro, B. G., and H. Gainer (1988). *J. Comp. Neurol.* 273:344–358. Identities, antigenic determinants, and topographic distributions of neurofilament proteins in the nervous systems of adult frogs and tadpoles of *Xenopus laevis.*

Szarski, H. (1976). *Int. Rev. Cytol.* 44:93–111. Cell size and nuclear DNA content in vertebrates.

Székely, G. (1954). *Acta Biol. Acad. Sci. Hung.* 5:157–167. Zur Ausbildung der lokalen funktionellen Spezifität der Retina.

Székely, G. (1957). *Arch. Entw.-Mech. Organ.* 150:48–60. Regulationstendenzen in der Ausbildung der "funktionellen Spezifität" der Retinaanlage bei Triturus vulgaris.

Székely, G. (1959a). *J. Embryol. Exp. Morphol.* 7:375–379. The apparent "corneal specificity" of sensory neurons.

Székely, G. (1959b). *Acta Biol. Acad. Sci. Hung.* 10:107–116. Functional specificity of cranial sensory neuroblasts in Urodela.

Székely, G. (1963). *J. Embryol. Exp. Morphol.* 11:431–444. Functional specificity of spinal cord segments in the control of limb movements.

Székely, G. (1966). *Adv. Morphogenesis* 5:181–219. Embryonic determination of neural connections.

Székely, G. (1968). Development of limb movements: embryological physiological and model studies, pp. 77–93. In *Growth of the Nervous System. A Ciba Foundation Symposium* (G. E. W. Wolstenholme, and M. O'Connor, eds.), Little, Brown, Boston.

Székely, G. (1971). *Vision Res.* Suppl. 3:269–279. The mesencephalic and diencephalic optic centres in the frog.

Székely, G. (1973). Anatomy and synaptology of the optic tectum, pp. 1–26. In *Handbook of Sensory Physiology*, Vol. VII/3B, (R. Jung, ed.), Springer-Verlag, Berlin.

Székely, G. (1974). Problems of neuronal specificity in the development of some behavior patterns in amphibia, pp. 115–150. In *Studies on the Development of Behavior and the Nervous System*, Vol. 2, *Aspects of Neurogenesis* (G. Gottlieb, ed.), Academic Press, New York.

Székely, G., and G. Czéh (1967). *Acta Physiol. Acad. Sci. Hung.* 32:3–18. Localization of motoneurones in the limb moving spinal cord segments of Amblystoma.

Székely, G., and F. Gallyas (1975). *Acta Biol. Acad. Scien. Hung.* 26:175–188. Intensification of cobaltous sulphide precipitate in frog nervous tissue.

Székely, G., and G. Lázár (1976). Cellular and synaptic architecture of the optic tectum, pp. 407–434. In *Frog Neurobiology* (R. Llinas, and W. Precht, eds.), Springer-Verlag, New York.

Székely, G., G. Czéh, and G. Vörös (1969). *Exp. Brain Res.* 9:53–62. The activity pattern of limb muscles in freely moving normal and deafferented newts.

Székely, G., G. Sétáló, and G. Lázár (1973). *J. Hirnforsch.* 14:189–225. Fine structure of the frog's optic tectum: Optic fibre termination layers.

Székely, G., K. Matesz, R. E. Baker, and M. Antal (1982). *Exp. Brain Res.* 45:19–28. The termination of cutaneous nerves in the dorsal horn of the spinal cord in normal and in skin-rotated frogs.

Szeligo, F., and C. P. Leblond (1977). *J. Comp. Neurol.* 172:247–264. Response of the three main types of glial cells of cortex and corpus callosum in rats handled during suckling or exposed to enriched, control and impoverished environments following weaning.

Szentágothai, J. (1948). *J. Comp. Neurol.* 88:207–220. The representation of facial and scalp muscles in the facial nucleus.

Szentágothai, J. (1949). *J. Comp. Neurol.* 90:111–120. Functional representation in the motor trigeminal nucleus.

Szentágothai, J. (1956). *Acta Biol. Acad. Sci. Hung.* 6:215–229. Zum Problem des Kreuzung von Nervenbahnen.

Szentágothai, J., and G. Székely (1956). *Acta Physiol. Acad. Sci. Hung.* 10:43–55. Elementary nervous mechanisms underlying optokinetic responses, analysed by contralateral eye grafts in urodele larvae.

Szepsenwol, J. (1947). *Anat. Rec.* 98:67–85. Electrical excitability and spontaneous activity in explants of skeletal and heart muscles of chick embryos.

Szymonowicz, W. (1895). *Arch. mikr. Anat. Bonn* 14:624–635. Beiträge zur Kenntniss der Nervenendigungen in Hautgebilden. Ueber Bau und Entwickelung der Nervenendigungen in der Schnauze des Schweines.

Taber Pierce, E. (1966). *J. Comp. Neurol.* 126:219–239. Histogenesis of the nuclei griseum pontis, corporis pontobulbaris and reticularis tegmenti pontis (Bechterew) in the mouse: An autoradiographic study.

Taber Pierce, E. (1967a). *J. Comp. Neurol.* 131:27–54. Histogenesis of the dorsal and ventral cochlear nuclei in the mouse: An autoradiographic study.

Taber Pierce, E. (1967b). *Anat. Rec.* 157:301. Histogenesis of deep cerebellar nuclei studied autoradiographically with thymidine-H^3 in the mouse.

Taber Pierce, E. (1973). *Prog. Brain Res.* 40:53–65. Time of origin of neurons in the brain stem of the mouse.

Tachibana, T., and T. Nawa (1980). *J. Anat. (London)* 131:145–155. Merkel cell differentiation in the labial mucous epithelium of the rabbit.

Tachibana, T., Y. Sakakura, K. Ishizeki, S. Iida, and T. Nawa (1983). *Arch. Histol. Jpn.* 46:469–477. An experimental study of the influence of sensory nerve fibers on Merkel cell differentiation in the labial mucosa of the rabbit.

Taghert, P. H., M. J. Bastiani, R. K. Ho, and C. S. Goodman (1982). *Dev. Biol.* 94:391–399. Guidance of pioneer growth cones: Filopodial contacts and coupling revealed with an antibody to Lucifer yellow.

Takada, Y., J. L. Strominger, and M. E. Hemler (1987). *Proc. Natl. Acad. Sci. U.S.A.* 84:3239–3243. The very late antigen family of heterodimers is part of a superfamily of molecules involved in adhesion and embryogenesis.

Takahashi, H., and R. I. Howes (1986). *Anat. Embryol.* 174:283–288. Binding pattern of ferritin-labeled lectins (RCA and WGA) during neural tube closure in the bantam embryo.

Takasaki, H., and H. Konishi (1989). *Dev. Growth. Differ.* 31:147–156. Dorsal blastomeres in the equatorial region of the 32-cell *Xenopus* embryo autonomously produce progeny committed to the organizer.

Takahashi, H., R. I. Howes and J. R. Anglin (1979). *Anat. Rec.* 193:758. Binding pattern of some fluorescent labeled lectins during neural tube closure in the chick embryo.

Takahashi, N., A. Roach, D. B. Teplow, S. B. Prusiner, and L. Hood (1985). *Cell* 42:139–148. Cloning and characterization of the myelin basic protein gene from mouse: One gene can encode both 14 kd and 18.5 kd MBPs by alternate use of exons.

Takahashi, T., Y. Nakajima, K. Hirosawa, S. Nakajima, and K. Onodera (1987). *J. Neurosci.* 7:473–481. Structure and physiology of developing neuromuscular synapses in culture.

Takeichi, M. (1988). *Development* 102:639–655. The cadherins: Cell-cell adhesion molecules controlling animal morphogenesis.

Tam, P. P. L., and R. S. P. Beddington (1987). *Development* 99:109–126. The formation of mesodermal tissues in the mouse embryo during gastrulation and early organogenesis.

Tam. P. P. L., S. Meier and A. G. Jacobson (1982). *Differentiation* 21:109–122. Differentiation of the metameric pattern in the embryonic axis of the mouse. II. Somitomeric organisation of the presomitic mesoderm.

Tan, S. S., and G. M. Morriss-Kay (1985). *Cell Tiss. Res.* 240:403–416. The development and distribution of the cranial neural crest in the rat embryo.

Tan, S. S., and G. M. Morriss-Kay (1986). *J. Embryol. Exp. Morph.* 98:21–58. Analysis of cranial neural crest cell migration and early fates in postimplantation rat chimaeras.

Tanaka, H. (1987). *Dev. Biol.* 124:347–357. Chronic application of curare does not increase the level of motoneuron survival-promoting activity in limb muscle extracts during the naturally occurring motoneuron cell death period.

Tanaka, H., and L. T. Landmesser (1986a). *J. Neurosci.* 6:2880–2888. Interspecies selective motoneuron projection patterns in chick-quail chimeras.

Tanaka, H., and L. T. Landmesser (1986b). *J. Neurosci.* 6:2889–2899. Cell death of lumbosacral motoneurons in chick, quail, and chick-quail chimera embryos: A test of the quantitative matching hypothesis of neuronal cell death.

Tanaka, H., and K. Obata (1982). *Dev. Brain Res.* 4:313–321. Survival and neurite outgrowth of chick embryo spinal cord cells in serum-free culture.

Taniuchi, M., and E. M. Johnson, Jr. (1985). *J. Cell Biol.* 101:1100–1106. Characterization of the binding properties and retrograde axonal transport of a monoclonal antibody directed against the rat nerve growth factor receptor.

Taniuchi, M, H. B. Clark, and E. M. Johnson, Jr. (1986a). *Proc. Natl. Acad. Sci. U.S.A.* 83:4094–4098. Induction of nerve growth factor receptor in Schwann cells after axotomy.

Taniuchi, M., J. B. Schweitzer, and E. M. Johnson, Jr. (1986b). *Proc. Natl. Acad. Sci. U.S.A.* 83:1950–1954. Nerve growth factor receptor molecules in the rat brain.

Taniuchi, M., H. B. Clark, J. B. Schweitzer, and E. M. Johnson, Jr. (1988). *J. Neurosci.* 8:664–681. Expression of nerve growth factor receptors by schwann cells of axotomized peripheral nerves: Ultrastructural location, suppression by axonal contact, and binding properties.

Tanner, J. M., R. H. Whitehouse, and M. Takaishi (1966). *Arch. Dis. Childh.* 41:613–635. Standards from birth to maturity for height, weight, height velocity and weight velocity: British children, 1965.

Tao-Cheng, J.-H., Z. Nagy, and M. Brightman (1986). *Int. J. Dev. Neurosci.* 4:Suppl. 1, S75. Cerebral endothelial tight junctions are modified *in vitro* by primary glial cultures.

Tapscott, S. J., G. S. Bennet, and H. Holtzer (1981a). *Nature* 292:836–838. Neuronal precursor cells in the chick neural tube express neurofilament proteins.

Tapscott, S. J., G. S. Bennet, Y. Toyama, F. Kleinbart, and H. Holtzer (1981b). *Dev. Biol.* 86:40–54. Intermediate filament proteins in the developing chick spinal cord.

Tarrab-Hazdai, R., A. Aharonov, I. Silman, and S. Fuchs (1975). *Nature* 256:128–130. Experimental autoimmune myasthenia induced in monkeys by purified acetylcholine receptor.

Tartakoff, A. M. (1982). *Trends Biochem. Sci.* 7:174–176. Simplifying the complex Golgi.

Tauc, L. (1955). *J. Physiol. Path. Gen.* 47:769–792. Etude de l'activité élémentaire des cellules du ganglion abdominal de l'Aplysie.

Tauchi, M., and R. H. Masland (1984). *Proc. Roy. Soc. (London) Ser. B.* 223:101–119. The shape and arrangement of the cholinergic neurones in the rabbit retina.

Taxi, J., and C. Sotelo (1973). *Brain Res.* 62:431–437. Cytological aspects of the axonal migration of catecholamines and of storage material.

Taxt, T., R. Ding, and J. K. S. Jansen (1983). *Acta Physiol. Scand.* 117:557–560. A note on the elimination of polyneuronal innervation of skeletal muscles in neonatal rats.

Taylor, A. C. (1943). *Anat. Rec.* 87:379–413. Development of the innervation pattern in the limb bud of the frog.

Taylor, A. C. (1944). *J. Exp. Zool.* 96:159–185. Selectivity of nerve fibers from the dorsal and ventral roots in the development of the frog limb.

Taylor, A. C., and J. J. Kollros (1946). *Anat. Rec.* 94:7–23. Stages in the normal development of *Rana pipiens* larvae.

Taylor, D. L., and J. S. Condeelis (1979). *Int. Rev. Cytol.* 56:57–144. Cytoplasmic structure and contractility in amoeboid cells.

Taylor, E. W. (1965). *J. Cell Biol.* 25:145–160. The mechanism of colchicine inhibition of mitosis. I. Kinetics of inhibition and the binding of H^3-colchicine.

Taylor, S., and J. Folkman (1982). *Nature* 297:307–312. Protamine is an inhibitor of angiogenesis.

Teichberg, S., and E. Holtzman (1973). *J. Cell Biol.* 57:88–108. Axonal granular reticulum and synaptic vesicles in cultured embryonic chick sympathetic neurons.

Teichberg, S., E. Holtzman, S. M. Crain, and E. R. Peterson (1975). *J. Cell Biol.* 67:215–230. Circulation and turnover of synaptic vesicle membrane in cultured fetal mammalian spinal cord neurons.

Teilhard de Chardin, P. (1965). *The Phenomenon of Man*, J. M. Cohen, transl. Harper and Row, New York.

Teillet, M.-A., C. Kalcheim, and N. M. Le Douarin (1987). 120:329–347. Formation of the dorsal root ganglia in the avian embryo: Segmental origin and migratory behavior of neural crest progenitor cells.

Tello, J. F. (1917). *Trab. Lab. Invest. Biol. Univ. Madrid* 15:101–199. Genesis de los terminaciones nerviosas motrices y sensitivas. I. En el sistema locomotor de los vertebrados superiores. Histogenesis muscular.

Tello, J. F. (1922a). *Trab. Lab. Invest. Biol. Univ. Madrid* 21:1–93. Les différenciations neuronales dans l'embryon des poulet pendent les premiers jours de l'incubation.

Tello, J. F. (1922b). *Z. Anat. Entw. Gesch. Organ.* 64:348–440. Die Entstehung der motorischen und sensiblen Nervenendigungen. I. In dem lokomotorischen system der hoheren Wirbeltiere: Muskulare histogenese.

Tello, J. F. (1925). *Trab. Lab. Invest. Biol. Univ. Madrid* 23:1–28. Sur la formation des chaines primaires et secondaires du grand sympathique dans l'embryon de poulet.

Tello, J. F. (1932). *Trab. Lab. Invest. Biol. Univ. Madrid* 28:1–58. Contribution a la connaissance des terminaisons sensitives dans les organes genitaux externes et de leur développement.

Tello, J. F. (1935). *Cajal y su labor histologica*. Tipographia Artistica, Madrid.

Temkin, O. (1946). *Bull. Hist. Med.* 20:322–327. Materialism in French and German physiology of the early nineteenth century.

Tennyson, V. M. (1965). *J. Comp. Neurol.* 124:267–318. Electron microscopic study of the developing neuroblast of the dorsal root ganglia of the rabbit embryo.

Tennyson, V. M. (1970). *J. Cell Biol.* **44**:62–79. The fine structure of the axon and growth cone of the dorsal root neuroblast of the rabbit embryo.

Tennyson, V. M., and G. D. Pappas (1962). *Z. Zellforsch. Mikroskop. Anat. Abt. Histochem.* **56**:595–618. An electron microscope study of ependymal cells of the fetal, early postnatal and adult rabbit.

Tennyson, V. M., and G. D. Pappas (1968). The fine structure of the choroid plexus: Adult and developmental stages, pp. 63–85. In *Progress in Brain Research,* vol. 29. Amsterdam, London, New York, Elsevier.

Tennyson, V. M., M. Brzin, and P. E. Duffy (1967). *J. Neuropathol. Exp. Neurol.* **26**:136–137. Cholinesterase localization in the dorsal root ganglion of the rabbit embryo by electron microscopic histochemistry.

Tennyson, V. M., T. D. Pham, T. P. Rothman, and M. D. Gershon (1986). *Anat. Rec.* **215**:267–281. Abnormalities of smooth muscle, basal laminae, and nerves in the aganglionic segments of the bowel of lethal spotted mutant mice.

Terashima, T., K. Inoue, Y. Inoue, K. Mikoshiba, and Y. Tsukada (1983). *J. Comp. Neurol.* **218**:314–326. Distribution and morphology of corticospinal tract neurons in reeler mouse cortex by the retrograde HRP method.

Terashima, T., K. Inoue, Y. Inoue, K. Mikoshiba, and Y. Tsukada (1985a). *J. Comp. Neurol.* **232**:83–98. Distribution and morphology of callosal commissural neurons within the motor cortex of normal and reeler mice.

Terashima, T., K. Inoue, Y. Inoue, K. Mikoshiba, and Y. Tsukada (1985b). *Dev. Brain Res.* **18**:103–112. Observations on Golgi epithelial cells and granule cells in the cerebellum of the reeler mutant mouse.

Terashima, T., K. Inoue, Y. Inoue, M. Yokoyama, and K. Mokoshiba (1986). *J. Comp. Neurol.* **252**:264–278. Observations on the cerebellum of normal-reeler mutant mouse chimera.

Terävänen, H. (1968). *Z. Zellforsch. Mikroskop. Anat. Abt. Histochem.* **87**:249–265. Development of the myoneural junction in the rat.

Tergast, P. (1873). *Arch. f. mikr. Anat.* **9**:36–46. Ueber das Verhältniss von Nerve und Muskel.

Ter Horst, J. (1947). *Arch. Entw.-Mech. Organ.* **143**:275–303. Differenzierungs und Induktionsleistungen verschiedener Abschnitte der Medullarplatte und des Urdarmdaches von Triton im Kombinat.

Terplan, K. L., E. C. Lopez, and H. B. Robinson (1970). *Am. J. Dis. Child.* **119**:228–235. Histologic structural anomalies in the brain in trisomy 18 syndrome.

Terry, R. J., and J. Gordon, Jr. (1960). *J. Exp. Zool.* **143**:245–257. The effects of unilateral and bilateral enucleation on optic lobe development and pigmentation of the skin in *Rana catesbeiana* larvae.

Tessier-Lavigne, M., M. Placzek, A. G. S. Lumsden, J. Dodd, and T. M. Jessell (1988). *Nature* **336**:775–778. Chemotropic guidance of developing axons in the mammalian central nervous system.

Tettenborn, U., R. Dofuku, and S. Ohno (1971). *Nature (New Biol.)* **234**:37–40. Noninducible phenotypes exhibited by a proportion of female mice heterozygous for the X-linked testicular feminization mutation.

Thaller, C., and G. Eichele (1987). *Nature* **327**:625–628.

Identification and spatial distribution of retinoids in the developing chick limb bud.

Thanos, S., and F. Bonhoeffer (1983). *J. Comp. Neurol.* **219**:420–430. Investigations on the development and topographic order of retinotectal axons: Anterograde and retrograde staining of axons and perikarya with rhodamine *in vivo*.

Thanos, S., and F. Bonhoeffer (1984). *J. Comp. Neurol.* **224**:407–414. Development of the transient ipsilateral retinotectal projection in the chick embryo: A numerical fluorescence microscopic analysis.

Thanos, S., and F. Bonhoeffer (1987). *J. Comp. Neurol.* **261**:155–164. Axonal arborization in the developing chick retinotectal system.

Thanos, S., and D. Dütting (1987). *Dev. Brain Res.* **32**:161–179. Outgrowth and directional specificity of fibers from embryonic retinal transplants in the chick optic tectum.

Thanos, S., M. Bähr, Y.-A. Barde, and J. Vanselow (1989). *Eur. J. Neurosci.* **1**:19–26. Survival and axonal elongation of adult rat retinal ganglion cells: *In vitro* effects of lesioned sciatic nerve and brain-derived neurotrophic factor (BDNF).

Thesleff, S. (1960). *Physiol. Rev.* **40**:734–752. Effects of motor innervation on the chemical sensitivity of skeletal muscle.

Thiébaud, C. H. (1983). *Dev. Biol.* **98**:245–249. A reliable new cell marker in *Xenopus*.

Thiery, J. P. (1984). *Cell Diff.* **15**:1–15. Mechanisms of cell migration in the vertebrate embryo.

Thiery, J. P., G. Blanc, A. Sobel, L. Stinus, and J. Glowinski (1973). *Science* **182**:499–501. Dopaminergic terminals in the rat cortex.

Thiery, J. P., R. Brackenbury, U. Rutishauser, and G. M. Edelman (1977). *J. Biol. Chem.* **252**:6841–6845. Adhesion among neural cells of the chick embryo. II. Purification and characterization of a cell molecule from neural retina.

Thiery, J. P., J.-L. Duband, and A. Delouvée (1982a). *Dev. Biol.* **93**:324–343. Pathways and mechanisms of avian trunk neural crest migration and localization.

Thiery, J. P., J.-L. Duband, U. Rutishauser, and G. M. Edelman (1982b). *Proc. Natl. Acad. Sci. U.S.A.* **79**:6737–6741. Cell adhesion molecules in early chick embryogenesis.

Thiery, J. P., A. Delouvée, W. J. Gallin, B. A. Cunningham, and G. M. Edelman (1983). *Dev. Biol.* **102**:61–78. Ontogenetic expression of cell adhesion molecules: L-CAM is found in epithelia derived from the three primary germ layers.

Thiery, J. P., G. C. Tucker and H. Aoyama (1984a). Gangliogenesis in the avian embryo: Migration and adhesion properties of neural crest cells. In *Molecular Basis of Neural Development* (G. M. Edelman, and W. E. Gall, eds.), John Wiley and Sons, New York.

Thiery, J. P., A. Delouvee, W. J. Gallin, B. A. Cunningham, and G. M. Edelman (1984b). *Dev. Biol.* **102**:61–78. Ontogenic expression of cell adhesion molecules: L-CAM is found in epithelia derived from the three primary germ layers.

Thiery, J. P., J.-L. Duband, and G. C. Tucker (1985). *Ann. Rev. Cell Biol.* **1**:91–113. Cell migration in the vertebrate embryo.

Thoa, N. B., G. F. Wooten, J. Axelrod, and I. J. Kopin (1972). *Proc. Nat. Acad. Sci. U.S.A.* **69**:520–522. Inhibition of release of dopamine-B-hydroxylase and norepinephrine from sympathetic nerves by colchicine, vinblastine or cytochalasin.

Thoenen, H. and Y.-A. Barde (1980). *Physiol. Rev.* 60:1284–1335. Physiology of nerve growth factor.

Thoenen, H., and D. Edgar (1985). *Science* 229:238–242. Neurotrophic factors.

Thoenen, H., and G. W. Kreutzberg (1981). *Neurosci. Res. Prog. Bull.* 20:45–55. The role of fast transport in the nervous system.

Thoenen, H., P. U. Angeletti, R. Levi-Montalcini, and R. Kettler (1971). *Proc. Natl. Acad. Sci. U.S.A.* 68:1598–1602. Selective induction by nerve growth factor of tyrosine hydroxylase and dopamine β-hydroxylase in the rat superior cervical ganglia.

Thoenen, H., A. Saner, R. Kettler, and P. U. Angeletti (1972). *Brain Res.* 44:593–602. Nerve growth factor and preganglionic cholinergic nerves; their relative importance to the development of the terminal adrenergic neuron.

Thoenen, H., C. Bandtlow, and R. Heumann (1987). *Rev. Physiol. Biochem. Pharmacol.* 109:145–178. The physiological function of nerve growth factor in the central nervous system: Comparison with the periphery.

Thom, R. (1975). *Structural Stability and Morphogenesis. An Outline of a General Theory of Models.* W. A. Benjamin, Inc., Reading, Mass.

Thomas, G. A. (1948). *J. Anat. (London)* 82:135–145. Quantitative histology of Wallerian degeneration, II. Nuclear population in two nerves of different fibre spectrum.

Thomas, P. K. (1955). *Proc. Roy. Soc. (London) Ser. B.* 143:380–391. Growth changes in myelin sheath of peripheral nerve fibers in fishes.

Thomas, P. K. (1970). *J. Anat. (London)* 106:463–470. The cellular response to nerve injury. III. The effect of repeated crush injuries.

Thomas, P. K., and J. Z. Young (1949). *J. Anat. (London)* 83:336–350. Internode lengths in nerves of fishes.

Thomas, W. A., and J. Yancey (1988). *Development* 103:37–48. Can retinal adhesion mechanisms determine cell-sorting patterns: A test of the differential adhesion hypothesis.

Thomas, Y. M., K. S. Bedi, C. A. Davies, and J. Dobbing (1979). *Early Hum. Dev.* 3/2:109–126. A stereological analysis of the neuronal and synaptic content of the frontal and cerebellar cortex of weanling rats undernourished from birth.

Thompson, C. C., C. Weinberger, R. Lebo, and R. M. Evans (1987). *Science* 237:1610–1614. Identification of a novel thyroid hormone receptor expressed in the mammalian central nervous system.

Thompson, H. (1899). *J. Comp. Neurol.* 9:113–140. The total number of functional nerve cells in the cerebral cortex of man.

Thompson, W. (1978). *Acta Physiol. Scand.* 103:81–91. Reinnervation of partially denervated rat soleus muscles.

Thompson, W. (1983). *Nature* 302:614–616. Synapse elimination in neonatal rat muscle is sensitive to pattern of muscle use.

Thompson, W. (1985). *Cell. Mol. Neurobiol.* 5:167–182. Activity and synapse elimination at the neuromuscular junction.

Thompson, W. J. (1983). *J. Physiol. (London)* 335:343–352.

Lack of segmental selectivity in elimination of synapses from soleus muscle of new-born rats.

Thorpe, W. H. (1961). *Bird-Song*, Columbia Univ. Press, Cambridge.

Thorpe, W. H. (1964). *Learning and Instinct in Animals.* Methuen and Co., London.

Threlfal, R. (1930). *Biol. Rev.* 5:357–361. The origin of the automatic microtome.

Thudichum, J. L. W. (1876). *Report Med. Off. Privy Council, n. s. 8, Appendix 6*, pp. 117–149. (On Kephalin and Myelin, p. 131).

Thudichum, J. L. W. (1884). *A Treatise on the Chemical Constitution of the Brain.* Baillière, Tindall and Cox, London.

Tickle, C., A. Crawley, and J. Farrar (1989). *Development* 106:691–705. Retinoic acid application to chick wing buds leads to a dose-dependent reorganization of the apical ectodermal ridge that is mediated by the mesenchyme.

Tiedemann, F. (1816). *Anatomie und Bildungsgeschichte des Gehirns im Foetus des Menschen nebst einer vergleichenden Darstellung des Hirnbaues in den Thieren.* Steinischen Buchhandlung, Nuremberg. (English transl. by W. Bennet, 1823, *The anatomy of the foetal brain*, Carfrae, Edinburgh).

Tiedemann, F. (1836). *Phil. Trans. Roy. Soc. (London) Ser. B.* 23:497–527. On the brain of the Negro compared with that of the European and the Orang-Outang.

Tiedemann, H. (1968). *J. Cell. Physiol.* 72:Suppl. 129–144. Factors determining embryonic differentiation.

Tiegs, O. W. (1927). *Aust. J. Exp. Biol. Med. Sci.* 4:193–212. A critical review of the evidence on which is based the theory of discontinuous synapses in the spinal cord.

Tiegs, O. W. (1953). *Physiol. Rev.* 33:90–144. Innervation of voluntary muscle.

Tigges, J., W. B. Spatz, and M. Tigges (1973). *J. Comp. Neurol.* 148:481–490. Reciprocal point-to-point connections between parastriate and striate cortex in the squirrel monkey (*Saimiri*).

Tilney, F. (1933). *Bull. Neurol. Inst. N.Y.* 3:252–358. Behavior in its relation to the development of the brain. Part II. Correlation between the development of the brain and behavior in the albino rat from embryonic states to maturity.

Tilney, F., and L. Casamajor (1924). *Arch. Neurol. Psychiat.* 12:1–6. Myelogeny as applied to the study of behavior.

Tilney, L. G., and S. Inoue (1982). *J. Cell Biol.* 93:820–827. Acrosomal reaction of *Thyone* sperm. II. The kinetics and possible mechanism of acrosomal process elogation.

Tilney, L. G., and M. Mooseker (1971). *Proc. Natl. Acad. Sci. U.S.A.* 68:2611–2615. Actin in the brush of epithelial cells of the chicken intestine.

Tilney, L. G., J. Bryan, D. J. Bush, K. Fujiwara, M. S. Mooseker, D. B. Murphy, and D. H. Snyder (1973) *J. Cell Biol.* 59:267–275. Microtubules: Evidence for 13 protofilaments.

Tilney, L. G., E. M. Bonder, and D. J. DeRosier (1981). *J. Cell Biol.* 90:485–494. Actin filaments elongate from their membrane-associated ends.

Timpe, L., E. Martz, and M. S. Steinberg (1978). *J. Cell Sci.* 30:293–304. Cell movement in a confluent monolayer are not caused by gaps: Evidence for direct contact inhibition of overlapping.

Timpl, R., and M. Dziadek (1986). *Int. Rev. Exp. Pathol.*

29:1–112. Structure, development, and molecular pathology of basement membrane.

Titchener, E. B. (1921). *Amer. J. Psychol.* 32:161–178, 575–580. Wilhelm Wundt.

Tizard, B. (1959). *Med. Hist.* 3:132–145. Theories of brain localization from Flourens to Lashley.

Tizard, J. (1974). *Br. Med. Bull.* 30:169–174. Early malnutrition, growth and mental development in man.

Tobet, S. A., and M. J. Baum (1987). *Horm. Behav.* 21:419–429. Role for prenatal estrogen in the development of masculine sexual behavior in the male ferret.

Tobet, S. A., D. J. Zahniser, and M. J. Baum (1986). *Brain Res.* 364:249–257. Sexual dimorphism in the preoptic/anterior hypothalamic area of ferrets: Effects of adult exposure to sex steroids.

Todd, P. H. (1982). *J. Theor. Biol.* 97:529–538. A geometric model for the cortical folding pattern of simple folded brains.

Togari, A., D. Baker, G. Dickens, and G. Guroff (1983). *Biochem. Biophys. Res. Comm.* 114:1189–1193. The neurite-promoting effect of fibroblast growth factor on PC12 cells.

Toivonen, S., and S. Saxén (1955a). *Exp. Cell Res. Suppl.* 3:346–357. The simultaneous inducing action of liver and bone-marrow of the guinea-pig in implantation and explantation experiments with embryos of triturus.

Toivonen, S., and L. Saxén (1955b). *Ann. Acad. Sci. Fenn. A.* 30:1–29. Ueber die Induktion des Neuralrohrs bei Trituruskeimen als simultane Leistungs des Leber- und Knochenmarkgewebes vom Meerschweinchen.

Toivonen, S., and L. Saxén (1968). *Science* 159:539–540. Morphogenetic interaction of presumptive neural and mesodermal cells mixed in different ratios.

Toivonen, S., D. Tarin, L. Saxén, P. J. Tarin, and J. Wartiovaara (1975). *Differentiation* 4:1–7. Transfilter studies on neural induction in the newt.

Toivonen, S., D. Tarin, and S. Saxén (1976). *Differentiation* 5:49–55. The transmission of morphogenetic signals from amphibian mesoderm to ectoderm in primary induction.

Tolbert, L. P., and L. A. Oland (1989). *Trends Neurosci.* 12:70–75. A role for glia in the development of organized neuropilar structures.

Tomanek, R. J., and D. L. Lund (1974). *J. Anat. (London)* 118:531–541. Degeneration of different types of skeletal muscles fibres. II. Immobilization.

Tomaselli, K. J., and L. F. Reichart (1988). *J. Neurosci. Res.* 21:275–285. Peripheral motoneuron interactions with laminin and schwann cell-derived neurite-promoting molecules: Developmental regulation of laminin receptor function.

Tomaselli, K. J., K. M. Neugebauer, J. L. Bixby, J. Lilien, and L. F. Reichardt (1988). *Neuron* 1:33–43. N-cadherin and integrins: Two receptor systems that mediate neuronal process outgrowth on astrocyte surfaces.

Tonge, D. A. (1974a). *J. Physiol. (London)* 236:22–23. Reinnervation of skeletal muscle in the mouse.

Tonge, D. A. (1974b). *J. Physiol. (London)* 239:96–97. Synaptic function in experimental dually innervated muscle in the mouse.

Tonge, D. A. (1974c). *J. Physiol. (London)* 241:141–153. Physiological characteristics of re-innervation of skeletal muscle in the mouse.

Tootell, R. B. H., and S. L. Hamilton (1989). *J. Neurosci.* 9:2620–2644. Functional anatomy of the second visual area (V2) in the macaque.

Tootell, R. B. H., M. S. Silverman, E. Switkes, and R. L. De Valois (1982). *Science* 218:902–904. Deoxyglucose analysis of retinotopic organization in primate striate cortex.

Tootell, R. B. H., M. S. Silverman, R. L. De Valois, and G. H. Jacobs (1983). *Science* 220:737–739. Functional organization of the second cortical visual area of primates.

Tootell, R. B. H., S. L. Hamilton, M. S. Silverman, and E. Switkes (1988a). *J. Neurosci.* 8:1500–1530. Functional anatomy of macaque striate cortex. I. Ocular dominance, baseline conditions, and binocular interactions.

Tootell, R. B. H., E. Switkes, M. S. Silverman, and S. L. Hamilton (1988b). *J. Neurosci.* 8:1531–1568. Functional anatomy of macaque striate cortex. II. Retinotopic organization.

Tootell, R. B. H., M. S. Silverman, S. L. Hamilton, R. L. De Valois, and E. Switkes (1988c). *J. Neurosci.* 8:1569–1593. Functional anatomy of macaque striate cortex. III. Color.

Tootell, R. B. H., S. L. Hamilton, and E. Switkes (1988d). *J. Neurosci.* 8:1594–1609. Functional anatomy of macaque striate cortex. IV. Contrast and magno/parvo streams.

Tootell, R. B. H., M. S. Silverman, S. L. Hamilton, E., Switkes, and R. L. De Valois (1988e). *J. Neurosci.* 8:1610–1624. Functional anatomy of macaque striate cortex. V. Spatial frequency.

Tooth, H. H. (1893). *The Gulstonian Lectures on Secondary Degenerations of the Spinal Cord.* Churchill, London.

Toran-Allerand, C. D. (1984). *Brain Res.* 61:63–97. On the genesis of sexual differentiation of the central nervous system: Morphogenetic consequences of steroidal exposure and possible role of alpha-fetoprotein.

Torrey, T. W. (1934). *J. Comp. Neurol.* 59:203–220. The relation of taste buds to their nerve fibers.

Torrey, T. W. (1936). *J. Comp. Neurol.* 64:325–336. The relation of nerves to degenerating taste buds.

Torrey, T. W. (1940). *Proc. Natl. Acad. Sci. U.S.A.* 26:627–634. The influence of nerve fibers upon taste buds during embryonic development.

Torvik, A. (1956). *J. Neuropathol. Exp. Neurol.* 15:119–145. Transneuronal changes in the inferior olive and pontine nuclei in kittens.

Torvik, A. (1972). *J. Neuropathol. Exp. Neurol.* 31:132–146. Phagocytosis of nerve cells during retrograde degeneration.

Torvik, A. (1975). *Acta Neuropathol.* 6:297–300. The relationship between microglia and brain macrophages. Experimental investigations.

Torvik, A. (1976). *Neuropathol. Appl. Neurobiol.* 2:423–432. Central chromatolysis and the axon reaction: A reappraisal.

Torvik, A., and A. Heding (1969). *Acta Neuropathol.* 14:62–71. Effect of actinomycin D on retrograde nerve cell reaction. Further observations.

Torvik, A., and F. Skjörten (1971a). *Acta Neuropathol.* 17:248–264. Electron microscopic observations on nerve cell regeneration and degeneration after axon lesions. I. Changes in the nerve cell cytoplasm.

Torvik, A., and F. Skjörten (1971b). *Acta Neuropathol.* 17:265–282. Electron microscopic observations on nerve cell regeneration and degeneration after axon lesions. II. Changes in the glial cells.

Torvik, A., and F. Skjörten (1974). *J. Neurocytol.* 3:87–97. The effect of actinomycin D. upon normal neurons and retrograde nerve cell reaction.

Torvik, A., and A. J. Söreide (1972). *J. Neuropathol. Exp. Neurol.* 31: 683–695. *Brain Res.* 95:519–529. The perineuronal glial reaction after axotomy.

Toschi, G., E. Dore, P. U. Angeletti, R. Levi-Montalcini, and C. H. Dehaën (1965). *J. Neurochem.* 13:539–544. Characteristics of labelled RNA from spinal ganglia of chick embryo and the action of a specific growth factor (NGF).

Tosney, K. W. (1982). *Dev. Biol.* 89:13–24. The segregation and early migration of cranial neural crest cells in the avian embryo.

Tosney, K. W., and L. T. Landmesser (1984). *J. Neurosci.* 4:2518–2527. Pattern and specificity of axonal outgrowth following varying degrees of chick limb bud ablation.

Tosney, K. W., and L. T. Landmesser (1985a). *J. Neurosci.* 5:2336–2344. Specificity of early motoneuron growth cone outgrowth in the chick embryo.

Tosney, K. W., and L. T. Landmesser (1985b). *J. Neurosci.* 5:2345–2358. Growth cone morphology and trajectory in the lumbosacral region of the chick embryo.

Tosney, K. W., and L. T. Landmesser (1985c). *Dev. Biol.* 109:193–214. Development of the major pathways for neurite outgrowth in the chick hindlimb.

Tosney, K. W., S. Schroeter, and J. A. Pokrzywinski (1988). *Dev. Biol.* 130:558–572. Cell death delineates axon pathways in the hindlimb and does so independently of neurite outgrowth.

Toth, L. E., K. L. Slavin, J. E. Pintar, and M. Chi Nguyen-Huu (1987). *Proc. Natl. Acad. Sci. U.S.A.* 84:6790–6794. Region-specific expression of mouse homeobox genes in the embryonic mesoderm and central nervous system.

Toulmin, S. (1967). *Amer. Sci.* 55:456–471. The evolutionary development of natural science.

Toulmin, S. (1972). *Human Understanding.* Clarendon Press, Oxford.

Towbin, H., T. Staehelin, and J. Gordon (1979). *Proc. Natl. Acad. Sci. U.S.A.* 76:4350–4354. Electorphoretic transfer of proteins from polyacrylamide gels to nitrocellulose sheets: Procedure and some applications.

Towe, A. L. (1975). *Brain Behav. Evol.* 11:16–47. Notes on the hypothesis of columnar organization in somatosensory cerebral cortex.

Tower, D. B. (1970). Johann Ludwig Wilhelm Thudichum (1829–1901), pp. 297–302. In *Founders of Neurology,* 2nd edn., (W. Haymaker, and F. Schiller, eds.), Thomas, Springfield, Illinois.

Tower, S. S. (1932). *Brain* 55:77–89. Atrophy and degeneration in the muscle spindle.

Tower, S. S. (1937a). *J. Comp. Neurol.* 67:109–131. Function and structure in the chronically isolated lumbo-sacral spinal cord of the dog.

Tower, S. S. (1937b). *J. Comp. Neurol.* 67:241–269. Trophic control of non-nervous tissues by the nervous system: A study of muscle and bone innervated from an isolated and quiescent region of spinal cord.

Townes, P. L., and J. Holtfreter (1955). *J. Exp. Zool.* 128:53–120. Directed movements and selective adhesions of embryonic amphibian cells.

Toynbee, A. J. (1954). *A Study of History,* Vol. 9, *Contacts Between Civilizations in Time (Renaissances).* Oxford Univ. Press, New York, 1962.

Trapp, B. D. (1988). *J. Cell Biol.* 107:675–685. Distribution of the myelin-associated glycoprotein and P_o protein during myelin compaction in quaking mouse peripheral nerve.

Trapp, B. D., and R. H. Quarles (1982). *J. Cell Biol.* 92:877–882. Presence of the myelin-associated glycoprotein correlates with alterations in the periodicity of peripheral myelin.

Trapp, B. D., and R. H. Quarles (1984). *J. Neuroimmunol.* 6:231–249. Immunocytochemical localization of the myelin-associated glycoprotein. Fact or artifact?

Trapp, B. D., Y. Itoyama, N. H. Sternberger, R. H. Quarles, and H. deF. Webster (1981). *J. Cell Biol.* 90:1–6. Immunocytochemical localization of P_o protein in Golgi complex membranes and myelin of developing rat Schwann cells.

Trapp, B. D., T. Moench, M. Pulley, E. Barbosa, G. Tennekoon, and J. Griffin (1987). *Proc. Natl. Acad. Sci. U.S.A.* 84:7773–7777. Spatial segregation of mRNA encoding myelin-specific proteins.

Trapp, B. D., P. Hauer, and G. Lemke (1988). *J. Neurosci.* 8:3515–3521. Axonal regulation of myelin protein mRNA levels in actively myelinating Schwann cells.

Traub, P. (1985). *Intermediate Filaments: A Review.* Springer-Verlag, Berlin.

Triarhou, L. C., and B. Ghetti (1986). *Neuroscience* 18:795–807. Monoaminergic nerve terminals in the cerebellar cortex of Purkinje cell degeneration mutant mice: Fine structural integrity and modification of cellular environs following loss of Purkinje and granule cells.

Trimble, W. S., and R. H. Scheller (1988). *Trends Neurosci.* 11:241–242. Molecular biology of synaptic vesicle-associated proteins.

Trimmer, P. A., P. J. Reier, T. H. Oh, and L. F. Eng (1982). *J. Neuroimmunol.* 2:235–260. An ultrastructural and immunocytochemical study of astrocytic differentiation *in vitro*.

Trinkaus, J. P. (1966). Morphogenetic cell movements, pp. 125–176. In *Major Problems in Developmental Biology* (M. Locke, ed.), Academic Press, New York.

Trinkaus, J. P. (1984). *Cells Into Organs. The Forces that Shape the Embryo.* 2nd edn. Prentice-Hall, New Jersey.

Trisler, D., and F. Collins (1987). *Science* 237:1208–1209. Corresponding spatial gradients of TOP molecules in the developing retina and optic tectum.

Trisler, G. D., M. D. Schneider, and M. Nirenberg (1981). *Proc. Natl. Acad. Sci. U.S.A.* 78:2145–2149. A topographic gradient of molecules in retina can be used to identify neuron position.

Troeltsch, E. (1922a). *Der Historismus und seine Probleme.* Tübingen.

Troeltsch, E. (1922b). *Die Neue Rundschau* 33:572–590. Die Krisis des Historismus.

Trujillo-Cenoz, O. (1962). *Z. Zellforsch. Mikroskop. Anat. Abt. Histochem.* 56:649–682. Some aspects of the structural organization of the arthropod ganglia.

Truman, J. W. (1983). *J. Comp. Neurol.* 216:445–452. Programmed cell death in the nervous system of an adult insect.

Truman, J. W. (1984). *Ann. Rev. Neurosci.* 7:171–188. Cell death in invertebrate nervous systems.

Truman, J. W., and L. M. Schwartz (1982). *Neurosci. Comm.* 1:66–72. Insect systems for the study of programmed neuronal death.

Trumpy, J. H. (1971). *Ergebn. Anat. Entwick.* 44:7–70. Transneuronal degeneration in the pontine nuclei of the cat. I. Neuronal changes in animals of varying ages.

Trune, D. R. (1982a). *J. Comp. Neurol.* 209:409–424. Influence of neonatal cochlear removal on the development of mouse cochlear nucleus. I. Number, size, and density of its neurons.

Trune, D. R. (1982b). *J. Comp. Neurol.* 209:425–434. Influence of neonatal cochlear removal on the development of mouse cochlear nucleus. II. Dendritic morphometry of its neurons.

Tsai, H. M., B. B. Garber, and L. M. H. Larramendi (1981). *J. Comp. Neurol.* 198:293–306. H-thymidine autoradiographic analysis of the telencephalic histogenesis in the chick embryo. II. Dynamic of neuronal migration displacement and aggregation.

Tsang, Y. (1937). *J. Comp. Neurol.* 66:211–261. Visual centers in blinded rats.

Tsang, Y. (1939). *J. Comp. Neurol.* 70:1–8. Ventral horn cells and polydactyly in mice.

Tschumi, P. A. (1957). *J. Anat. (London)* 91:149–173. The growth of the hindlimb bud of *Xenopus laevis* and its dependence upon the epidermis.

Tse, A. G. D., A. Barclay, A. Watts, and A. F. Williams (1985). *Science* 230:1003–1008. A glycophospholipid tail at the carboxyl terminus of the *Thy-1* glycoprotein of neurons and thymocytes.

Tsiang, H. (1979). *J. Neuropathol. Exp. Neurol.* 38:286–296. Evidence for an intra-axonal transport of fixed and street rabies virus.

Tsui, H.-C. T., K. L. Lankford, and W. L. Klein (1985). *Proc. Natl. Acad. Sci. U.S.A.* 82:8256–8260. Differentiation of neuronal growth cones: Specialization of filopodial tips for adhesive interactions.

Tsui, H.-C. T., D. Schubert, and W. L. Klein (1988). *J. Cell Biol.* 106:2095–2108. Molecular basis of growth cone adhesion: Anchoring of adheron-containing filaments at adhesive loci.

Tsui, H. T., H. Ris, and W. L. Klein (1983). *Proc. Natl. Acad. Sci. U.S.A.* 80:5779–5783. Ultrastructural networks in growth cones and neurites of cultured central nervous system neurons.

Tsukita, S., and H. Ishikawa (1980). *J. Cell Biol.* 84:513–530. The movement of membranous organelles in axons. Electron microscopic identification of anterogradely and retrogradely transported organelles.

Tucker, G. C., G. Ciment, and J. P. Thiery (1986). *Dev. Biol.* 116:439–450. Pathways of avian neural crest cell migration in the developing gut.

Tucker, R. P., and C. A. Erickson (1984). *Dev. Biol.* 104:390–405. Morphology and behavior of quail neural crest cells in artificial three-dimensional matrices.

Tucker, R. P., and C. A. Erickson (1986). *J. Embryol. Exp. Morph.* 97:141–168. The control of pigment cell pattern formation in the California newt, *Taricha torosa*.

Tucker, R. P., L. I. Binder, and A. I. Matus (1988a). *Dev. Brain Res.* 38:313–318. Differential localization of developmentally-regulated MAP2 isoforms in the retina.

Tucker, R. P., L. I. Binder, and A. I. Matus (1988b). *J. Comp. Neurol.* 271:44–55. Neuronal microtubule-associated proteins in the embryonic avian spinal cord.

Tucker, R. P., L. I. Binder, C. Viereck, B. A. Hemmings, and A. I. Matus (1988c). *J. Neurosci.* 8:4503–4512. The sequential appearance of low- and high-molecular-weight forms of MAP2 in the developing cerebellum.

Tucker, R. P., C. Viereck, and A. I. Matus (1988d). *Protoplasma* 145:195–199. The ontogeny and phylogenetic conservation of MAP2 forms.

Tucker, T. J., and A. Kling (1967). *Brain Res.* 5:377–389. Differential effects of early and late lesions of frontal granular cortex in the monkey.

Tuckett, F., and G. M. Morriss-Kay (1985). *J. Embryol. Exp. Morph.* 85:111–119. The kinetic behavior of the cranial neural epithelium during neurulation in the rat.

Tuffery, A. R. (1971). *J. Anat. (London)* 110:221–247. Growth and degeneration of motor end-plates in normal cat hind limb muscles.

Tumbleson, M. E. (1973). *Growth* 37:13–17. Brain weight, as a function of age, in miniature swine.

Tuohimaa, P., and R. Johansson (1971). *Endocrinology* 88:1159–1164. Decreased estradiol binding in the uterus and anterior hypothalamus of androgenized female rats.

Tuohimaa, P., and M. Niemi (1972). *Acta Endocrinol. (Kbh)* 71:45–54. *In vitro* uptake of tritiated sex steroids by the hypothalamus of adult male rats treated neonatally with an antiandrogen (cyproterone).

Türck, L. (1852). *Z. König. Kais. Gesellsch. Wien.* 2:511. Ueber secundäre Erkrankung einzelner Rückenmarksstränge und ihrer Fortsetzungen zum Gehirne.

Turing, A. (1952). *Phil. Trans. Roy. Soc. (London) Ser. B.* 237:37–72. The chemical basis of morphogenesis.

Turner, A. M., and W. T. Greenough (1985). *Brain Res.* 329:195–203. Differential rearing effects on rat visual cortex synapses. I. Synaptic and neuronal density and synapses per neuron.

Turner, B. B. (1978). *Am. Zool.* 18:461–475. Ontogeny of glucocorticoid binding in rodent brain.

Turner, D. L., and C. Cepko (1987a). *Soc. Neurosci. Abstr.* 13:700. Use of a retroviral vector-mediated gene transfer to study cell lineage and differentiation in rat retina.

Turner, D. L., and C. Cepko (1987b). *Nature* 328:131–136. A common progenitor for neuron and glia persists in the rat retina late in development.

Turner, P. T., and A. B. Harris (1974). *Brain Res.* 74:305–326. Ultrastructure of exogenous peroxidase in cerebral cortex.

Turner, W. (1891). *J. Anat. (London)* 25:105–153. The convolutions of the brain: A study in comparative anatomy.

Turpen, J. B., and C. M. Knudson (1982). *Dev. Biol.* 89:138–151. Ontogeny of hematopoietic cells in *Rana pipiens*: Precursor cell migration during embryogenesis.

Tweedle, C. D. (1978). *Neuroscience* 3:481–486. Ultrastructure of Merkel cell development in aneurogenic and control amphibian larvae (*Ambystoma*).

Twitty, V. C. (1932). *J. Exp. Zool.* 61:333–374. Influence of the eye on the growth of its associated structures, studied by means of heteroplastic transplantation.

Twitty, V. C. (1955). Organogenesis: The eye, pp. 402–414. In *Analysis of Development* (B. H. Willier, P. A. Weiss, and V. Hamburger, eds.), Saunders, Philadelphia.

Twitty, V. C., and J. L. Schwind (1931). *J. Exp. Zool.* 59:61–86. The growth of eyes and limbs transplanted heteroplastically between two species of *Amblystoma*.

Uchizono, K. (1965). *Nature* 207:642–643. Characteristics of excitatory and inhibitory synapses in the central nervous system of the cat.

Uchizono, K. (1966). *Jap. J. Physiol.* 16:570–575. Excitatory and inhibitory synapses in the cat spinal cord.

Udenfriend, S. (1966). *Harvey Lect.* 60:57–83. Biosynthesis of the sympathetic neurotransmitter, norepinephrine.

Udin, S. B. (1975). *Neurosci. Abstr.* 2:799. Retinotectal plasticity after half-tectum ablation in adult frogs.

Udin, S. B. (1976). *Neurosci. Abstr.* II/(2):1213. Progressive alterations in optic tract and retinotectal topography during optic nerve regeneration in *Rana pipiens*.

Udin, S. B. (1977). *J. Comp. Neurol.* 173:561–583. Rearrangement of the retinotectal projection in *Rana pipiens* after unilateral caudal half-tectum ablation.

Udin, S. B. (1983). *Nature* 301:336–338. Abnormal visual input leads to development of abnormal axon trajectories in frog.

Udin, S. B., and J. W. Fawcett (1988). *Ann. Rev. Neurosci.* 11:289–327. Formation of topographic maps.

Udin, S. B., and M. D. Fisher (1986). *Soc. Neurosci. Abstr.* 12:1028. Electron microscopy of crossed isthmotectal axons in *Xenopus laevis* frogs.

Udin, S. B., and M. J. Keating (1981). *J. Comp. Neurol.* 203:575–594. Plasticity in a central nervous pathway in *Xenopus:* Anatomical changes in the isthmotectal projection after larval eye rotation.

Udin, S. B., M. D. Fisher, and J. J. Norden (1990). *J. Comp. Neurol.* 292:246–254. Ultrastructure of the crossed isthmotectal projection in *Xenopus* frogs.

Ueda, S., H. Ito, H. Masai, and T. Kawahara (1979). *Brain Res.* 177:183–188. Abnormal organization of the cerebellar cortex in the mutant Japanese quail, *Coturnix coturnix japonica*.

Uga, S., and K. Hama (1967). *J. Electron Microsc.* 16:269–276. Electron microscopic studies on the synaptic region of the taste organ of carps and frogs.

Ugolini, G., H. G. J. M. Kuypers, and A. Simmons (1987). *Brain Res.* 422:242–256. Retrograde transneuronal transfer of herpes simplex virus 1 (HSV1) from motoneurons.

Ugolini, G., H. G. J. M. Kuypers, and P. L. Strick (1989). *Science* 243:89–91. Transneuronal transfer of herpes virus from peripheral nerves to cortex and brainstem.

Ulett, G., Jr., R. S. Dow, and O. Larsell (1944). *J. Comp. Neurol.* 80:1–10. The inception of conductivity in the corpus callosum and the cortico-pontocerebellar pathway of young rabbits with reference to myelination.

Ulfhake, B., and S. Cullheim (1986). *Neurosci. Lett.* 26:492. Direct contacts between dendrites and blood vessels in the cat spinal cord.

Ulfhake, B., and S. Cullheim (1988). *J. Comp. Neurol.* 278:88–102. Postnatal development of cat hind limb motoneurons. II: *In vivo* morphology of dendritic growth cones and the maturation of dendrite morphology.

Ulfhake, B., and J.-O Kellerth (1981). *J. Comp. Neurol.* 202:571–584. A quantitative light microscopic study of the dendrites of cat spinal alpha-motoneurons after intracellular staining with horseradish peroxidase.

Ulfhake, B., and J.-O. Kellerth (1983). *Brain Res.* 264:1–20. A quantitative morphological study of HRP-labeled cat alpha-motoneurones supplying different muscles.

Ulfhake, B., S. Cullheim, and P. Franson (1988). *J. Comp. Neurol.* 278:69–87. Postnatal development of cat hind limb motoneurons. I. Changes in length, branching structure, and spatial distribution of dendrites of cat triceps surae motoneurons.

Umansky, S. R. (1977). *J. Theor. Biol.* 97:591–602. The genetic program of cell death. Hypothesis and some applications: Transformation, carcinogenesis, aging.

Unna, P. G. (1890). *Monatsschr. Prak. Dermatol.* 11:366–367. Über die Taenzersche (Orcein-) Färbung des elastischen Gewebes.

Unna, P. G. (1891). *Z. wiss. Mikrosk* 8:475–487. Über die Reifung unserer Farbstoffe.

Unsicker, K., B. Krisch, J. Otten and H. Thoenen (1978). *Proc. Natl. Acad. Sci. U.S.A.* 75:3498–3502. Nerve growth factor-induced fiber outgrowth from isolated rat adrenal chromaffin cells: Impairment by glucocorticoids.

Unsicker, K., J. Vey, H. Hofmann, T. H. Mueller, and A. J. Wilson (1984). *Proc. Natl. Acad. Sci. U.S.A.* 81:2242–2246. C6 glioma cell-conditioned medium induces neurite outgrowth and survival of rat chromaffin cells *in vitro:* Comparison with the effects of nerve growth factor.

Unsicker, K., H. Reichert-Preibsch, R. Schmidt, B. Pettmann, G. Labourdette, and M. Sensenbrenner (1987). *Proc. Natl. Acad. Sci. U.S.A.* 84:5459–5463. Astroglial and fibroblast growth factors have neurotrophic functions for cultured peripheral and central nervous system neurons.

Unzer, J. A. (1771). *The Principles of Physiology,* Transl. T. Laycock (1851). The Sydenham Society, London.

Uray, N. J. (1985). *J. Comp. Neurol.* 232:129–142. Early stages in the formation of the cerebellum in the frog.

Uray, N. J., and A. G. Gona (1982). *J. Comp. Neurol.* 212:202–207. Golgi studies on Purkinje cell development in the frog during spontaneous metamorphosis. III. Axonal development.

Urbán, L., and G. Székely (1983). *J. Neurobiol.* 14:157–161. Intracellular staining of motoneurons with complex cobalt compounds in the frog.

Usowicz, M. M., V. Gallo, and S. G. Cull-Candy (1989). *Nature* 339:380–383. Multiple conductance channels in type-2 cerebellar astrocytes activated by excitatory amino acids.

Utset, M. F., A. Awgulewitsch, F. H. Ruddle and W. McGinnis (1987). *Science* 235:1379–1382. Region specific expression of two mouse homeo box genes.

Uylings, H. B. M., K. Kuypers, and W. A. M. Veltman (1978). *Prog. Brain Res.* 48: . Environmental influences on cortical development in later life.

Uylings, H. B. M., and G. J. Smit (1975). *Adv. Neurol.* 12:247–253. Ordering methods in quantitative analysis of branching structures of dendritic trees.

Uylings, H. B. M., K. Kuypers, and W. A. M. Veltman (1978). *Prog. Brain Res.* 48:261–274. Environmental influences on the neocortex in later life.

Uylings, H. B. M., R. W. H. Verwer, J. Van Pelt, and J. G. Parnavelas (1983). *ACTA Stereol.* 2:55–62. Topological analysis of dendritic growth at various stages of cerebral development.

Uzman, B. G., and E. T. Hedley-Whyte (1968). *J. Gen. Physiol.* 51:8–18. Myelin: Dynamic or stable?

Uzman, B. G., and G. M. Villegas (1960). *J. Biophys. Biochim. Cytol.* 7:761–762. A comparison of nodes of Ranvier in sciatic nerves with nodelike structures in optic nerves of the mouse.

Uzman, L. L. (1960). *J. Comp. Neurol.* 114:137–160. The histogenesis of the mouse cerebellum as studied by its tritiated thymidine uptake.

Vaage, S. (1969). *Ergeb. Anat. Entwicklungsgesch.* 41:1–88. The segmentation of the primitive neural tube in chick embryos. (*Gallus domesticus*). A morphological, histochemical and autoradiographical investigation.

Vaccaro, D. E., S. E. Leeman, and L. Reif-Lehrer (1979). *J. Neurochem.* 33:953–957. Glutamine synthetase activity *in vivo* and in primary cell cultures of rat hypothalamus.

Valat, J., A. Privat, and J. Fulcrand (1983). *Anat. Embryol.* 167:335–346. Multiplication and differentiation of glial cells in the optic nerve of the postnatal rat.

Valcana, T., and P. S. Timiras (1978). *Molec. Cell. Endocr.* 11:31–41. Nuclear triiodothyronine receptors in the developing rat brain.

Vale, R. D., B. J. Schnapp, T. S. Reese, and M. P. Sheetz (1985a). *Cell* 40:449–454. Movement of organelles along filaments dissociated from axoplasm of the squid giant axon.

Vale, R. D., B. J. Schnapp, T. S. Reese, and M. P. Sheetz (1985b). *Cell* 40:559–569. Organelle, bead and microtubule translocations promoted by soluble factors from the squid giant axon.

Vale, R. D., B. J. Schnapp, T. Mitchison, E. Steuer, T. S. Reese, and M. P. Sheetz (1985c). *Cell* 43:623–632. Different axoplasmic proteins generate movement in opposite directions along microtubules *in vitro*.

Valenstein, E. S. (1986). *Great and Desperate Cures. The Rise and Decline of Psychosurgery and Other Radical Treatments for Mental Illness*. Basic Books, New York.

Valentin, G. (1842). Gewebe des menschlichen und thierischen Körpers, p. 714. In *Handwörterbuch der Physiologie*, Vol. 1, (R. Wagner, ed.), Vieweg, Braunschweig.

Valentin, G. G. (1835). *Handbuch der Entwickelungsgeschichte des Menschen mit vergleichender Rücksicht der Entwickelung der Säugethiere und Vögel*. August Rücker, Berlin.

Valentin, G. G. (1836). *Nova Acta Physico-medica Academiae Caesareae Leopoldino-Carolinae Naturae Curiosorum* 18:51–240. Über den Verlauf und die letzten Enden der Nerven.

Valentin, G. G. (1838). *Repert. Anat. Physiol.* 3:72–80. Kritische Darstellung fremder und Ergebnisse eigener Forschung.

Valentin, G. G. (1839). *Arch. f. Anat. Physiol. wissensch. Med.* pp. 139–164. Ueber die Scheiden der Ganglienkugeln und deren Fortsetzungen.

Valentino, K. L., and E. G. Jones (1981). *Anat. Embryol.* 163:157–172. Morphological and immunocytochemical identification of macrophages in the developing corpus callosum.

Valentino, K. L., E. G. Jones, and S. A. Kane (1983). *Dev. Brain Res.* 9:319–336. Expression of GFAP immunoreactivity during development of long fiber tracts in the rats CNS.

Valinsky, J., and N. M. Le Douarin (1984). *Proc. Natl. Acad. Sci. U.S.A.*. Production of plasminogen activator by migrating cephalic neural crest cells.

Vallee, R. B., H. S. Shpetner, and B. M. Paschal (1989). *Trends Neurosci.* 12:66–70. The role of dynein in retrograde axonal transport.

Valverde, F. (1967). *Exp. Brain Res.* 3:337–352. Apical dendritic spines of the visual cortex and light deprivation in the mouse.

Valverde, F. (1968). *Exp. Brain Res.* 5:274–292. Structural changes in the area striata of the mouse after enucleation.

Valverde, F. (1970). The Golgi method. A tool for comparative structural analyses, pp. 11–31. In *Contemporary Research Methods in Neuroanatomy* (W. H. J. Nauta, and S. O. E. Ebbeson, eds.), Springer, New York.

Valverde, F. (1971) *Brain Res.* 33:1–11. Rate and extent of recovery from dark rearing in the visual cortex of the mouse.

Valverde, F., and M. E. Esteban (1968). *Brain Res.* 9:145–148. Peristriate cortex of mouse: Location and the effects of enucleation on the number of dendritic spines.

Valverde, F., and A. Ruiz-Marcos (1969). *Exp. Brain Res.* 8:269–383. Dendritic spines in the visual cortex of the mouse: Introduction to a mathematical model.

Valverde, F., M. V. Facal-Valverde, M. Santacana, and M. Heredia (1989). *J. Comp. Neurol.* 290:118–140. Development and differentiation of early generated cells of sublayer VIb in the somatosensory cortex of the rat: A correlated Golgi and autoradiographic study.

Van Buren, J. M. (1963). *J. Neurol. Neurosurg. Psychiatry* 26:402–409. Trans-synaptic retrograde degeneration in the visual system of primates.

Van Buren, J. M., and D. A. Maccubin (1962). *J. Neurosurg.* 19:811–839. An outline atlas of the human basal ganglia with estimation of anatomical variants.

Van Buskirk, C. (1945). *J. Comp. Neurol.* 82:303–333. The seventh nerve complex.

Van Campenhout, E. (1930a). *Quart. Rev. Biol.* 5:23–50; 217–234. Historical survey of the development of the sympathetic nervous system.

Van Campenhout, E. (1930b). *J. Exp. Zool.* 56:295–320. Contributions to the problem of the development of the sympathetic nervous system.

Van Campenhout, E. (1931). *Arch. Biol. (Paris)* 42:479–507. Le développement du systéme nerveux sympathique chez le poulet.

Van Campenhout, E. (1935). *J. Exp. Zool.* 72:175–193. Experimental researches on the origin of the acoustic ganglion in amphibian embryos.

Van Campenhout, E. (1937). *Arch. Biol. Liège* 48:611–666. Le développement du système nerveux crânien chez le poulet.

Vandenburg, S. G. (1966). *Psychol. Bull.* 66:327–352. Contributions of twin research to psychology.

van den Eijnden-Van Raaij, A. J. M., E. J. J. van Zoelent, K. van Nimmen, C. H. Koster, G. T. Snoek, A. J. Durston, and D. Huylebroeck. *Nature* 345:732–734. Acitvin-like factor from a *Xenopus laevis* cell line responsible for mesoderm induction.

Van der Loos, H. (1965). *Bull. Johns Hopkins Hosp.* 117:228–250. The "improperly" oriented pyramidal cell in the cerebral cortex and its possible bearing on problems of growth and cell orientation.

Van der Loos, H. (1967). The history of the neuron, pp. 1–47. In *The Neuron* (H. Hydén, ed.), Elsevier.

Van der Loos, H. (1976). *Neurosci. Lett.* 2:1–6. Barreloids in mouse somatosensory thalamus.

Van der Loos, H., and T. A. Woolsey (1973). *Science* 179:395–398. Somatosensory cortex: Structural alterations following early injury to sense organs.

Van Essen, D. (1982). Neuromuscular synapse elimination, pp. 333–376. In *Neuronal Development* (N. Spitzer, ed.), Plenum, New York.

Van Essen, D., and J. K. S. Jansen (1974). *Acta Physiol. Scand.* 91:571–573. Reinnervation of the rat diaphragm during perfusion with alpha-bungarotoxin.

Van Essen, D., and J. K. S. Jansen (1977). *J. Comp. Neurol.* 171:433–454. The specificity of re-innervation by identified sensory and motor neurons in the leech.

Van Essen, D., and J. Kelly (1973). *Nature* 241:403–405. Correlation of cell shape and function in the visual cortex of the cat.

van Gehuchten, A. (1890). *Cellule* 6:395. Contribution à l'étude de la muqueuse olfactive chez les mammifères.

Van Gehuchten, A. (1891). *Cellule* 7:81–122. La structure des centres nerveux. La moëlle épinière et le cervelet.

Van Gehuchten, A. (1891). *Cellule* 8:1–43. La structure des centres nerveux la moelle épinière et le cervelet.

Van Gehuchten, A. (1892a). *La Cellule* 8:1–43. La structure des lobes optiques chez l'embryon de poulet.

Van Gehuchten, A. (1892b). *Anat. Anz.* 7:341–348. Contributions à l'étude de l'innervation des poils.

Van Gehuchten, A. (1903). *Névraxe* 5:3. La dégénérescence dite rétrograde ou dégénérescence Wallérienne indirecte.

Van Gehuchten, A. (1906). *Anatomie du système nerveux de l'homme*, 4th Edn. A. Uystpruyst-Dieudonne, Louvain.

Van Gehuchten, A., and J. Martin (1891). *La Cellule* 7:205–237. Le bulbe Olfactif chez quelques mammifères.

Van Gieson, J. (1889). *N.Y. Med. J.* 50:57–60. Laboratory notes of technical methods for the nervous system.

Van Harreveld, A. (1945). *Am. J. Physiol.* 144:477–493. Reinnervation of denervated muscle fibers by adjacent functioning motor units.

Van Harreveld, A. (1947). *Am. J. Physiol.* 150:670–676. On the mechanism of the "spontaneous" re-innervation in paretic muscle.

Van Harreveld, A. (1972). The extracellular space in the vertebrate central nervous system, pp. 447–511. In *The Structure and Function of Nervous Tissue* (G. H. Bourne, ed.), Academic Press, New York.

Van Harreveld, A., and E. Fifková (1975). *Exp. Neurol.* 49:736–749. Swelling of dendritic spines in the fascia dentata after stimulation of the perforant fibers as a mechanism of post-tetanic potentiation.

Van Harreveld, A., and F. I. Khattab (1969). *J. Cell Sci.* 4:437–453. Changes in extracellular space of the mouse cerebral cortex during hydroxyadipaldehyde fixation and osmium tetroxide post-fixation.

Van Harreveld, A., and J. Steiner (1970). *Anat. Rec.* 166:117–130. Extracellular space in frozen and ethanol substituted central nervous tissue.

Van Harreveld, A., and J. Trubatch (1974). *Anat. Rec.* 178:587–598. Conditions affecting the extracellular space in the frog's forebrain.

Van Harreveld, A., J. Crowell, and S. K. Malhotra (1965). *J. Cell Biol.* 25:117–137. A study of extracellular space in central nervous tissue by freeze-substitution.

Van Harreveld, A., H. Collewijn, and S. K. Malhotra (1966). *Am. J. Physiol.* 210:251–256. Water, electrolytes, and extracellular space in hydrated and dehydrated brains.

Van Hooff, C. O. M., A. B. Oestreicher, P. N. E. De Graan, and W. H. Gispen (1989). *Mol. Neurobiol.* 3:101–133. Role of the growth cone in neuronal differentiation.

Van Huizen, F., H. J. Romijn, and A. M. M. C. Habets (1985). *Dev. Brain Res.* 19:67–80. Synaptogenesis in rat cerebral cortex cultures is affected during chronic blockade of spontaneous bioelectric activity by tetrodotoxin.

Van Pelt, J., and R. W. H. Verwer (1982). *Bull. Math. Biol.* 45:269–285. The exact probabilities of branching patterns under terminal and segmental growth hypothesis.

Van Pelt, J., and R. W. H. Verwer (1984). *J. Microsc.* 136:23–34. New classification methods of branching patterns.

Van Sluyters, R. C., and D. L. Stewart (1974). *Exp. Brain Res.* 19:196–204. Binocular neurons of the rabbit's visual cortex: Effects of monocular sensory deprivation.

Van Straaten, H. W. M., F. Thors, L. Wiertz-Hoessels, J. Hekking, and J. Drukker (1985). *Dev. Biol.* 110:247–254. Effect of a notochordal implant on the early morphogenesis of the neural tube and neuroblasts: Histometrical and histological results.

Van Straaten, H. W. M., J. W. M. Hekking, J. P. W. M. Beursgens, E. Terwindt-Rouwenhorst, and J. Drukker (1989). *Development* 107:793–803. Effect of the notochord on proliferation and differentiation in the neural tube of the chick embryo.

Van Valen, L. (1974). *Am. J. Phys. Anthropol.* 40:417–424. Brain size and intelligence in man.

Van Wijhe, J. W. (1882). *Verh. K. ned. Akad. Wet.* 22:1–50. Ueber die Mesodermsegmente und die Entwickelung der Nerven des Selachierkopfes.

Van Wijhe, J. W. (1886). *Zool. Anz.* 9:678–682. Uber die Kopfsegmente und die Phylogenese des Geruchsorgans der Wirbelthiere.

Vargas-Lizardi, P., and K. M. Lyser (1974). *Dev. Biol.* 38:220–228. Time of origin of Mauthner's neuron in *Xenopus laevis* embryos.

Varmas, H. E. (1984). *Ann. Rev. Genet.* 18:553–612. The molecular genetics of cellular oncogenes.

Varon, S., C. Raiborn, and P. A. Burnham (1974a). *Neurobiol.* 4:231–252. Selective potency of homologous ganglionic non-neuronal cells for the support of dissociated ganglionic neurons in culture.

Varon, S., C. Raiborn, and S. Norr (1974b). *Exp. Cell Res.* 88:247–256. Association of antibody to nerve growth factor with ganglionic non-neurons (glia) and consequent interference with their neuron-supportive action.

Vartanian, A. (1960). *La Mettrie's L' Homme Machine: A Study in the Origins of an Idea*, Princeton, Princeton.

Vaughn, J. E. (1969). *Z. Zellforsch. Mikroskop. Anat. Abt. Histochem.* 94:293–324. An electron microscopic analysis of gliogenesis in rat optic nerves.

Vaughn, J. E. (1980). Development of synaptic connections in the spinal cord, pp. 95–123. In *The Spinal Cord and Its Reaction to Traumatic Injury* (W. F. Windle, ed.), Marcel Dekker, Inc., New York.

Vaughn, J. E. (1989). *Synapse* 3:255–285. Review: Fine structure of synaptogenesis in the vertebrate central nervous system.

Vaughn, J. E., and J. A. Grieshaber (1973). *J. Comp. Neurol.* 148:177–210. A morphological investigation of an early reflex pathway in developing rat spinal cord.

Vaughn, J. E., and D. C. Pease (1970). *J. Comp. Neurol.* 140:207–226. Electron microscopic studies of Wallerian degeneration in rat optic nerve. II. Astrocytes, oligodendrocytes and adventitial cells.

Vaughn, J. E., and A. Peters (1967). *Am. J. Anat.* 121:131–152. Electron microscopy of the early postnatal development of fibrous astrocytes.

Vaughn, J. E., and A. Peters (1968). *J. Comp. Neurol.* 133:269–288. A third neuroglial cell type. An electron microscope study.

Vaughn, J. E., and A. Peters (1971). The morphology and development of neuroglial cells, pp. 103–140. In *Cellular*

Aspects of Growth and Differentiation, UCLA Forum Med. Sci. No. 14, (D.C. Pease, ed.), Univ. of California Press, Los Angeles.

Vaughn, J. E., and T. J. Sims (1978). *J. Neurocytol.* 7:337–363. Axonal growth cones and developing axonal collaterals form synaptic junctions in embryonic mouse spinal cord.

Vaughn, J. E., P. L. Hinds, and R. P. Skoff (1970). *J. Comp. Neurol.* 140:175–206. Electron microscopic studies of Wallerian degeneration in rat optic nerves. I. The multipotential glia.

Vaughn, J. E., C. K. Henrikson, and J. A. Grieshaber (1974). *J. Cell Biol.* 60:664–672. A quantitative study of synapses on motor neuron dendritic growth cones in developing mouse spinal cord.

Vaughn, J. E., C. K. Henrikson, C. R. Chernow, J. A. Grieshaber, and C. C. Wimer (1975). *J. Comp. Neurol.* 161:541–554. Genetically-associated variations in the development of reflex movements and synaptic junctions within an early reflex pathway of mouse spinal cord.

Vaughn, J. E., D. A. Matthews, R. P. Barber, C. C. Miner, and R. E. Wimer (1977). *J. Comp. Neurol.* 173:41–52. Genetically-associated variations in the development of hippocampal pyramidal neurons may produce differences in mossy fiber connectivity.

Vaughn, J. E., R. P. Barber, and T. J. Sims (1988). *Synapse* 2:69–78. Dendritic development and preferential growth into synaptogenic fields: A quantitative study of Golgi-impregnated spinal motor neurons.

Veit, O. (1947). *Über das Problem Wirbeltierkopf.* Thomas-Verlag, Kempen-Niederrhein.

Venable, J. H. (1966). *Am. J. Anat.* 119:271–302. Morphology of the cells of normal, testosterone-deprived, and testosterone-stimulated levator ani muscles.

Vendrely, R., and C. Vendrely (1956). *Int. Rev. Cytol.* 5:171–197. The results of cytophotometry in the study of the deoxyribonucleic acid (DNA) content of the nucleus.

Veneroni, G. (1968). *Anat. Rec.* 160:503. Formation *de novo* and development of neuromuscular junctions *in vitro.*

Veneroni, G., and M. R. Murray (1969). *J. Embryol. Exp. Morphol.* 21:369–382. Formation *de novo* and development of neuromuscular junctions *in vitro.*

Verbitskaya, L. B. (1969). Some aspects of the ontogenesis of the cerebellum, pp. 859–874. In *Neurobiology of Cerebellar Evolution and Development* (R. Llinás, ed.), A.M.A. Educ. and Res. Fdn., Chicago.

Vercelli-Retta, J., R. Silviera, F. Dejas, and D. Rodriguez (1976). *Acta Anat.* 96:534–546. Enzyme histochemistry of rat interfascicular oligodendroglia, with special reference to 5′-nucleotidase.

Verge, V. M. K., W. Tetzlaff, P. M. Richardson, and M. A. Bisby (1990). *J. Neurosci.* 10:926–934. Correlation between GAP43 and nerve growth factor receptors in rat sensory neurons.

Verhaagen, J., A. B. Oestreicher, W. H. Gispen, and F. L. Margolis (1989). *J. Neurosci.* 9:683–691. The expression of the growth associated protein B50/GAP43 in the olfactory system of neonatal and adult rats.

Verity, A. N., and A. T. Campagnoni (1988). *J. Neurosci. Res.* 21:238–248. Regional expression of myelin protein genes in the developing mouse brain: *In situ* hybridization studies.

Verley, R., and H. Axelrod (1977). *C. R. Acad. Sci. Paris* 284:1183–1185. Organisation en "barils" des cellules de la couched IV du cortex SI chez la souris: Effets des lésions ou de la privation des vibrisses mystaciales.

Verna, J.-M. (1985). *J. Embryol. Exp. Morph.* 86:53–70. *In vitro* analysis of interactions between sensory neurons and skin: Evidence for selective innervation of dermis and epidermis.

Vernadakis, A., and D. M. Woodbury (1965). *Arch. Neurol. (Chicago)* 12:284–293. Cellular and extracellular spaces in developing rat brain.

Vernadakis, A., and D. M. Woodbury (1971). Effects of cortisol on maturation of the central nervous system, pp. 85–97. In *Influence of Hormones on the Nervous System* (D. H. Ford, ed.), Karger, Basel.

Verney, C., B. Berger, J. Adrien, A. Vigny, and M. Gay (1982). *Dev. Brain Res.* 5:41–52. Development of the dopaminergic innervation of the rat cerebral cortex. A light microscopic immunocytochemical study using anti-tyrosine hydroxylase antibodies.

Vernon, J. A., and J. Butsch (1957). *Science* 125:1033–1034. Effect of tetraploidy on learning and retention in the salamander.

Vertes, M., A. Barnea, H. R. Lindner, and R. J. B. King (1973). *Adv. Exp. Med. Biol.* 36:137–173. Studies on androgen and estrogen uptake by rat hypothalamus.

Verwer, R. W. H., and J. Van Pelt (1983). *J. Neurosci. Meth.* 8:335–351. A new method for the topological analysis of neuronal tree structures.

Verwoerd, C. D. A., and G. G. van Oostrom (1979). *Adv. Anat. Embryol. Cell Biol.* 58:1–75. Cephalic neural crest and placodes.

Vidal-Sanz, M., G. M. Bray, M. P. Villegas-Perez, S. Thanos, and A. J. Aguayo (1987). *J. Neurosci.* 7:2894–2909. Axonal regeneration and synapse formation in the superior colliculus by retinal ganglion cells in the adult rat.

Viets, H. R. (1926). *Arch. Neurol. Psychiat.* 15:623–627. Obituary. Camillo Golgi 1843–1926.

Viglietti-Panzica, C., G. C. Panzica, M. G. Fiori, M. Calcagni, G. C. Anselmetti, and J. Balthazart (1986). *Neurosci. Lett.* 64:129–134. A sexually dimorphic nucleus in the quail preoptic area.

Vignal, W. (1888). *Arch. Physiol. Norm. Path. (Paris)* 4:228–254, 311–338. Recherches sur le développement des éléments des couches corticales du cerveau et du cervelet chez l'homme et les mammifères.

Vignal, W. (1889). *Développement des éléments du système nerveux cérébro-spinal.* Paris.

Vigny, M., J. Koenig, and F. Rieger (1976). *J. Neurochem.* 27:1347–1353. The motor end-plate specific form of acetylcholinesterase: Appearance during embryogenesis and re-innervation of rat muscle.

Vincent, M. and J.-P. Thiery (1984). *Dev. Biol.* 103:468–481. A cell surface marker for neural crest and placodal cells: Further evolution in peripheral and central nervous system.

Vincent, M., J. L. Duband and J.-P. Thiery (1983). *Dev. Brain Res.* 9:235–238. A cell surface determinant expressed early on migrating avian neural crest cells.

Virchow, R. (1846). *Allgem. Zeitschr. Psychiat.* 3:242–250. Über das granulirte Ansehen der Wandungen der Gehirnventrikel.

Virchow, R. (1854). *Arch. Path. Anat. Physiol. Klin. Med.* 6:562–572. Ueber die ausgebreitete Vorkommen einer dem Nervenmark analogen Substanz in den tierischen Geweben.

Virchow, R. (1858). *Cellularpathologie in ihre Begründung auf Physiologische und Pathologische Gewebelehre.* A. Hirschwald, Berlin, 440 pp. English translation by F. Chance (1863) based on 2nd German edition, J. B. Lippincott & Co., Philadelphia; Reprinted 1971, Dover, New York, 554 pp.

Virchow, R. (1867). *Virchow's Archiv.* 38:129. Kongenitale Encephalitis und Myelitis.

Virchow, R. (1885). *Arch. path. Anat. klin. Med.* 8:1–15. Cellular pathology.

Visintini, F., and R. Levi-Montalcini (1939). *Schweiz. Arch. Neurol. Neurochim. Psychiat.* 43:381–393; 44:119–150. Relazione tra differenziazione strutturale e funzionale dei centri e delle vie nervose nell' embrione di pollo.

Vitiello, F., and G. Gombos (1987). Cerebellar development and nutrition, pp. 99–130. In *Current Topics in Nutrition and Disease*, Vol. 16, *Basic and Clinical Aspects of Nutrition and Brain Development* (D. K. Rassin, B. Haber, and B. Drujan, eds.), Alan R. Liss, New York.

Vitiello, F., J. Clos, C. Di Benedetta, and G. Gombos (1989). *Int. J. Dev. Neurosci.* 7:335–341. Developing rat cerebellum. III. Effects of abnormal thyroid states and undernutrition on gangliosides.

Vito, C. C., and T. O. Fox (1979). *Science* 204:517–519. Embryonic rodent brain contains estrogen receptors.

Vito, C. C., M. J. Baum, C. Bloom, and T. O. Fox (1985). *J. Neurosci.* 5:268–274. Androgen and estrogen receptors in perinatal ferret brain.

Vitry, F. de, R. Picaret, C. Jacque, and A. Tixier-Vidal (1981). *Dev. Neurosci.* 4:457–460. Glial fibrillary acidic protein: A cellular marker of tanycytes in the mouse hypothalamus.

Vizoso, A. D. (1950). *J. Anat. (London)* 82:342–353. The relationship between internodal length and growth in human nerves.

Vizoso, A. D., and J. Z. Young (1948). *J. Anat. (London)* 82:110–134. Internode length and fiber diameter in developing and regenerating nerves.

Voeller, K., G. D. Pappas, and D. P. Purpura (1963). *Exp. Neurol.* 7:107–130. Electron microscope study of development of cat superficial neocortex.

Vogt, C., and O. Vogt (1902–1904). *Neurobiologische arbeiten. I. Zur Erforschung der Hirnfaserung. II. Die markreifung des Kindergehirn während der ersten vier Lebensmonate und ihre methodologische Bedeutung.* Verlag von Gustav Fischer, Jena.

Vogt, O. (1903). *J. Psychol. Neurol. Leipzig* 2:160–180. Zur anatomische Gliederung des Cortex cerebri.

Vogt, O. (1911). *J. Psychol. Neurol.* 18:379–390. Die myeloarchitektonik des Isocortex parietalis.

Vogt, O., and C. Vogt (1919). *J. Psychol. Neurol. Leipzig* 25:277–462. Ergebnisse unserer Hirnforschung.

Vogt, W. (1925). *Arch. Entw. Mech. Organ.* 106:542–610. Gestaltungsanalyse am Amphibienkeim mit örtlicher Vitalfärbung. I. Methodik und Wirkungsweise der ortlichen Vitalfärbung mit Agar als Farbträger.

Vogt, W. (1929). *Arch. Entw. Mech. Organ.* 120:384–706. Gestaltungsanalyse am Amphibienkeim mit örtliche Vitalfärbung. II. Gastrulation und Mesodermbildung bei Urodelen und Anuren.

Voigt, J., and H. Pakkenberg (1983). *Acta Anat.* 116:290–301. Brain weight of Danish children: A forensic material.

Voigt, T. (1989). *J. Comp. Neurol.* 289:74–88. Development of glial cells in the cerebral wall of ferrets: Direct tracing of their transformation from radial glia into astrocytes.

Voitkevich, A. A., and I. I. Dedov (1972). *Z. Zellforsch.* 124:311–319. Ultrastructural study of neurovascular contacts in the median eminence of the rat.

Volberg, T., B. Geiger, J. Kartenbeck, and W. W. Franke (1986). *J. Cell Biol.* 102:1832–1842. Changes of membrane-microfilament interaction in intercellular adherens junctions upon removal of extracellular Ca^{2+} ions.

Volkmann, R. (1893). *Beitr. Pathol. Anat.* 12:233–332. Über die Regeneration des quergestreiften Muskelgewebes beim Menschen und Saugethier.

Volkmar, F. R., and W. T. Greenough (1972). *Science* 176:1445–1447. Rearing complexity affects branching of dendrites in the visual cortex of the rat.

Vollmer, G. (1988). *Was können wir wissen?* Band 1: *Die Natur der Erkenntnis.* Band 2: *Die Erkenntnis der Natur.* S. Hirzel Verlag, Stuttgart.

vom Saal, F. S., W. M. Grant, C. W. McMullen, and K. S. Laves (1983). *Science* 220:1306–1309. High fetal estrogen concentrations: Correlation with increased adult sexual activity and decreased aggression in male mice.

Von Baer, K. E. (1828, 1837). *Über Entwickelungsgeschichte der Thiere, Beobachtung und Reflexion.* I Theil, 1828; II Theil, 1837. Gebrüder Bornträger, Königsberg.

Von Bonin, G. (1934). *J. Comp. Neurol.* 59:1–28. On the size of man's brain, as indicated by skull capacity.

Von Bonin, G. (1937). *J. Gen. Psychol.* 16:379–389. Brain-weight and body-weight in mammals.

Von Bonin, G. (1963). *The Evolution of the Human Brain.* Univ. Chicago Press, Chicago.

von der Malsburg, C., and D. J. Willshaw (1976). *Exp. Brain Res.* 1:463–469. A mechanism for producing continuous neural mappings: Ocularity dominance stripes and ordered retino-tectal projections.

Von Economo, C. (1926). *Deut. Klin. Wschr.* 5:593–595. Ein Koeffizient für Organisationshohe der Grosshirnrinde.

Von Economo, C., and G. N. Koskinas (1925). *Die Cytoarchitektonik der Hirnrinde des erwachsenen Menschen. Text und Atlas.* Springer, Berlin.

Vongdokmai, R. (1980). *J. Comp. Neurol.* 191:283–294. Effect of protein malnutrition on development of mouse cortical barrels.

Von Gudden, B. A. (1869). *Arch. Psychiat.* 2:693–723. Experimentaluntersuchungen uber das peripherische und centrale Nervensystem.

Von Knebel Doeberitz, C. (1986). *Neuroscience* 17:409–426. Destruction of meningeal cells over the newborn hamster cerebellum with 6-hydroxydopamine prevents foliation and lamination in the rostral cerebellum.

Von Kupffer, K. (1906). Die Morphogenie des Centralnervensystems, pp. 1–272. In *Handbuch der vergleichende und experimentelle Entwicklungslehre der Wirbeltiere*, Vol. 2, Part 3, (R. Hertwig, ed.). Fischer Verlag, Jena.

Von Szily, A. (1912). *Graefe's Arch.* 81:67–86. Ueber einleitende Vorgänge bei der ersten Entwicklung der Nervenfasern im N. opticus.

Von Vintschgau, M. (1880). *Arch. Ges. Physiol.* 23:1–13. Beobachtungen über die Veränderungen der Schmeckbecher nach Durchschneidung des N. glossopharyngeus.

Von Vintschgau, M., and J. Honigschmied (1876). *Arch. Ges.*

Physiol. 14:443–448. Nervus glossopharyngeus und Schmeckbecher.

Von Woellwarth, C. (1950). *Arch. Entw. Mech. Organ.* 144:178–256. Experimentelle untersuchungen über den Situs Inversus der Eingeweide und der Habenula des Zwischenhirns bei Amphibien.

Von Woellwarth, C. (1952). *Arch. Entw. Mech. Organ.* 145:582–668. Die Induktionsstufen des Gehirns.

Von Woellwarth, C. (1960). *Arch. Entw. Mech. Organ.* 152:602–631. Über das Anlagenmuster und die Kinematik des Ektoderms, im Neural- und Schwanzknospenstadium von *Triturus alpestris.*

Von Woellwarth, C. (1969). *Roux' Arch. Entw. Organismen* 162:336–340. Auslösung von Situs inversus durch Materialdefekte im lateralen Ektoderm der Gastrula bei *Triturus alpestris.*

Vorbrodt, A. W., A. S. Lossinski, D. H. Dobrogowska, and H. M. Wisniewski (1986a). *Dev. Brain Res.* 29:69–79. Distribution of anionic sites and glycoconjugates on the endothelial surfaces of the developing blood-brain barrier.

Vorbrodt, A. W., A. S. Lossinski, and H. M. Wisniewski (1986b). *Dev. Neurosci.* 8:1–13. Localization of alkaline phosphatase activity in endothelia of developing and mature mouse blood-brain barrier.

Voyvodic, J. T. (1987). *J. Neurosci.* 7:904–912. Development and regulation of dendrites in the rat superior cervical ganglion.

Voyvodic, J. T. (1989). *J. Neurosci.* 9:1997–2010. Peripheral target regulation of dendritic geometry in the rat superior cervical ganglion.

Vrbová, G. (1963a). *J. Physiol. (London)* 166:241–250. Changes in the motor reflexes produced by tenotomy.

Vrbová, G. (1963b). *J. Physiol. (London)* 169:513–526. The effect of motoneurone activity on the speed of contraction of striated muscle.

Vrensen, G., and D. de Groot (1974). *Brain Res.* 78:263–278. The effect of dark rearing and its recovery on synaptic terminals in the visual cortex of rabbits. A quantitative electron microscopic study.

Vulpian, A. (1868). *Arch. Physiol.* 1:443–448. Influence de l'abolition des fonctions des nerfs sur la région de la moelle épinière dans des cas d'amputation d'ancienne date.

Wachtler, F. and M. Jacob (1986). *Biblthca Anat.* 29:24–46. Origin and development of the cranial skeletal muscles.

Wada, J. A., R. Clarke, and A. Hamm (1975). *Arch. Neurol.* 32:239–246. Cerebral hemispheric asymmetry in humans.

Waddington, C. H. (1952). *The Epigenetics of Birds.* Cambridge Univ. Press, London.

Waddington, C. H. (1957). *The Strategy of the Genes.* Allen and Unwin, London.

Waddington, C. H. (1966). Fields and gradients, pp. 105–124. In *Major Problems in Developmental Biology* (M. Locke, ed.), Academic Press, New York.

Waddington, C. H. (1970). Concepts and theories of growth, development, differentiation and morphogenesis, pp. 177–197. In *Towards a Theoretical Biology,* Vol. 3, (C. H. Waddington, ed.), Aldine, Chicago.

Waddington, C. H., and E. M. Deuchar (1953). *J. Embryol. Exp. Morph.* 1:349–361. Studies on the mechanism of meristic segmentation.

Waddington, C. H., and M. M. Perry (1966). *Exp. Cell Res.* 41:691–693. A note on the mechanisms of cell deformation in the neural folds of amphibia.

Waechter, H. (1953). *Arch. Entw.-Mech. Organ.* 146:201–274. Die Induktionsfähigkeit der Gehirnplatte bei Urodelen und ihr medianlaterales Gefälle.

Waechter, R. V., and B. Jaensch (1972). *Brain Res.* 46:235–250. Generation times of the matrix cells during embryonic brain development: An autoradiographic study in rats.

Waganer, G. (1949). *Rev. Suisse Zool.* 56:519–619. Die Bedeutung der Neuralleiste für die Kopfgestaltung der Amphibienlarven. Untersuchungen an Chimaeren von *Triton* und *Bombinator.*

Wagner, R., (ed.) (1842–1853). *Handwörterbuch der Physiologie mit Rücksicht auf physiologische Pathologie,* 4 vols. in 5. F. Vieweg, Braunschweig.

Wagner, R. (1847). *Neue Untersuchungen über den Bau und die Endigungen der Nerven. und die Struktur der Ganglienzellen,* Leipzig.

Wagner, R. P. (1969). *Science* 163:1026–1031. Genetics and phenogenetics of mitochondria.

Wahn, H. L., L. E. Lightbody, T. T. Tchen, and J. D. Taylor (1975). *Science* 188:366–369. Induction of neural differentiation in cultures of amphibian undetermined presumptive epidermis by cyclic AMP derivatives.

Wakahara, M. (1989). *Dev. Growth Diff.* 31:197–207. Specification and establishment of dorsal-ventral polarity in eggs and embryos of *Xenopus laevis.*

Wake, K. (1976). *Cell Tissue Res.* 173:383–400. Formation of myoneural and myotendenous junctions in the chick.

Walberg, F. (1963). *Exp. Neurol.* 8:112–124. Role of normal dendrites in removal of degenerating terminal boutons.

Waldeyer, H. W. G. (1891). *Deutsch. Med. Wschr.* 17:1213–1218, 1244–1246, 1267–1269, 1287–1289, 1331–1332, 1352–1356. Über einige neuere Forschungen im Gebiete der Anatomie des Centralnervensystems.

Waldeyer, W. (1865). *Arch. Pathol. Anat. Physiol.* 34:473–514. Ueber die Veränderungen der quergestreiften Muskeln bei der Entzündung und dem Typhusprozess, sowie über die Regeneration derselben nach Substanzdefecten.

Walicke, P., W. M. Cowan, N. Ueno, A. Baird, and R. Guillemin (1986). *Proc. Natl. Acad. Sci. U.S.A.* 83:3012–3016. Fibroblast growth factor promotes survival of dissociated hippocampal neurons and enhances neurite extension.

Walicke, P. A. (1988). *J. Neurosci.* 8:2618–2627. Basic and acidic fibroblast growth factors have trophic effects on neurons from multiple CNS regions.

Walicke, P. A., and A. Baird (1988). *Dev. Brain Res.* 40:71–79. Neurotrophic effects of basic and acidic fibroblast growth factors are not mediated through glial cells.

Walker, A. E. (1942). *Arch. Neurol. Psychiat.* 48:13–29. Lissencephaly.

Walker, A. E. (1957). *Bull. Hist. Med.* 31:99–121. The development of the concept of cerebral localization in the nineteenth century.

Walker, B. E. (1960). *Am. J. Anat.* 107:95–105. Renewal of cell populations in the female mouse.

Walker, P. A., and J. Money (1972). *Hormones* 3:119–128. Prenatal androgenization of females.

Walker, S. F. (1980). *Br. J. Psychol.* 71:329–369. Lateralization of function in the vertebrate brain: A review.

Wall, J. T. (1988). *Trends Neurosci.* 11:549–557. Variable organization in cortical maps of the skin as an indication of the lifelong adaptive capacities of circuits in the mammalian brain.

Wall, J. T., C. G. Cusick, and J. H. Kaas (1981). *Neurosci. Abstr.* 7:758. Evidence for incomplete reorganization of the S-I foot representation following sciatic nerve section in the adult rat.

Wall, P. D. (1977). *Phil. Trans. Roy. Soc. (London) Ser. B.* 178:361–372. The presence of ineffective synapses and the circumstances which unmask them.

Wall, P. D., and M. Devor (1981). *Brain Res.* 209:95–111. The effects of peripheral nerve injury on dorsal root potentials and on transmission of afferent signals into the spinal cord.

Wall, P. D., and M. D. Egger (1971). *Nature* 232:542–545. Formation of new connections in adult rat brains after partial deafferentation.

Wallace, H. (1972). *J. Embryol. Exp. Morphol.* 28:419–435. The components of regrowing nerves which support the regeneration of irradiated salamander limbs.

Wallace, H. (1981). *Vertebrate Limb Regeneration.* John Wiley and Sons, New York.

Wallace, H. (1984). *J. Embryol. exp. Morph.* 84:303–307. The response of denervated axolotl arms to delayed amputation.

Wallace, L. J., and L. M. Partlow (1976). *Proc. Natl. Acad. Sci. U.S.A.* 73:4210–4214. α-Adrenergic regulation of secretion of mouse saliva rich in nerve growth factor.

Wallace, T. L., and E. M. Johnson, Jr. (1989). *J. Neurosci.* 9:115–124. Cytosine arabinoside kills postmitotic neurons: Evidence that deoxycytidine may have a role in neuronal survival that is independent of DNA synthesis.

Waller, A. (1850). *Phil. Trans. Roy. Soc. (London) Ser. B.* 140:423–429. Experiments on the section of the glossopharyngeal and hypoglossal nerves of the frog, and observations of the alterations produced thereby in the structure of their primitive fibres.

Waller, A. (1851a). *Edinburgh Med. Surg. J.* 76:369–376. Experiments on the section of the glosso-pharyngeal and hypoglossal nerves of the frog, and observations of the alterations produced thereby in the structure of their primitive fibres.

Waller, A. (1851b). *Compt. rend. Acad. Sci. Paris* 33:606–611. Nouvelle méthode pour l'étude du système nerveux applicable à l'investigation de la distribution anatomique des cordons nerveux.

Waller, A. (1852). *Arch. Anat. Physiol. (Liepzig)* 11:392–401. Sur la reproduction des nerfs et sur la structure et les fonctions des ganglions spinaux.

Walsh, C., and C. Cepko (1988). *Science* 241:1342–1345. Clonally related cortical cells show several migration patterns.

Walsh, C., and E. H. Polley (1985). *J. Neurosci.* 5:741–750. The topography of ganglion cell production in the cat's retina.

Walsh, R. N. (1981). *Int. J. Neurosci.* 12:33–51. Effects of environment complexity and deprivation on brain anatomy and histology: A review.

Walsh, R. N., O. E. Budtz-Olsen, A. Torok, and R. A. Cummins (1971). *Dev. Psychobiol.* 4:115–122. Environmentally induced changes in the rat cerebrum.

Walsh, R. N., R. A. Cummins, and O. E. Budtz-Olsen (1973). *Dev. Psychobiol.* 6:3–7. Environmentally induced changes in the dimension of the cerebrum: A replication and extension.

Walshe, F. M. R. (1943). *Brain* 66:104–139. On the mode of representation of movements in the motor cortex with special reference to 'convulsions beginning unilaterally'.

Walter, G. (1861). *Virchow's Arch. f. pathol. Anat. und Phys.* Berlin 22:241–259. Ueber den feineren Bau des Bulbus olfactorius.

Walter, J., S. Henke-Fahle, and F. Bonhoeffer (1987a). *Development* 101:909–913. Avoidance of posterior tectal membranes by temporal retinal axons.

Walter, J., B. Kern-Veits, J. Huf, B. Stolze, and F. Bonhoeffer (1987b). *Development* 101:685–696. Recognition of position-specific properties of tectal cell membranes by retinal axons *in vitro.*

Walz, M. A., R. W. Price, and A. L. Notkins (1974). *Science* 184:1185–1187. Latent ganglionic infection with herpes simplex virus types 1 and 2: Viral reactivation *in vivo* after neurectomy.

Wand, M., E. Zeuthen, and E. A. Evans (1967). *Science* 157:436–438. Tritiated thymidine: Effect of decomposition by self-radiolysis on specificity as a tracer for DNA synthesis.

Wanner, R. A., M. J. Edwards, and R. G. Wright (1976). *J. Pathol.* 118:235–244. The effect of hyperthermia on the neuroepithelium of the 21-day guinea-pig foetus: Histologic and ultrastructural study.

Warden, C. J. (1927). *Psychol. Rev.* 34:57–85, 135–168. The historical development of comparative psychology.

Ware, R. W., and V. LePresti (1975). *Int. Rev. Cytol.* 40: 325–440. Three-dimensional reconstruction from serial sections.

Warembourg, M. (1975). *Brain Res.* 89:61–70. Radioautographic study of the rat brain after injection of [1,2-³H] corticosterone.

Warembourg, M., U. Otten, and M. E. Schwab (1981). *Neuroscience* 6:1139–1143. Labelling of Schwann and satellite cells by [³H]-dexamethasone in rat sympathetic ganglion and sciatic nerve.

Warner, A. (1988). *J. Cell. Sci.* 89:1–7. The gap junction.

Warner, A. E. (1970). *J. Physiol. (London)* 210:150–151P. Electrical connexions between cells at neural stages of the axolotl.

Warner, A. E. (1973). *J. Physiol. (London)* 235:267–286. The electrical properties of the ectoderm in the amphibian embryo during induction and early development of the nervous system.

Warren, H. C. (1921). *A History of the Association Psychology,* Constable, London.

Warren, M. A., and K. S. Bedi (1982). *J. Comp. Neurol.* 210:59–64. Synapse-to-neuron ratios in the visual cortex of adult rats undernourished from about birth until 100 days of age.

Warren, M. A., and K. S. Bedi (1984). *J. Comp. Neurol.* 227:104–108. A quantitative assessment of the development of synapses and neurons in the visual cortex of control and undernourished rats.

Wartiovaara, J., S. Nordling, E. Lehtonen, and L. Saxen (1974). *J. Embryol. Exp. Morphol.* 31:667–682. Transfilter induction of kidney tubules: Correlation with cytoplasmic penetration into Nucleopore filters.

Warwick, R. (1978). *Anat. Rec.* 190:1–4. The future of Nomina anatomica—A personal view.

Wassef, M., and C. Sotelo (1984). *Neuroscience* 13:1217–1241. Asynchrony in the expression of guanosine 3':5'-phosphate dependent protein kinase by clusters of Purkinje cells during the perinatal development of rat cerebellum.

Wassef, M., J.-P. Zanetta, A. Brehier, and C. Sotelo (1985). *Dev. Biol.* 111:129–137. Transient biochemical compartmentalization of Purkinje cells during early cerebellar development.

Wassef, M., C. Sotelo, B. Cholley, A. Brehier, and M. Thomasset (1987). *Dev. Biol.* 124:379–389. Cerebellar mutations affecting the postnatal survival of Purkinje cells in the mouse disclose a longitudinal pattern of differentially sensitive cells.

Wassef, M., C. Sotelo, M. Thomasset, A.-C. Granholm, N. Leclerc, J. Rafrafi, and R. Hawkes (1990). *J. Comp. Neurol.* 294:223–234. Expression of compartmentation antigen zebrin I in cerebellar transplants.

Wassermann, F. (1965). The ground substance of connective tissue in a foreshortened historical perspective, pp. 177–192. In *Aus der Werkstatt der Anatomen* (W. Bargmann, ed.), Georg Thieme Verlag, Stuttgart.

Wässle, H. (1988). *Trends Neurosci.* 11:87–89. Dendritic maturation of retinal ganglion cells.

Wässle, H., B. B. Boycott, and R. B. Illing (1981a). *Proc. Roy. Soc. (London) Ser. B.* 212:177–195. Morphology and mosaic of on- and off-beta cells in the cat retina and some functional considerations.

Wässle, H., L. Peichl, and B. B. Boycott (1981b). *Nature* 292:344–345. Dendritic territories of cat retinal ganglion cells.

Wässle, H., L. Peichl, and B. B. Boycott (1981c). *Proc. Roy. Soc. (London) Ser. B.* 212:157–175. Morphology and topography of on- and off-alpha cells in cat retina.

Watanabe, I. (1965). *Tohoku J. Exp. Med.* 86:201–218. Enzyme histochemical study of the motor nerve cells in axonal reaction.

Watanabe, M., H. Ito, and H. Masai (1983). *J. Comp. Neurol.* 213:188–198. Cytoarchitecture and visual receptive neurons in the wulst of the Japanese quail (*Coturnix coturnix japonica*).

Watanabe, T., and M. C. Raff (1988). *Nature* 332:834–837. Retinal astrocytes are immigrants from the optic nerve.

Waterlow, J. C., J. Cravioto, and J. M. L. Stephen (1960). *Advances Protein Chem.* 15:131–238. Proteins malnutrition in man.

Watkins, D. W., J. R. Wilson, and S. M. Sherman (1978). *J. Neurophysiol.* 41:332–337. Receptive-field properties of neurons in binocular and monocular segments of striate cortex in cats raised with binocular lid suture.

Watkins, J. W. N. (1970). Against normal science, pp. 25–37. In *Falsification and the Methodology of Scientific Research Programmes* (I. Lakatos, and A. Musgrave, eds.), Cambridge Univ. Press, Cambridge.

Watson, J. B. (1903). *Chicago Univ. Contrib. Phil.* 4:90–111. Animal education. An experimental study of the psychical development of the white rat correlated with the growth of its nervous system.

Watson, W. E. (1965). *J. Physiol. (London)* 180:741–753. An autoradiographic study of the incorporation of nucleic acid precursors by neurones and glia during nerve regeneration.

Watson, W. E. (1968). *J. Physiol. (London)* 196:655–676. Observations on the nucleolar and total cell body nucleic acid of injured nerve cells.

Watson, W. E. (1969). *J. Physiol. (London)* 202:611–630. The response of motor neurones to intramuscular injection of botulinum toxin.

Watson, W. E. (1974a). *Brain Res.* 65:317–322. The binding of actinomycin D to the nuclei of axotomised neurons.

Watson, W. E. (1974b). *Physiol. Res.* 54:245–271. Physiology of neuroglia.

Watson, W. E. (1974c). *Br. Med. Bull.* 30:112–115. Cellular responses to axotomy and to related procedures.

Watterson, R. L., and I. Fowler (1953). *Anat. Rec.* 117:773–803. Regulative development in lateral halves of chick neural tubes.

Watterson, R. L., P. Veneziano, and A. Bartha (1956). *Anat. Rec.* 124:379. Absence of a true germinal zone in neural tubes of young chick embryos as demonstrated by the colchicine technique.

Waxman, S. G., and M. V. L. Bennett (1972). *Nature (New Biol.)* 238:217–219. Relative conduction velocities of small myelinated and non-myelinated fibres in the central nervous system.

Waxman, S. G., and G. D. Pappas (1969). *Brain Res.* 14:240–244. Pinocytosis at postsynaptic membranes: Electron microscopic evidence.

Waxman, S. G., and G. D. Pappas (1971). *J. Comp. Neurol.* 143:41–72. An electron microscopic study of synaptic morphology in the oculomotor nuclei of three inframamalian species.

Wayne, D. B., and M. B. Heaton (1988). *Dev. Biol.* 127:220–223. Retrograde transport of NGF by early chick embryo spinal cord motoneurons.

Weakley, J. N. (1980). *Brain Res.* 197:512–515. The number of endplates is dependent on the physical properties of twitch fibers in amphibian muscle.

Weatherbee, J. A. (1981). *Int. Rev. Cytol.* Suppl. 12:113–176. Membranes and cell movement: Interactions of membranes with the proteins of the cytoskeleton.

Weber, E. D., and D. J. Stelzner (1980). *Brain Res.* 185:17–37. Synaptogenesis in the intermediate gray region of the lumbar spinal cord in the postnatal rat.

Weber, K., and U. Groeschel-Stewart (1974). *Proc. Natl. Acad. Sci. U.S.A.* 70:750–754. Antibody to Myosin: The specific visualization of myosin-containing filaments in nonmuscle cells.

Weber, L., R. Pollack, and T. Bibring (1975). *Proc. Natl. Acad. Sci. U.S.A.* 72:459–463. Antibody against tubulin: The specific visualization of cytoplasmic microtubules in tissue culture cells.

Weber, R. (1962). *Experientia* 18:84–85. Induced metamorphosis in isolated tails of *Xenopus*.

Weber, R. (1964). *J. Cell Biol.* 22:481–487. Ultrastructural changes in regressing tail muscles of *Xenopus larvae* at metamorphosis.

Webster, H. deF. (1971). *J. Cell Biol.* 48:348–367. The geometry of peripheral myelin sheaths during their formation and growth in rat sciatic nerves.

Webster, H. deF., J. R. Martin, and M. F. O'Connell (1973). *Dev. Biol.* 32:401–416. The relationships between interphase Schwann cells and axons before myelination: A quantitative electron microscopic study.

Webster, M. J., C. J. Shatz, M. Kliot, and J. Silver (1988). *J. Comp. Neurol.* 269:592–611. Abnormal pigmentation and unusual morphogenesis of the optic stalk may be correlated with retinal axon misguidance in embryonic siamese cats.

Webster, W., M. Shimade, and J. Langman (1973). *Am. J. Anat.* 137:67–85. Effect of fluorodeoxyuridine, colcemid, and bromodeoxyuridine on developing neocortex of the mouse.

Wechsler, W. (1966a). *Z. Zellforsch. Mikroskop. Anat.* 74:232–251. Elektronenmikroskopischer Beitrag zur Histogenese der Weissen Substanz des Rückenmarks von Hühnerembryonen.

Wechsler, W. (1966b). *Z. Zellforsch. Mikroskop. Anat.* 74:401–422. Elektronenmikroskopischer Beitrag zur Nervenzelldifferenzierung und Histogenese der grauen Substanz des Rückenmarks von Hühnerembryonen.

Wechsler, W. (1966c). *Z. Zellforsch. Mikroskop. Anat.* 74:423–442. Elektronenmikroskopischer Beitrag zur Differenzierung des Ependyms am Rückenmark von Hühnerembryonen.

Wechsler, W. (1967). Electron microscopy of the cytodifferentiation in the developing brain of chick embryos, pp. 213–224. In *Evolution of the Forebrain* (R. Hassler, and H. Stephan, eds.), Plenum Press, New York.

Weddell, G., and E. Zander (1951). *J. Anat. (London)* 85:242–250. The fragility of non-myelinated nerve fibre terminals.

Weddell, G., L. Guttmann, and E. Guttmann (1941). *J. Neurol. Neurosurg. Psychiat.* 4(N.S.):206–225. The local extension of nerve fibers into denervated areas of skin.

Wedden, S. E., K. Pang, and G. Eichele (1989). *Development* 105:639–650. Expression pattern of homeobox containing genes during chick embryogenesis.

Weeks, D. L., and D. A. Melton (1987). *Proc. Natl. Acad. Sci. U.S.A.* 84:2798–2802. A maternal mRNA localized to the animal pole of *Xenopus* eggs encoder a subunit of mitochondrial ATPase.

Wegener, K., S. Hollweg, and W. Maurer (1963). *Naturwissenschaften* 50:738–739. Autoradiographische Bestimmung er Dauer des DNS-Verdopplung und der Generationszeit bei fetalen Zellen der Ratte.

Wegener, K., S. Hollweg, and W. Maurer (1964). *Z. Zellforsch. Mikroskop. Anat. Abt. Histochem.* 63:309–326. Autoradiographische bestimmung der DNS-verdopplungszeit und anderer Teil-Phasen des Zell-Zyklus bei fetalen Zellarten der Ratte.

Wehrmacher, W. H., and H. M. Hines (1945). *Fed. Proc.* 4:75–76. The recovery of skeletal muscle from the effects of partial denervation.

Weichsel, M. E., Jr. (1974). *Brain Res.* 78:455–465. Effect of thyroxine on DNA synthesis and thymidine kinase activity during cerebellar development.

Weigert, C. (1882). *Z. med. Wissench.* 20:753–757, 772–774. Ueber eine neue Untersuchungsmethode des Centralnervensystems.

Weigert, C. (1895). *Beiträge zur Kenntniss der normalen menschlichen Neuroglia.* Festschrift zum 50-jährigen Jubil. d. ärztl. Vereins zu Frankfurt a.M.

Weil, A., and H. A. Davenport (1933). *Arch. Neurol. Psychiat.* 30:175–178. Staining of oligodendroglia and microglia in celloidin sections.

Weinberg, C. B., and Z. W. Hall (1979). *Dev. Biol.* 68:631–635. Junctional form of acetylcholinesterase restored at nerve-free endplates.

Weinberg, C. B., J. R. Sanes, and Z. W. Hall (1981). *Dev. Biol.* 84:255–266. Formation of neuromuscular junctions in adult rats: Accumulation of acetylcholine receptors, acetylcholinesterase, and components of synaptic basal lamina.

Weinberg, H. J., and P. S. Spencer (1975). *J. Neurocytol.* 4:395–418. Studies on the control of myelinogenesis. I. Myelination of regenerating axons after entry into a foreign unmyelinated nerve.

Weinberg, H. J., and P. S. Spencer (1976). *Brain Res.* 113:363–378. Studies on the control of myelinogenesis. II. Evidence for neuronal regulation of myelin production.

Weindl, A. (1973). Neuroendocrine aspects of circumventricular organs, pp. 3–32. In *Frontiers in Neuroendocrinology* (W. F. Ganong, and L. Martini, eds.), Oxford Univ. Press, New York.

Weinstein, R. S., and C M. Cassidy (1981). *Fed. Proc.* 40:2570–2571. Nutritional anthropology: Theory and method.

Weis, P. (1970). *J. Embryol. Exp. Morph.* 24:381–392. The *in vitro* effect of the nerve growth factor in chick embryo spinal ganglia—A light microscopic evaluation.

Weis, P. (1971). *J. Comp. Neurol.* 141:117–132. The *in vitro* effect of the nerve growth factor on chick embryo spinal ganglia: An electron microscopic evaluation.

Weisblat, D. A., and S. S. Blair (1984). *Dev. Biol.* 101:326–335. Developmental indeterminacy in embryos of the leech *Helobdella triserialis.*

Weisblat, D. A., and M. Shankland (1985). *Phil. Trans. Roy. Soc. (London) Ser. B.* 312:39–56. Cell lineage and segmentation in the leech.

Weismann, A. (1891–1892). *Essays Upon Heredity and Kindred Biological Problems,* 2nd edn., 2 Vols. Clarendon Press, Oxford.

Weismann, A. (1892). *Das Keimplasma: Eine Theorie der Vererbung.* Verlag von Gustav Fischer, Jena.

Weismann, A. (1904). *The Evolution Theory* (Transl. of Vorträge über Descendenztheorie, Jena, 1902), 2 vols. Edward Arnold, London.

Weiss, G. M., and J. J. Pysh (1978). *Brain Res.* 154:219–230. Evidence for loss of Purkinje cell dendrites during late development: A morphometric Golgi analysis in the mouse.

Weiss, P. (1922). *Öst. Akad. Wiss. Math. Naturwiss. Klin. Abt. I.* 59:199–201. Die Funktion transplantierter Amphibienextremitäten.

Weiss, P. (1924). *Arch. Entw.-Mech. Organ.* 102:635–672. Die Funktion transplantierter Amphibienextremitäten. Aufstellung einer Resonanztheorie der motorischen Nerventätigkeit auf Grund abgestimmter Endorgane.

Weiss, P. (1928a). *Naturwissenschaften* 16:626–636. Eine neue theorie der Nervenfunktion. Nicht durch gesonderte Bahnen. Sondern durch spezifische Formen der Erregung schalter das Nervensystem mit den Muskeln.

Weiss, P. (1928b). *Ergeb. Biol.* 3:1–151. Erregungsspezifität und Erregungsresonanz.

Weiss, P. (1929). *Arch. Entw.-Mech. Organ.* 116:438–554. Erzwingung elementarer Strukturverschiedenheiten am *in vitro* wachsenden Gewebe.

Weiss, P. (1931). *Wien. Klin. Wochschr.* 39:1–17. Das Resonanzprinzip der Nerventätigkeit.

Weiss, P. (1933). *Am. Naturalist* 67:322–340. Functional adaptation and the role of group substances during development.

Weiss, P. (1934). *J. Exp. Zool.* 68:393–448. *In vitro* experiments on the factors determining the course of the outgrowing nerve fiber.

Weiss, P. (1935). *J. Comp. Neurol.* 61:135–174. Experimental innervation of muscles by the central ends of afferent nerves (establishment of one-neuron connection between receptor and effector organ), with functional tests.

Weiss, P. (1936). *Biol. Rev.* 11:494–531. Selectivity controlling the central- peripheral relations in the nervous system.

Weiss, P. (1937a). *J. Comp. Neurol.* 66:181–209. Further investigations on the phenomenon of homologous response in transplanted amphibian limbs. I. Functional observations.

Weiss, P. (1937b). *J. Comp. Neurol.* 66:481–535. Further experimental investigations on the phenomenon of homologous response in transplanted amphibian limbs. II. Nerve regeneration and the innervation of transplanted limbs.

Weiss, P. (1937c). *J. Comp. Neurol.* 66:537–548. Further experimental investigations on the phenomenon of homologous response in transplanted amphibian limbs. III. Homologous response in the absence of sensory innervation.

Weiss, P. (1937d). *J. Comp. Neurol.* 67:269–315. Further experimental investigations on the phenomenon of homologous response in transplanted amphibian limbs. IV. Reverse locomotion after the interchange of right and left limbs.

Weiss, P. (1939). *Principles of Development*, Henry Holt, New York.

Weiss, P. (1941a). *Third Growth Symposium* 5:163–203. Nerve patterns. The mechanics of nerve growth.

Weiss, P. (1941b). *Comp. Psychol. Monographs* 17:1–96. Self-differentiation of the basic patterns of coordination.

Weiss, P. (1942). *J. Comp. Neurol.* 77:131–169. Lid-closure reflex from eyes transplanted to atypical locations in Triturus torosus: Evidence of a peripheral origin of sensory specificity.

Weiss, P. (1947). *Yale J. Biol. Med.* 19:235–278. The problem of specificity in growth and development.

Weiss, P. (1950). *J. Exp. Zool.* 113:397–461. Deplantation of fragments of nervous system in amphibians. I. Central reorganization and the formation of nerves.

Weiss, P. (1952). *Res. Publ. Assoc. Res. Nerv. Ment. Dis.* 30:3–23. Central versus peripheral factors in the development of coordination.

Weiss, P. (1955). Nervous system, pp. 346–401. In *Analysis of Development* (B. H. Willier, P. Weiss, and V. Hamburger, eds.), Saunders, Philadelphia.

Weiss, P. (1963). Self-renewal and proximo-distal convection in nerve fibers, pp. 171–183. In *The Effect of Use and Disuse on Neuromuscular Functions* (E. Gutman, and P. Hnik, eds.), Czechoslovak Acad. Sci., Prague.

Weiss, P. (1964). *Proc. Natl. Acad. Sci. U.S.A.* 52:1024–1029. The dynamics of the membrane-bound incompressible body: A mechanism of cellular and subcellular motility.

Weiss, P. (1972). *Proc. Natl. Acad. Sci. U.S.A.* 69:1309–1312. Neuronal dynamics and axonal flow: Axonal peristalsis.

Weiss, P., and G. Andres (1952). *J. Exp. Zool.* 121:449–488. Experiments on the fate of embryonic cells (chick) disseminated by the vascular route.

Weiss, P., and M. V. Edds, Jr. (1945). *J. Neurophysiol.* 8:173–193. Sensory-motor nerve crosses in the rat.

Weiss, P., and M. V. Edds, Jr. (1946). *Am. J. Physiol.* 145:587–607. Spontaneous recovery of muscle following partial denervation.

Weiss, P., and H. B. Hiscoe (1948). *J. Exp. Zool.* 107:315–396. Experiments on the mechanism of nerve growth.

Weiss, P., and A. Hoag (1946). *J. Neurophysiol.* 9:413–418. Competitive reinnervation of rat muscles by their own and foreign nerves.

Weiss, P., and R. Mayr (1971). *Acta Neuropathol. (Suppl. (Berl.)* 5:198–206. Neuronal organelles in neuroplasmic ("axonal") flow II. Neurotubules.

Weiss, P., and A. Pillai (1965). *Proc. Natl. Acad. Sci. U.S.A.* 54:48–56. Convection and fate of mitochondria in nerve fibers: Axonal flow as vehicle.

Weiss, P., and F. Rossetti (1951). *Proc. Natl. Acad. Sci. U.S.A.* 37:540–556. Growth responses of opposite sign among different neuron types exposed to thyroid hormone.

Weiss, P., and A. C. Taylor (1944). *J. Exp. Zool.* 95:233–257. Further experimental evidence against "neurotropism" in nerve regeneration.

Weiss, P., and A. C. Taylor (1960). *Proc. Natl. Acad. Sci. U.S.A.* 46:1177–1185. Reconstitution of complete organs from single-cell suspensions of chick embryos in advanced stages of differentiation.

Weiss, P., and M. V. Edds, and M. Cavanaugh (1945a). *Anat. Rec.* 92:215–233. The effects of terminal connections on the caliber of nerve fibers.

Weiss, P., H. Wang, A. C. Taylor, and M. V. Edds, Jr. (1945b). *Am. J. Physiol.* 143:521–540. Proximo-distal fluid convection in the endoneurial spaces of peripheral nerves, demonstrated by colored and radioactive (isotope) tracers.

Weiss, P., A. C. Taylor, and P. A. Pillai (1962). *Science* 136:330. The nerve fiber as a system in continuous flow: Microcinematographic and electronmicroscopic demonstrations.

Welker, C. (1971). *Brain Res.* 26:259–276. Microelectrode delineation of fine grain somatotopic organization of SmI cerebral neocortex in albino rat.

Welker, C. (1973). *Anat. Rec.* 175:467–468. Organization of somatosensory cerebral neocortex in micrencephalic rat.

Welker, C. (1976). *J. Comp. Neurol.* 166:173–190. Receptive fields of barrels in the somatosensory neocortex of the rat.

Welker, C., and T. A. Woolsey (1974). *J. Comp. Neurol.* 158:437–454. Structure of layer IV in the somatosensory neocortex of the rat: Description and comparison with the mouse.

Welker, E., and H. van der Loos (1986). *J. Neurosci.* 6:3355–3373. Quantitative correlation between barrel-field size and the sensory innervation of the whiskerpad: A comparative study in six strains of mice bred for different patterns of mystacial vibrissae.

Welker, W. I., and G. B. Campos (1963). *J. Comp. Neurol.* 120:19–36. Physiological significance of sulci in somatic sensory cerebral cortex in mammals of the family Procyonidae.

Welker, W. I., and S. Seidenstein (1959). *J. Comp. Neurol.* 111:469–501. Somatic sensory representation in the cerebral cortex of the racoon (*Procyon Lotor*).

Welker, W. I., J. I. Johnson, Jr., and B. H. Pubols, Jr. (1964). *Am. Zool.* 4:75–94. Some morphological and physiological characteristics of the somatic sensory system in raccoons.

Weller, W. L., and J. I. Johnson (1975). *Brain Res.* 83:504–508. Barrels in cerebral cortex altered by receptor disruption in newborn, but not in five-day-old mice (*Cricetidae and Muridae*).

Wendell-Smith, C. P., M. J. Blunt, and F. Baldwin (1966). *J.*

Comp. Neurol. 127: 219–240. The ultrastructural characterization of macroglial cell types.

Wenger, E. L. (1950). *J. Exp. Zool.* 114:51–85. An experimental analysis of relations between parts of the brachial spinal cord of the embryonic chick.

Went, F. W. (1937). *Science* 86:127. Salt accumulation and polar transport of plant hormones.

Wenzel, J., C. Schmidt, G. Duwe, W. G. Skrebitz, and I. Kudrjats (1985). *J. Hirnfor.* 26:573–583. Stimulation-induced changes of the ultrastructure of synapses in hippocampus following posttetanic potentiation.

Werner, G. (1970). The topology of the body representation in the somatic afferent pathway. In *The Neurosciences: Second Study Program* (F. O. Schmitt, ed.), Rockefeller Univ. Press, New York.

Werner, G., and B. L. Whitsel (1967). *J. Physiol. (London)* 192:123–144. The topology of dermatomal projection in the medial lemniscal system.

Werner, G., and B. L. Whitsel (1968). *J. Neurophysiol.* 31:856–869. Topology of the body representation in somatosensory area 1 of primates.

Werner, J. K. (1973). *Exp. Neurol.* 41:214–217. Duration of normal innervation required for complete differentiation of muscle spindles in newborn rats.

Wernig, A., and A. A. Herrera (1986). *Prog. Neurobiol.* 27:251–291. Sprouting and remodelling at the nerve-muscle junction.

Wessells, N. K. (1965). *Dev. Biol.* 12:121–153. Morphology and proliferation during early feather development.

Wessells, N. K., and K. Roessner (1965). *Dev. Biol.* 12:419–433. Nonproliferation in dermal condensations of mouse vibrissae and pelage hairs.

Wessells, N. K., B. S. Spooner, J. F. Ash, M. O. Bradley, M. A. Luduena, E. L. Taylor, J. T. Wrenn, and K. M. Yamada (1971a). *Science* 171:135–143. Microfilaments in cellular and developmental processes.

Wessells, N. K., B. S. Spooner, J. F. Ash, M. A. Luduena, and J. T. Wrenn (1971b). *Science* 173:356–359. Cytochalasin B: Microfilaments and "contractile" processes.

West, J. M., and M. Del Cerro (1976). *J. Comp. Neurol.* 165:137–160. Early formation of synapses in the molecular layer of the fetal rat cerebellum.

West, M. J. (1990). *Prog. Brain Res.* 83:13–36. A quantitative comparison of the hippocampal subdivisions of diverse species including hedgehogs, laboratory rodents, wild mice and men.

West, M. J., and H. J. G. Gundersen (1990). *J. Comp. Neurol.* 296:1–22. Unbiased stereological estimation of the number of neurons in the human hippocampus.

Weston, J. A. (1963). *Dev. Biol.* 6:279–310. A radioautographic analysis of the migration and localization of trunk neural crest cells in the chick.

Weston, J. A. (1970). *Adv. Morphogen.* 8:41–114. The migration and differentiation of neural crest cells.

Weston, J. A. (1971). *U.C.L.A. Forum Med. Sci.* 14:1–19. Neural crest cell migration and differentiation.

Weston, J. A., and S. L. Butler (1966). *Dev. Biol.* 14:246–266. Temporal factors affecting localization of neural crest cells in the chicken embryo.

Weston, J. A., K. S. Vogel, and M. F. Marusich (1988). Identification and fate of neural crest cell subpopulations in early embryonic development, pp. 224–237. In *Message To Mind: Directions in Developmental Neurobiology* (S. Easter, K. F. Barald, and B. M. Carlson, eds.), Sinauer, Sunderland, MA.

Westrum, L. E., E. G. Gray, R. D. Burgoyne, and J. Barron (1983). *Cell Tissue Res.* 231:93–102. Synaptic development and microtubule organization.

Wetts, R., and S. E. Fraser (1988). *Science* 239:1142–1145. Multipotent precursors can give rise to cell major cell types of frog retina.

Wetts, R., and K. Herrup (1982a). *J. Embryol. exp. Morphol.* 68:87–98. Interaction of granule, Purkinje, and inferior olivary neurons in lurcher chimeric mice. I. Qualitative studies.

Wetts, R., and K. Herrup (1982b). *Brain Res.* 250:358–362. Interaction of granule, Purkinje, and inferior olivary neurons in lurcher chimeric mice. II. Granule cell death.

Wetts, R., and K. Herrup (1982c). *J. Neurosci.* 2:1494–1498. Cerebellar Purkinje cells are descended from a small number of progenitors committed during early development: Quantitative analysis of lurcher chimeric mice.

Wetts, R., and K. Herrup (1983). *Dev. Brain Res.* 10:41–47. Direct correlation between Purkinje and granule cell number in the cerebella of lurcher chimeras and wild-type mice.

Wetts, R., G. N. Serbedzija, and S. E. Fraser (1989). *Dev. Biol.* 136:254–263. Cell lineage analysis reveals multipotent precursors in the ciliary margin of the frog retina.

Weurker, R. B. (1970). *Tiss. Cell* 2:1–9. Neurofilaments and glial filaments.

Weurker, R. B., and S. L. Palay (1969). *Tiss. Cell* 1:387–402. Neurofilaments and microtubules in anterior horn cells of the rat.

Weyl, H. (1949). *Philosophy of Mathematics and Natural Science*, Princeton Univ. Press, Princeton, N.J.

Whalen, R. E., and W. G. Luttge (1971a). *Horm. Behav.* 2:117–125. Testosterone, androstenedione, and dihydrotestosterone: Effects of mating behavior of rats.

Whalen, R. E., and G. E. Luttge (1971b). *Endocrinol.* 89:1320–1322. Perinatal administration of dihydrotestosterone to female rats and the development of reproductive function.

Whalen, R. G., S. M. Sell, G. S. Butler-Browne, K. Schwartz, P. Bouveret, and I. Pinset-Härström (1981). *Nature* 292:805–809. Three myosin heavy-chain isoenzymes appear sequentially in rat muscle development.

Wheatley, D. N. (1982). *The Centriole: A Central Enigma of Cell Biology*. Elsevier, New York.

Wheeler, L. R. (1939). *Vitalism: Its History and Validity*. London.

Wheeler, W. M. (1891). *J. Morphol.* 4:337–343. Neuroblasts in the arthropod's embryo.

Wheeler, W. M. (1893). *J. Morphol.* 8:1–160. A contribution to insect morphology.

Whitaker, D. M. (1940a). *J. Cellular Comp. Physiol.* 15:173–188. The effects of ultracentrifuging and of pH on the development of Fucus eggs.

Whitaker, D. M. (1940b). *Growth Suppl.* 73–90. Physical factors of growth.

Whitaker, D. M. (1941). *J. Gen. Physiol.* 24:263–278. The effect of unilateral ultraviolet light on the development of the Fucus egg.

White, E. L. (1948). *J. Exp. Zool.* 108:439–469. An experimental study of the relationship between the size of the eye and the size of the optic tectum in the brain of the developing teleost, *Fundulus heteroclitus.*

White, E. L. (1976). *Brain Res.* 105:229–251. Ultrastructure and synaptic contacts in barrels of mouse SI cortex.

White, E. L., and F. D. Nolan (1974). *Anat. Rec.* 178:486. Absence of re-innervation in the chinchilla medial superior olive.

White, J. G., E. Southgate, J. N. Thomson, and S. Brenner (1974). *Phil. Trans. Roy. Soc. (London) Ser. B.* 275:327–348. The structure of the ventral nerve cord of *Caenorhabditis elegans.*

Whitear, M. (1974). *J. Zool. Lond.* 172:503–529. The nerves in frog skin.

Whitehead, M. C., M. E. Frank, T. P. Hettinger, L. T. Hou, and H. D. Nah (1987). *Brain Res.* 405:192–195. Persistence of taste buds in denervated fungiform papillae.

Whiting, H. P. (1957). *Quart. J. Microscop. Sci.* 98:163–178. Mauthner neurones in young larval lampreys (*Lampetra* spp.).

Whiting, P. W. (1932). *J. Comp. Psychol.* 14:345–363. Reproductive reactions of sex mosaics of a parasitic wasp *Habrobracon juglandis.*

Whitman, C. O. (1887). *J. Morphol.* 1:105–182. A contribution to the history of germ layers in Clepsine.

Whitsel, B. L., L. M. Petrucelli, and G. Werner (1969). *J. Neurophysiol.* 32:170–183. Symmetry and connectivity in the map of the body surface in somatosensory area II of primates.

Whittaker, J. R. (1973). *Proc. Natl. Acad. Sci. U.S.A.* 70:2096–2100. Segregation during ascidian embryogenesis of egg cytoplasmic information for tissue-specific enzyme development.

Whittaker, J. R. (1979). Cytoplasmic determinants of tissue differentiation in the ascidian egg, pp. 29–51. In *Determinants of Spatial Organization* (S. Subtelny, and I. R. Konigsberg, eds.), Academic Press, New York.

Whittaker, J. R. (1980). *J. Embryol. Exp. Morph.* 55:343–354. Acetylcholinesterase development in extra cells caused by changing the distribution of myoplasm in ascidian embryos.

Whittaker, J. R. (1982). *Dev. Biol.* 93:463–470. Muscle lineage cytoplasm can change the developmental expression in epidermal lineage cells of ascidian embryos.

Whittaker, J. R. (1983). *J. Embryol. Exp. Morph.* 76:235–250. Quantitative regulation of acetylcholinesterase development in the muscle lineage cells of cleavage-arrested ascidian embryos.

Whittemore, S. R., and A. Seiger (1987). *Brain Res. Rev.* 12:439–464. The expression, localization, and functional significance of β-nerve growth factor in the central nervous system.

Whittemore, S. R., T. Ebendal, L. Lärkfors, L. Olson, Å. Seiger, I. Strömberg, and H. Persson (1986). *Proc. Natl. Acad. Sci. U.S.A* 83:817–821. Development and regional expression of β nerve growth factor messenger RNA and protein in the rat central nervous system.

Whittemore, S. R., P. L. Friedman, D. Larhammar, H. Persson, M. Gonzalez-Carvajal, and V. R. Holets (1988). *J. Neurosci. Res.* 20:403–410. Rat β-nerve growth factor sequence and site of synthesis in the adult hippocampus.

Whitten, J. M. (1969). *Science* 163:1456–1457. Cell death during early morphogenesis: Parallels between insect limb and vertebrate limb development.

Whitteridge, G. (1964). *The Anatomical Lectures of William Harvey.* Livingstone, Edinburgh.

Whyte, L. L., A. G. Wilson and D. Wilson, eds. (1969). *Hierarchical Structures,* Am. Elsevier, New York.

Wickelgren, B. G., and P. Sterling (1969). *J. Neurophysiol.* 32:16–23. Influence of visual cortex on receptive fields in the superior colliculus of the cat.

Wiedersheim, R. (1890). *Anat. Anz.* 5. Über Bewegungserscheinungen im Gehirn von Leptodora hyalina.

Wieland, S. J., and T. O. Fox (1981). *J. Steroid Biochem.* 14:409–418. Androgen receptors from rat kidney and brain; DNA-binding properties of wild-type and Tfm mutant.

Wieman, H. L., and T. C. Nussmann (1929). *Physiol. Zool.* 2:99–124. Experimental modification of nerve development in *Amblystoma.*

Wiener, G. (1962). *J. Nerv. Ment. Dis.* 134:129–143. Psychological correlates of premature birth: A review.

Wiersma, C. A. G. (1931). *Arch. Neurol. Physiol.* 16:337–345. An experiment on the "resonance theory" of muscular activity.

Wiersma, C. A. G. (1957). *Acta Physiol. Pharmacol. Neerl.* 6:135–142. On the number of nerve cells in a crustacean central nervous system.

Wiesel, T. N., and D. H. Hubel (1963a). *J. Neurophysiol.* 26:978–993. Effects of visual deprivation on morphology and physiology of cells in the cat's lateral geniculate body.

Wiesel, T. N, and D. H. Hubel (1963b). *J. Neurophysiol.* 26:1003–1017. Single- cell responses in striate cortex of kittens deprived of vision in one eye.

Wiesel, T. N., and D. H. Hubel (1965a). *J. Neurophysiol.* 28:1029–1040. Comparison of the effects of unilateral and bilateral eye closure on cortical unit responses in kittens.

Wiesel, T. N., and D. H. Hubel (1965b). *J. Neurophysiol.* 28:1060–1072. Extent of recovery from the effects of visual deprivation in kittens.

Wiesel, T. N., and D. H. Hubel (1974). *J. Comp. Neurol.* 158:307–318. Ordered arrangement of orientation columns in monkeys lacking visual experience.

Wiesel, T. N., D. H. Hubel, and D. M. K. Lam (1974). *Brain Res.* 79:273–279. Autoradiographic demonstration of ocular dominance columns in the monkey striate cortex by means of transneuronal transport.

Wiest, W. D., and J. Hallervorden (1958). *Deutsch. Z. Nervenheilk.* 178:224–238. Migrationshemmung in Gross- und Kleinhirn.

Wigger, H. (1939). *Z. Morphol. Oekol. Tiere* 36:1–20. Vergleichende Untersuchungen am Auge von Wild und Hausschwein unter besonderer Berücksichtigung der Retina.

Wiggins, R. C. (1982). *Brain Res. Rev.* 4:151–175. Myelin development and nutritional insufficiency.

Wiggins, R. C., and G. N. Fuller (1979). *Brain Res.* 162:103–112. Relative synthesis of myelin in different brain regions of postnatally undernourished rats.

Wiggins, R. C., S. L. Miller, J. A. Benjamins, M. R. Krigman, and P. Morell (1976). *Brain Res.* 107:257–273. Myelin synthesis during postnatal nutritional deprivation and subsequent rehabilitation.

Wigglesworth, V. B. (1959). *The Control of Growth and Form: A Study of the Epidermal Cell in an Insect.* Cornell Univ. Press. Ithaca, New York.

Wigston, D. J. (1989). *J. Neurosci.* 9:639–647. Remodeling of neuromuscular junctions in adult mouse soleus.

Wigston, D. J., and P. R. Kennedy (1987). *J. Neurosci.* 7:1857–1865. Selective reinnervation of transplanted muscles by their original motoneurons in the axolotl.

Wikler, K. C., G. Perez, and B. L. Finlay (1989). *J. Comp. Neurol.* 285:157–176. Duration of retinogenesis: Its relationship to retinal organization in two cricetine rodents.

Wilder, B. (1897). *J. Comp. Neurol.* 6:216–352. Neural terms.

Wileman, T., C. Harding, and P. Stahl (1982). *Biochem. J.* 232:1–14. Receptor mediated endocytosis.

Wiley, R. G., and T. N. Oeltmann (1986). *J. Neurosci. Meth.* 17:43–53. Anatomically selective peripheral nerve ablation using intraneural ricin injection.

Wiley, R. G., W. W. Blessing, and D. J. Reis (1982). *Science* 216:889–890. Suicide transport: Destruction of neurons by retrograde transport of ricin, abrin and modeccin.

Wilkin, G. P., D. R. Marriott, and A. J. Cholewinski (1990). *Trends Neurosci.* 13:43–45. Astrocyte heterogeneity.

Wilkinson, D. G. (1990). *Seminars Dev. Biol.* 1:127–134. Segmental gene expression in the developing mouse brain.

Wilkinson, D. G., and R. Krumlauf (1990). *Trends Neurosci.* 13:335–339. Molecular approaches to the segmentation of the hindbrain.

Wilkinson, D. G., S. Bhatt, P. Chavier, R. Bravo, and P. Charnay (1989a). *Nature* 337:461–464. Segment-specific expression of a zinc-finger gene in the developing nervous system of the mouse.

Wilkinson, D. G., S. Bhatt, M. Cook, E. Boncinelli, and R. Krumlauf (1989b). *Nature* 341:405–409. Segmental expression of Hox-2 homoeobox-containing genes in the developing mouse hindbrain.

Willard, M. (1977). *J. Cell Biol.* 75:1–11. The identification of two intra-axonally transported polypeptides resembling myosin in some respects in the rabbit visual system.

Willard, M., and C. Simon (1981). *J. Cell Biol.* 89:198–205. Antibody decoration of neurofilaments.

Willard, M., and C. Simon (1983). *Cell* 35:551–559. Modulations of neurofilament axonal transport during the development of rabbit retinal ganglion cells.

Wille, W., and E. Trenkner (1981). *J. Neurochem.* 37:443–446. Changes in particulate neuraminidase activity during normal and staggerer mutant mouse development.

Willerman, L., and J. A. Churchill (1967). *Child Dev.* 38:623–629. Intelligence and birth weight in identical twins.

Willey, A. (1894). *Amphioxus and the Ancestry of the Vertebrates.* Macmillan, New York and London.

Williams, A. F. (1987). *Immunol. Today* 8:298–303. A year in the life of the immunoglobulin superfamily.

Williams, B. P., E. R. Abney, and M. C. Raff (1985). *Dev. Biol.* 112:126–134. Macroglial cell development in embryonic rat brain: Studies using monoclonal antibodies, fluorescence activated cell sorting and cell culture.

Williams, C., G. Wohlenberg, and M. J. O'Donovan (1987). *Dev. Brain Res.* 34:215–221. Regional variations in the extent and timing of motoneuron cell death in the lumbosacral spinal cord of the chick embryo.

Williams, L. R., S. Varon, G. M. Peterson, K. Wictorin, W. Fischer, A. Bjorklund, and F. H. Gage (1986). *Proc. Natl. Acad. Sci. U.S.A.* 83:9231–9236. Continuous infusion of nerve growth factor prevents basal forebrain neuronal death after fimbria fornix transection.

Williams, L. T. (1989). *Science* 243:1564–1570. Signal transduction by the platelet-derived growth factor receptor.

Williams, P. L., and S. M. Hall (1971). *J. Anat. (London)* 108:397–408. Prolonged *in vivo* observations of normal peripheral nerve fibres and their acute reactions to crush and deliberate trauma.

Williams, R. W., and L. M. Chalupa (1982). *J. Neurosci.* 2:604–622. Prenatal development of retino-collicular projections in the cat: An anterograde tracer transport study.

Williams, R. W., and K. Herrup (1988). *Ann. Rev. Neurosci.* 11:423–453. The control of neuron number.

Williams, R. W., and P. Rakic (1988). *J. Comp. Neurol.* 278:344–352. Three-dimensional counting: An accurate and direct method to estimate numbers of cells in sectioned material.

Williams, R. W., and P. Rakic (1989). *J. Comp. Neurol.* 281:335. Erratum and Addendum. Three-dimensional counting: An accurate and direct method to estimate numbers of cells in sectioned material.

Williams, R. W., M. J. Bastiani, and L. M. Chalupa (1983). *J. Neurosci.* 3:133–144. Loss of axons in the cat optic nerve following fetal unilateral enucleation: An electron microscopic analysis.

Willinger, M., and D. M. Margolis (1985a). *Dev. Biol.* 107:156–172. Effect of the weaver (*wv*) mutation on cerebellar neuron differentiation. I. Qualitative observations of neuron behavior in culture.

Willinger, M., and D. M. Margolis (1985b). *Dev. Biol.* 107:173–179. Effect of the weaver (*wv*) mutation on cerebellar neuron differentation. II. Quantitation of neuron behavior in culture.

Willinger, M., D. M. Margolis, and R. L. Sidman (1981). *J. Supermolec. Struct.* 17:79–86. Neuronal differentiation in cultures of weaver mutant mouse cerebellum.

Willingham, M. C., and I. Pastan (1984). *Int. Rev. Cytol.* 92:51–92. Endocytosis and exocytosis; current concepts of vesicle traffic in animal cells.

Willison, H. J., A. I. Ilyas, D. J. O'Shannessy, M. J. Pulley, B. D. Trapp, and R. H. Quarles (1987). *J. Neurochem.* 49:1853–1862. Myelin-associated glycoprotein and related glycoconjugates in developing cat peripheral nerve: A correlative biochemical and morphometric study.

Willison, H. J., B. D. Trapp, J. D. Bacher, and R. H. Quarles (1988). *Brain Res.* 444:10–16. The expression of myelin-associated glycoprotein during remyelination in cat sciatic nerve.

Willison, J. G., and E. L. Engel (1976). *J. Neurocytol.* 5:605–615. Peripheral nerve glycoproteins and myelin fine structure during development of the rat sciatic nerve.

Willshaw, D. J., and C. von der Malsburg (1976). *Proc. Roy. Soc. (London) Ser. B.* 194:431–445. How patterned neural connections can be set up by self-organization.

Willshaw, D. J., J. W. Fawcett, and R. M. Gaze (1983). *J. Embryol. Exp. Morphol.* 74:29–45. The visuotectal projection made by *Xenopus* 'pie slice' compound eyes.

Wilson, D. B. (1972). *Am. J. Anat.* 135:549–560. Effects of embryonic overgrowth on the avian optic tectum.

Wilson, D. B. (1973). *J. Embryol. Exp. Morphol.* 29:745–751. Chronological changes in the cell cycle of chick neuroepithelial cells.

Wilson, D. B. (1974). *Brain Res.* 69:41–48. The cell cycle of ventricular cells in the overgrown optic tectum.

Wilson, D. B. (1975). *Experientia* 31:220–221. Brain abnormalities in the lurcher (*Lc*) mutant mouse.

Wilson, D. B. (1976). *J. Neuropath. Exp. Neurol.* 35:40–45. Histological defects in the cerebellum of adult lurcher (*Lc*) mice.

Wilson, D. B. (1982). *Dev. Brain. Res.* 2:420–424. The cell cycle during closure of the neural folds in the C57BL mouse.

Wilson, G. F., and S. Y. Chiu (1990). *J. Neurosci.* 10:1615–1625. Potassium channel regulation in schwann cells during early developmental myelinogenesis.

Wilson, H. V. (1907). *J. Exp. Zool.* 5:245–258. On some phenomena of coalescence and regeneration in sponges.

Wilson, J. R., and S. M. Sherman (1976). *J. Neurophysiol.* 39:512–533. Receptive-field characteristics of neurons in cat striate cortex: Changes with visual field eccentricity.

Wilson, L., J. Bryan, A. Ruby, and D. Mazia (1970). *Proc. Natl. Acad. Sci. U.S.A.* 66:807–814. Precipitation of proteins by vinblastine and calcium ions.

Wilson, L., J. R. Bamburg, S. B. Mizel, L. M. Grisham, and K. M. Creswell (1974). *Fed. Proc.* 33:158–166. Interaction of drugs with microtubule proteins.

Wilson, M. A. (1971). *J. Exp. Physiol.* 56:83–91. Optic nerve fibre counts and retinal ganglion cell counts during development of *Xenopus laevis (Daudin)*.

Wilson S., D. A. Tonge, and N. Holder (1989). *Development* 106:707–715. Homing behaviour of regenerating axons in the amphibian limb.

Wilt, F. H. (1959). *Dev. Biol.* 1:199–233. The differentiation of visual pigments in metamorphosing larvae of *Rana catesbeiana*.

Wilt, F. H., and M. Anderson (1972). *Dev. Biol.* 28:443–447. The action of 5-bromodeoxyuridine on differentiation.

Wimer, C. C., and R. E. Wimer (1989). *Dev. Brain Res.* 48:167–176. On the sources of strain and sex differences in granule cell number in the dentate area of house mice.

Wimer, R. E., and C. C. Wimer (1982). *Dev. Brain Res.* 2:129–140. A biometrical-genetic analysis of granule cell number in the area dentata of house mice.

Wimer, R. E., and C. C. Wimer (1985). *Brain Res.* 328:105–109. Three sex dimorphisms in the granule cell layer of the hippocampus in house mice.

Wimer, R. E., and C. C. Wimer, J. E. Vaughn, R. P. Barber, B. A. Balvanz, and C. R. Chernow (1976). *Brain Res.* 118:219–243. The genetic organization of neuron number in Ammon's horns of house mice.

Wimer, R. E., C. C. Wimer, J. E. Vaughn, R. P. Barber, B. A. Balvanz, and C. R. Chernow (1978). *Brain Res.* 157:105–122. The genetic organization of neuron number in the granule cell layer of the area dentata in house mice.

Wimer, R. E., C. C. Wimer, C. R. Chernow, and C. A. Balvanz (1980). *Brain Res.* 196:59–77. The genetic organization of neuron number in the pyramidal cell layer of hippocampal region superior in house mice.

Wimer, R. E., C. C. Wimer, and L. A. Alameddine (1988). *Dev. Brain Res.* 42:191–197. On the development of strain and sex differences in granule cell number in the area dentata in house mice.

Wimsatt, W. C. (1970). *Stud. Hist. Phil. Sci.* 3:1–80. Teleology and the logical structure of function statements.

Windle, W. F. (1958). *Biology of Neuroglia*, 340 pp. C. C. Thomas, Springfield.

Windle, W. F., and D. W. Orr (1934). *J. Comp. Neurol.* 60:287–307. The development of behavior in chick embryos: Spinal cord structure correlated with early somatic motility.

Windle, W. F., M. W. Fish, and J. E. O'Donnell (1934). *J. Comp. Neurol.* 59:139–165. Myelogeny of the cat as related to development of fiber tracts and prenatal behavior patterns.

Windle, W. F., W. L. Minear, M. F. Austin, and D. W. Orr (1935). *Physiol. Zool.* 8:156–185. The origin and early development of somatic behavior in the albino rat.

Windrem, M. S., S. Jan de Beur, and B. L. Finlay (1988). *Dev. Brain Res.* 43:13–22. Control of cell number in the developing neocortex. II. Effects of corpus callosum section.

Wine, J. J. (1973). *Exp. Neurol.* 38:157–169. Invertebrate central neurons: Orthorgrade degeneration and retrograde changes after axonotomy.

Winfield, D. A. (1981). *Brain Res.* 206:166–171. The postnatal development of synapses in the visual cortex of the cat and the effects of eyelid suture.

Winick, M. (1967). *J. Pediatr.* 71:390–395. Cellular growth of the human placenta. III. Intrauterine growth failure.

Winick, M. (1969). *J. Pediat.* 74:667–679. Malnutrition and brain development.

Winick, M. (1970a). *Pediatr. Clin. N. Am.* 17:69–78. Cellular growth in intrauterine malnutrition.

Winick, M. (1970b). *Exp. Neurol.* 26:393–400. Cellular growth of cerebrum, cerebellum, and brain stem in normal and marasmic children.

Winick, M., and R. E. Greenberg (1965a). *Nature* 205:180–181. Chemical control of sensory ganglia during a critical period of development.

Winick, M., and R. E. Greenberg (1965b). *Pediatrics* 35:221–228. Appearance and localization of a nerve growth-promoting protein during development.

Winick, M., and A. Noble (1965). *Dev. Biol.* 12:451–466. Quantitative changes in DNA, RNA and protein during prenatal and postnatal growth in the rat.

Winick, M., and P. Rosso (1969). *Pediat. Res.* 3:181–184. Effects of severe early malnutrition on cellular growth of human brain.

Winick, M., K. K. Meyer, and R. C. Harris (1975). *Science* 190:1173–1175. Malnutrition and environmental enrichment by early adoption.

Winkel, G. K., and R. A. Pedersen (1988). *Dev. Biol.* 127:143–156. Fate of the inner cell mass in mouse embryos as studied by microinjection of lineage tracers.

Winkelmann, R. K. (1977). *J. Invest. Dermatol.* 69:41–46. The Merkel cell system and a comparison between it and the neurosecretory or APUD cell system.

Winkelmann, R. K., and A. S. Breathnach (1973). *J. Invest. Dermatol.* 60:2–15. The Merkel cell.

Wion, D., C. Perret, N. Frechin, A. Keller, G. Behar, P. Brachet, and C. Auggray (1986). *FEBS Lett.* 203:82–86. Molecular cloning of the avian β-nerve growth factor gene: Transcription in brain.

Wischik, C. M., R. A. Crowther, M. Stewart, and M. Roth (1985). *J. Cell Biol.* 100:1905–1912. Subunit structure of paired helical filaments in Alzheimer's disease.

Wise, S. P., and M. Godschalk (1987). *Trends Neurosci.* 10:449–450. Functional fractionation of frontal fields.

Wise, S. P., and E. D Jones (1976). *J. Comp. Neurol.* 168:313–344. The organization and postnatal development of the commisural projections of the rat somatic sensory cortex.

Wise, S. P., and E. D. Jones (1978). *J. Comp. Neurol.* 178:187–208. Developmental studies of thalamocortical and commissural connections in the rat somatic sensory cortex.

Wise, S. P., J. W. Fleshman, Jr., and E. G. Jones (1979). *Neuroscience* 4:1275–1298. Maturation of pyramidal cell form in relation to developing afferent and efferent connections of rat somatic sensory cortex.

Wislocki, G. B., and E. H. Leduc (1952). *J. Comp. Neurol.* 96:371–413. Vital staining of the hematoencephalic barrier by silver nitrate and trypan blue, and the cytological comparison of the neurohypophysis, pineal body, area postrema intercolumnar tubercle, and supraoptic crest.

Witelson, S. F. (1976). *Science* 193:425–427. Sex and the single hemisphere: Specialization of the right hemisphere for spatial processing.

Witelson, S. F. (1985). *Science* 229:665–668. The brain connection: The corpus callosum is larger in left-handers.

Wittenberg, C., and S. I. Reed (1988). *Cell* 54:1061–1072. Control of the yeast cell cycle is associated with assembly/disassembly of the cdc28 protein kinase complex.

Wittenberger, B., D. Raben, M. A. Lieberman, and L. Glaser (1978). *Proc. Natl. Acad. Sci. U.S.A.* 75:5457–5461. Inhibition of growth of 3T3 cells by extract of surface membranes.

Wittgenstein, L. (1977). *Vermischte Bemerkungen.* Suhrkamp Verlag, Frankfurt am Main.

Wittman, K. S., P. L. Krupa, I. Pesetsky, and M. Hamburgh (1972). *Dev. Biol.* 27:419–424. Electron microscopy and histochemistry of tail regression in the Brachyury mouse.

Wlassak, R. (1889). *Arch. Entw. Mech. Organ.* 6:453–493. Die Herkunft des Myelins.

Wolf, M. K. (1964). *J. Cell Biol.* 22:259–279. Differentiation of neuronal types and synapses in myelinating cultures of mouse cerebellum.

Wolf, M. K., and M. Dubois-Dalcq (1970). *J. Comp. Neurol.* 140:261–280. Anatomy of cultured mouse cerebellum. I. Golgi and electron microscopic demonstrations of granule cells, their afferent and efferent synapses.

Wolfe, A. (1952). *A History of Science, Technology and Philosophy in the Eighteenth Century.* 2nd ed. rev. by D. McKie. London

Wolff, J. R., and M. Rickmann (1977). *Folia morph.* 25:235–237. Cytological characteristics of early stages of glial differentiation in neocortex.

Wolff, J. R., C. Goerz, T. Bär, and F. H. Guldner (1975). *Microvasc. Res.* 10:373–395. Common morphogenetic aspects of various organotypic microvascular systems.

Wolff, J. R., S. Eins, M. Holzgraefe, and L. Záborszky (1981). *Cell Tissue Res.* 214:303–321. The temporo-spatial course of degeneration after cutting cortico-cortical connections in adult rats.

Wolff, J. R., V. J. Balcar, T. Zetzsche, H. Bottcher, D. E. Schmechel, and B. M. Chronwall (1984). Development of Gabaergic system in rat visual cortex, pp. 215–239. In *Gene Expression and Cell-Cell Interaction* (J. M. Lauder, and P. G. Nelson, eds.), Plenum, New York.

Wolff, M. (1905). *J. Psychol. Neurol.* 4:144–157. Zur Kenntnis des Heldschen Nervenendfüsse.

Wolpert, L. (1969). *J. Theor. Biol.* 25:1–47. Positional information and the spatial pattern of cellular differentiation.

Wolpert, L. (1971). *Curr. Top. Dev. Biol.* 6:183–224. Positional information and pattern formation.

Wolpert, L. (1974). *Lect. Math. Life Sci.* 6:29–41. Positional information and the development of pattern and form.

Wolswijk, G., and M. Noble (1989). *Development* 105:387–400. Identification of an adult-specific glial progenitor cell.

Wong, K. C., and L.-T. Wu (1936). *History of Chinese Medicine,* 2nd edn. China National Quarantine Service, Shanghai.

Wong-Riley, M. T. T. (1972). *J. Comp. Neurol.* 144:61–92. Terminal degeneration and glial reactions in the lateral geniculate nucleus of squirrel monkey after eye removal.

Wong-Riley, M. T. T. (1979). *Brain Res.* 171:11–28. Changes in the visual system of monocularly sutured or enucleated cats demonstrable with cytochrome oxidase histochemistry.

Wong-Riley, M. T. T. (1989). *Trends Neurosci.* 12:94–101. Cytochrome oxidase: An endogenous metabolic marker for neuronal activity.

Wong-Riley, M. T. T., and D. Riley (1983). *Brain Res.* 261:185–193. The effect of impulse blockage on cytochrome oxidase activity in the cat visual system.

Wong-Riley, M. T. T., and C. Welt (1980). *Proc. Natl. Acad. Sci. U.S.A.* 77:2333–2337. Histochemical changes in cytochrome oxidase or cortical barrels after vibrissal removal in neonatal and adult mice.

Wong, R. O. L., and A. Hughes (1987a). *J. Comp. Neurol.* 255:159–177. The morphology, number and distribution of a large population of confirmed displaced amacrine cells in the adult cat retina.

Wong, R. O. L., and A. Hughes (1987b). *J. Comp. Neurol.* 262:473–495. Developing neuronal population of the cat retinal ganglion cell layer.

Wong, R. O. L., and A. Hughes (1987c). *J. Comp. Neurol.* 262:496–511. Role of cell death in the topogenesis of neuronal distributions in the developing cat retinal ganglion cell layer.

Woo, H. H., L. S. Jen, and K.-F. So (1985). *Dev. Brain Res.* 20:1–13. The postnatal development of retinocollicular projections in normal hamsters and in hamsters following neonatal monocular enucleations: A horseradish peroxidase tracing study.

Wood, J. C., and N. King (1971). *Nature* 229:56–57. Turnover of basic protein of rat brain.

Wood, J. G., S. S. Mirra, N. J. Pollock, and L. I. Binder (1986). *Proc. Natl. Acad. Sci. U.S.A* 83:4040–4043. Neurofibrillary tangles of Alzheimer disease share antigenic determinants with the axonal microtubule-associated protein tau.

Wood, J. N., and B. H. Anderton (1981). *Biosci. Rep.* 1:263–268. Monoclonal antibodies to mammalian neurofilaments.

Wood, P., and R. P. Bunge (1984). The biology of the oligodendrocyte, pp. 1–46. In *Oligodendroglia, Advances In Neurochemistry,* Vol. 5, (W. T. Norton, ed.) Plenum, New York.

Wood, P. M., and R. P. Bunge (1975). *Nature* 256:662–664. Evidence that sensory axons are mitogenic for Schwann cells.

Woodard, J. S. (1960). *J. Comp. Neurol.* 115:65–73. Origin of the external granule layer of the cerebellar cortex.

Woods, J. E., G. W. De Vries, and R. C. Thommes (1971). *Gen. Comp. Endocrinol.* 17:407–415. Ontogenesis of the pituitary-adrenal axis in the chick embryo.

Woodward, D. J., B. J. Hoffer, G. R. Siggins, and F. E. Bloom (1971). *Brain Res.* 34:73–97. The ontogenetic development of synaptic junctions, synaptic activation and responsiveness to neurotransmitter substances in rat cerebellar Purkinje cells.

Woodward, D. J., B. J. Hoffer, and J. Altman (1974). *J. Neurobiol.* 5:283–304. Physiological and pharmacological properties of Purkinje cells in rat cerebellum degranulated by postnatal X-irradiation.

Woolsey, C. N. (1943). *Fed. Proc.* 2:55–56. 'Second' somatic receiving areas in the cerebral cortex of cat, dog and monkey.

Woolsey, C. N. (1958). Organization of somatic sensory and motor areas of the cerebral cortex, pp. 63–81. In *Biological and Biochemical Bases of Behavior* (H. F. Harlow, and C. N. Woolsey, eds.), Madison: Univ. Wisc. Press.

Woolsey, C. N., P. H. Settlage, D. R. Meyer, W. Sencer, T. P. Hamuy, and A. M. Travis (1952). *Res. Publ. Assoc. Res. Nerv. Ment. Dis.* 30:238–264. Patterns of localization in precentral and 'supplementary' motor areas and their relation to the concept of a premotor area.

Woolsey, C. N., A. M. Travis, J. W. Barnard, and R. S. Ostenso (1953). *Fed. Proc.* 12:160. Motor representation in the postcentral gyrus after chronic ablation of precental and supplementary motor areas.

Woolsey, T. A. (1967). *Johns Hopkins Med. J.* 121:91–112. Somatosensory, auditory and visual cortical areas of the mouse.

Woolsey, T. A., and H. Van der Loos (1970). *Brain Res.* 17:205–242. The structural organization of layer IV in the somatosensory region (SI) of the mouse cerebral cortex. The description of a cortical field composed of discrete cytoarchitectonic units.

Woolsey, T. A., and J. R. Wann (1976). *J. Comp. Neurol.* 170:53–66. Areal changes in mouse cortical barrels following vibrissal damage at different postnatal ages.

Woolsey, T. A., M. L. Dierker, and D. F. Wann (1975a). *Proc. Natl. Acad. Sci. U.S.A.* 72:2165–2169. Mouse SmI cortex: Qualitative and quantitative classification of Golgi-impregnated barrel neurons.

Woolsey, T. A., C. Welker, and R. H. Schwartz (1975b). *J. Comp. Neurol.* 164:79–94. Comparative anatomical studies of the Sml face cortex with special reference to the occurrence of "barrels" in layer IV.

Wree, A., K. Zilles, and A. Schleicher (1981). *Anat. Embryol.* 161:419–431. Growth of fresh volumes and spontaneous cell death in the nuclei habenulai of albino rats during ontogenesis.

Wree, A., K. Zilles, and A. Schleicher (1983). *Anat. Embryol.* 166:333–353. A quantitative approach to cytoarchitectonics. VIII. The Areal pattern of the cortex of the albino mouse.

Wright, B. A., and J. M. Spink (1959). *Gerontologia* 3:277–287. A study of the loss of nerve cells in the central nervous system in relation to age.

Wright, L. L. (1981). *J. Comp. Neurol.* 199:125–132. Time of cell origin and cell death in the avian dorsal motor nucleus of the vagus.

Wright, L. L. (1982). *Dev. Brain Res.* 1:283–286. Cell survival in the chick embryo ciliary ganglion is reduced by chronic ganglion blockade.

Wright, L. L., and A. J. Smolen (1983a). *Dev. Brain Res.* 8:145–153. Neonatal testosterone treatment increases neuron and synapses numbers in male rat superior cervical ganglion.

Wright, L. L., and A. J. Smolen (1983b). *Dev. Brain Res.* 6:299–303. Effects of 17-beta-estradiol on developing superior cervical ganglion neurons and synapses.

Wright, L. L., and A. J. Smolen (1985). *Dev. Brain Res.* 20:314–316. Effects of neonatal castration or treatment with dihydrotestosterone on numbers of neurons in the rat superior cervical sympathetic ganglion.

Wright, L. L., and A. J. Smolen (1987). *Int. J. Dev. Neurosci.* 5:305–311. The role of neuron death in the development of the gender difference in the number of neurons in the rat superior cervical ganglion.

Wright, L. L., T. J. Cunningham, and A. J. Smolen (1981). *Anat. Rec.* 199:283A. Neuronal degeneration in the rat superior cervical ganglion.

Wright, M. R. (1964). *J. Exp. Zool.* 156:377–390. Taste organs in tongue-to-liver grafts in the newt, *Triturus viridescens.*

Wright, N., and D. Appleton (1980). *Cell Tiss. Kinet.* 13:643–664. The metaphase arrest technique: A critical review.

Wu, C. (1964). *Arch. Biochem. Biophys.* 106:394–401. Glutamine synthetase. III. Factors controlling its activity in the developing rat.

Wuerker, R. B., and J. B. Kirkpatrick (1972). *Int. Rev. Cytol.* 33:45–75. Neuronal microtubules, neurofilaments, and microfilaments.

Wuerker, R. B., and S. L. Palay (1969). *Tiss. Cell* 1:387–402. Neurofilaments and microtubules in anterior horn cells of the rat.

Wuerker, R. B., A. M. McPhedran, and E. Henneman (1965). *J. Neurophysiol.* 28:85–99. Properties of motor units in a homogeneous pale muscle (*M. gastrocnemius*) of the cat.

Wujek, J. R., and R. J. Lasek (1983). *J. Neurosci.* 3:243–251. Correlation of axonal regeneration and slow component b in two branches of a single axon.

Wundt, W. (1904). *Principles of Physiological Psychology, Vol. 1,* Translated from the Fifth German Edition (1902) by E. B. Titchener. Swan Sonnenschein, Macmillan, New York.

Wye-Dvorak, J. (1984). *J. Comp. Neurol.* 228:491–508. Postnatal development of primary visual projections in the tammar wallaby (*Macropus eugenii*).

Wyllie, A. H., J. F. R. Kerr, and A. R. Currie (1980). *Int. Rev. Cytol.* 68:251–306. Cell death: The significance of apoptosis.

Wyllie, A. H., G. J. Beattie, and A. D. Hargreaves (1981). *Histochem. J.* 13:681–692. Chromatin changes in apoptosis.

Xeros, N. (1962). *Nature* 194:682–683. Deoxyriboside control and synchronization of mitosis.

Xue, Z. G., J. Smith, and N. M. Le Douarin (1985). *Proc. Natl. Acad. Sci. U.S.A* 82:8800–8804. Differentiation of catecholaminergic cells in cultures of embryonic avian sensory ganglia.

Yakovlev, P. I., and A.-R. Lecours (1967). The myelogenetic cycles of regional maturation of the brain, pp. 3–64. In *Regional Development of the Brain in Early Life* (A. Minkowski, ed.), Blackwell, Oxford.

Yaktin, J. S., and D. S. McLaren (1970). *J. Ment. Defic. Res.* 14:25–32. The behavioral development of infants recovering from severe malnutrition.

Yamada, K. M., and D. W. Kennedy (1984). *J. Cell Biol.* 99:29–36. Dualistic nature of adhesive protein function:

Fibronectin and its biologically active peptide fragments can auto inhibit fibronectin function.

Yamada, K. M., and N. K. Wessels (1971). *Exp. Cell Res.* 66:346–352. Axon elongation: Effect of nerve growth factor on microtubule protein.

Yamada, K. M., B. S. Spooner, and N. K. Wessels (1970). *Proc. Natl. Acad. Sci. U.S.A.* 66:1206–1212. Axon growth: Roles of microfilaments and microtubules.

Yamada, K. M., B. S. Spooner, and N. K. Wessells (1971). *J. Cell Biol.* 49:614–635. Ultrastructure and function of growth cones and axons of cultured nerve cells.

Yamada, T. (1950). *Embryologia* 1:1–20. Regional differentiation of the isolated ectoderm of the *Triturus gastrula* induced through a protein extract.

Yamada, T. (1958). *Experientia* 14:81–87. Induction of specific differentiation by samples of proteins and nucleoproteins in the isolated ectoderm of *Triturus* gastrulae.

Yamamoto, T., Y. Iwasaki, and H. Konno (1983). *Brain Res.* 274:325–328. Retrograde axoplasmic transport of toxin lectins is useful for transganglionic tracings of the peripheral nerve.

Yamamoto, T., Y. Iwasaki, and H. Konno (1984). *J. Neurosurg.* 60:108–114. Experimental sensory ganglionectomy by way of sciatic axoplasmic transport.

Yan, Q., and E. M. Johnson, Jr. (1987). *Dev. Biol.* 121:139–148. A quantitative study of the developmental expression of nerve growth factor (NGF) receptor in rats.

Yan, Q., and E. M. Johnson, Jr. (1988). *J. Neurosci.* 8:3481–3498. An immunohistochemical study of the nerve growth factor receptor in developing rats.

Yan, Q., and E. M. Johnson, Jr. (1989). *J. Comp. Neurol.* 290:585–598. Immunohistochemical localization and biochemical characterization of nerve growth factor receptor in adult rat brain.

Yan, Q., W. D. Snider, J. J. Pinzone, and E. M. Johnson, Jr. (1988). *Neuron* 1:335–343. Retrograde transport of nerve growth gactor (NGF) in motoneurons of developing rats: Assessment of potential neurotrophic effects.

Yankner, B. A., E. M. Shooter (1979). *Proc. Natl. Acad. Sci. U.S.A.* 76:1269–1273. Nerve growth factor in the nucleus: Interaction with receptors on the nuclear membrane.

Yankner, B. A., and E. M. Shooter (1982). *Ann. Rev. Biochem.* 51:845–868. The biology and mechanism of action of nerve growth factor.

Yasargil, G. M., L. Macintyre, R. Doucette, B. Visheau, M. Holmes, and J. Diamond (1988). *J. Comp. Neurol.* 270:301–312. Axonal domains within shared touch domes in the rat: A comparison of their fate during conditions favoring collateral sprouting and following axonal regeneration.

Yates, R. D. (1961). *J. Exp. Zool.* 147:167–182. A study of division in chick embryonic ganglia.

Yawa, H. (1987). *J. Neurosci.* 7:3703–3711. Changes in the dendritic geometry of mouse superior cervical ganglion cells following postganglionic axotomy.

Yellin, H. (1967a). *Anat. Rec.* 157:345. Muscle fiber plasticity and the creation of localized motor units.

Yellin, H. (1967b). *Exp. Neurol.* 19:92–103. Neural regulation of enzymes in muscle fibers of red and white muscle.

Yew, D. T. (1979). *Neurosci. Lett.* 13:173–176. Cell kinetic in retinal cell morphogenesis.

Yin, H. L. (1987). *BioEssays* 7:176–179. Gelsolin: Calcium-and polyphosphoinositide-regulated actin-modulating protein.

Yip, H. K., and B. Grafstein (1982). *Brain Res.* 238:329–339. Effect of nerve growth factor on regeneration of goldfish optic axons.

Yip, H. K., and E. M. Johnson, Jr. (1984). *Proc. Natl. Acad. Sci. U.S.A.* 81:6245–6249. Developing dorsal root ganglion neurons require trophic support from their central processes: Evidence for a role of retrogradely transported nerve growth factor from the central nervous system to the periphery.

Yisraeli, J. K., S. Sokol, and D. A. Melton (1990). *Development* 108:289–298. A two-step model for the localization of maternal mRNA in *Xenopus* oocytes: involvement of microtubules and microfilaments in the translation and anchoring of Vg1 mRNA.

Yntema, C. L. (1943). *J. Exp. Zool.* 94:319–349. Deficient efferent innervation of the extremities following removal of neural crest in *Amblystoma*.

Yntema, C. L., and W. S. Hammond (1945). *J. Exp. Zool.* 100:237–263. Depletions and abnormalities in the cervical sympathetic system of the chick following extirpation of the neural crest.

Yntema, C. L., and W. S. Hammond (1947). *Biol. Rev.* 22:344–359. The development of the autonomic nervous system.

Yntema, C. L., and W. S. Hammond (1954). *J. Comp. Neurol.* 101:515–541. The origin of intrinsic ganglia of trunk viscera from vagal neural crest in the chick embryo.

Yodlowski, M. L, J. R. Fredieu, and S. C. Landis (1984). *J. Neurosci.* 4:1535–1548. Neonatal 6-hydroxydopamine treatment eliminates cholinergic sympathetic innervation and induces sensory sprouting in rat sweat glands.

Yolton, L. W. (1923). *Proc. Natl. Acad. Sci. U.S.A.* 9:383–395. The effects of cutting the giant fibers in the earthworm *Eisenia foetida* (Sav.).

Yonezawa, T., M. B. Bornstein, E. R. Peterson, and M. R. Murray (1962). *J. Neuropath. Exp. Neurol.* 21:479–487. A histochemical study of oxidative enzymes in myelinating cultures of central and peripheral nervous tissue.

Yoon, M. G. (1971). *Exp. Neurol.* 33:395–411. Reorganization of retinotectal projection following surgical operations on the optic tectum in goldfish.

Yoon, M. G. (1972a). *Exp. Neurol.* 37:451–462. Transposition of the visual projection from the nasal hemiretina onto the foreign rostral zone of the optic tectum in goldfish.

Yoon, M. G. (1972b). *Exp. Neurol.* 35:565–577. Reversibility of the reorganization of retinotectal projection in goldfish.

Yoon, M. G. (1975a). *J. Physiol. (London)* 252:137–158. Readjustment of retinotectal projection following reimplantation of a rotated or inverted tectal tissue in adult goldfish.

Yoon, M. G. (1975b). *Cold Spring Harbor Symp. Quant. Biol.* 15:503–509. Topographic polarity of the optic tectum studied by reimplantation of tectal tissue in adult goldfish.

Yoon, M. G. (1976). *J. Physiol. (London)* 257:621–643. Progress of topographic regulation of the visual projection in the halved optic tectum of adult goldfish.

Yoon, M. G. (1977). *J. Physiol. (London)* 264:379–410. Induction of compression in the re-established visual projections on to a rotated tectal reimplant that retains its original topographic polarity within the halved optic tectum of adult goldfish.

Yoon, M. G. (1980). *J. Physiol. (London)* 308:197–215. Retention of topographic addresses by reciprocally translocated tectal re-implants in adult goldfish.

Yoshida-Noro, C., N. Suzuki, and M. Takeichi (1984). *Dev. Biol.* 101:19–27. Molecular nature of the calcium-dependent cell-cell adhesion system in mouse teratocarcinoma and embryonic cells studied with a monoclonal antibody.

Yoshikami, D., and L. M. Okun (1984). *Nature* 310:53–56. Staining of living presynaptic nerve terminals with selective fluorescent dyes.

Young, D. (1972). *J. Exp. Biol.* 57:305–316. Specific reinnervation of limb transplanted between segments in the cockroach, *Periplaneta americana*.

Young, D. (1973). Specificity and regeneration in insect motor neurons, pp. 179–202. In *Developmental Neurobiology of Arthropods* (D. Young, ed.), Cambridge Univ. Press, London.

Young, H. S., and M. M. Poo (1983). *Nature* 305:634–637. Spontaneous release of transmitter from growth cones of embryonic neurons.

Young, J. Z. (1932). *Quart. J. Microscop. Sci.* 75:1–49. On the cytology of the neurons of cephalopods.

Young, J. Z. (1942). *Physiol. Rev.* 22:318–374. The functional repair of nervous tissue.

Young, J. Z. (1944). *Nature* 153:333. Contraction, turgor and the cytoskeleton of nerve fibers.

Young, J. Z. (1945). The history of the shape of a nerve fiber, pp. 41–94. In *Essays on Growth and Form* (W. E. Le Gros Clark, and P. B. Medawar, eds.), Clarendon Press, Oxford.

Young, J. Z. (1951). *Proc. Roy. Soc. (London) Ser. B.* 139:18–37. Growth and plasticity in the nervous system.

Young, J. Z. (1963). *Proc. Zool. Soc. London* 140:229–254. The number and sizes of nerve cells in octopus.

Young, J. Z. (1964). *A Model of the Brain*, Clarendon Press, Oxford.

Young, M., J. Oger, M. H. Blanchard, H. Asdourian, H. Amos, and B. G. W. Arnason (1975). *Science* 187:361–362. Secretion of a nerve growth factor by primary chick fibroblast cultures.

Young, M. B. (1977). *J. Neuropath. Exp. Neurol.* 36:465–473. H³T-labelled blood cells in the CNS response to axotomies at various times after isotope injection.

Young, R. M. (1970). *Mind, Brain and Adaptation in the Nineteenth Century*. Clarendon Press, Oxford.

Young, R. W. (1984). *J. Comp. Neurol.* 229:362–373. Cell death during differentiation of the retina in the mouse.

Yu, W. (1977). *Am. J. Anat.* 150:89–108. The effects of 5-bromodeoxyuridine on the postnatal development of the rat cerebellum: Morphologic and radioautographic studies.

Yuan, J., and H. R. Horvitz (1990). *Dev. Biol.* 138:33–41. The *Caenorhabditis elegans* genes *ced-3* and *ced-4* act cell autonomously to cause programmed cell death.

Yurchenco, P. D., and J. C. Schittny (1990). *FASEB J.* 4:1577–1590. Molecular architecture of basement membranes.

Yurkewicz, L., J. M. Lander, M. Marchi, and E. Giacobini (1981). *J. Comp. Neurol.* 203:257–267. ³H-thymidine long survival autoradiography as a method for dating the time of neuronal origin in the chick embryo: The locus coeruleus and cerebellar Purkinje cells.

Yusuf, H. K. M., and J. W. T. Dickerson (1979). *J. Neurochem.* 33:815–818. Effect of chronic undernutrition in the rat on the development of myelin.

Zacharias, L. R. (1938). *J. Exp. Zool.* 78:135–157. An analysis of cellular proliferation in grafted segments of embryonic spinal cords.

Zacks, S. I., and A. Saito (1969). *J. Histochem. Cytochem.* 17:161–170. Uptake of exogenous horseradish peroxidase by coated vesicles in mouse neuromuscular junctions.

Zagon, I. S. (1975). *Exp. Neurol.* 46:69–77. Prolonged gestation and cerebellar development in the rat.

Zagon, I. S., and P. J. McLaughlin (1986). *Brain Res.* 28:233–246. Opioid antagonist-induced modulation of cerebral and hippocampal development: Histological and morphometric studies.

Zagoren, J. C., and S. Fedoroff (1984). *The Node of Ranvier.* Academic Press, New York.

Zahm, D., and B. Munger (1983). *J. Comp. Neurol.* 219:36–51. Fetal development of primate chemosensory corpuscles. II. Synaptic relationships in early gestation.

Zaimis, E. (1964). *J. Physiol. (London)* 177:35–36. The immunosympathectomized animal: A valuable tool in physiological and pharmacological research.

Zaimis, E., L. Berk, and B. A. Callingham (1965). *Nature* 206:1220–1222. Morphological, biochemical and functional changes in the sympathetic nervous system of rats treated with nerve growth factor-antiserum.

Zalc, B., M. Monge, P. Dupouey, J. J. Hauw, and N. A. Baumann (1981). *Brain Res.* 211:341–354. Immunohistochemical localization of galactosyl and sulfogalactosyl ceramide in the brain of the 30-day-old mouse.

Zalewski, A. A. (1968). *Exp. Neurol.* 22:40–51. Changes in phosphatase enzymes following denervation of the vallate papilla of the rat.

Zalewski, A. A. (1969a). *Exp. Neurol.* 23:18–28. Role of nerve and epithelium in the regulation of alkaline phosphatase activity in gustatory papillae.

Zalewski, A. A. (1969b). *J. Neurobiol.* 1:123–132. Neurotrophic-hormonal interaction in the regulation of taste buds in the rat's vallate papilla.

Zalewski, A. A. (1969c). *Exp. Neurol.* 24:285–297. Combined effects of testosterone and motor, sensory, or gustatory nerve reinnervation on the regeneration of taste buds.

Zalewski, A. A. (1970a). *Exp. Neurol.* 26:621–629. Regeneration of taste buds in the lingual epithelium after excision of the vallate papilla.

Zalewski, A. A. (1970b). *Exp. Neurol.* 29:462–467. Trophic influence of *in vivo* transplanted sensory neurons on taste buds.

Zalewski, A. A. (1970c). *Am. J. Physiol.* 219:1675–1679. Effects of reinnervation of denervated skeletal muscle by axons of motor, sensory, and sympathetic neurons.

Zalewski, A. A. (1972). *Exp. Neurol.* 35:519–528. Regeneration of taste buds after transplantation of tongue and ganglia grafts to the anterior chamber of the eye.

Zalewski, A. A. (1973). *Exp. Neurol.* 40:161–169. Regeneration of taste buds in tongue grafts after reinnervation by neurons in transplanted lumbar sensory neurons.

Zalewski, A. A. (1974a). *Ann. N.Y. Acad. Sci.* 228:344–349. Neuronal and tissue specifications involved in taste bud formation.

Zalewski, A. A. (1974b). *Exp. Neurol.* 45:189–193. Trophic function of neurons in transplanted neonatal ganglia.

Zalewski, A. A. (1976). *Exp. Neurol.* 52:565–580. The neural induction of taste buds in the salivary ducts of the lingual gland of Von Ebner.

Zalewski, A. A. (1980). *Exp. Neurol.* 68:390–394. Survival, regeneration and trophic function of neurons in 1-year transplants of sensory ganglia.

Zalewski, A. A. (1981). *J. Comp. Neurol.* 200:309–314. Regeneration of taste buds after reinnervation of a denervated tongue papilla by a normally nongustatory nerve.

Zamenhof, S. (1941). *Growth* 5:123–139. Stimulation of the proliferation of neurons by growth hormone: I. Experiments on tadpoles.

Zamenhof, S. (1942). *Physiol. Zool.* 15:281–292. Stimulation of cortical-cell proliferation by the growth hormone. III. Experiments on the albino rats.

Zamenhof, S. (1976). *Brain Res.* 109:392–394. Final number of Purkinje and other large cells in the chick cerebellum influenced by incubation temperatures during their proliferation.

Zamenhof, S., and E. Van Marthens (1971). Hormonal and nutritional aspects of prenatal brain development, pp. 329–359. In *Cellular Aspects of Neural Growth and Differentiation* (D.C. Pease, ed.), Univ. Calif. Press, Berkeley.

Zamenhof, S., H. Bursztyn, K. Rich, and P. J. Zamenhof (1964). *J. Neurochem.* 11:505–509. The determination of deoxyribonucleic acid and of cell number in brain.

Zamenhof, S., J. Mosley, and E. Schuller (1966). *Science* 152:1396–1397. Stimulation of the proliferation of cortical neurons by prenatal treatment with growth hormone.

Zamenhof, S., E. van Marthens, and F. L. Margolis (1968). *Science* 160:322–323. DNA (cell number) and protein in neonatal brain: Alteration by maternal dietary protein restriction.

Zamenhof, S., L. Grauel, and E. van Marthens (1971a). *Biol. Neonate.* 18:140–145. Study of possible correlations between prenatal brain development and placental weight.

Zamenhof, S., L. Grauel, and E. van Marthens (1971b) *Res. Commun. Chem. Pathol. Pharmacol.* 2:261–270. The effect of thymidine and 5-bromodeoxyuridine on developing chick embryo brain.

Zamenhof, S., E. van Marthens, and H. Bursztyn (1971c). The effect of hormones on DNA synthesis and cell number in the developing chick and rat brain, pp. 101–119. In *Hormones in Development* (M. Hamburgh, and E. J. W. Barrington, eds.), Appleton-Century-Crofts, New York.

Zamenhof, S., E. van Marthens, and L. Grauel (1971d). *J. Nutr.* 9:1265–1270. DNA (cell number) and protein in neonatal rat brain: Alterations by timing of maternal dietary protein restriction.

Zamenhof, S., E. van Marthens, and L. Grauel (1971e). *Science* 172:850–851. DNA (cell number) in neonatal brain: Second generation (F_2) alteration by maternal (F_0) dietary protein restriction.

Zamenhof, S., E. van Marthens, and L. Grauel (1971f). *Science* 174:954–955. Prenatal cerebral development: Effect of restricted diet, reversal by growth hormone.

Zamora, A. J., and M. Mutin (1988). *Neuroscience* 27:279–288. Vimentin and glial fibrillary acidic protein filaments in radial glia of the adult urodele spinal cord.

Zander, E., and G. Weddell (1951). *J. Anat. (London)* 85:66–99. Observations on the innervation of the cornea.

Zangwill, O. L. (1963–1964). *Adv. Sci.* 20:335–344. The cerebral localization of psychological functions.

Zanini, A., P. Angeletti, and R. Levi-Montalcini (1968). *Proc. Nat. Acad. Sci. U.S.A.* 61:835–842. Immunochemical properties of the nerve growth factor.

Zanobio, B. (1959). *Physis* 1:307–320. Le osservazioni microscopiche di Felice Fontana sulla struttura dei nervi.

Zanobio, B. (1975). Golgian memorabilia in the museum for the history of the University of Pavia, pp. 650–655. In *Golgi centennial symposium* (M. Santini, ed.), Raven Press, New York.

Zecevic, N., and P. Rakic (1976). *J. Comp. Neurol.* 167:27–48. Differentiation of Purkinje cells and their relationship to other components of developing cerebellar cortex in man.

Zecevic, N. R., and M. E. Molliver (1978). *Brain Res.* 150:387–397. The origin of the monoaminergic innervation of immature rat neocortex. An ultrastructural analysis following lesions.

Zelená, J. (1957). *J. Embryol. Exp. Morphol.* 5:283–292. The morphogenetic influence of innervation on the ontogenetic development of muscle spindles.

Zelená, J. (1963). *Physiol. Bohemoslov.* 12:30–36. Development of muscle receptors after tenotomy.

Zelená, J. (1964). *Prog. Brain Res.* 13:175–213. Development, degeneration and regeneration of receptor organs.

Zelená, J. (1965). *Cesk. Fysiol.* 14:377–378. The influence of fusimotor innervation upon the development of muscle spindles.

Zelená, J. (1968). *Z. Zellforsch. Mikroskop. Anat.* 92:186–196. Bidirectional movements of mitochondria along axons of an isolated nerve segment.

Zelená, J. (1972a). *Z. Zellforsch. Mikrosk. Anat.* 124:217–220. Ribosomes in myelinated axons of dorsal root ganglia.

Zelená, J. (1972b). *Folia Morphol. (Praha)* 20:91–93. Ribosomes in the axoplasm of myelinated nerve fibers.

Zelená, J. (1975). The role of sensory innervation in the development of mechanoreceptors, pp. 59–64. In *Somatosensory and Visceral Receptor Mechanisms* (A. Iggo, and O. B. Ilyinsky, eds.), Elsevier, Amsterdam.

Zelená, J. (1976). *J. Neurocytol.* 5:447–463. Sensory terminals on extrafusal muscle fibres in myotendinous regions of developing rat muscles.

Zelená, J. (1978). *J. Neurocytol.* 7:71–91. The development of Pacinian corpuscles.

Zelená, J. (1980). *Brain Res.* 187:97–111. Rapid degeneration of developing rat Pacinian corpuscles after denervation.

Zelená, J. (1982). *Cell Tissue Res.* 224:673–683. Survival of Pacinian corpuscles after denervation in adult rats.

Zelená, J. (1984). *J. Neurocytol.* 13:665–684. Multiple axon terminals in reinnervated Pacinian corpuscles of adult rat.

Zelená, J., and I. Jirmanová (1988). *Brain Res.* 438:165–174. Grafts of Pacinian corpuscles reinnervated by dorsal root axons.

Zelená, J., and M. Sobotková (1971). *Physiol. Bohemoslov.* 20:433–439. Absence of muscle spindles in regenerated muscles of the rat.

Zelená, J., and T. Soukup (1973). *Z. Zellforsch. Mikrosk. Anat.* 144:435–452. Development of muscle spindles deprived of fusimotor innervation.

Zelená, J., and T. Soukup (1974a). *Cell Tissue Res.* 153:115–136. The differentiation of intrafusal fibre types in rat muscle spindles after motor denervation.

Zelená, J., and T. Soukup (1974b). *Folia Morphol. (Praha)* 22:268–269. Ultrastructural differentiation of muscle spindles after de-efferentation.

Zelená, J., and T. Soukup (1977). *J. Neurocytol.* 6:171–194. The development of Golgi tendon organs.

Zelená, J., L. Lubinska, and E. Gutmann (1968). *Z. Zellforsch. Mikroskop. Anat.* 91:200–219. Accumulation of organelles at the ends of interrupted axons.

Zelená, J., M. Sobotková, and H. Zelená (1978). *Physiologia Bohemoslovaca* 27:437–443. Age-modulated dependence of Pacinian corpuscles upon their sensory innervation.

Zeller, N. K., M. J. Hunkeler, A. T. Campagnoni, J. Sprague, and R. A Lazzarini (1984). *Proc. Natl. Acad. Sci. U.S.A.* 81:18–22. Characterization of mouse myelin basic protein messenger RNAs with a myelin basic protein cDNA clone.

Zeller, N. K., T. N. Behar, M. E. Dubois-Dalcq, and R. A. Lazzarini (1985). *J. Neurosci.* 5:2955–2962. The timely expression of myelin basic protein gene in cultured rat brain oligodendrocytes is independent of continuous neuronal influences.

Zeman, F. J., and E. C. Stanbrough (1969). *J. Nutr.* 99:274–282. Effect of maternal protein deficiency on cellular development in the fetal rat.

Zenker, W., and E. Hohberg (1973). *Z. Anat. Entwicklungsgesch.* 139:163–172. α-Motorische Nervenfaser: Axonquerschnittsflache von Stammfaser und Endasten.

Ziegler, H. E. (1908). *Jena z. Med. Naturw.* 43:653–684. Die phylogenetische Entwickelung des Kopfes der Wirbeltiere.

Zigmond, R. E., R. Nottebohm, and D. W. Pfaff (1973). *Science* 179:1005–1007. Androgen-concentrating cells in the midbrain of a songbird.

Zigmond, S. H. (1974). *Nature* 249:450–452. Mechanisms of sensing chemical gradients by polymorphonuclear leukocytes.

Ziller, C., E. Dupin, P. Brazeau, D. Paulin, and N. M. Le Douarin (1983). *Cell* 32:627–638. Early segregation of a neuronal precursor cell line in the neural crest as revealed by culture in a chemically defined medium.

Ziller, C., M. Fauquet, C. Kalcheim, J. Smith,. and N. M. Le Douarin (1987). *Dev. Biol.* 120:101–111. Cell lineages in peripheral nervous system ontogeny: Medium-induced modulation of neuronal phenotypic expression in neural crest cell cultures.

Zilles, K., B. Zilles, and A. Schleicher (1980). *Anat. Embryol.* 159:335–360. A quantitative approach to cytoarchitectonics. VI. The areal pattern of the cortex of the albino rat.

Zilles, K., C. M. Becker, and A. Schleicher (1981). *Anat. Embryol.* 163:87–123. Transmission blockade during neuronal development: Observations on the trochlear nucleus with quantitative histological methods and with ultrastructural and axonal transport studies in the chick embryo.

Zilles, K., H. Stephan, and A. Schleicher (1982). Quantitative cytoarchitectonics of the cerebral cortices of several prosimian species. In *Primate brain evolution: Methods and Concepts* (Armstrong, E., and D. Falk, eds.), Plenum Publishing Corporation, New York.

Zimmerman, A., and A. Sutter (1983). *EMBO J.* 2:879–885. β-Nerve growth factor (βNGF) receptors on glial cells. Cell-cell interaction between neurones and Schwann cells in cultures of chick ensory ganglia.

Zimmerman, T. R., and W. Cammer (1982). *J. Neurosci. Res.* 8:73–81. ATPase activities in myelin and oligodendrocytes isolated from the brains of developing rats and from bovine brain white matter.

Ziskind-Conhaim, L. (1988). *Dev. Biol.* 128:21–29. Electrical properties of motoneurons in the spinal cord of rat embryos.

Ziskind-Conhaim, L., and J. I. Bennett (1982). *Dev. Biol.* 90:185–197. The effects of electrical inactivity and denervation on the distribution of acetylcholine receptors in developing rat muscle.

Zottoli, S. J. (1981). *J. Comp. Physiol.* 143:541–553. Electrophysiological and morphological characterization of the winter flounder mauthner cell.

Zottoli, S. J., and D. S. Faber (1979). *Brain Res.* 174:319–323. Properties and distribution of anterior VIIIth nerve excitatory inputs to the goldfish Mauthner cell.

Zottoli, S. J., D. H. Hangen, and D. S. Faber (1984). *J. Comp. Neurol.* 230:497–516. The axon reaction of the goldfish mauthner cell and factors that influence its morphological variability.

Zucker, E., and W. I. Welker (1969). *Brain Res.* 12:138–156. Coding of somatic input by vibrissae neurons in the rat's trigeminal ganglion.

Zukin, S. R., A. B. Young, and S. H. Snyder (1975). *Brain Res.* 83:525–530. Development of the synaptic glycine receptor in chick embryo spinal cord.

Zwaan, J., P. R. Bryan, Jr., and T. L. Pearce (1969). *J. Embryol. Exp. Morphol.* 21:71–83. Interkinetic nuclear migration during the early stages of lens formation in the chicken embryo.

Index